ACID-BASE BALANCE

Acidosis, 267

CELLULAR REGULATION

Breast Cancer, 1433
Cirrhosis, 1156
Hypothryroidism, 1250
Osteoporosis, 984
Prostate Cancer, 1479

CLOTTING

Venous Thromboembolism, 720

COGNITION

Alzheimer's Disease, 844
Traumatic Brain Injury, 912

COMFORT

End-of-Life, 136

ELIMINATION

Benign Prostatic Hyperplasia, 1470
Chronic Kidney Disease, 1383
Urinary Incontinence, 1326
Intestinal Obstruction, 1111
Pyelonephritis, 1356

FLUID AND ELECTROLYTE BALANCE

Dehydration, 246
Hypercortisolism, 1240

GAS EXCHANGE

Chronic Obstructive Pulmonary Disease, 542
Obstructive Sleep Apnea, 517
Pneumonia, 570
Pulmonary Embolism, 587

GLUCOSE REGULATION

Diabetes Mellitus, 1266

IMMUNITY

HIV Infection and AIDS (HIV-III), 323
Leukemia and Preleukemia, 802
Multiple Sclerosis, 872
Rheumatoid Arthritis, 1017
Systemic Lupus Erythematosus, 353

INFECTION

Hepatitis, 1166
Pelvic Inflammatory Disease, 1518
Peptic Ulcer Disease (PUD), 1096
Peritonitis, 1132
Pulmonary Tuberculosis, 575
Sepsis and Septic Shock, 740

INFLAMMATION

Acute Pancreatitis, 1182
Ulcerative Colitis, 1137
Cholecystitis, 1177

MOBILITY

Fracture, 1029
Osteoarthritis, 1002
Parkinson Disease, 853
Spinal Cord Injury, 877

NUTRITION

Gastroesophageal Reflux Disease (GERD), 1081
Obesity, 1209
Undernutrition, 1201

PAIN

Pelvic Inflammatory Disease, 1518

PERFUSION

Acute Coronary Syndrome, 750
Amputation, 1046
Atrial Fibrillation, 652
Heart Failure, 666
Hypertension, 698

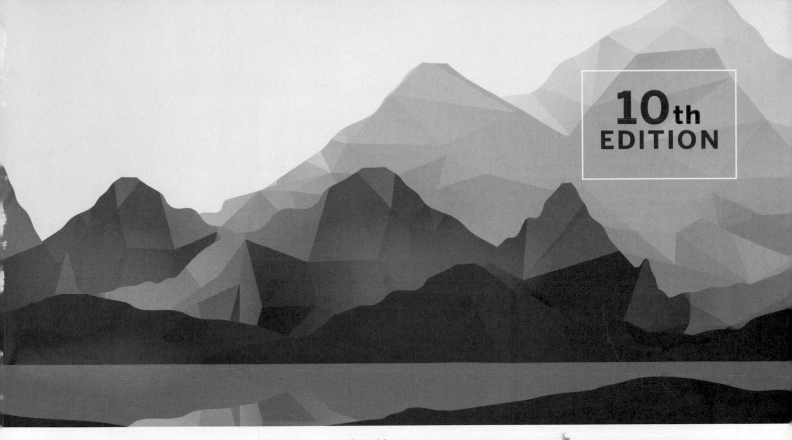

10th EDITION

MEDICAL-SURGICAL NURSING
CONCEPTS FOR INTERPROFESSIONAL COLLABORATIVE CARE

Donna D. Ignatavicius,
MS, RN, CNE, CNEcl, ANEF
Speaker and Nursing Education Consultant;
Founder, Boot Camp for Nurse Educators;
President, DI Associates, Inc.
Littleton, Colorado

M. Linda Workman,
PhD, RN, FAAN
Author and Consultant
Visiting Professor and Former Endowed Professor
Frances Payne Bolton School of Nursing
Case Western Reserve University
Cleveland, Ohio

Cherie R. Rebar,
PhD, MBA, RN, COI
Subject Matter Expert and Nursing Education Consultant
Beavercreek, Ohio;
Professor of Nursing
Wittenberg University
Springfield, Ohio

Nicole M. Heimgartner,
DNP, RN, COI
Subject Matter Expert and Nursing Education Consultant
Louisville, Kentucky;
Adjunct Faculty
American Sentinel University
Aurora, Colorado

ELSEVIER

Elsevier
3251 Riverport Lane
St. Louis, Missouri 63043

Notice

Practitioners and researchers must always rely on their own experience and knowledge in evaluating
and using any information, methods, compounds or experiments described herein. Because of rapid
advances in the medical sciences, in particular, independent verification of diagnoses and drug dosages
should be made. To the fullest extent of the law, no responsibility is assumed by Elsevier, authors, editors
or contributors for any injury and/or damage to persons or property as a matter of products liability,
negligence or otherwise, or from any use or operation of any methods, products, instructions, or ideas
contained in the material herein.

Previous editions copyrighted 2018, 2016, 2013, 2010, 2006, 2002, 1999, 1995, 1991

International Standard Book Number (single volume): 978-0-323-61242-5
International Standard Book Number (2-volume set): 978-0-323-61241-8

Executive Content Strategist: Lee Henderson
Director, Content Development: Laurie Gower
Senior Content Development Specialist: Laura Goodrich
Publishing Services Manager: Julie Eddy
Senior Project Manager: Jodi M. Willard
Design Direction: Brian Salisbury

Printed in Canada

Last digit is the print number: 9   8   7   6   5   4   3   2   1

Working together
to grow libraries in
developing countries

www.elsevier.com • www.bookaid.org

Marie Bashaw, DNP, RN, NEA-BC
Professor and Director of Nursing
Department of Nursing
Wittenberg University
Springfield, Ohio

Cecilia Bidigare, MSN
Professor
Nursing
Sinclair Community College
Dayton, Ohio

Maureen Bishop, MSN, RN, CCRN, CCNS
Clinical Nurse Specialist
Lakeland University
Lakeland Health
St. Joseph, Michigan

Andrea A. Borchers, PhD, RN
Assistant Professor
School of Nursing
Northern Arizona University
Flagstaff, Arizona

Samuel A. Borchers, OD
Optometrist
Vision Clinic
Northern Arizona VA Healthcare System
Prescott, Arizona

Katherine Byar, MSN, ANP, BC, BMTCN
Nurse Practitioner
Hematological Malignancy
Nebraska Medicine
Omaha, Nebraska

Michelle Camicia, PhD, CRRN, CCM, NEA-BC, FAHA
Director of Operations
Kaiser Foundation Rehabilitation Center
Kaiser Permanente
Vallejo, California

Lara Carver, PhD, MSN, RN, CNE
Director
College of Health Professions
Western Governors University
Salt Lake City, Utah

Keelin C. Cromar, MSN, RN
Subject Matter Expert
Nursing Consultant
Wichita County Public Health District
Wichita Falls, Texas

Laura M. Dechant, DNP, CCNS, CCRN
Clinical Nurse Specialist
Heart, Vascular and Interventional Services
Christiana Care Health System
Newark, Pennsylvania

Stephanie M. Fox, PsyD
Clinical Psychologist
Littleton, Colorado

Carolyn J. Gersch, PhD, MSN, RN, CNE
Professor
Wittenberg University
Springfield, Ohio

Darla Green, RN, DNP, FNP-C
Assistant Professor
Del Mar College
Department of Nurse Education
Corpus Christi, Texas

Charity Hacker, RN, MSN-Ed
Assistant Professor
Nursing
Ivy Tech Community College
Madison, Indiana;
Adjunct Faculty
Nursing
Indiana University Purdue University
Columbus (IUPUC)
Columbus, Indiana

Linda Laskowski-Jones, MS, APRN, ACNS-BC, CEN, FAWM, FAAN
Vice President
Emergency & Trauma Services
Christiana Care Health System
Newark, Delaware

Cheryl L. Leksan, MSN, MEd, BSN
Formerly, Teaching Professor
School of Nursing
Xavier University
Cincinnati, Ohio

Hannah Lopez, MSN, RN, OCN, CBCN
Clinical Nurse Manager
Hematology/Oncology & Supportive and
Palliative Care
Baylor Scott & White Health
Round Rock, Texas

Robyn Mitchell, APRN-CNP, MSN, CCRN, CSC, CMC, AGACNP AG, AGACNP-BC, ACNP
Critical Care House Officer
Cleveland Clinic
Cleveland, Ohio

Jennifer Dawn Powers, FNP-BC, MSN, BSN
Adjunct Faculty
Department of Nursing
National University
Henderson, Nevada

Harry Rees III, MSN, APRN-CNP
Trauma, Critical Care, and Burn
The Ohio State University Wexner Medical
Center
Columbus, Ohio

Jonathon Rospierski, MSN, BS, RN-BC
Nursing Professional Development
Specialist/Nurse Residency Program
Coordinator
Lakeland University
Lakeland Health
St. Joseph, Michigan

James G. Sampson, DNP, RN
Infectious Disease
Denver Health Medical Center
Denver, Colorado

Karen L. Toulson, DNP, MBA, CEN, NE-BC
Director, Clinical Operations
Emergency Department
Christiana Care Health System
Newark, Delaware

Sharon A. Watts, DNP, MSN, BSN
Endocrinology
Veterans Health Administration
Cleveland, Ohio

CONTRIBUTORS TO TEACHING/LEARNING RESOURCES

PowerPoint Slides

Nicole M. Heimgartner, DNP, RN, COI
Subject Matter Expert and Nursing
   Education Consultant
Louisville, Kentucky;
Adjunct Faculty
American Sentinel University
Aurora, Colorado

Cherie R. Rebar, PhD, MBA, RN, COI
Subject Matter Expert and Nursing
   Education Consultant
Beavercreek, Ohio;
Professor of Nursing
Wittenberg University
Springfield, Ohio

Teach® for Nurses Lesson Plans

Nicole M. Heimgartner, DNP, RN, COI
Subject Matter Expert and Nursing
   Education Consultant
Louisville, Kentucky;
Adjunct Faculty
American Sentinel University
Aurora, Colorado

Cherie R. Rebar, PhD, MBA, RN, COI
Subject Matter Expert and Nursing
   Education Consultant
Beavercreek, Ohio;
Professor of Nursing
Wittenberg University
Springfield, Ohio

Test Bank

Meg Blair, PhD, MSN, RN, CEN
Professor
Nursing Division
Nebraska Methodist College
Omaha, Nebraska

Donna D. Ignatavicius, MS, RN, CNE, CNEcl, ANEF
Speaker and Nursing Education Consultant;
Founder, Boot Camp for Nurse Educators;
President, DI Associates, Inc.
Littleton, Colorado

Case Studies

Tami Kathleen Little, DNP, RN, CNE
Corporate Director of Nursing
Vista College
Richardson, Texas

Review Questions for the NCLEX® Examination

Donna D. Ignatavicius, MS, RN, CNE, CNEcl, ANEF
Speaker and Nursing Education Consultant;
Founder, Boot Camp for Nurse Educators;
President, DI Associates, Inc.
Littleton, Colorado

M. Linda Workman, PhD, RN, FAAN
Author and Consultant
Visiting Professor and Former Endowed
   Professor
Frances Payne Bolton School of Nursing
Case Western Reserve University
Cleveland, Ohio

Cherie R. Rebar, PhD, MBA, RN, COI
Subject Matter Expert and Nursing
   Education Consultant
Beavercreek, Ohio;
Professor of Nursing
Wittenberg University
Springfield, Ohio

Nicole M. Heimgartner, DNP, RN, COI
Subject Matter Expert and Nursing
   Education Consultant
Louisville, Kentucky;
Adjunct Faculty
American Sentinel University
Aurora, Colorado

Rosalinda Alfaro-Lefevre, MSN, RN, ANEF
President
Teaching Smart/Learning Easy
Stuart, Florida

Nell Britton, MSN, RN, CNE
Adjunct Nursing Instructor
Anderson University
Anderson, South Carolina

Mary Dolansky, PhD, RN, FAAN
Associate Professor
Frances Payne Bolton School of Nursing;
Assistant Professor
Department of Population and Quantitative Health Sciences
School of Medicine;
Director, QSEN Institute
Frances Payne Bolton School of Nursing;
Senior Faculty Scholar
VA Quality Scholars Program
Case Western Reserve University
Cleveland, Ohio

Claudia Grobbel, DNP, RN
Associate Professor
Oakland University
Rochester, Michigan

Michael J. Rebar, DO, DPM
Hospitalist
Miami Valley Hospital
Dayton, Ohio

Christy Roberts, MSN, BSN, APRN, FNP-C
Family Nurse Practitioner
One Medical
Mount Washington, Kentucky

Jeffrey Schultz, MS, APRN, ACNP-BC, CCNS, RN-BC, CCRN, CEN, NE-BC, NR-P
Senior APP-CVICU
Cardiothoracic Surgery
North Florida Regional Medical Center
Gainesville, Florida;
Flight Nurse
University of Florida Health
ShandsCair Critical Care Transport Program
Gainesville, Florida

The first edition of this textbook, entitled *Medical-Surgical Nursing: A Nursing Process Approach,* was a groundbreaking work in many ways. The following nine editions built on that achievement and further solidified the book's position as a major trendsetter for the practice of evidence-based adult health nursing. Now in its tenth edition, "Iggy" again charts the cutting-edge approach for the future of adult nursing practice—an approach reflected in its current title: *Medical-Surgical Nursing: Concepts for Interprofessional Collaborative Care.* The focus of this new edition continues to help students learn how to utilize clinical judgment skills to provide safe, quality nursing care that is patient-centered, evidence-based, and interprofessionally collaborative. In addition to print formats as single- and two-volume texts, this edition is available in a variety of electronic formats.

KEY COMPONENTS OF THE TENTH EDITION

Similar to the last edition's conceptual learning approach, the tenth edition organizes the content in each chapter by the most important *professional nursing and/or health concepts* and then presents commonly occurring *exemplars* for each concept. The key components for this edition that strengthen the text's conceptual focus are consistent with the Quality and Safety Education for Nurses' (QSEN) competencies and include *clinical judgment, safety, quality care,* and *patient-centeredness.* Further information about these components are described below.

- **Enhanced Emphasis on Professional Nursing and Health Concepts.** This edition uniquely balances a focus on nursing concepts with a conceptual approach to teaching and learning. Prelicensure programs that embrace the concept-based nursing curriculum, system-focused curriculum, or a hybrid or modified approach will find this edition easy to use. To help students connect previously learned concepts with new information in the text, Chapters 1 and 3 review the main concepts used in this edition, giving a working definition on which the students will reflect and build as they learn new material. These unique features build on basic concepts learned in nursing fundamentals courses, such as gas exchange and safety, to help students make connections between foundational concepts and interprofessional care for patients with medical-surgical conditions. For continuity and reinforcement, a list of specific Priority and Interrelated Nursing Concepts is highlighted at the beginning of each chapter. This placement is specifically designed to help students better understand the priority and associated needs that the nurse will address when providing safe, evidence-based, patient-centered care for individuals with selected health problems.
- **Emphasis on Common Exemplars.** For each priority concept listed in the beginning of the Nursing Care chapters, the authors have identified common or major exemplars. The nursing and interprofessional collaborative care for patients experiencing these exemplar diseases and illnesses is discussed through the lens of the priority and interrelated concepts. In addition, patient problems are presented as a collaborative problem list.
- **Focus on Clinical Judgment.** Stressing the importance of clinical judgment helps to prepare students for professional nursing practice and the current and Next-Generation NCLEX® (NGN) Examination for nursing licensure. A new chapter in this edition (Chapter 2), entitled *Clinical Judgment and Systems Thinking,* focuses on how nurses use clinical judgment in practice. Systems thinking allows the nurse to look beyond an individual action for additional or enhanced methods to promote safety and increase quality of care, which drives more favorable patient outcomes. Inversely, the nurse can look at interventions that have served populations and then navigate ways to bring those to the individual patient level.

    In addition to the new chapter, most chapters in this edition present **Clinical Judgment Challenges** that describe complex clinical situations and require the students to use clinical judgment skills based on the NCSBN's Clinical Judgment Measurement Model (CJMM). This model is the basis for the new test item types on the Next-Generation NCLEX® Examination. Suggested answer guidelines for these Clinical Judgment Challenges are provided on the companion Evolve website (http://evolve.elsevier.com/Iggy/).

    In the tenth edition, the six cognitive skills of the NCSBN's CJMM can be aligned with each nursing process step. The authors use this alignment to help students and faculty transition from the basic foundation of the nursing process to the critical thinking and clinical reasoning required for clinical judgment as follows:
    - Assessment: Recognize Cues
    - Analysis: Analyze Cues and Prioritize Hypotheses
    - Planning and Implementation: Generate Solutions and Take Action
    - Evaluation: Evaluate Outcomes
- **Emphasis on Patient Safety.** Patient safety is emphasized throughout this edition, not only in the narrative but also in **Nursing Safety Priority boxes** that enable students to immediately identify the most important care needed for patients with specific health problems. These highlighted features are further classified as an Action Alert, Drug Alert, or Critical Rescue. We also continue to include our leading-edge **Best Practice for Patient Safety & Quality Care boxes** to emphasize the most important nursing care.
- **Highlight on Quality Care.** The QSEN Institute emphasizes, and clinical practice agencies require, that all nurses have *quality improvement* knowledge, skills, attitudes, and abilities. To help prepare students for that role, this edition includes unique **Systems Thinking and Quality Improvement boxes.** Each box summarizes a quality improvement project published in the literature and discusses the implications of the project's success in improving nursing care.

The inclusion of these boxes disseminates information and research and helps students understand that quality improvement begins at the bedside as the nurse identifies potential evidence-based solutions to practice problems.

- **Enhanced Focus on Patient-Centered Care.** Patient-centered care is enhanced in this tenth edition in several ways. This edition continues to use the term "patient" instead of "client" throughout. Although the use of these terms remains a subject of discussion among nursing educators, we have not defined the patient as a dependent person. Rather, the patient can be an individual, a family, or a group—all of whom have rights that are respected in a mutually trusting nurse-patient relationship. Most health care agencies and professional organizations use "patient" in their practice and publications, and most professional nursing organizations support the term. To help illustrate the importance of Patient-Centered Care, this text incorporates the following special boxes:
  - Patient-Centered Care: Older Adult Considerations
  - Patient-Centered Care: Veterans Health Considerations
  - Patient-Centered Care: Cultural/Spiritual Considerations
  - Patient-Centered Care: Genetic/Genomic Considerations
  - Patient-Centered Care: Gender Health Considerations

  In addition, specific differences in patient values, preferences, and beliefs are addressed in **Chapter 68, Concepts of Care for Transgender Patients**. Along with other individuals in the LGBTQ population, the health needs of transgender patients have gained national attention through their inclusion in *Healthy People 2020* and The Joint Commission's Standards affecting transgender patients. This chapter, first introduced in the eighth edition, continues to provide tools to help prepare students and faculty to provide safe, evidence-based, patient-centered care for transgender patients who are considering, currently undergoing, or have undergone the gender transition process.

- **Emphasis on Evidence-Based Practice.** The tenth edition focuses again on the importance of *using best current evidence in nursing practice* and how to locate and use this information to improve patient care. **Evidence-Based Practice boxes** offer a solid foundation in this essential component of nursing practice. Each box summarizes a useful research article, explains the implications of its findings for nursing practice and further research, and rates the level of evidence based on a well-respected scale.

- **Continued Emphasis on Preparation for the NCLEX® Examination.** An enhanced emphasis on the NCLEX® Examination and consistency with the 2019 NCLEX-RN® test plan has been refined in this edition. The tenth edition emphasizes "readiness"—readiness for the NCLEX® Examination, readiness for disaster and mass casualty events, readiness for safe drug administration, and readiness for the continually evolving world of genetics and genomics. An increased number of new **NCLEX Examination Challenges** are interspersed throughout the text to allow students the opportunity to practice test-taking and decision making. **NCLEX Mastery Questions**, new to the tenth edition, are at the end of each chapter. Answers to these Challenges are provided in the back of the book, and their rationales are provided on the Evolve website (http://evolve.elsevier.com/Iggy). In a world that needs more nurses than ever before, it is critical that students be ready to pass the licensure examination on the first try. To help students and faculty achieve that goal, **Learning Outcomes** at the beginning of each chapter continue to be consistent with the competencies outlined in the 2019 NCLEX-RN® Test Plan. The tenth edition continues to include an innovative end-of-chapter feature called **Get Ready for the Next-Generation NCLEX® Examination!** This unique and effective learning aid consists of a list of **Key Points** *organized by Client Needs Category* as found in the NCLEX-RN® Test Plan. Relevant QSEN and Nurse of the Future competency categories are identified for selected Key Points.

- **Focus on Care Coordination and Transition Management.** Similar to the ninth edition, the tenth edition includes a priority focus on continuity of care via a Care Coordination and Transition Management section in each Nursing Care chapter. Literature continues to emphasize the importance of care coordination and transition management between acute care and community-based care. To help students prepare for this role, this edition of our text provides content focusing on Home Care Management, Self-Management Education, and Health Care Resources.

CLINICAL CURRENCY AND ACCURACY

To ensure currency and accuracy, we listened to students and faculty who have used the previous editions, hearing their impressions of and experiences with the book. A thorough literature search of current best evidence regarding nursing education and clinical practice helped us validate best practices and national health care trends that have shaped the focus of the tenth edition. Further cumulative efforts are reflected in this edition:

- Strong, consistent focus on NCLEX-RN® Examination preparation, clinical judgment, safe patient-centered interprofessional care, pathophysiology, drug therapy, quality improvement, evidence-based clinical practice, and care coordination and transition management
- Foundation of relevant research and best practice guidelines
- Emphasis on critical "need-to-know" information that entry-level nurses must master to provide safe patient care

With the amount of information that continues to evolve in health care practice and education, it is easy for a book to become larger with each new edition. The reality is that today's nursing students have a limited time to absorb and apply essential information to provide safe medical-surgical nursing care. Materials in this edition were carefully scrutinized to determine the essential information that students will actively *use* when providing safe, patient-centered, interprofessional, quality nursing care for adults.

OUTSTANDING READABILITY

Today's students must maximize their study time to read information and quickly understand it. The average reading level of today's learner is 10th to 11th grade. To achieve this level of readability without reducing the quality or depth of material that students need to know, this text uses a direct-address style (where appropriate) that speaks directly to the reader. Sentences are as short as possible without sacrificing essential content. The new edition has continued to improve within consistency among chapters. The result of our efforts is a medical-surgical text of consistently outstanding readability in which content is clear, focused, and accessible.

EASE OF ACCESS

To make this text as easy to use as possible, we have maintained our approach of having smaller chapters of more uniform length. Consistent with our focus on "need-to-know" material, we chose exemplars to illustrate concepts of care versus detailing every health disorder. The focused tenth edition contains 69 chapters. To help decrease the number of chapters and stay focused on essential "need-to-know" content, several changes were made, including:

- Combining the content on skin disorders and burns into one chapter instead of two separate chapters
- Deleting the chapter on Intraoperative Care, a specialized area of expertise that is no longer tested on the NCLEX-RN® Examination
- Combining the preoperative and postoperative content from two chapters into one chapter (Chapter 9: Concepts of Care for Perioperative Patients)
- Deleting the chapter on arthritis and connective tissue disorders but moving essential content into appropriate chapters, including a new chapter in the musculoskeletal section (Chapter 46: Concepts of Care for Patients with Arthritis and Total Joint Arthroplasty)
- Combining the two chapters on disorders of the oral cavity and esophagus into one chapter (Chapter 49) to prevent duplication of content

The overall presentation of the tenth edition has been updated, including more current, high-quality photographs for realism. Design changes have been made to improve accessibility of material. There is appropriate placement of display elements (e.g., figures, tables, and boxes) for a chapter flow that enhances text reading without splintering content or confusing the reader. Instead of including a glossary at the end of the text, each chapter's key terms are now defined at the beginning of the chapters for quick reference. To increase the smoothness of flow and reader concentration, side-turned tables and charts or tables and charts that span multiple pages are infrequently used.

We have maintained the unit structure of previous editions, with larger vital body systems appearing earlier in the book. However, in the tenth edition we expanded complex care content in separate critical care chapters for patients with coronary artery disease, respiratory health problems, and neurologic health problems.

To break up long blocks of text and highlight key information, we continue to include streamlined yet eye-catching headings, bulleted lists, tables, boxes, and in-text highlights. Current references at the end of each chapter include research articles, nationally accepted clinical guidelines, and other sources of evidence when available for each chapter. Classic sources from before 2015 are noted with an asterisk (*).

A PATIENT-CENTERED, INTERPROFESSIONAL COLLABORATIVE CARE APPROACH

As in previous editions, we maintain in this edition a collaborative, interprofessional care approach to patient care. In the real world of health care, nurses, patients, and all other providers who are part of the interprofessional team *share* responsibility for the management of patients and their health problems. Thus we present information in a collaborative framework with an increased emphasis on the interprofessional nature of care. In this framework we make no *artificial* distinctions between medical treatment and nursing care. Instead, under each Interprofessional Collaborative Care heading we discuss how the nurse coordinates care and transition management while interacting with members of the interprofessional team. A new feature for the tenth edition is **Interprofessional Collaboration boxes** that present helpful content on how nurses can collaborate with the interprofessional health care team to help meet optimal patient outcomes. Each box identifies the Interprofessional Education Collaborative (IPEC) Expert Panel's Competency of Roles and Responsibilities that aligns with its content.

Although our approach has a focus on interprofessional care, the text is first and foremost a *nursing* text. We therefore use a nursing process/clinical judgment approach as a tool to organize discussions of patient health problems and their management. Discussions of *major* health problems follow a full nursing process format using this structure:

[Health problem]
Pathophysiology Review
    Etiology (and Genetic Risk when appropriate)
    Incidence and Prevalence
Health Promotion and Maintenance (when appropriate)
Interprofessional Collaborative Care
    Assessment: Recognize Cues
    Analysis: Analyze Cues and Prioritize Hypotheses
    Planning and Implementation: Generate Solutions and Take Action
        [Collaborative Intervention Statement (based on priority patient problems)]
      Planning: Expected Outcomes
      Interventions
    Care Coordination and Transition Management
      Home Care Management
      Self-Management Education
      Health Care Resources
    Evaluation: Evaluate Outcomes

Discussions of less common (but important) or less complex disorders follow a similar yet abbreviated format: a discussion of the problem itself (including pertinent review information on pathophysiology) followed by a section on interprofessional collaborative care of patients with the disorder. To demonstrate our commitment to providing the content foundational to nursing education, and consistent with the recommendations of Benner and colleagues through the Carnegie Foundation for the Future of Nursing Education, we highlight essential pathophysiologic concepts that are key to understanding the basis for collaborative management.

Integral to the interprofessional care approach is a narrative of who on the health care team is involved in the care of the patient. When a responsibility is primarily the nurse's, the text says so. When a decision must be made jointly by various members of the team (e.g., by the patient, nurse, primary health care provider, and physical therapist), this is clearly stated. When health care practitioners in different care settings are involved in the patient's care, this is noted.

ORGANIZATION

The 69 chapters of *Medical-Surgical Nursing: Concepts for Interprofessional Collaborative Care* are grouped into 15 units. Unit I, Concepts for Medical-Surgical Nursing, provides fundamental information for the health care concepts incorporated throughout the text. Unit II consists of three chapters on concepts of emergency care and disaster preparedness.

Unit III consists of three chapters on the management of patients with fluid, electrolyte, and acid-base imbalances. Chapters 13 and 14 review key assessments associated with fluid and electrolyte balance, acid-base balance, and related patient care in a clear, concise discussion. The chapter on infusion therapy (Chapter 15) is supplemented with an online Fluids & Electrolytes Tutorial on the companion Evolve website.

Unit IV provides core content on health problems related to immunity. This material includes information on inflammation and the immune response, altered cell growth and cancer development, and interventions for patients with connective tissue disease, HIV infection, and other immunologic disorders, cancers, and infections.

The remaining 11 units focus on medical-surgical content by body system. Each of these units begins with an Assessment chapter and continues with one or more Nursing Care chapters for patients with selected health problems, highlighted via exemplars, in that body system. This framework is familiar to students who learn the body systems in preclinical foundational science courses such as anatomy and physiology.

MULTINATIONAL, MULTICULTURAL, MULTIGENERATIONAL FOCUS

To reflect the increasing diversity of our society, *Medical-Surgical Nursing: Concepts for Interprofessional Collaborative Care* takes a multinational, multicultural, and multigenerational focus. Addressing the needs of both U.S. and Canadian readers, we have included U.S. and international units for normal values of selected laboratory tests. When appropriate, we identify specific Canadian health care resources, including their websites. In many areas, Canadian health statistics are combined with those of the United States to provide an accurate "North American" picture.

To help nurses provide quality care for patients whose preferences, beliefs, and values may differ from their own, numerous **Patient-Centered Care: Cultural/Spiritual Considerations** and **Patient-Centered Care: Gender Health Considerations boxes** highlight important aspects of culturally competent care. Chapter 68 is dedicated to the special health care needs of transgender patients.

Increases in life expectancy and aging of the baby-boom generation contribute to a steadily increasing older adult population. To help nurses care for this population, the tenth edition continues to provide thorough coverage of the care of older adults. Chapter 4 offers content on the role of the nurse and interprofessional team in promoting health for this population, with coverage of common health problems that older adults may experience, such as falls and inadequate nutrition. **Patient-Centered Care: Considerations for Older Adults boxes** that specify normal physiologic changes to expect in the older population are found in each Assessment chapter. In the Nursing Care chapters, these boxes also present key points for the student to consider when caring for these patients. A new feature for the ninth edition was **Patient-Centered Care: Veterans Health Considerations**. The tenth edition increases emphasis on the special health needs of this population. An increasing number of veterans have multiple physical and mental health concerns that require special attention in today's environment of care.

AN INTEGRATED MULTIMEDIA RESOURCE BASED ON PROVEN STRATEGIES FOR STUDENT ENGAGEMENT AND LEARNING

Medical-Surgical Nursing: Concepts for Interprofessional Collaborative Care, 10th edition, is the centerpiece of a comprehensive package of electronic and print learning resources that break new ground in the application of proven strategies for student engagement, learning, and evidence-based educational practice. This integrated multimedia resource actively engages the student in problem solving and using clinical judgment to make important clinical decisions.

Resources for Instructors

For the convenience of faculty, all Instructor Resources are available on a streamlined, secure instructor area of the Evolve website (http://evolve.elsevier.com/Iggy/). All ancillaries for this edition were developed with direct involvement of the textbook authors. Included among these Instructor Resources are the *TEACH® for Nurses* **Lesson Plans.** These Lesson Plans focus on the most important content from each chapter and provide innovative strategies for student engagement and learning. This tenth edition *TEACH for Nurses* product incorporates numerous interprofessional activities that give students an opportunity to practice as an integral part of the health care team. Lesson Plans are provided for each chapter and are categorized into several parts:

Learning Outcomes

Teaching Focus

Key Terms

Nursing Curriculum Standards

    QSEN

    Concepts

    BSN Essentials

Student Chapter Resources
Instructor Chapter Resources
Teaching Strategies

Additional Instructor Resources provided on the Evolve website include:

- A completely revised, updated, high-quality **Test Bank** consisting of more than 1509 items, both traditional multiple-choice and NCLEX-RN® "alternate-item" types. Each question is coded for correct answer, rationale, cognitive level, NCLEX Integrated Process, NCLEX Client Needs Category, and new key words to facilitate question searches. Page references are provided for Remembering (Knowledge)-level and Understanding (Comprehension)-level questions. (Questions at the Applying [Application] and above cognitive level require the student to draw on understanding of multiple or broader concepts not limited to a single textbook page, so page cross references are not provided for these higher-level critical thinking questions.) The Test Bank is provided in the Evolve Assessment Manager and in ExamView and ParTest formats. New to this edition, 75 Next-Generation NCLEX® Examination Review questions are provided within an interactive application for further testing options.
- An electronic **Image Collection** containing all images from the book (approximately 550 images), delivered in a format that makes incorporation into lectures, presentations, and online courses easier than ever.
- A completely revised collection of more than 2000 **PowerPoint slides** corresponding to each chapter in the text and highlighting key materials with integrated images and Unfolding Case Studies. Audience Response System Questions (three discussion-oriented questions per chapter for use with iClicker and other audience response systems) are included in these slide presentations. Answers and rationales to the Audience Response System Questions and Unfolding Case Studies are found in the "Notes" section of each slide.

Also available for adoption and separate purchase:

- Corresponding chapter-by-chapter to the textbook, *Elsevier Adaptive Quizzing (EAQ)* integrates seamlessly into your course to help students of all skill levels focus their study time and effectively prepare for class, course exams, and the NCLEX® certification exam. *EAQ* is comprised of a bank of high-quality practice questions that allows students to advance at their own pace—based on their performance—through multiple mastery levels for each chapter. A comprehensive dashboard allows students to view their progress and stay motivated. The educator dashboard, grade book, and reporting capabilities enable faculty to monitor the activity of individual students, assess overall class performance, and identify areas of strength and weakness, ultimately helping to achieve improved learning outcomes.
- *Simulation Learning System (SLS) for Medical-Surgical Nursing* is an online toolkit designed to help you effectively incorporate simulation into your nursing curriculum, with scenarios that promote and enhance the clinical decision-making skills of students at all levels. It offers detailed instructions

for preparation and implementation of the simulation experience, debriefing questions that encourage critical thinking, and learning resources to reinforce student comprehension. Modularized simulation scenarios correspond to Elsevier's leading medical-surgical nursing texts, reinforcing students' classroom knowledge base, synthesizing lecture and clinicals, and offering the remediation content that is critical to debriefing.

Resources for Students

Resources for students include a revised, updated, and retitled Study Guide, a Clinical Companion, Elsevier Adaptive Learning (EAL), Virtual Clinical Excursions (VCE), and Evolve Learning Resources.

The *Study Guide* has been completely revised and updated and features a fresh emphasis on clinical decision making, priorities of delegation, management of care, and pharmacology. Unlike earlier editions, the rationales are provided along with the correct responses to allow students the opportunity to enhance their understanding of content and increase their test-taking skills.

The pocket-sized *Clinical Companion* is a handy clinical resource that retains its easy-to-use alphabetical organization and streamlined format, with completely revised content for ease of use and on-the-go care. The bulleted format is integrated with key elements of the NCSBN Clinical Judgment Measurement Model. It includes "Critical Rescue," "Drug Alert," and "Action Alert" highlights throughout based on the Nursing Safety Priority features in the textbook. National Patient Safety Goals highlights have been expanded as a QSEN feature, focusing on one of six QSEN core competencies while still underscoring the importance of observing vital patient safety standards. Increased use of illustrations facilitates clinical application of key content. This "pocket-sized Iggy" has been tailored to the special needs of students preparing for clinicals and clinical practice.

Corresponding chapter-by-chapter to the textbook, *Elsevier Adaptive Learning (EAL)* combines the power of brain science with sophisticated, patented Cerego algorithms to help students to learn faster and remember longer. It's fun, it's engaging, and it constantly tracks and adapts to student performance to deliver content precisely when it's needed to ensure core information is transformed into lasting knowledge.

Virtual Clinical Excursions, featuring an updated and easy-to-navigate "virtual" clinical setting, is once again available for the tenth edition. This unique learning tool guides students through a virtual clinical environment and helps them "learn by doing" in the safety of a "virtual" hospital.

Also available for students is a dynamic collection of Evolve Student Resources, available at http://evolve.elsevier.com/Iggy/. The Evolve Student Resources include the following:

- Review Questions—NCLEX® Examination
- Review Questions—Next-Generation NCLEX® Examination
- Answer Guidelines for Next-Generation NCLEX® Examination and Clinical Judgment Challenges
- Interactive Case Studies
- Concept Maps

- Concept Map Creator (a handy tool for creating customized Concept Maps)
- Fluid & Electrolyte Tutorial (a complete self-paced tutorial on this perennially difficult content)
- Key Points (downloadable expanded chapter reviews for each chapter)
- Audio Glossary
- Audio Clips and Video Clips

In summary, *Medical-Surgical Nursing: Concepts for Interprofessional Collaborative Care,* tenth edition, together with its fully integrated multimedia ancillary package, provides the tools you will need to equip nursing students to meet the opportunities and challenges of nursing practice both now and in an evolving health care environment. The only elements that remain to be added to this package are those that you uniquely provide—your passion, your commitment, your innovation, *your nursing expertise.*

Donna D. Ignatavicius
M. Linda Workman
Cherie R. Rebar
Nicole M. Heimgartner

*We are dedicating this landmark tenth edition to our parents. These wonderful
women and men were our first teachers, believed in our dreams, and instilled in us
the fortitude to reach high to accomplish our professional and personal goals.
It is with love and gratefulness that we honor and remember:*

Donna's parents
Mary P. Dennis (1929-1972)
Barney J. Dennis, Jr. (1923-1985)

Linda's parents
M. Eunice R. Workman (1929-2019)
Homer D. Workman (1928-1992)

Cherie's parents
Ruth (Whitt) Carnes (1933-2019)
Charles R. Carnes, Jr. (1930-2008)

Nicole's parents
Edna Surles (1944-2018)
Logan Surles, Jr. (living)

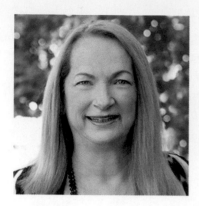

Donna D. Ignatavicius received her diploma in nursing from the Peninsula General School of Nursing in Salisbury, Maryland. After working as a charge nurse in medical-surgical nursing, she became an instructor in staff development at the University of Maryland Medical Center. She then received her BSN from the University of Maryland School of Nursing. For 5 years she taught in several schools of nursing while working toward her MS in Nursing, which she received in 1981. Donna then taught in the BSN program at the University of Maryland, after which she continued to pursue her interest in gerontology and accepted the position of Director of Nursing of a major skilled-nursing facility in her home state of Maryland. Since that time, she has served as an instructor in several associate degree nursing programs. Through her consulting activities, faculty development workshops, and international nursing education conferences (such as Boot Camp for Nurse Educators®), Donna is nationally recognized as an expert in nursing education. She is currently the President of DI Associates, Inc. (http://www.diassociates.com/), a company dedicated to improving health care through education and consultation for faculty. In recognition of her contributions to the field, she was inducted as a charter Fellow of the prestigious Academy of Nursing Education in 2007, received her Certified Nurse Educator credential in 2016, and obtained her Academic Clinical Nurse Educator certification in 2020.

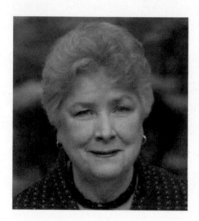

M. Linda Workman, a native of Canada, received her BSN from the University of Cincinnati College of Nursing and Health. After serving in the U.S. Army Nurse Corps and working as an Assistant Head Nurse and Head Nurse in civilian hospitals, Linda earned her MSN from the University of Cincinnati College of Nursing and a PhD in Developmental Biology from the University of Cincinnati College of Arts and Sciences. Linda's 30-plus years of academic experience include teaching at the diploma, associate degree, baccalaureate, master's, and doctoral levels. Her areas of teaching expertise include medical-surgical nursing, physiology, pathophysiology, genetics, oncology, and immunology. Linda has been recognized nationally and internationally for her teaching expertise and was inducted as a Fellow into the American Academy of Nursing in 1992. She received Excellence in Teaching awards at the University of Cincinnati and at Case Western Reserve University. She is a former American Cancer Society Professor of Oncology Nursing and occupied an endowed chair in oncology for 5 years. She has authored several additional textbooks and continues to serve as a consultant for major universities.

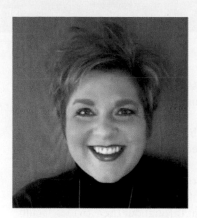

Cherie R. Rebar earned her first degree in education from Morehead State University in Morehead, Kentucky. She returned to school to earn an Associate of Science degree in Nursing from Kettering College, MSN and MBA degrees from the University of Phoenix, a post-masters certificate in Family Nurse Practitioner studies from the University of Massachusetts—Boston, a Psychiatric-Mental Health Nurse Practitioner post-masters certificate from the University of Cincinnati College of Nursing, and a PhD in Psychology (Health Behaviors) from Northcentral University. Combining her loves of nursing and education, Cherie continues to teach students in prelicensure and graduate nursing programs. She has served in numerous leadership positions over the years, including Chair of ASN, BSN Completion, and BSN Prelicensure Nursing Programs, and Director of Nursing. She currently is a Professor of Nursing at Wittenberg University and an Adjunct Faculty Member at Indiana Wesleyan University and Mercy College of Ohio. Her years of clinical practice include medical-surgical, acute care, ear/nose/throat surgery and allergy, community, and psychiatric-mental health nursing. A frequent presenter at national and state nursing conferences, Cherie serves as a consultant to nursing programs and faculty, contributes regularly to professional publications, and holds student success at the heart of all she does.

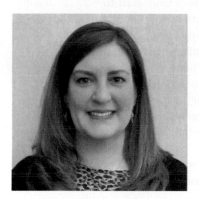

Nicole M. Heimgartner received her BSN from Spalding University in Louisville, Kentucky, her MSN with an emphasis in education from the University of Phoenix, and her Doctorate of Nursing Practice in Educational Leadership from American Sentinel University in Aurora, Colorado. Nicole is also certified in online education.

Nicole has a very diverse clinical background, with extensive practice experience in cardiovascular, medical-surgical, and community nursing. As her love for the nursing profession grew, Nicole started teaching in undergraduate and graduate degree programs. Nicole now has over 17 years of experience as an educator, focusing on innovative educational strategy, nursing leadership, and incorporating online learning into nursing education. Her expertise includes currency in clinical practice as well as teaching and designing curriculum at the undergraduate and graduate levels of nursing education. Nicole also presents at the state and national level on best nursing practice, serves as a consultant with nursing programs and faculty, contributes regularly to professional publications, and is passionate about current practice and engaging the adult learner.

ACKNOWLEDGMENTS

Publishing a textbook and ancillary package of this magnitude would not be possible without the combined efforts of many people. With that in mind, we would like to extend our deepest gratitude to many people who were such an integral part of this journey.

For the tenth edition, we welcomed Nicole M. Heimgartner as a full member of the author and editor team. Nicole has worked with our team previously in contributor, section editor, and ancillary roles over the past editions.

Our contributing authors once again provided excellent manuscripts to underscore the clinical relevancy of this publication. Our reviewers—expert clinicians and instructors from around the United States and Canada—provided invaluable suggestions and encouragement throughout the development of book.

The staff of Elsevier has, as always, provided us with meaningful guidance and support throughout every step of the planning, writing, revision, and production of the tenth edition. Executive Content Strategist Lee Henderson worked closely with us from the early stages of this edition to help us hone and focus our revision plan while coordinating the project from start to finish. Senior Content Development Specialist Laura Goodrich then worked with us to bring the logistics of the tenth edition from vision to publication. Laura also held the reins of our complex ancillary package and worked with the authors and a gifted group of writers and content experts to provide an outstanding library of resources to complement and enhance the text.

Senior Project Manager Jodi Willard was, as always, an absolute joy with whom to work. If the mark of a good editor is that his or her work is invisible to the reader, then Jodi is the consummate editor. Her unwavering attention to detail, flexibility, and conscientiousness helped to make the tenth edition consistently readable, while making the production process incredibly smooth. Also, a special thanks to Publishing Services Manager Julie Eddy.

Designer Brian Salisbury is responsible for the beautiful cover and the new interior design of the tenth edition. Brian's work on this edition has cast important features in exactly the right light, contributing to the readability and colorful beauty of this edition.

Our acknowledgments would not be complete without recognizing our dedicated team of Educational Solutions Consultants and other key members of the Sales and Marketing staff who helped to put this book into your hands.

Donna D. Ignatavicius
M. Linda Workman
Cherie R. Rebar
Nicole M. Heimgartner

CONTENTS

Asterisk (*) denotes a Concept Exemplar.

UNIT IV Interprofessional Collaboration for Patients With Problems of Immunity

GUIDE TO SPECIAL FEATURES

COMMON EXAMPLES OF DRUG THERAPY

EVIDENCE-BASED PRACTICE

FOCUSED ASSESSMENT

HOME CARE CONSIDERATIONS

KEY FEATURES

LABORATORY PROFILE

PATIENT AND FAMILY EDUCATION: PREPARING FOR SELF-MANAGEMENT

SYSTEMS THINKING AND QUALITY IMPROVEMENT

Assessment and Concepts of Care for Patients With Eye and Vision Problems

Cherie R. Rebar, Samuel A. Borchers, Andrea A. Borchers

http://evolve.elsevier.com/Iggy/

LEARNING OUTCOMES

1. Collaborate with the interprofessional team to perform assessments of eyes and vision.
2. Prioritize evidence-based care for patients having an eye assessment or treatment for eye or vision problems that affect **sensory perception.**
3. Teach evidence-based way for adults to protect their eyes from injury or infection to preserve **sensory perception.**
4. Explain how physiologic aging changes of the eyes and vision affect **sensory perception.**
5. Teach patients who need vision assistive devices how to use them.
6. Implement nursing interventions to decrease the psychosocial impact for the patient undergoing eye assessment or treatment for eye or vision problems.
7. Apply knowledge of anatomy and physiology, genetic risk, and principles of aging to perform a focused assessment of the eyes and vision.
8. Use clinical judgment to analyze assessment findings and diagnostic data in the care of patients with an eye or vision problem.
9. Plan care coordination and transition management for patients with an eye or vision problem.

KEY TERMS

arcus senilis An opaque, bluish-white ring within the outer edge of the cornea.

cataract A lens opacity that distorts the image projected onto the retina.

enucleation Surgical removal of the entire eyeball.

glaucoma A condition in the eye that occurs with increased pressure and resulting hypoxia of photoreceptors and their synapsing nerve fibers.

hyperopia Farsightedness.

keratitis Inflammation of the cornea.

keratoconus Degeneration of the cornea.

keratoplasty Corneal transplant. The surgical removal of diseased corneal tissue and replacement with tissue from a human donor cornea.

myopia Nearsightedness.

nystagmus An involuntary and rapid twitching of the eyeball.

photophobia Sensitivity to light.

primary angle-closure glaucoma (PACG) A form of glaucoma that can have a sudden onset and is an emergency; it is characterized by a forward displacement of the iris, which presses against the cornea and closes the chamber angle, suddenly preventing outflow of aqueous humor. Also called *closed-angle glaucoma, narrow-angle glaucoma,* or *acute glaucoma.*

primary open-angle glaucoma (POAG) The most common form of primary glaucoma; characterized by reduced outflow of aqueous humor through the chamber angle. Because the fluid cannot leave the eye at the same rate it is produced, intraocular pressure gradually increases.

retinal detachment The separation of the retina from the epithelium.

retinal hole a break in the retina, often caused by trauma or aging.

retina tear A jagged and irregularly shaped break in the retina, which can result from traction on the retina.

Sensory perception is the ability to perceive and interpret sensory input into one or more meaningful responses (see Chapter 3). Many adults think of vision as their most important sense because it assesses surroundings, allows independence, warns of danger, appreciates beauty, and helps them work, play, and interact with others. Changes in the eye and vision can provide information about the patient's general health status and problems that might occur in self-care.

ANATOMY AND PHYSIOLOGY REVIEW

Visual *sensory perception* takes place when the eye and brain work together. Vision begins when light is changed into nerve impulses in the eye and the impulses are sent on to the brain to fully perceive images (McCance et al., 2019). Systemic conditions and eye problems can change vision temporarily or permanently.

Structure

The eyeball, a round, ball-shaped organ, is located in the front part of the eye orbit. The orbit is the bony socket of the skull that surrounds and protects the eye along with the attached muscles, nerves, vessels, and tear-producing glands.

Layers of the Eyeball. The eye has three layers (Fig. 42.1). The external layer is the sclera (the "white" of the eye) and the transparent cornea on the front of the eye.

The middle layer, or **uvea,** is heavily pigmented and consists of the choroid, the ciliary body, and the iris. The choroid, a dark brown membrane between the sclera and the retina, lines most of the sclera. It has many blood vessels that supply nutrients to the retina.

The ciliary body connects the choroid with the iris and secretes aqueous humor. The **iris** is the colored portion of the external eye; its center opening is the *pupil.* The muscles of the iris contract and relax to control pupil size and the amount of light entering the eye.

The innermost layer is the *retina,* a thin, delicate structure made up of sensory photoreceptors that begin the transmission of impulses to the optic nerve (McCance et al., 2019). The retina contains blood vessels and two types of photoreceptors called *rods* and *cones.* The rods work at low light levels and provide peripheral vision. The cones are active at bright light levels and provide color and central vision.

The *optic fundus* is the area at the inside back of the eye that can be seen with an ophthalmoscope. This area contains the *optic disc,* a pinkish-orange or white depressed area where the nerve fibers that synapse with the photoreceptors join together to form the optic nerve and exit the eyeball. The optic disc contains only nerve fibers and no photoreceptor cells. To one side of the optic disc is a small, yellowish pink area called the *macula lutea.* The center of the macula is the *fovea centralis,* where vision is most acute.

Refractive Structures and Media. Light waves pass through the cornea, aqueous humor, lens, and vitreous humor on the way to the retina. Each structure bends *(refracts)* the light waves to focus images on the retina. Together these structures are the eye's *refracting media.*

The *cornea* is the clear layer that forms the external bump on the front of the eye (see Fig. 42.1). The *aqueous humor* is a clear,

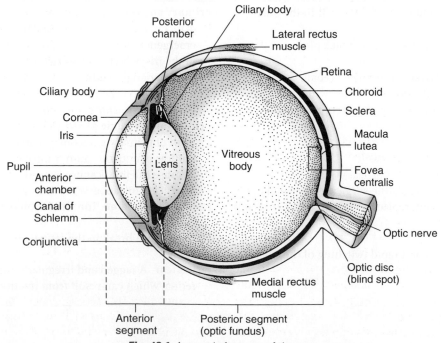

Fig. 42.1 Anatomic features of the eye.

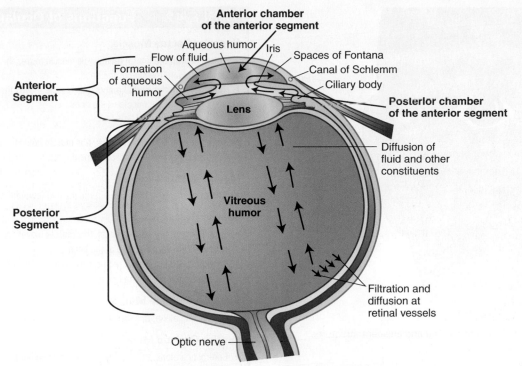

Fig. 42.2 Flow of aqueous humor.

watery fluid that fills the anterior and posterior chambers of the eye. This fluid is continually produced by the ciliary processes and passes from the posterior chamber, through the pupil, and into the anterior chamber. This fluid drains through the canal of Schlemm into the blood to maintain a balanced intraocular pressure (IOP), the pressure within the eye (Fig. 42.2).

The *lens* is a circular, convex structure that lies behind the iris and in front of the vitreous body. It is transparent and bends the light rays entering through the pupil to focus properly on the retina. The curve of the lens changes to focus on near or distant objects. A cataract is a lens opacity that distorts the image projected onto the retina.

The *vitreous body* is a clear, thick gel that fills the large vitreous chamber (the space between the lens and the retina). This gel transmits light and maintains eye shape.

The eye is a hollow organ and must be kept in the shape of a ball for vision to occur. To maintain this shape, the vitreous humor gel in the posterior segment and the aqueous humor in the anterior segment must be present in set amounts that apply pressure inside the eye to keep it inflated. This pressure is the *intraocular pressure* or *IOP*. IOP has to be precisely accurate. If the pressure is too low, the eyeball is soft and collapses, preventing light from getting to the photoreceptors on the retina in the back of the eye. If the pressure becomes too high, the extra pressure compresses capillaries in the eye and nerve fibers. Pressure on retinal blood vessels prevents blood from flowing through them; therefore, the photoreceptors and nerve fibers become hypoxic. Compression of the fine nerve fibers prevents intracellular fluid flow, which also reduces nourishment to the distal portions of these thin nerve fibers. Glaucoma occurs with increased pressure and resulting hypoxia of photoreceptors and their synapsing nerve fibers. Continued retinal hypoxia results

in necrosis and death of photoreceptors, as well as permanent nerve fiber damage. When extensive photoreceptor and nerve fiber loss occur, vision is lost, and the person is permanently blind (Bagheri & Wajda, 2017).

External Structures. The eyelids are thin, movable skinfolds that protect the eyes and keep the cornea moist. The *canthus* is the place where the two eyelids meet at the corner of the eye.

The *conjunctivae* are the mucous membranes of the eye. The palpebral conjunctiva is a thick membrane with many blood vessels that lines the undersurface of each eyelid. The thin, transparent bulbar conjunctiva covers the entire front of the eye.

A small *lacrimal gland,* which is located in the upper outer part of each orbit (Fig. 42.3), produces tears. Tears flow across the front of the eye, toward the nose, and into the inner canthus. They drain through the *punctum* (an opening at the nasal side of the lid edges) into the lacrimal duct and sac and then into the nose through the nasolacrimal duct.

Muscles, Nerves, and Blood Vessels. Six voluntary muscles rotate the eye and coordinate eye movements (Fig. 42.4 and Table 42.1). Coordinated eye movements ensure that both eyes receive an image at the same time so that only a single image is seen.

The muscles around the eye are innervated by cranial nerves (CNs) III (oculomotor), IV (trochlear), and VI (abducens). The *optic nerve* (CN II) is the nerve of sight, connecting the optic disc to the brain. The trigeminal nerve (CN V) stimulates the blink reflex when the cornea is touched. The facial nerve (CN VII) innervates the lacrimal glands and muscles for lid closure.

The ophthalmic artery brings oxygenated blood to the eye and the orbit. It branches to supply blood to the retina. The ciliary arteries supply the sclera, choroid, ciliary body, and iris.

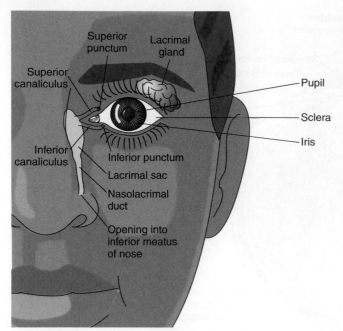

Fig. 42.3 Front view of the eye and adjacent structures.

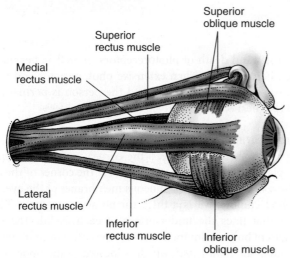

Fig. 42.4 Extraocular muscles.

Outflow moves through several venous pathways that empty into the superior ophthalmic vein.

Function

The four eye functions that provide clear images and vision are refraction, pupillary constriction, accommodation, and convergence.

Refraction bends light rays from the outside into the eye through curved surfaces and refractive media and finally to the retina. Each surface and media bend (refract) light differently to focus an image on the retina. *Emmetropia* is the perfect refraction of the eye in which light rays from a distant source are focused into a sharp image on the retina. Fig. 42.5 shows the normal refraction of light within the eye. Images fall on the retina inverted and reversed left to right. For example, an object in the lower nasal visual field strikes the upper outer area of the retina.

TABLE 42.1 Functions of Ocular Muscles

Superior Rectus Muscle
- Together with the lateral rectus, this muscle moves the eye diagonally upward toward the side of the head.
- Together with the medial rectus, this muscle moves the eye diagonally upward toward the middle of the head.

Lateral Rectus Muscle
- Together with the medial rectus, this muscle holds the eye straight.
- Contracting alone, this muscle turns the eye toward the side of the head.

Medial Rectus Muscle
- Contracting alone, this muscle turns the eye toward the nose.

Inferior Rectus Muscle
- Together with the lateral rectus, this muscle moves the eye diagonally downward toward the side of the head.
- Together with the medial rectus, this muscle moves the eye diagonally downward toward the middle of the head.

Superior Oblique Muscle
- Contracting alone, this muscle pulls the eye downward.

Inferior Oblique Muscle
- Contracting alone, this muscle pulls the eye upward.

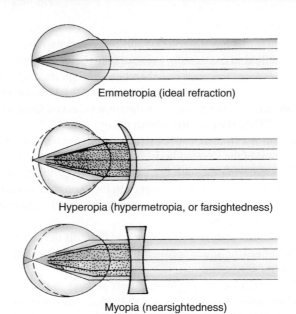

Fig. 42.5 Refraction and correction in emmetropia, hyperopia, and myopia.

Errors of refraction are common. **Hyperopia** (farsightedness) occurs when the eye does not refract light enough. As a result, images actually converge behind the retina (see Fig. 42.5). In hyperopia, distant vision is normal, but near vision is poor. It is corrected with a convex lens in eyeglasses or contact lenses.

Myopia (nearsightedness) occurs when the eye overbends the light and images converge in front of the retina (see Fig. 42.5). Near vision is normal, but distance vision is poor. Myopia is corrected with a concave lens in eyeglasses or contact lenses.

Astigmatism is a refractive error caused by unevenly curved surfaces on or in the eye, especially the cornea. These uneven surfaces distort vision.

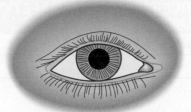 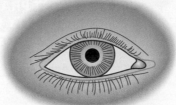 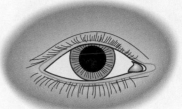

Normal pupil slightly dilated for moderate light

Miosis—pupil constricted when exposed to increased light or close work, such as reading

Mydriasis—pupil dilated when exposed to reduced light or when looking at a distance

Fig. 42.6 Miosis and mydriasis.

PATIENT-CENTERED CARE: OLDER ADULT CONSIDERATIONS (QSEN)

Changes in the Eye and Vision Related to Aging

Structure/ Function	Change	Implication
Appearance	Eyes appear "sunken." Arcus senilis forms. Sclera yellows or appears blue.	Do not use eye appearance as an indicator for hydration status. Reassure patient that this change does not affect vision. Do not use sclera to assess for jaundice.
Cornea	Cornea flattens, which blurs vision and can cause or worsen astigmatism.	Encourage older adults to have regular eye examinations and wear prescribed corrective lenses for best vision.
Ocular muscles	Muscle strength is reduced, making it more difficult to maintain an upward gaze or a focus on a single image.	Reassure patient that this is a normal finding and to refocus gaze frequently to maintain a single image.
Lens	Elasticity is lost, increasing the near point of vision (making the near point of best vision farther away). Lens hardens, compacts, and forms a cataract.	Encourage use of corrective lenses for reading. Emphasize the importance of annual vision checks and monitoring.
Iris and pupil	Decrease in ability to dilate results in small pupil size and poor adaptation to darkness.	Teach that good lighting is needed to avoid bumping into objects, tripping, and falling.
Color vision	Discrimination among greens, blues, and violets decreases.	The patient may not be able to use color-indicator monitors of health status.
Tears	Tear production is reduced, resulting in dry eyes, discomfort, and increased risk for corneal damage or eye infections.	Teach the proper use of saline eyedrops to reduce dryness. Teach to increase humidity in the home.

Pupillary constriction (miosis) and pupillary dilation (mydriasis) (Fig. 42.6) control the amount of light that enters the eye. If the level of light to one or both eyes is increased, both pupils constrict (become smaller). The amount of constriction depends on how much light is available and how well the retina can adapt to light changes. Certain drugs can alter pupillary constriction.

The process of maintaining a clear visual image when the gaze is shifted from a distant to a near object is known as *accommodation.* The healthy eye can adjust its focus by changing the curve of the lens.

Convergence is the ability to turn both eyes inward toward the nose at the same time. This action helps ensure that only a single image of close objects is seen.

Eye Changes Associated With Aging

Visual acuity decreases with age due to changes inside the eye (Touhy & Jett, 2018). Age-related changes of the nervous system and in the eye support structures also reduce visual function (see the Patient Centered Care: Older Adult Considerations: Changes in the Eye and Vision Related to Aging box).

Structural changes occur with aging, including decreased eye muscle tone that reduces the ability to keep the gaze focused on a single object. The lower eyelid may relax and fall away from the eye *(ectropion),* leading to dry eye signs and symptoms.

Arcus senilis, an opaque, bluish-white ring within the outer edge of the cornea, is caused by fat deposits (Fig. 42.7). This change does not affect vision.

Fatty deposits cause the sclera to develop a yellowish tinge. A bluish color may be seen as the sclera thins. With age, the iris has less ability to dilate, which leads to difficulty in adapting to dark environments. Older adults may benefit from additional light for reading and other "close-up" work and to avoid tripping over objects.

Functional changes also occur with aging. The lens yellows, hardens, shrinks, and loses elasticity, which reduces accommodation. The **near point of vision** (i.e., the closest distance at which the eye can see an object clearly) increases. Near objects,

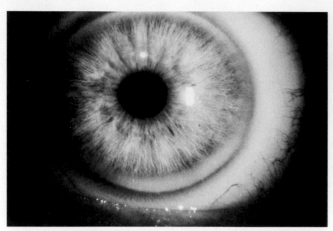

Fig. 42.7 Arcus senilis of the iris.

Basic Eye Examination Frequency

Age	Recommended Frequency
20-39 African-American	Every 2-4 years
20-39 Caucasian	Every 3-5 years
40-64 (any race)	Every 2-4 years
65 years and over (of any race)	Every 1-2 years
People with special risks (e.g., diabetes, eye surgery or trauma, glaucoma)	As recommended by the eye care provider (may be more frequent)

Adapted from American Academy of Ophthalmology. (2019). Eye exam and vision testing basics. Retrieved from https://www.aao.org/eye-health/tips-prevention/eye-exams-101; and PreventBlindness.org. (2020). How often should I have an eye examination? Retrieved from https://www.preventblindness.org/how-often-should-i-have-eye-exam.

especially reading material, must be placed farther from the eye to be seen clearly (**presbyopia**). The **far point** (i.e., the farthest point at which an object can be distinguished) decreases. Together these changes narrow the visual field of an older adult.

General color perception decreases, especially for green, blue, and violet. More light is needed to stimulate the visual receptors. Intraocular pressure (IOP) is slightly higher in older adults.

Health Promotion and Maintenance

Impairment of vision impacts physical and psychological well-being and is identified as one of the top 10 disabilities in the United States (Quaranta et al., 2016). Many vision and eye problems can be avoided, and others can be corrected or managed if found early. Teach adults about eye-protection methods, adequate nutrition that supports eye health, and the importance of regular eye examinations.

The risks for cataract formation and for cancer of the eye (ocular melanoma) increase with exposure to ultraviolet (UV) light. Teach adults to protect the eyes by using sunglasses that filter UV light whenever they are outdoors, at tanning salons, and when work involves UV exposure.

Vision can be affected by eye injury, which increases the risk for cataract formation and glaucoma. Teach adults to wear eye and head protection when working with particulate matter, fluid or blood spatter, high temperatures, or sparks. Protection should also be worn during participation in sports or any activity that increases the risk for the eye being hit by objects in motion. Teach adults to avoid rubbing the eyes to avoid trauma to outer eye surfaces.

Eye infections can lead to vision loss. Although the eye surface is not sterile, the sclera and cornea have no separate blood supply and thus are at risk for infection. Teach adults to wash their hands before touching the eye or eyelid. Teach patients who use eyedrops about the proper technique to use these drugs and to not share eyedrops with others. If an eye has a discharge, teach the patient to use a separate eyedrop bottle for this eye and to wash the unaffected eye before washing the affected eye.

Other health problems, especially diabetes and hypertension, can seriously affect visual *sensory perception.* Teach patients with these conditions about the importance of controlling blood glucose levels and managing blood pressure to reduce the risk for vision loss. Annual evaluation by an eye care provider is needed prevent eye complications and detect problems early. See the Best Practice for Patient Safety & Quality Care: Basic Eye Examination Frequency box for specific recommendations about how often patients should be seen by an eye care provider for a general eye examination.

Eye care providers may recommend that adults older than 40 years have an eye examination annually that includes assessment of intraocular pressure and visual fields because the risk for both glaucoma and cataract formation increases with age.

Action Alert

Teach adults to see a health care provider immediately when an eye injury occurs or an eye infection is suspected.

NCLEX EXAMINATION CHALLENGE 42.1

Health Promotion and Maintenance

What is the appropriate nursing response when a 66-year-old healthy client asks how often a visit to the eye care provider is recommended?
A. "Annually."
B. "Every 6 months."
C. "Only if you have vision problems."
D. "Every 3 to 5 years if you have no eye problems."

◆ ASSESSMENT: RECOGNIZE CUES

Patient History

Collect information to determine whether problems with the eye or vision have an impact on ADLs or other daily functions.

Age is an important factor to consider when assessing visual *sensory perception* and eye structure. The incidence of glaucoma and cataract formation increases with aging. Presbyopia commonly begins in the 40s.

TABLE 42.2 Systemic Conditions and Common Drugs Affecting the Eye and Vision

Systemic Conditions and Disorders	Drugs
• Diabetes mellitus • Hypertension • Lupus erythematosus • Sarcoidosis • Thyroid problems • HIV-III (acquired immune deficiency syndrome) • Cardiac disease • Multiple sclerosis • Pregnancy	• Antihistamines[a] • Decongestants[a] • Antibiotics • Opioids • Anticholinergics • Cholinergic agonists • Adrenergic agonists • Adrenergic antagonists (beta blockers) • Oral contraceptives • Chemotherapy agents • Corticosteroids[a]

[a]Prescription and over-the-counter.

Gender may be important. Retinal detachments occur more often in men, and dry eye syndromes occur more often in women.

Occupation and leisure activities can affect visual **sensory perception.** Ask about how the eyes are used at work, because those who frequently use computers may experience eyestrain. Machine operators are at risk for injury because of high speeds at which particles can be thrown at the eye. Chronic exposure to infrared or UV light may cause photophobia and cataract formation. A blow to the face or head near the eye when playing sports such as baseball can damage external structures, the eye, the connections with the brain, or the area of the brain where vision is perceived. Teach all people to wear eye protection that is in keeping with their chosen occupation or sport.

Social habits such as smoking or vaping can be a significant risk factor for developing eye problems. Specifically, airborne formaldehyde can cause burning and watering of the eyes. Inquire about whether a patient smokes or vapes, and collect pertinent history regarding this practice.

Systemic health problems can affect vision. Check whether the patient has any condition listed in Table 42.2. Ask about past accidents, injuries, surgeries (including laser surgeries), or blows to the head that may have led to the present problem.

Drugs can also affect vision and the eye (see Table 42.2). Ask about the use of any prescription or over-the-counter drugs, especially decongestants and antihistamines, which cause eye dryness and may increase intraocular pressure. Document the name, strength, dose, and scheduling for all drugs the patient uses. Ocular effects from drugs include itching, foreign body sensation, redness, tearing, **photophobia** (sensitivity to light), and development of cataracts or glaucoma.

Nutrition History. Some eye problems are caused or worsened by vitamin deficiencies, so ask the patient about food choices. Vitamin A deficiency can cause eye dryness, keratomalacia, and blindness. Some nutrients and antioxidants, such as lutein, zeaxanthin, and beta carotene, help maintain retinal function (Eisenhauer, Natoli, Liew, & Flood, 2017). A diet rich in fruit and red, orange, and dark green vegetables is important to eye health.

Family History and Genetic Risk. Ask about a family history of eye problems because some conditions have a familial tendency and some genetic problems lead to visual impairment.

Current Health Problems. Ask the patient about the onset of visual changes. Question whether the change occurred rapidly or slowly. Determine whether the signs and symptoms are present to the same degree in both eyes. If eye injury or trauma is involved, also ask:
- How long ago did the injury occur?
- What was the patient doing when it happened?
- If a foreign body was involved, what was its source?
- Was any first aid administered at the scene? If so, what kind, and what other actions were taken?

! NURSING SAFETY PRIORITY (QSEN)

Critical Rescue

Recognize that a sudden or persistent loss of visual **sensory perception** within the past 48 hours, eye trauma, a foreign body in the eye, or sudden ocular pain is an emergency. Respond by notifying the eye care provider immediately.

Physical Assessment

Inspection. Look for head tilting, squinting, or other actions that indicate that the patient is trying to attain clear vision. For example, patients with double vision may cock the head to the side to focus the two images into one, or they may close one eye to see clearly.

Assess for symmetry in the appearance of the eyes. Determine whether they are equally distant from the nose, are the same size, and have the same degree of prominence. Assess for their placement in the orbits and for symmetry of movement. *Exophthalmos (proptosis)* is protrusion of the eye. *Enophthalmos* is the sunken appearance of the eye.

Examine the eyebrows and eyelashes for hair distribution and determine the direction of the eyelashes. Eyelashes normally point outward and away from the eyelid. Assess the eyelids for **ptosis** (drooping), redness, lesions, or swelling. The lids normally close completely, with the lid edges touching. When the eyes are open, the upper lid covers a small portion of the iris. The edge of the lower lid lies at the iris. No sclera should be visible between the eyelid and the iris.

Scleral and corneal assessment require a penlight. Examine the sclera for color; it is usually white. In patients with light skin, a yellow color may indicate jaundice or systemic problems. In adults with dark skin, the normal sclera may appear yellow; and small, pigmented dots may be visible (Jarvis, 2020).

The cornea is best seen by directing a light at it from the side. It should be transparent, smooth, shiny, and bright. Any cloudy areas or specks may indicate injury.

Assess the blink reflex by bringing a hand quickly toward the patient's face. Use extreme caution when performing this maneuver, especially with confused patients. Patients with vision will blink.

Pupillary assessment involves examining each pupil separately and comparing the results. The pupils are usually round and of equal size, between 3 and 5 mm in diameter. About 20% of adults normally have a noticeable difference in the size of their pupils, which is known as anisocoria (Merck Manual, 2019). Pupil size varies in adults exposed to the same amount of light. Pupils are smaller in older adults, which reduces vision in low light conditions. Patients with myopia have larger pupils, whereas those with hyperopia have smaller pupils.

Observe pupils for response to light. Increasing light causes constriction, whereas decreasing light causes dilation. Constriction of both pupils is the normal response to direct light and to accommodation. Assess pupillary reaction to light by asking the patient to look straight ahead while you quickly bring the beam of a penlight in from the side and direct it at the right pupil. Constriction of the right pupil is a direct response to shining the penlight into that eye. Constriction of the left pupil when light is shined at the right pupil is known as a *consensual response*. Assess the responses for each eye. (You may see the abbreviation "PERRLA" in the electronic health record, which stands for **p**upils **e**qual, **r**ound, **r**eactive to **l**ight, and **a**ccommodation.)

Evaluate each pupil for speed of reaction. The pupil should immediately constrict when a light is directed at it (i.e., a *brisk* response). If the pupil takes more than 1 second to constrict, the response is *sluggish*. Pupils that fail to react are *nonreactive* or *fixed*. Compare the reactivity speed of right and left pupils and document any difference.

Assess for accommodation by holding your finger about 18 degrees cm from the patient's nose and move it toward the nose. The patient's eyes normally converge during this movement, and the pupils constrict equally.

Vision Testing. Visual *sensory perception* is measured by first testing each eye separately and then testing both eyes together. Patients who wear corrective lenses are tested without and with their lenses. The eye care provider usually conducts this type of testing, which includes:

- Visual acuity testing to measure distance and near vision
- Use of the *Snellen eye chart* to assess distance vision
- Use of the Rosenbaum Pocket Vision Screener or Jaeger card to assess near vision
- Testing for light perception
- Testing the visual field for degree of peripheral vision
- Assessment of extraocular muscle function (Fig. 42.8) and eye alignment, and assessment of color vision via *Ishihara color plates* (Fig. 42.9).

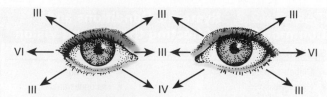

Fig. 42.8 Checking extraocular movements in the six cardinal positions indicates the functioning of cranial nerves III, IV, and VI.

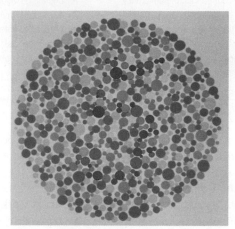

Fig. 42.9 An Ishihara color plate for testing color vision.

Psychosocial Assessment

A patient with changes in visual *sensory perception* may be anxious about possible vision loss. Patients with severe visual defects may be unable to perform ADLs. Dependency from reduced vision can affect self-esteem. Ask the patient how he or she feels about vision changes. Assess available family support, and the patient's coping techniques. Provide information about local resources and services as needed.

Diagnostic Assessment

Laboratory Assessment. Results of corneal cultures or conjunctival swabs and scrapings can help diagnose infections. If a culture is ordered, obtain a sample of the exudate from the conjunctiva or an ulcerated or inflamed area before antibiotics or topical anesthetics are instilled.

Imaging Assessment. *CT* is useful for assessing the eyes, the bony structures around the eyes, and the extraocular muscles. It can also detect tumors in the orbital space. A contrast agent is used unless trauma is suspected.

MRI is often used to examine the orbits and optic nerves and to evaluate ocular tumors. It cannot be used to evaluate injuries involving metal in the eyes. *Metal in the eye is an absolute contraindication for MRI.*

Radioisotope scanning is used to locate tumors and lesions. This test requires that the patient sign an informed consent, and sedation may be used for those who are very anxious. A tracer dose of the radioactive isotope is given orally or by injection, and then the patient must lie still. The scanner measures the radioactivity emitted by the radioactive atoms concentrated in the area being studied. No special follow-up care is required.

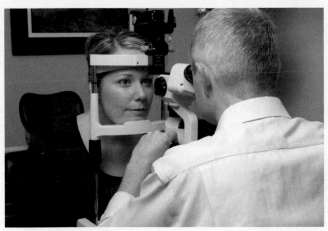

Fig. 42.10 Slit-lamp ocular examination. (From deWit, S. C., Stromberg, H. K., & Dallred, C. V. [2017]. *Medical-surgical nursing* [3rd ed.]). St. Louis: Elsevier.)

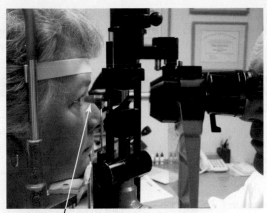

Goldmann applanation tonometer

Fig. 42.11 Use of Goldmann applanation tonometer and a slit lamp to measure intraocular pressure.

Ultrasonography is used to examine the orbit and eye with high-frequency sound waves. This noninvasive test helps diagnose trauma, intraorbital tumors, proptosis, and choroidal or retinal detachments. It is also used to determine the length of the eye and any gross outline changes in the eye and the orbit in patients with cloudy corneas or lenses that reduce direct examination of the fundus.

Inform the patient that this test is painless. It is performed with the eyes closed or, when the eyes must remain open, with anesthetic eyedrops instilled first. The patient is usually positioned upright with the chin in the chin rest, although the test can be done with the patient lying back. The probe is touched against the patient's anesthetized cornea, and sound waves are bounced through the eye. The sound waves create a reflective pattern on a computer screen that can be examined for abnormalities. No special follow-up care is needed. Remind the patient not to rub or touch the eye until the anesthetic agent has worn off.

Other Diagnostic Assessment. Many tests are used to examine specific eye structures when patients have risks, signs and symptoms, or exposures. These tests are performed only by health care providers.

Slit-lamp examination magnifies the anterior eye structures (Fig. 42.10). The patient leans on a chin rest to stabilize the head. A narrow beam (slit) of light is aimed so that only a segment of the eye is brightly lit. The eye care provider can then locate the position of any abnormality in the cornea, lens, or anterior vitreous humor.

Corneal staining consists of placing fluorescein or other topical dye into the conjunctival sac, and then the eye is viewed through a blue filter. The procedure is noninvasive and is performed under aseptic conditions. The dye outlines corneal surface irregularities in a bright green color. This test is used to assess corneal trauma, problems caused by a contact lens, or the presence of foreign bodies, abrasions, ulcers, or other corneal disorders.

Tonometry measures intraocular pressure (IOP) using a tonometer, which applies pressure to the outside of the eye until

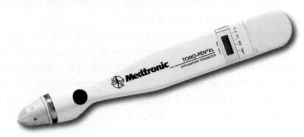

Fig. 42.12 The Tono-Pen XL. (Courtesy Medtronic Ophthalmics, Minneapolis, Minn.)

it equals the pressure inside the eye. The thickness of the cornea affects how much pressure must be applied before indentation occurs. Tonometer readings are indicated for all patients older than 40 years of age. Adults with a family history of glaucoma should have their IOP measured once or twice a year. Normal readings range from 10 to 20 mm Hg (Gudgel, 2018). IOP varies throughout the day and typically peaks at certain times of the day. Therefore always document the type and time of measurement.

The most common instrument used by eye care providers to measure IOP is the Goldmann applanation tonometer used with a slit lamp (Fig. 42.11). This method involves direct eye contact. Another instrument, the Tono-Pen XL (Fig. 42.12), is designed for use by eye care providers in extended care or long-term care facilities or for other patients unable to be positioned behind a slit lamp. Evidence shows that the Goldmann tonometer remains the most reliable method of IOP assessment (Wong et al., 2018).

Ophthalmoscopy allows viewing of the eye's external and interior structures with an *ophthalmoscope*. The health care provider positions the ophthalmoscope to see the patient's eye through the sight hole (Fig. 42.13). A *red reflex* is usually seen in the pupil as a reflection of the light off of the retina. An absent red reflex in an adult may indicate a lens opacity or cloudiness of the vitreous. The provider can also examine the retina, optic disc, optic vessels, fundus, and macula with this tool. Table 42.3 lists the features that can be observed in each structure.

The use of an ophthalmoscope may raise anxiety in some patients. When working with a patient with confusion or a patient who does not speak the language used at the agency, use an interpreter service to ensure understanding and cooperation with the examination.

! NURSING SAFETY PRIORITY (QSEN)

Action Alert

Avoid using an ophthalmoscope with a confused patient or one who does not understand the language spoken at the facility to prevent accidental injury to the eye.

Fluorescein angiography, which is performed by a health care provider, provides a detailed image of eye circulation. Digital pictures are taken in rapid succession after the dye is given IV. This test helps to assess problems of retinal circulation (e.g., diabetic retinopathy, retinal hemorrhage, and macular degeneration) or to diagnose intraocular tumors.

Explain the procedure to the patient, check that the patient has signed informed consent, and instill mydriatic eyedrops (cause pupil dilation) 1 hour before the test. Teach that the dye may cause the skin to appear yellow for several hours after the test. The stain is eliminated through the urine, which may be green in appearance.

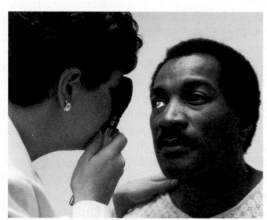

Fig. 42.13 Proper technique for direct ophthalmoscopic visualization of the retina.

TABLE 42.3	**Structures Assessed by Direct Ophthalmoscopy**
Red Reflex • Presence or absence **Optic Disc** • Color • Margins (sharp or blurred) • Cup size • Presence of rings or crescents **Optic Blood Vessels** • Size • Color • Kinks or tangles • Light reflection • Narrowing • Nicking at arteriovenous crossings	**Fundus** • Color • Tears or holes • Lesions • Bleeding **Macula** • Presence of blood vessels • Color • Lesions • Bleeding

Encourage patients to drink fluids to help eliminate the dye. Remind them that any staining of the skin will disappear in a few hours. Instruct the patient to wear dark glasses and avoid direct sunlight until pupil dilation returns to normal because the bright light will cause eye discomfort.

Electroretinography graphs the retina's response to light stimulation. This test is helpful in detecting and evaluating blood vessel changes from disease or drugs. The graph is obtained by placing an electrode on an anesthetized cornea. Lights at varying speeds and intensities are flashed, and the neural response is graphed. The measurement from the cornea is identical to the response that would be obtained if electrodes were placed directly on the retina.

Gonioscopy is a test performed when a high IOP is found and determines whether open-angle or closed-angle glaucoma is present. It uses a special lens that eliminates the corneal curve, is painless, and allows visualization of the angle where the iris meets the cornea.

Ultrasonic imaging of the retina and optic nerve (ocular coherence tomography) creates a three-dimensional view of the back of the eye. It is often used for patients with ocular hypertension or who are at risk for glaucoma because of other health problems.

✳ SENSORY PERCEPTION CONCEPT EXEMPLAR: CATARACT

Pathophysiology Review

The lens is a transparent, elastic structure suspended behind the iris that focuses images onto the retina. A **cataract** is a lens opacity that distorts the image (Fig. 42.14). As people age, the lens gradually loses water and increases in density (Touhy & Jett, 2018). Lens density increases with drying and compression of older lens fibers and production of new fibers and lens crystals. With time, as lens density increases and transparency is lost, visual *sensory perception* is greatly reduced. Both eyes may have cataracts, but the rate of progression is different in each eye.

Etiology and Genetic Risk. Cataracts may be present at birth or develop at any time. They may be age related or caused by

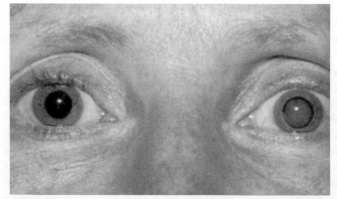

Fig. 42.14 Appearance of an eye with a mature cataract. (From Patton, K. T., & Thibodeau, G. A. [2016]. *Anatomy and physiology* [9th ed.]. St. Louis: Mosby.)

TABLE 42.4	Common Causes of Cataracts
Age • Lens water loss and fiber compaction **Trauma** • Blunt injury to eye or head • Penetrating eye injury • Intraocular foreign bodies • Radiation exposure, therapy **Toxin Exposure** • Corticosteroids • Phenothiazine derivatives • Miotic agents	**Health Conditions** • Diabetes mellitus • Hypoparathyroidism • Down syndrome • Chronic sunlight exposure **Complications** • Retinitis pigmentosa • Glaucoma • Retinal detachment

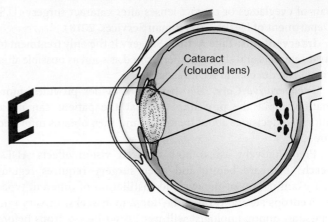

Fig. 42.15 Visual impairment produced by the presence of a cataract.

trauma or exposure to toxic agents. They also occur with other diseases and eye disorders (Table 42.4).

Incidence and Prevalence. The age-related cataract is the most common type. By age 75, more than half of all Americans have had a cataract (American Academy of Ophthalmology, 2020).

Health Promotion and Maintenance

Although most cases of cataracts in North America are age related, the onset of cataract formation occurs earlier with heavy sun exposure or exposure to other sources of ultraviolet (UV) light. Teach adults to reduce the risk for cataracts by wearing sunglasses that limit exposure to UV light whenever they are outdoors in the daytime. Cataracts also may result from direct eye injury. Urge adults to wear eye and head protection during sports, such as baseball, or any activity that increases the risk for the eye being hit. Individuals who smoke are at higher risk for development of cataracts versus nonsmokers (Boyd, 2020).

❖ Interprofessional Collaborative Care

Care for the patient with cataracts occurs in the community, with the exception of the surgical procedure, which takes place in an ambulatory surgical setting.

◆ Assessment: Recognize Cues

History. Age is important because cataracts are most prevalent in the older adult. Ask about these other predisposing factors:
- Recent or past trauma to the eye
- Exposure to radioactive materials, x-rays, or UV light
- Prolonged use of corticosteroids, chlorpromazine, or beta blockers
- Presence of intraocular disease (e.g., recurrent uveitis)
- Presence of systemic disease (e.g., diabetes mellitus, hypoparathyroidism, hypertension)
- Previous cataract, or family history of cataracts
- History of smoking

Ask the patient to describe his or her vision. For example, you might say, "Tell me what you can see well and what you have difficulty seeing."

Physical Assessment/Clinical Signs and Symptoms. Early signs and symptoms of cataracts are slightly blurred vision and decreased color perception. At first the patient may think

that his or her glasses are smudged, or contacts are not fitting correctly. As lens cloudiness continues, blurred and/or double vision occurs and the patient may have difficulty with ADLs. Patients commonly report increasing difficulty seeing at night, especially while driving. Without surgical intervention, visual impairment progresses to blindness. *No pain or eye redness is associated with age-related cataract formation.*

Unless a cataract has matured, it is not always visible to the naked eye upon examination. Visual *sensory perception* is tested using an eye chart and brightness acuity testing. The health care provider will examine the lens with an ophthalmoscope and note any observed densities by size, shape, and location. A slit lamp can also be used to visualize the cornea, iris (and space between the cornea and iris), and lens. A retinal examination will also likely be performed to clearly see the back of the eye. As a cataract matures, the opacity makes it difficult to see the retina, and the red reflex may be absent. When this occurs, the pupil is bluish white (Fig. 42.15).

Psychosocial Assessment. Loss of vision is gradual, and the patient may not be aware of it until reading or driving is affected. The patient may have anxiety about loss of independence. Encourage the patient and family to express concerns about reduced vision.

◆ Analysis: Analyze Cues and Prioritize Hypotheses. The priority collaborative problem for patients with cataracts is:
1. Impaired visual *sensory perception* due to cataracts

◆ Planning and Implementation: Generate Solutions and Take Action. The priority problem for the patient with cataracts is impaired visual *sensory perception,* which is a safety risk. Patients often live with reduced vision for years before the cataract is removed.

Improving Vision

Planning: Generate Solutions. As long as a patient does not have cognitive deficits, he or she is expected to recognize when ADLs cannot be performed safely and independently due to cataracts. At that time, surgery is indicated. For patients on Medicare, coverage is provided for an intraocular lens that is implanted during cataract surgery; the cost of the facility, provider, and supplies needed to perform the surgery; and one pair of eyeglasses or contact lenses after cataract surgery (U.S. Department of Health and Human Services, 2018).

Interventions: Take Action. Surgery is the only treatment to treat cataracts and should be performed as soon as possible after vision is reduced and ADLs are affected.

Preoperative Care. The eye care provider provides information about the procedure so that the patient can make informed decisions about treatment and then obtains informed consent.

Preoperatively, assess how reduced vision affects ADLs. Teach that care before and after surgery requires regular self-examination of the eye and instillation of different types of eyedrops several times a day for 2 to 4 weeks. In very rare cases, an ophthalmologist will not prescribe eyedrops before surgery; advise the patient to clarify with the ophthalmologist whether there is a need, or lack of need, to use them before the procedure (American Academy of Ophthalmology, 2017). If the patient is unable to instill the drops, help him or her make arrangements for this care.

Ask whether the patient takes any drugs that affect blood clotting, such as aspirin, warfarin, clopidogrel, and dabigatran. Communicate this information to the surgeon because, for some patients, these drugs may need to be discontinued before cataract surgery.

A series of ophthalmic drugs are instilled just before surgery to dilate the pupils and cause vasoconstriction. Other eyedrops are instilled to induce paralysis to prevent lens movement. When the patient is in the surgical area, a local anesthetic is injected into the muscle cone behind the eye for anesthesia and eye paralysis.

Operative Procedures. The lens is often extracted by *phacoemulsification* (Fig. 42.16), in which a probe is inserted through the capsule and high-frequency sound waves break the lens into small pieces, which are then removed by suction. The replacement intraocular lens

Sound wave and suctioning probe

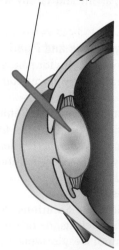

Sound waves break up the lens, pieces are sucked out, and the capsule remains largely intact

Fig. 42.16 Cataract removal by phacoemulsification.

---

❷ CLINICAL JUDGMENT CHALLENGE 42.1
Patient-Centered Care

A 66-year-old female client is taking part in a community health fair, which offers free vision screenings. The nurse takes a brief history, noting that the client reports having type 2 diabetes, hypertension, and a history of seasonal allergies related to pollen and mold. She lives in a one-bedroom apartment in a city. Social history reveals that the client smokes one pack of cigarettes per day and consumes an occasional glass of wine at celebratory events two to three times per year. The client reports that over the past few months, she has noticed that it is becoming harder to see clearly out of her right eye and difficult to see at night when she drives. She finds herself squinting in an attempt to clear her vision, yet the field does not seem to change. While performing an assessment, the nurse does not observe any unusual findings in either eye.

1. **Recognize Cues:** What assessment information in this client situation is the most important and immediate concern for the nurse? (Hint: Identify the **relevant** information *first* to determine what is most important.)
2. **Analyze Cues:** What client conditions are consistent with the **most relevant** information? (Hint: Think about priority collaborative problems that support and contradict the information presented in this situation.)
3. **Prioritize Hypotheses:** Which possibilities or explanations are **most likely** to be present in this client situation? Which possibilities or explanations are the most serious? (Hint: Consider all possibilities and determine their urgency and risk for this client.)
4. **Generate Solutions:** What interventions would most likely achieve the desired outcomes for this client? Which interventions should be **avoided** or are **potentially harmful**? (Hint: Determine the desired outcomes first to decide which interventions are appropriate and those that should be avoided.)
5. **Take Action:** Which interventions are the most appropriate, and how should they be implemented? In what **priority order** should they be implemented? (Hint: Consider health teaching, documentation, requested health care provider orders or prescriptions, nursing skills, collaboration with or referral to health team members, etc.)
6. **Evaluate Outcomes:** What client assessment would indicate that the nurse's interventions were **effective**? (Hint: Think about signs that would indicate an improvement, decline, or unchanged client condition.)

(IOL) is placed inside the capsule to be positioned so that light rays are focused in the retina. The IOL is a small, clear, plastic lens. Different types are available, and one is selected by the surgeon and patient to allow correction of a specific refractive error. Some patients have distant vision restored to 20/20 and may need glasses only for reading or close work. Some replacement lenses have multiple focal planes and may correct vision to the extent that glasses or contact lenses may not be needed.

Postoperative Care. Immediately after surgery, antibiotic and steroid ointments are instilled. The patient is usually discharged within an hour after surgery, after stabilization and monitoring. Instruct him or her to wear dark glasses outdoors or in brightly lit environments until the pupil responds to light. Teach the patient and family members how to instill the prescribed eyedrops. Help them create a written schedule for the timing and the order of eyedrops administration. Remind the patient that vision in that eye will be blurred and to not drive or operate heavy machinery until the ointment is removed. Stress the importance of keeping all follow-up appointments.

TABLE 42.5 Activities That Increase Intraocular Pressure
• Bending from the waist
• Lifting objects weighing more than 10 lb.
• Sneezing, coughing
• Blowing the nose
• Straining to have a bowel movement
• Vomiting
• Having sexual intercourse
• Keeping the head in a dependent position
• Wearing tight shirt collars

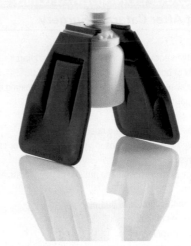

Fig. 42.17 Autosqueeze, a mechanism for self-administering eyedrops. (Courtesy Owen Mumford, Marietta, Ga.)

Remind the patient that mild eye itching is normal, as is a "bloodshot appearance." The eyelid may be slightly swollen. However, significant swelling or bruising is abnormal. Cool compresses may be beneficial. Discomfort at the site is controlled with acetaminophen or acetaminophen with oxycodone as prescribed. Aspirin is avoided because of its effects on blood clotting.

Pain early after surgery may indicate increased intraocular pressure (IOP) or hemorrhage. Instruct patients to contact the surgeon if pain occurs with nausea or vomiting.

To prevent increases in IOP, teach the patient and family about activity restrictions. Activities that can cause a sudden rise in IOP are listed in Table 42.5.

Infection is a potential and serious complication. Teach the patient and family to observe for increasing eye redness, a decrease in vision, or an increase in tears and photophobia. Creamy white, dry, crusty drainage on the eyelids and lashes is normal. However, yellow or green drainage indicates infection and must be reported. Stress the importance of proper handwashing to reduce the potential for infection.

Patients usually experience a dramatic improvement in vision within a day of surgery. Remind them that final best vision will not occur until 4 to 6 weeks after surgery.

! NURSING SAFETY PRIORITY (QSEN)

Action Alert

Instruct the patient who has had cataract surgery to immediately report any reduction of vision in the eye that just had the cataract removed.

Care Coordination and Transition Management. Because the patient is usually discharged within an hour after cataract surgery, nursing interventions focus on helping the patient and family plan the eyedrop schedule and daily home eye examination.

Home Care Management. If the patient has difficulty instilling eyedrops, a supportive neighbor, friend, or family member can be taught the procedure. Adaptive equipment that positions the bottle of eyedrops directly over the eye can also be purchased (Fig. 42.17).

Self-Management Education. To achieve best results of cataract removal, the patient must be taught to closely adhere to

the eyedrop regimen after surgery. Providing the patient or family with accurate information and demonstration of needed skills are nursing priorities. Before discharge, review these complications with the patient and family. Although complications are not anticipated, teach the patient to immediately report any of these symptoms following cataract surgery:

• Sharp, sudden pain in the eye
• Bleeding or increased discharge from the eye
• Green or yellow, thick drainage from the eye
• Eyelid swelling of the eye
• Reappearance of a bloodshot sclera after the initial appearance has cleared
• Decreased vision in the eye that had surgery
• Flashes of light or floating shapes seen in the eye

Remind the patient to avoid activities that can increase IOP (see Table 42.5). Some patients are prescribed to wear a light eye patch at night to prevent accidental rubbing. Instruct the patient to avoid getting water in the eye for 3 to 7 days after surgery.

Teach the patient about activity restrictions. Cooking and light housekeeping are permitted, but vacuuming should be avoided for several weeks because of the forward flexion involved and the rapid, jerky movements required. Advise the patient to refrain from driving until vision is clear. The Home Care Considerations: The Patient After Cataract Surgery box lists items to cover in the focused assessment of a patient at home after cataract surgery.

Health Care Resources. If the patient lives alone and has no support, arrange for a home care nurse to assess him or her and the home situation.

◆ **Evaluation: Evaluate Outcomes.** Evaluate the care of the patient with cataracts on the basis of improving visual *sensory perception.* The expected outcomes include that the patient will have improved visual *sensory perception* following surgery and recognize signs and symptoms of complications.

🏠 HOME CARE CONSIDERATIONS

The Patient After Cataract Surgery

Assess:
- Visual acuity in both eyes using a handheld eye chart
- Visual fields of both eyes
- Presence or absence of redness, tearing, and/or draining in the operative eye in comparison with the nonoperative eye

Ask the patient:
- If there is pain in or around the operative eye
- If there have been any changes in vision (decreased or improved) in the operative eye
- Whether any of these have been noticed in the operative eye:
  - Dark spots
  - Increase in the number of floaters
  - Bright flashes of light

Assess the home environment for:
- Safety hazards (especially tripping and falling hazards)
- Level of room lighting

Assess patient adherence to, and understanding of, treatment and limitations, such as:
- Signs and symptoms to report
- Drug regimen
- Activity restrictions
- Ability to perform ADLs

NCLEX EXAMINATION CHALLENGE 42.3

Physiological Adaptation: Reduction of Risk Potential

Which client statement affirms that nurse teaching about instillation of multiple different eyedrops has been effective? **Select all that apply.**
A. "It will be very easy for me to instill all of the drops at one time."
B. "A schedule will help me remember when to instill the eyedrops."
C. "If I have trouble instilling the drops, there are devices that can be helpful."
D. "I can label the eyedrops by color to help me easily distinguish which one is which."
E. "I will not touch the droppers to my eyes as this can cause contamination and infection."

✳ SENSORY PERCEPTION CONCEPT EXEMPLAR: GLAUCOMA

Pathophysiology Review

Glaucoma is a group of eye disorders resulting in increased intraocular pressure (IOP). As described earlier in this chapter, the eye is a hollow organ. For proper eye function, the gel in the posterior segment (vitreous humor) and the fluid in the anterior segment (aqueous humor) must be present in set amounts that apply pressure inside the eye to keep it ball shaped.

In adults, the volume of the vitreous humor does not change. However, the aqueous humor is continuously made from blood plasma by the ciliary bodies located behind the iris and just in front of the lens (see Fig. 42.2). The fluid flows through the pupil into the bulging area in front of the iris. At

TABLE 42.6	**Common Causes of Glaucoma**
Primary Glaucoma	**Secondary Glaucoma**
• Aging	• Uveitis
• Heredity	• Iritis
Associated Glaucoma	• Neovascular disorders
• Diabetes mellitus	• Trauma
• Hypertension	• Ocular tumors
• Severe myopia	• Degenerative disease
• Retinal detachment	• Eye surgery
	• Central retinal vein occlusion

the outer edges of the iris beneath the cornea, blood vessels collect fluid and return it to the blood. Usually about 1 mL of aqueous humor is always present, but it is continuously made and reabsorbed at a rate of about 5 mL daily. A normal IOP requires a balance between production and outflow of aqueous humor (McCance et al., 2019). If the IOP becomes too high, the extra pressure compresses retinal blood vessels and photoreceptors and their synapsing nerve fibers. This compression results in poorly oxygenated photoreceptors and nerve fibers. These sensitive nerve tissues become ischemic and die. When too many have died, vision is lost permanently. Tissue damage starts in the periphery and moves inward toward the fovea centralis. Untreated, glaucoma can lead to complete loss of visual *sensory perception*. Glaucoma is usually painless, and the patient may be unaware of gradual vision reduction.

There are several causes and types of glaucoma (Table 42.6), classified as primary, secondary, or associated. The most common type is primary glaucoma. **Primary open-angle glaucoma (POAG)**, the most common form of primary glaucoma, usually affects both eyes and has no signs or symptoms in the early stages. It develops slowly, with gradual loss of visual fields that may go unnoticed because central vision at first is unaffected. At times, vision is foggy and the patient has mild eye aching or headaches. Late signs and symptoms occur after irreversible damage to optic nerve function and include seeing halos around lights, losing peripheral vision, and having decreased visual *sensory perception* that does not improve with eyeglasses. Outflow of aqueous humor through the chamber angle is reduced. Because the fluid cannot leave the eye at the same rate that it is produced, IOP gradually increases. **Primary angle-closure glaucoma (PACG)** or *acute glaucoma* has a sudden onset and is an emergency. The problem is a forward displacement of the iris, which presses against the cornea and closes the chamber angle, suddenly preventing outflow of aqueous humor.

Etiology and Genetic Risk. Anyone can develop glaucoma, although some adults are at higher risk, such as African Americans or Hispanic/Latino Americans over 40 years of age, any individual over 60 years of age, those who have a family history of glaucoma, and adults who have high eye pressure, corneal thinness, and abnormality of the optic nerve (National Eye Institute, 2020).

Incidence and Prevalence. Glaucoma is a common cause of blindness in North America. It is usually age related, occurring in about 3 million adults in the United States (Centers for Disease Control and Prevention, 2018a).

Health Promotion and Maintenance

At this time, there are no known ways to prevent glaucoma. The best prevention against damage that glaucoma can cause is for adults to have eye examinations with glaucoma checks done every 2 to 4 years before age 40, every 1 to 3 years between ages 40 and 54, every 1 to 2 years between ages 55 and 64, and every 6 to 12 months over the age of 65 (Glaucoma Research Foundation, 2017).

❖ Interprofessional Collaborative Care

Care for the patient with glaucoma generally takes place in the community setting. Members of the interprofessional team who collaborate most closely to care for this patient include the eye care provider and the nurse. For patients who experience psychosocial concerns related to decreased visual *sensory perception,* collaborate with the mental health provider (see the Interprofessional Collaboration: The Patient With Glaucoma box).

👥 INTERPROFESSIONAL COLLABORATION
The Patient With Glaucoma

The possibility or reality of the loss of vision can be distressing for patients. Numerous studies have identified a connection between glaucoma and anxiety and depression (Quaranta et al., 2016). For patients who experience anxiety or depression related to changes in their sight, collaborate with a mental health professional. You can support the patient at regular visits, and the mental health professional can provide ongoing counseling and support to the patient during this time of transition. According to the Interprofessional Education Collaborative (IPEC) Expert Panel's Competency of Roles and Responsibilities, using the unique and complementary abilities of other team members optimizes health and patient care (IPEC, 2016; Slusser et al., 2019).

◆ Assessment: Recognize Cues

History. Ask about visual symptoms that have developed suddenly or over time. Symptoms of acute angle-closure glaucoma include a sudden visual loss, pain, conjunctival erythema, and corneal edema (Jacobs, 2019). In POAG, patients are often asymptomatic in the early stages. The visual fields first show a small loss of peripheral vision that gradually progresses to a larger loss.

Physical Assessment/Clinical Signs and Symptoms. Ophthalmoscopic examination shows cupping and atrophy of the optic disc. It becomes wider and deeper and turns white or gray. The sclera may appear reddened, and the cornea foggy. Ophthalmoscopic examination reveals a shallow anterior chamber, a cloudy aqueous humor, and a moderately dilated, nonreactive pupil.

Diagnostic Assessment. An elevated intraocular pressure (IOP) is measured by tonometry. In open-angle glaucoma, the tonometry reading is often between 22 and 32 mm Hg (normal is 10 to 20 mm Hg [Gudgel, 2018]). In angle-closure glaucoma, the tonometry reading may be 30 mm Hg or higher. Visual field testing by perimetry is performed, as is visualization by gonioscopy to determine whether the angle is open or closed. Usually the optic nerve is imaged to determine to what degree nerve damage is present.

◆ Analysis: Analyze Cues and Prioritize Hypotheses. The priority collaborative problems for patients with glaucoma include:
1. Impaired visual *sensory perception* due to glaucoma
2. Need for health teaching due to treatment regimen for glaucoma

◆ Planning and Implementation: Generate Solutions and Take Action

Supporting Visual Acuity via Health Teaching
Planning: Generate Solutions. With proper intervention, the patient is expected to maintain optimum visual acuity as long as possible by adhering to the treatment regimen.

Interventions: Take Action

Nonsurgical Management. Teach the patient that loss of visual *sensory perception* from glaucoma can be prevented by early detection, lifelong treatment, and close monitoring. Use of ophthalmic drugs that reduce ocular pressure can delay or prevent damage. The Patient-Centered Care: Older Adult Considerations: Promote Independent Living in Patients With Impaired Vision box lists ways to help the older-adult patient with reduced visual *sensory perception* to remain as independent as possible. The Best Practice for Patient Safety & Quality Care: Care of the Patient With Reduced Vision box provides a list of interventions to care for any patient who has reduced vision. These interventions can be very helpful when you care for hospitalized patients who have other disorders yet also have sight problems.

Drug therapy for glaucoma works to reduce IOP in several ways. Eyedrops can reduce the production of or increase the absorption of aqueous humor or constrict the pupil so that the ciliary muscle is contracted, allowing better circulation of the aqueous humor to the site of absorption. These drugs do not improve lost vision but prevent further damage by decreasing IOP. Close adherence to the prescribed dosage schedule is essential to receiving the maximum therapeutic effect of the eyedrops, so teach the patient to be dedicated to the regular timing of administration.

The prostaglandin agonist drugs reduce IOP by dilating blood vessels in the trabecular mesh, which then collects and drains aqueous humor at a faster rate. The adrenergic agonists and beta-adrenergic blockers reduce IOP by limiting the production of aqueous humor and by dilating the pupil, which improves the flow of the fluid to its absorption site. Cholinergic agonists reduce IOP by limiting the production of aqueous humor and making more room between the iris and the lens, which improves fluid outflow. Carbonic anhydrase inhibitors directly and strongly inhibit production of aqueous humor. They do not affect the flow or absorption of the fluid. Most eyedrops cause tearing, mild burning, blurred vision, and a reddened sclera for a few minutes after instilling the drug. Specific nursing implications related to drug therapy for glaucoma are listed in the Common Examples of

PATIENT-CENTERED CARE: OLDER ADULT CONSIDERATIONS (QSEN)

Promote Independent Living in Patients With Impaired Vision

Drugs
- Having a neighbor, relative, friend, or home health nurse visit weekly to organize the proper drugs for each day may be helpful.
- If the patient is to take drugs more than once each day, use a container of a different shape (with a lid) each time. For example, if the patient is to take drugs at 9 AM, 3 PM, and 9 PM, the 9 AM drugs would be placed in a round container, the 3 PM drugs in a square container, and the 9 PM drugs in a triangular container.
- Place each day's drug containers in a separate box with raised letters on the side of the box spelling out the day.
- "Talking clocks" are available for the patient with low vision.
- Some drug boxes have alarms that can be set for different times.

Communication
- Telephones with large, raised block numbers are helpful. Those with black numbers on a white phone or white numbers on a black phone are most easily seen by a patient with low vision.
- Telephones that recognize vocal commands or have programmable automatic dialing feature ("speed dial") are very helpful. Programmed numbers should include those for the fire department, police, relatives, friends, neighbors, and 911.

Safety
- It is best to leave furniture the way the patient wants it and not move it.
- Throw rugs should be eliminated, as these increase the risk for falls.
- Appliance cords should be short and kept out of walkways.
- Chairs with built-in footrests are preferable to footstools.
- Unbreakable dishes, cups, and glasses are preferable to breakable ones.
- Cleansers and other toxic agents should be labeled with large, raised letters.

Food Preparation
- Meals on Wheels America is a service that many older adults appreciate. This service is delivered at the local level and brings food at mealtime, cooked and ready to eat. The cost of this service varies, depending on the patient's ability to pay. Some seniors do not have to pay anything to receive this valuable service.
- Many grocery stores offer a delivery service. Customers can create a cart online or shop by telephone. The store gathers the ordered food and either has it ready for pick-up when a customer arrives or gives it to others who provide a delivery service to the patient's door. Costs vary for this service; some stores charge for each delivery, while others are more affordable by offering an annual subscription fee.
- A microwave oven is a safer means of cooking than a standard stove, although some older patients are afraid of microwave ovens. If the patient has and will use a microwave oven, others can prepare and label meals ahead of time and freeze them for later use. Also, many complete frozen dinners that comply with a variety of dietary restrictions are available to warm in the microwave.
- Friends or relatives may be able to help with food preparation. Often relatives do not know what to give an older adult for birthdays or other gift-giving occasions. One suggestion is a homemade prepackaged frozen dinner that the patient enjoys.

Personal Care
- Handgrips should be installed in bathrooms.
- The tub floor should have a nonskid surface.
- Patients who shave should use an electric shaver rather than a razor.
- Have the patient choose a hairstyle that is becoming but easy to care for; this promotes self-care.
- Home hair-care services are available in some areas.

Diversional Activity
- Some patients can read large-print books, newspapers, and magazines (available through local libraries and vision services).
- Books, magazines, and some newspapers are available on audiotape or by streaming.
- Card games, dominoes, and some board games are available in large, high-contrast print.

BEST PRACTICE (QSEN) PATIENT SAFETY & QUALITY CARE

Care of the Patient With Reduced Vision

- Always knock or announce your entrance into the patient's room or area and introduce yourself.
- Ensure that all members of the health care team also use this courtesy of announcement and introduction.
- Ensure that the patient's reduced vision is noted in the electronic health record, communicated to all staff, marked on the call board, and identified on the door of the patient's room.
- Determine to what degree the patient can see.
- Orient the patient to the environment, counting steps with him or her to the bathroom.
- Help the patient place objects on the bedside table and do not move them without the patient's permission.
- Remove all obstacles and clutter between the patient's bed and the bathroom.
- Ask the patient what type of assistance is preferred for grooming, toileting, eating, and ambulating; communicate these preferences with staff.
- Describe food placement on a plate in terms of a clock face.
- Open milk cartons; open salt, pepper, and condiment packages; and remove lids from cups and bowls.
- Unless the patient also has a hearing problem, use a normal tone of voice when speaking.
- When walking with the patient, offer him or her your arm and walk a step ahead.

Drug Therapy (Eyedrops): Glaucoma box. It is important to teach the patient about potential interactions that may exist between medications and systemic effects that may occur when using these drugs.

The priority nursing intervention for the patient with glaucoma is teaching. Teach the patient that the benefit of drug therapy occurs only when the drugs are used on the prescribed schedule; therefore, patients must instill drops on time and not skip doses. When more than one drug is prescribed, teach the patient to wait 5 to 10 minutes between drug instillations to prevent one drug from diluting another drug. Stress the need for good handwashing, keeping the eyedrop container

COMMON EXAMPLES OF DRUG THERAPY (EYEDROPS)

Glaucoma

Drug Category	Nursing Implications
Prostaglandin Agonists	
Bimatoprost	Teach the patient to check the cornea for abrasions or trauma. *Drugs should not be used when the cornea is not intact.*
Latanoprost	Teach the patient that eye color darkens, and eyelashes elongate, over time in the eye receiving the drug. *Knowing the side effects in*
Travoprost	*advance reassures the patient that their presence is expected and normal.*
	If only one eye is to be treated, teach the patient *not* to place drops in the other eye to try to make the eye colors similar. *Using the drug in an eye with normal IOP can cause a **lower**-than-normal IOP, which reduces vision.*
	Warn the patient that using more drops than prescribed reduces drug effectiveness. *Drug action is based on blocking receptors, which can increase in number when the drug is overused.*
Adrenergic Agonists	
Apraclonidine	Ask whether the patient is taking any antidepressants from the MAO inhibitor class. *These enzyme inhibitors increase blood pressure,*
Brimonidine tartrate	*as do the adrenergic agonists. When taken together, the patient may experience hypertensive crisis.*
	Teach the patient to wear dark glasses outdoors and also indoors when lighting is bright. *The pupil dilates (mydriasis) and remains dilated, even when there is plenty of light, causing discomfort.*
	Teach the patient not to use the eyedrops with contact lenses in place and to wait 15 minutes after using the drug to put in contact lenses, if worn. *These drugs are absorbed by the contact lens, which can become discolored or cloudy.*
Beta-Adrenergic Blockers	
Betaxolol hydrochloride	Ask whether the patient has moderate-to-severe asthma or COPD. *If these drugs are absorbed systemically, they constrict pulmonary*
Carteolol	*smooth muscle and narrow airways.*
Levobunolol	Teach patients with diabetes to check their blood glucose levels more often when taking these drugs. *These drugs induce hypoglycemia*
Timolol	*and can mask the hypoglycemic symptoms.*
	Teach patients who also take oral beta blockers to check their pulse at least twice per day and to notify the primary health care and eye care providers if the pulse is consistently below 60 beats/min. *These drugs potentiate the effects of systemic beta blockers and can cause an unsafe drop in heart rate and blood pressure.*
Cholinergic Agonists	
Carbachol	Teach the patient not to administer more eyedrops than are prescribed and to report increased salivation or drooling to the primary
Echothiophate	health care and eye care providers. *These drugs are readily absorbed by conjunctival mucous membranes and can cause systemic*
Pilocarpine	*side effects of headache, flushing, increased saliva, and sweating.*
	Teach the patient to use good light when reading and to turn lights on in rooms. *The pupil of the eye will not open more to let in more light, and it may be harder to see objects in dim light. This can increase the risk for falls.*
Carbonic Anhydrase Inhibitors	
Brinzolamide	Ask whether the patient has an allergy to sulfonamide antibacterial drugs. *Drugs are similar to the sulfonamides; if a patient is allergic*
Dorzolamide	*to the sulfonamides, an allergy is likely with these drugs.*
	Teach the patient to shake the drug before applying. *Drug separates on standing.*
	Teach the patient not to use the eyedrops with contact lenses in place and to wait 15 minutes after using the drug to put in the lenses. *These drugs are absorbed by the contact lens, which can become discolored or cloudy.*
Combination Drug	
Brimonidine tartrate and timolol maleate	Same as for each drug alone.

COPD, Chronic obstructive pulmonary disease; *IOP,* intraocular pressure; *MAO,* monoamine oxidase.

tip clean, and avoiding touching the tip to any part of the eye. Also teach the technique of punctal occlusion (placing pressure on the corner of the eye near the nose) immediately after eyedrop instillation to prevent systemic absorption of the drug (Fig. 42.18).

 NURSING SAFETY PRIORITY (QSEN)

Drug Alert

Most eyedrops used for glaucoma therapy can be absorbed systemically and cause systemic problems. It is critical to teach punctal occlusion to patients using eyedrops for glaucoma therapy (see Fig. 42.18).

Systemic osmotic drugs like IV mannitol may be given for angle-closure glaucoma to rapidly reduce IOP.

Surgical Management. Surgery can be performed when drugs for open-angle glaucoma are not effective at controlling IOP. Two common procedures are laser trabeculoplasty and trabeculectomy. A *laser trabeculoplasty* burns the trabecular meshwork, scarring it and causing the meshwork fibers to tighten. Tight fibers increase the size of the spaces between the fibers, improving outflow of aqueous humor and reducing IOP. *Trabeculectomy* is a surgical procedure that creates a new channel for fluid outflow. Both are ambulatory surgery procedures.

If glaucoma fails to respond to common approaches, an implanted shunt procedure may be used. A small tube or

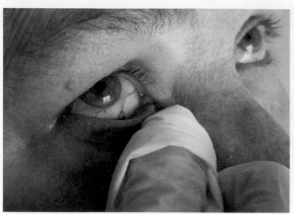

Fig. 42.18 Applying punctal occlusion to prevent systemic absorption of eyedrops. (From Workman, M. L., & LaCharity, L. [2016]. *Understanding pharmacology* [2nd ed.]. St. Louis: Saunders.)

◆ **Evaluation: Evaluate Outcomes.** Evaluate the care of the patient with glaucoma based on the identified priority patient problem. The primary expected outcome is that the patient will have optimum visual acuity as long as possible as demonstrated by adherence to the treatment regimen.

CORNEAL DISORDERS

For a sharp retinal image, the cornea must be transparent and intact. Corneal problems may be caused by inflammation of the cornea (keratitis), degeneration of the cornea (keratoconus), or deposits in the cornea. All corneal problems reduce visual *sensory perception,* and some can lead to blindness.

CORNEAL ABRASION, ULCERATION, AND INFECTION
Pathophysiology Review

A corneal abrasion is a scrape or scratch injury of the cornea. This painful condition can be caused by a small foreign body, trauma, contact lens use, malnutrition, dry eye syndromes, and certain cancer therapies. The abrasion allows organisms to enter, leading to corneal infection. Bacterial, protozoal, and fungal infections can lead to *corneal ulceration,* a deeper injury. This problem is an emergency because the cornea has no separate blood supply and infections that can permanently impair vision develop rapidly.

❖ **Interprofessional Collaborative Care**

The patient with a corneal disorder has pain, reduced vision, photophobia, and eye secretions. Cloudy or purulent fluid may be present on the eyelids or lashes. Care for patients with a corneal disorder usually takes place in the community setting. Members of the interprofessional team who collaborate most closely to care for this patient include the eye care provider and the nurse.

◆ **Assessment: Recognize Cues.** Wear gloves when examining the eye. Anticipate the cornea to look hazy or cloudy with a patchy area of ulceration. When fluorescein stain is used, the patchy area appears green. Corneal scrapings (done by an eye care provider after anesthetizing the cornea with a topical agent) and microbial cultures are used to determine the causative organism. For culture, obtain swabs from the ulcer and its edges.

filament is connected to a flat plate that is positioned on the outside of the eye in the eye orbit. The open part of the fine tube is placed into the front chamber of the eye. The fluid then drains through or around the tube into the area around the flat plate, where it collects and is reabsorbed into the bloodstream. Potential complications of glaucoma surgery include choroidal hemorrhage and choroidal detachment.

Care Coordination and Transition Management

Home Care Management. Similar to management of cataracts, the patient with glaucoma will need to instill eyedrops regularly as part of home care. If the patient is unable or resistant to instilling his or her own eyedrops, teach the caregiver the proper technique or recommend adaptive equipment (see Fig. 42.17).

Self-Management Education. The patient with glaucoma is usually managed in the outpatient setting and seen every 1 to 3 months, depending on how well controlled their IOP is. Teach the importance of good handwashing and keeping the tip of the eyedrop container clean. Remind the patient to instill eyedrops on time as recommended by the eye care provider and not to skip doses.

For the patient who has had surgical management, teach the signs and symptoms of choroidal detachment and hemorrhage. These can occur during or after coughing, sneezing, straining at stools, or Valsalva maneuver. Serous detachment involves some degree of vision loss yet is usually painless. Hemorrhagic detachment involves an immediate loss of vision with sudden, excruciating, throbbing pain. Any vision loss, particularly when accompanied by pain, should be reported immediately to the eye care provider.

Health Care Resources. If needed, refer the patient and family to care services that can assist in the home. Support groups for individuals with vision impairment may also be helpful.

◆**Interventions: Take Action.** Anti-infective therapy is started before the organism is identified because of the high risk for vision loss. A broad-spectrum antibiotic is prescribed first and may be changed when culture results are known. Steroids may be used with antibiotics to reduce the eye inflammation. Drugs can be given topically as eyedrops or injected subconjunctivally or intravenously. The nursing priorities are to begin the drug therapy, to ensure patient understanding of the drug-therapy regimen, and to prevent infection spread.

Often the anti-infective therapy involves instilling eyedrops *every hour* for the first 24 hours. Teach the patient or family member how to instill the eyedrops correctly.

If the eye infection occurs only in one eye, teach the patient not to use the drug in the unaffected eye. Reinforce the importance of handwashing after touching the affected eye and before touching or doing anything to the healthy eye. If both eyes are infected, separate bottles of drugs are needed for each eye. Teach the patient to clearly label the bottles "right eye" and "left eye" and not to switch the drugs from eye to eye. Remind the patient not to wear contact lenses during the entire time that these drugs are being used because the eye is more vulnerable to infection or injury, and the drugs can cloud or damage the contact lenses.

> ⚠ **NURSING SAFETY PRIORITY** (QSEN)
>
> **Action Alert**
>
> Teach the importance of applying the drug as often as prescribed, even at night, and to complete the entire course of antibiotic therapy. Treating the infection can save the vision in the infected eye. Remind the patient to make and keep all follow-up appointments.

Drug therapy may continue for weeks to ensure eradication of the infection. Teach patients to avoid using makeup around the eye until the infection has cleared. Instruct them to discard all open containers of contact lens solutions and bottles of eyedrops because these may be contaminated. Patients should not wear contact lenses for weeks to months until the infection is gone and the ulcer is healed.

> ⚠ **NURSING SAFETY PRIORITY** (QSEN)
>
> **Drug Alert**
>
> Check the route of administration for ophthalmic drugs. Most are administered by the eye instillation route, not orally. Administering these drugs orally can cause systemic side effects and will not therapeutically treat the eye condition. Be sure to reinforce the correct route when teaching the patient.

KERATOCONUS

Pathophysiology Review

The cornea can permanently lose it shape, become scarred or cloudy, or become thinner, reducing useful visual *sensory perception.* Keratoconus, the degeneration of corneal tissue resulting in abnormal corneal shape, can occur with trauma or may

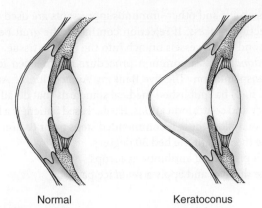

Normal   Keratoconus

Fig. 42.19 Profile of a normal cornea and one with keratoconus.

be an inherited disorder (Fig. 42.19). Inadequately treated corneal infection and severe trauma can scar the cornea and lead to severe visual impairment that can be improved only by surgical interventions.

❖ Interprofessional Collaborative Care

Keratoplasty (corneal transplant) is a surgical procedure to improve clarity for a permanent corneal disorder that obscures vision. The diseased corneal tissue is removed and replaced with tissue from a cornea donated by a human who has passed away.

Postoperative care involves comprehensive patient teaching. Local antibiotics are injected or instilled. Usually the eye is covered with a pressure patch and a protective shield until the patient returns to the surgeon.

Instruct the patient to lie on the nonoperative side to reduce intraocular pressure (IOP). If a patch is to be used for more than a day, teach application processes. Instruct the patient to wear the shield at night for the first month after surgery and whenever around small children or pets to avoid injury. Instruct him or her *not* to use an ice pack on the eye. Complications after surgery include bleeding, wound leakage, infection, and graft rejection. Teach the patient how to instill eyedrops. Teach him or her to examine the eye (or have a family member examine it) daily for the presence of infection or graft rejection. Stress that the presence of purulent discharge, a continuous leak of clear fluid from around the graft site (not tears), or excessive bleeding needs to be reported immediately to the surgeon. Other complications include decreased vision, increased reddening of the eye, pain, increased sensitivity to light, and the presence of light flashes or "floaters" in the field of vision. These concerns should be reported to the surgeon if they develop after the first 48 hours and persist for more than 6 hours.

The eye should be protected from any activity that can increase the pressure on, around, or inside the eye. Teach the patient to avoid jogging, running, dancing, and any other activity that promotes rapid or jerky head motions for several weeks after surgery. Other activities that may raise IOP and should be avoided are listed in Table 42.5.

Graft rejection can occur and starts as inflammation in the cornea near the graft edge that moves toward the center. Vision is reduced, and the cornea becomes cloudy. Topical corticosteroids and other immunosuppressants are used to stop the rejection process. If rejection continues, the graft becomes opaque and blood vessels branch into the opaque tissue.

Eye donation is a common procedure and needed for corneal transplantation. The Eye Banking Association of America (EBAA, n.d.) has published medical standards that detail donor eligibility and contraindications. If a deceased patient is a known eye donor, follow these recommended steps prior to donation:

- Raise the head of the bed 30 degrees.
- Instill prescribed antibiotic eyedrops.
- Close the eyes and apply a *small* ice pack.

RETINAL DISORDERS

MACULAR DEGENERATION

Pathophysiology Review

Macular degeneration, also known as *age-related macular degeneration* (AMD), is the deterioration of the macula (the area of central vision) and can be age related or exudative. It is the leading cause of blindness in individuals in the United States who are 65 years of age and older (Centers for Disease Control and Prevention, 2018b). There are two types of age-related macular degeneration (AMD): *dry* and *wet.*

Dry AMD is the more common type of this condition. It is caused by a slow and gradual blockage of retinal capillaries by pigmented residue and photoreceptor waste products in the retina, allowing retinal cells in the macula to become ischemic and necrotic. Central vision declines, and patients describe mild blurring and distortion at first. Night vision is impacted, and the ability to see clearly when reading is impaired. Eventually the patient loses all central vision.

Dry AMD progresses at a faster rate among smokers than among nonsmokers. Individuals with diabetes, hypertension, and high cholesterol are at risk for developing this condition. Other risk factors include being older than 60 years old, being Caucasian, and having a family history of AMD (National Eye Institute, 2019).

Wet (exudative) AMD progresses quickly. Patients experience a sudden decrease in vision after a detachment of pigment epithelium in the macula. Newly formed blood vessels, which have very thin walls, invade this injured area and cause fluid and blood to collect under the macula (like a blister), with scar formation and visual distortion. Wet (exudative) AMD can occur at any age, in only one eye or in both eyes. The patient with dry AMD can also develop wet (exudative) macular degeneration.

❖ **Interprofessional Collaborative Care**

◆ **Assessment: Recognize Cues.** An eye care provider will likely conduct indirect ophthalmoscopy to assess for gross macular changes, opacities, retinal concerns, and hemorrhage (Rebar & Rebar, 2019). IV fluorescein angiography may be performed by the eye care provider to locate leaking vessels, and Amsler's grid test may be conducted to demonstrate central visual field loss (Rebar & Rebar, 2019).

◆ **Interventions: Take Action.** Dry AMD has no cure. Management in the community setting is focused on slowing the progression of the vision loss and helping the patient maximize remaining vision and quality of life. The risk for dry AMD can be reduced by increasing long-term dietary intake of the carotenoids *lutein* and *zeaxanthin* (American Optometric Association, 2020).

Central vision loss reduces the ability to read, write, recognize safety hazards, and drive. Suggest alternatives (e.g., large-print books, public transportation) and refer to community resources that provide adaptive equipment.

Management of patients with wet (exudative) AMD involves slowing the process and identifying further changes in visual perception. Fluid and blood may reabsorb in some patients. Laser therapy to seal the leaking blood vessels can limit the extent of the damage. Ocular injections with the vascular endothelial growth factor inhibitors (VEGFIs), such as bevacizumab or ranibizumab, can improve vision for the patient with wet AMD.

NCLEX EXAMINATION CHALLENGE 42.5
Physiological Integrity

Which patient does the nurse identify at **highest** risk for development of dry age-related macular degeneration (AMD)?

A. 55-year-old client who recently began wearing glasses
B. 59-year-old client who has controlled hypertension
C. 62-year-old client with hypothyroidism
D. 65-year-old client with diabetes

RETINAL HOLES, TEARS, AND DETACHMENTS

Pathophysiology Review

A retinal hole is a break in the retina caused by trauma or that occurs with aging. A retinal tear is a jagged and irregularly shaped break in the retina, which can result from traction on the retina. A retinal detachment is the separation of the retina from the epithelium. Detachments are classified by the type and cause of their development.

One common cause of retinal holes, tears, and detachments is a *posterior vitreous detachment* (PVD). With aging, the vitreous gel often shrinks or thickens, causing it to pull away from the retina. The patient may experience small flashes of light seen as "shooting stars" or thin "lightning streaks" in one eye, most visible in a dark environment. These flashes of light may be accompanied by "floaters." In addition to aging, risk factors for PVD include extreme myopia, inflammation inside the eye, and cataract or eye laser surgery. When the PVD does not cause a retinal tear or detachment, no treatment is needed.

❖ **Interprofessional Collaborative Care**

◆ **Assessment Recognize Cues.** The onset of a retinal detachment is usually sudden and painless. Patients may report suddenly seeing bright flashes of light (*photopsia*) or floating dark spots in the affected eye. During the initial phase of the detachment or if the detachment is partial, the patient may describe the sensation of a curtain being pulled over part of the visual field. The visual field loss corresponds to the area of detachment. Patients who report this type of concern to a telehealth triage nurse should be cautioned to have another individual drive them to their eye care provider of choice.

The eye care provider will perform an ophthalmoscopic examination. Detachments are seen as gray bulges or folds in the retina. Sometimes a hole or tear may be seen at the edge of the detachment.

◆ **Interventions: Take Action.** If a retinal hole or tear is discovered before it causes a detachment, the defect may be closed or sealed. Closure prevents fluid from collecting under the retina and reduces the risk for a detachment. Treatment involves creating a scar with laser photocoagulation or a freezing probe (*cryopexy*) that will bind the retina and choroid together around the break.

Spontaneous reattachment of a totally detached retina is rare. Surgical repair—called *scleral buckling*—is needed to place the retina in contact with the underlying structures.

Preoperative Care. Most patients are anxious and fearful about the possible permanent loss of vision. Nursing priorities include providing information and support.

Instruct the patient to restrict activity and head movement before surgery to prevent further tearing or detachment. An eye patch is placed over the affected eye to reduce eye movement. Topical drugs are given before surgery to inhibit pupil constriction and accommodation.

Operative Procedures. Surgery is performed with the patient under general anesthesia. In scleral buckling, the eye surgeon repairs wrinkles or folds in the retina and indents the eye surface to relieve the tugging pressure on the retina. The indentation or "buckling" is performed by placing a small piece of silicone against the outside of the sclera and holding it in place with an encircling band. This device keeps the retina in contact with the choroid for reattachment. Any fluid under the retina is drained.

Silicone oil or gas is placed inside the eye to promote retinal reattachment. These agents float up and against the retina to hold it in place until healing occurs.

Postoperative Care. After surgery an eye patch and shield are usually applied. Monitor the patient's vital signs, and check the eye patch and shield for drainage.

Activity after surgery varies. If oil or gas has been placed in the eye, teach the patient to keep his or her head in the position instructed by the surgeon to promote reattachment. Teach the patient to report sudden increase in pain or pain occurring with nausea to the surgeon immediately. Remind him or her to avoid activities that increase intraocular pressure (IOP) (see Table 42.5).

Instruct the patient to avoid reading, writing, and work that requires close vision in the first week after surgery because these activities cause rapid eye movements and detachment. Teach the signs and symptoms of infection and detachment (sudden reduced visual acuity, eye pain, pupil that *does not constrict* in response to light) and to notify the surgeon immediately if these symptoms occur.

REFRACTIVE ERRORS

Pathophysiology Review

The ability of the eye to focus images on the retina depends on the length of the eye from front to back and the refractive power of the lens system. **Refraction** is the bending of light rays. Problems in either eye length or refraction can result in refractive errors.

Myopia is nearsightedness, in which the eye overrefracts the light and the bent images fall in front of, not on, the retina. **Hyperopia**, also called *hypermetropia,* is farsightedness, in which refraction is too weak, causing images to be focused behind the retina. **Presbyopia** is the age-related problem in which the lens loses its elasticity and is less able to change shape to focus the eye for close work. As a result, images fall behind the retina. This problem usually begins in adults in their 40s. **Astigmatism** occurs when the curve of the cornea is uneven. Because light rays are not refracted equally in all directions, the image does not focus on the retina.

❖ Interprofessional Collaborative Care

◆ **Assessment: Recognize Cues.** Refractive errors are diagnosed through a refraction test. The patient is asked to view an eye chart while lenses of different strengths are systematically placed in front of the eye. With each lens strength, he or she is asked whether the lenses sharpen or worsen vision. The strength of the lens needed to focus the image on the retina is expressed in measurements called *diopters.*

◆ **Interventions: Take Action**

Nonsurgical Management. Refractive errors are corrected with eyeglasses or contact lenses that focus light rays on the retina (see Fig. 42.5). Hyperopic vision is corrected with a convex lens that moves the image forward. Myopic vision is corrected with a concave lens that moves the image back to the retina.

Surgical Management. Surgery can correct some refractive errors and enhance vision. The most common vision-enhancing surgery is laser in-situ keratomileusis (LASIK). This procedure can correct nearsightedness, farsightedness, and astigmatism. The superficial layers of the cornea are lifted temporarily as a flap, and powerful laser pulses reshape the deeper corneal layers. After reshaping is complete, the corneal flap is placed back into its original position.

Usually both eyes are treated at the same time, which is convenient for the patient, although this practice has risks. Many patients have improved vision within an hour after surgery, and complete healing takes up to 4 weeks. The outer corneal layer is not damaged, and pain is minimal.

Complications of LASIK include infection, corneal clouding, chronic dry eyes, and refractive errors. Some patients have developed blurred vision, halos around lights, and other refractive errors months to years after this surgery as a result of excessive laser-thinning of the cornea. The cornea then becomes unstable and does not refract appropriately.

Aher procedure, corneal ring placement, can enhance vision for nearsightedness, although this procedure is usually performed for keratoconus.

TRAUMA

Trauma to the eye or orbital area can result from almost any activity. Care varies, depending on the area of the eye affected, whether the globe of the eye has been penetrated, and the mechanism of trauma.

Foreign Bodies

Eyelashes, dust, dirt, and airborne particles can come in contact with the conjunctiva or cornea and irritate or abrade the surface. If nothing is seen on the cornea or conjunctiva, the eyelid is everted to examine the conjunctivae. The patient usually has a feeling of something being in the eye and may have blurred vision. Pain occurs if the corneal surface is injured. Tearing and photophobia may be present.

Visual *sensory perception* is assessed before treatment. The eye is examined with fluorescein, followed by irrigation with normal saline (0.9%) to gently remove the particles. Ocular irrigation is discussed in the Best Practice for Patient Safety & Quality Care: Ocular Irrigation box. Remember, if both eyes are affected, irrigate them simultaneously using separate personnel and equipment.

If an eye dressing or patch is applied after the foreign body is removed, tell the patient how long this must be left in place. Follow-up as directed by the eye care provider is needed to confirm that appropriate healing is taking place.

Lacerations

Lacerations are caused by sharp objects and projectiles. The injury occurs most commonly to the eyelids and cornea, although any part of the eye can be lacerated. The patient with a laceration should receive medical attention right away. *Corneal lacerations are an emergency because eye contents may prolapse through the laceration.* Symptoms include severe eye pain, photophobia, tearing, decreased vision, and inability to open the eyelid. If the laceration is the result of a penetrating injury, an object may be seen protruding from the eye.

Minor lacerations of the eyelid can be sutured in an emergency department, an urgent care center, or an eye care provider's office. A microscope is needed in the operating room if the patient has a laceration that involves the eyelid margin, affects the lacrimal system, involves a large area, or has jagged edges.

! NURSING SAFETY PRIORITY (QSEN)

Action Alert

An object protruding from the eye is removed only by an eye care provider because it may be holding the eye structures in place. Improper removal can cause structures to prolapse out of the eye.

BEST PRACTICE FOR PATIENT SAFETY & QUALITY CARE (QSEN)

Ocular Irrigation

1. Assemble equipment:
   - Normal saline IV (1000-mL bag)
   - Macrodrip IV tubing
   - IV pole
   - Eyelid speculum
   - Topical anesthetic (as prescribed)
   - Gloves
   - Collection receptacle (emesis basin works well)
   - Towels
   - pH paper
2. Quickly obtain a history from the patient while flushing the tubing with normal saline, including:
   - Nature and time of the injury
   - Type of irritant or chemical (if known)
   - Type of first aid administered at the scene
   - Any allergies to the "caine" family of medications
3. Evaluate the patient's visual acuity *before* treatment:
   - Ask the patient to read your name tag with the affected eye while covering the good eye.
   - Ask the patient to "count fingers" with the affected eye while covering the good eye.
4. Wash hands and don gloves.
5. Remove contact lenses, if worn, before irrigation.
6. Place a strip of pH paper in the cul-de-sac of the patient's affected eye to test the pH of the agent splashed into the eye and to know when it has been washed out.
7. Instill topical anesthetic eyedrops as prescribed.
8. Place the patient in a supine position with the head turned slightly toward the affected eye.
9. Have the patient hold the affected eye open or position an eyelid speculum.
10. Direct the flow of normal saline across the affected eye from the nasal corner of the eye toward the outer corner of the eye.
11. Assess the patient's comfort during the procedure.

Data from Gwenhure, T. (2020). Procedure for eye irrigation to treat ocular chemical injury. *Nursing Times [online], 116*(2), 46-48.

Antibiotics are given to reduce the risk for infection. Depending on the depth of the laceration, scarring may develop. If the scar alters vision, a corneal transplant may be needed later. If the eye contents have prolapsed through the laceration or if the injury is severe, **enucleation** (surgical eyeball removal) may be indicated.

Penetrating Injuries

A penetrating eye injury often leads to permanent loss of visual *sensory perception.* Glass, high-speed metal or wood particles, BB pellets, and bullets are common causes of penetrating injuries. The particles can enter the eye and lodge in or behind the eyeball. A wound may be visible. Depending on where the object enters and rests within the eye, vision may be affected. Never remove an object protruding from the eye; the health care provider will assess the immediate condition and determine how to proceed.

X-rays and CT scans of the orbit are usually performed. MRI is contraindicated because the procedure may move any metal-containing projectile and cause more injury.

Surgery is usually needed to remove the foreign object, and sometimes vitreal removal is needed. IV antibiotics are started before surgery, and a tetanus booster is given if necessary.

! NURSING SAFETY PRIORITY (QSEN)
Action Alert

An object protruding from the eye is removed only by an eye care provider because it may be holding the eye structures in place. Improper removal can cause structures to prolapse out of the eye.

GET READY FOR THE NEXT-GENERATION NCLEX® EXAMINATION!

Key Points

Review these Key Points for each NCLEX Examination Client Needs Category.

Safe and Effective Care Environment

- Wash hands and don gloves before touching a patient's eyes or lids or instilling eyedrops. **QSEN: Safety**
- If a patient has discharge from one eye, examine the eye without the discharge first. **QSEN: Safety**
- Avoid performing an ophthalmoscopic examination on a patient with confusion. **QSEN: Safety**
- Use and teach aseptic technique when instilling drugs into the eye. **QSEN: Safety**
- Orient the patient with reduced vision to immediate surroundings. **QSEN: Safety**
- Identify the room of a patient with reduced vision with a sign. **QSEN: Safety**

Health Promotion and Maintenance

- Teach patients to avoid rubbing their eyes. **QSEN: Safety**
- Identify patients at risk for eye injury as a result of occupation or leisure activities. **QSEN: Safety**
- Teach adults to wear eye protection in any environment in which drops or particulate matter is airborne. **QSEN: Safety**
- Teach adults to wear sunglasses that filter UV light outdoors in sunlight. **QSEN: Evidence-Based Practice**
- Teach patients to wash their hands before and after touching the eyes. **QSEN: Safety**
- Encourage adults older than 40 years of age and patients with chronic disorders to have an eye examination with measurement of intraocular pressure (IOP) at least annually. **QSEN: Safety**

Psychosocial Integrity

- Fully explain diagnostic and therapeutic procedures, restrictions, and follow-up care. **QSEN: Patient-Centered Care**
- Provide opportunities for expression of concerns about a change in visual *sensory perception*. **Ethics**
- Refer the patient with reduced visual *sensory perception* to local services, resources, and support groups for those with impaired vision. **QSEN: Patient-Centered Care**

Physiological Integrity

- Ask about a family history of vision problems because some conditions have a genetic component. **QSEN: Evidence-Based Practice**
- Test the vision of both eyes immediately if a patient has experienced an eye injury or any sudden change in vision. **QSEN: Safety**
- Stress the importance of completing an antibiotic regimen for an eye infection. **QSEN: Evidence-Based Practice**
- Teach patients who are at risk for increased IOP which activities to avoid and how to use glaucoma drops exactly as prescribed. **QSEN: Safety**
- Instruct the patient who had cataract surgery to immediately report any vision reduction after surgery. **QSEN: Safety**
- Never attempt to remove any object protruding from the eye. **QSEN: Safety**
- Collaborate with the interprofessional team to increase the patient's independence and safety within the home and community. **QSEN: Teamwork and Collaboration**

MASTERY QUESTIONS

1. Which symptom will the nurse teach the client who just had surgery to correct a retinal detachment to immediately report to the eye care provider? **Select all that apply.**
   A. Pain in the affected eye
   B. Pus in the affected eye
   C. Decreased visual acuity
   D. Temperature of 99.0°F
   E. Pupil that constricts in response to light

2. Which assessment data do the nurse anticipate when a client presents to the emergency department reporting the sensation of a foreign body in the eye? **Select all that apply.**
   A. Pain
   B. Fever
   C. Tearing
   D. Photophobia
   E. Blurred vision

REFERENCES

American Academy of Ophthalmology. (2017). *Are eye drops always necessary before cataract surgery?*. Retrieved from https://www.aao.org/eye-health/ask-ophthalmologist-q/are-eye-drops-always-necessary-before-cataract-sur.

American Academy of Ophthalmology. (2020). *Eye health statistics.* Retrieved from https://www.aao.org/newsroom/eye-health-statistics#_edn1.

American Optometric Association. (2020). *Lutein & zeaxanthin.* Retrieved from https://www.aoa.org/patients-and-public/caring-for-your-vision/diet-and-nutrition/lutein.

Bagheri, N., & Wajda, B. N. (Eds.). (2017). *The Wills eye manual: Office and emergency room diagnosis and treatment of eye disease* (7th ed.) Philadelphia: Lippincott Williams & Wilkins.

Boyd, K. (2020). *Smoking and eye disease. American Academy of Ophthalmology.* Retrieved from https://www.aao.org/eye-health/tips-prevention/smokers.

Centers for Disease Control and Prevention. (2018a). *Don't let glaucoma steal your sight!.* Retrieved from https://www.cdc.gov/features/glaucoma-awareness/index.html.

Centers for Disease Control and Prevention. (2018b). *Learn about age-related macular degeneration.* Retrieved from https://www.cdc.gov/features/healthyvisionmonth/index.html.

Eisenhauer, B., Natoli, S., Liew, G., & Flood, V. M. (2017). Lutein and zeaxanthin: Food sources, bioavailability and dietary variety in age-related macular degeneration protection. *Nutrition, 9*(120), 1–14. https://doi.org/10.3390/nu9020.

Eye Banking Association of America (EBAA). (n.d.). Medical standards/procedures manual. http://restoresight.org/what-we-do/publications/medical-standards-procedures-manual/.

Glaucoma Research Foundation. (2017). What can I do to prevent glaucoma? http://www.glaucoma.org/gleams/what-can-i-do-to-prevent-glaucoma.php.

Gudgel, D. (2018). *Eye pressure.* Retrieved from https://www.aao.org/eye-health/anatomy/eye-pressure.

Gwenhure, T. (2020). Procedure for eye irrigation to treat ocular chemical injury. *Nursing Times [online], 116*(2), 46–48.

Interprofessional Education Collaborative. (2016). Core competencies for interprofessional collaborative practice: 2016 update. Retrieved from https://nebula.wsimg.com/2f68a39520b03336b-41038c370497473?AccessKeyId=DC06780E69ED19E2B3A5&disposition=0&alloworigin=1.

Jacobs, D. (2019). *Open-angle glaucoma: Epidemiology, clinical presentation, and diagnosis.* In *UpToDate,* M. Gardiner (Ed.). Waltham, MA.

Jarvis, C. (2020). *Physical examination & health assessment* (8th ed.). St. Louis: Elsevier.

McCance, K., Huether, S., Brashers, V., & Rote, N. (2019). *Pathophysiology: The biologic basis for disease in adults and children* (8th ed.). St. Louis: Mosby.

Merck Manual. (2019). *Professional version.* Anisocoria. Retrieved from https://www.merckmanuals.com/professional/eye-disorders/symptoms-of-ophthalmologic-disorders/anisocoria.

National Eye Institute of the National Institutes of Health. (2019). *Facts about age-related macular degeneration.* Retrieved from https://nei.nih.gov/health/maculardegen/armd_facts.

National Eye Institute of the National Institutes of Health. (2020). *Facts about glaucoma.* https://nei.nih.gov/health/glaucoma/glaucoma_facts.

PreventBlindnessorg. (2020). How often should I have an eye examination? . Retrieved from https://www.preventblindness.org/how-often-should-i-have-eye-exam.

Quaranta, L., et al. (2016). Quality of life in glaucoma: A review of the literature. *Advanced Therapies, 33,* 959–981. https://doi.org/10.1007/s12325-016-0333-6.

Rebar, C., & Rebar, M. (2019). *L. Willis's Professional Guide to Pathophysiology* (4th ed.). Philadelphia, PA: Wolters Kluwer. Authors for Chapter 15: Sensory System.

Slusser, M., et al. (2019). *Foundations of interprofessional collaborative practice* (1st ed.). St. Louis: Elsevier.

Touhy, T., & Jett, K. (2018). *Ebersole and Hess' gerontological nursing and healthy aging* (5th ed.). St. Louis: Mosby.

U.S. Department of Health and Human Services. (2018). *Medicare Learning Network: Medicare vision services.* Retrieved from https://www.cms.gov/outreach-and-education/medicare-learning-network-mln/mlnproducts/downloads/visionservices_factsheet_icn907165.pdf.

Wong, B., et al. (2018). Comparison of Disposable Goldmann applanation tonometer, ICare ic100, and Tonopen XL to standards of care Goldmann Nondisposable applanation tonometer for measuring intraocular pressure. *Journal of Glaucoma, 27*(12), 1119–1124.

Assessment and Concepts of Care for Patients With Ear and Hearing Problems

Cherie R. Rebar, Andrea A. Borchers

http://evolve.elsevier.com/Iggy/

LEARNING OUTCOMES

1. Collaborate with the interprofessional team to perform assessments of ears and hearing.
2. Prioritize evidence-based care for patients having assessment or treatment for ear or hearing problems that affect **sensory perception.**
3. Teach evidence-based ways for adults to protect their ears from injury or infection to preserve **sensory perception.**
4. Explain how physiologic aging changes of the ears and hearing affect **sensory perception.**
5. Teach patients who need hearing assistive devices how to use them.
6. Implement nursing interventions to decrease the psychosocial impact on the patient undergoing ear assessment or treatment for ear or hearing problems.
7. Apply knowledge of anatomy and physiology, genetic risk, and principles of aging to perform a focused assessment of the ears and hearing.
8. Use clinical judgment to analyze assessment findings and diagnostic data in the care of patients with an ear or hearing problem.
9. Plan care coordination and transition management for patients with an ear or hearing problem.

KEY TERMS

cerumen The wax produced by glands within the external ear canal; helps protect and lubricate the ear canal.

conductive hearing loss Hearing loss that results from any physical obstruction of sound wave transmission (e.g., a foreign body in the external canal, a retracted or bulging tympanic membrane, or fused bony ossicles)

external otitis A painful irritation or infection of the skin of the external ear, with resulting allergic response or inflammation. When it occurs in patients who participate in water sports, external otitis is called *swimmer's ear.*

frequency The highness or lowness of tones (expressed in hertz). The greater the number of vibrations per second, the higher the frequency (pitch) of the sound; the lower the number of vibrations per second, and the lower the pitch.

grommet A polyethylene tube that is surgically placed through the tympanic membrane to allow continuous drainage of middle ear fluids in the patient with otitis media.

intensity A quality of sound expressed in decibels (dB).

labyrinthectomy Surgical removal of the labyrinth.

mastoiditis An acute or chronic infection of the mastoid air cells caused by progressive otitis media.

Ménière disease Tinnitus, one-sided sensorineural hearing loss, and vertigo that is related to overproduction or decreased reabsorption of endolymphatic fluid, causing a distortion of the entire inner canal system.

mixed conductive-sensorineural hearing loss A profound hearing loss that results from a combination of both conductive and sensorineural types of hearing loss.

myringoplasty Simple surgical reconstruction of the eardrum.

myringotomy The surgical creation of a hole in the eardrum; performed to drain middle ear fluids and relieve pain in the patient with otitis media (middle ear infection).

nystagmus Involuntary eye movements.

ossiculoplasty Replacement of the ossicles within the middle ear.

otoscope An instrument used to examine the ear; consists of a light, a handle, a magnifying lens, and a pneumatic bulb for injecting air into the external canal to test eardrum mobility.

ototoxic Having a toxic effect on the inner ear structures.

presbycusis Sensorineural hearing loss, especially for high-pitched sounds; occurs as a result of aging.

sensorineural hearing loss Hearing loss that results from damage to the inner ear or auditory nerve (cranial nerve VIII).

swimmer's ear See *external otitis.*

threshold The lowest level of intensity at which pure tones and speech are heard by a patient about 50% of the time.

tinnitus A continuous ringing or noise perception in the ear.

vertigo A sense of whirling or turning in space.

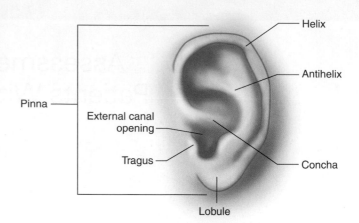

FIG. 43.1 Anatomic features of the external ear.

Used to assess surroundings, promote independence, warn of danger, appreciate music, and communicate with others, hearing is one of the five senses that allow *sensory perception.* Because ear and hearing problems are common in adults, assessment is an important skill for nurses practicing in any environment of care. Certain hearing problems develop over long periods and may be affected by drugs or systemic health problems; others occur suddenly, and immediately affect auditory *sensory perception.* These problems reduce the ability to fully communicate with the world and can lead to confusion, mistrust, and social isolation.

ANATOMY AND PHYSIOLOGY REVIEW

Structure

The external ear, the middle ear, and the inner ear make up the ear's three divisions.

External Ear. The external ear develops in the embryo at the same time as the kidneys and urinary tract. Any adult with a defect of the external ear should be examined for possible problems of the kidney and urinary systems, also.

The *pinna* is the part of the external ear that is composed of cartilage covered by skin and attached to the head at about a 10-degree angle at the level of the eyes. The external ear extends from the pinna through the external ear canal to the *tympanic membrane* (eardrum) (Fig. 43.1). It includes the *mastoid process,* which is the bony ridge located over the temporal bone behind the pinna. The ear canal is slightly S shaped and is lined with cerumen-producing glands, oil glands, and hair follicles. Cerumen (ear wax) helps protect and lubricate the ear canal. The distance from the opening of the ear canal to the eardrum in an adult is 1 to 1½ inches (2.5 to 3.75 cm).

Middle Ear. The eardrum separates the external ear and the middle ear. The middle ear consists of a compartment called the *epitympanum.* Located in the epitympanum are the top opening of the eustachian tube and three small bones known as the *bony ossicles,* which are the *malleus* (hammer), the *incus* (anvil), and the *stapes* (stirrup) (Fig. 43.2). The bony ossicles are joined loosely, thereby moving with vibrations created when sound waves hit the eardrum.

The eardrum is a thick sheet of tissue; is transparent, opaque, or pearly gray; and moves when air is injected into the external canal. The landmarks on the eardrum include the *annulus,* the *pars flaccida,* and the *pars tensa.* These correspond to the parts of the malleus that can be seen through the transparent eardrum. The eardrum is attached to the first bony ossicle, the malleus, at the umbo (Fig. 43.3). The umbo is seen through the eardrum membrane as a white dot and is one end of the long process of the malleus. The pars flaccida is that portion of the eardrum above the short process of the malleus. The pars tensa is that portion surrounding the long process of the malleus.

The middle ear is separated from the inner ear by the round window and the oval window. The eustachian tube begins at the floor of the middle ear and extends to the throat. The tube opening in the throat is surrounded by adenoid lymphatic tissue (Fig. 43.4). The eustachian tube allows the pressure on both sides of the eardrum to equalize. Secretions from the middle ear drain through the tube into the throat.

Inner Ear. The inner ear is on the other side of the oval window and contains the semicircular canals, the cochlea, the vestibule, and the distal end of the eighth cranial nerve (see Fig. 43.2). The *semicircular canals* are tubes made of cartilage and contain fluid and hair cells. These canals are connected to the sensory nerve fibers of the vestibular portion of the eighth cranial nerve. The fluid and hair cells within the canals help maintain the sense of balance.

The *cochlea,* the spiral organ of hearing, is divided into the scala tympani, the scala media, and the scala vestibuli. The scala media is filled with *endolymph,* and the scala tympani and scala vestibuli are filled with *perilymph.* These fluids protect the cochlea and the semicircular canals by allowing these structures to "float" in the fluids and be cushioned against abrupt head movements.

The *organ of Corti* is the receptor of hearing located on the membrane of the cochlea. The cochlear hair cells detect vibration from sound and stimulate the eighth cranial nerve.

The *vestibule* is a small, oval, bony chamber between the semicircular canals and the cochlea. It contains the utricle and the saccule, organs that are important for balance.

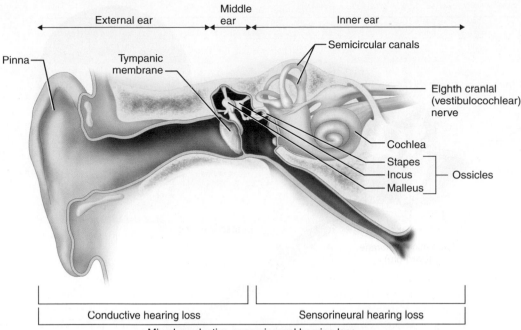

FIG. 43.2 Anatomic features of the middle and inner ear and areas involved in the three types of hearing loss.

Right tympanic membrane

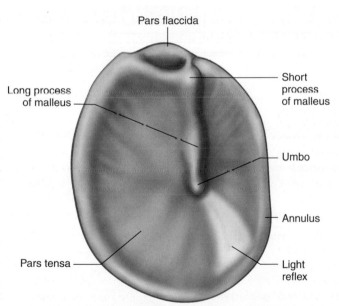

FIG. 43.3 Landmarks on the tympanic membrane.

Function

The ear's function is to promote auditory *sensory perception,* which occurs when sound is delivered through the air to the external ear canal. The sound waves strike the movable eardrum, creating vibrations. The eardrum is connected to the first bony ossicle, which allows the sound wave vibrations to be transferred from the eardrum to the malleus, the incus, and the stapes. From the stapes, the vibrations are transmitted to the cochlea. Receptors at the cochlea transduce (change) the vibrations into action potentials. The action potentials are conducted to the brain as nerve impulses by the cochlear portion of the eighth cranial (auditory) nerve. The nerve impulses are processed and interpreted as sound by the brain in the auditory cortex of the temporal lobe.

Ear and Hearing Changes Associated With Aging. All older adults should be screened for hearing acuity. Ear and hearing changes related to aging, and associated nursing adaptations and actions, are listed in the Patient Centered Care: Older Adult Considerations: Age-Related Changes in the Ear and Hearing box. Some of the ear changes do not cause harm; others affect the hearing ability of older adults.

✳ SENSORY PERCEPTION CONCEPT EXEMPLAR: HEARING LOSS

Pathophysiology Review

Loss of auditory *sensory perception* is common and may be conductive, sensorineural, or a combination of the two (see Fig. 43.2). **Conductive hearing loss** results from obstruction of sound wave transmission such as a foreign body in the external canal, a retracted or bulging tympanic membrane, or fused bony ossicles. Tumors, scar tissue, and overgrowth of soft bony tissue (**otosclerosis**) on the ossicles from previous middle ear surgery also lead to conductive hearing loss.

Sensorineural hearing loss occurs when the inner ear or auditory nerve (cranial nerve VIII) is damaged. Prolonged exposure to loud noise damages the hair cells of the cochlea.

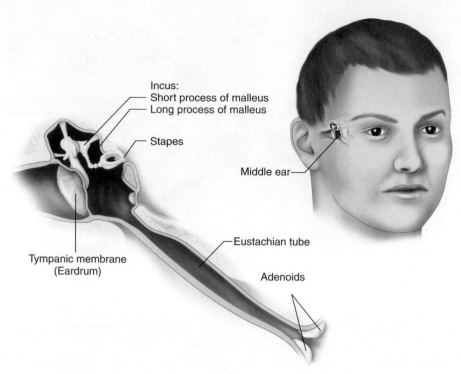

Fig. 43.4 Anatomic features and attached structures of the middle ear.

TABLE 43.1 Comparison of Features of Conductive and Sensorineural Hearing Loss	
Conductive Hearing Loss	**Sensorineural Hearing Loss**
Causes	*Causes*
Cerumen	Prolonged exposure to noise
Foreign body	Presbycusis
Perforation of the tympanic membrane	Ototoxic substance
Edema	Ménière disease
Infection of the external ear or middle ear	Acoustic neuroma
Tumor	Diabetes mellitus
Otosclerosis	Labyrinthitis
	Infection
	Myxedema
Assessment Findings	*Assessment Findings*
Evidence of obstruction with otoscope	Normal appearance of external canal and tympanic membrane
Abnormality in tympanic membrane	Tinnitus common
Speaking softly	Occasional dizziness
Hearing best in a noisy environment	Speaking loudly
Rinne test: air conduction greater than bone conduction	Hearing poorly in loud environment
Weber test: lateralization to affected ear	Rinne test: air conduction less than bone conduction
	Weber test: lateralization to unaffected ear

Many drugs are toxic to the inner ear structures, and their effects on hearing can be transient or permanent.

The differences in conductive and sensorineural hearing loss are listed in Table 43.1. Disorders that cause conductive hearing loss are often corrected with minimal or no permanent damage. Sensorineural hearing loss is often permanent.

Presbycusis is a sensorineural hearing loss that occurs with aging (McCance et al., 2019). It is caused by degeneration of cochlear nerve cells, loss of elasticity of the basilar membrane, or a decreased blood supply to the inner ear. Deficiencies of vitamin B_{12} and folic acid increase the risk for presbycusis (Curhan et al., 2018).

PATIENT-CENTERED CARE: OLDER ADULT CONSIDERATIONS (QSEN)

Age-Related Changes in the Ear and Hearing

Ear or Hearing Change	Nursing Adaptations and Actions
Pinna becomes elongated because of loss of subcutaneous tissues and decreased elasticity.	Reassure the patient that this is normal. When positioning a patient on the side, do not "fold" the ear under the head.
Hair in the canal becomes coarser and longer, especially in men.	Reassure the patient that this is normal. More frequent ear irrigation may be needed to prevent cerumen attaching to hairs.
Cerumen is drier and becomes impacted more easily, reducing hearing function.	Teach the patient and caregiver to irrigate the ear canal weekly or whenever he or she notices a change in hearing.
Tympanic membrane loses elasticity and may appear dull and retracted.	Although this can indicate otitis media, do not use this as the only sign of this condition in older adults.
Hearing acuity decreases (in some people).	Assess hearing with the voice test or the watch test. If a deficit is present, refer the patient to a specialist to further assess hearing loss and recommend appropriate intervention. Do not assume that all older adults have a hearing loss!
The ability to hear high-frequency sounds is lost first. Older adults may have particular problems hearing the *f, s, sh,* and *pa* sounds.	Provide a quiet environment when speaking (close the door to the hallway) and face the patient. Avoid standing or sitting in front of bright lights or windows, which may interfere with the patient's ability to see your lips move. If the patient wears glasses, be sure that he or she is using them to enhance speech understanding. Speak slowly, clearly, and in a deeper voice and emphasize beginning word sounds. Some patients with an uncorrected hearing loss may benefit from wearing a stethoscope while listening to you speak.

Data from Touhy, T., & Jett, K. (2018). *Ebersole and Hess' gerontological nursing healthy aging* (5th ed.). St. Louis: Mosby.

Any type of hearing loss can impact quality of life, as noted in the Evidence-Based Practice box.

Etiology and Genetic Risk. Family history is important in determining genetic risk for hearing loss. Although most hearing loss resulting from a genetic mutation is noticed in childhood, some genetic problems can lead to progressive hearing loss in adults. For example, most people with Down syndrome develop hearing loss as adults. Assess who in the family experienced hearing problems (and whether problems were present in one gender versus another), at what age the hearing loss was diagnosed, and whether both ears were affected.

EVIDENCE-BASED PRACTICE (QSEN)

Hearing Loss and Its Impact on Residents of Long-Term Care Facilities

Punch, R., & Horstmanshof, L. (2019). Hearing loss and its impact on residents in long term care facilities: A systematic review of literature. *Geriatric Nursing, 40*(2), 138-147.

With the desire to maximize quality of life for older adults living in long-term care facilities, this systematic review was conducted to determine:
- If there was an association between residents' hearing and quality of life
- Barriers to and facilitators for achieving optimal hearing for these residents
- Barriers to and facilitators for using hearing aids or other assistive devices in long-term care
- Interventions that have been tried or implemented to improve residents' ability to hear

After initial consideration of more than 200 original articles, 22 articles were determined to be useful for this systematic review. Most studies were quantitative in nature; only three were purely qualitative, and four studies used mixed methods. Correlation was demonstrated between hearing loss and quality of life related to communication, social interaction, and psychological well-being. It was noted in many studies that the physical and social environment of the long-term care facility had significant bearing on the residents' abilities to communicate and engage socially.

Very few locations had sound-absorbent materials, quiet rooms, or optimal placement of furniture to facilitate communication. Even in the presence of locations attempting to provide a hearing-friendly environment, background noises including television, music, and loud staff contributed to communication difficulty for residents. Hearing loss was underestimated or unrecognized by staff in some patients, particularly those with dementia. Furthermore, in articles that indicated hearing aids were used by residents, staff members reported having a lack of training to implement and maintain these devices.

Level of Evidence: 1
This research was designed as a systematic review.

Commentary: Implications for Practice and Research
It is important for nurses to recognize hearing difficulties in all patients, especially older adults who may live in residential facilities where noise is not always controlled. The authors of this systematic review noted that the findings strongly suggest the need for environmental optimization with a focus placed on reducing background noises. When possible, sound-absorbent materials should be put in place, and quiet areas should be identified where people can talk together without the distraction of background sounds. Staff need greater training in the use and care of hearing aids and assistive hearing devices; without such, they may not engage residents (or patients) in the ongoing use of these items, which can greatly improve communication and therefore quality of life.

PATIENT-CENTERED CARE: GENETIC/GENOMIC CONSIDERATIONS (QSEN)

Mutations in several different genes are associated with hearing loss. One type of hearing loss among adults has a genetic basis with a mutation in gene *GJB2* (Online Mendelian Inheritance in Man [OMIM], 2016). This mutation causes poor production of the protein connexin 26, which has a role in the function of cochlear hair cells. Other genetic variations in some of the genes for drug-metabolizing enzymes (cytochrome P-450 family) slow the metabolism and excretion of drugs, including ototoxic drugs. This allows ototoxic drugs to remain in the body longer, thus increasing the risk for hearing loss.

Incidence/Prevalence. Because hearing loss may be gradual and affect only some aspects of hearing, many adults are unaware that their hearing is impaired. The prevalence of adult hearing loss in the United States is estimated to be approximately 15% of the adult population between 20 and 69 years of age; this amount increases among people in their 70s and 80s (National Institute on Deafness and Other Communication Disorders, 2016).

Health Promotion and Maintenance. When the ears are properly cared for, hearing can be preserved to the greatest extent possible. Encourage patients to have simple hearing testing performed as part of their annual health assessment.

Teach adults the danger in using objects such as hairpins, ear candles, cotton swabs, or toothpicks to clean the ear canal. These can scrape the skin of the canal, push cerumen up against the eardrum, and puncture the eardrum. If cerumen buildup is a problem, teach the patient the adhere only to the method of removal recommended by the primary health care provider.

Teach about the use of protective ear devices, such as over-the-ear headsets or foam ear inserts, when exposed to persistent loud noises. To prevent infections, suggest using earplugs when engaging in water sports and using an over-the-counter product such as Swim-Ear to help dry the ears after swimming.

❖ Interprofessional Collaborative Care

You will care for many patients with hearing loss who are seeking treatment for other conditions in a variety of inpatient and outpatient settings. Use the best practices strategies listed in the Best Practice for Patient Safety & Quality Care: Communicating With a Patient Who Is Hearing-Impaired box.

◆ Assessment: Recognize Cues

History. During the interview, sit in adequate light and face the patient to allow him or her to see you speak. The patient's posture and responses can provide information about hearing acuity. Tilting the head to one side or leaning forward when listening to another person speak may indicate the presence of a hearing problem. Other indicators of hearing difficulty include asking the speaker to repeat statements or frequently saying, "What?" or "Huh?" Note whether the patient responds to whispered questions or startles when an unexpected sound occurs in the environment. Assess whether the patient's responses match the question asked. For example, when you ask, "How old are you?" does the patient respond with an age or state, "No, I am not cold."

Obtain data on age, demographics, personal and family history, socioeconomic status, occupational history, current health problems, and the use of remedies for ear problems. The patient's gender is important as some hearing disorders such as otosclerosis are more common in women.

Personal history includes past or current signs and symptoms of ear pain or discharge, **vertigo** (spinning sensation), **tinnitus** (ringing), decreased hearing, and difficulty understanding others when they talk. Ask about:

- Changes in hearing, and when these began
- Head or ear trauma or surgery
- Past ear infections or perforations
- Excessive cerumen
- Type and pattern of ear hygiene
- Drugs used (for any condition), as some are **ototoxic** (having a toxic effect on the inner ear structures), such as NSAIDs, certain antibiotics (e.g., aminoglycosides), diuretics, quinine-based medications, and certain cancer medications (American Tinnitus Association, 2019)
- Exposure to loud noise or music during work or leisure activities
- Air travel (especially in unpressurized aircraft)
- Social or occupational habits that may affect hearing
- Health history of allergies, upper respiratory infections, cancer, hypothyroidism, atherosclerosis, human immune deficiency virus (HIV) disease, or diabetes.

Physical Assessment/Signs and Symptoms. Techniques for assessment of patients with suspected loss of auditory *sensory perception* are found in the Focused Assessment: The Patient With Suspected Hearing Loss box. Remember to use Contact Precautions when assessing the ear because drainage may be present.

BEST PRACTICE FOR PATIENT SAFETY & QUALITY CARE (QSEN)

Communicating With a Patient Who Is Hearing-Impaired

- Position yourself directly in front of the patient.
- Ensure that you are not sitting or standing in front of a bright light or window, which can interfere with the patient's ability to see your lips move.
- Make sure that the room is well lighted.
- Get the patient's attention before you begin to speak.
- Move closer to the better-hearing ear.
- Speak clearly and slowly.
- Do not shout (shouting often makes understanding more difficult).
- Keep hands and other objects away from your mouth when talking to the patient.
- Have conversations in a quiet room with minimal distractions.
- Have the patient repeat your statements, not just indicate assent.
- Rephrase sentences and repeat information to aid understanding.
- Use appropriate hand motions.
- Write messages on paper if the patient is able to read.
- Obtain the assistance of an interpreter if needed, and ensure that all members of the interprofessional team use this service.

📋 FOCUSED ASSESSMENT

The Patient With Suspected Hearing Loss

Assess the ability to hear high-frequency consonants (*s, sh, f, th,* and *ch* sounds)
Assess visible ear structures:
- Position, size, and condition of the pinna; abnormalities include redness, excessive warmth, crusting, scaling, nodules, and pain (Jarvis, 2020).
- Patency of the external canal; presence of cerumen or foreign bodies, edema, or inflammation
- Condition of the tympanic membrane: intact, edema, fluid, inflammation
- Mastoid process, which should be free from pain, redness and swelling

Assess functional ability, including:
- Frequency of asking people to repeat statements
- Withdrawal from social interactions or large groups
- Shouting in conversation
- Failing to respond when not looking in the direction of the sound
- Answering questions incorrectly

Assess hearing aids (if present) for cracks, debris, proper fit

Tuning fork tests performed by the primary health care provider can help diagnose hearing loss. *Otoscopic examination,* performed by the primary health care provider with an otoscope, is used to assess the ear canal, eardrum, and middle ear structures that can be seen through the eardrum. Findings vary depending on the cause of the hearing loss. The purpose of a brief otoscopic examination is to assess the patency of the external canal, identify lesions or excessive cerumen in the canal, and assess whether the tympanic membrane (eardrum) is intact or inflamed (Jarvis, 2020).

! NURSING SAFETY PRIORITY (QSEN)

Action Alert

Do not use an otoscope to examine the ears of any patient who is unable to hold his or her head still during the examination or who is confused.

Psychosocial Assessment. For patients with a loss of auditory *sensory perception,* communication can be a struggle. They may isolate themselves because of the difficulty in talking, listening, and interpreting what is said to them. Social and work isolation can lead to depression. Encourage the patient and family to express their feelings and concerns about an actual or potential hearing loss.

NCLEX EXAMINATION CHALLENGE 43.1

Safe and Effective Care Environment

When caring for four clients, which client does the nurse report to the health care provider who should **not** receive an otoscopic examination?

A. 25-year-old with throat and ear pain
B. 39-year-old experiencing dizziness
C. 46-year-old who has type 2 diabetes
D. 60-year-old experiencing delirium

Imaging Assessment. Imaging assessment can determine some problems affecting hearing ability. Skull x-rays determine bony involvement in otitis media and the location of otosclerotic lesions. CT and MRI are used to determine soft-tissue involvement and the presence and location of tumors.

Other Diagnostic Assessment. Diagnostic assessments of hearing and balance can be useful in isolating the degree of hearing loss and, in some cases, the cause (Table 43.2).

Audiometry. Audiometry, performed by an audiologist, is the most reliable method of measuring the acuity of auditory *sensory perception.* Frequency is the highness or lowness of tones (expressed in hertz). The greater the number of vibrations per second, the higher the frequency (pitch) of the sound. The fewer the vibrations per second, the lower the frequency (pitch). Intensity of sound is expressed in decibels (dB). Threshold is the lowest level of intensity at which pure tones and speech are heard by a patient about 50% of the time. The lowest intensity at which a healthy ear can detect sound about 50% of the time is 0 dB. Conversational speech is around 60 dB, and a soft whisper is around 20 dB (Table 43.3). Sound at 110 dB is so intense (loud) that it can be painful for most people with normal hearing; this type of sound is akin to being near the speakers at a loud rock concert. With a hearing loss of 45 to 50 dB, a hearing aid may be necessary to hear normal speech. Someone with a hearing loss of 90 dB may not be able to hear speech even with a hearing aid.

◆ **Analysis: Analyze Cues and Prioritize Hypotheses.** The priority collaborative problems for the patient with any degree of hearing impairment include:

1. Decreased hearing ability due to obstruction, *infection,* damage to the middle ear, or damage to the auditory nerve
2. Decreased communication due to difficulty hearing

◆ **Planning and Implementation: Generate Solutions and Take Action**

Increasing Hearing. Nursing care priorities focus on teaching the patient about the use of any prescribed drug therapy and appropriate assistive devices, helping the patient and family to maintain or increase communication, and helping patients find community agency support.

Nonsurgical Management. Interventions include early detection of impaired auditory *sensory perception,* use of appropriate therapy, and use of assistive devices to augment the patient's usable hearing.

Early detection helps correct the problem causing the hearing loss. Assess for indications of hearing loss as covered in the Focused Assessment: The Patient With Suspected Hearing Loss box.

Drug therapy, if appropriate, is focused on correcting the underlying problem or reducing the side effects of problems occurring with hearing loss. Antibiotic therapy is used to manage external otitis and other ear infections. Teach the patient the importance of taking the drug or drugs exactly as prescribed. Caution him or her to not stop the drug just because signs and symptoms have improved. By treating the *infection,* antibiotics reduce local edema and improve hearing. When *pain* is also present, analgesics are used. Many ear disorders induce vertigo and dizziness with nausea and vomiting. Antiemetic, antihistamine, and antivertiginous drugs can be prescribed to reduce these problems.

Assistive devices are useful for patients with permanent hearing loss. Amplifiers increase telephone volume, allowing the caller to speak in a normal voice. Some phones also have a video display of words that are being spoken by the caller. Flashing lights activated by a ringing telephone or doorbell provides a visual alert. Video doorbell systems allow visualization of people outside. Some patients may have a service dog to alert them to sounds. Personal sound amplification products (PSAPs) offer solutions to situational activities that require a sound boost when a patient does not wish to have a hearing aid. These devices can help amplify sounds from a television or voices from people sitting at a table. Some devices are accessible via a headset or earpiece with Bluetooth capability, allowing a patient to take calls or listen to music directly through their smartphone.

A hearing aid is a small electronic amplifier that assists patients with conductive hearing loss but is less effective for sensorineural hearing loss (Fig. 43.5). The styles vary by size, placement, and the degree to which they amplify sound. Most common hearing aids are small. Some are attached to the wearer's glasses and are visible to other people. Another type fits into the ear and is less noticeable. Newer devices fit completely in the canal with only a fine, clear filament visible. The cost of smaller hearing aids varies with size and quality. The audiologist will teach the patient how to wear and acclimate to the hearing aid that is selected.

TABLE 43.2 Diagnostic Studies and Associated Nursing Care

Test	Purpose	Associated Nursing Care
Audiometry	*Pure tone audiometry* is used to assess hearing acuity (and demonstrates hearing loss). The test is done in a soundproof area and requires the patient to respond when a sound is heard. Speech audiometry is used to assess how intense (or loud) a simple speech stimulus must be before the patient can hear it well enough to repeat it correctly at least 50% of the time.	Describe procedure and confirm that no special preparation is needed.
Auditory brainstem evoked response (ABR)	Used to assess hearing in patients who are unable to indicate their recognition of sound stimuli during standard hearing tests. Can be used to diagnose conductive and sensorineural hearing losses.	Describe procedure. Teach that electrodes will be placed on the scalp, so no lotions, moisturizers, or oils should be on the face. Small red spots may remain on the areas where the electrodes were placed, but these will resolve. Teach that that hair should be cleaned afterward to remove electrode gel.
Auditory evoked potential (AEP)	Used to detect and estimate a patient's hearing level or degree of impairment.	Describe procedure, explaining that it is similar to an electroencephalogram (EEG). Teach that electrodes will be placed on the scalp, and that hair should be cleaned afterward to remove electrode gel.
Computerized dynamic posturography (CDP)	Used to measure whether a person can maintain steady balance as conditions (such as a visual field or the platform on which the patient stands) are manipulated.	Describe test and confirm that no special preparation is needed. Teach that a body sling may be used to promote safety.
Electronystagmography (ENG)	Used to assess for central and peripheral disease of the vestibular system in the ear by detecting and recording nystagmus.	Describe test. Remind to confirm which medications should be taken (or avoided) the day of the test. Teach that water and air will be introduced into the ear as part of caloric testing; cold water may be uncomfortable. Teach that dizziness, nausea, and vomiting during the test may occur. Teach to have an adult present after testing to drive home.
Imaging assessment	CT (with or without contrast)—used to assess ear structures in great detail; very helpful in diagnosing acoustic tumors. MRI—used to assess soft tissue changes.	Describe test. Teach to report claustrophobia prior to testing, as a mild sedative may be prescribed. Open MRI is an option for those who need this test.
Laboratory tests	Used to assess whether an infection is present; microbial culture and antibiotic sensitivity can be performed for specific causative organism and the antibiotic that will best manage the infection.	Describe test and confirm that no special preparation is needed.
Tympanometry	Used to assess eardrum mobility by changing air pressure in the external air canal. Used to assess middle ear problems (and recovery after treatment and/or surgery), eustachian tube patency, eardrum perforation, and/or fluid and wax accumulation.	Describe procedure and confirm that no special preparation is needed. Teach that there may be some discomfort while a probe is in the ear, and that sounds heard during the procedure may be loud.

TABLE 43.3 Decibel Intensity and Safe Exposure Time for Common Sounds

Sound	Decibel Intensity (dB)	Safe Exposure Time[a]
Threshold of hearing	0	
Whispering	20	
Average residence or office	40	
Conversational speech	60	
Car traffic	70	>8 hr
Motorcycle	90	8 hr
Chain saw	100	2 hr
Rock concert, front row	120	3 min
Jet engine	140	Immediate danger
Rocket launching pad	180	Immediate danger

[a]For every 5-dB increase in intensity, the safe exposure time is cut in half.

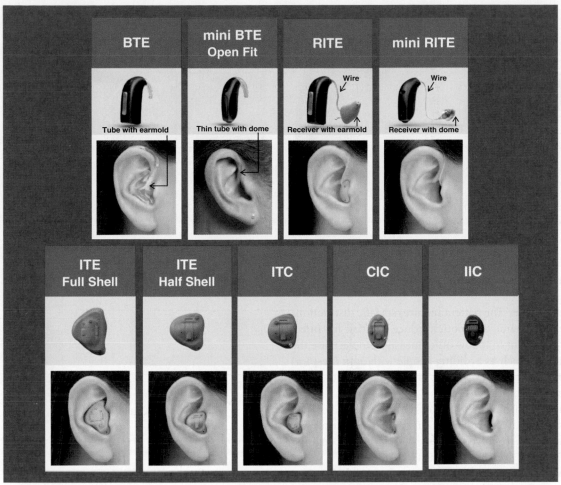

FIG. 43.5 Types of hearing aids. (From Oticon, Inc., Somerset, NJ. In Cifu, D.X., Lew, H.L., & Oh-Park, M. [2018]. *Geriatric rehabilitation*. Philadelphia: Elsevier.)

Teach the patient how to care for the hearing aid (see the Patient and Family Education: Preparing for Self-Management: Hearing Aid Care box). Hearing aids are delicate devices that should be handled only by people who know how to care for them properly.

Cochlear implantation may help patients with sensorineural hearing loss. Although a superficial surgical procedure is needed to implant the device, the procedure does not enter the inner ear and thus is not considered a surgical correction for hearing impairment (Fig. 43.6). A small computer converts sound waves into electronic impulses. Electrodes are placed near the internal ear, with the computer attached to the external ear. The electronic impulses then directly stimulate nerve fibers.

! NURSING SAFETY PRIORITY (QSEN)

Action Alert

Teach patients the safe way to clean their ears, stressing that nothing smaller than his or her own fingertip should be inserted into the canal.

Surgical Management. If nonsurgical management is not effective, various surgical interventions are available for patients with specific disorders that have contributed to hearing loss.

Tympanoplasty. Tympanoplasty (Fig. 43.7) reconstructs the middle ear to improve conductive hearing loss. The procedures

PATIENT AND FAMILY EDUCATION: PREPARING FOR SELF-MANAGEMENT

Hearing Aid Care

- Keep the hearing aid dry.
- Clean the ear mold with mild soap and water while avoiding excessive wetting.
- Using a soft toothbrush or the brush that came with the device, clean debris from the hole in the middle of the part that goes into your ear.
- Turn off the hearing aid when not in use.
- Check and replace the battery frequently.
- Keep extra batteries on hand.
- Keep the hearing aid in a safe place.
- Avoid dropping the hearing aid or exposing it to temperature extremes.
- Adjust the volume to the lowest setting that allows you to hear to prevent feedback squeaking.
- Avoid using hair spray, cosmetics, oils, or other hair and face products that might come into contact with the receiver.
- Check with your audiology provider to determine whether you can swim with your particular hearing aid(s). Some are water-resistant (and do not tolerate submersion), others are waterproof (and can be used while swimming).
- If the hearing aid does not work:
  - Change the battery.
  - Check the connection between the ear mold and the receiver.
  - Check the on/off switch.
  - Clean the sound hole.
  - Adjust the volume.
  - Take the hearing aid to an authorized service center for repair.

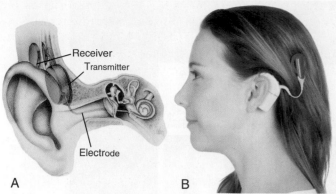

FIG. 43.6 Cochlear implant. (From Leonard, P.C. [2020]. *Quick and easy medical terminology*. [9th ed.]. St. Louis: Elsevier.)

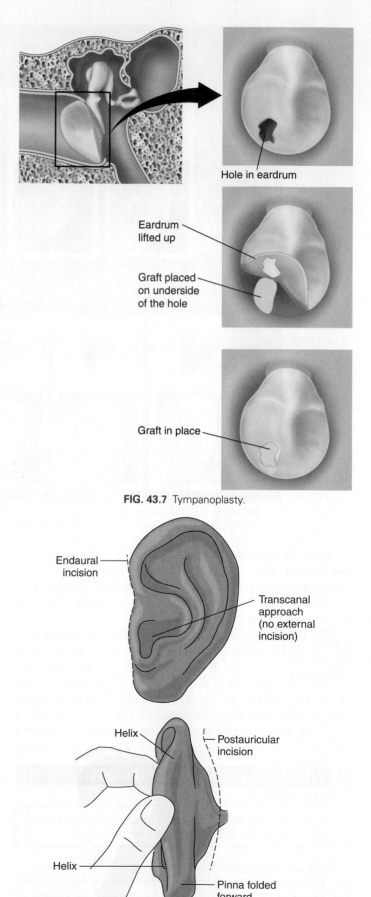

FIG. 43.7 Tympanoplasty.

FIG. 43.8 Surgical approaches for repair of the ear and hearing structures.

vary from simple reconstruction of the eardrum (**myringoplasty**) to replacement of the ossicles within the middle ear (**ossiculoplasty**).

Preoperative care. The patient requires specific instructions before surgery. Systemic antibiotics reduce the risk for *infection*. Teach the patient to follow other measures to decrease the risks for infection, such as avoiding people with upper respiratory infections, getting adequate rest, eating a balanced diet, and drinking adequate amounts of fluid.

Assure the patient that hearing loss immediately after surgery is normal because of canal packing and that hearing will improve when it is removed. Stress that forceful coughing increases middle ear pressure and must be avoided.

Operative procedures. Surgery is performed only when the middle ear is free of infection. If an infection is present, the graft is more likely to become infected and not heal. Surgery of the eardrum and ossicles requires the use of a microscope and is a delicate procedure. Local anesthesia can be used, although general anesthesia is often used to prevent the patient from moving.

The surgeon can repair the eardrum with many materials, including tissue from a vein or muscle sheath. If the ossicles are damaged, more extensive surgery is needed for repair or replacement. The ossicles can be reached in several ways—through the ear canal, with an endaural incision, or by an incision behind the ear (Fig. 43.8).

The surgeon removes diseased tissue and cleans the middle ear cavity. The patient's cartilage or bone, cadaver ossicles, stainless steel wire, or special polymers (Teflon) are used to repair or replace the ossicles.

Postoperative care. Iodoform gauze, which is soaked in antiseptic, is packed in the ear canal. If a skin incision is used, a dressing is placed over it. Keep the dressing clean and dry, using sterile technique for changes. Keep the patient flat, with the head turned to the side and the operative ear facing up for at least 12 hours after surgery. Give prescribed antibiotics to prevent *infection.*

Patients often report hearing improvement after removal of the canal packing. Until that time, communicate as with a patient who is hearing impaired, directing conversation to the unaffected ear. Instruct the patient in care and activity restrictions (see the Patient and Family Education: Preparing for Self-Management: Recovery From Ear Surgery box).

Stapedectomy. A partial or complete stapedectomy with a prosthesis can correct some hearing loss, especially in patients with hearing loss related to otosclerosis. Although hearing usually improves after primary stapes surgery, some patients redevelop conductive hearing loss after surgery, and revision surgery is needed.

Preoperative care. To prevent *infection*, the patient must be free from external otitis at surgery. Teach the patient to follow measures that prevent middle ear or external ear infections as noted in the Patient and Family Education: Preparing for Self-Management: Prevention of Ear Infection or Trauma box.

The surgeon will review the expected outcomes and possible complications of the surgery with the patient. The success rate of this procedure is high. However, there is always a risk for failure that might lead to total deafness on the affected side. Surgery is performed first on the ear with the greater hearing loss. If the surgery does not improve hearing, patients must decide to either attempt surgical correction of the other ear or continue to use an amplification device.

Other possible complications include vertigo, infection, and facial nerve damage. Remind the patient that hearing is initially worse after a stapedectomy.

Operative procedures. A stapedectomy is usually performed through the external ear canal with the patient under local anesthesia. After removal of the affected ossicles, a piston-shaped prosthesis is connected between the incus and the footplate (Fig. 43.9). Because the prosthesis vibrates with sound as the stapes did, most patients have restoration of functional hearing.

Postoperative care. Remind the patient that improvement in hearing may not occur until 6 weeks after surgery. Drugs for *pain* help reduce discomfort, and antibiotics are used to prevent infection. Teach the patient about the precautions in the Patient and Family Education: Preparing for Self-Management: Recovery From Ear Surgery box.

The surgical procedure is performed in an area where cranial nerves VII, VIII, and X can be damaged by trauma or by swelling after surgery. *Assess for facial nerve damage or muscle weakness. Indications include an asymmetric appearance or drooping of features on the affected side of the face. Ask the patient about changes in facial perception of touch and in taste.* Vertigo, nausea, and vomiting usually occur after surgery because of the nearness to inner ear structures.

Antivertiginous drugs (such as meclizine) and antiemetic drugs (such as ondansetron) may be prescribed. Prevent falls by assisting as needed and instructing the patient to move slowly from a sitting to a standing position.

PATIENT AND FAMILY EDUCATION: PREPARING FOR SELF-MANAGEMENT

Recovery From Ear Surgery

- Avoid straining when you have a bowel movement.
- Avoid drinking through a straw for 2 to 3 weeks.
- Avoid air travel for 2 to 3 weeks.
- Avoid excessive coughing for 2 to 3 weeks.
- Avoid people with respiratory infections.
- When blowing your nose, blow gently, without blocking either nostril, and with your mouth open.
- Avoid getting your head wet or washing your hair for several days.
- You may shower; before doing so, place a ball of cotton coated with petroleum jelly (e.g., Vaseline) in the ear, or use a waterproof earplug.
- Avoid rapidly moving the head, bouncing, and bending over for 3 weeks.
- If you have a dressing, change it every 24 hours or as directed.
- Report excessive drainage immediately to your primary health care provider.

PATIENT AND FAMILY EDUCATION: PREPARING FOR SELF-MANAGEMENT

Prevention of Ear Infection or Trauma

- Do not use small objects, such as cotton-tipped applicators, matches, toothpicks, keys, or hairpins, to clean your external ear canal.
- Wash your external ear and canal daily in the shower or while washing your hair.
- Blow your nose gently.
- Do not block one nostril while blowing your nose.
- Sneeze with your mouth open.
- Wear sound protection around loud or continuous noises.
- Avoid or wear head and ear protection during activities with high risk for head or ear trauma, such as wrestling, boxing, motorcycle riding, and skateboarding.
- Keep the volume on head receivers at the lowest setting that allows you to hear.
- Frequently clean objects that come into contact with your ear (e.g., headphones, telephone receivers).
- Avoid environmental conditions with rapid changes in air pressure.

! NURSING SAFETY PRIORITY (QSEN)

Action Alert

Prevent injury by assisting the patient with ambulation during the first 1 to 2 days after stapedectomy. Keep top bed side rails up and remind the patient to move the head slowly to avoid vertigo.

Totally Implanted Devices. Totally implanted devices, such as the Esteem, can improve bilateral moderate-to-severe sensorineural hearing loss without any visible part (Envoy Medical, 2020). These devices have three totally implanted components: a sound processor, a sensor, and a computer. Vibrations of the eardrum and ossicles are picked up by the sensor and converted to electric signals that are processed by the sound processor. The processor is programmed to the patient's specific hearing pathology. The processor filters out some background noise and amplifies the desired sound signal. The signal is transferred to the computer, which then converts the processed signal into

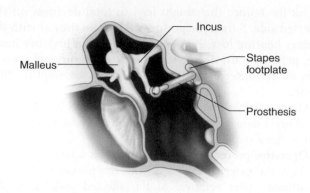

FIG. 43.9 Prosthesis used with stapedectomy. The stapes is removed, leaving the footplate. A metal or plastic prosthesis is connected to the incus and inserted through the hole to act as an artificial stapes.

vibrations that are transmitted to the inner ear for auditory *sensory perception.*

Patient criteria for totally implantable devices include:
- Bilateral stable sensorineural hearing loss
- Speech discrimination score of 40% or higher
- Healthy tympanic membrane, eustachian tube, and ossicles of the middle ear
- Large enough ear cavity to fit the device components
- At least 30 days of experience with an appropriate hearing aid
- Absence of middle ear, inner ear, or mastoid infection
- Absence of Ménière disease or recurring vertigo
- Absence of sensitivity to device materials

The devices and the surgery may lead to possible complications, including temporary facial paralysis, changes in taste sensation, and ongoing or new-onset tinnitus. Unlike cochlear implants, the middle ear is entered, and it is considered a surgical procedure. Care before and after surgery is similar to that required with stapedectomy. The cost of the implant and procedure can be very high; currently this type of implantable device is not covered by Medicare or Medicaid, and only by select private insurers.

Maximizing Communication

Nonsurgical Management. Nursing priorities focus on facilitating communication and reducing anxiety. For communicating, use best practices that are listed in the Best Practice for Patient Safety & Quality Care: Communicating With a Patient Who Is Hearing-Impaired box. Do not shout at the patient because the sound may be projected at a higher frequency, making him or her less able to understand. Communicate by writing (if he or she is able to see, read, and write) or with pictures of familiar phrases and objects. Many television programs are now closed captioned or video described (subtitled).

Collaborate with members of the interprofessional team, such as the audiologist, who can help with maximizing hearing, which can improve communication.

⚡ ETHICAL/LEGAL CONSIDERATIONS

Remember that you have a legal and ethical responsibility to make sure that you communicate effectively so that the patient receives the best care possible (National Association of the Deaf, 2020). Use all appropriate resources, based on the individual patient's abilities and needs, to ensure proper communication.

Lip-reading and *sign language* can increase communication. Patients are taught special cues to look for when lip-reading and how to understand body language. However, the best lip-reader still misses more than half of what is being said. Because even minimal lip-reading assists hearing, urge patients to wear their eyeglasses when talking with someone to see lip movement.

Sign languages, such as American Sign Language (ASL), combine speech with hand movements that signify letters, words, and phrases. These languages take time and effort to learn, and many people are unable to use them effectively.

Managing anxiety can increase the effectiveness of communication efforts. One source of anxiety is the possibility of permanent hearing loss. Provide accurate information about the likelihood of hearing returning. When the hearing impairment is likely to be permanent, reassure patients that communication and social interaction can be maintained with some practical modification.

Help patients use resources and communication to make social contact satisfying. Identify the patient's most satisfying activities and social interactions and determine the effort necessary to continue them. The patient can alter activities to improve satisfaction. Instead of large gatherings, the patient might choose smaller groups. A meal at home with friends can substitute for dining out, or consider requesting a table in a quiet area of a restaurant.

Care Coordination and Transition Management. Lengthy hospitalization is rare for ear and hearing disorders. If surgery is needed and the procedure is completed without complications, it may be performed in an ambulatory surgery center.

Home Care Management. Patients who have persistent vertigo are in danger of falling. Assess the home for potential hazards and to determine whether family or significant others are available to assist with meal preparation and other ADLs.

Self-Management Education. Provide written instructions to the patient and family about how to take drugs and when to return for follow-up care, if needed. Follow-up hearing tests may be scheduled routinely or are scheduled when surgical lesions are well healed in about 6 to 8 weeks. Audiograms done before and after treatment are compared, and evaluation for further intervention to improve hearing begins.

Teach patients how to instill eardrops and irrigate the ears and obtain a return demonstration.

To prevent *infection* after surgery, instruct patients to follow the information located in the Patient and Family Education: Preparing for Self-Management: Prevention of Ear Infection or Trauma box. Teach patients who use a hearing aid and their caregivers how to use it effectively.

Health Care Resources. A nurse case manager can coordinate with the patient, caregiver, and home care nurse to determine how to best maintain adequate self-care abilities, maintain a safe environment, decide about assistance needs, and obtain needed care. Support groups organized for patients with hearing problems can also be most helpful.

Costs to the patient with a hearing impairment can be extensive. Information and support can come from public and private agencies that specialize in counseling patients with disorders affecting auditory *sensory perception.*

◆ **Evaluation: Evaluate Outcomes.** Evaluate the care of the patient with hearing loss based on the identified priority patient problems. The expected outcomes include that the patient will:
- Maintain as much hearing as possible and/or use appropriate hearing compensation behaviors
- Successfully use (a) method(s) of communication that works best for the individual
- Successfully use assistive devices as needed

OTITIS MEDIA

Pathophysiology Review

The common forms of otitis media are acute otitis media, chronic otitis media, and serous otitis media. Each type affects the middle ear but has different causes and pathologic changes. If otitis progresses or is untreated, permanent conductive hearing loss may occur.

Acute otitis media and chronic otitis media are similar. An infecting agent in the middle ear causes inflammation of the mucosa, leading to swelling and irritation of the ossicles within the middle ear, followed by purulent inflammatory exudate. The acute form has a sudden onset and lasts 3 weeks or less. Chronic otitis media often follows repeated acute episodes, has a longer duration, and causes greater middle ear injury. It may be a result of the continuing presence of a biofilm in the middle ear. A *biofilm* is a community of bacteria working together to overcome host defense mechanisms to continue to survive and proliferate (see Chapter 21 for more information about biofilms). Therapy for complications associated with chronic otitis media usually involves surgical intervention.

The eustachian tube and mastoid, connected to the middle ear by a sheet of cells, are also affected by the *infection.* If the eardrum membrane perforates, the infection can thicken and scar the eardrum and middle ear if left untreated. Necrosis of the ossicles destroys middle ear structures and causes hearing loss.

❖ Interprofessional Collaborative Care

◆ **Assessment: Recognize Cues.** The patient with acute or chronic otitis media has ear *pain.* Acute otitis media causes more intense pain from increased pressure in the middle ear. Conductive hearing is reduced and distorted as sound-wave transmission is obstructed. The patient may notice tinnitus in the form of a low hum or a low-pitched sound. Headaches, malaise, fever, nausea, and vomiting can occur. As the pressure on the middle ear pushes against the inner ear, the patient may have dizziness.

Otoscopic examination findings vary, depending on the stage of the condition. The eardrum is initially retracted, which allows landmarks of the ear to be seen clearly. At this early stage, the patient may only have vague ear discomfort. As the condition progresses, the eardrum's blood vessels dilate and appear red (Fig. 43.10). Later the eardrum becomes red, thickened, and bulging, with loss of landmarks. Decreased eardrum mobility is

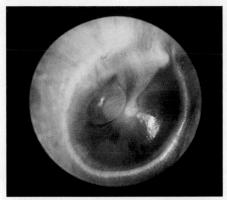

FIG. 43.10 Otoscopic view of otitis media.

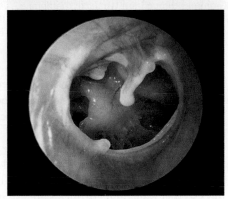

FIG. 43.11 Otoscopic view of a perforated tympanic membrane.

evident on inspection with a pneumatic otoscope. Pus may be seen behind the membrane.

With progression, the eardrum spontaneously perforates, and pus or blood drains from the ear (Fig. 43.11). The patient usually has a marked decrease in pain as the pressure on middle ear structures is relieved. Eardrum perforations often heal if the underlying problem is controlled. Simple central perforation does not interfere with hearing unless the ossicles are damaged or the perforation is large. Repeated perforations with extensive scarring cause hearing loss.

◆ **Interventions: Take Action**

Nonsurgical Management. Bedrest limits head movements that intensify the *pain.* Application of low heat may help reduce pain. Systemic antibiotic therapy is needed to address the *infection.* Teach the patient to complete the antibiotic therapy as prescribed and to not stop taking the drug even when he or she begins to feel better. Analgesics such as ibuprofen and acetaminophen can be used to relieve pain and reduce fever. For severe pain, opioid analgesics may be prescribed. Antihistamines and decongestants can also be prescribed to decrease fluid in the middle ear.

Surgical Management. If *pain* persists after antibiotic therapy and the eardrum continues to bulge, a myringotomy (surgical opening of the eardrum) may be performed. This procedure drains middle ear fluids and immediately relieves pain.

The procedure requires only a small surgical incision, which is often performed in an office or clinic under local anesthesia, yet can also be done in a surgical suite under general anesthesia. The incision heals rapidly. For relief of pressure caused by

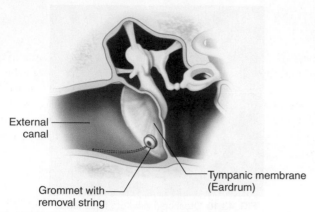

FIG. 43.12 Grommet through the tympanic membrane. A small grommet is placed through the tympanic membrane away from the margins, which allows prolonged drainage of fluids from the middle ear.

serous otitis media and for patients who have repeated episodes of otitis media, a small **grommet** (polyethylene tube) may be surgically placed through the eardrum to allow continuous drainage of middle ear fluids (Fig. 43.12).

Priority care after surgery includes teaching the patient to keep the external ear and canal clean and dry while the incision is healing. Hair-washing and showering should be avoided for several days so that water and chemicals are not introduced into the ear. Other instructions after surgery are listed in the Patient and Family Education: Preparing for Self-Management: Recovery from Ear Surgery box earlier in this chapter.

EXTERNAL OTITIS

Pathophysiology Review

External otitis (Fig. 43.13) is a painful condition caused when irritating or infective agents come into contact with the skin of the external ear. The result is an allergic response or inflammation with or without *infection*. Affected skin becomes red, swollen, and tender to touch or movement. Swelling of the ear canal can lead to temporary hearing loss from obstruction. Allergic external otitis is often caused by contact with cosmetics, hair sprays, earphones, earrings, or hearing aids. The most common infectious organisms are *Pseudomonas aeruginosa*, *Proteus vulgaris*, *Staphylococcus aureus*, and *Escherichia coli* (Kesser, 2019).

External otitis occurs more often in hot, humid environments, especially in the summer, and is known as **swimmer's ear** because it often occurs in people involved in water sports. Patients who have traumatized their external ear canal with sharp or small objects (e.g., hairpins, cotton-tipped applicators) or with headphones also are more susceptible to external otitis. Others at risk include people with general allergies, psoriasis, eczema, and seborrheic dermatitis (Kesser, 2019).

Necrotizing or *malignant otitis* is the most virulent form of external otitis. This extremely rare condition occurs most often in patients who are immunocompromised. Organisms spread beyond the external ear canal into the ear and skull. Death from complications such as meningitis, brain abscess, and destruction of cranial nerve VII is possible.

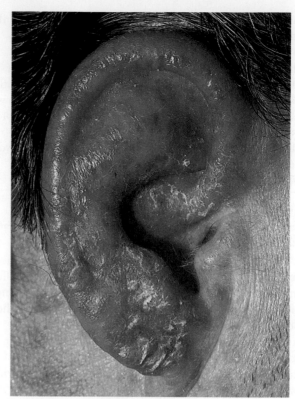

FIG. 43.13 External otitis. (From Habif, T.P. [2016]. *Clinical dermatology* [6th ed.]. Philadelphia: Elsevier.)

❖ Interprofessional Collaborative Care

◆ **Assessment: Recognize Cues.** Signs and symptoms of external otitis range from mild itching to *pain* with movement of the pinna or tragus, particularly when upward pressure is applied to the external canal. Patients report feeling as if the ear is plugged and hearing is reduced. The temporary hearing loss can be severe when inflammation obstructs the canal and prevents sounds from reaching the eardrum.

◆ **Interventions: Take Action.** Treatment focuses on reducing inflammation, edema, and *pain*. Cleaning is the first step, as cerumen, desquamated skin, and other purulent material must be removed from the ear canal (Goguen, 2019). The primary health care provider will conduct the cleaning through an otoscope. Once the ear canal is clean, eardrops will be much more effective.

Nursing priorities include enhancing comfort measures, such as applying heat to the ear for 20 minutes three times a day. This can be accomplished by using towels warmed with water and then wrapped in a plastic bag or by using a heating pad placed on the lowest setting. Teach the patient that minimizing head movements reduces pain.

Topical antibiotic and steroid therapies are generally prescribed to decrease inflammation and pain. Watch the patient or caregiver administer the eardrops to make sure that proper technique is used. Oral or IV antibiotics are used in severe cases, especially when *infection* spreads to surrounding tissue or when area lymph nodes are enlarged.

Analgesics, including opioids, may be needed for *pain* relief during the initial days of treatment. Ibuprofen or acetaminophen can relieve less severe pain. Teach the patient to place a cotton ball coated with petroleum jelly into the ear when showering. The patient must be taught to avoid water sports, ear buds, and hearing aid for at least 7 to 10 days. People who swim should be taught to wear earplugs when swimming. Finally, teach the patient to use preventive measures for minimizing ear canal moisture, trauma, or exposure to materials that lead to local irritation or contact dermatitis.

CERUMEN OR FOREIGN BODIES

Pathophysiology Review

Cerumen (earwax) is the most common cause of an impacted ear canal. Foreign bodies, such as small vegetables, beads, pencil erasers, and insects, can also be impacting. Although uncomfortable, cerumen or foreign bodies are rarely emergencies and can be removed carefully by a health care professional. Cerumen impaction in the older adult is common, and removal of the cerumen from older adults often improves hearing.

❖ Interprofessional Collaborative Care

◆ **Assessment: Recognize Cues.** Patients may report a sensation of fullness in the ear, with or without hearing loss, and may have ear *pain,* itching, dizziness, or bleeding from the ear. Cerumen or the foreign body may be visible with direct inspection.

◆ **Interventions: Take Action.** When the occluding material is cerumen, management options include watchful waiting, manual removal, or the use of ceruminolytic agents followed by manual removal or irrigation.

If the cerumen is thick and dry or cannot be removed easily, the primary health care provider may recommend use of a ceruminolytic product such as Cerumenex or Debrox to soften the wax before removal. Another recommendation may include adding 2 or 3 drops of mineral oil to the ear at bedtime. After a few days of this practice, a curette or cerumen spoon may then be used by the health care professional to remove the wax. In some cases, irrigation may be considered, only if the patient does not have an eardrum perforation or otitis media. Caution patients to avoid self-treatment without consultation with the primary health care provider.

Insects are killed before removal unless they can be coaxed out by a flashlight. A topical anesthetic can be placed in the ear canal for pain relief. Mineral oil or diluted alcohol instilled into the ear can suffocate the insect, which is then removed by the primary health care provider with ear forceps. If a foreign body cannot be removed in the outpatient setting, surgical removal under general anesthetic may be required.

! NURSING SAFETY PRIORITY (QSEN)

Action Alert

Do not irrigate an ear with an eardrum perforation or otitis media because this may spread the *infection* to the inner ear. Also, do not irrigate the ear when the foreign object is vegetable matter because this material expands when wet, making the impaction worse. An experienced health care professional performs removal of vegetable matter.

MASTOIDITIS

Pathophysiology Review

The lining of the middle ear is continuous with the lining of the mastoid air cells, which are embedded in the temporal bone. Mastoiditis is an *infection* of the mastoid air cells caused by progressive otitis media. Antibiotic therapy is used to treat the middle ear infection before it progresses to mastoiditis. If mastoiditis is not managed appropriately, it can lead to brain abscess, meningitis, and death.

❖ Interprofessional Collaborative Care

◆ **Assessment: Recognize Cues.** The signs and symptoms of mastoiditis include swelling behind the ear and *pain* when moving the ear or the head. Pain is *not* relieved by myringotomy. Cellulitis develops on the skin or external scalp over the mastoid process, pushing the ear sideways and down. The eardrum is red, dull, thick, and immobile. Perforation may or may not be present. Lymph nodes behind the ear are tender and enlarged. Patients may have low-grade fever, malaise, and ear drainage. Hearing loss occurs, and CT scans show fluid in the air cells of the mastoid process. If intracranial complications are anticipated, an MRI will be ordered instead of a CT scan (Lustig et al., 2018).

◆ **Interventions: Take Action.** Interventions focus on halting the *infection* before it spreads to other structures. IV antibiotics are used but do not easily penetrate the infected bony structure of the mastoid. Cultures of the ear drainage determine which antibiotics should be most effective. Surgical removal of the infected tissue is needed if the infection does not respond to antibiotic therapy within a few days. A simple or modified radical mastoidectomy with tympanoplasty is the most common treatment. All infected tissue must be removed so the infection does not spread to other structures. A tympanoplasty is then performed to reconstruct the ossicles and the eardrum to restore hearing (see the Tympanoplasty section).

TINNITUS

Tinnitus (continuous ringing or noise perception in the ear) is a common ear problem that can occur in one or both ears. Diagnostic testing cannot confirm tinnitus; however, testing is performed to assess hearing and rule out other disorders. A Tinnitus and Hearing Survey (Henry et al., 2015) may be used to help patients and clinicians determine whether intervention for tinnitus is warranted.

Signs and symptoms range from mild ringing, which can go unnoticed during the day, to a loud roaring in the ear, which can seriously interfere with thinking and attention span. Factors that contribute to tinnitus include age, sclerosis of the ossicles, Ménière disease, certain drugs (aspirin, NSAIDs, high-ceiling diuretics, quinine, aminoglycoside antibiotics), exposure to loud noise, and other inner ear problems.

The problem and its management vary with the underlying cause. When no cause can be found or the disorder is untreatable, therapy focuses on ways to mask the tinnitus with background sound, noisemakers, and music during sleeping hours. Ear-mold hearing aids can amplify sounds to dampen tinnitus during the day. A drug that is helpful to some patients is pramipexole, an antiparkinson drug. The American Tinnitus Association helps patients cope with tinnitus. Refer patients with tinnitus to local and online support groups as needed.

PATIENT-CENTERED CARE: VETERANS HEALTH CONSIDERATIONS (QSEN)

Veterans who have served are often exposed to noise, particularly if they have been around gunfire, detonation of weapons, explosives, or aircraft. Tinnitus and hearing loss are the top two compensated service-related disabilities and affect over 3.1 million veterans (U.S. Department of Veterans Affairs, 2018). Nurses must remember to assess patients for veteran status and inquire about occupational exposure (Elliott, 2019). Provide a quiet and private environment for care, be mindful of coexisting conditions that the veteran may have, and communicate with a multimodal approach using visual handouts and demonstrations (Elliott, 2019).

NCLEX EXAMINATION CHALLENGE 43.2
Physiological Integrity

Which client statement regarding a new diagnosis of tinnitus requires nursing teaching? **Select all that apply.**
A. "I am so glad this condition will go away permanently."
B. "It is important that I do not drive when I have tinnitus."
C. "Watching my diet will make a difference in my condition."
D. "Surgery is the only treatment that is available for tinnitus."
E. "I have found a couple of support groups that I like to attend."

MÉNIÈRE DISEASE

Pathophysiology Review

Ménière disease is a condition that includes a classic trio of symptoms—episodic **vertigo**, tinnitus, and hearing loss (Moskowitz & Dinces, 2020). Symptoms usually occur in adults between the ages of 20 and 60 years (Moskowitz & Dinces, 2020; National Institute on Deafness and Other Communication Disorders, 2017). Episodes, also called "attacks," can last several days, although some patients report ongoing symptoms of varying intensity at all times. Patients can be almost to totally incapacitated during an attack, and recovery can take hours to days. Although most patients have a window of forewarning when an attack is beginning, others experience Tumarkin otolithic crises, known as *sudden drop attacks* in which the patient falls to the ground with no warning (Wu et al., 2019).

The pathophysiology leading to this condition is not fully understood. However, it is known that Ménière disease is progressive, leading to an excess of endolymphatic fluid that builds up within the inner ear (Pullen, 2017) causing distortion and distention of portions of the labyrinth system (Moskowitz & Dinces, 2020). This distortion decreases hearing by dilating the cochlear duct, causes vertigo because of damage to the vestibular system, and stimulates tinnitus. At first, hearing loss is reversible, but repeated damage to the cochlea from increased fluid pressure can lead to permanent hearing loss.

❖ Interprofessional Collaborative Care

◆ **Assessment: Recognize Cues.** Signs and symptoms include vertigo, hearing loss, and tinnitus. Vertigo is often accompanied by nausea, vomiting, headache, and nystagmus (rapid eye movements). Blood pressure, pulse, and respirations may be elevated. Hearing loss occurs first with the low-frequency tones; in some patients, it progresses to include all levels and eventually becomes permanent. Patients may describe the tinnitus as having variable pitch and intensity, which may fluctuate or remain continuous.

◆ **Interventions: Take Action.** Nonpharmacologic treatment for Ménière disease includes diet and lifestyle adjustments, as some patients with this condition are sensitive to triggers such as high salt intake, caffeine, monosodium glutamate (MSG), alcohol, nicotine, stress, and allergens (Moskowitz & Dinces, 2020). Teach patients how to modify their diet accordingly. It is also important to teach the client to avoid activities that place them at risk of experiencing vertigo, such as standing on chairs or ladders. Patients with sudden drop attacks should not drive, and may be subject to having a driver's license suspended for safety purposes (Wu et al., 2019).

Teach patients to move the head slowly to prevent worsening of the vertigo. Institute and teach fall precautions to all patients with Ménière disease.

Vestibular rehabilitation therapy uses exercise activities to improve balance, which can be helpful. Pharmacologic treatment is used to reduce symptoms. Betahistine (in Canada) or diuretics can be prescribed to decrease endolymph volume, which reduces vertigo, hearing loss, tinnitus, and aural fullness. Other drugs, such as vestibular suppressants and antiemetics, may be used to address symptoms that occur during attacks. For patients who do not respond to pharmacologic intervention, systemic glucocorticoids may be used; if this fails, intratympanic glucocorticoid therapy or intratympanic gentamicin may be attempted (Moskowitz & Dinces, 2020).

When drug therapy is not effective in controlling symptoms or attacks, other procedures may be considered. Decompression and/or shunting of the endolymphatic sac has been shown to have favorable outcomes in controlling vertigo. Finally, **labyrinthectomy** can be done in extreme cases in which the patient already has significant hearing loss or continuous disabling vertigo. This surgical procedure destroys the bony and membranous labyrinth by removal of the neuroepithelium, resulting in total hearing loss on the operative side.

NCLEX EXAMINATION CHALLENGE 43.3
Physiological Integrity

What teaching will the nurse provide to a client who continues to experience more frequent episodes associated with Ménière disease? **Select all that apply.**
A. Reducing activity can reduce frequency of episodes.
B. Episodes will eventually decrease in severity and number.
C. Reducing sodium, caffeine, and alcohol intake can be beneficial.
D. The only treatment that is effective is to undergo labyrinthectomy.
E. When moving from sitting to standing, be cautious and take your time.

👤 CLINICAL JUDGMENT CHALLENGE 43.1

Safety; Patient-Centered Care

A 45-year-old female client has been admitted for observation after coming to the emergency department reporting dizziness, nausea, and vomiting. She states, "I can't seem to get rid of the flu. This is the third time I've had it recently." She reports being at home earlier in the day and having a sensation of spinning come over her suddenly. When she fell to the floor, her partner brought her immediately to the emergency department. Now, several hours later, she reports feeling somewhat better but still has the spinning sensation and is nauseated. She says that she also has ringing in her ears. On assessment, vital signs include BP 140/90 mm Hg, pulse 100 beats/min, and respirations 20 breaths/min. Nystagmus is noted. When someone stands on the left side of the client, she does not respond to questions or dialogue.

1. **Recognize Cues:** What assessment information in this client situation is the most important and immediate concern for the nurse? (Hint: Identify the **relevant** information *first* to determine what is most important.)

2. **Analyze Cues:** What client conditions are consistent with the **most relevant** information? (Hint: Think about priority collaborative problems that support and contradict the information presented in this situation.)

3. **Prioritize Hypotheses:** Which possibilities or explanations are **most likely** to be present in this client situation? Which possibilities or explanations are the most serious? (Hint: Consider all possibilities and determine their urgency and risk for this client.)

4. **Generate Solutions:** What actions would most likely achieve the desired outcomes for this client? Which actions should be **avoided** or are **potentially harmful**? (Hint: Determine the desired outcomes first to decide which interventions are appropriate and those that should be avoided.)

5. **Take Action:** Which actions are the most appropriate and how should they be implemented? In what **priority order** should they be implemented? (Hint: Consider health teaching, documentation, requested health care provider orders or prescriptions, nursing skills, collaboration with or referral to health team members, etc.)

6. **Evaluate Outcomes:** What client assessment would indicate that the nurse's actions were **effective**? (Hint: Think about signs that would indicate an improvement, decline, or unchanged client condition.)

ACOUSTIC NEUROMA

An *acoustic neuroma* is a benign tumor of the vestibulocochlear nerve (cranial nerve VIII) that often damages other structures as it grows. Depending on the size and exact location of the tumor, damage to hearing, facial movements, and sensation can occur. An acoustic neuroma can cause neurologic signs and symptoms as the tumor enlarges in the brain.

Signs and symptoms begin with tinnitus and progress to gradual sensorineural hearing loss. Later, patients have constant mild-to-moderate vertigo. As the tumor enlarges, nearby cranial nerves are damaged.

The tumor is diagnosed with an MRI. If the patient cannot tolerate an MRI, high-resolution CT with or without contrast can be used (Park, 2020). Treatment involves surgery, radiation, or watchful observation. If surgery is performed, risks include hearing loss, facial weakness, persistent headaches, and/or vestibular disturbances (Park, 2020). Because these tumors grow very slowly, even patients who have had surgery need prolonged follow-up.

▌ GET READY FOR THE NEXT-GENERATION NCLEX® EXAMINATION!

Key Points

Review these Key Points for each NCLEX Examination Client Needs Category.

Safe and Effective Care Environment

- Use Contact Precautions with any patient who has ear drainage. **QSEN: Safety**
- Do not perform an otoscopic examination on a patient who is confused. **QSEN: Safety**
- Protect the patient with vertigo or dizziness from injury by assisting with ambulation. **QSEN: Safety**
- Raise upper side rails for the patient experiencing dizziness or vertigo. **QSEN: Safety**
- Teach patients to move the head slowly after ear surgery to prevent dizziness or vertigo. **QSEN: Safety**

Health Promotion and Maintenance

- Identify adults at risk for hearing impairment based on occupational and leisure activities. **QSEN: Safety**

- Teach adults ways to protect hearing before loss occurs. **QSEN: Safety**
- Use best practices to enhance communication with a patient who is hearing-impaired. **QSEN: Patient-Centered Care**
- Ensure that all members of the interprofessional team use a medical interpreter as needed for the patient who cannot hear. **QSEN: Patient-Centered Care**
- Teach patients the proper way to clean their ears and safely remove cerumen. **QSEN: Evidence-Based Practice**
- If ordered, teach patients and caregivers the proper techniques for self-instillation of eardrops. **QSEN: Evidence-Based Practice**
- Teach patients and caregivers how to properly care for hearing aids. **QSEN: Safety**

Psychosocial Integrity

- Allow the patient the opportunity to express fear or anxiety about hearing concerns. **QSEN: Patient-Centered Care**

- Assess the degree to which hearing problems interfere with the patient's ability to interact with others. **Clinical Judgment**
- Refer patients newly diagnosed with hearing impairment to appropriate local resources and support groups. **QSEN: Teamwork and Collaboration**

Physiological Integrity

- Perform a thorough family history because some hearing problems have a genetic component. **QSEN: Evidence-Based Practice**

- Ask the patient about current and past drug use (prescribed, over-the-counter) and evaluate for the possibility of ototoxicity. **QSEN: Safety**
- Avoid ear canal irrigation if the eardrum is perforated or if the canal contains vegetable matter. **QSEN: Safety**
- Stress the importance of completing an antibiotic regimen for an ear *infection*. **QSEN: Evidence-Based Practice**
- Remind patients having ear surgery that hearing in the affected ear may be reduced because of packing, swelling, or surgical manipulation. **QSEN: Patient-Centered Care**

▌ MASTERY QUESTIONS

1. Which communication method is appropriate when the nurse is interacting with a client who is deaf?
   A. Use pictures and writing
   B. Speak with enunciated words
   C. Ask client to read the nurse's lips
   D. Dialogue with the client's caregivers
2. When teaching a community group of older adults, what information will the nurse include regarding normal hearing changes associated with aging? **Select all that apply.**
   A. Hair in the ear thins and falls out
   B. Hearing acuity changes in all older adults
   C. Cerumen dries and becomes impacted more easily
   D. The ability to hear low-frequency pitches diminishes first
   E. Sounds such as *f, s, sh,* and *pa* may be more difficult to discern

3. What teaching will the nurse provide to a client who has just been fitted for new hearing aids?
   A. Turn off the hearing aid when not using it.
   B. Immerse the ear mold in alcohol to fully clean it.
   C. Store the hearing aid in a warm, humid bathroom when not in use.
   D. Avoid using hair spray, makeup, and personal care products around the device.

REFERENCES

American Tinnitus Association. (2019). Causes. https://www.ata.org/understanding-facts/causes.

Curhan, S. G., Wang, M., Eavey, R. D., Stampfer, M. J., & Curhan, G. C. (2018). Adherence to healthful dietary patterns is associated with lower risk of hearing loss in women. *Journal of Nutrition, 143*(6), 944–951.

Elliott, B. (2019). Tinnitus and hearing impairment in the veteran population. *MedSurg Matters!, 38*(3), 8–10.

Envoy Medical. (2020). *Esteem.* http://esteemhearing.com/.

Goguen, L. (2019). External otitis: Treatment. In D. Deschler, & M. Edwards (Eds.), *UpToDate.* Waltham, MA.

Henry, J. A., Griest, S., Zaugg, T. L., Thielman, E., Kaelin, C., Galvez, G., et al. (2015). Tinnitus and hearing survey: A screening tool to differentiate bothersome tinnitus from hearing difficulties. *American Journal of Audiology, 24,* 66–77.

Jarvis, C. (2020). *Physical examination & health assessment* (8th ed.). St. Louis: Saunders.

Kesser, B. (2019). *External otitis (acute). Merck manual: Professional version.* Retrieved from https://www.merckmanuals.com/professional/ear,-nose,-and-throat-disorders/external-ear-disorders/external-otitis-acute.

Lustig, L., et al. (2018). Chronic otitis media, cholesteatoma, and mastoiditis in adults. In D. Descher (Ed.), *UpToDate.* Waltham, MA.

McCance, K., Huether, S., Brashers, V., & Rote, N. (2019). *Pathophysiology: The biologic basis for disease in adults and children* (8th ed.). St. Louis: Mosby.

Moskowitz, H., & Dinces, E. (2020). Meniere disease: Evaluation, diagnosis and management. In D. Deschler (Ed.), *UpToDate.* Waltham, MA.

National Association of the Deaf. (2020). *Hospitals and other health care facilities.* Retrieved from https://www.nad.org/resources/health-care-and-mental-health-services/health-care-providers/hospitals-and-other-health-care-facilities/.

National Institute Deafness and Other Communication Disorders (NIDCD). (2016). *Quick statistics about hearing.* http://www.nidcd.nih.gov/health/statistics/Pages/quick.aspx.

National Institute Deafness and Other Communication Disorders (NIDCD). (2017). *Meniere's disease.* Retrieved from https://www.nidcd.nih.gov/health/menieres-disease.

Online Mendelian Inheritance in Man (OMIM). (2020). *Gap junction proteins, beta-2.* GJB2. www.omim.org/entry/121011.

Park, J., et al. (2020). Vestibular schwannoma (acoustic neuroma). In Loeffler, J., & Wen, P. (Eds.). *UpToDate.* Waltham, MA.

Pullen, R. (2017). Navigating the challenges of Ménière disease. *Nursing 2017, 38*–45.

Touhy, T., & Jett, K. (2018). *Ebersole and Hess' gerontological nursing healthy aging* (5th ed.). St. Louis: Mosby.

U.S. Department of Veterans Affairs. (2018). *Veterans benefits administration annual benefits report: Fiscal year 2018.* Retrieved from https://www.benefits.va.gov/reports/abr.

Wu, V., et al. (2019). Approach to Ménière disease management. *Canadian Family Physician, 65*(7), 463–467.

Assessment of the Musculoskeletal System

Donna D. Ignatavicius

http://evolve.elsevier.com/Iggy/

LEARNING OUTCOMES

1. Identify evidence-based health promotion activities to help prevent musculoskeletal health problems or trauma.
2. Apply knowledge of common physiologic changes associated with aging to accurately interpret musculoskeletal assessment findings and plan interventions to ensure patient safety.
3. Identify potential patient reactions to musculoskeletal health problems or injuries.
4. Apply knowledge of anatomy and physiology for a focused musculoskeletal assessment to assess patients for *mobility, pain*, and *sensory perception.*
5. Use clinical judgment to interpret assessment findings in a patient with a musculoskeletal health problem.
6. Plan patient-centered health teaching for preparation and follow-up care for selected musculoskeletal diagnostic testing.

KEY TERMS

arthralgias Joint aches and discomfort.

arthritis Joint inflammation.

arthrogram An x-ray study of a joint after contrast medium (air or solution) has been injected to enhance its visualization.

arthroscopy A diagnostic or surgical procedure in which a fiberoptic tube is inserted into a joint for direct visualization of the ligaments, menisci, and articular surfaces of the joint.

bone scan A radionuclide test in which radioactive material is injected for viewing the entire skeleton.

bursitis Inflammation of bursae, which are small sacs lined with synovial membrane located at joints and bony prominences to prevent friction between bone and structures next to bone.

dermatomyositis Polymyositis which occurs with a purplish skin rash.

effusion Fluid accumulation, such as in a joint.

fascia Dense fibrous tissue that surrounds skeletal muscle, which contains the muscle's blood, lymph, and nerve supply.

goniometer A tool that may be used by rehabilitation therapists or nurses to provide an exact measurement of joint flexion and extension or joint range of motion.

gout A genetically linked arthritis caused by an inborn error of purine metabolism.

kyphosis Outward curvature of the thoracic spine causing a "humped back."

lordosis An inward abnormal curvature of the lumbar spine.

muscle atrophy Skeletal muscle deterioration that results when muscles are not regularly exercised and they deteriorate from disuse.

muscular dystrophy A group of genetically linked diseases that cause chronic skeletal muscle weakness and organ dysfunction due to smooth muscle involvement.

myopathy A problem in muscle tissue often resulting in weakness.

neuropathy A problem in nerve tissue often resulting in weakness and decreased *sensory perception.*

neurovascular assessment (also called a *circ check*) An assessment that includes palpation of pulses in the extremities below the level of injury and assessment of sensation, movement, color, temperature, and pain in the injured part.

osteoblasts Bone-forming cells.

osteoclasts Bone-destroying cells.

osteomalacia Softening of bone in adults due to inadequate vitamin D.

osteopenia Decreased bone density (bone loss) that occurs as one ages.

osteoporosis A chronic disease of *cellular regulation* in which bone loss causes significant decreased density and possible fracture.

Paget disease A chronic metabolic disorder that causes bone to become fragile and misshapen.

polymyositis An uncommon chronic rheumatic disease that is characterized by inflammation of multiple muscles.

scoliosis An abnormal lateral curvature of the spine.

synovial joints Body joints that are lined with synovium, a membrane that secretes synovial fluid for lubrication and shock absorption.

✳ PRIORITY AND INTERRELATED CONCEPTS

The priority concepts for this chapter are:
- *Mobility*
- *Pain*

The interrelated concept for this chapter is:
- *Sensory Perception*

The musculoskeletal system is the second largest body system. It includes the bones, joints, and skeletal muscles, as well as the supporting structures needed to move them. *Mobility* is a basic human need that is essential for performing ADLs. When a patient cannot move to perform ADLs or other daily routines, self-esteem and a sense of self-worth can be diminished. Chapter 3 reviews this concept.

Disease, surgery, and trauma can affect one or more parts of the musculoskeletal system, often leading to decreased mobility. When *mobility* is impaired for a long time, other body systems are affected. For example, prolonged immobility can lead to skin breakdown, constipation, and venous thromboembolism. If nerves are damaged by trauma or disease, patients may also have both impaired *sensory perception* and *pain* (see Chapter 3 for a review of these health concepts).

ANATOMY AND PHYSIOLOGY REVIEW

Skeletal System

The skeletal system consists of 206 bones and multiple joints. The growth and development of these structures occur during childhood and adolescence and are not discussed in this text. Common physical skeletal differences among selected racial/ethnic groups are listed in Table 44.1.

Bones

Types and Structure. Bone can be classified in two ways: by *shape* and by structure. For example, *long bones,* such as the femur, are cylindric with rounded ends and often bear weight. *Short bones,* such as the phalanges, are small and bear little or no weight.

The second way bone is classified is by *structure* or composition. As shown in Fig. 44.1, the outer layer of bone, or cortex, is composed of dense, compact bone tissue. The inner layer, in the medulla, contains spongy, cancellous tissue. Almost every bone has both tissue types but in varying quantities.

The structural unit of the cortical compact bone is the haversian system, which is detailed in Fig. 44.1. The haversian

TABLE 44.1 Musculoskeletal Differences in Selected Ethnic Groups	
Group	**Musculoskeletal Differences**
African Americans	Greater bone density than Europeans, Asians, and Hispanics
	Accounts for decreased incidence of osteoporosis
Amish	Greater incidence of dwarfism than in other populations
Chinese Americans	Bones shorter and smaller with less bone density
	Increased incidence of osteoporosis
Egyptian Americans	Shorter in stature than Euro-Americans and African Americans
Filipino/Vietnamese	Short in stature; adult height about 5 feet
Irish Americans	Taller and broader than other Euro-Americans
	Less bone density than African Americans
Navajo American Indians	Taller and thinner than other American Indians

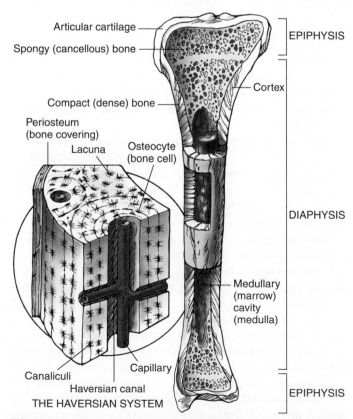

FIG. 44.1 Structure of a typical long bone. The cortex, or outer layer, is composed of dense, compact tissue. The microscopic structure of this compact cortical tissue is the haversian system.

system is a complex canal network containing microscopic blood vessels that supply nutrients and oxygen to bone and lacunae, which are small cavities that house osteocytes (bone cells). The canals run vertically within the hard cortical bone tissue.

The softer cancellous tissue contains large spaces, or trabeculae, which are filled with red and yellow marrow. Hematopoiesis (production of blood cells) occurs in the red marrow. The yellow marrow contains fat cells, which can be dislodged and enter the bloodstream to cause *fat embolism syndrome (FES)*, a life-threatening complication. Volkmann canals connect bone marrow vessels with the haversian system and periosteum, the outermost covering of the bone. In the deepest layer of the periosteum are osteogenic cells, which later differentiate into osteoblasts (bone-forming cells) and osteoclasts (bone-destroying cells) (McCance et al., 2019).

Bone is a very vascular tissue. Each bone has a main nutrient artery, which enters near the middle of the shaft and branches into ascending and descending vessels. These vessels supply the cortex, the marrow, and the haversian system. Very few nerve fibers are connected to bone. Sympathetic nerve fibers control dilation of blood vessels. Sensory nerve fibers transmit pain signals experienced by patients who have primary lesions of the bone, such as bone tumors.

Function. The skeletal system:

- Provides a framework for the body and allows the body to be weight bearing, or upright
- Supports the surrounding tissues (e.g., muscle and tendons)
- Assists in movement through muscle attachment and joint formation
- Protects vital organs, such as the heart and lungs
- Manufactures blood cells in red bone marrow
- Provides storage for mineral salts (e.g., calcium and phosphorus)

After puberty, bone reaches its maturity and maximum growth. Bone is a dynamic tissue. It undergoes a continuous process of formation and resorption, or destruction, at equal rates until the age of 35 years. In later years, bone resorption increases, decreasing bone mass and predisposing patients to injury, especially older women.

Bone accounts for about 99% of the *calcium* in the body and 90% of the *phosphorus*. In healthy adults, the serum concentrations of calcium and phosphorus maintain an inverse relationship. As calcium levels rise, phosphorus levels decrease. When serum levels are altered, calcitonin and parathyroid hormone (PTH) work to maintain equilibrium. If the calcium in the blood is decreased, the bone, which stores calcium, releases calcium into the bloodstream in response to PTH stimulation. Chapter 13 describes these electrolytes in more detail.

Calcitonin is produced by the thyroid gland and *decreases* the serum calcium concentration if it is increased above its normal level. Calcitonin inhibits bone resorption and increases renal excretion of calcium and phosphorus as needed to maintain balance in the body.

Vitamin D and its metabolites are produced in the body and transported in the blood to promote the absorption of calcium and phosphorus from the small intestine. They also seem to enhance PTH activity to release calcium from the bone. A decrease in the body's vitamin D level can result in osteomalacia (softening of bone) in the adult.

When serum calcium levels are lowered, *parathyroid hormone* (PTH, or parathormone) secretion increases and stimulates bone to promote osteoclastic activity and *release* calcium to the blood. PTH reduces the renal excretion of calcium and facilitates its absorption from the intestine. If serum calcium levels increase, PTH secretion diminishes to preserve the bone calcium supply. This process is an example of the feedback loop system of the endocrine system.

Growth hormone secreted by the anterior lobe of the pituitary gland is responsible for increasing bone length and determining the amount of bone matrix formed before puberty. During childhood, an increased secretion results in gigantism, and a decreased secretion results in dwarfism. In the adult, an increase causes acromegaly, which is characterized by bone and soft-tissue deformities.

Adrenal glucocorticoids regulate protein metabolism, either increasing or decreasing catabolism to reduce or intensify the organic matrix of bone. They also aid in regulating intestinal calcium and phosphorus absorption.

Estrogens stimulate osteoblastic activity and inhibit PTH. When estrogen levels decline at menopause, women are susceptible to low serum calcium levels with increased bone loss (osteoporosis). *Androgens,* such as testosterone in men, promote anabolism (body tissue building) and increase bone mass.

Thyroxine (T_4) is one of the principal hormones secreted by the thyroid gland. Its primary function is to increase the rate of protein synthesis in all types of tissue, including bone. *Insulin* works together with growth hormone to build and maintain healthy bone tissue. More information about these hormones can be found in the endocrine health problem chapters of this text.

Joints. A *joint* is a space in which two or more bones come together. This is also referred to as articulation of the joint. The major function of a joint is to provide movement and flexibility in the body.

There are three types of joints in the body:

- Synarthrodial, or completely immovable, joints (e.g., in the cranium)
- Amphiarthrodial, or slightly movable, joints (e.g., in the pelvis)
- Diarthrodial (synovial), or freely movable, joints (e.g., the elbow and knee)

Although any of these joints can be affected by disease or injury, the synovial joints are most commonly involved, as discussed in Chapter 46. The diarthrodial, or synovial, joint is

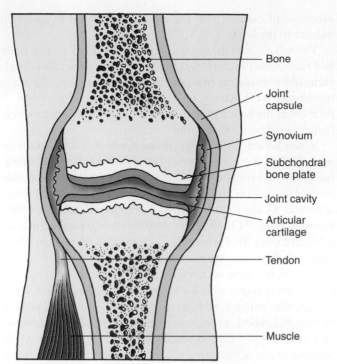

Bone

Joint capsule

Synovium

Subchondral bone plate

Joint cavity

Articular cartilage

Tendon

Muscle

FIG. 44.2 Structure of a synovial joint. Synovium lines the joint capsule but does not extend into the articular cartilage.

the most common type of joint in the body. **Synovial joints** are the only type lined with synovium, a membrane that secretes synovial fluid for lubrication and shock absorption. As shown in Fig. 44.2, the synovium lines the internal portion of the joint capsule but does not normally extend onto the surface of the cartilage at the spongy bone ends. Articular cartilage consists of a collagen fiber matrix impregnated with a complex ground substance. Patients with **arthritis** (joint inflammation) often have synovitis (synovial inflammation) and breakdown of the cartilage. Bursae, small sacs lined with synovial membrane, are located at joints and bony prominences to prevent friction between bone and structures next to bone. These structures can also become inflamed, causing painful **bursitis.**

Synovial joints are described by their anatomic structures. For example, *ball-and-socket* joints (shoulder, hip) permit movement in any direction. *Hinge* joints (elbow) allow motion in one plane—flexion and extension. The knee is often classified as a hinge joint, but it rotates slightly, as well as flexes and extends. It is best described as a *condylar* type of synovial joint.

Muscular System

There are three types of muscle in the body: smooth muscle, cardiac muscle, and skeletal muscle. Smooth, or non-striated, involuntary muscle is responsible for contractions of organs and blood vessels and is controlled by the autonomic nervous system. Cardiac or striated involuntary muscle is also controlled by the autonomic nervous system. The smooth and cardiac muscles are discussed in the

assessment chapters, along with the body systems to which they belong.

In contrast to smooth and cardiac muscle, skeletal muscle is striated voluntary muscle controlled by the central and peripheral nervous systems. The junction of a peripheral motor nerve and the muscle cells that it supplies is sometimes referred to as a *motor end plate.* Muscle fibers are held in place by connective tissue in bundles, or fasciculi. The entire muscle is surrounded by dense fibrous tissue, or **fascia,** which contains the muscle's blood, lymph, and nerve supply.

The main function of skeletal muscle is *movement* of the body and its parts. When bones, joints, and supporting structures are adversely affected by injury or disease, the adjacent muscle tissue is often involved, limiting **mobility.** During the aging process, muscle fibers decrease in size and number, even in well-conditioned adults. **Muscle atrophy** results when muscles are not regularly exercised, and they deteriorate from disuse.

Supporting structures for the muscular system are very susceptible to injury. They include tendons (bands of tough, fibrous tissue that attach muscles to bones) and ligaments, which attach bones to other bones at joints.

Musculoskeletal Changes Associated With Aging

Osteopenia, or decreased bone density (bone loss), occurs as one ages. Many older adults, especially white, thin women, have *severe* osteopenia, a disease called **osteoporosis.** This condition can cause **kyphosis** (outward curvature of the thoracic spine causing a "humped back") and gait changes, which predispose the person to fractures (Jarvis, 2020). Chapter 45 discusses this health problem in detail.

Synovial joint cartilage can become less elastic and compressible as a person ages. As a result of these cartilage changes and continued use of joints, the joint cartilage becomes damaged, leading to osteoarthritis (OA). Genetic defects in cartilage may also contribute to joint disease. The most common joints affected are the weight-bearing joints of the hip, knee, and cervical and lumbar spine, but joints in the shoulder and upper extremity, feet, and hands also can be affected. Refer to Chapter 46 for a complete discussion of OA.

As one ages, muscle tissue atrophies. Increased activity and exercise can slow the progression of atrophy and restore muscle strength. Musculoskeletal changes cause decreased coordination, loss of muscle strength, gait changes, and a risk for falls with injury. (See Chapter 4 for discussion on fall prevention.) The Patient-Centered Care: Older Adult Considerations: Changes in the Musculoskeletal System Related to Aging box lists the major anatomic and physiologic changes and related nursing interventions to ensure patient safety.

Health Promotion and Maintenance

Many health problems of the musculoskeletal system can be prevented through health promotion strategies and avoidance

PATIENT-CENTERED CARE: OLDER ADULT CONSIDERATIONS (QSEN)

Changes in the Musculoskeletal System Related to Aging

Physiologic Change	Nursing Interventions	Rationales
Decreased bone density	Teach safety tips to prevent falls (see Chapter 4).	Porous bones are more likely to fracture.
	Reinforce need to exercise, especially weight-bearing exercise.	Exercise slows bone loss.
Increased bone prominence	Prevent pressure on bone prominences.	There is less soft tissue to prevent skin breakdown.
Kyphosis and widened gait, shift in the center of gravity, which could cause imbalance and falls	Teach proper body mechanics; instruct the patient to sit in supportive chairs with arms. Assess need for ambulatory device, such as cane or walker; ensure use of supportive shoes.	Correction of posture problems prevents further deformity; the patient should have support to ensure improved balance.
Cartilage degeneration (osteoarthritis [OA]) (see Chapter 46)	Provide moist heat, such as a shower or warm, moist compresses or heating pad.	Moist heat increases blood flow to the area and promotes *mobility*.
Decreased range of motion (ROM)	Assess the patient's ability to perform ADLs and *mobility*.	The patient may need assistance with ADLs and ambulation.
Muscle atrophy, decreased strength	Teach isometric and isotonic exercises.	Exercises increase muscle strength.
Slowed movement	Do not rush the person; be patient.	The patient may become frustrated if hurried or sustain a fall.

of risky lifestyle behaviors. For example, women can slow the process of bone loss by taking vitamin D and calcium supplements and increasing these nutrients in their diet. Weight-bearing activities, such as walking and strengthening exercises, can reduce risk factors for osteoporosis and maintain muscle strength (McCance et al., 2019).

Accidents, illnesses, lifestyle, and substance abuse can contribute to the occurrence of musculoskeletal injury. Young men are at the greatest risk for trauma related to motor vehicle or scooter crashes. Older adults are at the greatest risk for falls that result in fractures and soft-tissue injury. High-impact sports, such as excessive jogging or running, can cause musculoskeletal injury to soft tissues and bone.

Tobacco smoking also has negative effects on the musculoskeletal system (see the Evidence-Based Practice box). The nicotine in tobacco is the primary cause of these effects (Smith & Jackson, 2018).

EVIDENCE-BASED PRACTICE (QSEN)

What Is the Effect of Smoking on Musculoskeletal Health?

AL-Bashaireh, A.M., Haddad, L.G., Weaver, M., Kelly, D.L., Chengguo, X., & Yoon, S. (2018). The effect of tobacco smoking on musculoskeletal health: A systematic review. *Journal of Environmental and Public Health*, July 11. Doi:10.1155/2018/4184190.

The authors conducted a systematic study to determine the effect of tobacco smoking on the health of the musculoskeletal system. After a thorough review of the literature, 243 research articles were selected for inclusion and used for data abstraction. Findings of the systematic review include that the nicotine in cigarettes is associated with negative musculoskeletal effects, including:
- Decreased bone mineral density, which could lead to fractures
- Decreased immunity, which could delay fracture healing
- Muscle atrophy
- Deterioration in joint cartilage, especially in the knees

Level of Evidence: 1
The research was a systematic review of the literature that included multiple studies to determine the negative effects of tobacco smoking on musculoskeletal health.

Commentary: Implications for Practice and Research
This research provides evidence that not only does smoking cause cardiovascular and pulmonary health problems, but cigarette nicotine has negative effects on the musculoskeletal and immune systems. Nurses need to provide information on smoking cessation to help patients quit and improve health.

Excessive alcohol intake can decrease vitamins and nutrients that the person needs for bone and muscle tissue growth. Develop a patient-centered health promotion plan for each patient to help promote bone health and prevent musculoskeletal injury. Additional health promotion strategies can be found in other chapters of this unit related to specific health problems of the musculoskeletal system.

NCLEX EXAMINATION CHALLENGE 44.1

Health Promotion and Maintenance

A nurse is performing a musculoskeletal assessment on an older adult. What normal physiologic changes of aging does the nurse expect? **Select all that apply.**
A. Muscle atrophy
B. Slowed movement
C. Kyphosis
D. Arthritis
E. Widened gait
F. Decreased joint range of motion

ASSESSMENT: RECOGNIZE CUES

Patient History

In the assessment of a patient with an actual or potential musculoskeletal problem, a detailed and accurate history is helpful in identifying priority problems and nursing interventions. The history reveals information about the patient that can direct the physical assessment.

When taking a personal health history, question the patient about any traumatic injuries and sports activities, no matter when they occurred. An injury to the lumbar spine 30 years ago may have caused a patient's current low back pain. A motor vehicle crash or sports injury can cause osteoarthritis years after the event. Ask the patient if he or she is following a pain management plan, including the use of opioids or other substances such as cannabis (marijuana).

Previous or current illness or disease may affect musculoskeletal status. For example, a patient with diabetes who is treated for a foot ulcer is at high risk for acute or chronic osteomyelitis (bone infection). In addition, diabetes slows the healing process. Ask the patient about any previous hospitalizations and illnesses or complications. Inquire about his or her ability to perform ADLs independently or if assistive-adaptive devices are used.

Current lifestyle also contributes to musculoskeletal health. When assessing a patient with a possible musculoskeletal alteration, inquire about occupation or work life. A person's occupation can cause or contribute to an injury. For instance, fractures are not uncommon in patients whose jobs require manual labor, such as housekeepers, mechanics, and industrial workers. Certain occupations, such as computer-related jobs, may predispose a person to carpal tunnel syndrome (entrapment of the median nerve in the wrist) or neck pain.

Ask about allergies, particularly allergy to dairy products, and previous and current use of drugs (prescribed, over-the-counter, and illicit). Allergy to dairy products could cause decreased calcium intake. Some drugs, such as steroids, can negatively affect calcium metabolism and promote bone loss. Other drugs may be taken to relieve musculoskeletal pain. Inquire about herbs, vitamin and mineral supplements, or biologic compounds that may be used for arthritis and other musculoskeletal problems, such as glucosamine and chondroitin. These integrative therapies are commonly used by patients with various types of arthritis and **arthralgias** (joint aches and discomfort).

Nutrition History. A brief review of the patient's nutrition history helps determine any risks for inadequate nutrient intake. For example, most people, especially women, do not get enough calcium in their diet. Determine if the patient has had a significant weight gain or loss and whether the weight change was expected.

Ask the patient to recall a typical day of food intake to help identify deficiencies and excesses in the diet. Lactose intolerance is a common problem that can cause inadequate calcium intake. People who cannot afford to buy food are especially at risk for undernutrition. Some older adults and others are not financially able to buy the proper foods for adequate nutrition.

Inadequate protein or insufficient vitamin C or D in the diet slows bone and tissue healing. Obesity places excess stress and strain on bones and joints, with resulting trauma to joint cartilage. In addition, obesity inhibits *mobility* in patients with musculoskeletal problems, which predisposes them to complications such as respiratory and circulatory problems. People with eating disorders such as anorexia nervosa and bulimia nervosa are also at risk for osteoporosis related to decreased intake of calcium and vitamin D.

Family History and Genetic Risk. Obtaining a family history helps to identify disorders that have a familial or genetic tendency. For example, **osteoporosis** and **gout** (a genetically linked arthritis caused by an inborn error of purine metabolism) often occur in several generations of a family. Positive family history of these types of disorders can increase risks to the patient. Chapters 45 and 46 provide a more complete description of musculoskeletal problems that have strong genetic links.

Current Health Problems. The most common reports of people with a musculoskeletal problem are *pain* and/or weakness, either of which can impair *mobility*. Collect data pertinent to the patient's presenting health problem:

- Date and time of onset
- Factors that cause or exacerbate (worsen) the problem
- Course of the problem (e.g., intermittent or continuous)
- Signs and symptoms (as expressed by the patient) and the pattern of their occurrence
- Measures that improve signs and symptoms (e.g., heat, ice)

Assessment of pain can present many challenges. *Pain* can be related to bone, muscle, or joint problems. It may be described as acute or chronic, depending on the onset and duration. Pain with movement could indicate a fracture and/or muscle or joint injury. Assess the intensity of pain by using a pain scale and asking the patient to rate the level that he or she is experiencing. Quality of pain may be described as dull, burning, aching, or stabbing. Determine the location of pain and areas to which it radiates. With any assessment, it is always best if the patient describes the pain in his or her own words and points to its location, if possible. Chapter 5 describes acute and persistent pain in detail.

Weakness may be related to individual muscles or muscle groups. Determine if weakness occurs in proximal or distal muscles or muscle groups. Proximal weakness (near trunk of body) may indicate myopathy (a problem in muscle tissue), whereas distal weakness and impaired *sensory perception* (especially in lower extremities) may indicate neuropathy (a problem in nerve tissue). Muscle weakness in the lower extremities may increase the risk for falls and injury. Weakness in the upper extremities may interfere with *mobility* and functional ability.

Assessment of the Skeletal System

Although bones, joints, and muscles are usually assessed during a head-to-toe approach, each subsystem is described separately for emphasis and understanding. For physical assessment of the musculoskeletal system, use inspection, palpation, and range of motion (ROM). A general assessment is described in this chapter. More specific assessment techniques are discussed in the musculoskeletal problem chapters in this unit.

General Inspection. Observe the patient's posture, gait, and general *mobility* for gross deformities and impairment. Note unusual findings and coordinate with the physical or occupational therapist for an in-depth physical assessment.

Posture and Gait. Posture includes the person's body build and alignment when standing and walking. Assess the curvature of the spine and the length, shape, and symmetry of extremities. Fig. 44.3 illustrates several common spinal deformities. Lordosis (an inward abnormal curvature of the lumbar spine) is a common finding in adults who have abdominal obesity. During screening for scoliosis (an abnormal lateral curvature of the spine), ask the patient to flex forward from the hips and

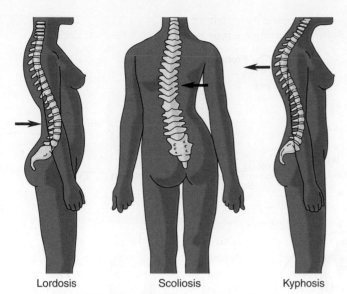

FIG. 44.3 Common spinal deformities.

Lordosis   Scoliosis   Kyphosis

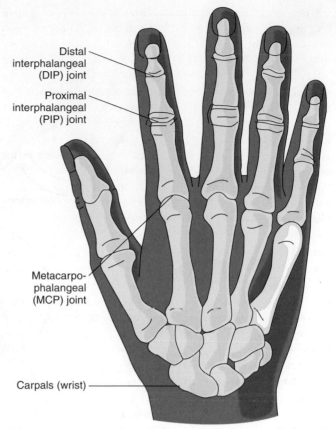

FIG. 44.4 Small joints of the hand.

inspect for the classic lateral curve in the spine. Inspect muscle mass for size and symmetry (Jarvis, 2020).

Most patients with musculoskeletal problems eventually have a problem with *gait.* The nurse or therapist evaluates the patient's balance, steadiness, and ease and length of stride. Any limp or other asymmetric leg movement or deformity is noted.

If the extremities are affected by a musculoskeletal problem, assess arms or legs at the same time for side-to-side comparisons. For example, inspect and palpate both shoulders for size, swelling, deformity, poor alignment, tenderness or pain, and **mobility.** A shoulder injury may prevent the patient from combing his or her hair with the affected arm, but severe arthritis may inhibit movement in both arms. Assess the elbows and wrists in a similar way.

Because the hand has multiple joints in a single digit, assessment of hand function is perhaps the most critical part of the examination. If the hands are affected, inspect and palpate the metacarpophalangeal (MCP), proximal interphalangeal (PIP), and distal interphalangeal (DIP) joints (Fig. 44.4). The same digits are compared on the right and left hands. Determine the range of motion (ROM) for each joint by observing active movement. If movement is not possible, evaluate passive motion. For a quick and easy assessment of ROM, ask the patient to make a fist and then appose each finger to the thumb. If he or she can perform these maneuvers, ROM of the hand is not seriously restricted.

Mobility and Functional Assessment. In collaboration with the physical or occupational therapist, assess the patient's need for ambulatory devices, such as canes and walkers, during transfer from bed to chair and while walking and climbing stairs. Observe his or her ability to perform ADLs, such as dressing and bathing. *Pain,* deformity, and/or impaired **sensory perception** may limit physical **mobility** and function. Coordinate with the physical and occupational therapists to assess the patient's functional status. A discussion of functional assessment is found in Chapter 7.

Assess major bones, joints, and muscles by inspection, palpation, and determination of ROM. Pay special attention to areas that are affected or may be affected, according to the patient's history or current problem.

A **goniometer** is a tool that may be used by rehabilitation therapists or nurses to provide an exact measurement of flexion and extension or joint ROM. Active range of motion (AROM) can be evaluated by asking the patient to move each joint through the ROM himself or herself. If the patient cannot actively move a joint through ROM, ask him or her to relax the muscles in the extremity. Hold the part with one hand above and one hand below the joint to be evaluated and allow passive range of motion (PROM) to evaluate joint **mobility.** Movements shown in Fig. 44.5 may be used to evaluate AROM and PROM. Circumduction is a movement that can also be evaluated in the shoulder by having the patient move the arm in circles from the shoulder joint. As long as the patient can function to meet personal needs, a limitation in ROM may not be significant. For each anatomic location, observe the skin for color, elasticity, and lesions that may relate to musculoskeletal dysfunction. For instance, redness or warmth may indicate an inflammatory process and/or pressure injury to skin.

Evaluation of the hip joint relies primarily on determination of its degree of mobility because the joint is deep and difficult to inspect or palpate. *The patient with hip joint pain usually experiences it in the groin or has pain that radiates to the knee or lower back.* The knee is readily accessible for physical assessment, particularly when the patient is sitting and the knee is flexed. Fluid accumulation, or **effusion,** is easily detected in the knee joint. Limitations in movement with accompanying pain are common findings. The knees may be poorly aligned, as in genu valgum ("knock-knee") or genu varum ("bowlegged") deformities (Jarvis, 2020).

The ankles and feet are often neglected in the physical examination. However, they contain multiple bones and joints that can

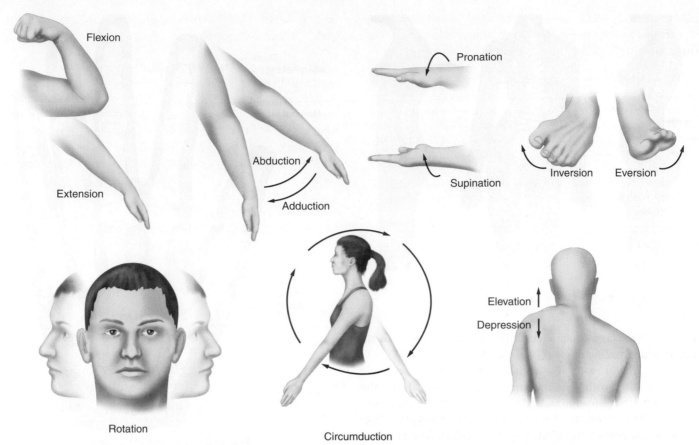

FIG. 44.5 Movements of the skeletal muscles.

be affected by disease and injury. Observe and palpate each joint and test for ROM if feet are affected by musculoskeletal problems.

Neurovascular Assessment. While completing a physical assessment of the musculoskeletal system, perform an assessment of peripheral vascular and nerve integrity. Beginning with the injured side, always compare one extremity with the other.

> ⚠ **NURSING SAFETY PRIORITY** (QSEN)
> ### Action Alert
> Perform a complete neurovascular assessment (also called a *circ check*), which includes palpation of pulses in the extremities below the level of injury and assessment of sensation, movement, color, temperature, and pain in the injured part. If pulses are not palpable, use a Doppler to find pulses in the extremities.

Assessment of the Muscular System

During the skeletal assessment, note the size, shape, tone, and strength of major skeletal muscles. The circumference of each muscle may be measured and compared for symmetry for an estimation of muscle mass if abnormalities are observed.

Ask the patient to demonstrate muscle strength. Apply resistance by holding the extremity and asking the patient to move against resistance. As an option, place your hands on the patient's upper arms and ask him or her to try to raise the arms. Although movement against resistance is not easily quantified, several scales used by nurses and therapists are available for

TABLE 44.2 **Common Scale for Grading Muscle Strength**	
Rating	**Description**
5	Normal: ROM unimpaired against gravity with full resistance
4	Good: can complete ROM against gravity with some resistance
3	Fair: can complete ROM against gravity
2	Poor: can complete ROM with gravity eliminated
1	Trace: no joint motion and slight evidence of muscle contractility
0	Zero: no evidence of muscle contractility

ROM, Range of motion.

grading the patient's strength. A commonly used scale is shown in Table 44.2.

Psychosocial Assessment

The data from the history and physical assessment provide clues for anticipating psychosocial problems. For instance, prolonged absence from employment or permanent disability may cause job or career loss. Further stress may be experienced if chronic pain continues and the patient cannot cope with numerous stressors. Anxiety and depression are common when patients have chronic pain. Deformities resulting from musculoskeletal disease or injury, such as an amputation, can affect a person's body image and self-concept. Help the patient identify support systems and coping mechanisms that may be useful if he or she has long-term musculoskeletal health problems. Encourage him or her to verbalize feelings related to loss and body image changes. Refer the patient and family for psychological or spiritual counseling if needed and if it is culturally appropriate.

Diagnostic Assessment

Laboratory Assessment. The common laboratory tests used in assessing patients with musculoskeletal disorders are outlined in the Laboratory Profile: Musculoskeletal Assessment box (Pagana & Pagana, 2018; Pagana et al., 2019). There is no special patient preparation or follow-up care for any of these tests. Teach the patient about the purpose of the test and the procedure that can be expected. Additional tests performed for patients with connective tissue diseases, such as rheumatoid arthritis, are described in Chapter 46.

Disorders of bone and the parathyroid gland are often reflected in an alteration of the serum calcium or phosphorus level. Therefore these electrolytes, especially calcium, are monitored. A decrease in serum calcium could indicate bone density loss.

Alkaline phosphatase (ALP) is an enzyme normally present in blood. The concentration of ALP increases with bone or liver damage. In metabolic bone disease and bone cancer, the enzyme concentration rises in proportion to the osteoblastic activity, which indicates bone formation. The level of ALP is normally slightly increased in older adults (Pagana & Pagana, 2018).

The major *muscle enzymes* affected in skeletal muscle disease or injuries are:
- Creatine kinase (CK-MM)
- Lactate dehydrogenase (LDH)
- Aspartate aminotransferase (AST)
- Aldolase (ALD)

⚑ LABORATORY PROFILE

Musculoskeletal Assessment

Test	Normal Range for Adults	Significance of Abnormal Findings
Serum calcium	9.0-10.5 mg/dL (2.10-2.50 mmol/L) *Older adults:* decreased	*Hypercalcemia* (increased calcium) • Metastatic cancers of the bone • Paget disease • Bone fractures in healing stage *Hypocalcemia* (decreased calcium) • **Osteoporosis** • **Osteomalacia**
Serum phosphorus (phosphate)	3.0-4.5 mg/dL (0.97-1.45 mmol/L) *Older adults:* decreased	*Hyperphosphatemia* (increased phosphorus) • Bone fractures in healing stage • Bone tumors *Hypophosphatemia* (decreased phosphorus) • **Osteomalacia**
Alkaline phosphatase (ALP)	30-120 units/L (40-160 IU/L) *Older adults:* slightly increased	*Elevations* may indicate: • Metastatic cancers of the bone or liver • **Paget's disease** (a chronic metabolic disorder that causes bone to become fragile and misshapen) • **Osteomalacia**
Serum muscle enzymes Creatine kinase (CK-MM)	Total CK: *Men:* 55-170 units/L (20-215 IU/L) *Women:* 30-135 units/L (20-160 IU/L) CK-MM: 96%-100%	*Elevations* may indicate: • Muscle trauma • **Muscular dystrophy** (a group of genetically linked diseases that cause chronic skeletal muscle weakness and organ dysfunction due to smooth muscle involvement) • Effects of electromyography
Lactate dehydrogenase (LDH)	Total LDH: 100-190 units/L (45-90 IU/L) *Older adults:* slightly increased LDH₁: 17%-27% LDH₂: 27%-37% LDH₃: 18%-25% LDH₄: 3%-8% LDH₅: 0%-5%	*Elevations* may indicate: • Skeletal muscle necrosis (cell death) • Extensive cancer • **Muscular dystrophy**
Aspartate aminotransferase (AST)	0-35 units/L 97-40 IU/L *Older adults:* slightly increased	*Elevations* may indicate: • Skeletal muscle trauma • **Muscular dystrophy**
Aldolase (ALD)	3.0-8.2 units/dL (less than 8 U/L)	*Elevations* may indicate: • **Polymyositis** (an uncommon chronic rheumatic disease that is characterized by inflammation of multiple muscles) and **dermatomyositis** (polymyositis which occurs with a purplish skin rash) • **Muscular dystrophy**

As a result of damage, the muscle tissue releases additional amounts of these enzymes, which increases serum levels.

❓ CLINICAL JUDGMENT CHALLENGE 44.1

Patient-Centered Care

A 33-year-old woman visits her primary health care provider with concerns about new-onset muscle weakness in her left arm. She also reports numbness and tingling in both hands and occasional pain in some of her finger joints. Currently she states that her pain is a 3/10 (3 on a 1-10 pain intensity scale). The nurse records this additional assessment.

- Works full-time as the main teller in a bank requiring long hours using the computer and other machines
- Client's mother has a history of osteoarthritis and carpal tunnel syndrome
- Has two small children (ages 1 and 3) who attend day care while the client is at work
- Single mother with little support from family or friends
- Has health insurance through her work
- Has been taking ibuprofen with some relief of pain

1. **Recognize Cues:** What assessment information in this client situation is the most important and immediate concern for the nurse? (Hint: Identify the **relevant** information *first* to determine what is most important.)
2. **Analyze Cues:** What client conditions are consistent with the **most relevant** information? (Hint: Think about priority collaborative problems that support and contradict the information presented in this situation.)

Imaging Assessment. The skeleton is very visible on *standard x-rays.* Anteroposterior and lateral projections are the initial screening views used most often. Other approaches, such as oblique or stress views, depend on the part of the skeleton to be evaluated and the reason for the x-ray.

Radiography. Bone density, alignment, swelling, and intactness can be seen on x-ray. The conditions of joints can be determined, including the size of the joint space, the smoothness of articular cartilage, and synovial swelling. Soft-tissue involvement may be evident but not clearly differentiated.

Inform the patient that the x-ray table is hard and cold, and instruct him or her to remain still during the filming process. Coordinate with the radiology department or clinic to keep older adults and those at risk for hypothermia as warm as possible (e.g., by using blankets).

CT has gained wide acceptance for detecting musculoskeletal problems, particularly those of the vertebral column and joints. The scanned images can be used to create additional images from other angles or to create three-dimensional images and view complex structures from any position. The nurse or radiology technologist should ask the patient about iodine-based contrast allergies.

Nuclear Scans. The bone scan is a radionuclide test in which radioactive material is injected for viewing the entire skeleton. It may be used primarily to detect tumors, arthritis, osteomyelitis (bone infection), osteoporosis, vertebral compression fractures, and unexplained bone *pain.* Bone scans are used less commonly today as more sophisticated MRI equipment becomes more available. However, it may be very useful for detecting hairline fractures in patients with unexplained bone pain and diffuse metastatic bone disease. Gallium citrate (^{67}Ga) is the radioisotope most commonly used. This substance also migrates to the brain, liver, and breast tissue and therefore is used in examination of these structures when disease is suspected.

For patients with osteosarcoma (type of primary bone cancer), thallium (^{201}Tl) is better than gallium or technetium for diagnosing the extent of the disease. Thallium has traditionally been used for the diagnosis of myocardial infarctions but can be used for additional evaluation of cancers of the bone.

Because bone takes up gallium slowly, the nuclear medicine physician or technician administers the isotope 4 to 6 hours before scanning. Other tests that require contrast media or other isotopes cannot be given during this time.

Instruct the patient that the radioactive material poses no threat because it readily deteriorates in the body. Because gallium is excreted through the intestinal tract, it tends to collect in feces after the scanning procedure.

Depending on the tissue to be examined, the patient is taken to the nuclear medicine department 4 to 6 hours after injection. The procedure takes 30 to 60 minutes, during which time the patient must lie still for accurate test results to be achieved. The scan may be repeated at 24, 48, and/or 72 hours. Mild sedation may be necessary to facilitate relaxation and cooperation during the procedure for confused older adults or those in severe pain.

No special care is required after the test. The radioisotope is excreted in stool and urine, but no precautions are taken in handling the excreta. Remind the patient to push fluids to facilitate urinary excretion.

Magnetic Resonance Imaging. MRI, with or without the use of contrast media, is commonly used to diagnose musculoskeletal disorders. It is more accurate than CT for many spinal and knee problems. MRI is most appropriate for joints, soft tissue, and bony tumors that involve soft tissue. CT is still the test of choice for injuries or pathology that involves only bone.

The image is produced through the interaction of magnetic fields, radio waves, and atomic nuclei showing hydrogen density. Simply put, the radio waves "bounce" off the body tissues being examined. Because each tissue has its own density, the computer image clearly distinguishes normal and abnormal tissues. For some tissues, the cross-sectional image is better than that produced by radiography or CT. The lack of hydrogen ions in cortical bone makes it easily distinguishable from soft tissues. The test is particularly useful in identifying problems with muscles, tendons, and ligaments.

Ensure that the patient removes all metal objects and checks for clothing zippers and metal fasteners. Many large facilities and those focused on sports medicine have orthopedic-type MRI machines that have an open design and are vertically oriented (upright) to make the examination more comfortable. The Best Practice for Patient Safety & Quality Care: Preparing the Patient for Magnetic Resonance Imaging box lists questions that the nurse or technician should consider in preparing the patient for MRI.

Preparing the Patient for Magnetic Resonance Imaging

- Is the patient pregnant?
- Does the patient have ferromagnetic fragments or implants, such as an older-style aneurysm clip?
- Does the patient have a cardiac pacemaker, metal stent, or electronic implant, such as a medication pump?
- Does the patient have chronic kidney disease? (Gadolinium contrast agents may cause severe systemic complications if the kidneys do not function.)
- Can the patient lie still in the supine position for 45 to 60 minutes (unless using an upright or vertically oriented machine)?
- Does the patient need life-support equipment available?
- Can the patient communicate clearly and understand verbal communication?
- Does the patient have a cochlear implant?
- Is the patient claustrophobic? (Ask this question for closed MRI units; open MRI units do not cause claustrophobia.)

MR arthrography combines arthrography and MRI. It is particularly useful for diagnosing problems of the shoulder and the type and degree of rotator cuff tears. The patient's shoulder is injected with gadolinium contrast medium under fluoroscopy. Then the patient is taken for an MRI, where the shoulder is examined.

Ultrasonography. Sound waves produce an image of the tissue in ultrasonography. An ultrasound procedure may be used to view:

- Soft-tissue disorders, such as masses and fluid accumulation
- Traumatic joint injuries
- Osteomyelitis (bone infection)
- Surgical hardware placement

A jelly-like substance applied to the skin over the site to be examined promotes the movement of a metal probe. No special preparation or posttest care is necessary. A quantitative ultrasound (QUS) may be done for determining fractures or bone density. Bone-density testing is discussed in Chapter 46.

Other Diagnostic Assessment

Biopsies. In a bone biopsy, the physician extracts a specimen of the bone tissue for microscopic examination. This invasive test may confirm the presence of infection or neoplasm, but it is not commonly done today. One of two techniques may be used to retrieve the specimen: needle (closed) biopsy or incisional (open) biopsy.

! NURSING SAFETY PRIORITY (QSEN)

Action Alert

After a bone biopsy, watch for bleeding from the puncture site and for tenderness, redness, or warmth that could indicate infection. Mild analgesics may be used.

Muscle biopsy is done for the diagnosis of atrophy (as in muscular dystrophy) and inflammation (as in polymyositis). The procedure and care for patients undergoing muscle biopsy are the same as those for patients undergoing bone biopsy.

Arthroscopy. Arthroscopy may be used as a diagnostic test or a surgical procedure. An arthroscope is a fiberoptic tube inserted

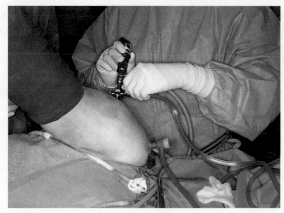

FIG. 44.6 An arthroscope is used in the diagnosis of pathologic changes in the joints. This patient is undergoing arthroscopy of the shoulder.

into a joint for direct visualization of the ligaments, menisci, and articular surfaces of the joint. The knee and shoulder are most commonly evaluated. In addition, synovial biopsy and surgery to repair traumatic injury can be done through the arthroscope as an ambulatory care or same-day surgical procedure.

Patient Preparation. Arthroscopy is performed on an ambulatory care basis or as same-day surgery. The patient must have *mobility* in the joint being examined. Those who cannot move the joint or who have an infected joint are not candidates for the procedure.

If the procedure is done for surgical repair, the patient may have a physical therapy consultation before arthroscopy to learn the exercises that are necessary after the test. ROM exercises are also taught but may not be allowed immediately after arthroscopic surgery. The nurse in the surgeon's office or at the surgical center can teach these exercises or reinforce the information provided by the physical therapist. The nurse also reinforces the explanation of the procedure and posttest care and ensures that the patient has signed an informed consent form.

Procedure. The patient is usually given local, light general, or epidural anesthesia, depending on the purpose of the procedure. As shown in Fig. 44.6, the arthroscope is inserted through a small incision shorter than ¼ inch (0.6 cm). Multiple incisions may be required to allow inspection at a variety of angles. After the procedure, a dressing may be applied, depending on the amount of manipulation during the test or surgery.

Follow-up Care. The immediate care after arthroscopy is the same for patients having the procedure for diagnostic purposes as for those having it for surgical intervention.

! NURSING SAFETY PRIORITY (QSEN)

Action Alert

The priority for postprocedure care after arthroscopy is to assess the neurovascular status of the patient's affected limb every hour or according to agency or surgeon protocol. Monitor and document distal pulses, warmth, color, capillary refill, *pain,* movement, and sensation of the affected extremity.

Encourage the patient to perform exercises as taught before the procedure, if appropriate. For the mild discomfort experienced after the diagnostic arthroscopy, the primary health care provider prescribes a mild analgesic, such as acetaminophen. If postoperative, the patient may have short-term activity restrictions, depending on the musculoskeletal problem. Ice is often used for 24 hours, and the extremity should be elevated for 12 to 24 hours. When arthroscopic surgery is performed, the primary health care provider usually prescribes a short-term opioid-analgesic combination, such as oxycodone and acetaminophen.

Although complications are not common, monitor and teach the patient to observe for:
- Swelling
- Increased joint pain attributable to mechanical injury
- Thrombophlebitis
- Infection

Severe joint or limb pain after discharge may indicate a possible complication. Teach the patient to immediately contact the primary health care provider, who usually sees the patient about 1 week after the procedure to check for complications.

NCLEX EXAMINATION CHALLENGE 44.2
Safe and Effective Care Environment

A client returns to the postanesthesia care unit (PACU) after an arthroscopy to repair a shoulder injury. What is the nurse's **priority** when caring for this client?
A. Keep the affected arm elevated and immobilized.
B. Ensure that the client uses the patient-controlled analgesia (PCA) pump.
C. Check the neurovascular status of the affected arm.
D. Instruct the client to stay in bed for 24 hours.

GET READY FOR THE NEXT-GENERATION NCLEX® EXAMINATION!

Key Points
Review these Key Points for each NCLEX Examination Client Needs Category.

Safe and Effective Care Environment
- Perform a focused musculoskeletal assessment, including gait, muscle strength, *pain,* and *mobility* status as indicated by the patient's signs and symptoms. **Clinical Judgment**

Health Promotion and Maintenance
- Be aware that older adults have physiologic changes that affect their musculoskeletal system, such as decreased bone density and joint cartilage degeneration; plan nursing interventions to ensure patient safety. **QSEN: Patient-Centered Care; Safety**

Psychosocial Integrity
- Recall that potential patient reactions to musculoskeletal trauma or disease can include anxiety, depression, and/or altered body image and self-concept. **QSEN: Patient-Centered Care**

Physiological Integrity
- Perform a thorough *pain* assessment, including pain intensity, quality, duration, and location. **Clinical Judgment**
- Interpret the patient's laboratory values that are related to musculoskeletal disease. **Clinical Judgment**
- Instruct the patient to report swelling, infection, and increased pain after an arthroscopy. **QSEN: Safety**
- Ask the patient questions to ensure safety before an MRI. **QSEN: Safety**
- Ask the patient about allergy to contrast media before diagnostic testing such as CT scans. **QSEN: Safety**
- Evaluate the neurovascular status of the patient's affected extremity after an arthroscopic procedure as the *priority for care.* **QSEN: Safety**

MASTERY QUESTIONS

1. The nurse is preparing to teach a client about how to promote musculoskeletal health. Which statements will the nurse include in the teaching plan? **Select all that apply.**
   A. "If you smoke, you need a smoking cessation plan."
   B. "Avoid drinking excessive alcohol."
   C. "Be sure to take in enough calcium and vitamin D."
   D. "Avoid high-risk activities that could cause an accident."
   E. "Include weight-bearing exercise like walking on a regular basis."

2. Which serum laboratory finding is of concern for the nurse and should be reported to the primary health care provider?
   A. Calcium = 9 mg/dL (2.10 mmol/L)
   B. Phosphorus = 4.5 mg/dL (1.45 mmol/L)
   C. Lactate dehydrogenase = 150 units/L (150 IU/L)
   D. Alkaline phosphatase = 210 units/L (210 IU/L)

REFERENCES

AL-Bashaireh, A. M., Haddad, L. G., Weaver, M., Kelly, D. L., Chengguo, X., & Yoon, S. (2018). The effect of tobacco smoking on musculoskeletal health: A systematic review. *Journal of Environmental and Public Health.* https://doi.org/10.1155/2018/4184190. July 11.

Jarvis, C. (2020). *Physical examination & health assessment* (8th ed.). St. Louis: Elsevier Saunders.

McCance, K., Huether, S., Brashers, V., & Rote, N. (2019). *Pathophysiology: The biologic basis for disease in adults and children* (8th ed.). St. Louis: Mosby.

Pagana, K. D., & Pagana, T. J. (2018). *Mosby's manual of diagnostic and laboratory tests* (6th ed.). St. Louis: Mosby.

Pagana, K. D., Pagana, T. J., & Pike-MacDonald, S. A. (2019). *Mosby's Canadian manual of diagnostic and laboratory tests* (2nd ed.). St. Louis: Mosby.

Smith, M. A., & Jackson, A. (2018). Tobacco use, tobacco cessation, & musculoskeletal health. *Orthopaedic Nursing, 37*(5), 280–284.

45

Concepts of Care for Patients With Musculoskeletal Problems

Donna D. Ignatavicius

http://evolve.elsevier.com/Iggy/

LEARNING OUTCOMES

1. Prioritize collaborative evidence-based care for patients with common musculoskeletal problems affecting mobility, perfusion, and cellular regulation.
2. Identify community resources for patients with common musculoskeletal problems.
3. Teach adults how to decrease the risk for osteoporosis.
4. Assess the psychosocial impact for patients experiencing common musculoskeletal health problems.
5. Apply knowledge of pathophysiology to assess patients with common musculoskeletal problems caused by impaired *cellular regulation* and *infection.*
6. Plan health teaching for the patient and caregiver(s) about common drugs used for common musculoskeletal problems, including those used for *pain* control.

KEY TERMS

bone mineral density (BMD) The amount of mineral in bone that determines bone strength and peaks between 25 and 30 years of age.

bunionectomy Surgical removal of the first metatarsal bony overgrowth and bursa with realignment to manage *Pain.*

dual x-ray absorptiometry (DXA) A noninvasive radiographic scan to assess bone mineral density.

Dupuytren contracture (or deformity) A slowly progressive thickening of the palmar fascia, resulting in flexion contracture of the fourth (ring) and fifth (little) fingers of the hand.

fragility fracture A fracture caused by osteoporosis.

ganglion A round, benign cyst, often found on a wrist or foot joint or tendon.

hallux valgus deformity A common foot problem in which the great toe drifts laterally at the first metatarsophalangeal (MTP) joint.

kyphosis Outward curvature of the thoracic spine causing a "humped back."

osteomalacia Loss of bone related to lack of vitamin D, which causes bone softening.

osteomyelitis *Infection* in bone caused by bacteria (most often), viruses, parasites, or fungi; the infection may be acute or chronic.

osteonecrosis (also known as *avascular necrosis*); bone death secondary to lack of or disruption in blood supply to the affected bone, usually from trauma or chronic steroid therapy.

osteopenia Loss of bone mass.

osteoporosis A chronic disease of *cellular regulation* in which bone loss causes significant decreased density and possible fracture.

plantar fasciitis An inflammation of the plantar fascia, which is located in the area of the arch of the foot, causing pain.

✳ PRIORITY AND INTERRELATED CONCEPTS

The priority concepts for this chapter are:
- *Mobility*
- *Infection*
- *Cellular Regulation*

The *Cellular Regulation* concept exemplar for this chapter is Osteoporosis.

The interrelated concepts for this chapter are:
- *Pain*
- *Perfusion*

Musculoskeletal disorders include diseases of *cellular regulation* (e.g., osteoporosis), bone tumors, bone *infection,* and a variety of deformities and syndromes. Older adults are at the greatest risk for most of these problems, although *primary* bone cancer is most often found in adolescents and young adults.

Almost all musculoskeletal health problems result in decreased *mobility,* acute or persistent (chronic) *pain,* and/or impaired *perfusion.* These concepts are reviewed in Chapter 3. This chapter focuses on selected adult musculoskeletal health disorders not covered in Chapter 46 on arthritis and Chapter 47 on musculoskeletal trauma. Musculoskeletal problems that are seen most often in children, such as scoliosis and progressive muscular dystrophies, are not included in this chapter because they are included in pediatric textbooks.

✳ CELLULAR REGULATION CONCEPT EXEMPLAR: OSTEOPOROSIS

Pathophysiology Review

Osteoporosis is a chronic disease of *cellular regulation* in which bone loss causes significant decreased density and possible fracture. It is often referred to as a *silent disease* or *silent thief* because the first sign of osteoporosis in most people follows some kind of a fracture.

Euro-American postmenopausal women have a 50% chance of having a fragility fracture (fracture caused by osteoporosis; sometimes referred to as a "bone attack") in their lifetime (National Osteoporosis Foundation [NOF], 2018). A woman who experiences a hip fracture has a greater risk for a second fracture. Fractures as a result of osteoporosis and falling can decrease a patient's *mobility* and quality of life. The mortality rate for older patients with hip fractures is very high, especially within the first 6 to 12 months, and the debilitating effects can be devastating (also see Chapter 47 on fractures).

Osteoporosis is a major global health problem. In less affluent or famine countries, many people have both osteoporosis *and* osteomalacia as a result of dietary deficiencies. Osteomalacia is loss of bone related to lack of vitamin D, which causes bone softening. Vitamin D is needed for calcium absorption in the small intestine. As a result of vitamin D deficiency, normal bone building is disrupted, and calcification does not occur to harden the bone. Table 45.1 compares these two bone diseases.

Bone is a living, changing tissue that is constantly undergoing changes in a process referred to as *bone remodeling*, a type of *cellular regulation.* Osteoporosis and osteopenia (loss of bone mass) occur when osteoclastic (bone resorption) activity is greater than osteoblastic (bone-building) activity. The result is a decreased bone mineral density (BMD). BMD is the amount of mineral that determines bone strength and peaks between 25 and 30 years of age. Before and during the peak years, osteoclastic activity and osteoblastic activity work at the same rate. After the peak years, osteoclastic activity exceeds bone-building activity, and bone density decreases. BMD decreases most rapidly in postmenopausal women as serum estrogen levels diminish. Although estrogen does not build bone, it helps prevent bone loss. *Trabecular,* or *cancellous* (spongy), bone is lost first, followed by loss of *cortical* (compact) bone. The hip, wrist, and spinal column have the highest amount of cancellous bone and are therefore the most likely to fracture first.

Standards for the diagnosis of osteoporosis are based on BMD testing that provides a T-score for the patient. A T-score represents the number of standard deviations above or below (designated with a minus sign) the average BMD for young, healthy adults. The T-score in a healthy 30-year-old adult is 0. *Osteopenia is present when the T-score is at −1 and above −2.5. Osteoporosis is diagnosed in a person who has a T-score at or lower than −2.5* (NOF, 2018). *Severe or established osteoporosis is defined as the presence of osteoporosis plus one or more fractures.*

Osteoporosis can be classified as generalized or regional. *Generalized* osteoporosis involves many structures in the skeleton and is further divided into two categories: primary and secondary. *Primary* osteoporosis is more common and occurs in postmenopausal women and in men in their seventh or eighth decade of life. *Secondary* osteoporosis may result from other medical conditions, such as hyperparathyroidism; long-term drug therapy, such as with corticosteroids; or prolonged decreased *mobility,* such as that seen with spinal cord injury (Table 45.2). Treatment of the secondary type is directed toward the cause of the osteoporosis when possible.

Regional (localized) osteoporosis, an example of secondary disease, can occur when a limb is immobilized related to a fracture, injury, or paralysis. Decreased *mobility* for longer than 8 to 12 weeks can result in this type of osteoporosis. Bone loss also

TABLE 45.2	Common Causes of Secondary Osteoporosis	
Diseases and Conditions	**Drugs (Chronic Use)**
• Diabetes mellitus	• Corticosteroids
• Hyperthyroidism	• Antiepileptic drugs (AEDs) (e.g.,
• Hyperparathyroidism	phenytoin)
• Cushing syndrome	• Barbiturates (e.g., phenobarbital)
• Growth hormone deficiency	• Ethanol (alcohol)
• Metabolic acidosis	• Drugs that induce hypogonadism
• Female hypogonadism	(decreased levels of sex hormones)
• Rheumatoid arthritis	• High levels of thyroid hormone
• Prolonged immobilization	• Cytotoxic agents
• Bone cancer	• Immunosuppressants
• Cirrhosis	• Loop diuretics
• HIV infection	• Aluminum-based antacids

TABLE 45.1	Differential Features of Osteoporosis and Osteomalacia	
Characteristic	**Osteoporosis**	**Osteomalacia**
Definition	Decreased bone mass caused by multiple factors	Bone softening caused by lack of calcification
Primary etiology	Lack of calcium and estrogen or testosterone	Lack of vitamin D
Radiographic findings	Osteopenia (bone loss), fractures	Fractures
Calcium level	Low or normal	Low or normal
Phosphate level	Normal	Low or normal
Parathyroid hormone	Normal	High or normal
Alkaline phosphatase	Normal	High

occurs when people spend prolonged time in a gravity-free or weightless environment (e.g., astronauts).

Etiology and Genetic Risk. Primary osteoporosis is caused by a combination of genetic, lifestyle, and environmental factors. The Best Practice for Patient Safety & Quality Care: Assessing Risk Factors for Primary Osteoporosis box lists the major modifiable and nonmodifiable risk factors that contribute to the development of this disease (Capriotti & Scanlon, 2018).

PATIENT-CENTERED CARE: GENETIC/ GENOMIC CONSIDERATIONS (QSEN)

The genetic and immune factors that cause osteoporosis are very complex. Strong evidence demonstrates that genetics is a significant factor. Many genetic changes have been identified as possible causative factors, but there is no agreement about which ones are most important or constant in all patients. For example, changes in the vitamin D_3 receptor *(VDR)* gene and calcitonin receptor *(CTR)* gene have been found in some patients with the disease. Receptors are essential for the uptake and use of these substances by the cells (McCance et al., 2019).

The bone morphogenetic protein 2 *(BMP-2)* gene has a key role in bone formation and maintenance. Some osteoporotic patients who had fractures have changes in their *BMP-2* gene. Alterations in the growth hormone 1 *(GH-1)* gene have been discovered in petite Asian-American women (i.e., those who are predisposed to developing osteoporosis.)

Hormones, tumor necrosis factor (TNF), interleukins, and other substances in the body help control osteoclasts in a very complex pathway. The identification of the importance of the cytokine receptor activator of nuclear factor kappa-B ligand (RANKL), its receptor RANK, and its decoy receptor osteoprotegerin (OPG) has helped researchers understand more about the activity of osteoclasts in metabolic bone disease. Disruptions in the RANKL,

BEST PRACTICE FOR PATIENT SAFETY & QUALITY CARE (QSEN)

Assessing Risk Factors for Primary Osteoporosis

Assess for these *nonmodifiable* risk factors:
- Older age (over 50 years of age)
- Menopause or history of total hysterectomy, including removal of ovaries
- Parental history of osteoporosis, especially mother
- Euro-Caucasian or Asian ethnicity
- Eating disorders, such as anorexia nervosa
- Rheumatoid arthritis
- History of low-trauma fracture after age 50 years

Assess for these *modifiable* risk factors:
- Low body weight, thin build
- Chronic low calcium and/or vitamin D intake
- Estrogen or androgen deficiency
- Current smoking (active or passive)
- High alcohol intake (two or more drinks a day)
- Drug therapy, such as chronic steroid therapy (also see Table 45.2)
- Poor nutrition
- Lack of physical exercise or prolonged decreased *mobility*

RANK, and OPG system can lead to increased osteoclast activity in which bone is rapidly broken down (McCance et al., 2019). Knowledge of these physiologic changes has contributed to the development of new drugs to manage osteoporosis (see the Drug Therapy section later in this chapter).

PATIENT-CENTERED CARE: GENDER HEALTH CONSIDERATIONS (QSEN)

Primary osteoporosis most often occurs in women after menopause or removal of both ovaries as a result of decreased estrogen levels. Obese women can store estrogen in their tissues for use as necessary to maintain a normal level of serum calcium better than thinner women and are therefore less likely to develop osteoporosis and resulting fractures.

Men also develop osteoporosis as they age because their testosterone levels decrease. Testosterone is the major sex hormone that builds bone tissue. Older men are often underdiagnosed.

The relationship of osteoporosis to nutrition is well established. For example, excessive caffeine in the diet can cause calcium loss in the urine. A diet lacking enough calcium and vitamin D stimulates the parathyroid gland to produce parathyroid hormone (PTH). PTH triggers the release of calcium from the bony matrix. Activated vitamin D is needed for calcium uptake in the body. Malabsorption of nutrients in the small intestine also contributes to low serum calcium levels. Institutionalized or homebound patients who are not exposed to sunlight may be at a higher risk because they do not receive adequate vitamin D for the metabolism of calcium (NOF, 2018).

Calcium loss occurs at a more rapid rate when phosphorus intake is high. (Chapter 13 describes the usual relationship between calcium and phosphorus in the body.) People who drink large amounts of carbonated beverages each day (over 40 ounces [1200 mL]) are at high risk for calcium loss and subsequent osteoporosis, regardless of age or gender.

Protein deficiency may also affect *cellular regulation.* Because 50% of serum calcium is protein bound, protein is needed to use calcium. However, excessive protein intake may increase calcium loss in the urine. For example, people who are on high-protein, low-carbohydrate diets, such as the Atkins diet, may consume too much protein to replace other foods that are not allowed.

Incidence and Prevalence. Osteoporosis is a health problem for more than 44 million Americans. About 10 million people in the United States have the disease, and about 34 million people

PATIENT-CENTERED CARE: CULTURAL/ SPIRITUAL CONSIDERATIONS (QSEN)

Body build, weight, and race/ethnicity seem to influence who gets the disease. Osteoporosis occurs most often in older, lean-built Euro-American and Asian women, particularly those who do not exercise regularly. However, African Americans are at risk for decreased vitamin D, which is needed for adequate calcium absorption in the small intestines. Dietary preferences or intolerances, sun avoidance, or the inability to afford high-nutrient food may influence anyone's rate of bone loss. For example, many blacks have lactose intolerance and cannot drink regular milk or eat other dairy-based foods (NOF, 2018). As an alternative, lactose-free milk, almond milk, or soy milk provides calcium. Milk and cheese are good sources of protein, a nutrient needed to bind calcium for use by the body.

50 years of age and older have osteopenia and are at risk for development of osteoporosis (NOF, 2018). As "baby boomers" age, these numbers are expected to increase dramatically.

Health Promotion and Maintenance

Peak bone mass is achieved by about 30 years of age in most women. *Building strong bone as a young person may be the best defense against osteoporosis in later adulthood.* Young women need to be aware of appropriate health and lifestyle practices that can prevent this potentially disabling disease. Patient-centered teaching should begin with young women because they begin to lose bone after 30 years of age. Nurses can play a vital role in patient education for women of any age to prevent and manage osteoporosis (Evenson & Sanders, 2016).

The focus of evidence-based osteoporosis prevention is to decrease modifiable risk factors to promote patient safety. For example, teach patients who do not include enough dietary calcium which foods to eat, such as dairy products and dark green leafy vegetables. Teach them to read food labels for sources of calcium content. Explain the importance of sun exposure (but not so much as to get sunburned) and adequate vitamin D in the diet. The National Osteoporosis Foundation recommends that all adults take a vitamin D_3 supplement, but strong evidence to support this recommendation is lacking or controversial (NOF, 2018; Reid, 2017).

Teach people at high risk for bone loss the importance of smoking cessation (if needed), weight loss (if needed), and avoidance of excessive alcohol use. Teach them the need to limit the amount of carbonated beverages consumed each day. Remind patients who have sedentary lifestyles about the importance of exercise and which types of exercise build bone tissue. Weight-bearing exercises, such as regularly scheduled walking, are preferred. Teach people at high risk to avoid activities that cause jarring, such as horseback riding and jogging, to prevent potential vertebral compression fractures.

❖ Interprofessional Collaborative Care

◆ Assessment: Recognize Cues

History. A complete health history with assessment of risk factors is important in the prevention, early detection, and treatment of osteoporosis. Patients who have risk factors for osteoporosis are at increased risk for fractures when falls occur. In some cases, the fracture occurs before the fall. Include a fall risk assessment in the health history, especially for older adults. Assess for fall risk factors as described in Chapter 4.

Physical Assessment/Signs and Symptoms. When performing a musculoskeletal assessment, inspect the vertebral column. The classic "dowager's hump," or kyphosis (outward curvature of the thoracic spine causing a "humped back"), is often present (Fig. 45.1). The older patient may state that he or she has gotten shorter, perhaps as much as 2 to 3 inches (5 to 7.5 cm), within the previous 20 years. Take or delegate the taking of height and weight measurements and compare with previous measurements if they are available (Jarvis, 2020).

The patient may have back pain, which often occurs after lifting, bending, or stooping. The pain may be sharp and acute or persistent (chronic). *Pain* is worse with activity and is often reduced by rest. Back pain accompanied by tenderness and voluntary restriction of spinal movement suggests one or more compression vertebral fractures (i.e., one of the most common types of osteoporotic or fragility fracture). Movement restriction and spinal deformity may result in constipation, abdominal distention, reflux esophagitis, and respiratory compromise in severe cases. The most likely area for spinal fracture is between T8 and L3, the most movable part of the vertebral column.

Fractures are also common in the distal end of the radius (wrist) and the upper third of the femur (hip). Ask the patient to locate all areas that are painful and observe for signs and symptoms of fractures, such as swelling and malalignment. Signs and symptoms of fractures are discussed in Chapter 47.

NCLEX EXAMINATION CHALLENGE 45.1
Physiological Integrity

Which assessment data are factors that increase the risk for osteoporosis for an older Euro-American female? **Select all that apply.**
A. Drinks 3 to 4 glasses of wine each day
B. Sits at a desk all day at her job
C. Smokes a pack of cigarettes a day
D. Takes a mile-long walk 5 days a week
E. Takes 1000 mg acetaminophen for arthritis daily
F. Weighs 110 lb (50 kg)

Psychosocial Assessment. Women associate osteoporosis with menopause, getting older, and becoming less independent. The disease can result in decreased *mobility,* deformity, and disability that can affect the patient's well-being and life satisfaction. Quality of life may be further affected by persistent (chronic) *pain,* insomnia, depression, and fear of falling (Touhy & Jett, 2018).

Assess the patient's concept of body image, especially if he or she is severely kyphotic. For example, the patient may have difficulty finding clothes that fit properly. Social interactions may be avoided because of a change in appearance or the physical limitations of being unable to sit in chairs in restaurants, movie theaters, and other places. Changes in sexuality may occur as a result of poor self-esteem or the discomfort caused by positioning during intercourse.

Because osteoporosis poses a risk for fractures, teach the patient to be extremely cautious about activities. As a result, the

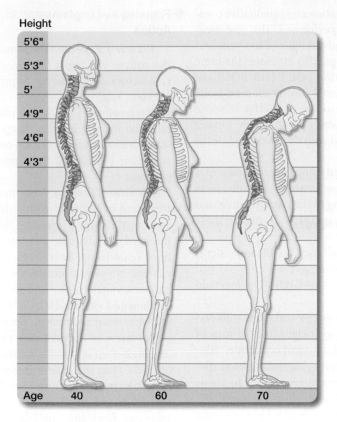

FIG. 45.1 Normal spine at age 40 years and osteoporotic changes at ages 60 and 70 years. These changes can cause a loss of as much as 6 inches in height and can result in the so-called *dowager's hump (far right)* in the upper thoracic vertebrae.

threat of fracture can create anxiety and fear and result in further limitation of social or physical activities. Assess for these feelings to assist in treatment decisions and health teaching. For example, the patient may not exercise as prescribed for fear that a fracture will occur.

Laboratory Assessment. Serum calcium and vitamin D_3 levels should be routinely monitored (at least once a year) for all women and for men older than 50 years who are at a high risk for the disease. Serum calcium should be between 9.0 and 10.5 mg/dL (2.10 and 2.50 mmol/L). Total 25-hydroxyvitamin D (D_2 plus D_3) levels should be between 25 and 80 ng/mL (75 and 200 nmol/L) (Pagana & Pagana 2018; Pagana et al., 2019). These results can help determine the need for supplements and preventive measures to slow bone loss. No definitive laboratory tests confirm a diagnosis of primary osteoporosis, although a number of *bone turnover markers* can provide information about bone resorption and formation activity. Although not commonly tested, these markers are sensitive to bone changes and can be used to monitor effectiveness of treatment for osteoporosis or to detect bone changes early in the disease process. Examples of these markers are osteocalcin and bone-specific alkaline phosphatase (BSAP).

Imaging Assessment. Conventional x-rays of the spine and long bones show decreased bone density, but only after a large amount of bone loss has occurred. Fractures can also be seen on x-rays. According to the National Osteoporosis Foundation (NOF, 2018), all postmenopausal women and men age 50 and older should be evaluated for osteoporosis risk to determine the need for BMD testing and/or vertebral imaging.

The most commonly used screening and diagnostic radiographic test for measuring bone mineral density (BMD) is dual x-ray absorptiometry (DXA). The spine and hip are most often assessed when central DXA (cDXA) scan is performed. If spinal deformity is present, the wrist may also be assessed. Many primary health care providers recommend that women in their 40s have a baseline screening DXA scan so later bone changes can be detected and compared. DXA is a noninvasive, painless scan that emits less radiation than a chest x-ray. It is the most common test currently used but has limitations. First, BMD alone explains only part of the bone change and provides no information on cellular activity. Second, there are variations among different DXA systems. In addition, DXA is not useful for very tall or very obese patients.

Tell patients that their height is measured before a DXA scan. The patient stays dressed but is asked to remove any metallic objects such as belt buckles, coins, keys, or jewelry that might interfere with the test. The results are displayed on a computer graph, and a T-score is calculated. No special follow-up care for the test is required. However, the patient needs to discuss the results with the primary health care provider for any decisions about possible preventive or management interventions. Patients who have osteopenia usually have follow-up DXA scans every 2 years.

For some patients, *CT-based absorptiometry* (qualitative computed tomography [QCT]) may be performed. This test measures the volume of bone density and strength of the vertebral spine and hip. The peripheral QCT (pQCT) measures the same at the forearm or tibia. High-resolution pQCT (HR-pQCT) of the radius and tibia provides additional information on bone structure and architecture. These tests are predictive of spine and/or hip fractures in women; however, they require greater amounts of radiation when compared with the more traditional DXA.

Vertebral imaging can be performed using lateral spine x-rays or lateral vertebral fracture assessment, which is available as part of most DXA systems. According to the clinical guidelines outlined by NOF (2018), vertebral imaging is indicated for these groups:

- All women age 70 and older and all men age 80 and older if BMD is less than or equal to a T-score of 1.0
- Women age 65 to 69 and men age 70 to 79 if BMD is less than or equal to a T-score of 1.5
- Postmenopausal women and men age 50 and older with certain risk factors, such as significant height loss, history of low-trauma fracture, or being on long-term corticosteroids

The most promising imaging test for diagnosing bone disease is the use of *magnetic resonance imaging (MRI)* to assess bone marrow composition (see Chapter 44 for procedure). MRI does not involve radiation and can be used to view bone in ways that other techniques cannot. To determine the presence of osteoporosis, quantitative MRI procedures provide information about yellow bone marrow content, diffusion, and perfusion to the bone. **Perfusion** to osteoporotic bone is lower than to bone of normal bone density. Fat marrow content, sometimes referred to as *bone marrow adipose tissue (BMAT),* is higher in patients with bone loss compared with those with normal BMD (Xiaojuan & Schwartz, 2020). These tests are more reliable and offer more information about bone change than BMD measurements alone but are very expensive and not widely used.

Several imaging tests are available for community-based screening because these devices are more portable. However, they lack the preciseness and reliability of the previously discussed imaging procedures. Examples include the peripheral DXA (pDXA) and the peripheral quantitative ultrasound densitometry (pQUS). The *pDXA scan* assesses BMD of the heel, forearm, or finger. It is often used for large-scale screening purposes. The *pQUS* is an effective and low-cost screening tool that can detect osteoporosis and predict risk for hip fracture. The heel, tibia, and patella are most commonly tested. This procedure requires no special preparation, is quick, and has no radiation exposure or specific follow-up care (Pagana & Pagana, 2018). Both tests are commonly used for screening at community health fairs, skilled nursing facilities, and women's health centers.

◆ Analysis: Analyze Cues and Prioritize Hypotheses

The priority problem for patients with osteoporosis or osteopenia is *Potential for fractures due to weak, porous bone tissue.*

◆ Planning and Implementation: Generate Solutions and Take Action

Planning: Expected Outcomes. The expected outcome is that the patient will avoid fractures by preventing falls, managing risk factors, and adhering to preventive or treatment measures for bone loss.

Interventions. Because the patient is predisposed to fractures, nutrition therapy, lifestyle changes, and drug therapy are used to slow bone resorption and form new bone tissue. Self-management education (SME) can help prevent osteoporosis or slow the progress.

Nutrition Therapy. The nutritional considerations for the treatment of a patient with a diagnosis of osteoporosis are the same as those for preventing the disease. Teach patients about the need for adequate amounts of calcium and vitamin D for bone remodeling. Instruct them to avoid excessive alcohol and caffeine consumption. People who are lactose intolerant can choose a variety of soy and rice products that are fortified with calcium and vitamin D. In addition, calcium and vitamin D are added to many fruit juices, bread, and cereal products.

A variety of nutrients are needed to maintain bone health. *The promotion of a single nutrient will not prevent or treat osteoporosis.* Help the patient develop a nutrition plan that is most beneficial in maintaining bone health; the plan should emphasize fruits and vegetables, low-fat dairy and protein sources, increased fiber, and moderation in alcohol and caffeine (NOF, 2018).

Lifestyle Changes. Exercise is important in the prevention and management of osteoporosis. It also plays a vital role in **pain** management, cardiovascular function, and an improved sense of well-being.

In collaboration with the primary health care provider, the physical therapist may prescribe exercises for strengthening the abdominal and back muscles for those at risk for vertebral fractures. These exercises improve posture and support for the spine. Abdominal muscle tightening, deep breathing, and pectoral stretching are stressed to increase lung capacity. Exercises for the extremity muscles include muscle-tightening, resistive, and range-of-motion (ROM) exercises to improve **mobility.** Muscle strengthening also helps to prevent falls and promote balance. Swimming and yoga provides overall muscle exercise.

In addition to exercises for muscle strengthening, a general weight-bearing exercise program should be implemented. Teach patients that walking for 30 minutes three to five times a week is the single most effective exercise for osteoporosis prevention. Remind them to avoid any activity that would cause jarring of the body, such as jogging and horseback riding. These activities can cause compression fractures of the vertebral column.

In addition to nutrition and exercise, other lifestyle changes may be needed. Teach the patient to avoid tobacco in any form, especially active or passive cigarette smoking (NOF, 2018). Remind women not to consume more than one alcoholic drink per day (5 ounces each); instruct men not to have more than two alcoholic drinks per day.

Drug Therapy. The evidence shows that drug therapy should be used for postmenopausal women and men age 50 and older when the BMD T-score for the hip or lumbar spine is below or equal to –2.5 with no other risk factors, or when the T-score is below –1.5 with risk factors or previous fracture. Anyone age 50 or older who had a hip or vertebral fracture should also be treated (NOF, 2018). The primary health care provider may prescribe calcium and vitamin D_3 supplements, bisphosphonates, estrogen agonists/antagonists (formerly called *selective estrogen receptor modulators* [SERMS]), parathyroid hormone (PTH), RANKL inhibitor, or a combination of several drugs to treat or prevent osteoporosis (see the Common Examples of Drug Therapy: Osteoporosis box).

Calcium and Activated Vitamin D (D_3). Intake of *calcium* alone is not a treatment for osteoporosis, but calcium is an important part of any program to promote bone health. Many people cannot or do not have enough calcium in their diet; therefore calcium supplements may be needed. NOF (2018) supports the National Academy of Medicine's research recommendation of 1000 mg daily for all postmenopausal women and men between ages 50 and 70, and 1200 mg for both women and men 71 years of age and older (NOF, 2018). Teach women to start taking supplements in young adulthood to help maintain peak bone mass. Because vitamin D is needed for calcium absorption by the body, vitamin D_3 supplementation is also indicated. Laboratory tests to measure serum calcium and vitamin D_3 may be done to monitor the effectiveness of these supplements.

Bisphosphonates. Bisphosphonates slow bone resorption by binding with crystal elements in bone, especially spongy, cancellous bone tissue. They are the most common drugs used for osteoporosis, but some are also approved for Paget disease and hypercalcemia caused by cancer. Three Food and Drug Administration (FDA)–approved bisphosphonates (alendronate, ibandronate, and risedronate) are commonly used for the *prevention and treatment* of osteoporosis (Burchum & Rosenthal, 2019). These drugs are available as oral preparations; ibandronate is also available as an IV preparation.

COMMON EXAMPLES OF DRUG THERAPY

Osteoporosis

Drug Category	Nursing Implications
Calcium (With Vitamin D)	
Calcium and vitamin D_3 may be taken separately or in combination	Take a third of the daily dose at bedtime *because no weight-bearing activity to build bone occurs while sleeping.*
	Encourage increased fluids, unless medically contraindicated, *to help prevent urinary calculi (stones).*
	Teach patient to take the drugs with 6-8 ounces of water *to help dissolve them.*
	Assess for a history of urinary stones before giving calcium.
	Monitor calcium level to determine drug effectiveness.
	Observe for signs of hypercalcemia, such as calcium deposits under the skin, cardiac dysrhythmias, changes in skeletal muscle tone, and urinary stones, *which may indicate calcium excess.*
	Teach patients to check with their primary health care providers about recommended doses to take.
Bisphosphonates	
Common examples of bisphosphonates: • Alendronate • Ibandronate • Risedronate • Pamidronate (IV) • Zoledronic acid (IV)	Teach patients to take drug on an empty stomach first thing in the morning with a full glass of water *to help prevent esophagitis, esophageal ulcers, and gastric ulcers.*
	Remind patients to take drug 30 minutes before food, drink, and other drugs *to prevent interactions.*
	Instruct the patient to remain upright, sitting or standing, for 30 minutes after taking the drug *to help prevent esophagitis (esophageal inflammation).*
	Instruct the patient to have a dental examination before starting the drug because it can cause jaw and maxillary osteonecrosis, particular if oral hygiene is poor.
	Do not give the drug to patients who are sensitive to aspirin *because bronchoconstriction may occur.*
	For IV drug, infuse over 15-30 min to prevent rare complications such as atrial fibrillation.
	For IV drugs, check the patient's serum creatinine before and after administering the medication *because it can cause renal insufficiency or acute kidney injury.*
Estrogen Agonists/Antagonists	
Example of estrogen agonist/antagonists: • Raloxifene	Teach the patient the signs and symptoms of venous thromboembolism (VTE), especially in the first 4 months of therapy, *because these drugs can cause VTE.*
	Monitor liver function tests (LFTs) in collaboration with the primary health care provider *because the drug can increase LFT values.*
RANKL Inhibitors	
Common examples of RANKL inhibitors: • Denosumab • Romosozumab	Teach patients to report new musculoskeletal pain, especially in the back, and skin reactions, not just at the injection site.
	Teach patients to report signs and symptoms of infection, *a common adverse effect.*
	Monitor levels of calcium, magnesium, and phosphorus *because the drug can cause severe hypocalcemia;* patients with impaired renal function are especially at risk.
	Instruct the patient to have a dental examination before starting the drug *because it can cause jaw and maxillary osteonecrosis, particularly if oral hygiene is poor.*

The most recent additions to the bisphosphonates are IV zoledronic acid and IV pamidronate. For management of osteoporosis, zoledronic acid is needed only once a year, and pamidronate is given every 3 to 6 months. Both drugs have been linked to a complication called jaw osteonecrosis (also known as *avascular necrosis*, or *bone death*), in which infection and necrosis of the mandible or maxilla occur (Burchum & Rosenthal, 2019). The incidence of this serious problem is low, but it can be a complication of this infusion therapy.

! NURSING SAFETY PRIORITY (QSEN)
Drug Alert

Do not confuse Fosamax (U.S. trade name for alendronate) with Flomax (U.S. trade name for tamsulosin), a selective alpha-adrenergic blocker used for benign prostatic hyperplasia (BPH). To promote safety, teach patients to take bisphosphonates early in the morning with 8 ounces of water and wait 30 to 60 minutes in an upright position before eating. If chest discomfort (a symptom of esophageal irritation) occurs, instruct patients to discontinue the drug and contact their health care provider. Patients with poor renal function, hypocalcemia, or gastroesophageal reflux disease (GERD) should not take bisphosphonates. *Teach patients to have an oral assessment and preventive dentistry before beginning any bisphosphonate therapy.* To promote safety, instruct them to inform any dentist who is planning invasive treatment, such as a tooth extraction or implant, that they are taking a bisphosphonate drug.

Teach patients that they should not take bisphosphonates continuously as lifelong management owing to long-term adverse effects such as esophageal cancer, atrial fibrillation, jaw osteonecrosis, and severe musculoskeletal pain. The decision to continue the drug after 2 years is made based on follow-up DXA scan results. If bone loss is maintained or bone density increases, the bisphosphonate is discontinued. If bone loss continues to occur, the drug can be continued for up to 5 years (Burchum & Rosenthal, 2019).

Other Drugs. Formerly called the *selective estrogen receptor modulators (SERMs)*, estrogen agonist/antagonists are a class of drugs designed to mimic estrogen in some parts of the body while blocking its effect elsewhere. Raloxifene is currently the only approved drug in this class and is used for *prevention and treatment* of osteoporosis in postmenopausal women. Raloxifene increases bone mineral density (BMD), reduces bone resorption, and reduces the incidence of osteoporotic vertebral fractures. The drug should not be given to women who have a history of venous thromboembolism (VTE) because it can cause deep vein thrombosis and pulmonary embolism.

A newer drug class is *RANKL (receptor activator of nuclear factor kappa-B ligand) inhibitors*, such as denosumab and romosozumab. These drugs are approved for treatment of osteoporosis when other drugs are not effective (Burchum & Rosenthal, 2019). By preventing the protein from activating its receptor, the drug decreases bone loss. The drug is given subcutaneously twice a year by a health care professional.

Teriparatide and abaloparatide are *parathyroid hormone–related protein drugs* that build bone and may not be used long-term. These drugs are available as daily subcutaneous injections and are indicated for patients who had a previous fracture or have multiple risk factors. After the drug is stopped, the patient is usually started on a bisphosphonate (NOF, 2018).

Salmon *calcitonin* (Miacalcin or Fortical) is approved for osteoporosis in women who are at least 5 years postmenopausal when alternative drug therapy is not appropriate. Two preparations are available: an intranasal spray or a subcutaneous injection. Intranasal calcitonin can cause rhinitis and epistaxis (nosebleeds). In a few patients, malignancies have been attributed to the use of calcitonin. For others, allergic responses to salmon may prevent the drug from being used or continued. Patients are usually tested for this allergy before they begin the drug. Calcitonin is less commonly used than other drugs to prevent bone loss and fractures (Burchum & Rosenthal, 2019).

Care Coordination and Transition Management

Home Care Management. Patients with osteoporosis are usually managed at home unless they have major fragility fractures. Some patients do not know that they have osteoporosis until they experience a fall and have one or more fractures.

Remind patients to have follow up DXA scans as prescribed to determine the effectiveness of drug therapy. For example, some patients maintain or gain bone mass and can discontinue their prescribed drug as directed by their primary health care provider. After discontinuation of medication, follow-up scans determine whether drug therapy needs to be restarted or another drug prescribed. This process helps to reduce the potential adverse effects that are associated with certain drug classifications.

Part of your responsibility is to collaborate with members of the interprofessional health team to ensure that the patient's home is safe and hazard free to help prevent falling. In some cases, home modifications may be needed, such as ramps instead of stairs or handrails near toilets and bathtubs and showers. Teach patients to prevent clutter in the home for clear pathways, avoid slippery floors, wear rubber-soled shoes, and avoid scatter rugs. Chapter 4 describes fall prevention in detail.

Self-Management Education. Teach patients about lifestyle practices that can help prevent additional bone loss. For example, to help prevent vitamin D deficiency, daily sun exposure (at least 5 minutes each day) is the most important source of vitamin D. If vitamin D levels remain low, teach patients to take their vitamin D_3 and calcium supplements as described earlier. Increase calcium and vitamin D sources in the diet.

Some people are lactose intolerant or do not use dairy products because of their vegan diets. However, many products are available for people who avoid dairy products. Soy and rice milk, tofu, and soy products are substitutes, but they are expensive. Teach patients to choose products that are fortified with vitamin D. Other foods rich in the vitamin are eggs, swordfish, chicken, liver, and enriched cereals and bread products.

If the patient is on drug therapy for osteopenia or osteoporosis, teach him or her to adhere to the medication regimen and take the prescribed drug(s) as instructed. Lack of adherence to long-term therapy for osteoporosis and bone health promotion practices is a major problem that results in increased fractures, hospital stays, and health care costs.

Health Care Resources. Refer patients to the National Osteoporosis Foundation (www.nof.org) in the United States for information regarding the disease and its treatment. The Osteoporosis Society of Canada (www.osteoporosis.ca) has similar services. Large health care systems often have osteoporosis specialty clinics and support groups for patients with osteoporosis.

◆ **Evaluation: Evaluate Outcomes**

Evaluate the care of the patient with osteoporosis or at risk for osteoporosis based on the identified priority patient problem. Expected outcomes are that the patient:

- Continues to follow up with DXA screenings as recommended to assess ongoing bone health
- Makes necessary changes in lifestyle to help prevent further bone loss
- Does not experience a fragility fracture due to bone loss

OSTEOMYELITIS

Pathophysiology Review

Infection in bony tissue can be a severe and difficult-to-treat problem. Bone infection can result in chronic recurrence, loss of function, persistent (chronic) *pain,* amputation, or even death due to sepsis.

Bacteria (most common), viruses, parasites, or fungi can cause ***infection*** in bone, known as osteomyelitis. Invasion by one or more pathogenic microorganisms stimulates the inflammatory response in bone tissue. The inflammation produces an increased vascular leak and edema, often involving the surrounding soft tissues. Once inflammation is established, the vessels in the area become thrombosed and release exudate (pus) into bony tissue. Ischemia of bone tissue follows and results in necrotic bone. This area of necrotic bone separates from surrounding bone tissue, and *sequestrum* is formed. The presence of sequestrum prevents bone healing and causes superimposed infection, often in the form of bone abscess which can lead to chronic osteomyelitis (McCance et al., 2019). As shown in Fig. 45.2, the cycle repeats itself as the new infection leads to further inflammation, vessel thromboses, and necrosis. Because bone is a dynamic tissue and attempts to heal itself, osteoblasts often lay new bone tissue over the infected tissue, making it difficult for drug therapy to penetrate into the infected bone.

Osteomyelitis may be categorized as *exogenous,* in which infectious organisms enter from outside the body as in an open fracture or after surgery, or *endogenous (hematogenous),* in which organisms are carried by the bloodstream from other areas of infection in the body. A third category is *contiguous,* in which bone infection results from skin infection of adjacent

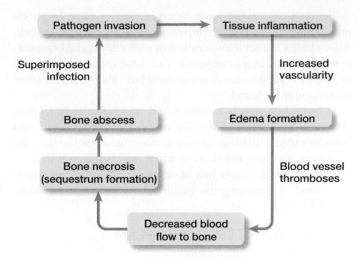

FIG. 45.2 Infection cycle of osteomyelitis.

tissues. Osteomyelitis can be further divided into two major types: acute and chronic (McCance et al., 2019).

Each type of bone infection has its own causative factors. Pathogenic microbes favor bone that has a rich blood supply and a marrow cavity. *Acute hematogenous infection* results from bacteremia, underlying disease, or nonpenetrating trauma. Urinary tract infections, particularly in older men, tend to spread to the lower vertebrae. Long-term IV catheters can be primary sources of infection. Patients undergoing long-term hemodialysis and IV drug users are also at risk for osteomyelitis. *Salmonella* infections of the GI tract may spread to bone. Patients with sickle cell disease and other hemoglobinopathies often have multiple episodes of salmonellosis, which can cause bone infection (McCance et al., 2019).

Poor dental hygiene and periodontal (gum) infection can be causative factors in *contiguous* osteomyelitis in facial bones. Minimal nonpenetrating trauma can cause hemorrhages or small-vessel occlusions, leading to bone necrosis. Regardless of the source of infection, many infections are caused by *Staphylococcus aureus.* Treatment of infection may be complicated further by the presence of *methicillin-resistant Staphylococcus aureus* (MRSA) or other multidrug-resistant organisms (MDROs), which are very common in hospitalized and other institutionalized patients as discussed in Chapter 21. The most common causes of MRSA in patients with musculoskeletal health problems are postoperative surgical site infections (SSIs) and infections from surgically implanted devices, such as an open reduction, internal fixation device.

PATIENT-CENTERED CARE: OLDER ADULT CONSIDERATIONS (QSEN)

Malignant external otitis media involving the base of the skull is sometimes seen in older adults with diabetes. However, the most common cause of contiguous spread in older adults is found in those who have slow-healing foot ulcers. Multiple organisms tend to be responsible for the resulting osteomyelitis (McCance et al., 2019).

Penetrating trauma leads to acute osteomyelitis by direct inoculation. A soft-tissue *infection* may be present as well. Animal bites, puncture wounds, skin ulcerations, and bone surgery can result in osteomyelitis. The most common offending organism is *Pseudomonas aeruginosa,* but other gram-negative bacteria may be found.

If bone *infection* is misdiagnosed or inadequately treated, *chronic osteomyelitis* may develop, especially in older adults who have foot ulcers. Inadequate care management results when the treatment period is too short or when the treatment is delayed or inappropriate. About half of cases of chronic osteomyelitis are caused by gram-negative bacteria, especially in older adults (McCance et al., 2019).

❖ Interprofessional Collaborative Care

◆ Assessment: Recognize Cues

Bone *pain,* with or without other signs and symptoms, is a common concern of patients with osteomyelitis. The pain is often described as a constant, localized, pulsating sensation that worsens with movement. Perform a complete pain assessment as described in Chapter 5.

The patient with acute osteomyelitis has fever, usually with temperature higher than 101°F (38.3°C). Older adults may not have an extreme temperature elevation because of a lower core body temperature and compromised immune system that occur with normal aging. The area around the infected bone swells and is tender when palpated. Erythema (redness) and heat may also be present. Fever, swelling, and erythema are less common in those with chronic osteomyelitis (see the Key Features: Acute Versus Chronic Osteomyelitis box). When vascular compromise is severe, patients may not experience **pain** because of nerve damage from lack of adequate **perfusion.**

When vascular insufficiency is suspected, assess circulation in the distal extremities. Ulcerations may be present on the feet or hands, indicating inadequate healing ability as a result of impaired *perfusion.*

The patient with osteomyelitis may have an elevated white blood cell (leukocyte) count, which may be double the normal value. The erythrocyte sedimentation rate (ESR) may be normal early in the course of the disease but may rise as the condition

progresses. It may remain elevated for as long as 3 months after drug therapy is discontinued.

If bacteremia (bacteria in the bloodstream that could lead to septic shock) is present, a blood culture identifies the offending organisms to determine which antibiotics should be used in treatment. Both aerobic and anaerobic blood cultures are collected before drug therapy begins. Further diagnostic testing using a variety of radionuclide scans or MRI may be performed to assess the extent of the infection and *perfusion* in the affected area.

◆ Interventions: Take Action

The specific treatment for osteomyelitis depends on the type and number of microbes present in the infected tissue. If other measures fail to resolve the infectious process, surgical management may be needed.

Nonsurgical Management. The primary health care provider typically prescribes at least 4 to 6 weeks of antimicrobial therapy as soon as possible for *acute* osteomyelitis based on the wound culture and sensitivity results. In the presence of copious wound drainage, follow Contact Precautions to prevent the spread of the offending organism to other patients and health care personnel. Teach patients, visitors, and staff members how to use these precautions. (See Chapter 21 for a discussion of Contact Precautions.)

More than one antimicrobial agent may be needed to combat multiple types of organisms. The hospital or home care nurse gives the drugs at specifically prescribed times so therapeutic serum levels are achieved. Observe for the actions, side effects, and toxicity of these drugs. Teach family members or other caregivers in the home setting how to administer drug therapy if they are continued after hospital discharge or are used only at home. Some patients may need to be admitted to a skilled nursing facility (SNF) for IV drug therapy. For patients with MRSA infection, IV vancomycin or linezolid (IV or oral) may be used. Oral linezolid allows older patients to remain at home or in assisted living rather than being admitted to an SNF (Burchum & Rosenthal, 2019).

The optimal drug regimen for patients with *chronic* osteomyelitis is not well established. Prolonged therapy for more than 3 months is typically needed to eliminate the *infection.* Patients are usually cared for in the home or skilled care setting with long-term vascular access catheters, such as a peripherally inserted central catheter (PICC). After discontinuation of IV drugs, oral therapy may be needed. Patients and families must understand the complications of inadequate treatment or failure to follow up with their primary health care provider.

▶▶ KEY FEATURES

Acute Versus Chronic Osteomyelitis

Acute Osteomyelitis
- Fever; temperature usually above 101°F (38.3°C)
- Swelling around the affected area
- Possible erythema and heat in the affected area
- Tenderness of the affected area
- Bone pain that is constant, localized, and pulsating; worsens with movement

Chronic Osteomyelitis
- Foot ulcer(s) or bone surgery (most commonly)
- Sinus tract formation
- Localized *pain*
- Drainage from the affected area (usually due to bone abscess)

❗ NURSING SAFETY PRIORITY (QSEN)

Drug Alert

Even when symptoms of osteomyelitis appear to be improved, teach the patient and family that the full course of IV and/or oral antimicrobials must be completed to ensure that the *infection* is resolved.

In addition to systemic drug therapy, if a wound is present it may be irrigated, either continuously or intermittently, with one or more antimicrobial solutions. A medical technique in which beads made of bone cement are impregnated with an antibiotic and packed into the wound can provide direct contact of the antibiotic with the offending organism.

Drugs are also needed to manage *pain.* Patients often experience acute and persistent (chronic) pain and must receive a regimen of drug therapy for control. Chapter 5 describes pharmacologic and nonpharmacologic interventions for both acute and persistent (chronic) pain.

A treatment to increase tissue *perfusion* for patients with chronic, unremitting osteomyelitis is the use of a hyperbaric chamber or portable device to administer hyperbaric oxygen (HBO) therapy. These devices are usually available in large tertiary care centers and may not be accessible to all patients who might benefit from them. With HBO therapy, the affected area is exposed daily to a high concentration of oxygen that diffuses into the tissues to promote healing. In conjunction with high-dose drug therapy and surgical débridement, HBO has proven very useful in treating a number of anaerobic infections. Other wound-management therapies are described in Chapter 23.

Surgical Management. Antimicrobial therapy alone may not meet the desired outcome of treatment. Surgical techniques include incision and drainage of skin and subcutaneous infection, wound débridement, and bone excision.

Because bone cannot heal in the presence of necrotic tissue, a *sequestrectomy* may be performed to remove the necrotic bone and allow revascularization of tissue. The excision of dead and infected bone often results in a sizable cavity, or bone defect. Bone *grafts* to repair bone defects are also widely used.

When infected bone is extensively resected, reconstruction with *microvascular bone transfers* or bone graft from donor bone may be done. This procedure is reserved for larger skeletal defects. The most common donor sites are the patient's fibula and iliac crest. Nursing care of the patient after surgery is similar to that for any postoperative patient (see Chapter 9). However, the important difference is that neurovascular assessments must be done frequently because the patient experiences increased swelling after the surgical procedure. Elevate the affected extremity to increase venous return and thus control swelling. Assess and document the patient's neurovascular status, including:

- Pain
- Movement
- Sensation
- Warmth
- Temperature
- Distal pulses
- Capillary refill (not as reliable as the above indicators)

When the previously described surgical procedures are not appropriate or successful and as a last resort, the affected limb may need to be amputated. The physical and psychological care for a patient who has undergone an amputation is discussed in Chapter 47.

CLINICAL JUDGMENT CHALLENGE 45.1
Patient-Centered Care; Safety

A 25-year-old obese man has received 2 weeks of a 6-week course of IV antibiotic therapy for acute osteomyelitis resulting from three knee surgeries for a sports injury. He visits his nurse practitioner but is initially assessed by the office nurse, who documents the following physical assessment changes:

- Reports increased difficulty when climbing stairs to his third-floor apartment when compared with last week (no elevator in building)
- States that the affected knee pain has increased from a 3 to a 7 on a 0-10 pain scale regardless of when he takes his analgesic
- States that he has noticed purulent, odorous drainage present when he changes his knee dressings daily
- Reports that he feels hot every evening but does not own a thermometer
- Reports increased fatigue and inability to concentrate while working remotely on his computer
- Oral temperature = 100.8°F (38.2°C)
- Radial pulse = 88 beats/min
- Blood pressure = 124/76 mm Hg
- WBCs = 18,500/mm³ (drawn 3 days ago)

1. **Recognize Cues:** What assessment information in this client situation is the most important and immediate concern for the nurse? (Hint: Identify the **relevant** information *first* to determine what is most important.)
2. **Analyze Cues:** What client conditions are consistent with the **most relevant** information? (Hint: Think about priority collaborative problems that support and contradict the information presented in this situation.)
3. **Prioritize Hypotheses:** Which possibilities or explanations are **most likely** to be present in this client situation? Which possibilities or explanations are the most serious? (Hint: Consider all possibilities and determine their urgency and risk for this client.)
4. **Generate Solutions:** What actions would most likely achieve the desired outcomes for this client? Which actions should be **avoided** or are **potentially harmful**? (Hint: Determine the desired outcomes first to decide which interventions are appropriate and those that should be avoided.)
5. **Take Action:** Which actions are the most appropriate and how should they be implemented? In what **priority order** should they be implemented? (Hint: Consider health teaching, documentation, requested health care provider orders or prescriptions, nursing skills, collaboration with or referral to health team members, etc.)
6. **Evaluate Outcomes:** What client assessment would indicate that the nurse's actions were **effective**? (Hint: Think about signs that would indicate an improvement, decline, or unchanged client condition.)

BONE TUMORS

Pathophysiology Review
Benign Bone Tumors

Bone tumors may be classified as benign (noncancerous) or malignant (cancerous). *Benign* bone tumors are often asymptomatic and may be discovered on routine x-ray examination or as the cause of pathologic fractures. The cause of benign bone tumors is not known. Tumors may arise from several types of tissue. The major classifications include *chondrogenic* tumors (from cartilage), *osteogenic* tumors (from bone), and *fibrogenic* tumors (from fibrous tissue and found most often in children).

The most common benign bone tumor is the *osteochondroma.* Although its onset is usually in childhood, the tumor grows until skeletal maturity and may not be diagnosed until adulthood. The tumor may be a single growth or multiple growths and can occur in any bone. The femur and the tibia are most often involved (McCance et al., 2019).

Malignant Bone Tumors

Malignant (cancerous) bone tumors may be primary (those that begin in bone) or secondary (those that originate in other tissues and metastasize [spread] to bone). *Primary tumors* occur most often in people between 10 and 30 years of age and make up a small percentage of bone cancers. As with other forms of cancer, the exact cause of bone cancer is unknown, but genetic and environmental factors are likely causes. *Metastatic lesions* most often occur in the older age-group and account for most bone cancers in adults (McCance et al., 2019).

Osteosarcoma, or osteogenic sarcoma, is the most common type of *primary* malignant bone tumor. More than 50% of cases occur in the distal femur, followed in decreasing order of occurrence by the proximal tibia and humerus. The tumor is relatively large, causing acute *pain* and swelling. The involved area is usually warm because the blood flow to the site increases. The center of the tumor is sclerotic from increased osteoblastic activity. The periphery is soft, extending through the bone cortex in the classic sunburst appearance associated with the neoplasm (which is visible on x-ray). Osteosarcoma typically metastasizes (spreads), which results in death.

Although *Ewing sarcoma* is not as common as other tumors, it is the most malignant. Like other primary tumors, it causes *pain* and swelling. In addition, systemic signs and symptoms, particularly low-grade fever, leukocytosis, and anemia, are common. The pelvis and the lower extremity are most often affected. Pelvic involvement is a poor prognostic sign. It often extends into soft tissue. Death results from metastasis to the lungs and other bones. Although the tumor can be seen in patients of any age, it usually occurs in children and young adults in their 20s. Men are affected more often than women (McCance et al., 2019). The reason for this pattern is not known.

In contrast to the patient with osteosarcoma, the patient with *chondrosarcoma* experiences dull *pain* and swelling for a long period. The tumor typically affects the pelvis and proximal femur near the diaphysis. Arising from cartilaginous tissue, it destroys bone and often calcifies. The patient with this type of tumor has a better prognosis than one with osteogenic sarcoma. Chondrosarcoma occurs in middle-age and older people, with a slight predominance in men.

Arising from fibrous tissue, *fibrosarcomas* can be divided into subtypes, of which malignant fibrous histiocytoma (MFH) is the most malignant. Usually the clinical presentation of MFH is gradual, without specific symptoms. Local tenderness, with or without a palpable mass, occurs in the long bones of the lower extremity. As with other bone cancers, the lesion can metastasize to the lungs (McCance et al., 2019).

Primary tumors of the prostate, breast, kidney, thyroid, and lung are called *bone-seeking* cancers because they spread to the bone more often than other primary tumors. The vertebrae, pelvis, femur, and ribs are the bone sites commonly affected. Simply stated, primary tumor cells, or seeds, are carried to bone through the bloodstream. *Fragility fractures caused by metastatic bone are a major concern in patient care management.*

❖ Interprofessional Collaborative Care

◆ Assessment: Recognize Cues

Assess for *pain,* the most common symptom of most bone tumors. Pain can range from mild to severe. It can be caused by direct tumor invasion into soft tissue, compressed peripheral nerves, or a resulting pathologic or fragility fracture. Perform a complete pain assessment for the patient as a baseline to plan care as described in Chapter 5.

In addition, observe and palpate the suspected involved area. When the tumor affects the lower extremities or the small bones of the hands and feet, local swelling may be detected as the tumor enlarges. In some cases, muscle atrophy or muscle spasm may be present. Marked disability and impaired *mobility* may occur in those with advanced metastatic bone disease.

In performing a musculoskeletal assessment, inspect the involved area and palpate the mass, if possible, for size and tenderness. In collaboration with the physical and occupational therapists, assess the patient's ability to perform *mobility* tasks and ADLs.

In a patient with Ewing sarcoma, a low-grade fever may occur because of the systemic features of the neoplasm. For this reason, it may be confused with osteomyelitis. Fatigue and pallor resulting from anemia are also common.

Patients with malignant bone tumors may be young adults whose productive lives are just beginning. They need strong support systems to help cope with the diagnosis and its treatment. Family, significant others, and health care professionals are major components of the needed support. Determine which systems or resources are available.

Patients often experience a loss of control over their lives when a diagnosis of cancer is made. As a result, they become anxious and fearful about the outcome of their illness. Coping with the diagnosis becomes a challenge. As patients progress through the grieving process, there may be initial denial. Identify the anxiety level and assess the stage or stages of the grieving process. Explore any maladaptive behavior, indicating ineffective coping mechanisms. Chapter 20 further describes the psychosocial assessment for patients with cancer.

Routine x-rays are used to find bone tumors and bone metastasis. CT and MRI are useful for complex anatomic areas, such as the spinal column and sacrum. These tests are particularly helpful in evaluating the extent of soft-tissue involvement. Metastatic lesions may increase or decrease bone density, depending on the amount of osteoblastic and osteoclastic activity.

In some cases a needle bone biopsy may be performed, usually under fluoroscopy to guide the surgeon. Needle biopsy is an ambulatory care procedure with rare complications. After biopsy, the cancer is staged for size and degree of spread. One popular method is the TNM system, based on tumor size and number (T), the presence of cancer cells in lymph nodes (N), and metastasis (spread) to distant sites (M) (see Chapter 19 for further discussion).

The patient with a *malignant* bone tumor typically shows elevated serum alkaline phosphatase (ALP) levels, indicating the body's attempt to form new bone by increasing osteoblastic activity. The patient with Ewing sarcoma or metastatic bone cancer often has anemia and leukocytosis (increased white blood cells). The progression of Ewing sarcoma may be evaluated by elevated serum lactic dehydrogenase (LDH) levels.

In some patients with bone metastasis from the breast, kidney, or lung, the serum calcium level is elevated. Massive bone destruction stimulates release of the mineral into the bloodstream. In patients with Ewing sarcoma and bone metastasis, the erythrocyte sedimentation rate (ESR) may be elevated because of secondary tissue inflammation (Pagana & Pagana, 2018).

◆ Interventions: Take Action

Because *pain* is often due to direct primary tumor invasion, treatment is aimed at reducing the size of or removing the tumor. *Benign* or small primary malignant bone tumors are usually completely removed for a potential cure. The expected outcome of treating *metastatic* bone tumors is palliative rather than curative. Palliative therapies may prevent further bone destruction and improve patient function. A combination of nonsurgical and surgical management is used for bone cancer. Collaborate with members of the interprofessional health care team to plan high-quality care to achieve positive patient outcomes. The following discussion focuses on interventions for patients with malignant bone tumors or metastatic bone cancer.

Nonsurgical Management. In addition to analgesics for local *pain* relief, chemotherapy and radiation therapy are often given to shrink the malignant tumor. For patients with painful metastatic spinal involvement, bracing and short-term immobilization may be appropriate.

The primary health care provider may prescribe *chemotherapy* to be given alone or in combination with radiation or surgery. Certain proliferating tumors, such as Ewing sarcoma, are sensitive to cytotoxic drugs. Others, such as chondrosarcomas, are often totally drug resistant. Chemotherapy seems to work best for small, metastatic tumors and may be administered before or after surgery. In most cases the primary health care provider prescribes a combination of agents. The drugs selected are determined in part by the primary source of the cancer in metastatic disease. For example, when metastasis occurs from breast cancer, estrogen and progesterone blockers may be used. Chapter 20 describes the general nursing care of patients who receive chemotherapy. *Remember that all chemotherapeutic agents are categorized as high-alert medications* (Institute for Safe Medication Practices, 2020).

Other drugs are given for specific metastatic cancers, depending on the location of the primary site. For example, biologic agents, such as cytokines, are given to stimulate the immune system to recognize and destroy cancer cells, especially in patients with renal cancer. Zoledronic acid and pamidronate are two IV bisphosphonates that are approved for bone metastasis from the breast, lung, and prostate (Burchum & Rosenthal, 2019). These drugs help protect bones and prevent fractures. Although rare, inform patients that osteonecrosis of the jaw may also occur, especially in those who have invasive dental procedures. Monitor associated laboratory tests, such as serum creatinine and electrolytes, because these drugs can be toxic to the kidneys and cause acute kidney injury (AKI). Bisphosphonates are described earlier in the Osteoporosis section.

Denosumab is a RANKL inhibitor that is also approved for metastatic bone disease (Burchum & Rosenthal, 2019). The drug binds to a protein that is essential for the formation, function, and survival of osteoclasts. By preventing the protein from activating its receptor, the drug decreases bone loss and increases bone mass and strength.

Radiation therapy, either brachytherapy or external radiation, is used for selected types of malignant tumors. For patients with Ewing sarcoma and early osteosarcoma, radiation may be the treatment of choice in reducing tumor size and thus pain.

For patients with metastatic disease, radiation is given primarily for palliation. The therapy is directed toward the painful sites to provide a better quality of life. One or more treatments are given, depending on the extent of disease. With precise planning, radiation therapy can be used with minimal complications. The general nursing care for patients receiving radiation therapy is described in Chapter 20.

Interventional radiologists can perform several noninvasive procedures to help relieve *pain* in the patient with metastasis to the spinal column. For example, *microwave ablation (MWA)* can be done under moderate sedation or general anesthesia to kill the targeted tissue with heat using microwaves. Most patients have pain relief or control after this ambulatory care procedure.

Surgical Management. Primary malignant bone tumors are usually reduced or removed with surgery, and surgery may be combined with radiation or chemotherapy.

In addition to the nature, progression, and extent of the tumor, the patient's age and general health state are considered. Chemotherapy may be administered before surgery. As for any patient preparing for cancer surgery, the patient with bone cancer needs psychological support from the nurse and other members of the health care team.

👤 PATIENT-CENTERED CARE: CULTURAL/ SPIRITUAL CONSIDERATIONS (QSEN)

Assess the level of the patient's and family's understanding about the surgery and related treatments. Be present to establish a trusting relationship with the patient and be available for listening. As an advocate, encourage the patient and family to discuss concerns and questions and provide information regarding hospital routines and procedures. Provide hope but be realistic and accurate with information. Assess the patient to determine if religious and/ or spiritual support is important. Contact a member of the clergy or a spiritual leader or talk with a clergy member affiliated with the hospital based on the patient's preferences.

Anticipate postoperative needs as much as possible before the patient undergoes surgery. Remind him or her what to expect after surgery and how to help ensure adequate recovery.

Wide or radical resection procedures are used for patients with bone sarcomas to salvage the affected limb. Wide excision is removal of the lesion surrounded by an intact cuff of normal tissue and leads to cure of low-grade tumors only. A radical resection includes removal of the lesion, the entire muscle, bone, and other tissues directly involved. It is the procedure used for high-grade tumors.

Large bone defects that result from tumor removal may require either:

- Total joint replacements with prosthetic implants, either whole or partial
- Custom metallic implants
- Allografts from the iliac crest, rib, or fibula

As an alternative to total replacement, an allograft may be implanted with internal fixation for patients who do not have metastases. This is a common procedure for sarcomas of the proximal femur. Allograft procedures for the knee are also performed, particularly in young adults. Preoperative chemotherapy is given to enhance the likelihood of success. Allografts with adjacent tendons and ligaments are harvested from cadavers and can be frozen or freeze-dried for a prolonged period. The graft is fixed with a series of bolts, screws, or plates.

The surgical incision for a limb salvage procedure is often extensive. A pressure dressing with wound suction is typically maintained for several days. The patient who has undergone a limb salvage procedure has some degree of impaired physical *mobility* and a self-care deficit. The nature and extent of the alterations depend on the location and extent of the surgery.

⚠ NURSING SAFETY PRIORITY (QSEN)

Action Alert

> For patients who have allografts, monitor for signs of hemorrhage, infection, and fracture. After ensuring that the patient is safe, report these complications to the Rapid Response Team or surgeon immediately.

After upper extremity surgery, the patient can engage in active-assistive exercises by using the opposite hand to help achieve motions such as forward flexion and abduction of the shoulder. Continuous passive motion (CPM) using a CPM machine may be initiated as early as the first postoperative day for either upper extremity or lower extremity procedures.

After lower extremity surgery, the emphasis is on strengthening the quadriceps muscles by using passive and active motion when possible. Maintaining muscle tone is an important prerequisite to weight bearing, which progresses from toe touch or partial weight bearing to full weight bearing by 2 to 3 months after surgery. Coordinate the patient's plan of care for ambulation and muscle strengthening with the physical therapist.

The patient who has had a bone graft may have a cast or other supportive device for several months. Weight bearing is prohibited until there is evidence that the graft is incorporated into the adjacent bone tissue.

During the recovery phase, the patient may also need assistance with ADLs, particularly if the surgery involves the upper extremity. Assist if needed but, at the same time, encourage the patient to do as much as possible unaided. Some patients need assistive-adaptive devices for a short period while they are healing. Coordinate the patient's plan of care for promoting independence in ADLs with the occupational therapist.

Surrounding tissues, including nerves and blood vessels, may be removed during surgery. Vascular grafting is common, but the lost nerve(s) is (are) usually not replaced. Assess the neurovascular status of the affected extremity and hand or foot every 1 to 2 hours immediately after surgery. Splinting or casting of the limb may also cause neurovascular compromise and needs to be checked for proper placement.

In addition to needing emotional support to cope with physical disabilities, the patient may need help coping with the surgery and its effects. Help identify available support systems as soon as possible.

As a result of most of the surgical procedures, the patient experiences an altered body image. Suggest ways to minimize cosmetic changes. For example, a lowered shoulder can be covered by a custom-made pad worn under clothing. The patient can cover lower extremity defects with pants.

NCLEX EXAMINATION CHALLENGE 45.2

Physiological Integrity

> The nurse assesses a client recently diagnosed with metastatic vertebral bone cancer. Which intervention is the **priority** when caring for this client?
> A. Consultation with rehabilitative therapy
> B. Referral to hospice care
> C. Drug therapy to manage persistent pain
> D. Oxygen therapy to prevent dyspnea

Care Coordination and Transition Management

Home Care Management. After medical treatment for any type of primary bone tumor, the patient is usually managed at home with follow-up care. Hospice care at home is often needed for patients with metastatic disease. When home support is not available, the patient may be admitted to a long-term care facility for extended or hospice care. Coordinate the patient's transition and continuity of care with the case manager and other interprofessional health team members, depending on the patient's needs.

In collaboration with the occupational therapist, evaluate the patient's home environment for structural barriers that may hinder *mobility.* The patient may be discharged with a cast, walker, crutches, or a wheelchair. Assess his or her support system for availability of assistance if needed.

Accessibility to eating and toileting facilities is essential to promote ADL independence. Because the patient with metastatic disease is susceptible to pathologic fractures, potential hazards that may contribute to falls or injury should be removed.

For the patient receiving intermittent chemotherapy or radiation on an ambulatory care basis, emphasize the importance of keeping appointments. Review the expected side and toxic effects of the drugs with the patient and family. Teach how to treat less serious side effects and when to contact the primary health care provider. If the drugs are administered at home via long-term IV catheter, explain and demonstrate the care involved with daily dressing changes and potential catheter complications. Chapter 15 describes the health teaching required for a patient receiving infusion therapy at home.

If the patient has undergone surgery, he or she has a wound and the potential for impaired *mobility.* Teach the patient, family, and/or significant others how to care for the wound. Help the patient learn how to perform ADLs and mobility activities independently for self-management. Coordinate with the occupational therapist to assist in ADL teaching and provide or recommend assistive and adaptive devices, if necessary. The physical therapist can teach the proper use of any needed ambulatory aids, such as a walker or cane, and routine exercises.

Pain management can be a major challenge, particularly for the patient with metastatic bone disease. Discuss the various options for persistent pain relief, including relaxation and music therapy. Emphasize the importance of techniques that worked during hospitalization. See Chapter 5 for cancer pain assessment and management.

The patient with bone cancer may fear that the malignancy will return. Acknowledge this fear but reinforce confidence in the health care team and medical treatment chosen. Mutually establish realistic outcomes regarding returning to work and participating in recreational activities. Encourage the patient to resume a functional lifestyle but caution that it should be gradual. Certain activities, such as participating in sports, may be prohibited.

Help the patient with advanced metastatic bone disease prepare for death. The nurse and other support personnel assist the patient through the stages of death and dying. Identify resources that can help the patient write a will, visit with distant family members, or do whatever he or she thinks is needed for a peaceful death. Chapter 8 describes end-of-life care in detail.

In addition to family and significant others, cancer support groups are helpful to the patient with bone cancer. Some organizations, such as *I Can Cope,* provide information and emotional

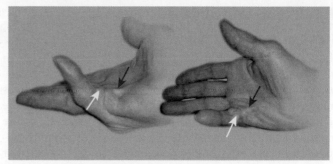

FIG. 45.3 Dupuytren contracture. (Courtesy of School of Medicine, SUNY Stony Brook, NY. In Wolfe, S.W., Hotchkiss, R.N., Pederson, W.C., & Kozin, S.H. [2011]. *Green's operative hand surgery* [6th ed.]. Philadelphia: Churchill Livingstone.)

support. Others, such as *CanSurmount,* are geared more toward patient and family education. The American Cancer Society (www.cancer.org) and the Canadian Cancer Society (www.cancer.ca) can also provide education and resources for patients and families.

DISORDERS OF THE HAND

Specific localized health problems affecting the hand or part of the hand may affect the musculoskeletal system. Two of these problems are discussed here. **Dupuytren contracture or deformity** is a slowly progressive thickening of the palmar fascia, resulting in flexion contracture of the fourth (ring) and fifth (little) fingers of the hand (Fig. 45.3). The third or middle finger is occasionally affected. Although Dupuytren contracture is a common problem, the cause is unknown. It usually occurs in older Euro-American men, tends to occur in families, is most common in people with diabetes, and can be bilateral.

When function becomes impaired, surgical release is required. A partial or selective fasciectomy (cutting of fascia) is performed. After removal of the surgical dressing, a splint may be used. Nursing care is similar to that for the patient with carpal tunnel repair (see Chapter 47).

A **ganglion** is a round, benign cyst, often found on a wrist or foot joint or tendon. The synovium surrounding the tendon degenerates, allowing the tendon sheath tissue to become weak and distended. Ganglia are painless on palpation, but they can cause joint discomfort after prolonged joint use or minor trauma or strain. The lesion can rapidly disappear and then recur. Ganglia are most likely to develop in people between 15 and 50 years of age. With local or regional anesthesia in a primary health care provider's office or clinic, the fluid within the cyst can be aspirated through a small needle. A cortisone injection may follow. If the cyst is very large, it is removed using a small incision. Teach patients to avoid strenuous activity for 48 hours after surgery and report any signs of inflammation to their primary health care provider.

DISORDERS OF THE FOOT

Common Foot Deformities

The **hallux valgus deformity** is a common foot problem in which the great toe drifts laterally at the first metatarsophalangeal (MTP) joint (Fig. 45.4). The first metatarsal head becomes enlarged, resulting in a *bunion*. As the deviation worsens, the bony enlargement causes pain, particularly when shoes are worn. Women are affected more often than men. Hallux valgus often occurs as a result of poorly fitted shoes, in particular those with narrow toes and high heels. Other causes include osteoarthritis, rheumatoid arthritis, foot and ankle surgery, and family history.

For some patients who are of advanced age or are not surgical candidates, custom-made shoes can be made to fit the deformed feet and provide comfort and support. A plaster mold is made to conform to each foot; shoes can be made from these molds. Teach the patient to consult with a podiatrist or foot clinic to be evaluated for custom shoes.

The surgical procedure, a simple **bunionectomy**, involves removal of the bony overgrowth and bursa and realignment to manage *pain.* When other toe deformities accompany the condition or if the bony overgrowth is large, several *osteotomies,* or bone resections, may be performed. Fusions may also be performed. Screws or wires are often inserted to stabilize the bones in the great toe and first metatarsal during the healing process. If both feet are affected, one foot is usually treated at a time. Surgery usually is performed as a same-day procedure. Be sure to assess neurovascular status and pain control before allowing the patient to be discharged.

Most patients are allowed partial weight bearing while wearing an orthopedic boot or shoe. Walking is difficult because the feet bear body weight. The healing time after surgery may be more than 6 to 12 weeks because the feet receive less blood flow than other parts of the body as a result of their distance from the heart.

Often patients have hammertoes and hallux valgus deformities at the same time. As shown in Fig. 45.4, a *hammertoe* is the dorsiflexion of any MTP joint with plantar flexion of the proximal interphalangeal (PIP) joint next to it. The second toe is most often affected. As the deformity worsens, uncomfortable corns may develop on the dorsal side of the toe, and calluses may appear on the plantar surface. Patients are uncomfortable when wearing shoes and walking.

Hammertoe may be treated by surgical correction of the deformity with osteotomies (bone resections) and the insertion of wires or screws for fixation. The postoperative course is similar to that for the patient with hallux valgus repair.

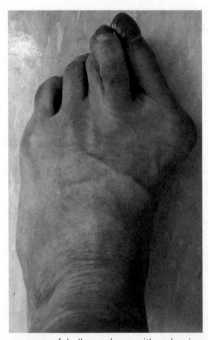

FIG. 45.4 Appearance of hallux valgus with a bunion and hammertoes. (From Federer, A.E., Tainter, D.M., Adams, S.B., & Schweitzer, K.M. [2018]. Conservative management of metatarsalgia and lesser toe deformities. *Foot and Ankle Clinics, 23*[1], 9–20. doi.org/10.1016/j.fcl.2017.09.003.)

NCLEX EXAMINATION CHALLENGE 45.3
Physiological Integrity

The nurse is caring for a client immediately after a bunionectomy. What is the nurse's **priority** action?

A. Relieve or reduce the client's pain.
B. Maintain the client's airway.
C. Assess neurovascular status in the surgical foot.
D. Apply a hot compress to the surgical area.

Plantar Fasciitis

Plantar fasciitis is an inflammation of the plantar fascia, which is located in the area of the arch of the foot. It is often seen in middle-age and older adults, as well as in athletes, especially runners. Obesity is also a contributing factor. Patients report severe *pain* in the arch of the foot, especially when getting out of bed. The pain is worsened with weight bearing. Although most patients have unilateral plantar fasciitis, the problem can affect both feet (McCance et al., 2019).

Most patients respond to conservative management, which includes rest, ice, stretching exercises, strapping of the foot to maintain the arch, shoes with good support, and orthotics. NSAIDs or steroids may be needed to control *pain* and inflammation. If conservative measures are unsuccessful, endoscopic surgery to remove the inflamed tissue may be required. Teach the patient about the importance of adhering to the treatment plan and to follow the physical therapist's instruction regarding exercise.

GET READY FOR THE NEXT-GENERATION NCLEX® EXAMINATION!

Key Points
Review these Key Points for each NCLEX Examination Client Needs Category.

Safe and Effective Care Environment
- Collaborate with interprofessional team members when assessing patients with osteoporosis for risk for falls. **QSEN: Teamwork and Collaboration**
- Teach the patient with *cellular regulation* problems (e.g., osteoporosis) and his or her family about evidence-based home safety modifications and the need to create a hazard-freeenvironment. **QSEN: Safety; Evidence-Based Practice**

Health Promotion and Maintenance
- Develop a teaching plan for patients at risk for osteoporosis to minimize risk factors, such as stopping smoking, decreasing alcohol intake, exercising regularly, and increasing dietary calcium and vitamin D foods. **QSEN: Patient-Centered Care**
- Remind patients at risk for osteoporosis to have regular screening tests, such as the DXA scan, as needed. **QSEN: Evidence-Based Practice; Safety**
- Refer patients with musculoskeletal problems to appropriate community resources, such as the National Osteoporosis Foundation (NOF). **QSEN: Patient-Centered Care**

Psychosocial Integrity
- Assess the patient's and family's responses to a diagnosis of bone disorders and treatment options. Be aware that they may experience fear and require referral. **QSEN: Teamwork and Collaboration**

Physiological Integrity
- Osteoporosis and osteomalacia cause bone loss and fragility fractures (see Table 45.1); recognize that osteoporosis can be primary or secondary (see Table 45.2). **QSEN: Safety**
- Remind patients taking bisphosphonates to take them early in the morning, at least 30 to 60 minutes before breakfast, with a full glass of water, and to remain sitting upright during that time to prevent esophagitis, a common complication of bisphosphonate therapy. **QSEN: Safety**
- Recall that most patients are unaware that they have osteoporosis until they experience a fracture, the most common complication of the disease. **QSEN: Safety**
- Assess for signs and symptoms of osteomyelitis, which differ based on type (acute versus chronic). **QSEN: Patient-Centered Care**
- Use clinical judgment to prioritize care for patients with osteomyelitis, including maintaining Contact Precautions for open wounds. For patients having surgical intervention, assess the affected extremity for neurovascular status to ensure adequate tissue *perfusion.* **Clinical Judgment**
- For patients who have surgery to remove benign or malignant bone tumors, report and document postoperative signs and symptoms of *infection,* dislocation, or neurovascular compromise to the surgeon promptly. **QSEN: Safety; Informatics**
- Remember that severe persistent *pain* is a priority for patients with metastatic bone disease. **QSEN: Patient-Centered Care; Evidence-Based Practice**
- In collaboration with the health care team (physical therapist, occupational therapist, neurologist), provide supportive care for patients with bone cancer to improve *mobility* and function. **QSEN: Teamwork and Collaboration**
- Foot disorders can be treated with custom-made shoes or surgery to repair deformities and promote *mobility.* **QSEN: Evidence-Based Practice; Safety**

MASTERY QUESTIONS

1. The nurse is teaching a client who has osteopenia about alendronate. Which statement by the client indicates a **need for further teaching?**
   A. "I will take this drug at night to prevent nausea."
   B. "I need a dental checkup before taking the drug."
   C. "I need to sit up for 30 minutes after taking the drug."
   D. "I will drink plenty of water after I take the drug."

2. The nurse is caring for a client who was admitted with a draining diabetic ulcer on the lower extremity. What personal protective equipment will the nurse teach the staff to use? **Select all that apply.**
   A. Gown
   B. Gloves
   C. Mask
   D. Foot covers
   E. Goggles

REFERENCES
Burchum, J. L. R., & Rosenthal, L. D. (2019). *Lehne's pharmacology for nursing care* (10th ed.). St. Louis: Elsevier.

Capriotti, T., & Scanlon, M. (2018). Osteoporosis: A clinical update for home healthcare clinicians. *Home Healthcare Now, 36*(4), 216–224.

Evenson, A. L., & Sanders, G. F. (2016). Educational intervention impact on osteoporosis knowledge, health beliefs, self-efficacy, dietary calcium, and vitamin D intakes in young adults. *Orthopaedic Nursing, 35*(1), 30–38.

Institute for Safe Medication Practices. (2020). *ISMPs list of high-alert medications.* www.ismp.org/Tools/highalertmedications.pdf.

Jarvis, C. (2020). *Physical examination & health assessment* (8th ed.). St. Louis: Elsevier Saunders.

McCance, K., Huether, S., Brashers, V., & Rote, N. (2019). *Pathophysiology: The biologic basis for disease in adults and children* (8th ed.). St. Louis: Mosby.

National Osteoporosis Foundation (NOF). (2018). *Clinician's guide to prevention and treatment of osteoporosis*. Washington, DC: Author.

Pagana, K. D., & Pagana, T. J. (2018). *Manual of diagnostic and laboratory tests* (6th ed.). St. Louis: Mosby.

Pagana, K. D., Pagana, T. J., & Pike-MacDonald, S. A. (2019). *Mosby's Canadian manual of diagnostic and laboratory tests* (2nd ed.). Toronto, ON: Elsevier.

Reid, I. R. (2017). Vitamin D effect on bone mineral density and fractures. *Endocrinology and Metabolism Clinics of North America, 46*(4), 935–945.

Touhy, T. A., & Jett, K. F. (2018). *Ebersole and Hess' gerontological nursing and healthy aging* (5th ed.). St. Louis: Elsevier.

Xiaojuan, L., & Schwartz, A. V. (2020). MRI assessment of bone marrow composition in osteoporosis. *Current Osteoporosis Reports, 18*, 57–66.

46

Concepts of Care for Patients With Arthritis and Total Joint Arthroplasty

Donna D. Ignatavicius

http://evolve.elsevier.com/Iggy/

LEARNING OUTCOMES

1. Collaborate with interprofessional team to coordinate high-quality care for patients with arthritis.
2. Use clinical judgment to prioritize collaborative interventions for patients with arthritis to promote *mobility,* reduce *inflammation,* and manage *pain.*
3. Describe the psychosocial impact for patients experiencing arthritis.
4. Teach the patient and caregiver(s) about common drugs used for rheumatoid arthritis (RA), including those used for *immunity* suppression.
5. Plan evidence-based preoperative and postoperative care for the patient having a total hip or knee arthroplasty.
6. Plan care coordination and transition management for patients with arthritis.

KEY TERMS

arthritis Inflammation of one or more joints.

arthrocentesis An invasive diagnostic procedure performed at the bedside or in a primary health care provider's office to aspirate a sample of synovial fluid for analysis and to relieve pressure caused by excess fluid.

arthrofibrosis The buildup of excessive scar tissue that restricts joint motion and functional ability.

crepitus A grating sound caused by loosened bone and cartilage in a synovial joint.

exacerbations Flare-ups of disease (that typically alternate with disease remissions).

gout A systemic disease in which urate crystals (the result of errors in purine metabolism) deposit in joints causing severe joint inflammation.

joint coach A care partner who can help the patient having a total joint arthroplasty through the perioperative period and assist with discharge needs.

joint effusion The presence of excess joint fluid, especially common in the knee.

osteoarthritis The progressive deterioration and loss of articular (joint) cartilage and bone in one or more joints.

osteonecrosis Bone death secondary to lack of or disruption in blood supply to the affected bone, usually from trauma or chronic steroid therapy.

osteophytes Bone spurs caused by irregular bony overgrowth.

paresthesias Burning and tingling sensations, especially in the extremities.

peripheral nerve block (PNB) A single injection or continuous infusion by a portable pump (e.g., continuous femoral nerve blockade or CFNB) to provide regional/local anesthesia during and/or after surgery.

primary arthroplasty First-time joint arthroplasty.

quadriceps-setting exercises ("quad sets") Postoperative exercises designed to decrease the risk of deep vein thrombosis by straightening the legs and pushing the back of the knees into the bed.

regenerative therapies Minimally invasive treatment modalities, such as stem cell therapy and platelet-rich plasma, that are used to repair joint cartilage.

revision arthroplasty An arthroplasty done to replace an implant that has loosened or failed.

Sjögren syndrome A condition in which the patient has dry eyes (keratoconjunctivitis sicca [KCS], or the sicca syndrome), dry mouth (xerostomia), and dry vagina (in some cases). This health problem may occur as a separate condition or be associated with late-stage rheumatoid arthritis or other autoimmune arthritis-related disease.

subcutaneous nodules Soft, round, movable nodules that often occur along the ulnar side of the arm in patients with advanced rheumatoid arthritis.

subluxation Partial joint dislocation.

synovitis Joint inflammation.

total joint arthroplasty (TJA) The surgical creation of a functional (synovial) joint using implants, also sometimes called a *total joint replacement (TJR).*

vasculitis Inflammation of blood vessel walls that can decrease arterial blood flow.

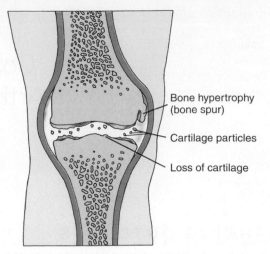

FIG. 46.1 Joint changes in osteoarthritis.

Arthritis means *inflammation* of one or more joints. However, in clinical practice arthritis is categorized as either noninflammatory or inflammatory. Although there are many types of arthritis and diseases in which arthritis occurs as a symptom, the two most common types are osteoarthritis and rheumatoid arthritis and are the focus of this chapter.

The major exemplar for the concept of *mobility* is osteoarthritis (OA), a noninflammatory, localized disorder. The major exemplar for *immunity* is rheumatoid arthritis (RA), a systemic, autoimmune inflammatory disorder. Both of these health problems can cause joint *pain* and stiffness. These priority concepts are reviewed briefly in Chapter 3. Other autoimmune disorders causing arthritis are discussed elsewhere in this text.

✳ MOBILITY CONCEPT EXEMPLAR: OSTEOARTHRITIS

Pathophysiology Review

Osteoarthritis is the most common arthritis and a major cause of impaired *mobility,* persistent *pain,* and disability among adults in the United States and the world. It is sometimes referred to as *osteoarthrosis* or *degenerative joint disease (DJD).*

Osteoarthritis is the progressive deterioration and loss of articular (joint) cartilage and bone in one or more joints. Articular cartilage contains water and a matrix of:
- Proteoglycans (glycoproteins containing chondroitin, keratin sulfate, and other substances)
- Collagen (elastic substance)
- Chondrocytes (cartilage-forming cells)

As people age or experience joint injury, proteoglycans and water decrease in the joint. The production of synovial fluid, which provides joint lubrication and nutrition, also declines because of the decreased synthesis of hyaluronic acid and less body fluid in older adults when compared with younger adults (McCance et al., 2019).

In patients of any age with OA, enzymes such as stromelysin break down the articular matrix. In early disease the cartilage changes from its normal bluish-white, translucent color to an opaque and yellowish-brown appearance. As cartilage and the bone beneath the cartilage begin to erode, the joint space narrows and osteophytes (bone spurs caused by irregular bony overgrowth) form (Fig. 46.1). As the disease progresses, fissures, calcifications, and ulcerations develop and the cartilage thins.

Inflammatory cytokines (enzymes) such as interleukin-1 (IL-1) may enhance this deterioration. The body's normal repair process cannot overcome the rapid process of degeneration (McCance et al., 2019). Secondary joint *inflammation* can occur when joint involvement is severe. Joint inflammation, also called synovitis, is evident when the joint is red, warm, painful, and swollen.

Eventually the cartilage disintegrates, and pieces of bone and cartilage "float" in the diseased joint, causing crepitus, a grating sound caused by the loosened bone and cartilage in a synovial joint. The resulting joint *pain* and stiffness can lead to decreased *mobility* and muscle atrophy. Muscle tissue helps support joints, particularly those that bear weight (e.g., hips, knees).

Etiology and Genetic Risk. The cause of OA is a combination of many factors. For patients with *primary* OA, the disease is caused by aging and genetic factors. Weight-bearing joints (hips and knees), the shoulders, the vertebral column, and the hands are most commonly affected, probably because they are used most often or bear the mechanical stress of body weight and many years of use.

Secondary OA occurs less often than primary disease and can result from joint injury and obesity. Injury to the joints from excessive use, trauma, or other joint disease (e.g., rheumatoid arthritis) predisposes a person to OA. Heavy manual occupations (e.g., carpet laying, construction, farming) cause high-intensity or repetitive stress to the joints. The risk for hip and knee OA is increased in professional and amateur athletes, especially football players, runners, and gymnasts. Fractures or other joint tissue injuries can lead to OA years after the trauma. Certain metabolic diseases (e.g., diabetes mellitus, Paget disease of the bone) and blood disorders (e.g., hemophilia, sickle cell disease) can also cause joint degeneration.

OA occurs in people who are obese much more commonly than in those who are not obese (Arthritis Foundation, 2019). Weight-bearing joints such as hips and knees are most often affected in obese individuals.

Incidence and Prevalence. The prevalence of OA varies among different populations but is a universal problem. Most people older than 60 years have joint changes that can be seen on x-ray examination, although not all of these adults actually develop the disease. According to the Arthritis Foundation (2019) estimates, 31 million people in the United States have symptomatic OA. By 2050, 40 million people worldwide are expected to be severely disabled by OA and 130 million will have the disease (Saccomano, 2018). OA is the fifth most common cause of disability worldwide (Arthritis Foundation, 2019).

PATIENT-CENTERED CARE: GENDER HEALTH CONSIDERATIONS (QSEN)

More men than women younger than 55 years old have OA caused by athletic injuries. After age 55 women have the disease more often than men. Although the cause for this difference is not known, contributing factors may include increased obesity in women after having children and broader hips in women than men (Arthritis Foundation, 2019). Be sure to assess all patients in the hospital or community-based setting, particularly those who are older and obese, for signs and symptoms of OA.

PATIENT-CENTERED CARE: VETERANS HEALTH CONSIDERATIONS (QSEN)

Almost all OA that occurs among the military population is the result of combat injury. OA occurs twice as often among the military who are younger than 40 years of age compared with the general population (Arthritis Foundation, 2019).

Health Promotion and Maintenance. Based on the etiology of OA, teach adults to:

- Maintain proper nutrition to prevent obesity.
- Take care to avoid injuries, especially those that can occur from professional or amateur sports.
- Take adequate work breaks to rest joints in jobs where repetitive motion or joint stress is common.
- Stay active and maintain a healthy lifestyle.

❖ Interprofessional Collaborative Care

◆ Assessment: Recognize Cues

History. Patients with OA usually seek medical attention in ambulatory care settings for their joint pain. However, you will also care for those who have OA as a secondary diagnosis in acute and chronic care facilities. Ask the patient about the course of the disease. Collect information specifically related to OA such as the nature and location of joint pain and how much pain and suffering he or she is experiencing. *Remember that older patients may underreport pain, resulting in inadequate management.* Use a 0-to-10 scale or other assessment tool to assess pain intensity. Chapter 5 discusses pain assessment in detail.

Other questions to ask include:

- If joint stiffness has occurred, where and for how long?
- When and where has any joint swelling occurred?
- How much discomfort are you having?
- How much is your *pain* disrupting your daily life?
- What do you do to control the discomfort, *pain,* or stiffness?
- Do you have any loss of *mobility* or difficulty in performing ADLs?

Because this disease occurs more often in older women, age and gender are important factors for the nursing history. Ask patients about their occupation, nature of work, history of injury (including falls), weight history, and current or previous involvement in sports. A history of obesity is significant, even for those currently within the ideal range for body weight. Document any family history of arthritis. Determine whether the patient has a current or previous medical condition that may cause joint symptoms.

Physical Assessment/Signs and Symptoms. In the early stage of the disease the signs and symptoms of OA may appear similar to those of rheumatoid arthritis (RA) (discussed later in this chapter) or other types of arthritis. The distinction between OA and RA becomes more evident as the disease progresses. Table 46.1 compares the major characteristics of both diseases and their common drug therapy. Some patients have both types of arthritis or an additional type, such as gout. **Gout** is a systemic disease in which urate crystals (the result of errors in purine metabolism) deposit in joints, causing severe joint inflammation. Common joints typically affected are the smaller joints of the body (especially the great toe). This type of arthritis is usually well controlled with drug therapy.

The typical patient with OA is a middle-age or older woman who reports *persistent (chronic) joint **pain** and stiffness.* Early in the course of the disease, these symptoms are relieved after rest or sleep and worsen after extended activity. Later, they may occur with slight motion or even when at rest. Because cartilage has no nerve supply, the ***pain*** is caused by joint and soft-tissue involvement and spasms of the surrounding muscles, or secondary joint ***inflammation.*** During the joint examination the patient may have tenderness on palpation or when putting the joint through range of motion. **Crepitus** (a coarse grating sound caused by loosened bone and cartilage) may be felt or heard as the joint goes through range of motion. One or more joints may be affected. The patient may also report joint stiffness that usually lasts *less than* 30 minutes after a period of inactivity (McCance et al., 2019).

On inspection the joint is often enlarged because of bony hypertrophy (overgrowth) and osteophytes may be present. The joint feels hard on palpation. The presence of ***inflammation*** in patients with OA indicates a secondary synovitis. About half of patients with hand involvement have *Heberden nodes* (bony nodules at the distal interphalangeal [DIP] joints) and *Bouchard nodes* (bony nodules at the proximal interphalangeal [PIP] joints) (Fig. 46.2). Although OA is *not* typically a bilateral, symmetric disease, these large bony nodes appear on both hands, especially in women. The nodes may be painful and red. Some patients experience ***pain*** when developing nodes or when nodes are palpated. These deformities tend to be familial and are often a cosmetic concern to patients.

Joint effusions (excess joint fluid) are common when the knees are inflamed. Observe any *atrophy of skeletal muscle* from disuse. The vicious cycle of the disease discourages the movement of painful joints, which may result in contractures, muscle atrophy, and further ***pain.*** *Loss of function* or decreased ***mobility*** may result, depending on which joints are involved. Hip or knee pain may cause the patient to limp and restrict walking distance.

TABLE 46.1   Differential Features of Rheumatoid Arthritis and Osteoarthritis

Characteristic	Rheumatoid Arthritis	Osteoarthritis
Typical onset (age)	35-45 yr	Older than 60 yr
Gender affected	Female (2-3:1)	Female (2:1)
Risk factors or cause	Autoimmune (genetic basis) Emotional stress (triggers exacerbation) Environmental factors	Aging Genetic factor (possible) Obesity Trauma Occupation
Disease process	Inflammatory	Likely degenerative with secondary *inflammation*
Disease pattern	Bilateral, symmetric, multiple joints Usually affects upper extremities first Distal interphalangeal joints of hands spared Systemic	May be unilateral, single joint Affects weight-bearing joints and hands, spine Metacarpophalangeal joints spared Nonsystemic
Laboratory findings	Elevated rheumatoid factor, antinuclear antibody, and ESR	Normal or slightly elevated ESR
Common drug therapy	NSAIDs (short-term use) Methotrexate Leflunomide Biological response modifiers Other immunosuppressive agents	NSAIDs (short-term use) Acetaminophen Other analgesics

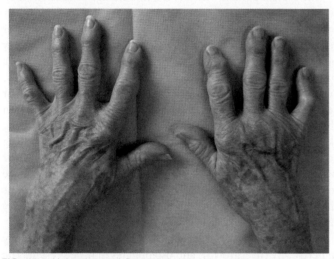

FIG. 46.2 Heberden and Bouchard nodes are enlarged bony nodules affecting the joints of the hand. (From Firestein, G.S., Budd, R.C., Gabriel, S.E., McInnes, I.B., & O'Dell, J.R. [2017]. *Kelley and Firestein's textbook of rheumatology* [10th ed.]. Philadelphia: Elsevier.)

OA can affect the spine, especially the lumbar region at the L3-4 level or the cervical region at C4-6 (neck). Compression of spinal nerve roots may occur as a result of vertebral facet bone spurs. The patient typically reports radiating pain, stiffness, and muscle spasms in one or both extremities (McCance et al., 2019).

Severe *pain* and deformity often interfere with ambulation and self-care. In addition to performing a musculoskeletal assessment, collaborate with the physical and occupational therapists to assess functional ability. Assess the patient's *mobility* and ability to perform ADLs. Chapter 7 describes functional assessment.

Psychosocial Assessment. OA is a chronic condition that may cause permanent changes in lifestyle. An inability to care for oneself in advanced disease can result in role changes and other losses. Persistent *pain* interferes with quality of life, including sexuality. Patients may not have the energy for sexual intercourse or may find positioning uncomfortable.

Patients with continuous *pain* from arthritis may develop depression or anxiety. The patient may also have a role change in the family, workplace, or both. To identify changes that have been or need to be made, ask about his or her roles before the disease developed. Identify coping strategies to help live with the disease. Ask the patient about his or her expectations regarding treatment for OA.

In addition to role changes, joint deformities and bony nodules often alter body image and self-esteem. Observe the patient's response to body changes. Does he or she ignore them or seem overly occupied with them? Ask patients directly how they perceive their body image. Document your assessment findings in the interprofessional health record per agency policy.

Laboratory Assessment. The primary health care provider uses the history and physical examination to make the diagnosis of OA. The results of routine laboratory tests are usually normal but can be helpful in screening for associated conditions. For example, an examination of aspirated joint fluid can show urate crystals, which indicates gout. The erythrocyte sedimentation rate (ESR) and high-sensitivity C-reactive protein (hsCRP) may be slightly elevated when secondary synovitis occurs. The ESR also tends to rise with age and *infection.*

Imaging Assessment. Routine x-rays are useful in determining structural joint changes. Specialized views are obtained when the disease cannot be visualized on standard x-ray film but is suspected. Magnetic resonance imaging (MRI) may be used to determine vertebral or knee involvement.

◆ **Analysis: Analyze Cues and Prioritize Hypotheses.** The priority collaborative problems for patients with osteoarthritis (OA) include:

1. Persistent *pain* due to joint swelling, cartilage deterioration, and/or secondary joint *inflammation*
2. Potential for decreased *mobility* due to joint *pain* and muscle atrophy

◆ **Planning and Implementation:Generate Solutions and Take Action.** In 2010 the Osteoarthritis Research Society International (OARSI) committee updated its evidence-based expert consensus guidelines for patients with knee, hand, and hip OA (Zhang et al., 2010). These interprofessional best practice guidelines remain the most current except for nonsurgical management for OA of the knee, which were updated in 2014 (McAlindon et al., 2014). The OARSI clinical guidelines have major implications for nursing care as described in the following section.

Managing Persistent Pain

Planning: Expected Outcomes. The patient with OA is expected to have a *pain* level that is acceptable to the patient (e.g., at a 3 or less on a pain intensity scale of 0 to 10).

Interventions. No drug therapy can influence the course of OA. Optimal management of patients with OA requires a multimodal approach (combination of therapies) to manage persistent *pain*. Perform a pain assessment before and after implementing interventions (see Chapter 5).

Nonsurgical Management. Management of persistent joint *pain* can be challenging for both the patient and the health care professional. Drug therapy and a variety of nonpharmacologic therapies are used to manage the patient with OA. Chapter 5 elaborates on interventions for persistent noncancer pain.

Drug therapy. The purpose of drug therapy is to reduce *pain* and *inflammation* caused by cartilage destruction, muscle spasm, and/or synovitis. The American Pain Society, American Geriatrics Society, and OARSI committee recommend regular *acetaminophen* as the primary drug of choice because OA is not a primary anti-inflammatory disorder (Burchum & Rosenthal, 2019).

! NURSING SAFETY PRIORITY (QSEN)

Drug Alert

The standard ceiling dose of acetaminophen is 4000 mg each day. However, patients may be at risk for liver damage if they take more than 3000 mg daily, have alcoholism, or have liver disease. *Older adults are particularly at risk because of normal changes of aging such as slowed excretion of drug metabolites.* Remind patients to read the labels of over-the-counter (OTC) or prescription drugs that could contain acetaminophen before taking them. Teach them that their liver enzyme levels may be monitored while taking this drug.

Topical drug applications may help with temporary relief of mild *pain*. Prescription lidocaine 5% patches have been approved by the U.S. Federal Drug Administration (FDA) for postherpetic neuralgia (nerve pain) but may also relieve joint pain (especially the knee) for some patients. Teach the patient to apply the patch on clean, intact skin for 12 hours each day. Up to three patches may be applied to painful joints at one time, but skin irritation may result. Teach the patient that the lidocaine patch is contraindicated in patients taking class I antidysrhythmics. Topical salicylates, such as OTC patches, gels, or creams, are useful for some patients as a temporary pain reliever, especially for knee pain.

If acetaminophen or topical agents do not relieve discomfort, other oral *NSAIDs* may be prescribed if the patient can tolerate them. These traditional drugs supported by OARSI guidelines include oral COX-2 nonselective and selective NSAIDs.

Before beginning oral NSAID therapy, baseline laboratory information is obtained, including a complete blood count (CBC) and complete metabolic panel (CMP). Celecoxib, a COX-2 inhibitor, is the preferred drug choice unless the patient has hypertension, kidney disease, or cardiovascular disease.

! NURSING SAFETY PRIORITY (QSEN)

Drug Alert

All of the COX-2 inhibiting drugs are thought to cause cardiovascular disease, such as myocardial infarction and hypertension, due to vasoconstriction and increased platelet aggregation (clumping). All NSAIDs can cause GI side effects, bleeding, and acute kidney injury if used long term (Burchum & Rosenthal, 2019). Therefore they are prescribed at the lowest effective dose. Remind patients to take celecoxib with food to decrease GI distress. Teach your patient about potential adverse effects and the need to report them to his or her primary health care provider. Examples include having dark, tarry stools; shortness of breath; edema; frequent dyspepsia; hematemesis (bloody vomitus), and changes in urinary output.

Topical NSAIDs are considered to be safer and effective nonsystemic drugs for pain relief. For example, the diclofenac-epolamine patch and diclofenac 1% gel may be used for patients with signs and symptoms associated with knee OA. However, diclofenac has the same two *black box warnings* as other NSAIDs in that they can cause cardiovascular or gastrointestinal adverse effects.

Weak opioid drugs such as tramadol may also be given for patients with OA. This drug should be used with caution in older adults because it can cause acute confusion. Remind any patient not to drive or operate dangerous machinery when taking any type of opioid. Chapter 5 discusses drug therapy for **pain** relief in more detail.

Nonpharmacologic interventions. In addition to analgesics, many nonpharmacologic measures can be used for patients with OA, such as rest balanced with exercise, joint positioning, heat or cold applications, weight control, and a variety of complementary and integrative therapies. Minimally invasive *regenerative therapies,* such as stem cell

NCLEX EXAMINATION CHALLENGE 46.1

Physiological Integrity

The primary health care provider prescribes daily celecoxib for a client experiencing persistent joint pain in both knees. Which health teaching will the nurse provide for the client regarding this drug for long-term pain control?
Select all that apply.
A. "Take the prescribed drug before breakfast each day."
B. "Report any sign of bleeding, including bloody or dark, tarry stool."
C. "Do not take other NSAIDs while on celecoxib."
D. "Report any major changes in the amount of urine you excrete each day."
E. "Follow up with lab tests to assess liver function."

therapy and platelet-rich plasma (PRP), are being used for knee OA to delay surgery. PRP has shown very effective results in treating knee OA because it is rich in growth factor, which stimulates regeneration of knee cartilage, reduces pain, and improves joint function (Mogoi et al., 2019). More studies are needed to provide additional evidence for the use of regenerative therapies in clients who have OA (Zhao et al., 2018).

Teach the patient to *position joints in their functional position.* For example, when in a supine position (recumbent), he or she should use a small pillow under the head or neck but avoid the use of other pillows. The use of large pillows under the knees or head may result in flexion contractures. Remind him or her to use proper posture when standing and sitting to reduce undue strain on the vertebral column. Teach the patient to wear supportive shoes; foot insoles may help relieve pressure on painful metatarsal joints. Collaborate with the physical therapist (PT) to plan a program for muscle-strengthening exercises to better support the joints.

Many patients apply *heat* or *cold* for temporary relief of *pain.* Heat may help decrease the muscle tension around the tender joint and thereby decrease pain and stiffness. Suggest hot showers and baths, hot packs or compresses, and moist heating pads. *Regardless of treatment, teach him or her to check that the heat source is not too heavy or so hot that it causes burns.* A temperature just above body temperature is adequate to promote comfort.

If needed, collaborate with the PT to provide special heat treatments, such as paraffin dips, diathermy (using electrical current), and ultrasonography (using sound waves). A 15- to 20-minute application is usually sufficient to temporarily reduce pain, spasm, and stiffness. Cold packs or gels that feel hot and cold at the same time may also be used.

Cold therapy has limited use for most patients in promoting comfort. Cold works by numbing nerve endings and decreasing secondary joint *inflammation,* if present.

Gradual *weight loss* for obese patients may lessen the stress on weight-bearing joints, decrease *pain,* and perhaps slow joint degeneration. If needed, collaborate with the registered dietitian nutritionist to provide more in-depth teaching and meal planning or make referrals to community resources for weight reduction.

Complementary and integrative health. Some patients with OA report that a variety of integrative therapies are useful.

However, the evidence supporting their effectiveness is often inconsistent and inconclusive.

Topical *capsaicin* products are safe over-the-counter (OTC) drugs. They work by blocking or modifying substance P and other neurotransmitters for *pain.* Tell the patient using capsaicin to expect a burning sensation for a short time after applying it. Recommend the use of plastic gloves for application. To prevent burning of eyes or other body areas, wash hands immediately after applying the substance.

Dietary supplements may complement traditional drug therapies. Glucosamine and chondroitin are widely used and are the most effective nonprescription supplements taken to decrease pain and improve functional ability. However, the evidence to support their use is inconsistent (Arthritis Foundation, 2019). These natural products are found in and around bone cartilage for repair and maintenance. Glucosamine may decrease *inflammation,* and chondroitin may play a role in strengthening cartilage. However, most national medical guidelines do not currently recommend these supplements (Gourdine, 2019).

Medical marijuana (cannabis). Medical marijuana (cannabis) has been used for many years to assist in pain management. Patients with osteoarthritis pain have reported the effectiveness of cannabinoids, and there is a growing body of scientific evidence that supports these reports. Both plant-based and man-made cannabinoids may be effective for pain control (O'Brien & McDougall, 2018).

Surgical Management. Surgery may be indicated when conservative measures and/or drug therapy no longer provide *pain* control, when *mobility* becomes so restricted that the patient cannot participate in activities he or she enjoys, and when he or she cannot maintain the desired quality of life. The most common surgical procedure for OA is **total joint arthroplasty (TJA)** (surgical creation of a functional [synovial] joint using implants), also known as *total joint replacement (TJR).* Almost any synovial joint of the body can be replaced with a prosthetic system that consists of at least two implants—one for each joint surface. The hip and knee are most often replaced, but shoulder and ankle arthroplasties are becoming increasingly common as a result of advances in technology. TJAs are expected to increase as baby boomers age over the next 20 years.

TJA is a procedure used most often to manage the pain of OA and improve *mobility,* although other conditions causing cartilage and bone destruction may require the surgery. These disorders include rheumatoid arthritis (RA), congenital anomalies, trauma, and osteonecrosis (Bodden & Coppola, 2018). Osteonecrosis is bone death secondary to lack of or disruption in blood supply to the affected bone, usually from trauma or chronic steroid therapy. The affected bone site is most commonly the femoral or humeral head, distal femur, and proximal tibia.

The *contraindications* for TJA are active *infection* anywhere in the body and rapidly progressive *inflammation.* An active infection elsewhere in the body or from the joint being replaced can result in an infected TJA and subsequent prosthetic failure. Severe medical problems, such as uncontrolled diabetes or hypertension, put the patient at risk for major postoperative complications and possible death. Therefore these problems should be stabilized before surgery (Hohler, 2018).

Total hip arthroplasty. The number of total hip arthroplasty (THA) procedures (also known as *total hip replacement [THR]*) has steadily increased over the past 40 years. If the patient has a joint replacement for the first time, it is referred to as **primary arthroplasty.** If the implant loosens or fails for any reason, **revision arthroplasty** may be performed to replace the previous one. Availability of improved joint implant materials and better custom design features allow longer life of a THA. Although adult patients of any age can undergo THA, the procedure is performed most often in those older than 60 years. *The special needs and normal physiologic changes of older adults often complicate the perioperative period and may result in additional postoperative complications.*

Preoperative care. As with any surgery, preoperative care begins with assessing the patient's level of understanding about the surgery and his or her ability to participate in the postoperative plan of care. Identifying a **joint coach** (care partner) can help the patient through the perioperative period and assist with discharge needs. The surgeon explains the procedure and postoperative expectations (including possible complications) during the office visit, but this *patient education* may have occurred weeks or months before the scheduled elective surgery. Research is needed to determine the best time for preoperative education (Bodden & Coppola, 2018). Information may be provided in a notebook, pamphlet, DVD format, or online so that the patient can review it at home and share with the joint coach and other family members. This review is particularly useful to patients with inadequate reading skills or poor memory.

PATIENT-CENTERED CARE: CULTURAL/ SPIRITUAL CONSIDERATIONS (QSEN)

Written materials or other media provided in the language appropriate for the patient's educational level and culture are essential. If an interpreter is needed to be sure that the information is understood, one needs to be provided at each appointment, while in the hospital, and when discharged with home or inpatient rehabilitation services.

Preoperative rehabilitation, or "prehab," is essential to prevent functional decline after surgery and provide a quicker functional recovery. As part of prehab, the patient and joint coach learn postoperative exercises, transfer and positioning techniques, and ambulation with a walker or crutches, depending on the patient's age and stability. Other best practices for preoperative patient and family education are summarized in the Patient and Family Education: Preparing for Self-Management: Preoperative Care and Education for Patients Having a Total Hip Arthroplasty box (Bodden & Coppola, 2018).

In addition to the care and patient education outlined in the Patient and Family Education: Preparing for Self-Management box, patients preparing for elective orthopedic surgery may be screened for their risk of postoperative *delirium.* Jones and Taylor (2019) described a quality improvement initiative for identifying delirium risk to anticipate the need for safety sitters to prevent patient falls. Delirium is discussed in Chapter 3 and in mental health textbooks.

PATIENT AND FAMILY EDUCATION: PREPARING FOR SELF-MANAGEMENT

Preoperative Care and Education for Patients Having a Total Hip Arthroplasty

Teaching Area	Health Teaching
Nutrition Assessment	Stress the need for preoperative assessment for clinical malnutrition, which is associated with prolonged postoperative rehabilitation and surgical complications.
	Collaborate with the registered dietitian nutritionist for nutritional assessment.
Pain Assessment and Management	Assess for use of opioids for persistent pain before surgery.
	Teach the patient and joint coach about multimodal pain management options.
Venous Thromboembolism (VTE) Prevention	Teach the need for anticoagulant drug therapy, which should start within 24 hours after surgery and continue for at least 14 days after surgery.
	For patients taking anticoagulants or antiplatelet drugs before surgery, plan for interruption of these drugs for several days before surgery.
	Teach the need for frequent mobilization after surgery; early mobility also helps to prevent constipation.
	Teach the need for compression stockings and/or sequential compression devices during the hospital stay.
Infection Prevention	Teach the patient that he or she will receive an IV antibiotic before surgery and possibly up to 24 hours after surgery.
	Teach the importance of screening for nares (nose) colonization of *Staphylococcus aureus* 2-4 weeks before surgery.
	Teach the need to use nasal mupirocin ointment twice a day for 1 week (or longer depending on the nasal culture) before surgery.
	Teach the need to bathe with chlorhexidine gluconate solution (CHG) for at least the night before and the morning of surgery (a longer period of time may be needed depending on agency or surgeon protocol).
	Teach the patient to sleep on clean linens and not use lotions or powders after the CHG baths; remind the patient to avoid sleeping with pets in the bed.

For patients not at risk for delirium, *Enhanced Recovery After Surgery (ERAS) programs,* also called "fast track," "accelerated track," or "rapid recovery" programs, are common in Total Joint Replacement Centers to improve patient outcomes, such as a shortened hospital length of stay (LOS), improved patient experiences, and enhanced functional outcomes. Patients who participate in this type of program also have fewer hospital readmissions (Bodden & Coppola, 2018).

In addition to usual preoperative laboratory tests and x-rays, the surgeon may ask the patient with RA to have a cervical spine x-ray if he or she is having general anesthesia. Those with RA often have cervical spine disease that can lead to **subluxation** (partial joint dislocation) during intubation. A CT scan and/or MRI may be done to assess the operative joint and surrounding soft tissues, especially if the patient is undergoing a robotic-assisted THA. Chapter 9 discusses general preoperative care in detail.

Operative procedures. Similar to other orthopedic surgeries, the patient receives an *IV antibiotic,* usually a cephalosporin such as cefazolin or cefuroxime, within an hour before the initial surgical incision per the Surgical Care Improvement Project (SCIP) Core Measures to help prevent infection. If the patient has a beta-lactum allergy, vancomycin or clindamycin is administered 2 hours before the initial incision (Bodden & Coppola, 2018).

Several different types of anesthesia are used for THA surgeries and are administered by an anesthesiologist or nurse anesthetist. These options include general anesthesia, neuraxial (spinal or epidural) anesthesia, regional nerve blocks, or a combination of these agents. Patients receiving neuraxial or regional anesthetics may also be given IV moderate sedation to keep them unaware of their environment during the procedure. The benefit of a regional block is that the patient may receive extended **pain** relief, often up to 24 hours after surgery. Chapter 9 describes complications and nursing implications associated with varying types of anesthesia.

For most patients, *tranexamic acid (TXA)* is used to reduce blood loss during the THA surgical procedure. TXA is an antifibrinolytic agent that improves postoperative hemoglobin and hematocrit and decreases the need for blood transfusions (Hohler, 2018). Preventing hypothermia is another important goal during THA surgery because it is associated with increased blood loss, increased risk for infection, and increased risk for a cardiac event. Patients with a low body mass index (BMI) are at the highest risk for hypothermia (Bodden & Coppola, 2018).

Some patients are candidates for *minimally invasive surgery (MIS)* using a small incision (usually 4 inches [10.16 cm] instead of 6 to 12 inches [15.24 to 30.48 cm] for traditional surgery) with special instruments, cameras, and computers to reduce muscle cutting and stretching. This newer technique cannot be used for patients who are obese or those with osteoporosis. It is done only for primary THAs, not for revision surgeries. Like those of any MIS, the benefits of minimally invasive THA are decreased soft tissue damage, blood loss, and postoperative **pain.** Patients usually have a shorter hospital stay and quicker recovery. They are generally satisfied with the cosmetic appearance of the incision because there is less scarring. Postoperative complications are not as common in patients having minimally invasive ("mini") hip arthroplasty compared with those having the traditional technique.

Hip resurfacing is an alternative to total hip replacement surgery. This procedure is most often performed for younger patients or for those with early-stage cartilage loss of the weight-bearing surface of the femoral head. Instead of completely removing the femoral head and inserting the stem into the femoral canal, the surgeon removes the cartilage from the surface and an artificial cap is placed over the existing natural femoral head.

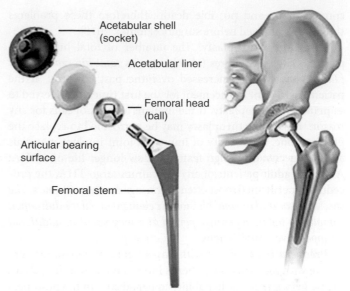

Acetabular shell (socket)

Acetabular liner

Femoral head (ball)

Articular bearing surface

Femoral stem

FIG. 46.3 Two major components of total hip arthroplasty. (From Zhang, Y., Zhu, J., Wang, Z., Zhou, Y., & Zhang, X. [2015]. Constructing a 3D-printable, bioceramic sheathed articular spacer assembly for infected hip arthroplasty. *Journal of Medical Hypotheses and Ideas, 9*[1], 13–19.)

Two components are used in the THA—the acetabular implant and the femoral implant (Fig. 46.3). A noncemented prosthesis is commonly used for younger patients. Bone surfaces are smoothed as they are prepared to receive the artificial implants. The noncemented components are press-fitted into the prepared bone. The acetabular cup may be placed using computer- or robotic-assisted guidance. For cemented prostheses, polymethyl methacrylate (an acrylic fixating substance) is typically used. It often contains an antibiotic to reduce the risk of **infection.** The hybrid surgical technique usually involves a cemented femoral component and a noncemented acetabular component. A closed wound drainage system is not commonly used today for a THA because it can contribute to increased blood loss and cause hematoma formation (Bodden & Coppola, 2018). A surgical pressure dressing is applied before the patient is discharged to the postanesthesia care unit (PACU).

Considerations of a noncemented prosthesis include protection of weight-bearing status to allow bone to grow into the prosthesis and decreased problems with loosening of the prosthesis. With a cemented prosthesis, cement can fracture or deteriorate over time, leading to loosening of the prosthesis. These problems cause **pain** and can lead to the need for a revision arthroplasty. In revision arthroplasty the old prosthesis is removed and new implants are placed. Bone graft may be added if bone loss is significant. Outcomes from revision arthroplasty may not be as positive as with primary arthroplasty, particularly for obese patients.

Three surgical approaches are commonly used to perform a THA. Nursing care and patient education differ slightly depending on which approach is used. Be sure to confirm the surgeon's surgical method for each patient. For the *anterior approach,* the hip joint can be exposed without detaching surrounding muscles. Therefore this approach has the least likely chance of postoperative hip dislocation and may have the quickest postoperative recovery.

Both of the other surgical methods, *direct lateral* and *posterolateral approaches,* require detaching and/or cutting into large skeletal muscles, which can cause severe postoperative *pain* and a high risk for hip dislocation. The posterolateral approach has the highest risk for dislocation and is therefore used less commonly today (Hohler, 2018).

Postoperative care. The typical hospital stay for the patient having a traditional THA is 3 days unless the patient participates in an ERAS program. Some younger patients only stay in the hospital overnight. The goal for rapid recovery programs is for the patients to have same-day THA surgery.

In addition to providing the routine postoperative care discussed in Chapter 9, assess for and help prevent possible postoperative complications. One of the most common complications after a THA is hip dislocation. Other complications include venous thromboembolism, *infection,* and complications of decreased *mobility.*

Preventing Hip Dislocation. As described earlier, the risk for hip dislocation depends on the operative approach used by the surgeon.

⚠ NURSING SAFETY PRIORITY (QSEN)

Action Alert

Teach patients to maintain correct positioning of the hip joint and leg at all times. When the patient returns from the postanesthesia care unit (PACU), place him or her in a supine position with the head slightly elevated. One or two regular bed pillows are used in most cases to remind patients to keep their legs abducted if they had one of the two lateral surgical approaches. *For abduction devices with straps, be sure to loosen the straps every 2 hours and check the patient's skin for irritation or breakdown.* Place and support the affected leg in neutral rotation. The procedure for postoperative turning is not universal and is specified by agency policy or surgeon preference. Turning the patient to the operative side provides "splinting" of the operative hip but may be too painful for some patients. If the patient is turned to the nonoperative side, the operative leg needs to be fully supported with pillows to prevent slipping of the leg into an adducted position that can lead to dislocation. Teach the patient and family about other precautions to prevent hip dislocation.

Older adults may have difficulty understanding health teaching because they often become acutely confused after a THA as a result of surgery, anesthesia, and/or unfamiliar environments. The Patient Centered Care: Older Adult Considerations: Special Postoperative Care of the Older Adult With a Total Hip Arthroplasty box highlights special nursing care of older adults in the postoperative period.

Observe the patient carefully for signs and symptoms of hip dislocation, including report of sudden intense *pain* or sudden agitation for the patient who is unable to communicate, affected leg rotation, and/or leg shortening. If the surgical hip becomes dislocated, the surgeon may be able to manipulate and relocate it after the patient receives moderate sedation. If the hip does not reduce into position, the patient may have surgical reduction in the operating room (OR). Following reduction, the hip is usually immobilized by an abduction splint or other device until healing occurs—usually in about 6 weeks.

👤 PATIENT-CENTERED CARE: OLDER ADULT CONSIDERATIONS (QSEN)

Special Postoperative Care of the Older Adult With a Total Hip Arthroplasty

- For patients who had a *posterolateral or direct lateral surgical approach,* use an abduction pillow or splint (rather than bed pillows) to keep their legs apart and prevent adduction, especially if the patient is very restless or has an altered mental state. Hip adduction can cause the surgical hip to become partially or completely dislocated.
- Keep the patient's heels off the bed to prevent pressure injuries.
- Do not rely on fever as a sign of *infection;* older patients often have infection without fever. Be alert to decreasing mental status and/or elevated white blood cell count as indicators of infection.
- When assisting the patient out of bed, move him or her slowly to prevent orthostatic (postural) hypotension. Allow the patient to sit on the side of the bed for a brief period of time before standing; have him or her stand for a brief period before beginning ambulation.
- Encourage the patient to deep breathe and cough and to use the incentive spirometer every 2 hours to prevent atelectasis and pneumonia.
- As soon as permitted, get the patient out of bed to a recliner chair to prevent complications of decreased *mobility.*
- Anticipate the patient's need for pain medication, especially if he or she cannot verbalize the need for *pain* control. For patients on a multimodal pain protocol, assess the need to medicate for breakthrough pain (see Chapter 5).
- Expect a temporary change in mental state immediately after surgery as a result of the anesthetic and unfamiliar sensory stimuli. Reorient the patient frequently.

⚠ NURSING SAFETY PRIORITY (QSEN)

Action Alert

As with other musculoskeletal surgery, *monitor neurovascular assessments* frequently for a possible compromise in circulation to the affected distal extremity following a THA. Check and document color, temperature, distal pulses, capillary refill, movement, and sensation. The procedure for performing a thorough lower-extremity neurovascular assessment is described in detail in Chapter 44. Remember to compare the operative leg with the nonoperative leg. These assessments are performed at the same time the vital signs are checked. Report any changes in neurovascular assessment to the surgeon and carefully monitor for changes. Early detection of changes in neurovascular status can prevent permanent tissue damage.

Preventing Postoperative Complications. The most potentially life-threatening and commonly occurring complication after THA is venous thromboembolism (VTE), which includes deep venous thrombosis (DVT) and pulmonary embolism (PE). *Older patients are especially at increased risk for VTE because of age and decreased circulation before surgery. Obese patients, patients who currently smoke, and those with a history of VTE are also at high risk for thrombi.*

Preventive evidence-based postoperative interventions include a combination of *p*harmacology, *a*mbulation, and *c*ompression (PAC) (Tubog, 2019; Wilson et al., 2018). *Anticoagulants* such as subcutaneous low-molecular-weight heparin (LMWH) or factor Xa inhibitors are effective drugs in preventing VTE to patients having a THA. Patients are usually on anticoagulants for 10 days to several weeks after surgery, depending on surgeon preference and the patient's response and risk factors.

The use of subcutaneous LMWH, such as enoxaparin and dalteparin, is common for patients with total hip or knee arthroplasty. As an alternative to LMWH, subcutaneous fondaparinux, a factor Xa inhibiting agent, may be prescribed for some patients undergoing these surgeries. A newer Xa inhibitor, rivaroxaban, can be given orally once a day. Recently oral apixaban has received FDA approval for VTE prophylaxis in patients having a THA. You do not need to monitor the PT or INR for patients receiving these drugs because they do not affect coagulation values. However, for other older anticoagulants such as warfarin, patients are at risk for bleeding due to impaired *clotting.* A complete discussion of nursing care associated with patients taking anticoagulants is found in Chapter 33.

Early *ambulation* and exercise also help prevent VTE. Wilson et al. (2018) reported the results of establishing best practices for VTE prevention, which included a requirement for ambulation at least three times a day for all patients who were allowed to be out of bed. Teach the patient about leg exercises, which should begin in the immediate postoperative period and continue through the rehabilitation period. These exercises include plantar flexion and dorsiflexion (heel pumping), circumduction (circles) of the feet, gluteal and quadriceps muscle setting, and straight-leg raises (SLRs). Teach the patient to perform gluteal exercises by pushing the heels into the bed and achieve quadriceps-setting exercises ("quad sets") by straightening the legs and pushing the back of the knees into the bed. In addition to preventing clots, these exercises improve muscle tone, which helps restore the function of the extremity.

Intermittent pneumatic *compression* devices, also called bilateral sequential compression devices (SCDs), are also important in preventing VTE by increasing venous blood flow during periods of inactivity (Wilson et al., 2018). However, clients often report that these devices are hot and bulky to wear, which affects their willingness to use them. Some surgeons prescribe antiembolism stockings, which are not as effective but are more widely accepted by clients.

Monitor the surgical incision and vital signs carefully—every 4 hours for the first 24 hours and every 8 to 12 hours thereafter, following facility and surgeon protocols. Observe for signs of *infection,* such as an elevated temperature, increased redness around the incision, and excessive or foul-smelling drainage from the incision. These signs and symptoms may be seen as early as 2 to 3 days after surgery. *An older patient may not have a fever with infection but instead may experience an altered mental state, especially delirium.* If you suspect this problem, obtain a sample of any drainage for culture and sensitivity to determine the causative organisms and the antibiotics that may be needed for treatment.

Managing Postoperative Pain. Although hip arthroplasty is performed to relieve joint *pain,* patients experience varying levels of pain related to the surgical procedure. Pain control

protocols vary, depending on the region of the country, anesthesiologist/nurse anesthetist, and surgeon. Many patients equate pain control with opioids (Morland, 2019). However, in view of the opioid crisis, a *multimodal pain management* approach is best practice for patients having a major joint arthroplasty.

Immediate pain control may be achieved by short-term patient-controlled analgesia (PCA), or IV push, typically with morphine or hydromorphone. Pizzi et al. (2020) demonstrated that oral patient-controlled analgesia with oxycodone is effective in managing pain for patients having total joint arthroplasty. Nonopioid drugs are used as part of the multimodal analgesic approach because they act at different pain receptor sites. Examples of these drugs include (Bodden & Coppola, 2018; Goode et al., 2019):

- Continuous peripheral nerve block (e.g., bupivacaine, ropivacaine)
- NSAIDs (e.g., ketorolac, celecoxib)
- NMDA receptor antagonists (e.g., ketamine)
- Gabapentinoids (e.g., gabapentin, pregabalin)

Chapter 5 contains information on the nursing care associated with these medications.

Nonpharmacologic methods for acute and chronic pain control, such as cryotherapy and music therapy, can also be used to decrease the amount of drug therapy used. Chapter 5 describes these methods in detail. Also see the Evidence-Based Practice box in the section on total knee arthroplasty (TKA) later in this chapter.

Promoting Postoperative Mobility and Activity. Depending on the time of day that the surgery is performed, the patient with a THA gets out of bed with assistance the night of surgery to prevent problems related to decreased *mobility* (e.g., atelectasis, pneumonia), especially in older adults.

❗ NURSING SAFETY PRIORITY (QSEN)

Action Alert

Be sure to assist the patient the first time he or she gets out of bed to prevent falls and observe for dizziness. When getting the patient out of bed, put a gait belt on him or her and then stand on the same side of the bed as the affected leg. After the patient sits on the side of the bed, remind him or her to stand on the unaffected leg and pivot to the chair with guidance. *To avoid injury, do not lift the patient!*

The surgeon, type of prosthesis, and surgical procedure determine the amount of weight bearing that can be applied to the affected leg. A patient with a cemented implant is usually allowed immediate weight bearing as tolerated (WBAT). Typically only "toe-touch" or minimal weight bearing is initially permitted for patients with noncemented prostheses. When x-ray evidence of bony ingrowth can be seen, the patient can progress to partial weight bearing (PWB) and then to full weight bearing (FWB) over a period of weeks.

In collaboration with the physical therapist (PT), teach the patient how to follow weight-bearing restrictions. Most patients use a walker, but younger adults may use crutches. They are usually advanced to a single cane or crutch if they can walk without a severe limp 4 to 6 weeks after surgery. When the limp disappears, they no longer need an ambulatory/assistive device and may be permitted to sit in chairs of normal height, use regular toilets, and drive a car. Timing of driving may be slightly longer in a patient who has had surgery on the right hip because of patient safety concerns.

NCLEX EXAMINATION CHALLENGE 46.2

Physiological Integrity

A client had a left noncemented posterolateral total hip arthroplasty 2 days ago. Which statements will the nurse include in health teaching for the client?
Select all that apply.
A. "Practice leg exercises each day as instructed."
B. "Take deep breaths and use incentive spirometry every 2 hours."
C. "Be sure to cross your legs to be more comfortable in a chair."
D. "Report sudden increased hip pain or rotation immediately to the nurse."
E. "Stand on your right leg and pivot into the chair when getting out of bed."

Promoting Postoperative Self Management. With the increase in ERAS programs that emphasize a structured approach and rapid recovery, the length of stay in the acute care hospital is typically less than 3 days if there are no postoperative complications. McCann-Spry et al. (2016) reported a quality improvement project in which the patient's length of stay was reduced to 2.5 days for a 2-night stay rather than the typical 3-night stay (see the Systems Thinking and Quality Improvement box). Patients experiencing postoperative complications often stay longer. Medicare patients need a 3-day qualifying hospital stay to receive rehabilitation in a skilled inpatient unit. Discharge from the acute care facility may be to the home, a rehabilitation unit, a transitional care unit, or a skilled unit or long-term care facility for continued rehabilitation before discharge to home. The interprofessional team provides written instructions for posthospital care and reviews them with patients and their joint coaches. Be sure to provide a copy of these instructions for the patient.

Acute rehabilitation usually takes several weeks, depending on the patient's age and progress and the type of prosthesis used. However, it often takes 6 weeks or longer for complete recovery. Patients who are discharged to their home are able to attend physical therapy sessions in an office or ambulatory care setting. Others have no means or cannot use community resources and need physical therapy in the home, depending on their health insurance coverage. *Collaborate with the case manager to determine which option is best for your patient.* The Patient and Family Education: Preparing for Self-Management: Care of Patients With Total Hip Arthroplasty After Hospital Discharge box outlines the most important health teaching for you to provide to the patient being discharged after a THA.

SYSTEMS THINKING AND QUALITY IMPROVEMENT (QSEN)

Can Hospital Length of Stay Be Shortened for Patients Having Joint Replacements?

McCann-Spry, L., Pelton, J., Grandy, G., & Newell, D. (2016). An interdisciplinary approach to reducing length of stay in joint replacement patients. *Orthopaedic Nursing, 35*(5), 279–300.

Demand for total joint replacement surgeries is increasing as baby boomers become older adults. One large hospital in a northern U.S. state developed a process for decreasing postoperative hospital length of stay (LOS) using an interprofessional collaborative approach. Four interventions were implemented: (1) improve communication for primary health care providers (surgeons), including a letter explaining the goal of reducing LOS from 3 nights to 2 nights; (2) develop a script for staff conversations with the patient and family for each hospital day; (3) standardize the risk assessment and prediction for reducing LOS; and (4) initiate physical therapy the day of surgery. As a result of this quality improvement project, patient LOS was reduced an average of 0.5 days per patient for primary hip and knee replacement surgeries. This reduction was very cost-effective without negatively affecting patient and family satisfaction.

Commentary: Implications for Research and Practice

This QI project was very successful at improving financial outcomes and increasing collaboration and communication among interprofessional health care team members and improving staff-patient communication. Nurses play a major role in care coordination and discharge teaching for patients and their families. More QI projects and interventions are needed in additional joint replacement centers to achieve these positive outcomes and promote systems thinking.

Hospital readmission after THA. The most common complications of THA surgery that cause readmission to the hospital include thromboembolic problems, such as DVT and stroke; surgical site infection (SSI); and systemic infections, including pneumonia and sepsis. Men of advanced age and those with comorbidities, such as heart failure and diabetes, are at the highest risk for hospital re-admission after a THA (Bodden & Coppola, 2018).

Total knee arthroplasty. As the population ages, more adults are undergoing total knee arthroplasty (TKA, also known as *total knee replacement [TKR]*). The increased demand for TKA in the United States is due to the osteoarthritis and obesity, a contributing factor to OA in weight-bearing joints. Osteoarthritis is discussed earlier in this chapter. Patients who have rheumatoid arthritis or posttraumatic arthritis caused by a physical injury may also need a TKA (Mori & Ribsam, 2018). Similar to the THA, patients who experience a failed primary TKA have **revision arthroplasty.**

TKAs are most often performed as unilateral procedures, meaning that *one* knee is replaced during surgery. However, a growing number of patients chose to have *both* knees done at one time or within 3 months of each other. This procedure is referred to as bilateral total knee arthroplasty (BTKA). BTKA is sometimes done for patients who have moderate to severe arthritis in both knees. Two types of BTKA may be performed—a one-stage or two-stage procedure. In a one-stage procedure, both knees are replaced during the same surgery. This surgery is most

PATIENT AND FAMILY EDUCATION: PREPARING FOR SELF-MANAGEMENT

Care of Patients With Total Hip Arthroplasty After Hospital Discharge

Hip Precautions
- Do not sit or stand for prolonged periods.
- Do not cross your legs beyond the midline of your body.
- For *posterolateral or direct lateral surgical approach* patients: Do not bend your hips more than 90 degrees.
- For *anterior surgical approach* patients: Do not hyperextend your operative leg behind you.
- Do not twist your body when standing.
- Use the prescribed ambulatory aid such as a walker when walking.
- Use assistive/adaptive devices as needed (e.g., sock aids, shoehorns, dressing sticks, extenders [also see Chapter 7]).
- Do not put more weight on your affected leg than allowed and instructed.
- Call 911 if you experience any signs and symptoms of hip dislocation, including sudden difficulty bearing weight on the surgical leg, leg shortening or rotation, or a feeling that the hip has "popped" with immediate intense **pain.**
- Resume sexual intercourse as usual on the advice of your surgeon.

Pain Management
- Report increased hip or anterior thigh pain to the surgeon immediately.
- Take oral analgesics as prescribed and only as needed.
- Do not overexert yourself; take frequent rests.
- Use ice as needed to operative hip to decrease or prevent swelling and minimize pain.

Incisional Care
- Follow the instructions provided regarding dressing changes, if needed. Some surgeons use specialty clear dressings that do not need to be changed. No dressing may be needed if a skin sealant was used.
- Inspect your hip incision every day for redness, heat, or drainage; if any of these are present, call your surgeon immediately.
- Do not bathe the incision or apply anything directly to the incision unless instructed to do so. Shower according to the surgeon's instructions.

Other Care
- Continue walking and performing the leg exercises as you learned them in the hospital. Do not increase the amount of activity unless instructed to do so by the therapist or surgeon.
- Do not cross your legs to help prevent blood clots.
- Report pain, redness, or swelling in your legs to your surgeon immediately.
- Call 911 for acute chest pain or shortness of breath (could indicate pulmonary embolus).
- If you are taking an anticoagulant, follow the precautions learned in the hospital to prevent bleeding; avoid using a straight razor, avoid injuries, and report bleeding or excessive bruising to your surgeon immediately.
- Be sure to follow up with outpatient physical therapy for your exercise and ambulation program to build strength, **mobility,** and endurance.
- Follow up with visits to the surgeon's office as instructed.

commonly performed for *younger* patients. In a two-stage procedure, two surgeries are done either during the same hospital stay or within 3 months of each other (Pietsch et al., 2018).

Partial knee replacements are used for patients with minimal cartilage loss in specified areas of the involved knee and are typically done more often in younger patients. Minimally invasive surgery (MIS) is also an option for either partial or total knee arthroplasty for this population. Severe bone loss, obesity, and previous knee surgeries are contraindications for this type of surgery. Patients who have MIS procedures have less **pain** and blood loss and greater range of motion to promote a faster postoperative recovery.

Preoperative care. TKA is performed when joint **pain** can no longer be managed by conservative measures. When limited **mobility** severely prevents patients from participating in work or activities they enjoy, this procedure can restore a high quality of life. The preoperative care and teaching for patients undergoing a TKA are similar to that for THA. However, precautions for positioning are not the same because joint dislocation is not a common complication. Differences in patient and family teaching depend on the procedure used by the orthopedic surgeon and established best practices.

The use of Enhanced Recovery After Surgery (ERAS) programs for many types of surgery has improved outcomes for patients having a TKA. As part of this program, patients have a screening to determine their *nutritional status,* including identifying those who are malnourished and/or obese. Obesity is linked to health problems, such as heart disease, diabetes, hypertension, and stroke, and can impair bone and wound healing. Patients who have had bariatric surgery may have chronic anemia and bone loss due to insufficient nutrients. Bone health is a concern for adults of any age who have a history of bariatric surgery (Chicoski, 2018). Chapter 55 discusses obesity and bariatric surgery in detail.

Planning for postdischarge *transitions of care* begins before surgery, including identifying a **joint coach** (care partner) who plays an active role in patient care through the perioperative care (Mori & Ribsam, 2018). *Preoperative rehabilitation* ("prehab") is important to enhance functional ability and provide a quicker postoperative recovery. All patients are given verbal and either written or video preoperative instructions, which include the activity protocol to follow after surgery. The PT and OT provide information about transfers, ambulation, postoperative exercises, and ADL assistance. Patients should practice walking with walkers or crutches to prepare them for ambulation after TKA. Teach patients about the possible need for assistive/adaptive devices to assist with ADLs, including an elevated toilet seat, safety handrails, and dressing devices like a long-handled shoehorn. Some third-party payers may cover these devices, depending on the patient's condition and age. Teach the patient and family how and where this equipment can be obtained to have it available after surgery. Case managers or social workers may arrange for needed items to be delivered to the patient's room before discharge.

A *pain management* assessment and plan before surgery are essential to promote a satisfactory postoperative patient experience. Patients with persistent preoperative pain may have mental health problems, such as anxiety, depression, and/or substance use disorder. Some patients have been treated with long-term analgesics, including opioids, for many years before surgery. These factors place patients having major joint arthroplasty at high risk for severe postoperative pain that can be challenging to manage (Mori & Ribsam, 2018; Jackman, 2019).

Best practices for postoperative management of persistent pain patients include to (Jackman, 2019):

- Identify at-risk patients preoperatively.
- Establish trust and discuss the postoperative pain management plan.
- Perform a comprehensive preoperative and postoperative assessment of pain and reassessment.
- Use multimodal and alternative pain management modalities.
- Consult the pain management team if needed and available.
- Manage mental health/psychological disorders that may be present.
- Plan continuing pain management for and after discharge.

Teach patients that they will need to shower with a chlorhexidine gluconate (CHG) body wash the night before and the morning of surgery to decrease bacteria on the skin that could cause *infection.* Remind them to wear clean nightwear, sleep on clean linen, and avoid having pets in their bed. All patients having a TKA should be treated for at least a week with nasal mupirocin ointment to prevent surgical site infection from *Staphylococcus aureus* (Mori & Ribsam, 2018).

Ask patients to check with their surgeon about which drugs they can take the morning of surgery with a small amount of water, including antihypertensives, thyroid hormone supplements, and antidiabetic agents. Some drugs, such as NSAIDs and anticoagulant/antiplatelets, are discontinued 5 to 10 days before surgery to prevent surgical bleeding. See Chapter 9 for additional general preoperative care interventions and teaching.

Operative procedures. As with the hip, the knee can be replaced with the patient under a variety of anesthetic agents, including general or neuraxial (epidural or spinal) anesthesia. One of the more recent advances in postoperative pain management for TKA is the use of a **peripheral nerve block (PNB),** most commonly a femoral nerve block (FNB) using a local anesthetic. An IV moderate sedation agent is used in addition to the neuraxial or PNB drug. PNB may be either a single injection or continuous infusion by a portable pump (e.g., continuous femoral nerve blockade or CFNB). In addition, other local medications may be injected into the knee or surrounding tissues to assist in the reduction of severe pain that usually occurs after knee surgery and to minimize perioperative bleeding. Sasse et al. (2020) reported that adding a ketorolac periarticular injection decreased pain and improved postoperative mobility for patients having a TKS.

An antibiotic, usually an IV cephalosporin (cefazolin or cefuroxime), is given within 60 minutes before the surgical incision and proximal tourniquet inflation per the SCIP Core Measures to aid in the prevention of *infection.* If giving a fluoroquinolone or vancomycin, the infusion should begin 2 hours (120 minutes) before the incision and tourniquet inflation (Mori & Ribsam, 2018). In the *traditional surgery,* the surgeon makes a central longitudinal incision about 6 to 8 inches (15.24 to 20.32 cm) long. Osteotomies of the femoral and tibial condyles and of the posterior patella are performed, and the surfaces are prepared for the prosthesis. The femoral prosthesis is often noncemented (using a press-fit) with the tibial component being cemented.

Total knee arthroplasties require multiple bone incisions and extensive soft tissue involvement, which can result in significant blood loss. Interventions that may reduce blood loss include:

- Tourniquet use during surgery
- Surgical drains (used less commonly today)
- Fibrin sealants
- Transexamic acid (TXA), an antifibrinolytic agent

While these interventions may be effective, most of them also have disadvantages. For example, using an operative tourniquet can increase postoperative pain. The strongest evidence supports TXA use during surgery for blood loss reduction (Mori & Ribsam, 2018). This drug improves postoperative hemoglobin and hematocrit and decreases the need for blood transfusions. The surgeon also applies a compression (pressure) dressing from the toes to the thigh to decrease edema and bleeding.

Minimally invasive TKA may be performed using a shorter incision and special instruments to spare muscle and other soft tissue. Computer-guided or robotic equipment may be used to ensure accurate positioning of the knee implants.

Postoperative care. Provide the usual postoperative care needed for any patient who has surgery (see Chapter 9). Specific nursing care of the patient with a TKA is similar to that for the patient with a total hip arthroplasty as described in the previous section.

! NURSING SAFETY PRIORITY **QSEN**

Critical Rescue

If the patient has a continuous femoral nerve blockade (CFNB), perform and document neurovascular assessment every 2 to 4 hours, or according to hospital protocol. Be sure that patients can perform dorsiflexion and plantar flexion motions of the affected foot without pain in the lower leg. In addition, monitor these patients for signs and symptoms that indicate absorption of the local anesthetic into the patient's system, including:

- Metallic taste
- Tinnitus
- Nervousness
- Slurred speech
- Bradycardia
- Hypotension
- Decreased respirations
- Seizures

Document and report these new-onset signs and symptoms to the surgeon, anesthesiologist/nurse anesthetist, or Rapid Response Team immediately and carefully continue to monitor the patient for any changes.

Since joint dislocation is rare after TKA, there are no special positioning precautions required to prevent adduction. Maintain the operative leg in a neutral position, avoiding both internal and external rotation. Do not place a pillow under the replaced knee or hyperextend the knee.

Although not as commonly used today, the surgeon may prescribe a continuous passive motion (CPM) machine, which can be applied in the postanesthesia care unit (PACU) or soon after the patient is admitted to the postoperative unit (Fig. 46.4). For some patients, the CPM is prescribed for home use after the patient is discharged. The CPM machine keeps the prosthetic knee in motion

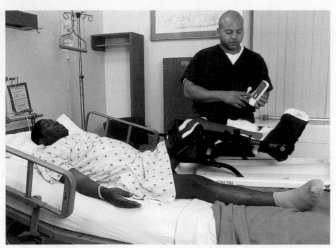

FIG. 46.4 A continuous passive motion (CPM) machine in use.

BEST PRACTICE FOR PATIENT SAFETY & QUALITY CARE (QSEN)

The Patient Using a Continuous Passive Motion (CPM) Machine

- Ensure that the machine is well padded.
- Check the cycle and range-of-motion settings at least once every 8 hours.
- Ensure that the joint being moved is properly positioned on the machine.
- If the patient is confused, place the controls to the machine out of his or her reach.
- Assess the patient's response to the machine.
- Turn off the machine while the patient is having a meal in bed.
- When the machine is not in use, do not store it on the floor.

EVIDENCE-BASED PRACTICE (QSEN)

Is Music Therapy Effective to Promote Comfort for Patients Having a Total Joint Arthroplasty?

Gallagher, L.M., Gardner, V., Bates, D., Mason, S., Nemecek, J., DiFiore, D.B., et al. (2018). Impact of music therapy on hospitalized patients post-elective orthopaedic surgery: A randomized controlled trial. *Orthopaedic Nursing, 37*(2), 124-135.

The purpose of this randomized controlled study was to determine the impact of music therapy (MT) sessions on promoting comfort for patients who had total joint arthroplasty. Comfort outcomes included pain, mood, nausea, anxiety, and use of opioids. Data on hospital length of stay were also collected. The majority of the 163 subjects had either hip or knee arthroplasties and were randomly assigned to either a control or experimental group. The patients in the experimental group received an MT session by a board-certified music therapist each hospital day. The patients in the control group received the usual postarthroplasty care.

Results showed that the experimental group had better outcomes related to pain, anxiety, and mood on Day 1. By Day 2, all comfort measures were better for the experimental group when compared with the control group. The researchers concluded that structured music therapy was effective in improving pain, mood, nausea, anxiety, and use of opioids. However, no significant differences were noted between groups related to hospital length of stay and opioid use.

Level of Evidence: 1
The study was a randomized controlled trial with multiple subjects.

Commentary: Implications for Practice and Research
This study demonstrated that music therapy can be an effective nonpharmacologic modality for improving patient comfort after total joint arthroplasty. More research is needed to focus more specifically on the role of nonpharmacologic interventions on pain management and the use of analgesic medications.

and may prevent the formation of scar tissue, which could decrease knee *mobility* and increase postoperative pain. Observe and document the patient's response to the device and follow the surgeon's protocol for settings. The Best Practice for Patient Safety & Quality Care: The Patient Using a Continuous Passive Motion (CPM) Machine box outlines your responsibility when caring for a patient using the CPM machine. This device may also be used for other types of orthopedic surgery, including toe, ankle, and shoulder ligament and cartilage repair.

Managing Postoperative Pain. In the immediate postoperative period, the surgeon prescribes some form of cryotherapy (cold application) to decrease swelling, hematoma formation, and *pain* at the surgical site. The affected knee is typically very swollen and discolored for a number of weeks after surgery. These problems are more common with this type of surgery than with hip surgery. Several types of cryotherapy are used, including ice/gel pack compression and circulating cold water cryotherapy devices. A recent study comparing these two cryotherapy methods for 100 randomized subjects found that the less expensive ice-gel packs were as effective as the circulating cold water devices in managing pain and swelling. Patient satisfaction was the same for both study groups (Schinsky et al., 2016).

In general, *pain* control measures for patients with TKA are similar to those with total hip arthroplasty. Many patients report high ratings on the pain intensity scale and require

analgesic medications longer than patients with THA, particularly if they have had bilateral knee surgery. Similar to best practices for managing pain in patients having a THA, a multimodal analgesic approach including a variety of opioid and nonopioid drugs is used (see earlier discussion in this chapter). For some younger patients, IV acetaminophen may be effective in managing TKA pain.

Nonpharmacologic pain modalities are becoming an integral part of the comprehensive pain management plan. For example, music therapy has been found to be an effective strategy for postoperative patients having a TKA (see the Evidence-Based Practice box).

Preventing Postoperative Complications. Some complications that affect patients with THA may also affect those having unilateral or bilateral TKA, such as venous thromboembolism (VTE) and *infection*. Complications generally depend on the overall health of the patient.

Average-risk patients begin anticoagulant therapy within 24 hours after surgery and continue for at least 14 days. Common drugs used include fondaparinux, apixaban, dabigatran, rivaroxaban, low-dose unfractionated heparin, and low-molecular-weight heparin. Mechanical VTE prevention includes pneumatic or sequential compression devices and/or compression stockings that are applied before surgery and worn during the hospital stay.

A recent integrative literature review to determine evidence-based nursing practices to prevent complications for patients with bilateral TKA found a lack of clinical practice guidelines for both nursing and surgeon care (Pietsch et al., 2018). Assessments and interventions associated with impaired *clotting* and *infection* are described in the Postoperative Care section of the discussion of Total Hip Arthroplasty.

Promoting Postoperative Self-Management. The desired outcome for discharge from the acute hospital unit is that the patient can walk with crutches or a walker and has adequate flexion in the operative knee for ambulation, including walking up and down stairs. Patients are able to bear weight as tolerated unless the prosthesis is not cemented. Patients may be discharged to their home or to an acute rehabilitation unit, transitional care unit, or skilled unit in a long-term care facility for therapy after 1 to 3 days in acute care. Patients participating in enhanced recovery (ERAS) programs have a shorter hospital length of stay and fewer complications or readmissions.

For some patients, home care services may provide physical therapy and nursing care for 1 to 2 weeks followed by outpatient therapy. *Collaborate with the case manager to determine which option is best for your patient.* During the home rehabilitation phase, the use of a stationary bicycle or CPM machine may help gain flexion. These patients typically return to work and other usual activities in 6 weeks, depending on their age, type of surgery, and other health status factors. Total recovery from a TKA surgery takes 6 weeks or longer, especially for those older than 75 years.

Hospital readmission after TKA. The primary causes of readmission after a TKA are *infection,* DVT, and arthrofibrosis. Arthrofibrosis is the buildup of excessive scar tissue that restricts joint motion and functional ability (Cheuy et al., 2017). Women who had a longer postoperative hospital stay and were discharged to an inpatient rehabilitation facility or skilled nursing facility are at the greatest risk for these complications (Causey-Upton et al., 2019).

NCLEX EXAMINATION CHALLENGE 46.3

Safe and Effective Care Environment

Assistive personnel (AP) are assigned to care for a client who had a cemented total knee arthroplasty yesterday. Which observation by the AP indicates a need for follow-up by the nurse?

A. "The client's surgical knee is very swollen and discolored."
B. "The client states that the surgical knee is very painful when moving it."
C. "The client's lower leg on the surgical side is painful and red."
D. "The client needs assistance with walking to the bathroom."

Other joint arthroplasties. The shoulder and other upper-extremity joints do not bear weight and therefore tend to have less degeneration and subsequent pain. Preoperative teaching for patients having any of these surgeries depends on the surgeon's technique and postoperative protocols.

Total shoulder arthroplasty (TSA) has gained popularity as newer prostheses and technology have been developed. This procedure usually decreases arthritic or traumatic pain and increases the patient's ability to perform ADLs. Because the shoulder joint is complex and has many articulations (joint surfaces), subluxation or complete dislocation is a major potential complication. Usually the glenohumeral joint, created by the glenoid cavity of the shoulder blade (scapula) and the head of the humerus, is replaced because it moves the most and is therefore most affected by arthritis. A cemented or noncemented hemiarthroplasty (replacement of part of the joint), typically the humeral component, may be performed as an alternative to TSA.

After surgery the patient may be placed in an abduction immobilizer or pillow device to protect the joint from excessive motion until rehabilitation therapy begins. *Do not remove these devices unless instructed to do so by the surgeon.*

In addition to the potential for dislocation, postoperative complications are similar to those for other total joint replacements and include infection and neurovascular compromise. *As for any other total joint arthroplasty, perform frequent neurovascular assessments at least every 4 to 8 hours.* The procedure for performing a thorough upper-extremity neurovascular assessment is described in detail in Chapter 44. Document and report any significant changes to the surgeon immediately. The hospital stay for TSA is shorter than for a total hip or knee replacement and may be performed as a same-day procedure. Rehabilitation with an OT generally takes several months.

Improving Mobility

Planning: Expected Outcomes. The patient with osteoarthritis (OA) is expected to maintain or improve a level of *mobility* and activity that allows him or her to function independently with or without an assistive ambulatory device.

Interventions. Management of the patient with OA often requires an interprofessional health team effort. If needed, consult and collaborate with the physical therapist (PT) and occupational therapist (OT) to meet the outcome of independent function and *mobility.* Major interventions include therapeutic exercise and the promotion of ADLs and ambulation by teaching about health and the use of assistive devices.

Certain recreational activities may also be therapeutic, such as swimming to enhance chest and arm muscles. Aerobic exercises (e.g., walking, biking, swimming, aerobic dance) are also recommended. Exercises may be prescribed by rehabilitation therapists for the patient with OA, but you will need to reinforce their techniques and principles. The ideal time for exercise is immediately after the application of heat. To prevent further joint damage, teach patients to carefully follow the instructions for exercise outlined in the Patient and Family Education: Preparing for Self-Management: Exercises for Patients With Osteoarthritis box.

Collaborate with the PT to evaluate the patient's need for ambulatory aids, such as canes or walkers. Although some patients do not like to use these aids or may forget how to use them, they can help prevent further joint deterioration and pain. Collaborate with the OT, if needed, to provide suggestions and devices for assistance for ADLs. Chapter 7 discusses rehabilitation therapies in more detail.

PATIENT AND FAMILY EDUCATION: PREPARING FOR SELF-MANAGEMENT

Exercises for Patients With Osteoarthritis

- Follow the exercise instructions that have been prescribed specifically for you. There are no universal exercises; your exercises have been specifically tailored to your needs.
- Do your exercises on both "good" and "bad" days. Consistency is important.
- Respect pain. Reduce the number of repetitions when the inflammation is severe and you have more pain.
- Use active rather than active-assist or passive exercise whenever possible.
- Do not substitute your normal activities or household tasks for the prescribed exercises.
- Avoid resistive exercises when your joints are severely inflamed.

PATIENT AND FAMILY EDUCATION: PREPARING FOR SELF-MANAGEMENT

Evidence-Based Instructions for Joint Protection

- Use large joints instead of small ones; for example, place your purse strap over your shoulder instead of grasping the purse with your hand.
- Do not turn a doorknob clockwise. Turn it counterclockwise to avoid twisting your arm and promoting ulnar deviation (especially for patients who also have rheumatoid arthritis).
- Use two hands instead of one to hold objects.
- Sit in a chair that has a high, straight back.
- When getting out of bed, do not push off with your fingers; use the entire palm of both hands.
- Do not bend at your waist; instead, bend your knees while keeping your back straight.
- Use long-handled devices, such as a hairbrush with an extended handle.
- Use assistive/adaptive devices, such as Velcro closures and built-up utensil handles to protect your joints.
- Do not use pillows in bed except a small one under your head.
- Avoid twisting or wringing your hands; use a device or rubber grip to open jars or bottles.

Care Coordination and Transition Management. The patient with OA is not usually hospitalized for the disease itself but may be admitted for surgical management. Expect that any patient older than 60 years will have some degree of arthritis and possibly persistent *pain* that needs to be managed.

Home Care Management. If weight-bearing joints are severely involved, the patient may have difficulty going up or down stairs. Making arrangements to live on one floor with accessibility to all rooms is often the best solution. A home care nurse or case manager may collaborate with a rehabilitation therapist to assess the need for structural alterations to the home to accommodate ambulatory aids and enable the patient to perform ADLs. For example, a kitchen counter may need to be lowered, or a seat and handrails may need to be installed in the shower. If the patient has undergone a total hip or knee arthroplasty, an elevated toilet seat is necessary for several weeks after surgery to prevent excessive hip flexion. Throw rugs and other environmental hazards should be removed to prevent tripping and falls.

Self-Management Education. Self-management education (SME) is an effective psychosocially focused nonpharmacologic intervention. Learning how to protect joints is the most important part of patient and family education. Preventing further damage to joints slows the progression of OA and minimizes *pain.* Explain the general principles of joint protection and give practical examples as outlined in the Patient and Family Education: Preparing for Self-Management: Evidence-Based Instructions for Joint Protection box.

As with other diseases in which drugs and nutrition therapy are used, teach the patient and family the drug therapy protocol, desired effects and potential side effects, and toxic effects. Emphasize the importance of reducing weight and eating a well-balanced diet to promote tissue healing.

Many patients with arthritis look for a cure after becoming frustrated and desperate about the course of the disease and treatment. Better control of arthritis is possible, but cure is not yet available. Unfortunately, tabloids, books, media, and the Internet often report "curative" remedies. People spend billions of dollars each year on quackery, including liniments, special diets, and copper bracelets. More hazardous substances such as snake oil and industrial cleaners are also advertised as remedies.

Refer the patient to the Arthritis Foundation for up-to-date information about these "cures." The practice of wearing a copper bracelet will not cure arthritis, but it will not cause harm. However, if the patient is using a potentially harmful substance or method, reinforce the need to avoid the unproven remedy and explain why it should not be used. Respect the patient's preferences, values, and beliefs for using benign remedies that do not cause harm.

With most types of arthritis, patients must live with a persistent, unpredictable, and painful disorder. Their roles, self-esteem, and body image may be affected by these diseases. Body image is usually not as devastating in OA as in the inflammatory arthritic diseases such as RA. The psychosocial component associated with having arthritis is discussed in more detail later in this chapter in the Rheumatoid Arthritis section.

Health Care Resources. The patient who has undergone surgery may need help from community resources. After an arthroplasty, he or she may need assistance with *mobility.* The patient may be discharged to home or an inpatient rehabilitation unit. Collaborate with the case manager and surgeon to determine the best placement. If the patient is discharged to home, home care nurses may be approved for third-party payment for several visits, depending on the presence of any existing systemic diseases. A home care aide may visit the home to help with hygiene-related needs, and a PT may work with ambulatory and *mobility* skills. For older patients, a family member, significant other, or other caregiver should be in the home for at least the first few weeks when the patient needs the most assistance. Emphasize the need for patient safety, especially interventions to prevent falls as described in Chapter 4.

Provide written instructions about the required care, regardless of whether the patient goes home or to another inpatient facility. *As required by The Joint Commission's National Patient Safety Goals (NPSGs) and other health care accrediting organizations, hand-off communication with the new care provider is essential for seamless continuity of care and care coordination.*

The Arthritis Foundation (www.arthritis.org) is an important community resource for all patients with all types of arthritis. This organization provides information to lay people and health care professionals and refers patients and their families to other resources as needed. Local support groups can help them cope with these diseases.

◆ **Evaluation: Evaluate Outcomes.** Evaluate the care of the patient with OA on the basis of the identified priority problems. The expected outcomes are that he or she:

- Achieves pain control to a pain intensity level of 2 to 3 on a scale of 0 to 10 or at a level that is acceptable to the patient
- Does not experience complications associated with total joint arthroplasty (if performed)
- Moves and functions in his or her own environment independently with or without assistive devices

✴ IMMUNITY CONCEPT EXEMPLAR: RHEUMATOID ARTHRITIS

Pathophysiology Review

Rheumatoid arthritis (RA) is a chronic, progressive, systemic inflammatory autoimmune disease process that affects primarily the synovial joints. *Systemic* means this disease can affect any or all parts of the body while affecting many joints.

In patients with RA, transformed autoantibodies (rheumatoid factors [RFs]) that attack healthy tissue, especially synovium, are formed, causing *inflammation*. The disease then begins to involve the articular cartilage, joint capsule, and surrounding ligaments and tendons. *Immunity* and inflammatory factors cause cartilage damage in patients with RA (McCance et al., 2019):

- CD4 helper T-cells and other immune cells in synovial fluid promote cytokine release, especially interleukin-1 (IL-1) and tumor necrosis factor–alpha (TNFA), which attack cartilage.
- Neutrophils and other inflammatory cells in the joint are activated and break down the cartilage.
- Immune complexes deposit in synovium, and osteoclasts are activated.
- B- and T-lymphocytes of the immune system are stimulated and increase the inflammatory response. (Also see Chapter 16 for a complete discussion of the inflammatory response.)

The synovium then thickens and becomes hyperemic, fluid accumulates in the joint space, and a pannus forms. The pannus is vascular granulation tissue composed of inflammatory cells; it erodes articular cartilage and eventually destroys bone. As a result, in late disease, fibrous adhesions, bony ankyloses (abnormal fusion of bones in the joint), and calcifications occur. Bone loses density, and secondary osteoporosis exists.

Permanent joint changes may be avoided if RA is diagnosed early. Early and aggressive treatment to suppress synovitis may lead to a remission. RA is a disease characterized by natural remissions and exacerbations (flare-ups). Interprofessional health care team management helps control the disease to decrease the intensity and number of exacerbations. Preventing flares helps prevent joint erosion and permanent joint damage.

Because RA is a systemic disease, areas of the body besides the synovial joints can be affected. Inflammatory responses similar to those occurring in synovial tissue may occur in any organ or body system in which connective tissue is prevalent. If blood vessel *inflammation* (vasculitis) occurs, the organ supplied by that vessel can be affected, leading to eventual failure of the organ or system in late disease.

Etiology and Genetic Risk. The etiology of RA remains unclear, but research suggests a *combination of environmental and genetic factors*. Some researchers also suspect that female reproductive hormones influence the development of RA because it affects women more often than men—usually young to middle-age women. Others suspect that infectious organisms may play a role, particularly the Epstein-Barr virus (McCance et al., 2019). Physical and emotional stresses have been linked to exacerbations of the disorder and may be contributing factors or "triggers" to its development.

👤 PATIENT-CENTERED CARE: GENETIC/GENOMIC CONSIDERATIONS (QSEN)

Research has shown that there is a strong association between RA and several human leukocyte antigen (HLA)–*DR* alleles. The cause of this association is not clear, but most HLA diseases are autoimmune (McCance et al., 2019). *DR* alleles, especially *DR4* and *DRB1*, are the primary genetic factors contributing to the development of RA. *DR4* is associated with more severe forms of the disease. Other contributing factors are being researched.

Incidence and Prevalence. RA affects over 1.5 million people, and Euro-Americans have the disease more often than other groups. Women are two to three times more likely to have RA compared with men (Arthritis Foundation, 2019). The cause for these trends is not known.

❖ Interprofessional Collaborative Care

◆ **Assessment: Recognize Cues.** The onset of rheumatoid arthritis (RA) may be acute and severe or slow and progressive; patients may have vague symptoms that last for several months before diagnosis. The onset of the disease is more common in the winter months than in the warmer months. The signs and symptoms of RA can be categorized as early or late disease and as joint (articular) or systemic (extra-articular), as summarized in the Key Features: The Patient With Rheumatoid Arthritis box.

Physical Assessment/Signs and Symptoms

Early Signs and Symptoms. In the early stage of RA the patient typically reports joint *inflammation,* generalized weakness, and fatigue. Anorexia, weight loss of about 2 to 3 lb (1 kg), and persistent low-grade fever are common. In patients with early disease, the upper-extremity joints are involved initially—often the proximal interphalangeal (PIP) and metacarpophalangeal (MCP) joints of the hands. These

➤➤ KEY FEATURES

The Patient With Rheumatoid Arthritis

Early Signs and Symptoms (Early Disease)	Late Signs and Symptoms (Advanced Disease)
Joint	**Joint**
• Inflammation	• Deformities (e.g., swan neck or ulnar deviation)
Systemic	• Moderate-to-severe **pain** and morning stiffness
• Low-grade fever	**Systemic**
• Fatigue	• Osteoporosis
• Weakness	• Severe fatigue
• Anorexia	• Anemia
• Paresthesias	• Weight loss
	• Subcutaneous nodules
	• Peripheral neuropathy
	• Vasculitis
	• Pericarditis
	• Fibrotic lung disease
	• Sjögren syndrome
	• Kidney disease
	• Felty syndrome

joints may be slightly reddened, warm, stiff, swollen, and tender or painful, particularly on palpation (caused by synovitis). The typical pattern of joint involvement in RA is bilateral and symmetric (e.g., both wrists). The number of joints involved usually increases as the disease progresses.

The presence of only *one* hot, swollen, painful joint (out of proportion to the other joints) may mean that the joint is infected. *Refer the patient to the primary health care provider (generally the rheumatologist) immediately if this is the case.* Single hot, swollen joints are considered infected until proven otherwise and require immediate long-term antibiotic treatment.

Late Signs and Symptoms. As the disease advances, the joints become progressively inflamed and very painful. The patient usually has frequent morning stiffness, which can last for several hours after awakening. On palpation the joints feel soft and look puffy because of synovitis and effusions. The fingers often appear spindle-like. Note any muscle atrophy (which can result from disuse secondary to joint pain) and a decreased range of motion in the affected joints.

Most or all synovial joints are eventually affected. The temporomandibular joint (TMJ) may be involved in severe disease, but such involvement is uncommon. When the TMJ is affected, the patient may have pain when chewing or opening the mouth.

When the spinal column is involved, the cervical joints are most likely to be affected. During clinical examination, gently palpate the posterior cervical spine and identify it as cervical pain, tenderness, or loss of motion.

⚠ NURSING SAFETY PRIORITY (QSEN)

Critical Rescue

Cervical RA may result in **subluxation**, especially of the first and second vertebrae. This complication may be life threatening because branches of the phrenic nerve that supply the diaphragm are restricted and respiratory function may be compromised. The patient is also in danger of becoming quadriparetic (weak in all extremities) or quadriplegic (paralyzed in all extremities). If cervical pain (may radiate down one arm) or loss of range of motion is present in the cervical spine, keep the neck straight in a neutral position to prevent permanent damage to the spinal cord or spinal nerves. *Notify the primary health care provider immediately about these neurologic changes!*

Joint deformity occurs as a late, articular manifestation, and secondary osteoporosis can cause bone fractures. Observe common deformities, especially in the hands and feet (Fig. 46.5). Extensive wrist involvement can result in carpal tunnel syndrome (see Chapter 47 for assessment and management of carpal tunnel syndrome).

Gently palpate the tissues around the joints to elicit pain or tenderness associated with other rheumatoid complications, unless the patient is having severe joint **pain.** For example, Baker cysts (enlarged popliteal bursae behind the knee) may occur and cause tissue compression and pain. Tendon rupture is also possible, particularly rupture of the Achilles tendon.

Numerous extra-articular signs and symptoms are associated with advanced disease. Assess the patient to ascertain systemic involvement. In addition to increased joint swelling and tenderness, *moderate-to-severe weight loss, fever,* and *extreme fatigue* are common in late disease **exacerbations,** often called *flare-ups.* Some patients have the characteristic soft, round, movable **subcutaneous nodules,** which usually appear on the ulnar surface of the arm, on the fingers, or along the Achilles tendon. These nodules can disappear and reappear at any time and are associated with severe, destructive disease. Rheumatoid nodules are usually not a problem themselves; however, they occasionally open and become infected and may interfere with ADLs. Accidentally bumping the nodules may cause discomfort. Occasionally nodules occur in the lungs.

Inflammation of the blood vessels results in **vasculitis,** particularly of small to medium-size vessels. When arterial involvement occurs, major organs can become ischemic and malfunction. Assess for ischemic skin lesions that appear in groups as small, brownish spots, most commonly around the nail bed. Monitor the number of lesions, note their location each day, and report vascular changes to the health care provider. Increased lesions indicate increased vasculitis, and a decreased number indicates decreased vasculitis. Also carefully assess any larger lesions that appear on the lower extremities. These lesions can lead to ulcerations, which heal slowly as a result of decreased circulation. Peripheral neuropathy associated with decreased circulation can cause footdrop and **paresthesias** (burning and tingling sensations), usually in older adults.

Respiratory complications may manifest as *pleurisy, pneumonitis, diffuse interstitial fibrosis,* and *pulmonary hypertension.* Cardiac complications include *pericarditis* and *myocarditis.* These health problems are discussed elsewhere in this text.

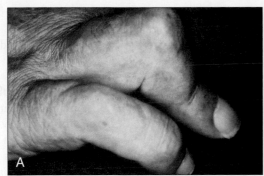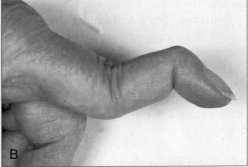

FIG. 46.5 Common joint deformities seen in rheumatoid arthritis. **A,** Boutonniere deformity; **B,** Swan neck deformity. (From Hochberg, M. C., Gravallese, E. M., Silman, A. J., et al. [2019]. *Rheumatology* [7th ed.]. Philadelphia: Elsevier.)

Assess for eye involvement, which typically manifests as *iritis* and *scleritis.* If either of these complications is present, the sclera of one or both eyes is reddened and the pupils have an irregular shape. Visual disturbances may occur.

Several syndromes are seen in patients with advanced RA. The most common is **Sjögren syndrome,** which includes a triad of:

- Dry eyes (keratoconjunctivitis sicca [KCS], or the sicca syndrome)
- Dry mouth (xerostomia)
- Dry vagina (in some cases)

Note the patient's report of dry mouth or dry eyes. Some patients state that their eyes feel "gritty," as if sand is in their eyes. Inspect the mouth for dry, sticky membranes and the eyes for redness and lack of tearing.

Psychosocial Assessment. Rheumatoid arthritis (RA) and other inflammatory types of arthritis are chronic diseases that can be disabling if not well controlled. Fear of becoming dependent, uncertainty about the disease process, altered body image, devaluation of self, frustration, and depression are common psychosocial problems. Physical limitations and persistent *pain* may limit the patient's *mobility.* These limitations can result in role changes in the family and society. For example, the person may not be able to cook for the family or be an active sexual partner. In addition, extreme fatigue often causes patients to desire an early bedtime and napping and may result in a reluctance to socialize.

Body changes caused by joint changes and drug therapy (if used) may also cause poor self-esteem and body image. Because many societies value people with physically fit, attractive bodies, the patient with RA may be embarrassed to be seen in public places. The patient may grieve or experience degrees of depression. He or she may have feelings of helplessness caused by a loss of control over a disease that can "consume" the body. Fortunately, newer drugs have improved the treatment of RA and provide the patient with hope and better disease control. Only a small percentage of patients with RA become wheelchair dependent.

Living with a chronic disease and its associated *pain* is difficult for the patient and family. Chronic suffering and pain affect quality of life. Assess the patient's emotional and mental status in relation to the disease and its problems. Evaluate his or her

support systems and resources. Patients who are knowledgeable about their disease and treatment options feel emotionally stronger to cope with their disease and better able to discuss treatment options with their primary health care provider.

Laboratory Assessment. Laboratory tests help support a diagnosis of RA, but no single test or group of tests can confirm it. The test for *rheumatoid factor (RF)* measures the presence of unusual antibodies of the immunoglobulins G (IgG) and M (IgM) types that develop in a number of connective tissue diseases. Many patients with RA have a positive titer (greater than 1:80), *especially in older adults* (Pagana & Pagana, 2018). However, the presence of RF is not diagnostic for RA.

The newest laboratory test called the *anticyclic citrullinated peptide (anti-CCP)* is very specific and sensitive in detecting early RA. The presence of anti-CCP is also a marker for aggressive and erosive late-stage disease.

The *antinuclear antibody (ANA)* test measures the titer of a group of antibodies that destroy the nuclei of cells and cause tissue death in patients with autoimmune disease. The fluorescent method is sometimes referred to as *FANA.* If this test result is positive (a value higher than 1:40), various subtypes of this antibody are identified and measured.

An elevated *erythrocyte sedimentation rate (ESR),* or "sed rate," (greater than 20 mm/hr) can confirm **inflammation** or infection anywhere in the body. An elevated ESR helps support a diagnosis of an unspecified inflammatory disease. The test is most useful to monitor the course of a disease, especially for inflammatory autoimmune diseases. In general the more severe the disease gets, the higher the ESR rises; as the disease improves or goes into remission, the ESR level decreases.

The *high-sensitivity C-reactive protein,* or *hsCRP,* is another useful test to measure **inflammation** and may be done with or instead of the ESR. As the name implies, it is more sensitive to inflammatory changes than the ESR. It is also very useful for detecting **infection** anywhere in the body.

The presence of most chronic diseases usually causes mild-to-moderate anemia, which contributes to the patient's fatigue. Therefore monitor the patient's complete blood count (CBC) for a low hemoglobin, hematocrit, and red blood cell (RBC) count. An increase in white blood cell (WBC) count is consistent with an inflammatory response. A decrease in the WBC count may indicate Felty syndrome, a pulmonary complication associated with late RA. Thrombocytosis (increased platelets) can also occur in patients with late RA. Additional laboratory tests may be performed, depending on the body systems and organs that may be affected by the disease. For example, if heart involvement is suspected, the primary health care provider may request cardiac enzyme testing.

Other Diagnostic Assessment. A standard x-ray is used to visualize the joint changes and deformities typical of RA. A CT scan may help determine the presence and degree of cervical spine involvement.

An **arthrocentesis** is an invasive diagnostic procedure that may be used for patients with joint swelling caused by excess synovial fluid (effusion). It may be performed at the bedside or in a health care provider's office or clinic. After administering a local anesthetic, the provider inserts a large-gauge needle into the joint (usually the knee) to aspirate a sample of synovial fluid and to relieve pressure caused by excess fluid. The fluid is analyzed for inflammatory cells and immune complexes, including RF. Fluid from patients with RA typically reveals increased WBCs, cloudiness, and volume.

Teach the patient to use ice and rest the affected joint for 24 hours after arthrocentesis. Often the primary health care provider will recommend acetaminophen as needed for discomfort. If increased pain or swelling occurs, teach the patient or family to notify the primary health care provider immediately.

! NURSING SAFETY PRIORITY (QSEN)

Action Alert

After an arthrocentesis, monitor the insertion site for bleeding or leakage of synovial fluid. Notify the primary health care provider if either of these problems occurs.

A bone scan or joint scan can also assess the extent of joint involvement. MRI may be performed to assess spinal column disease or other joint involvement.

Because RA can affect multiple body systems, tests to diagnose specific systemic manifestations are performed as needed. For example, nerve conduction studies help confirm peripheral neuropathy. Pulmonary function tests help determine the presence of lung involvement.

NCLEX EXAMINATION CHALLENGE 46.4

Physiological Integrity

Which assessment findings will the nurse expect for the client with **early-stage** rheumatoid arthritis? **Select all that apply.**
A. Joint inflammation
B. Subcutaneous nodules
C. Severe weight loss
D. Fatigue
E. Thrombocytosis
F. Anorexia

◆ **Analysis: Analyze Cues and Prioritize Hypotheses.** The priority collaborative problems for patients with rheumatoid arthritis (RA) include:

1. Chronic *inflammation* and persistent *pain* due to systemic autoimmune disease process

2. Potential for decreased *mobility* due to joint deformity, muscle atrophy, and fatigue
3. Potential for decreased self-esteem image due to joint deformity

◆ **Planning and Implementation: Generate Solutions and Take Action.** Patients who have RA are managed in the community under the supervision of a qualified primary health care provider. The expected outcome for management is that the disease goes into remission and its progression slows to decrease *pain*, prevent joint destruction, and increase *mobility*. When patients with RA are admitted to the inpatient acute care or long-term care facility, it is usually for health problems other than for complications of arthritis. Whether the patient is in a facility or community, be sure to plan interventions to manage his or her persistent *pain* and *inflammation*, as well as the potential for decreased *mobility* and decreased self-esteem.

Managing Chronic Inflammation and Pain

Planning: Expected Outcomes. The patient with RA is expected to have a *pain* level that is acceptable to the patient (e.g., at a 3 on a pain intensity scale of 0 to 10). A major focus of pain management is drug therapy to modify or prevent the progression of the disease, thereby decreasing joint and systemic *inflammation*.

Interventions. As in other types of arthritis, the interprofessional health care team manages *pain* by using a combination of pharmacologic and nonpharmacologic measures. A synovectomy to remove inflamed synovium may be needed for joints such as the knee or elbow. Total joint arthroplasty (TJA) may be indicated when other measures fail to relieve pain. TJA is discussed in the Osteoarthritis section of this chapter.

Drug Therapy. Some drugs prescribed for RA have anti-inflammatory and/or analgesic actions. For example, NSAIDs are sometimes used for RA to help and decrease pain and inflammation. The choice of which one to prescribe depends on the patient's needs and tolerance and the scientific evidence supporting the drug therapy. To decrease GI problems, the NSAID may be given with an H2-blocking agent such as famotidine. If there is no clinical change after 6 to 8 weeks, the primary health care provider may discontinue the current NSAID and try another one or change to a different drug class.

It was once thought that celecoxib, a COX-2 inhibiting NSAID, should be given rather than the older NSAIDs such as ibuprofen. However, all COX-2 inhibiting drugs have recently been associated with cardiovascular disease such as myocardial infarction, and some have been taken off the market. The risk for GI bleeding is also high in patients taking celecoxib, and the drug cannot be given to those who have had recent open-heart surgery.

Other drugs affect *immunity* through immunosuppression, thus modifying the progress of the disease. As a result, these drugs may cause remission of the illness and prevent erosive joint changes. *Biological response modifiers* make up the newest class of disease-modifying drugs that help reduce signals for the immune system to cause *inflammation*. Patients with inflammatory diseases other than RA are also using various biological response–modifying drugs successfully. Although

RA is a chronic disease and no cure is yet available, drugs now used can better control the disease and prevent further deterioration. Adjustments in drug therapy are recommended every 3 to 6 months until the expected outcome or disease remission is met.

The primary health care provider, often a rheumatologist, makes decisions about appropriate drug therapy for patients with rheumatoid disease based on the severity of the disease. Initially most patients are managed with *disease-modifying antirheumatic drugs (DMARDs)*. As the name implies, these drugs are given to slow the progression of the disease. For best results, they should be started early in the disease process.

First-line disease-modifying antirheumatic drugs. Methotrexate (MTX), an immunosuppressive medication, in a low, once-a-week dose is the mainstay of therapy for RA because it is effective and relatively inexpensive. It is a slow-acting drug, taking 4 to 6 weeks to begin to control joint *inflammation* (Burchum & Rosenthal, 2019). Observe for desired therapeutic drug effects such as a decrease in joint *pain* and swelling.

Monitor patients for potential adverse effects such as decreasing WBCs and platelets (as a result of bone marrow suppression) or elevations in liver enzymes or serum creatinine.

> **! NURSING SAFETY PRIORITY** (QSEN)
>
> ***Drug Alert***
>
> Patients taking MTX are at risk for *infection* caused by impaired or decreased drug-induced *immunity*. Teach them to avoid crowds and people who are ill. Remind patients to avoid alcoholic beverages while taking MTX to prevent liver toxicity. Teach them to observe and report other side and toxic effects, which include mouth sores and acute dyspnea from pneumonitis. Although not commonly occurring, lymph node tumor (lymphoma) and pneumonitis (lung *inflammation*) have been associated in those who have RA and are taking MTX. Folic acid, one of the B vitamins, is often given to those who are taking MTX to help decrease some of the drug's side effects.

Pregnancy is not recommended while taking methotrexate because birth defects are possible. *Strict birth control is recommended for childbearing women who are in need of MTX to control their RA.* If pregnancy is ever desired, instruct the patient to consult the rheumatologist and an obstetric/gynecologic (OB/GYN) health care provider. Generally the primary health care provider will discontinue the drug at least 3 months before planned pregnancy. MTX may be restarted after birth if the patient does not breast-feed (Burchum & Rosenthal, 2019).

Leflunomide may be prescribed for some patients. It is a slow-acting immune-modulating drug that helps diminish inflammatory symptoms of joint swelling and stiffness and improves *mobility.* The drug is generally prescribed as a loading dose for 3 days followed by a lower dose daily thereafter. Inform the patient that leflunomide takes 4 to 6 weeks and sometimes up to 3 months before maximum benefit is realized.

> **! NURSING SAFETY PRIORITY** (QSEN)
>
> ***Drug Alert***
>
> Leflunomide is a potent drug that is generally tolerated, but side effects of hair loss, diarrhea, decreased WBCs and platelets, or increased liver enzymes have been reported.
>
> Teach patients to report these changes and monitor laboratory results carefully. Remind them to avoid alcohol. Inform them that leflunomide can cause birth defects; therefore recommend strict birth control to women of childbearing age. Tell patients to contact their primary health care provider immediately if pregnancy occurs while taking the drug.

Another DMARD sometimes used for RA is hydroxychloroquine. This drug slows the progression of mild rheumatoid disease before it worsens. It is an antimalarial drug that helps suppress the immune response to decrease joint and muscle *pain.* Patients generally tolerate hydroxychloroquine quite well. In a few cases mild stomach discomfort, light-headedness, or headache has been reported. The drug should not be used for patients who have known cardiac disease or dysrhythmias (Burchum & Rosenthal, 2019).

> **! NURSING SAFETY PRIORITY** (QSEN)
>
> ***Drug Alert***
>
> The most serious adverse effect of hydroxychloroquine is retinal damage. Teach patients to report blurred vision or headache. Remind them to have an eye examination before taking the drug and every 6 months to detect changes in the cornea, lens, or retina. If this rare complication occurs, the primary health care provider discontinues the drug (Burchum & Rosenthal, 2019).

Biological response modifiers. As a group, *biological response modifiers (BRMs)*, sometimes called biologics, are one of the newest classes of DMARDs. Most BRMs neutralize the biologic activity of tumor necrosis factor–alpha (TNFA) by inhibiting its binding with TNF receptors. Any one of the BRMs may be tried. If one drug is not effective, the primary health care provider prescribes another drug in the same class. All these drugs are extremely expensive, and insurance companies may not completely pay for their use.

Teach patients receiving any one of the BRMs that they are at a high risk for developing impaired *immunity* and subsequent *infection*. Instruct them to stay away from people with infections and to avoid large crowds if possible. Remind patients with multiple sclerosis (MS), tuberculosis (TB), or a positive TB test that they should not receive TNF inhibitors because they make patients susceptible to flare-ups of these diseases. Determine whether the patient has had a recent negative purified protein derivative (PPD) test for TB. If not, a PPD skin test is typically administered and the selected BRM is not started until a negative test result is confirmed (Burchum & Rosenthal, 2019). Collaborate with the primary health care provider to ensure that this process is complete. The Common Examples of Drug Therapy: Biological Response Modifiers Used for Rheumatoid Arthritis and Other Chronic Autoimmune Diseases box provides specific examples of BRMs and associated nursing implications. Most of these drugs are given parenterally and require health teaching for self-administration.

COMMON EXAMPLES OF DRUG THERAPY

Biological Response Modifiers Used for Rheumatoid Arthritis and Other Chronic Autoimmune Diseases

Common Drugs	Purpose of Drug/Drug Classification	Nursing Implications
For *all* biological response modifiers (BRMs) (also called *biologics*)	Neutralize biologic activity of tumor necrosis factor–alpha (TNFA), interleukins (IL), T-lymphocytes, or tyrosine kinase (TK) to decrease immune response and inflammation	Do not give BRMs if patient has a serious ***infection,*** TB, or MS *because they may exacerbate these health problems.* Teach patients taking BRMs to avoid getting live vaccines. Teach patient to avoid crowds and people with infections *because serious infections, especially respiratory infections, can lead to hospitalization or cause death.*
Etanercept	TNFA inhibitor	Teach patient to report site reaction, *which may indicate a local allergic response and cause pain.* Teach patient how to self-administer drug.
Infliximab	TNFA inhibitor	Refrigerate all BRMs, except infliximab, *to prevent drug decomposition.* Teach patient to report chest pain or difficulty breathing during infusion, *which could indicate a severe allergic response;* monitor blood pressure and infusion site.
Adalimumab	TNFA inhibitor	Teach patient to report site reaction, *which may indicate local allergic response.*
Anakinra	IL-1 receptor antagonist	Teach patient to monitor site for reaction (occurs more commonly when compared with other BRMs). Monitor WBC count *because the drug can cause a severe decrease in WBC count and make the patient very susceptible to infection.* Teach the patient to report respiratory symptoms, such as cough and fever. Teach him or her that malignancies can result from taking this drug.
Abatacept	Selective T-lymphocyte co-stimulator modulator (T-cell inhibitor)	Report cough, dizziness, and sore throat; do not receive live vaccines while taking the drug. Monitor for dyspnea, wheezing, flushing, itching, *which may indicate a mild-to-moderate allergic reaction.*
Rituximab	Monoclonal antibody	Observe for infusion reaction as for etanercept. *Drug has a **black box warning** about serious infections from opportunistic pathogens that can lead to hospitalizations or death.*
Golimumab	TNFA inhibitor	Teach patient to report signs and symptoms of ***infection,*** including fever and malaise; teach patient to avoid live vaccines while taking drug. Teach patient about adverse drug effects, including hypertension, GI distress, and ***infection*** from opportunistic pathogens; report signs and symptoms of these problems to the primary health care provider.
Tocilizumab	IL-6 inhibitor	Teach patient the importance of having frequent WBC, platelet, and liver enzyme testing. *This drug can cause decreased WBCs and platelets and liver dysfunction.*

MS, Multiple sclerosis; *TB,* tuberculosis; *TNF,* tumor necrosis factor; *WBC,* white blood cell.

Other drugs. A few drugs may be given in combination with or instead of the previously described drugs. It is not unusual for a patient to be taking several disease-modifying drugs such as methotrexate, a BRM, and an adjunct medication. Each drug works differently to relieve symptoms and slow the progression of the disease. For example, sulfasalazine, a sulfa drug, may be given in combination with other drugs to reduce inflammation and pain. Be aware that this drug should not be used for patients who have a sulfa allergy. Common side effects of sulfasalazine include nausea, vomiting, and skin rash (Burchum & Rosenthal, 2019).

Glucocorticoids (steroids)—usually prednisone—may be given for their fast-acting anti-inflammatory and immunosuppressive effects. Prednisone may be given in high dose for short duration (pulse therapy) or as a low chronic dose. Moderate-dose short-term tapering bridge therapy may be used when inflammation is symptomatic and other RA medications are insufficient or have not yet had an effect.

Chronic steroid therapy can result in numerous complications such as:

- Diabetes mellitus
- Impaired or decreased ***immunity***

- Fluid and electrolyte imbalances
- Hypertension
- Osteoporosis
- Glaucoma

Some drug effects are dose related, whereas others are not. Observe the patient for complications associated with chronic steroid therapy and report them to the primary health care provider. For example, if blood pressure becomes elevated or significant laboratory values change, notify the primary health care provider.

Patients with RA may experience one or a few joints that have more *pain* and *inflammation* than the others. Cortisone injections in single joints may be used to temporarily relieve local *pain* and *inflammation*. Have the patient ice and rest the joint for 24 hours after the procedure. Oral analgesics are also sometimes needed during that time.

Nonpharmacologic Interventions. Adequate rest, proper positioning, and ice and heat applications are important in pain management. If acute inflammation is present, ice packs may be applied to "hot" joints for pain relief until the inflammation lessens. The ice pack should not be too heavy. At home the patient can use a small bag of frozen peas or corn as an ice pack.

Heated paraffin (wax) dips may help increase comfort of arthritic hands. Finger and hand exercises are often done more easily after paraffin treatment. To relieve morning stiffness or the pain of late-stage disease, recommend a hot shower rather than a sponge bath or a tub bath. It is often difficult for the patient with RA to get into and out of a bathtub, although special hydraulic lifts, tub chairs, and walk-in bathtubs are available to allow him or her to bathe. Safety (grab) bars and nonskid tread in the tub or shower floor are important safety features to discuss with all patients. Some older adults prefer using shower chairs and a walk-in shower that does not have a ledge that could cause falls.

Hot packs applied directly to involved joints may be beneficial. Most physical therapy departments have machines that keep hot packs ready anytime they are needed. Teach patients to use the microwave or stovetop heating instructions to warm heat packs at home. Remind them to follow the instructions given with each heating device used.

Plasmapheresis (sometimes called *plasma exchange*) is an in-hospital procedure prescribed by a primary health care provider in which the patient's plasma is treated to remove the antibodies causing the disease. Although not commonly done, this procedure may be combined with steroid pulse therapy for patients with severe, life-threatening disease.

Complementary and Integrative Health. Some patients may have *pain* relief from hypnosis, acupuncture, imagery, music therapy, or other techniques. Stress management is also popular as a pain relief intervention. Chapter 5 discusses these therapies in more detail.

Adequate nutrition is an important part of the management of RA. Obesity should be avoided or treated if present. The inflammatory state may place a greater burden on the metabolism of some essential nutrients. This catabolic state may be related to increased cytokine production, specifically tumor necrosis factor.

According to the Arthritis Foundation (2019), no one food causes or cures RA; however, healthy nutrition in general is important. Refer the patient to the Arthritis Foundation's publications regarding diet and arthritis. Refer him or her to the registered dietitian nutritionist for vitamin- and nutrition-specific questions or recommendations. Teach patients to take any herbal or nutrition supplement under the supervision of a qualified health care provider to prevent adverse events and drug-food or drug-drug interactions.

Other integrative therapies are safe and have been scientifically proven to be effective to help control RA *pain* for most people. Examples include mind-body therapies such as relaxation techniques, imagery, and spiritual practices. For information about these techniques, see Chapter 5.

Promoting Mobility

Planning: Expected Outcomes. Patients with RA often have decreased *mobility* related to multiple joint deformities and muscle atrophy. Fatigue and generalized weakness also contribute to decreased mobility. The expected outcome is that the patient will be able to independently perform ADLs with or without ambulatory and assistive devices.

Interventions. Although the physical appearance of a patient with severe RA may create the image that ADL independence is not possible, a number of alternative and creative methods can be used to perform these activities. *Do not perform these activities for the patient unless asked. Those with RA do not want to be dependent.* For example, hand deformities often prevent a patient from opening packages of food such as a box of crackers; however, he or she may prefer to use the teeth to open the crackers rather than depend on someone else.

In the hospital or long-term care facility, a patient may not eat because of the barriers of heavy plate covers, milk cartons, small packages of condiments, and heavy containers. Styrofoam or paper cups may bend and collapse as he or she attempts to hold them. A china or heavy plastic cup with handles may be easier to manipulate. Collaborate with the registered dietitian nutritionist to help with access to food and total independence in eating.

When fine-motor activities (e.g., squeezing a tube of toothpaste) become impossible, larger joints or body surfaces can substitute for smaller ones. For example, teach how to use the palm of the hand to press the paste onto the brush. Devices such as long-handled brushes can help patients brush their hair; dressing sticks can assist with putting on pants. These examples illustrate the need to assess the problem area, suggest alternative methods, and refer the patient to an OT or PT for special assistive and adaptive devices if necessary.

Additional nursing interventions depend in part on identifying the factors contributing to fatigue. For example, persistent *pain,* sleep disturbances, and weakness are associated with increased fatigue. Anemia may also be a contributing factor and may be treated with iron (if an iron deficiency anemia is present), folic acid, or vitamin supplements prescribed by the primary health care provider. Chronic normochromic or chronic hypochromic anemia often occurs in most chronic systemic diseases. Assess for drug-related blood loss such as that caused by NSAIDs by checking the stool for gross or occult blood. *Older white women are the most likely to experience GI bleeding as a result of taking these medications* (Burchum & Rosenthal, 2019).

PATIENT AND FAMILY EDUCATION: PREPARING FOR SELF-MANAGEMENT

Energy Conservation for the Patient With Arthritis

- Balance activity with rest. Take one or two naps each day.
- Pace yourself; do not plan too much for one day.
- Set priorities. Determine which activities are most important and do them first.
- Delegate responsibilities and tasks to your family and friends.
- Plan ahead to prevent last-minute rushing and stress.
- Learn your own activity tolerance and do not exceed it.

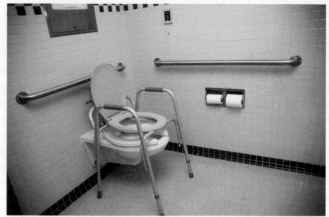

FIG. 46.6 Handrails and an elevated toilet seat make transfers easier for the patient.

If fatigue and decreased *mobility* result from muscle atrophy, the primary health care provider prescribes an aggressive physical therapy program to strengthen muscles and prevent further atrophy. Patients also experience increased fatigue when *pain* prevents them from getting adequate rest and sleep. Measures to facilitate sleep include promoting a quiet environment, giving warm beverages, and administering hypnotics or relaxants as prescribed if necessary.

In addition to identifying and managing specific reasons for fatigue, determine the patient's usual daily activities and teach principles of *energy conservation,* including:

- Pacing activities
- Allowing rest periods
- Setting priorities
- Obtaining assistance when needed

The Patient and Family Education: Preparing for Self-Management: Energy Conservation for the Patient With Arthritis box provides specific suggestions for conserving energy and thus increasing activity tolerance and *mobility.*

Enhancing Self Esteem

Planning: Expected Outcome. The patient with RA often has multiple joints that are inflamed or deformed, causing a potential for decreased self-esteem. Therefore the expected outcome is that the patient will verbalize a positive perception of self as a result of interprofessional interventions.

Interventions. Body image and self-esteem may be affected by the disease process. Determine the patient's perception of these changes and the impact of the reactions of family and significant others. The most important intervention is communicating acceptance of the patient. When a trusting relationship is established, encourage him or her to express personal feelings.

As a reaction to body changes and joint deformity and the presence of a chronic, painful disease, some patients display behaviors indicative of loss. They may use coping strategies that range from denial or fear to anger or depression. In an attempt to regain control over the effects of the disease process, they may appear to be "manipulative and demanding" and sometimes may be referred to as having an "arthritis personality." *This personality, which represents a negative label, is a myth; avoid using these terms.* Patients are trying to cope with the effects of their illness and should be treated with patience and understanding. Continually assess and accept these behaviors but remain realistic in discussing goals to improve self-esteem and body image. Emphasize their strengths and help them identify

previously successful coping strategies. If needed, consult with mental health professionals or religious/spiritual leaders to help patients cope with this potentially debilitating chronic disease.

Care Coordination and Transition Management. Patients with rheumatoid arthritis (RA) are usually managed at home but in a few cases may be institutionalized in a long-term care facility if they become restricted to bed or a wheelchair. Some patients may be transferred to a rehabilitation facility for several weeks to help develop strategies, techniques, and skills for independent living at home. Chapter 7 discusses the rehabilitation process in detail.

Home Care Management. The amount of home care preparation depends on the severity of the disease. Structural changes may be necessary if there are deficits in performing ADLs or *mobility.* Doors must be wide enough to accommodate a wheelchair or walker if one is used. Ramps are needed to prevent the patient in a wheelchair from becoming homebound. If the person cannot use stairs, he or she must have access to facilities for all ADLs on one floor. Handrails should be available in the bathroom and halls.

To promote continued homemaking functions, countertops and appliances may require structural changes. The patient may also require handrails and elevated chairs and toilet seats, which facilitate transfers (Fig. 46.6). *These devices are especially important for older adults with arthritis.*

Self-Management Education. Self-management education (SME) is a vital role for nurses in collaborative management of arthritis. Many people have signs and symptoms of joint *inflammation* but do not seek medical attention. Teach them to seek professional health care to reduce *pain* and prevent disability.

Teach patients to discuss any questions with their primary health care provider before trying any over-the-counter or home remedies. Some remedies may be harmful. Check with the Arthritis Foundation for the latest information on arthritis myths and quackery (www.arthritis.org).

Provide information to the patient and family about drug therapy, joint protection, energy conservation, rest, and exercise as summarized in the boxes presented earlier in the RA section.

Assess the patient's coping strategies. The patient with RA often reports being on an "emotional roller coaster" from coping with a chronic illness every day. Control over one's life is an important human need. The patient with an unpredictable chronic disease may lose this control, and this lowers self-esteem. Health care providers must allow the patient to make decisions about care. Families and significant others must also include him or her in decision making. Although the patient's behavior may be perceived as demanding or manipulative, his or her self-esteem cannot be improved without this important aspect of interpersonal relationships.

Increased dependency also affects a sense of control and self-esteem. Some people ignore their health needs and portray a tough image for others by insisting that they need no assistance. Emphasize to the patient and family that asking for help may be the best decision at times to prevent further joint damage and disease progression.

RA may also affect work and social roles. The patient may have physical difficulty doing tasks that require lifting, climbing, grasp, or gross- or fine-motor activities. The severity of RA disease may cause difficulty with total number of hours worked. Some people with RA can do their jobs well without problem; others may have varying degrees of difficulty. Those who can no longer do their job at work may need to discuss with their employer having a lighter workload, but some may need to file for disability with their company and U.S. Social Security office.

Health Care Resources. The need for health care resources for the patient with RA is similar to that for the patient with osteoarthritis. A home care nurse or aide, physical therapist, or occupational therapist may be needed during severe exacerbations or as the disease progresses. In collaboration with the case manager, identify these resources and make sure that they are available as needed. The Arthritis Foundation is an excellent source of information and support.

Arthritis support groups and self-help courses provide the education and support that patients, families, and friends need. Refer the patient to a psychological counselor or religious or spiritual leader for emotional support and guidance during times of crisis or as needed. Identify and recommend other support systems within the family and community when necessary.

◆ **Evaluation: Evaluate Outcomes.** Evaluate the care of the patient with RA on the basis of the identified priority problems. The expected outcomes are that he or she:

- Achieves *pain* control to a pain intensity level of 2 to 3 or less on a scale of 0 to 10 or at a level that is acceptable to the patient
- Moves and functions in his or her own environment independently with or without assistive devices
- Verbalizes increased self-esteem and positive perception of self

---

⚉ CLINICAL JUDGMENT CHALLENGE 46.1

Safety; Teamwork and Collaboration

A 70-year-old woman is admitted to the hospital with suspected streptococcal pneumonia. She continues to have an occasional cough, mild dyspnea, and a fever over 100° F (37.8° C) after a week of treatment with amoxicillin at home. The hospitalist prescribes IV levofloxacin 750 mg daily. The admitting nurse documents the following history and physical assessment data:

- Has a 25-year history of rheumatoid arthritis (RA) and osteoarthritis
- Was diagnosed with diabetes mellitus type 2 last year, which is controlled by diet
- Has a history of atrial fibrillation
- Is retired and lives alone in a senior housing apartment
- Volunteers twice a week in the local library
- Current medications include:
  - Etanercept 50 mg subcutaneously each week (self-administered) for RA
  - Leflunomide 10 mg orally each day for RA
  - Clopidogrel 75 mg orally each day for atrial fibrillation
  - Acetaminophen 500 mg orally as needed twice a day for OA pain
- Has two children who live locally
- Is able to perform ADLs independently, although she has ulnar deviation and finger deformities in both hands
- Uses a cane when not at home
- Drives short distances to the grocery store and bank
- Is alert and oriented
- Reports occasional constipation
- Reports current joint pain level is a 5 on a 0-10 pain scale; most painful joints are her feet and knees (states that her usual pain level is a 1-2 before hospital admission)
- Reports occasional paresthesias in both feet
- Has 1+ nonpitting edema in both feet

- Current oral temperature = 100.8° F (38.2° C)
- Current apical pulse = 82
- Resting respiratory rate = 32 breaths/min
- Current blood pressure = 138/88
- Admitting WBC = 15,500/mm³

1. **Recognize Cues:** What assessment information in this client situation is the most important and immediate concern for the nurse? (Hint: Identify the **relevant** information *first* to determine what is most important.)
2. **Analyze Cues:** What client conditions are consistent with the **most relevant** information? (Hint: Think about priority collaborative problems that support and contradict the information presented in this situation.)
3. **Prioritize Hypotheses:** Which possibilities or explanations are **most likely** to be present in this client situation? Which possibilities or explanations are the most serious? (Hint: Consider all possibilities and determine their urgency and risk for this client.)
4. **Generate Solutions:** What actions would most likely achieve the desired outcomes for this client? Which actions should be **avoided** or are **potentially harmful**? (Hint: Determine the desired outcomes first to decide which interventions are appropriate and those that should be avoided.)
5. **Take Action:** Which actions are the most appropriate and how should they be implemented? In what **priority order** should they be implemented? (Hint: Consider health teaching, documentation, requested health care provider orders or prescriptions, nursing skills, collaboration with or referral to health team members, etc.)
6. **Evaluate Outcomes:** What client assessment would indicate that the nurse's actions were **effective**? (Hint: Think about signs that would indicate an improvement, decline, or unchanged client condition.)

GET READY FOR THE NEXT-GENERATION NCLEX® EXAMINATION!

Key Points

Review these Key Points for each NCLEX Examination Client Needs Category.

Safe and Effective Care Environment

- Collaborate with the health care team to manage chronic pain and increase *mobility* for patients with arthritis. **QSEN: Teamwork and Collaboration**
- Prioritize care for patients having a total joint arthroplasty to prevent complications, such as dislocation, *infection,* and venous thromboembolism. **QSEN: Safety**

Health Promotion and Maintenance

- Provide information about community resources for patients with arthritis, especially professional organizations such as the Arthritis Foundation. **QSEN: Patient-Centered Care**
- Teach patients to prevent joint trauma and reduce weight as needed to help prevent osteoarthritis. **QSEN: Evidence-Based Practice**
- Recall that a combination of environmental, genetic, and immune risk factors can cause rheumatoid arthritis (RA). **QSEN: Patient-Centered Care**
- Reinforce the importance of good health practices, such as adequate sleep, proper nutrition, regular exercise, and stress-management techniques for patients with arthritis. **QSEN: Patient-Centered Care**
- Provide patients and their families with discharge instructions to prevent complications and promote *mobility* after total hip or knee arthroplasty. **QSEN: Safety, Evidence-Based Practice**
- Teach patients with arthritis about appropriate exercises, joint protection techniques, and energy conservation guidelines. **QSEN: Evidence-Based Practice**

Psychosocial Integrity

- Recognize that patients with rheumatoid arthritis (RA) may have body image disturbance as a result of potentially deforming joint involvement and nodules. **QSEN: Patient-Centered Care**
- Encourage patients with arthritis to discuss their chronic illness and identify coping strategies that have previously been successful. **QSEN: Patient-Centered Care**
- Be aware that chronic, painful diseases affect the patient's quality of life and role performance. **QSEN: Patient-Centered Care**

Physiological Integrity

- Differentiate OA as primarily a joint problem that can affect one or more joints and RA as a systemic disease that presents as a bilateral symmetric joint *inflammation.* Both diseases can impact the patient's *mobility.* **Clinical Judgment**
- Realize that older patients have OA more than younger patients; younger patients have RA more than older adults. Both diseases cause persistent joint *pain* that needs to be managed. **Clinical Judgment**
- Teach patients who have osteoarthritis (OA) or are prone to the disease to lose weight (if obese), avoid trauma, and limit strenuous weight-bearing activities. **QSEN: Evidence-Based Practice**
- Instruct patients with arthritic pain to use multiple modalities for *pain* relief, including ice/heat, rest, positioning, integrative therapies, and drug therapy as prescribed. **QSEN: Evidence-Based Practice**
- Teach patients to monitor and report side and adverse effects of drugs used to treat OA and RA. **QSEN: Safety**
- Teach patients who are taking hydroxychloroquine to have frequent (every 6 months) eye examinations to monitor for retinal changes. **QSEN: Safety**
- Remind patients to avoid crowds and other possible sources of infection when they are taking drugs that decrease *immunity.* **QSEN: Safety**
- Implement interventions for patients having total joint arthroplasty (TJA) to prevent venous thromboembolism (e.g., anticoagulants, exercises, sequential compression devices); observe the patient for bleeding when he or she is taking anticoagulants. **Clinical Judgment**
- Be careful when positioning a patient after a total hip arthroplasty (THA) to prevent dislocation; do not hyperflex the hips or adduct the legs, especially for patients who had a posterolateral surgical approach. **QSEN: Safety**
- Recognize the surgical site for a TKA is typically very swollen and discolored for several weeks after surgery; teach the patient to use cold applications to reduce swelling. **QSEN: Patient-Centered Care**
- Be aware that disease-modifying antirheumatic drugs (DMARDs) and biological response modifiers (BRMs) slow the progression of autoimmune diseases such as RA. **QSEN: Evidence-Based Practice**
- Teach patients receiving BRMs and other disease-modifying agents to avoid crowds and people with infections; opportunistic pathogens may cause serious infections or death. Check the patient's PPD test or history of tuberculosis before starting any of these drugs. **QSEN: Safety**

MASTERY QUESTIONS

1. The nurse is caring for a client with severe osteoarthritis. What will the nurse anticipate as the client's **priority** problem?
   A. Joint pain
   B. ADL dependence
   C. Risk for falls
   D. Muscle stiffness

2. The nurse is caring for a client who had an anterior total hip arthroplasty yesterday. For which **commonly occurring** postoperative complication will the nurse monitor for this client?
   A. Pneumonia
   B. Paralytic ileus
   C. Wound dehiscence
   D. Venous thromboembolism

3. The nurse is assessing a client who has **late-stage** rheumatoid arthritis. Which assessment findings would the nurse expect for this client? **Select all that apply.**
   A. Joint inflammation
   B. Severe weight loss
   C. Bony nodules
   D. Joint deformities
   E. Sjögren syndrome

REFERENCES

Asterisk (*) indicates a classic or definitive work on this subject.

Arthritis Foundation. (2019). *Arthritis by the numbers: Book of trusted facts and figures*. Atlanta, GA: Arthritis Foundation.

Bodden, J., & Coppola, C. (2018). *Best practice guideline: Total hip replacement (arthroplasty)*. Chicago, IL: SmithBucklin (for the National Association of Orthopaedic Nursing).

Burchum, J. L. R., & Rosenthal, L. D. (2019). *Lehne's pharmacology for nursing care* (9th ed.). St. Louis: Elsevier.

Causey-Upton, R., Howell, D. M., Kitzman, P. H., Custer, M. G., & Dressler, E. V. (2019). Factors influencing discharge readiness after total knee replacement. *Orthopaedic Nursing, 38*(1), 6–14.

Cheuy, V. A., Foran, J. R. H., Paxton, R. J., Bade, M. J., Zeni, J. A., & Stevens-Lapsley, J. E. (2017). Arthrofibrosis associated with total knee arthroplasty. *The Journal of Arthroplasty, 32*, 2604–2611.

Chicoski, A. S. (2018). Caring for the orthopaedic patient with a history of bariatric surgery. *Orthopaedic Nursing, 37*(2), 106–112.

Gallagher, L. M., Gardner, V., Bates, D., Mason, S., Nemecek, J., DiFiore, D. B., et al. (2018). Impact of music therapy on hospitalized patients post-elective orthopaedic surgery: A randomized controlled trial. *Orthopaedic Nursing, 37*(2), 124–135.

Goode, V. M., Morgan, B., Muckler, V. C., Cary, M. P., Jr., Zbed, C. E., & Zychowicz, M. (2019). Multimodal pain management for major joint replacement surgery. *Orthopaedic Nursing, 38*(2), 150–156.

Gourdine, J. (2019). Review of nonsurgical treatment guidelines for lower extremity osteoarthritis. *Orthopaedic Nursing, 38*(5), 303–308.

Hohler, S. E. (2018). Walk patients through total hip arthroplasty. *Nursing, 48*(9), 24–31.

Jackman, C. (2019). Perioperative pain management for the chronic pain patient with long-term opioid use. *Orthopaedic Nursing, 38*(2), 159–163.

Jones, L., & Taylor, T. (2019). Identifying acute delirium on acute care units. *Medsurg Nursing, 28*, 172–175 181.

*McAlindon, T. E., Bannuru, R. R., Sullivan, M. C., Arden, N. K., Berenbaum, F., Bierma-Zeinstra, S. M., et al. (2014). OARSI guidelines for the non-surgical management of knee osteoarthritis. *Osteoarthritis and Cartilage, 22*, 363–388.

McCance, K., Huether, S., Brashers, V., & Rote, N. (2019). *Pathophysiology: The biologic basis for disease in adults and children* (8th ed.). St. Louis: Mosby.

McCann-Spry, L., Pelton, J., Grandy, G., & Newell, D. (2016). An interdisciplinary approach to reducing length of stay in joint replacement patients. *Orthopaedic Nursing, 35*(5), 279–300.

Mogoi, V., Elder, B., Hayes, K., & Huhman, D. (2019). Effectiveness of platelet-rich plasma in management of knee osteoarthritis in a rural clinic. *Orthopaedic Nursing, 38*(3), 193–198.

Mori, C., & Ribsam, V. (2018). *Best practice guideline: Total knee replacement (arthroplasty)*. SmithBucklin (for the National Association of Orthopaedic Nursing).

Morland, R. (2019). Evolution of the national opioid crisis. *Nursing2019, 39*(5), 51–56.

O'Brien, M., & McDougall, J. J. (2018). Cannabis and joints: Scientific evidence for the alleviation of osteoarthritis pain. *Current Opinion in Pharmacology, 40*, 104–109.

Pietsch, T., David, J., & Vergara, F. (2018). Integrative review for patients with bilateral total knee replacement: A call for nursing practice guidelines. *Orthopaedic Nursing, 37*(4), 237–243.

Pizzi, L. J., Bates, M., Chelly, J. E., & Goodrich, C. J. (2020). A prospective randomized trial of an oral patient-controlled analgesia deice versus usual care following total hip arthroplasty. *Orthopaedic Nursing, 39*(1), 37–46.

Saccomano, S. J. (2018). Osteoarthritis treatment: Decreasing pain, increasing mobility. *The Nurse Practitioner, 43*(9), 49–55.

Sasse, L., Laessig-Stary, B., & Abitz, T. (2020). Periarticular ketorolac improves outcomes for patients with joint replacements. *Orthopaedic Nursing, 39*(1), 47–50.

Schinsky, M. F., McCune, C., & Bonomi, J. (2016). Multifaceted comparison of two cryotherapy devices used after total knee arthroplasty: Cryotherapy device comparison. *Orthopaedic Nursing, 35*(5), 317–324.

Tubog, T. D. (2019). Combined intermittent pneumatic leg compression and pharmacological prophylaxis for prevention of venous thromboembolism. *Orthopaedic Nursing, 38*(4), 270–272.

Wilson, K., Devito, D., Zavotsky, K. E., Rusay, M., Allen, M., & Huang, S. (2018). Keep it moving and remember to P.A.C. (Pharmacology, Ambulation, and Compression) for venous thromboembolism prevention. *Orthopeadic Nursing, 37*(6), 339–345.

*Zhang, W. W., Nuki, G., Moskowitz, R., Abramson, S., Altman, R. D., Arden, N. K., et al. (2010). OARSI recommendations for the management of hip and knee osteoarthritis, Part III: Changes in evidence following systematic cumulative update of research published through January 2009. *Osteoarthritis and Cartilage, 18*(4), 476–499.

Zhao, L., Kaye, A. D., & Abd-Elsayed, A. (2018). Stem cells for the treatment of knee osteoarthritis: A comprehensive review. *Pain Physician, 21*(3), 229–242.

47

Concepts of Care for Patients With Musculoskeletal Trauma

Donna D. Ignatavicius

http://evolve.elsevier.com/Iggy/

LEARNING OUTCOMES

1. Collaborate with the interprofessional team to manage quality care for patients with impaired *mobility* caused by caused by musculoskeletal trauma, including fractures and amputation.
2. Identify community resources for families and patients recovering from musculoskeletal trauma.
3. Apply knowledge of pathophysiology of fracture and amputation to identify common assessment findings, including actual or risk for impaired *sensory perception*, *tissue integrity*, and *perfusion.*
4. Prioritize evidence-based nursing interventions for patients with musculoskeletal trauma to promote *mobility,* maintain *perfusion,* manage *pain,* and protect *tissue integrity.*
5. Plan transition management and care coordination for patients with fractures and amputations, including health teaching about complications such as *infection* and altered *sensory perception.*

KEY TERMS

acute compartment syndrome (ACS) A serious but uncommon limb-threatening condition in which increased pressure within one or more compartments (that contain muscle, blood vessels, and nerves) reduces circulation to the lower leg or forearm.

amputation The removal of a part of the body.

ankle-brachial index A measure of blood flow in the lower extremities. It is calculated by dividing ankle systolic pressure by brachial systolic pressure. A normal ABI is 0.9 or higher.

avascular necrosis (also known as *osteonecrosis*) The death of bone tissue.

bone reduction Realignment of the bone ends for proper healing that is accomplished by a *closed* (nonsurgical) method or an *open* (surgical) procedure.

cast A rigid device (synthetic, or less commonly, plaster) that immobilizes the affected body part while allowing other body parts to move.

closed (simple) fracture A fracture that does not extend through the skin (no visible wound).

complex regional pain syndrome (CRPS) A poorly understood dysfunction of the central and peripheral nervous systems that leads to severe, persistent *pain.*

ergonomics The study of how equipment and furniture can be arranged so that people can do work or other activities more efficiently and comfortably without injury.

external fixation A surgical procedure in which pins or wires are inserted through the skin and affected bone and then connected to a rigid external frame outside the body to immobilize the fracture during healing.

fascia iliaca compartment block (FICB) A regional anesthetic technique to manage pain for patients who have a fractured hip. The anesthetic agent (such as levobupivacaine) blocks the femoral, lateral cutaneous, and obturator nerves while avoiding the risk of injury to the femoral artery and vein.

fasciotomy A procedure for acute compartment syndrome in which the surgeon cuts through fascia to relieve pressure and tension on vital blood vessels and nerves.

fat embolism syndrome (FES) A serious but uncommon complication of fractures in which fat globules are released from the yellow bone marrow into the bloodstream within 12 to 48 hours after injury. These globules clog small blood vessels that supply vital organs, most commonly the lungs, and impair organ *perfusion.*

fracture A break or disruption in the continuity of a bone that often affects *mobility* and causes *pain.*

fragility fracture A fracture caused by osteoporosis or other disease that weakens bone.

internal fixation A surgical procedure in which metal pins, screws, rods, plates, or prostheses are inserted inside the body to immobilize a fracture during healing.

neuroma A sensitive tumor consisting of damaged nerve cells that forms most often in patients with amputations of the upper extremity but can occur anywhere.

open (compound) fracture A fracture that extends through the skin, causing a visible wound.

opioid-induced constipation (OIC) Constipation that can result from taking opioids for a long period of time.

phantom limb pain (PLP) A persistent altered *sensory perception* in the amputated body part that is unpleasant or painful.

repetitive stress injury (RSI) A fast-growing occupational injury, which occurs in people whose jobs require repetitive hand activities, such as pinching or grasping during wrist flexion; carpal tunnel syndrome (CTS) is the most common RSI.

subcutaneous emphysema The appearance of bubbles under the skin because of air trapping.

traction The application of a pulling force to a part of the body to provide bone alignment or relief of muscle spasm.

✴ PRIORITY AND INTERRELATED CONCEPTS

The priority concepts for this chapter are:
- *Mobility*
- *Perfusion*

The *Mobility* concept exemplar for this chapter is Fracture.
The *Perfusion* concept exemplar for this chapter is Amputation.

The interrelated concepts for this chapter are:
- *Pain*
- *Tissue Integrity*
- *Sensory Perception*
- *Infection*

Musculoskeletal trauma accounts for about two thirds of all injuries and is one of the primary causes of disability in the United States. It includes health problems that range from simple muscle strain to multiple bone fractures with severe soft-tissue damage. This chapter focuses on the most common types of musculoskeletal trauma.

Fractures and other musculoskeletal trauma impair a patient's *mobility* in varying degrees, depending on the severity and extent of the injury. These injuries can also result in severe *pain*, altered *sensory perception*, and *infection*. Amputations result in impaired *tissue integrity* and are often performed because of inadequate arterial *perfusion* caused by chronic disease. These health concepts are reviewed in Chapter 3 of this text. In some cases, bleeding from traumatic injuries can lead to hemorrhage and hypovolemic shock, described elsewhere in this text.

✴ MOBILITY CONCEPT EXEMPLAR: FRACTURE

Pathophysiology Review

A fracture is a break or disruption in the continuity of a bone that often affects *mobility* and causes *pain*. It can occur anywhere in the body and at any age. All fractures have the same basic pathophysiologic mechanism and require similar patient-centered, interprofessional collaborative care, regardless of fracture type or location.

Classification of Fractures. A fracture can be classified by the extent of the break:
- *Complete fracture.* The break is across the entire width of the bone in such a way that the bone is divided into two distinct sections. If bone alignment is altered or disrupted, the fracture is also referred to as a *displaced* fracture. The ends of bone sections of a displaced fracture are more likely to damage surrounding nerves, blood vessels, and other soft tissues.

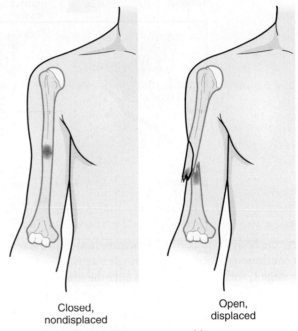

Closed, nondisplaced

Open, displaced

FIG. 47.1 Common types of fractures.

- *Incomplete fracture.* The fracture does not divide the bone into two portions because the break is through only part of the bone. This type of fracture is not typically displaced.

A fracture can also be described by the extent of associated soft-tissue damage: **open** (or **compound**) or **closed** (or **simple**) (Fig. 47.1). The skin surface over the broken bone is disrupted in a *compound* fracture, which causes an external wound. These fractures are often graded to define the extent of tissue damage. A *simple* fracture does not extend through the skin and therefore has no visible wound.

In addition to being identified by type, fractures are described by their cause. A *fragility fracture* (also known as a *pathologic* or *spontaneous fracture*) occurs after minimal trauma to a bone that has been weakened by disease. For example, a patient with bone cancer or osteoporosis can easily have a fragility fracture (see Chapter 45 for a discussion of these disorders). A *fatigue (stress) fracture* results from excessive strain and stress on the bone. This problem is commonly seen in recreational and professional athletes. *Compression fractures* are produced by a loading force applied to the long axis of cancellous bone. They commonly occur in the vertebrae of older patients with osteoporosis and are extremely painful.

Stages of Bone Healing. When a bone is fractured, the body immediately begins the healing process to repair the injury and

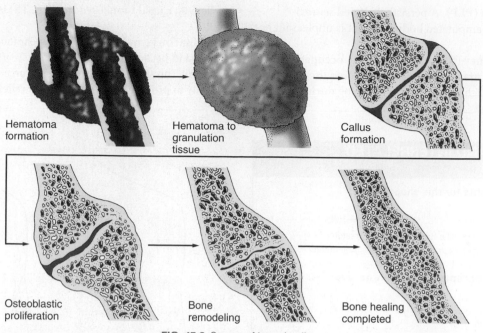

Hematoma formation

Hematoma to granulation tissue

Callus formation

Osteoblastic proliferation

Bone remodeling

Bone healing completed

FIG. 47.2 Stages of bone healing.

restore the body's equilibrium. Fractures heal in five stages that are a continuous process and not single stages.

- In stage 1, within 24 to 72 hours after the injury, a hematoma forms at the site of the fracture because bone is extremely vascular.
- Stage 2 occurs in 3 days to 2 weeks when granulation tissue begins to invade the hematoma. This then prompts the formation of fibrocartilage, providing the foundation for bone healing.
- Stage 3 of bone healing occurs as a result of vascular and cellular proliferation. The fracture site is surrounded by new vascular tissue known as a *callus* (within 3 to 6 weeks). *Callus* formation is the beginning of a nonbony union.
- As healing continues in stage 4, the callus is gradually resorbed and transformed into bone. This stage usually takes 3 to 8 weeks.
- During the fifth and final stage of healing, consolidation and remodeling of bone continue to meet mechanical demands. This process may start as early as 4 to 6 weeks after fracture and can continue for up to 1 year, depending on the severity of the injury and the age and health of the patient. Fig. 47.2 summarizes the stages of bone healing.

In young, healthy adult bone, healing takes about 4 to 6 weeks. In the older person who has reduced bone mass, healing time is lengthened. Complete healing may take 3 months or longer in people who are older than 70 years. Other factors, such as the severity of the trauma, the type of bone injured, how the fracture is managed, and/or the presence of infection or avascular necrosis (AVN), also called *osteonecrosis,* can also impact healing.

Complications of Fractures. Regardless of the type or location of the fracture, several limb- and life-threatening acute and chronic complications can result from the injury. Signs and symptoms of beginning complications must be treated early to prevent serious consequences. In some cases, careful monitoring

and assessment by the nurse can prevent these complications from occurring or worsening.

Acute Complications of Fractures. Common acute complications of fractures include venous thromboembolism (VTE) and bone or soft tissue *infection. Venous thromboembolism (VTE)* includes deep vein thrombosis (DVT) and its major complication, pulmonary embolism (PE). It is the most common complication of lower-extremity surgery or trauma and the most often fatal complication of musculoskeletal surgery. Chapter 33 discusses VTE, including prevention and management, in detail.

Whenever there is trauma to tissues, the body's defense system is disrupted. Wound infections are the most common type of *infection* resulting from orthopedic trauma. They range from superficial skin infections to deep wound abscesses. Infection can also be caused by implanted hardware used to repair a fracture surgically, such as screws, pins, plates, or rods. Clostridia infections can result in gas gangrene or tetanus and can prevent the bone from healing properly.

Bone *infection,* or osteomyelitis, is most common with open fractures in which *tissue integrity* is altered and after surgical repair of a fracture (see Chapter 45 for discussion of osteomyelitis). For patients experiencing this type of trauma, the risk for health care agency–acquired infections is increased. These infections are common, and many result from multidrug-resistant organisms, such as methicillin-resistant *Staphylococcus aureus* (MRSA). Reducing MRSA infection is a primary desired outcome for all health care agencies. Chapter 21 discusses prevention and management of **infection** in detail.

Several complications of fractures are more rare but are potentially life-threatening, including acute compartment syndrome and fat embolism syndrome. **Acute compartment syndrome (ACS)** is a serious, limb-threatening condition in which increased pressure within one or more compartments (that contain muscle, blood vessels, and nerves) reduces circulation to the lower leg or forearm.

The pathophysiologic changes of increased compartment pressure are sometimes referred to as the *ischemia-edema cycle*. Capillaries within the muscle dilate, which raises capillary (arterial) and venous pressure. Capillaries become more permeable because of the release of histamine by the ischemic muscle tissue, and venous drainage decreases. As a result, plasma proteins leak into the interstitial fluid space and edema occurs. Edema increases pressure on nerve endings and causes severe pain. The pain experienced is greater than expected for the nature of the injury. **Perfusion** to the area is reduced, and further ischemia results. **Sensory perception** deficits or paresthesia generally appears before changes in vascular or motor signs. The color of the tissue pales, and pulses begin to weaken but rarely disappear. The affected area is usually palpably tense, and acute severe **pain** occurs with passive motion of the extremity. If the condition is not treated, cyanosis, tingling, numbness, paresis, and necrosis

can occur. The Key Features: Acute Compartment Syndrome box summarizes the sequence of pathophysiologic events in compartment syndrome and the associated clinical assessment findings.

The pressure to the compartment can be from an external or internal source, but fracture is present in most cases of ACS. Tight, bulky dressings and casts are examples of *external* pressure causes. Blood or fluid accumulation in the compartment is a common source of *internal* pressure. ACS is not limited to patients with musculoskeletal problems. It can also occur in those with severe burns, extensive insect bites or snakebites, or massive infiltration of IV fluids. In these situations, edema increases internal pressure in one or more compartments. Patients with ACS may need a surgical procedure known as a **fasciotomy**. In this procedure, the surgeon cuts through the fascia to relieve pressure and tension on vital blood vessels and nerves. The wound remains open and requires care to begin to heal from the inside out. The surgeon usually closes the wound with a skin graft in several days. Wound care is described in Chapter 23 and in basic nursing fundamentals textbooks.

Long-term problems resulting from compartment syndrome include **infection,** persistent motor weakness in the affected extremity, contracture, and myoglobinuric renal failure. In extreme cases, amputation becomes necessary.

Fat embolism syndrome (FES) is another serious complication of fractures in which fat globules are released from the yellow bone marrow into the bloodstream within 12 to 48 hours after an injury. These globules clog small blood vessels that supply vital organs, most commonly the lungs, and impair organ **perfusion**. FES usually results from fractures or fracture repair but may also occur, although less often, in patients experiencing pancreatitis, osteomyelitis, blunt trauma, or sickle cell disease.

The earliest signs and symptoms of FES are a low arterial oxygen level (hypoxemia), dyspnea, and tachypnea (increased respirations). Headache, lethargy, agitation, confusion, decreased level of consciousness, seizures, and vision changes may follow. Nonpalpable, red-brown *petechiae*—a macular, measles-like rash—may appear over the neck, upper arms, and/or chest. This rash is a classic manifestation but is usually the last sign to develop (McCance et al., 2019).

Abnormal laboratory findings include:

- Decreased PaO_2 level (often below 60 mm Hg)
- Increased erythrocyte sedimentation rate (ESR)
- Decreased serum calcium levels
- Decreased red blood cell and platelet counts
- Increased serum level of lipids

These changes in blood values are poorly understood, but they aid in diagnosis of the condition.

The chest x-ray often shows bilateral infiltrates but may be normal. The chest CT often reveals a patchy distribution of opacities. An MRI of the brain can show evidence of neurologic deficits from hypoxemia. FES can result in respiratory failure or death, often from pulmonary edema. When the lungs are affected, the complication may be misdiagnosed as a pulmonary embolism from a blood clot (Table 47.1).

Chronic Complications of Fractures. Avascular necrosis, delayed bone healing, and chronic regional pain syndrome are later chronic complications of musculoskeletal trauma. Blood supply to the bone may be disrupted, causing decreased **perfusion**

▶▶ KEY FEATURES
Acute Compartment Syndrome

Physiologic Change	Clinical Findings
Increased compartment pressure	No change
Increased capillary permeability	Edema
Release of histamine	Increased edema
Increased blood flow to area	Pulses present Pink tissue
Pressure on nerve endings	Acute pain
Increased tissue pressure	Referred pain to compartment(s)
Decreased tissue perfusion	Increased edema
Decreased oxygen to tissues	Pallor
Increased production of lactic acid	Unequal pulses Flexed posture
Anaerobic metabolism	Cyanosis
Vasodilation	Increased edema
Increased blood flow	Tense muscle swelling
Increased tissue pressure	Tingling Numbness
Increased edema	Paresthesia
Muscle ischemia	Severe pain unrelieved by drugs
Tissue necrosis	Paresis/paralysis

TABLE 47.1 Fat Embolism Versus Blood Clot (Pulmonary) Embolism

Fat Embolism	Blood Clot Embolism
Definition	
Obstruction of the pulmonary (or other organ) vascular bed by fat globules	Obstruction of the pulmonary artery by a blood clot or clots
Origin	
Most from fractures of the long bones; occurs usually within 48 hr of injury	Most from deep vein thrombosis in the legs or pelvis; can occur anytime
Assessment Findings	
Altered mental status (earliest sign)	Same as for fat embolism, except no petechiae
Increased respirations, pulse, temperature	
Chest pain	
Dyspnea	
Crackles	
Decreased Sao$_2$	
Petechiae (not present in all patients)	
Mild thrombocytopenia	
Treatment	
Bedrest	Preventive measures (e.g., leg exercises, antiembolism stockings, SCDs)
Gentle handling	
Oxygen	Bedrest
Hydration (IV fluids)	Oxygen
Possibly steroid therapy	Possibly mechanical ventilation
Fracture immobilization	Anticoagulants
	Thrombolytics
	Possible surgery: pulmonary embolectomy, vena cava umbrella

Sao$_2$, Arterial oxygen saturation; *SCD,* sequential compression device.

and death of bone tissue, or **avascular necrosis.** This problem is most often a complication of hip fractures or any fracture in which there is displacement of bone. Surgical repair of fractures also can cause necrosis because the hardware can interfere with circulation. Patients on long-term corticosteroid therapy, such as prednisone, are also at high risk for ischemic necrosis.

Delayed union is a fracture that has not healed within 6 months of injury. Some fractures never achieve union; that is, they never completely heal *(nonunion).* Others heal incorrectly *(malunion).* These problems are most common in patients with tibial fractures, fractures that involve many treatment techniques (e.g., cast, traction), and pathologic fractures. Union may also be delayed or not achieved in the older patient due to poor bone health. If bone does not heal, he or she typically has persistent **pain** and decreased **mobility** from deformity.

Complex regional pain syndrome (CRPS), formerly called *reflex sympathetic dystrophy (RSD),* is a poorly understood dysfunction of the central and peripheral nervous systems that leads to severe, persistent **pain** and other symptoms. Genetic factors may play a role in the development of this devastating complication. CRPS most often results from fractures or other traumatic musculoskeletal injury and commonly occurs in the

feet and hands (Thurlow & Gray, 2018). In some cases, specific nerve injuries are present, but in others no injury can be identified. To facilitate soft tissue healing and *prevent* CRPS, the physical therapist asks the patient to frequently apply a variety of objects with varying surface types directly to the skin to desensitize it. These objects can be rough, smooth, hard, soft, sharp (but not enough to damage the skin), or dull.

When CRPS is present, a triad of signs and symptoms is present, including (Thurlow & Gray, 2018):
- Abnormalities of the autonomic nervous system (changes in color, temperature, and sensitivity of skin over the affected area, excessive sweating, edema)
- Motor symptoms (paresis, muscle spasms, loss of function)
- Altered *sensory perception* symptoms (intense burning pain that becomes intractable [unrelenting])

Etiology and Genetic Risk. The primary cause of a fracture is trauma from a motor vehicle crash or fall, especially in older adults. The trauma may be a direct blow to the bone or an indirect force from muscle contractions or pulling forces on the bone. Sports, vigorous exercise, and malnutrition are contributing factors. Bone diseases, such as osteoporosis, increase the risk for a fracture in older adults (see Chapter 45). Genetic factors that increase risk for fracture are discussed with these specific health problems throughout this text.

Incidence and Prevalence. The incidence of fractures depends on the location of the injury. Rib fractures are the most common type in the adult population. Femoral shaft fractures occur most often in young and middle-age adults.

PATIENT-CENTERED CARE: OLDER ADULT CONSIDERATIONS (QSEN)

The incidence of proximal femur (hip) fractures is highest in older adults. Humeral fractures are also common in older adults; the older the person, usually the more proximal is the fracture. Wrist (Colles) fractures are typically seen in middle and late adulthood and usually result from a fall. These fractures are sometimes referred to as *FOSH fractures* (fall out-stretched hand). Middle-age and older adults, especially women, have a higher incidence of osteoporosis, which increases the risk for fragility fractures.

Health Promotion and Maintenance

Airbags and seat belts have decreased the number of severe injuries and deaths, but they have *increased* the number of leg and ankle fractures, especially in older adults. Focus health teaching on risks for musculoskeletal injury, including:
- Osteoporosis screening and self-management education (see Chapter 45)
- Fall prevention (see Chapter 4)
- Home safety assessment and modification, if needed
- Dangers of substance use and driving
- Preventing overuse injuries for recreational and professional athletes
- Helmet use when riding bicycles, motorcycles, and other small motorized vehicles/devices

❖ Interprofessional Collaborative Care

◆ Assessment: Recognize Cues

History. The patient with a new fracture typically reports moderate-to-severe *pain.* Delay the detailed interview for a nursing history until he or she is more comfortable, and then ask about the cause of the fracture. Certain types of force (e.g., incisional, crush, acceleration, or deceleration), shearing, and friction lead to most musculoskeletal injuries. As a result, several body systems are often affected.

Incisional injuries, as from a knife wound, and *crush* injuries cause hemorrhage and decreased *perfusion* to major organs. *Acceleration or deceleration* injuries cause direct trauma to the spleen, brain, and kidneys when these organs are moved from their fixed locations in the body. *Shearing and friction* damage *tissue integrity* and cause a high level of wound contamination.

Asking about the events leading to the injury helps identify which forces were experienced and therefore which body systems or parts of the body to assess. For example, a forward fall often results in Colles fracture of the wrist because the person tries to catch himself or herself with an outstretched hand. Knowing the mechanism of injury also helps determine whether other types of injury, such as head and spinal cord injury, might be present.

Obtain a substance use history regardless of the patient's age. For example, a young adult may have had an excessive amount of alcohol and/or drugs, which contributed to a motor vehicle crash or a fall at the work site. Many older adults also consume alcohol and an assortment of prescribed and over-the-counter drugs, which can cause dizziness and loss of balance. *Assess adults of all ages about opioid use for persistent pain before the fracture. This information is essential for developing a pain management plan for the patient.*

Ask about the patient's occupation and recreational activities. Some occupations are more hazardous than others. For instance, construction work is potentially more physically dangerous than office work. Certain hobbies and recreational activities are also extremely hazardous, such as skiing. Contact sports, such as football and ice hockey, often result in musculoskeletal injuries, including fractures. Other activities do not have such an obvious potential for injury but can cause fractures nonetheless. For instance, daily jogging or running can lead to fatigue (stress) fractures.

Physical Assessment/Signs and Symptoms. The patient with a fracture often has trauma to other body systems. Therefore assess all major body systems *first* for life-threatening complications, especially when patients have head, chest, and/or abdominal trauma. Some fractures can cause internal organ damage resulting in hemorrhage. When a pelvic fracture is suspected, assess vital signs, skin color, and level of consciousness for indications of possible hypovolemic shock from internal blood loss. Remember that if there is one pelvic fracture, there is usually another fracture in the pelvis, even if it is small or hairline. Check the urine for blood, which indicates possible damage to the urinary system, often the bladder. If the patient cannot void, suspect that the bladder or urethra has been damaged. Complete assessment of organ function is described elsewhere in this text.

Patients with severe or multiple fractures of the arms, legs, or pelvis have severe *pain.* Vertebral compression fractures are also extremely painful. Patients *with a fractured hip may have groin pain or pain referred to the back of the knee or lower back. Pain* is usually caused by muscle spasm and edema that result from the fracture.

> **! NURSING SAFETY PRIORITY** (QSEN)
> **Action Alert**
>
> Patients with one or more fractured ribs have severe pain when they take deep breaths. Monitor respiratory status, which may be severely compromised from pain or pneumothorax (air in the pleural cavity). Assess the patient's *pain* level and manage pain *before* continuing the physical assessment.

For fractures of the shoulder and upper arm, the physical assessment is best done with the patient in a sitting or standing position, if possible, so shoulder drooping or other abnormal positioning can be seen. Support the affected arm and flex the elbow to promote comfort during the assessment. For more distal areas of the arm, perform the assessment with the patient in a supine position so that the extremity can be elevated to reduce swelling.

Place the patient in a supine position for assessment of the legs and pelvis. A patient with an impacted hip fracture may be able to walk for a short time after injury, although this is not recommended.

When inspecting the site of a possible fracture, look for a change in bone alignment. The bone may appear deformed, a limb may be internally or externally rotated, and/or one or more bones may also be dislocated (out of their joint capsules). Observe for extremity shortening or a change in bone shape.

If the skin is intact (closed fracture), the area over the fracture may be ecchymotic (bruised) from bleeding into the underlying soft tissues. Subcutaneous emphysema, the appearance of bubbles under the skin because of air trapping, may be present but is usually seen later.

> **! NURSING SAFETY PRIORITY** (QSEN)
> **Action Alert**
>
> Swelling at the fracture site is rapid and can result in marked neurovascular compromise as a result of decreased arterial *perfusion. Gently perform a thorough neurovascular assessment and compare extremities.* Assess skin color and temperature, *sensory perception, mobility, pain,* and pulses distal to the fracture site. If the fracture involves an extremity and the patient is not in severe pain, check the nails for capillary refill by applying pressure to the nail and observing for the speed of blood return (usually 3 to 5 seconds, depending on the patient's age). If nails are brittle or thick, assess the skin next to the nail. Checking for capillary refill is not as reliable as other indicators of *perfusion.*

The Best Practice for Patient Safety & Quality Care: Assessment of Neurovascular Status in Patients With Musculoskeletal Injury box describes the procedure for a neurovascular assessment, which evaluates <u>c</u>irculation, <u>m</u>ovement, and <u>s</u>ensation (CMS function).

BEST PRACTICE FOR PATIENT SAFETY & QUALITY CARE (QSEN)

Assessment of Neurovascular Status in Patients With Musculoskeletal Injury

Assessment Method	Normal Findings
Skin Color	
Inspect the area distal to the injury.	No change in pigmentation compared with other parts of the body.
Skin Temperature	
Palpate the area distal to the injury (the dorsum of the hands is most sensitive to temperature).	The skin is warm.
Movement	
Ask the patient to move the affected area or the area distal to the injury (active motion).	The patient can move without discomfort.
Move the area distal to the injury (passive motion).	No difference in comfort compared with active movement.
Sensation	
Ask the patient if numbness or tingling is present (paresthesia).	No numbness or tingling.
Palpate with a paper clip (especially the web space between the first and second toes or the web space between the thumb and forefinger).	No difference in sensation in the affected and unaffected extremities. (Loss of sensation in these areas indicates peroneal nerve or median nerve damage.)
Pulses	
Palpate the pulses distal to the injury.	Pulses are strong and easily palpated; no difference in the affected and unaffected extremities.
Capillary Refill (Least Reliable)	
Press the nail beds distal to the injury until blanching occurs (or the skin near the nail if nails are thick and brittle).	Blood returns (return to usual color) within 3 sec (5 sec for older patients).
Pain	
Ask the patient about the location, nature, and frequency of the pain.	Pain is usually localized and is often described as stabbing or throbbing. (Pain out of proportion to the injury and unrelieved by analgesics might indicate compartment syndrome.)

Psycosocial Assessment. The psychosocial status of a patient with a fracture depends on the extent of the injury, possible complications, coping ability, and availability of support systems. Hospitalization is not required for a single, uncomplicated fracture, and the patient returns to usual daily activities within a few days. Examples include a single fracture of a bone in the finger, wrist, foot, or toe.

In contrast, a patient suffering severe or multiple traumas may be hospitalized for weeks and may undergo many surgical procedures, treatments, and prolonged rehabilitation. These

PATIENT-CENTERED CARE: CULTURAL/SPIRITUAL CONSIDERATIONS (QSEN)

For patients experiencing long-term recovery from fractures and other trauma, stress, anxiety, and depression can affect relationships between the patient and family members or friends. Assess the patient's feelings and ask how he or she coped with previously experienced stressful events. Body image and sexuality may be altered by deformity, treatment modalities for fracture repair, or long-term immobilization. Establish a trusting relationship and determine the patient's spiritual beliefs and practices. Assess the availability of love and support systems, such as family, friends, church or temple, or community groups, who can help patients during the acute and rehabilitation phases when multiple or severe fractures occur.

disruptions in lifestyle can create a high level of stress, anxiety, and/or depression.

Active patients of any age or those who are older and live alone may become depressed during the healing process, especially if experiencing persistent *pain* that can decrease energy levels. Patients who were previously active and otherwise healthy often feel vulnerable and can become very anxious when they are not able to return to their usual level of activity. Provide hope that appropriate pain management will improve their comfort level and restore energy to return to their usual life habits. Some patients may benefit from counseling or psychotherapy services to help them with symptoms of depression and/or anxiety.

Laboratory Assessment. No special laboratory tests are available for assessment of fractures. Hemoglobin and hematocrit levels may often be low because of bleeding caused by the injury. If extensive soft-tissue damage is present, the erythrocyte sedimentation rate (ESR) may be elevated, which indicates the expected inflammatory response. If this value and the white blood cell (WBC) count increase during fracture healing, the patient may have a bone or soft tissue *infection.* During the healing stages, serum calcium and phosphorus levels may increase as the affected bone releases these elements into the blood.

Imaging Assessment. The primary health care provider requests standard *x-rays* to confirm a diagnosis of fracture, which often reveals bone disruption, malalignment, or deformity. If the x-ray does not show a fracture but the patient is symptomatic, the x-ray is usually repeated with additional views.

The *CT* scan is useful in detecting fractures of complex structures, such as the hip and pelvis. It also identifies compression fractures of the spine. *MRI* is useful in determining the amount of soft-tissue damage that may have occurred with the fracture.

◆ **Analysis: Analyze Cues and Prioritize Hypotheses.** The priority collaborative problems for patients with fractures include:
1. Acute *pain* due to fractured bone(s), soft-tissue damage, muscle spasm, and edema
2. Decreased *mobility* due to *pain,* muscle spasm, and soft-tissue damage
3. Potential for neurovascular compromise due to impaired tissue *perfusion*
4. Potential for *infection* due to impaired *tissue integrity* caused by an open fracture and/or extensive soft tissue damage

◆ **Planning and Implementation: Generate Solutions and Take Action**

Managing Acute Pain

Planning: Expected Outcomes. The patient with a fracture is expected to state that he or she has adequate *pain* control (a 2 to 3 on a pain scale of 0 to 10) after fracture reduction and immobilization.

Interventions. A fracture can happen anywhere and may be accompanied by multiple injuries to vital organs or major vessels (e.g., thoracic aorta dissection or tear). Interprofessional collaborative care depends on the severity and extent of the injury and the number of fractures the patient has.

Emergency Care: Fracture. For any patient who experiences trauma in the community, first call 911 and assess for **a**irway, **b**reathing, and **c**irculation (ABCs, or primary survey). Then provide lifesaving care if needed before being concerned about the fracture. If cardiopulmonary resuscitation (CPR) is needed, ensure circulation first, followed by airway and breathing (see the Best Practice for Patient Safety & Quality Care: Emergency Care of the Patient With an Extremity Fracture box).

After a head-to-toe assessment (secondary survey) and patient stabilization by the prehospital team, pain is often managed with short-term IV opioids such as fentanyl, hydromorphone, or morphine sulfate. Depending on the severity of the injury, other drugs to decrease opioid use, such as NSAIDs and regional nerve blocks, are also administered. Cardiac monitoring for patients who are older than 50 years is established before drug administration. In the emergency department (ED), primary health care provider office, or urgent care center, fracture management begins with reduction and immobilization of the fracture while attending to continued *pain* assessment and management.

Bone reduction, or realignment of the bone ends for proper healing, is accomplished by a closed method or an open (surgical) procedure. In some cases, dislocated bones are also

---

BEST PRACTICE FOR PATIENT SAFETY & QUALITY CARE (QSEN)

Emergency Care of the Patient With an Extremity Fracture

- Assess the patient's **a**irway, **b**reathing, and **c**irculation; establish any ABC that is affected by the injury.
- Perform a quick head-to-toe assessment.
- Remove the patient's clothing (cut if necessary) to inspect the affected area while supporting the area above and below the injury. Do not remove shoes because this can cause increased trauma unless the foot or ankle is injured.
- Apply direct pressure on the area if there is bleeding and pressure over the proximal artery nearest the fracture.
- Remove jewelry on the affected extremity in case of swelling.
- Keep the patient warm and in a supine position.
- Check the neurovascular status of the area distal to the fracture, including temperature, color, sensation, movement, and capillary refill. Compare affected and unaffected limbs.
- Immobilize the extremity by splinting; include joints above and below the fracture site. Recheck circulation after splinting.
- Cover any open areas with a dressing (preferably sterile).

---

reduced, such as when the distal tibia and fibula are dislocated with a fractured ankle. Immobilization is achieved by the use of bandages, casts, traction, internal fixation, or external fixation.

The primary health care provider selects the treatment method based on the type, location, and extent of the fracture. These interventions prevent further injury and reduce *pain.*

Nonsurgical Management. Nonsurgical management includes closed reduction and immobilization with a bandage, splint, boot, cast, or less commonly, traction. For some small, closed incomplete or "hairline" bone fractures in the hand or foot, reduction is not required. Immobilization with an orthotic device or special orthopedic shoe or boot may be the only management needed for healing to occur.

For each modality, the primary nursing concern is assessment and prevention of neurovascular dysfunction or compromise. Assess and document the patient's neurovascular status every hour for the first 24 hours and every 1 to 4 hours thereafter, depending on the injury and agency/primary health care provider protocol. Elevate the fractured extremity higher than the heart and apply ice for the first 24 to 48 hours as needed to reduce edema.

Closed reduction and immobilization. *Closed* reduction is the most common nonsurgical method for managing a simple fracture. While applying a manual pull, or traction, on the bone, the primary health care provider moves the bone ends so that they realign. Moderate sedation is used during this procedure for patient comfort. The nurse monitors the patient's oxygen saturation (and possibly end-tidal carbon dioxide [$ETCO_2$] level) to ensure adequate rate and depth of respirations during the procedure. *If the $ETCO_2$ becomes too low (30 mm Hg) and the respiratory rate falls to 10 breaths/min, rub the patient's sternum and encourage him or her to breathe.* An x-ray confirms that the bone ends are approximated (aligned) before the bone is immobilized, and a splint or other device is applied to keep the bone in alignment.

Splints and orthopedic boots/shoes. For certain areas of the body, such as the scapula (shoulder) and clavicle (collarbone), a commercial immobilizer may be used to keep the bone in place during healing. Because upper-extremity bones do not bear weight, splints may be sufficient to keep bone fragments in place for a closed fracture. Thermoplastic, a durable, flexible material for splinting, allows custom fitting to the patient's body part. Splints for lower extremities are also custom fitted using flexible materials and held in place with elastic bandages. When possible, splints are preferred over casts to prevent the complications that can occur with casting. Splints also allow room for extremity swelling without causing decreased arterial *perfusion.*

For foot or toe fractures, orthopedic shoes may be used to support the injured area during healing. For ankles or the lower part of the leg, padded orthopedic boots supported by multiple Velcro straps to hold the boot in place may be used (Fig. 47.3). These devices are especially useful when the patient is allowed to bear weight on the affected leg.

Casts. For more complex fractures or fractures of the lower extremity, the primary health care provider or orthopedic technician may apply a cast to hold bone fragments in place after reduction. A cast is a rigid device that immobilizes the affected body part while allowing other body parts to move. It also allows early *mobility* and reduces *pain*. Although its most common use is for fractures, a cast may be applied for correction of deformities (e.g., clubfoot) or for prevention of deformities (e.g., those seen in some patients with rheumatoid arthritis).

Fiberglass, a waterproof synthetic casting material, is used most often for fracture immobilization (Fig. 47.4). Fiberglass can dry and become rigid within minutes and decreases the risk for impaired *tissue integrity. Plaster* was the traditional material used for casts but is used less often today. When first applied, a plaster cast feels hot because an immediate chemical reaction occurs; it soon becomes damp and cool. This type of cast takes at least 24 hours to dry, depending on the size and location of the cast. A wet cast feels cold, smells musty, and is grayish. The cast is dry when it feels hard and firm, is odorless, and has a shiny white appearance.

If *tissue integrity* under the cast is impaired, the primary health care provider, orthopedic technician, or specially educated nurse cuts a window in the cast so that the wound can be observed and cared for. The piece of cast removed to make the window must be retained and replaced after wound care to prevent localized edema in the area. This is most important when a window is cut from a cast on an extremity. Tape or elastic bandage wrap may be used to keep the "window" in place. A window is also an access for taking pulses, removing wound drains, or preventing abdominal distention when the patient is in a body or spica cast.

If the cast is too tight, it may be cut with a cast cutter to relieve pressure or allow tissue swelling. The primary health care provider may choose to bivalve the cast (i.e., cut it lengthwise into two equal pieces). Either half of the cast can be removed for inspection or for provision of care. The two halves are then held in place by an elastic bandage wrap.

When a patient has an *arm cast,* teach him or her to elevate the arm above the heart to reduce swelling. The hand should be higher than the heart. Ice may be prescribed for the first 24 to 48 hours. When the patient is walking or standing, the arm is supported with a sling placed around the neck to alleviate fatigue caused by the weight of the cast. The sling should distribute the weight over a large area of the shoulders and trunk, not just the neck. Some primary health care providers prefer that the patient not use a sling after the first few days in an arm cast, particularly a short-arm cast. This encourages normal movement of the mobile joints and enhances bone healing. For many wrist fractures, a splint is used to immobilize the area instead of a cast to accommodate for edema formation.

A *leg cast* allows *mobility* and requires the patient to use ambulatory aids such as crutches or a walker. A cast shoe, sandal, or boot that attaches to the foot or a rubber walking pad attached to the sole of the cast assists in ambulation (if weight bearing is allowed) and helps prevent damage to the cast. Teach the patient to elevate the affected leg on several pillows to reduce swelling and to apply ice for the first 24 hours or as prescribed.

Before the cast is applied, explain its purpose and the procedure for its application. With a *plaster* cast, warn the patient about the heat that will be felt immediately after the wet cast is applied. *Do not cover a new plaster cast.* Allow for air-drying and handle the cast with the palms of the hand to prevent damage.

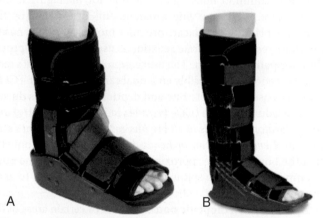

FIG. 47.3 A, Short boot. **B,** Long boot. (From Rizzone, K., & Gregory, A. [2013]. Using casts, splints, and braces in the emergency department. *Clinical Pediatric Emergency Medicine, 14*[4], 340–348. doi:10.1016/j.cpem.2013.11.003.)

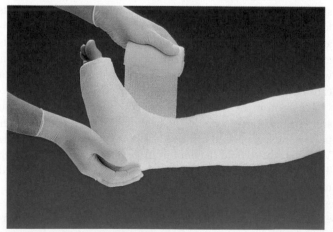

FIG. 47.4 Application of a fiberglass synthetic cast. (From Perry, A. G., Potter, P. A., & Elkin, M. K. [2012]. *Nursing interventions & clinical skills* [5th ed.]. St. Louis: Mosby.)

> **! NURSING SAFETY PRIORITY** (QSEN)
> **Action Alert**
>
> Check to ensure that any type of cast is not too tight and frequently monitor and document neurovascular status—usually every hour for the first 24 hours after application if the patient is hospitalized. You should be able to insert a finger between the cast and the skin. Teach the patient to apply ice for the first 24 to 36 hours to reduce swelling and inflammation.

Inspect the cast at least once every 8 to 12 hours for drainage, alignment, and fit. Plaster casts act like sponges and absorb drainage, whereas synthetic casts act like a wick pulling drainage away from the drainage site. Document the presence of any drainage on the cast. However, the evidence is not clear on whether drainage should be circled on the cast because it may increase anxiety and is not a reliable indicator of drainage amount. *Immediately report to the primary health care provider any sudden increases in the amount of drainage or change in the integrity of the cast.* After swelling decreases, it is not uncommon for the cast to become too loose and need replacement. If the patient is not admitted to the hospital, provide instructions regarding cast care.

During hospitalization, assess for other complications resulting from casting that can be serious and life threatening, such as infection, circulation impairment, and peripheral nerve damage. If the patient returns home after cast application, teach him or her how to monitor for these complications and when to notify the primary health care provider.

Infection most often results from impaired *tissue integrity* under the cast (pressure necrosis). If pressure necrosis occurs, the patient typically reports a very painful "hot spot" under the cast, and the cast may feel warmer in the affected area. Teach the patient or family to smell the area for mustiness or an unpleasant odor that would indicate infected material. If the infection progresses, a fever may develop. Teach the patient to never put anything down inside the cast, such as a hanger or pencil, to scratch an itch because this action can cause significant skin damage.

Circulation impairment causing decreased *perfusion* and *peripheral nerve damage* can result from tightness of the cast. Teach the patient to assess for circulation at least daily, including the ability to move the area distal to the extremity, numbness, and increased *pain*. Remind the patient to wiggle his or her toes and move them up and down.

The patient with a cast may be immobilized for a prolonged period, depending on the extent of the fracture and the type of cast. In this case, assess for complications of decreased *mobility,* such as skin breakdown, pneumonia, atelectasis, venous thromboembolism, and constipation. Before the cast is removed, inform the patient that the cast cutter will not injure the skin but that heat may be felt during the procedure.

Because of prolonged immobilization, a joint may become contracted, usually in a fixed state of flexion. Osteoarthritis and osteoporosis may develop from lack of weight bearing. Muscle can also atrophy from lack of exercise during prolonged immobilization of the affected body part, usually an extremity.

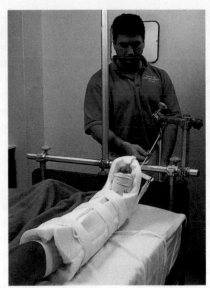

FIG. 47.5 Skin traction with a hook-and-loop fastener (Velcro) boot, commonly used for hip fractures. (Courtesy Smith & Nephew, Inc., Orthopaedics Divisions, Memphis, TN.)

that accompany hip and proximal femur fractures. A weight is used as a pulling force, which is limited to 5 to 10 lb (2.3 to 4.5 kg) to prevent injury to the skin (Duperouzel et al., 2018).

In *skeletal traction,* screws are surgically inserted directly into bone (e.g., femoral condyles for distal femur fractures). These allow the use of longer traction time and heavier weights, usually 15 to 30 lb (6.8 to 13.6 kg). Skeletal traction aids in bone realignment but impairs the patient's *mobility.* Use pressure-reduction measures and monitor for indications of impaired *tissue integrity.* Pin site care is also an important part of nursing management to prevent infection. Keep pin sites clean and document the nature of any drainage. Follow the agency's or primary health care provider's protocol for pin care.

NCLEX EXAMINATION CHALLENGE 47.1

Physiological Integrity

A client has a new synthetic leg cast for a right fractured tibia. What health teaching will the nurse include before discharge to home? **Select all that apply.**

A. "Elevate your right leg as often as possible to reduce swelling."
B. "Report increased pain or burning sensation under your cast."
C. "Use ice on the affected leg for the first 24-36 hours."
D. "Do not bear weight on the affected leg until instructed to do so."
E. "Do not cover the cast when you are in bed; keep it open to air to dry."

Traction. Traction is the application of a pulling force to a part of the body to provide bone reduction or as a last resort to decrease muscle spasm (thus reducing *pain*). A patient in traction is often hospitalized, but in some cases home care is possible even for skeletal traction.

Although not used as often today, the two major types of traction are skin and skeletal traction. *Skin traction* involves the use of a Velcro boot (Buck traction) (Fig. 47.5), belt, or halter, which is usually secured around the affected leg. The primary purpose of skin traction is to decrease painful muscle spasms

! NURSING SAFETY PRIORITY (QSEN)

Action Alert

When patients are in traction, weights are not removed without a prescription. They should not be lifted manually or allowed to rest on the floor. Weights should be freely hanging at all times. Teach this important point to assistive personnel on the unit, to other personnel such as those in the radiology department, and to visitors. Inspect the skin at least every 8 hours for signs of irritation or inflammation. When possible, remove the belt or boot that is used for skin traction every 8 hours to inspect under the device. Assess neurovascular status of the affected body part per agency or primary health care provider protocol to detect impaired *perfusion* and *tissue integrity.* The patient's circulation is usually monitored every hour for the first 24 hours after traction is applied and every 4 hours thereafter (Duperouzel et al., 2018).

Drug therapy. After fracture treatment, the patient often has *pain* for a prolonged time during the healing process. The primary health care provider commonly prescribes opioid and nonopioid analgesics, NSAIDs, and possibly, muscle relaxants.

For patients with severe persistent *pain,* opioid and nonopioid drugs are alternated or given together to manage pain both centrally in the brain and peripherally at the site of injury. For severe or multiple fractures, short-term patient-controlled analgesia (PCA) with morphine, fentanyl, or hydromorphone is used. Oxycodone and oxycodone with acetaminophen or hydrocodone with acetaminophen are common oral opioid drugs that are very effective for most patients with fracture pain. NSAIDs and other drugs are given to decrease associated tissue inflammation; however, they can slow bone healing.

For patients who have less severe injury, the analgesic may be given on an as-needed basis. Collaborate with the patient regarding the best times for the strong analgesics to be given (e.g., before a complex dressing change, after physical therapy sessions, or at bedtime). Assess the effectiveness of the analgesic and its side effects. Constipation is a common side effect of opioid therapy, especially for older adults. Assess for frequency of bowel movements and administer stool softeners or laxatives as needed for opioid-induced constipation (OIC). Encourage fluids, high-fiber foods, and activity as tolerated. Be aware that other drugs, such as anticholinergics, calcium channel blockers, antidepressants, and diuretics, may cause medication-induced constipation (MIC) (Turkowski, 2018).

Physical therapy. Collaborate with the physical therapist (PT) to assist with pain control and edema reduction by using ice/heat packs, electrical muscle stimulation ("e-stim"), and special treatments such as dexamethasone iontophoresis. Iontophoresis is a method for absorbing dexamethasone, a synthetic steroid, through the skin near the painful area to decrease inflammation and edema. A small device delivers a minute amount of electricity via electrodes that are placed on the skin. The patient may describe the sensation as a pinch or slight sting. The electrical current increases the ability of the skin to absorb the drug from a topical patch into the affected soft tissue.

When acute *pain* is not adequately controlled, some patients experience a chronic, intense burning pain and edema that are associated with complex regional pain syndrome (CRPS). This syndrome often results from fractures and other musculoskeletal trauma as described earlier in this chapter.

Surgical Management. For some types of fractures, closed reduction is not sufficient. Surgical intervention may be needed to realign the bone to enhance the healing process.

Preoperative care. Teach the patient and family what to expect during and after the surgery. The preoperative care for a patient undergoing orthopedic surgery is similar to that for anyone having surgery with general or epidural anesthesia. Some patients may also receive a regional nerve blockade, which promotes comfort immediately after surgery. (See Chapter 9 for a thorough discussion of general preoperative nursing care.)

Operative procedures. Open reduction with internal fixation (ORIF) is one of the most common methods of reducing and immobilizing a fracture. External fixation with closed reduction is used when patients have soft-tissue injury (open fracture). Although nurses do not decide which surgical technique is used, understanding the procedures enhances patient teaching and care.

Because ORIF permits early *mobility,* it is often the preferred surgical method. *Open* reduction allows the surgeon to directly view the fracture site. Internal fixation uses metal pins, screws, rods, plates, or prostheses inside the body to immobilize a fracture during healing. The surgeon makes one or more incisions to gain access to the broken bone(s) and implants one or more devices into bone tissue after each fracture is reduced. A cast, boot, or splint is placed to maintain immobilization during the healing process, depending on the body part affected.

After the bone achieves union, the metal hardware may be removed, depending on the location and type of fracture. Hardware is removed most frequently in ankle fractures, depending on the severity of the injury. If the metal implants are not bothersome, they may remain in place. Examples of internal fixation devices for fractured hips are discussed later in this chapter.

An alternative modality for the management of fractures is the external fixation apparatus, as shown in Fig. 47.6. External fixation is a surgical procedure in which pins or wires are inserted through the skin and affected bone and then connected to a rigid external frame outside the body to stabilize the fracture during healing (Georgiades, 2018). The system may be used for upper- or lower-extremity fractures or for fractures of the pelvis, especially for open fractures when wound management is needed. After a fixator is removed, the patient may be placed in a cast, boot, or splint until healing is complete or have internal fixation.

External fixation has several advantages over other surgical techniques:

- There is minimal blood loss compared with internal fixation.
- The device allows early ambulation and exercise of the affected body part while relieving pain.
- The device maintains alignment in closed fractures that will not maintain position in a cast and stabilizes comminuted fractures that require bone grafting.

A disadvantage of external fixation is an increased risk for pin-site *infection.* Pin-site infections can lead to osteomyelitis, which is serious and difficult to treat (see Chapter 45).

Postoperative care. The postoperative care for a patient undergoing ORIF or external fixation is similar to that provided for any patient undergoing surgery (see Chapter 9). Because bone is a vascular, dynamic body tissue, the patient is at risk

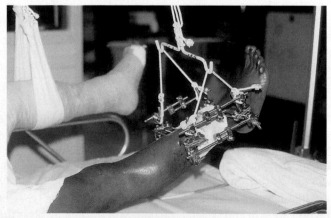

FIG. 47.6 Example of an external fixation device on the right leg. The left leg is in a splint. (From McCance, K. L., Huether, S. E., Brashers, V. L., & Rote, N. S. [2019]. *Pathophysiology: The biologic basis for disease in adults and children* [8th ed.]. St. Louis: Elsevier.)

for complications specific to fractures and musculoskeletal surgery. IV ketorolac is often given in the postanesthesia care unit (PACU) or soon after discharge to the postsurgical area to reduce inflammation and *pain.* Aggressive pain management starts as soon as possible after surgery to prevent the development of chronic pain and promote early *mobility.* Patients who had a regional nerve blockade typically have little or no pain immediately after surgery for about 18 to 24 hours. However, when the anesthetic begins to wear off, be sure that the patient is medicated to prevent severe pain. Use nonpharmacologic measures for pain management, such as imagery, distraction, music therapy, and other measures that the patient prefers and are allowed by agency policy to promote comfort.

Additional information about postoperative care may be found in the Selected Fractures of Specific Sites section later in this section. Depending on the fractures that are repaired, some ORIF procedures are performed as same-day surgeries. Patients stay in the hospital up to 23 hours after surgery.

For patients with an *external fixator,* assess the pin sites every 8 to 12 hours for drainage, color, odor, and severe redness, which indicate inflammation and possible *infection.* In the first 48 to 72 hours, *clear* fluid drainage or weeping is expected, which creates crusting around the pins. Although no standardized method or evidence-based protocol for pin-site care has been established, recommendations have been made based on current evidence. A systematic review of pin site care found that pin site crusts should not be removed because they protect the patient from infection (Georgiades, 2018).

The patient with an external fixator may have a disturbed body image. The frame may be large and bulky, and the affected area may have massive tissue damage with dressings. Be sensitive to this possibility in planning care. Teach about alterations to clothing that may be required while the fixator is in place.

Procedures for Nonunion. Some management techniques are not successful because the bone does not heal. Several additional options are available to the primary health care provider to promote bone union, such as electrical bone stimulation, bone grafting, and ultrasound fracture treatment.

For selected patients, *electrical bone stimulation* may be successful. This procedure is based on research showing that bone has electrical properties that are used in healing. The exact mechanism of action is unknown. A noninvasive, external system delivers a small continuous electrical charge directed toward the nonhealed bone. There are no known risks with this system, although patients with pacemakers cannot use this device on an arm. Implanted direct-current stimulators are placed directly in the fracture site and have no external apparatus. Both systems require several months of treatment.

Another method of treating nonunion is *bone grafting.* In most cases, chips of bone are taken from the iliac crest or other site and are packed or wired between the bone ends to facilitate union. Allografts from cadavers may also be used. These grafts are frozen or freeze-dried and stored under sterile conditions in a bone bank.

Bone banking from living donors is becoming increasingly popular. If qualified, patients undergoing total hip arthroplasty may donate their femoral heads to the bank for later use as bone grafts for others. Careful screening ensures that the bone is healthy and that the donor has no communicable disease. The bone cannot be donated without written consent.

One of the newest modalities for fracture healing is *low-intensity pulsed ultrasound.* Used for slow-healing fractures or for new fractures as an alternative to surgery, ultrasound treatment has had excellent results. The patient applies the treatment for about 20 minutes each day. It has no contraindications or adverse effects.

Increasing Mobility

Planning: Expected Outcomes. The patient with a fracture is expected to increase physical *mobility* and be free of complications associated with immobility. The patient is also expected to move purposefully in his or her own environment independently with or without an ambulatory device unless restricted by traction or other modality.

Interventions. The interventions necessary for this patient problem can be grouped into two types: those that help increase and promote *mobility* and those that prevent complications of decreased *mobility.* Interventions to prevent complications of decreased mobility are briefly summarized in Chapter 3. Additional information may be found in nursing fundamentals textbooks.

Many patients with musculoskeletal trauma, including fractures, are referred by their primary health care provider for rehabilitation therapy with a physical therapist (PT) (usually for lower-extremity injuries) and/or occupational therapist (OT) (usually for upper-extremity injuries). The timing for this referral depends on the nature, severity, and treatment modality of the fracture(s) or other musculoskeletal trauma.

For example, some patients who have an ORIF for an ankle fracture begin therapy when the incisional staples or wound closure strips are removed and an orthopedic boot is fitted. Based on the initial evaluation, the PT performs gentle manipulative exercises to increase range of motion. The therapist may also begin to help the patient with *laterality,* a concept to help the brain identify the injured foot from the uninjured foot. Computer programs and mirror-box therapy can help reprogram the brain as part of *cognitive retraining.* In mirror-box therapy for an injured foot, the patient covers his or her affected foot while looking at and moving the uninjured foot in front of the mirror. The brain often perceives the foot in the mirror as the injured foot.

Stimulation by touch also helps the brain acknowledge the injured foot. The PT teaches the patient to frequently touch the injured area and use various materials and objects against the skin to desensitize it. These interventions improve *mobility* and decrease the risk for complex regional pain syndrome, discussed earlier in this chapter.

The success of rehabilitation is affected by the patient's motivation and willingness to perform prescribed exercises and activities between PT visits. For example, rehabilitation for ankle surgery may take several months, depending on the severity of the injury and the age and general health of the patient.

When weight bearing begins for lower-extremity fractures about 6 weeks after surgery, the PT teaches the patient how to begin with toe-touch or partial weight bearing using crutches or a walker. Muscle-strengthening exercises of the affected leg help with ambulation because atrophy begins shortly after injury.

The use of crutches, knee-walker scooter, or a walker increases *mobility* and assists in ambulation. The patient may progress to a cane after the bone heals. *Crutches* are the most commonly used ambulatory aid for many types of lower-extremity musculoskeletal trauma (e.g., fractures, sprains, amputations). In most agencies, the physical therapist or emergency department/ambulatory care nurse fits the patient for crutches and teaches him or her how to ambulate with them. Reinforce those instructions and evaluate whether the patient is using the crutches correctly.

Walking with crutches or a knee-walker scooter requires strong arm muscles, balance, and coordination. For this reason, these ambulatory aids are not often used for older adults; traditional walkers and canes are preferred. Crutches can cause upper-extremity bursitis or axillary nerve damage if they are not fitted or used correctly. For that reason, the top of each crutch is padded. To prevent pressure on the axillary nerve, there should be two to three finger-breadths between the axilla and the top of the crutch when the crutch tip is at least 6 inches (15 cm) diagonally in front of the foot. The crutch is adjusted so that the elbow is flexed no more than 30 degrees when the palm is on the handle (Fig. 47.7). The distal tips of each crutch are rubber to prevent slipping.

There are several types of gaits for walking with crutches. The most common one for musculoskeletal injury is the three-point gait, which allows little weight bearing on the affected leg. The procedure for these gaits is discussed in fundamentals of nursing books.

A *walker* is most often used by the older patient who needs additional support for balance. The physical therapist assesses the strength of the upper extremities and the unaffected leg. Strength is improved with prescribed exercises as needed.

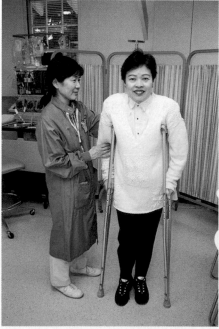

FIG. 47.7 Assisting the patient with crutch walking. Note how the therapist guards the patient and how the patient's elbows are at no more than 30 degrees of flexion.

A *cane* is sometimes used if the patient needs only minimal support for an affected leg. The straight cane offers the least support. A hemi-cane or quad-cane provides a broader base for the cane and therefore more support. The cane is placed on the *unaffected* side and should create no more than 30 degrees of flexion of the elbow. The top of the cane should be parallel to the greater trochanter of the femur or stylus of the wrist. Chapter 7 and fundamentals textbooks describe these ambulatory devices in more detail.

Preventing and Monitoring for Neurovascular Compromise

Planning: Expected Outcomes. The patient with a fracture is expected to have no compromise in neurovascular status as evidenced by adequate **perfusion** (circulation), **mobility** (movement), and **sensory perception** (sensation) (CMS). If severe compromise occurs, the patient is expected to have early and prompt emergency treatment to prevent severe tissue damage.

Interventions. Perform neurovascular (NV) assessments (also known as *"circ checks"* or *CMS assessments*) frequently before and after fracture treatment. Patients who have extremity casts, splints with elastic bandage wraps, and open reduction with internal fixation (ORIF) or external fixation are especially at risk for NV compromise. If **perfusion** to the distal extremity is impaired, the patient reports increased **pain,** impaired **mobility,** and decreased **sensory perception.** If these symptoms are allowed to progress, patients are at risk for acute compartment syndrome (ACS), as described earlier in this chapter.

> ### ! NURSING SAFETY PRIORITY (QSEN)
> #### Critical Rescue
>
> Monitor for and document early signs of ACS. Assess for the "six Ps" (i.e., **p**ain, **p**ressure, **p**aralysis, **p**aresthesia, **p**allor, and **p**ulselessness) (rare or late stage). **Pain** is increased even with passive motion and may seem out of proportion to the degree of injury. Analgesics that had controlled pain become less effective or noneffective. *Numbness and tingling (paresthesia) is often one of the first signs of the problem.* The affected extremity then becomes pale and cool as a result of decreased arterial perfusion to the affected area.
>
> If ACS is suspected, notify the primary health care provider immediately and, if possible, implement interventions to relieve the pressure. For example, for the patient with tight, bulky dressings, loosen the bandage or tape. If the patient has a cast, follow agency protocol about who may cut the cast. Do not elevate or ice the extremity because that could compromise blood flow.

In some cases, compartment pressure may be monitored on a one-time basis with a handheld device with a digital display, or pressure can be monitored continuously. Monitoring is recommended for comatose or unresponsive high-risk patients with multiple trauma and fractures.

Preventing Infection

Planning: Expected Outcomes. The patient with a fracture is expected to be free of wound or bone **infection** as evidenced by no fever, no increase in white blood cell count, and negative wound culture (if wound is present).

Interventions. When caring for a patient with an open fracture, use aseptic technique for dressing changes and wound irrigations. Check agency policy for specific protocols. *Immediately notify the primary health care provider if you observe inflammation and purulent drainage.* Other infections, such as pneumonia and urinary tract infection, may occur several days after the fracture.

Monitor the patient's vital signs every 4 to 8 hours because increases in temperature and pulse often indicate systemic *infection*.

👤 PATIENT-CENTERED CARE: OLDER ADULT CONSIDERATIONS (QSEN)

Older adults may not have a temperature elevation even in the presence of severe infection. An acute onset of confusion (delirium) often suggests an infection in the older-adult patient.

For most patients with an open fracture, the primary care provider prescribes one or more broad-spectrum antibiotics prophylactically and performs surgical débridement of any wounds as soon as possible after the injury. First-generation cephalosporins, clindamycin, and gentamycin are commonly used. In addition to systemic antibiotics, local antibiotic therapy through wound irrigation is commonly prescribed, especially during débridement.

A very effective treatment is negative-pressure wound therapy (e.g., vacuum-assisted closure [VAC] system) as a method of increasing the rate of wound healing for open fractures. This device allows quicker wound closure, which decreases the risk for *infection*.

Care Coordination and Transition Management. The patient with an *uncomplicated* fracture is usually discharged to home from the emergency department or urgent care center. Older adults with hip or other fractures or patients with multiple traumas are hospitalized and then transferred to home, a rehabilitation setting, or a long-term care facility for rehabilitation. Collaborate with the case manager or the discharge planner in the hospital to ensure care coordination. Be sure to communicate the plan of care clearly to the health care agency receiving the patient using situation-background-assessment recommendation or other communication method.

Home Care Management. If the patient is discharged to home, the nurse, rehabilitation therapist, or case manager (CM) may assess the home environment for structural barriers to *mobility* such as stairs. Be sure that the patient has easy access to the bathroom. Ask about small pets, scatter rugs, waxed floors, and walkway areas that could increase the risk for falls. If the patient needs to use a wheelchair or ambulatory aid, make sure that he or she can use it safely and that there is room in the house to ambulate with these devices. The physical therapist may teach the patient how to use stairs, but older adults or those using crutches may experience difficulty performing this task. Depending on the age and condition of the patient, a home health care nurse may make one or two visits to check that the home is safe and that the patient and family are able to follow the interprofessional plan of care.

Self-Management Education. The patient with a fracture may be discharged from the hospital, emergency department, office, or clinic with a bandage, splint, boot, or cast. Provide verbal and written instructions on the care of these devices.

The patient may also need to continue wound care at home. Instruct the patient and family about how to assess and dress the wound to promote healing and prevent *infection*. Teach them how to recognize complications and when and where to seek professional health care if complications occur. Additional educational needs depend on the type of fracture and fracture repair.

❓ CLINICAL JUDGMENT CHALLENGE 47.1
Evidence-Based Practice; Safety

A 24-year-old woman was a passenger in her boyfriend's car when their car was in a motor vehicle crash. The damage to her side of the car caused her right leg and arm to be severely injured. She was admitted yesterday to the hospital with a fracture of her tibia and fibula ("tib-fib" fracture), massive soft tissue and leg muscle damage, and a right wrist fracture. She also has multiple contusions and superficial lacerations. Both her leg and wrist are in temporary splints and elevated on pillows with ice packs until she is cleared for surgery. The client is right-handed. The night nurse reported that her parents are staying with her and that the client has been crying most of the night. The day nurse performs a shift assessment and notes the following:

- Reports that her pain level has increased from a 5 to a 9 even though she recently received morphine via IV push
- Reports numbness and tingling in her injured leg and foot
- Toes on her right foot are colder and more pale than those on the left foot
- Right pedal pulse not palpable or located via Doppler
- Oral temperature = 98.4° F (36.9° C)
- Apical pulse = 88 beats/min
- Respiratory rate = 28 breaths/min
- Blood pressure = 132/84 mm Hg
- States that she wish she had died in the accident
- Has difficulty answering questions because she is very emotional and crying
- Refuses to eat, stating that she is not hungry
- Has a urinary catheter in place, which is draining amber urine

1. **Recognize Cues:** What assessment information in this client situation is the most important and immediate concern for the nurse? (Hint: Identify the **relevant** information *first* to determine what is most important.)
2. **Analyze Cues:** What client conditions are consistent with the **most relevant** information? (Hint: Think about priority collaborative problems that support and contradict the information presented in this situation.)
3. **Prioritize Hypotheses:** Which possibilities or explanations are **most likely** to be present in this client situation? Which possibilities or explanations are the most serious? (Hint: Consider all possibilities and determine their urgency and risk for this client.)
4. **Generate Solutions:** What actions would most likely achieve the desired outcomes for this client? Which actions should be **avoided** or are **potentially harmful**? (Hint: Determine the desired outcomes first to decide which interventions are appropriate and those that should be avoided.)
5. **Take Action:** Which actions are the most appropriate and how should they be implemented? In what **priority order** should they be implemented? (Hint: Consider health teaching, documentation, requested health care provider orders or prescriptions, nursing skills, collaboration with or referral to health team members, etc.)
6. **Evaluate Outcomes:** What client assessment would indicate that the nurse's actions were **effective**? (Hint: Think about signs that would indicate an improvement, decline, or unchanged client condition.)

Encourage patients and their families to ensure adequate foods high in protein and calcium that are needed for bone and tissue healing. For patients with lower-extremity fractures, less weight bearing on long bones can cause anemia. The red bone marrow needs weight bearing to simulate red blood cell production. Encourage foods high in iron content. Teach the patient to take a daily iron-added multivitamin (take with food to prevent possible nausea) and a stool softener with a stimulant to prevent opioid-induced constipation.

Teach patients about the need for follow-up visits to the primary health care provider to assess bone healing and determine when casts or other devices can be discontinued. The Patient and Family Education: Preparing for Self-Management box describes care of the affected extremity after removal of the cast.

NCLEX EXAMINATION CHALLENGE 47.2

Physiological Integrity

A client had an open reduction internal fixation (ORIF) of the right wrist. What health teaching is appropriate for the nurse to provide for this client before returning home? **Select all that apply.**

A. "Keep your right arm below the level of your heart as often as possible."
B. "Use an ice pack for the first 24 hours to decrease tissue swelling."
C. "Report coolness or discoloration of your right hand to your doctor."
D. "Don't place any device under the cast to scratch the skin if it itches."
E. "Move the fingers of the right hand frequently to promote blood flow."

Health Care Resources. Arrange for follow-up care at home if needed. A social worker may need to help the patient apply for funds to pay medical bills. If there is severe bone and tissue damage, be realistic and help the patient and family understand the long-term nature of the recovery period. Multiple treatment techniques and surgical procedures required for complications can be mentally and emotionally draining for the patient and family. A vocational counselor may be needed to help the patient find a different type of job, depending on the extent of the fracture.

An older or incapacitated patient may need assistance with ADLs, which can be provided by home care aides if family or other caregivers are not available. In collaboration with the case manager, anticipate the patient's needs and arrange for these services.

◆ **Evaluation: Evaluate Outcomes.** Evaluate the care of the patient with one or more fractures based on the identified priority patient problems. The expected outcomes include that the patient:

- States that he or she has adequate *pain* control (a 2 to 3 on a 0 to 10 pain scale) to accomplish ADLs
- Ambulates independently with or without an assistive device (if not restricted by traction or other device)
- Is free of physiologic consequences of decreased *mobility*
- Has adequate blood flow to maintain tissue *perfusion* and function
- Is free of *infection* or other complication

LOWER EXTREMITY FRACTURES

Hip Fracture

Hip fracture is the most common injury in older adults and one of the most frequently seen injuries in any health care setting or community. It has a high mortality rate as a result of multiple complications related to surgery, depression, and decreased *mobility.* Over half of older adults experiencing a hip fracture are unable to live independently, and many die within the first year.

Hip fractures include those involving the upper third of the femur and are classified as *intracapsular* (within the joint capsule) or *extracapsular* (outside the joint capsule) (Hohler, 2018). These types are further divided according to fracture location (Fig. 47.8). In the area of the femoral neck, disruption of the blood supply to the head of the femur is a concern, which can result in ischemic or avascular necrosis (AVN) of the femoral head. AVN causes death and necrosis of bone tissue and results in pain and decreased *mobility.* This problem is most likely in patients with displaced fractures.

Osteoporosis is the biggest risk factor for hip fractures (see Chapter 45). This disease weakens the upper femur (hip), which causes it to break and lead to a fall. In some cases, a fall causes the fracture of the weakened hip, often referred to as a **fragility fracture.** The number of people with hip fracture is expected to continue to increase as the population ages, and the associated health care costs will be tremendous (Conley et al., 2020).

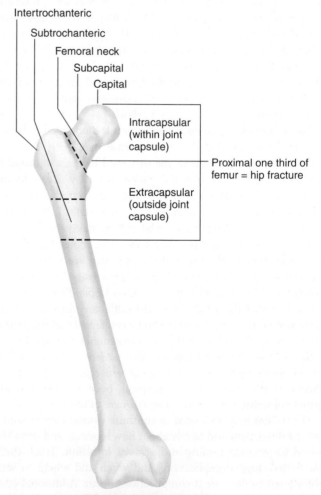

FIG. 47.8 Types of hip fractures.

PATIENT-CENTERED CARE: OLDER ADULT CONSIDERATIONS (QSEN)

Teach older adults about the risk factors for fragility hip fractures, including physiologic aging changes, disease processes, drug therapy, and environmental hazards. Physiologic changes include sensory changes such as diminished visual acuity and hearing; changes in gait, balance, and muscle strength; and joint stiffness. Disease processes such as osteoporosis, foot disorders, bony metastases, and changes in cardiac function increase the risk for fracture. These diseases are discussed elsewhere in this textbook. Drugs, such as diuretics, antihypertensives, antidepressants, sedatives, opioids, and alcohol, are factors that increase the risks for falling in older adults. Use of three or more drugs at the same time drastically increases the risk for falls. Throw rugs, loose carpeting, floor clutter, inadequate lighting, uneven walking surfaces or steps, and pets are environmental hazards that also cause falls.

The older adult with hip fracture usually reports groin pain or pain behind the knee on the affected side. In some cases, the patient has pain in the lower back or no pain at all. However, the patient is not able to stand without pain. X-ray or other imaging assessment confirms the diagnosis.

Preoperative Care. Patients usually receive IV morphine or hydromorphone after admission to the emergency department and may receive morphine or hydromorphone PCA or epidural analgesia after surgery. However, an integrative review of 38 research articles by Wennberg et al. (2018) found that first responders and emergency department staff do not adequately assess or manage pain among older adults who experience hip fracture. The authors recommended that nurses and other health professionals should continuously assess and better manage pain, which could improve cognition and patient satisfaction.

A major desired outcome for older adults experiencing a hip fracture is to achieve effective preoperative and postoperative pain management while avoiding adverse drug effects. A preoperative alternative to opioid administration is **fascia iliaca compartment block (FICB)**, a regional anesthetic technique using levobupivacaine or other drug to block femoral, lateral cutaneous, and obturator nerves. This procedure avoids the risk of injury to the femoral artery and vein. The benefits of FICB include effective pain relief without opioids and minimal cost (Williams et al., 2019).

Postoperative Care. The treatment of choice is surgical repair by ORIF, when possible, to reduce pain and allow the older patient to be out of bed and ambulatory. While not common, skin (Buck) traction may be applied before surgery to help decrease *pain* associated with muscle spasm. Depending on the exact location of the fracture, an ORIF may include an intramedullary rod, pins, prostheses (for femoral head or femoral neck fractures, also known as a *hemiarthroplasty*), or a compression screw. Figs. 47.9 and 47.10 illustrate examples of these devices. Epidural, spinal, or general anesthesia is used. Occasionally a patient will be so debilitated that surgery cannot be done. In these cases, nonsurgical options include pain management and bedrest to allow natural fracture healing.

Before and after a hip repair, older adults frequently experience acute confusion (delirium) (see Chapter 3). They may pull at tubes or the surgical dressing or attempt to climb out of bed, possibly falling and causing self-injury. Other patients stay awake all night and sleep during the day. Keep in mind that some patients have a quiet delirium. Monitor

the patient frequently to prevent falls. Use evidence-based fall prevention strategies and ask the family or other visitors to let staff know if the patient is attempting to get out of bed. Chapter 4 describes fall prevention strategies and delirium management in detail.

! NURSING SAFETY PRIORITY (QSEN)

Action Alert

Patients who have a *hemiarthroplasty* are at risk for hip dislocation or subluxation. Be sure to prevent hip adduction and rotation to keep the operative leg in proper alignment. Regular pillows or abduction devices can be used for patients who are confused or restless. If straps are used to hold the device in place, make sure that they are not too tight and check the skin every 2 hours for signs of pressure. Perform neurovascular assessments to ensure that the device is not interfering with arterial circulation or peripheral nerve conduction.

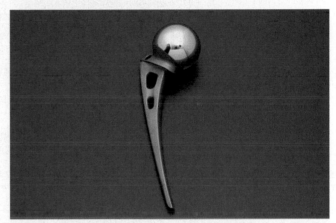

FIG. 47.9 Hip prosthesis used for femoral head or neck fractures (hemiarthroplasty). (Courtesy Smith & Nephew, Inc., Orthopaedics Divisions, Memphis, TN.)

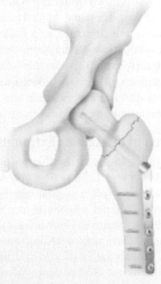

FIG. 47.10 Compression hip screw used for open reduction with internal fixation (ORIF) of the hip.

BEST PRACTICE FOR PATIENT SAFETY AND QUALITY CARE (QSEN)

Quality Indicators for Postoperative Nursing Care of Older Adults With Fragility Hip Fractures

Nursing Quality Indicator	Nursing Care Best Practice
Timing of Surgery	Ensure that the patient has surgery within 24-48 hours of the fracture, depending on the patient's condition.
Early and Frequent Mobility	Assist the patient to get out of the bed to stand, walk, or sit on the side of the bed on the day of surgery. Walk the patient 1-2 times a day on the first postoperative day.
Malnutrition Prevention	Conduct a nutritional screening on admission. Provide a diet as tolerated with daily oral nutritional supplements postoperatively.
Catheter-Associated Urinary Tract Infection (CAUTI) Prevention	Avoid the use of an indwelling urinary catheter, if possible. If a urinary catheter must be used, the catheter should be removed within 24 hours, if possible.
Pain Management	Use a multimodal pain management approach based on frequent pain assessments. Use geriatric drug dosing and regional nerve blocks if feasible.
Delirium	Complete cognitive screening on admission. Screen the patient each day for delirium.
Pneumonia Prevention	Keep the head of the patient's bed elevated to at least 30 degrees. Perform dysphagia screening and provide frequent mouth care.
Constipation Prevention	Assess daily for bowel movement. Implement an evidence-based bowel protocol, including preventive stool softeners and laxatives.
Venous Thromboembolism (VTE) Prevention	Implement an evidence-based VTE prevention protocol.
Pressure Injury Prevention	Perform a valid pressure injury risk assessment on admission. Perform daily skin assessments. Follow an evidence-based pressure injury prevention protocol/plan of care, including the need to keep the patient's heels off the bed to prevent breakdown.
Care Transitions/Preparing for Home	Provide patient self-management health teaching. Teach the need to follow up with the primary health care provider in 4-6 weeks after discharge.
Bone Health	Teach the patient the need to follow up on his or her bone health to prevent future fractures.

Best practices for care of patients with fragility hip fractures can be summarized by reviewing the 12 internationally accepted nursing quality indicators (MacDonald et al., 2018). These indicators and associated postoperative nursing care are outlined in the Best Practice for Patient Safety & Quality Care: Quality Indicators for Postoperative Nursing Care of Older Adults With Fragility Hip Fractures box.

Many patients recover fully from hip fracture repair and regain their functional ability. They are typically discharged to their home, rehabilitation unit or center, or a skilled nursing facility for physical and occupational therapy. However, some patients are not able to return to their prefracture ADLs and **mobility** level. Family caregivers often have unexpected responsibilities caring for patients during their recovery. Hip fracture resource centers can be very useful in providing caregiver support.

Other Fractures of the Lower Extremity

Other fractures of the lower extremity may or may not require hospitalization. However, if the patient has severe or multiple fractures, especially with soft-tissue damage, hospital admission is usually required. Patients who have surgery to repair their injury may also be hospitalized. Coordinate care with the physical and occupational therapists regarding transfers, positioning, and ambulation. Collaborate with the case manager regarding placement after discharge. Most patients go home unless there is

no support system or additional rehabilitation is needed. Health teaching and ensuring continuity of care are essential.

Fractures of the *lower two thirds of the femur* usually result from trauma, often from a motor vehicle crash. A femur fracture is seldom immobilized by casting because the powerful muscles of the thigh become spastic, which causes displacement of bone ends and significant pain. Extensive hemorrhage can occur with femur fracture.

Surgical treatment is ORIF with plates, nails, rods, or a compression screw. In a few cases in which extensive bone fragmentation or severe tissue trauma is found, external fixation may be used. Healing time for a femur fracture may be 6 months or longer. Skeletal traction, followed by a full-leg brace or cast, may be used in nonsurgical treatment.

Trauma to the lower leg most often causes fractures of both the *tibia* and the *fibula*, particularly the lower third, and is often referred to as a *tib-fib* fracture. The major treatment techniques are closed reduction with casting, internal fixation, and external fixation. If closed reduction is used, the patient may wear a cast for 6 to 10 weeks. Because of poor **perfusion** to parts of the tibia and fibula, delayed union is not unusual with this type of fracture. Internal fixation with nails or a plate and screws, followed by a long-leg cast for 4 to 6 weeks, is another option. Since the fibula is a non–weight-bearing bone, occasionally no fixation is required.

When the fractures cause extensive skin and soft-tissue damage, the initial treatment may be external fixation, often for 6 to 10 weeks, usually followed by application of a cast until the fracture is completely healed. The patient is typically non–weight bearing and uses ambulatory aids such as crutches.

Ankle fractures are described by their anatomic place of injury. For example, a bimalleolar (Pott) fracture involves the medial malleolus of the tibia and the lateral malleolus of the fibula. The small talus that makes up the rest of the ankle joint may also be broken. An ORIF is usually performed using two incisions: one on the medial (inside) aspect of the ankle and one on the lateral (outer) side. Several screws or nails are placed into the tibia, and a compression plate with multiple screws keeps the fibula in alignment. Weight bearing is restricted until the bone heals.

Treatment of fractures of the foot or phalanges (toes) is similar to that of other fractures. Phalangeal fractures may be more painful but are not as serious as most other types of fractures. Crutches are used for ambulation if weight bearing is restricted, but many patients can ambulate while wearing an orthopedic shoe or boot while the bone heals.

FRACTURES OF THE CHEST AND PELVIS

Chest trauma may cause fractures of the ribs or sternum. The major concern with rib and sternal fractures is the potential for puncture of the lungs, heart, or arteries by bone fragments or ends. *Assess airway, breathing, and circulation status* **first** *for any patient having chest trauma!* Fractures of the lower ribs may damage underlying organs, such as the liver, spleen, or kidneys. These fractures tend to heal on their own without surgical intervention. Patients are often uncomfortable during the healing process and require analgesia. They also have a high risk for pneumonia because of shallow breathing caused by **pain** on inspiration. Encourage them to breathe normally if possible and ensure that their pain is well managed.

Because the pelvis is very vascular and is close to major organs and blood vessels, associated internal damage is the major focus in fracture management. After head injuries, pelvic fractures are the second most common cause of death from trauma. In young adults, pelvic fractures typically result from motor vehicle crashes or falls from buildings. Falls are the most common cause in older adults. The major concern related to pelvic injury is venous oozing or arterial bleeding. Loss of blood volume leads to hypovolemic shock.

Assess for internal abdominal trauma by checking for blood in the urine and stool and by monitoring the abdomen for the development of rigidity or swelling. The trauma team may use peritoneal lavage, CT scanning, or ultrasound for assessment of hemorrhage. Ultrasound is noninvasive, rapid, reliable, and cost-effective, and it can be done at the bedside.

There are many classification systems for pelvic fractures. A system that is particularly useful divides fractures of the pelvis into two broad categories: non–weight-bearing fractures and weight-bearing fractures.

When a *non–weight-bearing* part of the pelvis is fractured, such as one of the pubic rami or the iliac crest, treatment can be as minimal as bedrest on a firm mattress or bed board. This type of fracture can be quite painful, and the patient may need stool softeners to facilitate bowel movements because of hesitancy to move. Well-stabilized fractures usually heal in 2 months.

A *weight-bearing* fracture, such as multiple fractures of the pelvic ring creating instability or a fractured acetabulum, necessitates external fixation or ORIF or both. Progression to weight bearing depends on the stability of the fracture after fixation. Some patients can fully bear weight within days of surgery, whereas others managed with traction may not be able to bear weight for as long as 12 weeks. For complex pelvic fractures with extensive soft-tissue damage, external fixation may be required.

COMPRESSION FRACTURES OF THE SPINE

Most vertebral fractures are caused by osteoporosis or metastatic bone cancer. Compression fractures result when trabecular or cancellous bone within the vertebra becomes weakened and causes the vertebral body to collapse. The patient has *severe pain* (especially when moving), deformity (kyphosis), and possible neurologic compromise. As discussed in the Osteoporosis section of Chapter 45, the patient's quality of life is reduced by the impact of this problem.

Nonsurgical management includes bedrest, analgesics, nerve blocks, and physical therapy to maintain muscle strength. Vertebral compression fractures (VCFs) that remain painful and impair **mobility** may be treated with **vertebroplasty** or kyphoplasty. These procedures are minimally invasive techniques in which bone cement is injected through the skin (percutaneously) directly into the fracture site to provide stability and immediate pain relief. In addition to vertebroplasty, radiologists and orthopedic surgeons may do a kyphoplasty (using a balloon) or the preferred vertebral augmentation (using a different cavity-creating device) to partially re-expand a compressed vertebral body.

Minimally invasive procedures can be done in an operating or interventional radiology suite by a surgeon or interventional radiologist. They can be done with moderate sedation or general anesthesia. IV ketorolac may be given before the procedure to reduce inflammation. Large-bore needles are placed into the fracture site using fluoroscopy or CT guidance. Then the deflated balloon is inserted through the needles and inflated in the fracture site, and the cement is injected.

Patients may have the procedures in an ambulatory care setting and return home after 2 to 4 hours or be admitted to the hospital for an overnight stay. The Best Practice for Patient Safety & Quality Care: Nursing Care for Patients Having Vertebroplasty or Kyphoplasty box outlines the preprocedure and postprocedure care for percutaneous interventions for vertebral compression fractures.

Before discharge, teach the patient to report any signs or symptoms of **infection** from puncture sites. Remind him or

Nursing Care for Patients Having Vertebroplasty or Kyphoplasty

Provide *preprocedure care*, including:

- Check the patient's coagulation laboratory test results; platelet count should be more than 100,000/mm³ (100 × 10⁹/L).
- Make sure that all anticoagulant drugs were discontinued as requested by the surgeon or interventional radiologist.
- Assess and document the patient's neurologic status, especially extremity movement and sensation.
- Assess the patient's pain level.
- Assess the patient's ability to lie prone for at least 1 hour.
- Establish an IV line in a size suitable for surgery and take vital signs.

Provide *postprocedure care*, including:

- Place the patient in a flat supine position for 1 to 2 hours or as requested by the surgeon or interventional radiologist.
- Monitor and record vital signs and frequent neurologic assessments; report any change immediately to the physician.
- Apply an ice pack to the puncture site if needed to relieve pain.
- Assess the patient's pain level and compare it with the preoperative level; give mild analgesic as needed.
- Monitor for complications, such as bleeding at the puncture site or shortness of breath; report these findings immediately if they occur.
- Assist the patient with ambulation.

Before discharge, teach the patient and family the following:

- Avoid driving or operating machinery for the first 24 hours because of drugs used during the procedure.
- Monitor the puncture site for signs of infection, such as redness, pain, swelling, or drainage.
- Keep the dressing dry and remove it the next day.
- Begin usual activities, including walking, the next day and should slowly increase activity level over the next few days.

her to not soak in a bath for 1 week, use analgesics as needed, resume activity, and contact the primary health care provider for questions or concerns. Surgery generally reduces preoperative pain significantly.

✳ PERFUSION CONCEPT EXEMPLAR: AMPUTATION

An **amputation** is the removal of a part of the body. Advances in microvascular surgical procedures, better use of antibiotic therapy, and improved surgical techniques for traumatic injury and bone cancer have reduced the number of elective amputations. The psychosocial aspects of the procedure are as devastating as the physical impairments that result. The loss is complete and permanent and causes a change in body image and self-esteem. Collaborate with members of the interprofessional team, including prosthetists, rehabilitation therapists, psychologists, case managers, and physiatrists (rehabilitation physicians), when providing care to the patient who has an amputation.

Pathophysiology Review

Types of Amputation. Amputations may be elective or traumatic. Most are *elective* and are related to complications of peripheral vascular disease (PVD) that result in decreased **perfusion** (ischemia) to distal areas of the lower extremity (Schrieber, 2017). Diabetes mellitus is often an underlying cause. Trauma to a limb is the second leading cause of amputation. Amputation is considered only after other interventions have not restored circulation to the lower extremity, sometimes referred to as *limb salvage procedures* (e.g., percutaneous transluminal angioplasty [PTA]). These procedures are discussed elsewhere in this text.

Traumatic amputations most often result from accidents or war and are the primary cause of *upper-extremity* amputation. A person may clean lawn mower blades or a snow blower without disconnecting the machine. A motor vehicle crash or industrial machine accident may also cause an amputation.

The number of traumatic amputations also increases during war as a result of hidden land mines (IEDs), bombs, and motor vehicle accidents (e.g., in Iraq and Afghanistan). Multiple limbs or parts of limbs may be amputated as a result of these devices. Thousands of veterans of war in the United States are amputees and have had to adjust to major changes in their lifestyles. Many veterans have multiple amputations that affect **mobility**, ADL functional ability, and psychosocial health.

Levels of Amputation. Elective lower-extremity (LE) amputations are performed much more frequently than upper-extremity amputations. Several types of LE amputations may be performed.

The loss of any or all of the small toes presents a minor disability. Loss of the great toe is significant because it affects balance, gait, and "push-off" ability during walking. Midfoot amputations and the Syme amputation are common procedures for peripheral vascular disease. In the Syme amputation, most of the foot is removed, but the ankle remains. The advantage of this surgery over traditional amputations below the knee is that weight bearing can occur without the use of a prosthesis and with reduced pain.

An intense effort is made to preserve knee joints with below-the-knee amputation (BKA). When the cause for the amputation extends beyond the knee, above-knee or higher amputations are performed. Hip disarticulation, or removal of the hip joint, and hemipelvectomy (removal of half of the pelvis with the leg) are more common in younger patients than in older ones who cannot easily handle the cumbersome prostheses required for ambulation. The higher the level of amputation, the more energy is required for **mobility**. These higher-level procedures are sometimes done for cancer of the bone, osteomyelitis, or trauma as a last resort.

An amputation of any part of the upper extremity is generally more incapacitating than one of the leg. The arms and hands are necessary for ADLs such as feeding, bathing, dressing, and driving a car. In the upper extremity, as much length as possible is saved to maintain function. Early replacement with a prosthetic device is vital for the patient with this type of amputation.

Complications of Amputation. The most common complications of amputations are:

- Hemorrhage leading to hypovolemic shock
- *Infection*
- Phantom limb *pain*
- Neuroma
- Flexion contractures

When a person loses part or all of an extremity either by surgery or by trauma, major blood vessels are severed, which causes *hemorrhage*. If the bleeding is uncontrolled, the patient is at risk for hypovolemic shock and possibly death.

As with any surgical procedure or trauma, infection can occur in the wound or the bone (osteomyelitis). The older adult who is malnourished and confused is at the greatest risk because excreta may soil the wound or he or she may remove the dressing and pick at the incision. Preventing *infection* is a major emphasis in hospitals and other health care settings.

Persistent *pain* is a frequent complication of amputation. This sensation is felt in the amputated part immediately after surgery and usually diminishes over time. When it persists and is unpleasant or painful, it is referred to as phantom limb pain (PLP). PLP is more common in patients who had chronic limb pain before surgery and less common in those who have traumatic amputations. The patient reports pain in the removed body part shortly after surgery, usually after an above-the-knee amputation (AKA). The *pain* is often described as intense burning, crushing, or cramping. Some patients report that the removed part is in a distorted, uncomfortable position. They experience numbness and tingling, referred to as *phantom limb sensation*, and pain. Others state that the most distal area of the removed part feels as if it is retracted into the residual limb end. For most patients, the pain is triggered by touching the residual limb or by temperature or barometric pressure changes, concurrent illness, fatigue, anxiety, or stress. Routine activities such as urination can trigger the pain. If *pain* is long-standing, especially if it existed before the amputation, any stimulus can cause it, including touching any part of the body.

Neuroma, a sensitive tumor consisting of damaged nerve cells, forms most often in amputations of the upper extremity but can occur anywhere. The patient may or may not have pain. It is diagnosed by sonography and can be treated either surgically or nonsurgically. Surgery to remove the neuroma may be performed, but it often regrows and is more painful than before the surgery. Nonsurgical modalities include peripheral nerve blocks, steroid injections, and cognitive therapies such as hypnosis.

Flexion contractures of the hip or knee are most frequently seen in patients with amputations of the lower extremity. This complication must be avoided so that the patient can ambulate with a prosthetic device. Proper positioning and active range-of-motion exercises in the early postoperative period help prevent this complication.

Health Promotion and Maintenance

The typical patient undergoing elective amputation is a middle-age or older man with diabetes and a lengthy history of smoking. He most likely has not cared for his feet properly, which has resulted in a nonhealing, infected foot ulcer and possibly gangrene. Therefore adherence to the disease management plan may help prevent the need for later amputation. Lifestyle habits such as maintaining a healthy weight, regular exercise, and avoiding smoking can help prevent chronic diseases such as diabetes and poor blood circulation.

The second largest group who has amputations consists of young men who have motorcycle or other vehicular crashes, are injured by industrial equipment, or have been in combat or accidents in war. These men may either experience a traumatic amputation or undergo a surgical amputation because of a severe crushing injury and massive soft-tissue damage. Teach young male adults the importance of taking safety precautions to prevent injury at work and to avoid speeding or driving while drinking alcohol. An increasing number of young women also tend to speed and drive while drinking, which endangers themselves and others around them.

❖ Interprofessional Collaborative Care
◆ Assessment: Recognize Cues

Physical Assessment/Signs and Symptoms. Monitor neurovascular status in the affected extremity that will be electively amputated. When the patient has peripheral vascular disease, check circulation in both legs. Assess skin color, temperature, sensation, and pulses in both affected and unaffected extremities. Capillary refill can be difficult to determine in the older adult related to thickened and opaque nails. In this situation, the skin near the nail bed can be used. Capillary refill is not as reliable as other indicators. Observe and document any discoloration of the skin, edema, ulcerations, presence of necrosis, and hair distribution on the lower extremities.

Psychosocial Assessment. People react differently to the loss of a body part. Be aware that an amputation of only a portion of one finger, especially the thumb, can be traumatic to the patient. The thumb is needed for hand activities. Therefore the loss must not be underestimated. Patients undergoing amputation face a complete, permanent loss. Evaluate their psychological preparation for a planned amputation and expect them to go through the grieving process. Adjusting to a traumatic, unexpected amputation is often more difficult than accepting a planned one.

PATIENT-CENTERED CARE: VETERANS HEALTH CONSIDERATIONS (QSEN)

The young veteran may be bitter, hostile, and depressed. In addition to loss of a body part, he or she may lose a job, the ability to participate in favorite recreational activities, or a social relationship if other people cannot accept the body change.

The patient having one or more amputations has an altered self-concept. The physical alterations that result affect body image and self-esteem. For example, a young male may think that an intimate relationship with a partner is no longer possible or desirable. An older adult may feel a loss of independence. Assess the patient's feelings about himself or herself to identify areas in which he or she needs emotional support. Consult with the certified hospital chaplain, other spiritual leader, or hospital social worker if the patient is hospitalized. Counseling resources are also available in the community and the Veterans' Administration health system in the United States.

Attempt to determine the patient's willingness and motivation to withstand prolonged rehabilitation after the amputation. Asking questions about how he or she has dealt with previous life crises can provide clues. Adjustment to the amputation and rehabilitation is less difficult if the patient is willing to make needed changes.

PATIENT-CENTERED CARE: CULTURAL/ SPIRITUAL CONSIDERATIONS (QSEN)

In addition to assessing the patient's psychosocial status, assess the family's reaction to the surgery or trauma. Their response usually correlates directly with the patient's progress during recovery and rehabilitation and his or her values and beliefs. Expect the family to grieve for the loss and allow them time to adjust to the change. Establish a trusting relationship and reassure the patient and family that you are available to listen to their concerns and needs.

Assess the patient's and family's coping abilities and help them identify personal strengths and weaknesses. Assess the patient's religious, spiritual, and cultural beliefs. Some groups (e.g., Jewish) require that the amputated body part be stored for later burial with the rest of the body or buried immediately. Other cultural customs and rituals may apply, depending on the group with which the patient associates.

Diagnostic Assessment. The surgeon determines which tests are performed to assess for viability of the limb based on blood flow. A large number of noninvasive techniques are available for this evaluation. For complete accuracy, the surgeon does not rely on any single test.

One procedure is measurement of segmental limb blood pressures, which can also be used by the nurse at the bedside. In this test, an **ankle-brachial index (ABI)** is calculated by dividing ankle systolic pressure by brachial systolic pressure. A normal ABI is 0.9 or higher.

Blood flow in an extremity can also be assessed by other noninvasive tests, including *Doppler* ultrasonography or laser Doppler flowmetry and transcutaneous oxygen pressure ($TcPO_2$). The ultrasonography and laser Doppler measure the speed of blood flow in the limb. The $TcPO_2$ measures oxygen pressure to indicate blood flow in the limb and has proven reliable for predicting healing.

◆ **Analysis: Analyze Cues and Prioritize Hypotheses**

The collaborative problems for patients with amputations include:

1. Potential for decreased tissue *perfusion* in residual limb due to soft tissue damage, edema, and/or bleeding
2. Acute and/or persistent *pain* due to soft-tissue damage, muscle spasm, and edema
3. Decreased *mobility* due to pain, muscle spasm, soft-tissue damage, and/or lack of balance due to a missing body part
4. Decreased self-esteem due to one or more ADL deficits, disturbed self-concept and body image, and/or lack of support systems

◆ **Planning and Implementation: Generate Solutions and Take Action**

Monitoring for Decreased Tissue Perfusion

Planning: Expected Outcomes. The patient with one or more amputations is expected to have adequate peripheral *perfusion* to the residual (surgical) limb(s) as evidenced by warm, usual-color skin.

Interventions. A *traumatic* amputation requires rapid emergency care to possibly save the severed body part for reattachment to promote *perfusion* and prevent hemorrhage.

Emergency Care: Traumatic vs. Elective Amputation. For a person who has a *traumatic amputation* in the community, first call 911. Assess the patient for airway or breathing problems. Examine the amputation site and apply direct pressure with layers of dry gauze or other cloth, using clean gloves if available. Many nurses carry gloves and first-aid kits for this type of emergency. Elevate the extremity above the patient's heart to decrease the bleeding. Do not remove the dressing to prevent dislodging the clot.

The fingers are the most likely part to be amputated and replanted. The current recommendation for prehospital care is to wrap the completely severed finger in dry sterile gauze (if available) or a clean cloth. Put the finger in a watertight, sealed plastic bag. *Place the bag in ice water, never directly on ice, at 1 part ice and 3 parts water.* Avoid contact between the finger and the water to prevent tissue damage. Do not remove any semidetached parts of the digit. Be sure that the part goes with the patient to the hospital.

For patients with a *planned surgical amputation*, the nurse's primary focus is to monitor for signs indicating that there is sufficient tissue *perfusion* and no hemorrhage. The skin flap at the end of the residual (remaining) limb should be pink in a light-skinned person and not discolored (lighter or darker than other usual skin pigmentation) in a dark-skinned patient. The area should be warm but not hot. Assess the closest proximal pulse for presence and strength and compare it with that in the other extremity. However, if the patient has bilateral vascular disease, comparison of limbs may not be an accurate way of measuring blood flow. Use a Doppler device to determine if the affected side is being perfused. Monitor vital signs per agency protocol.

! NURSING SAFETY PRIORITY (QSEN)
Critical Rescue

If the patient has decreased tissue **perfusion**, notify the surgeon or Rapid Response Team immediately to communicate your assessment findings! If the patient's blood pressure drops and the pulse increases, suspect covert (hidden) bleeding. To check for the presence of overt (obvious) bleeding, be sure to lift the residual limb and feel under the pressure dressing for dampness or drainage. If bleeding occurs, apply direct pressure and notify the Rapid Response Team or primary health care provider immediately. Continue to monitor the patient until help arrives.

Managing Acute and/or Persistent Pain

Planning: Expected Outcomes. The patient with an amputation is expected to state that he or she has adequate *pain* control after appropriate management.

Interventions. All patients experience *pain* as a result of either a traumatic or surgical (elective) amputation. Some patients also report pain in the missing body part (phantom limb pain [PLP]). Be sure to determine which type the patient has, because they are managed very differently.

! NURSING SAFETY PRIORITY (QSEN)
Action Alert

If the patient reports PLP, recognize that the *pain* is real and should be managed promptly and completely! It is *not* therapeutic to remind the patient that the limb cannot be hurting because it is missing. To prevent increased pain, handle the residual limb carefully when assessing the site or changing the dressing (Schreiber, 2017).

Opioid analgesics are not as effective for PLP as they are for residual limb pain. IV infusions of calcitonin during the week after amputation can reduce PLP. The primary health care provider prescribes other drugs on the basis of the type of PLP the patient experiences. For instance, beta-blocking agents such as propranolol are used for constant, dull, burning pain. Antiepileptic drugs such as pregabalin and gabapentin may be used for knifelike or sharp burning (neuropathic) pain. Antispasmodics such as baclofen may be prescribed for muscle spasms or cramping. Some patients improve with antidepressant drugs as adjuvant therapy.

Other pain management modalities are described in Chapter 5. Incorporate them into the plan of care if agreeable with the patient by collaborating with specialists who are trained to perform them. For example, physical therapists often use massage, heat, transcutaneous electrical nerve stimulation (TENS), mirror therapy, and ultrasound therapy for pain control. Yildirim & Sen (2020) found that mirror therapy, in which the patient regularly practices exercises with the affected and unaffected extremity in front of a mirror, helps to decrease phantom limb pain.

Consult with the certified hospital chaplain or social worker to provide emotional support based on the patient's preferences and beliefs. A psychologist may be needed to provide diagnostic assessment and/or psychotherapy.

Promoting Mobility

Planning: Expected Outcomes. The patient with an amputation is expected to have adequate *Mobility* and be free of complications associated with decreased mobility.

Interventions. Collaborate with the physical and/or occupational therapists to begin exercises as soon as possible after surgery. If the amputation is planned, the therapist may work with the patient before surgery to start muscle-strengthening exercises and evaluate the need for ambulatory aids, such as crutches. If the patient can practice with these devices before surgery, learning how to ambulate after surgery is much easier.

👥 INTERPROFESSIONAL COLLABORATION
Care of Patients Who Have an Amputation

Interprofessional collaborative care depends on the type and location of the amputation. For example, an above-the-knee amputation (AKA) has the potential for more postoperative complications than does a partial foot amputation. Regardless of where the amputation occurs, collaborate with the rehabilitation therapists to improve ambulation and/or enable the patient to be independent in ADLs. For many amputations, prostheses can be used to substitute for the missing body part.

According to the Interprofessional Education Collaborative (IPEC) Expert Panel's Competency of Roles and Responsibilities, using the unique and complementary abilities of other team members optimizes health and patient care (Slusser et al., 2019).

For patients with AKAs or BKAs, teach range-of-motion (ROM) exercises for prevention of flexion contractures, particularly of the hip and knee. A trapeze and an overhead frame aid in strengthening the arms and allow the patient to move independently in bed. Teach the patient how to perform ROM exercises. Be sure to turn the patient every 2 hours or teach him or her to turn independently. Move the patient slowly to prevent muscle spasms.

A firm mattress is essential for preventing contractures with a leg amputation. Assist the patient into a prone position every 3 to 4 hours for 20- to 30-minute periods if tolerated and not contraindicated. This position may be uncomfortable initially but helps prevent hip flexion contractures. Instruct the patient to pull the residual limb close to the other leg and contract the gluteal muscles of the buttocks for muscle strengthening. After staples are removed, the physical therapist may begin resistive exercises, which should also be done at home.

For above- and below-the-knee amputations, teach the patient how to push the residual limb down toward the bed while supporting it on a soft pillow at first. Then instruct him or her to continue this activity using a firmer pillow and then progress to a harder surface. This activity helps prepare the residual limb for prosthesis and reduces the incidence of phantom limb *pain* and sensation.

Elevation of a lower-leg residual limb on a pillow while the patient is in a supine position is controversial. Some practitioners advocate avoiding this practice at all times because it promotes hip or knee flexion contracture. Others allow elevation for the first 24 to 48 hours to reduce swelling and subsequent *pain.* Inspect the residual limb daily to ensure that it lies completely flat on the bed.

Before an elective amputation, the patient often sees a certified prosthetist-orthotist (CPO) so that planning can begin for the postoperative period. Arrangements for replacing an arm part are especially important for the patient to achieve self-management. Some patients are fitted with a temporary prosthesis at the time of surgery. Others, particularly older patients with vascular disease, are fitted after the residual limb has healed.

The patient being fitted for a leg prosthesis should bring a sturdy pair of shoes to the fitting. The prosthesis will be adjusted to that heel height.

Several devices help shape and shrink the residual limb in preparation for the prosthesis. Rigid, removable dressings are preferred because they decrease edema, protect and shape the limb, and allow easy access to the wound for inspection. An air splint, a plastic inflatable device, is sometimes used for this purpose. One of its disadvantages is air leakage and loss of compression. Wrapping with elastic bandages can also be effective in reducing edema, shrinking the limb, and holding the wound dressing in place.

For wrapping to be effective, reapply the bandages every 4 to 6 hours or more often if they become loose. *Figure-eight wrapping prevents restriction of blood flow. Decrease the tightness of the bandages while wrapping in a distal-to-proximal direction.* After wrapping, anchor the bandages to the highest joint, such as above the knee for BKAs.

The design of and materials for prostheses have improved dramatically over the years. Computer-assisted design and manufacturing (CAD-CAM) is used for a custom fit. One of the most important developments in lower-extremity prosthetics is the ankle-foot prosthesis, such as the Flex-Foot for more active amputees.

Promoting Self-Esteem

Planning: Expected Outcomes. The patient with an amputation is expected to adapt to the amputation to achieve a positive self-esteem and have an active and productive life.

Interventions. The patient often experiences feelings of inadequacy as a result of losing a body part, especially the older adult who was in poor health before surgery and men who are often the main providers for their families. If the patient is not able to adapt psychologically to the amputation, he or she may have difficulty adapting to a possible lifestyle change. If possible, arrange for him or her to meet with a rehabilitated, active amputee who is about the same age as the patient.

Freysteinson et al. (2016) studied a technique to help amputees get used to their body change as part of rehabilitation therapy. The authors asked the patients to view themselves in a mirror for repeated viewings. Four key themes emerged as a result of the study: mirror shock, mirror anguish, recognizing self, and acceptance as a new "normal." These themes are similar to other loss and grieving responses (see Chapter 8).

Use of the word *stump* for referring to the remaining portion of the limb (residual limb) continues to be controversial. Patients have reported feeling as if they were part of a tree when the term was used. However, some rehabilitation specialists who routinely work with amputees believe the term is appropriate because it forces the patient to realize what has happened and promotes adjustment to the amputation. *Assess the patient to determine which term he or she prefers.*

Assess the patient's verbal and nonverbal references to the affected area. Some patients behave euphorically (extremely happy) and seem to have accepted the loss. *Do not jump to the conclusion that acceptance has occurred.* Ask the patient to describe his or her feelings about changes in body image and self-esteem. He or she may verbalize acceptance but refuse to look at the area during a dressing change. This inconsistent behavior is not unusual and should be documented and shared with other health care team members.

With advancements in prostheses and surgical techniques, most patients can return to their jobs and other activities. Professional athletes who use prostheses are often quite successful in sports. Patients with amputations ski, hike, golf, bowl, and participate in other physically demanding activities. Many amputees participate actively in organized and recreational sports.

If a job or career change is necessary, collaborate with a social worker or vocational rehabilitation specialist to evaluate the patient's skills. A supportive family or significant other is important for the adjustment to this change. The patient may also think that an intimate relationship is no longer possible because of physical changes. Discuss sexuality issues with the patient and his or her partner as needed. Professional assistance from a sex therapist, intimacy coach, or psychologist may be needed.

Help the patient and family set realistic desired outcomes and take one day at a time. Help them recognize personal strengths. If the desired outcomes are not realistic, frustration and disappointment may decrease motivation during rehabilitation. Basic principles of rehabilitation are discussed in Chapter 7.

Care Coordination and Transition Management. The patient is discharged directly to home or to a skilled facility or rehabilitation facility, depending on the extent of the amputation. When rehabilitation is not feasible, as in the debilitated or demented older adult, he or she may be discharged to a long-term care facility. Coordinate this transfer with the case manager or discharge planner to ensure continuity of care.

Home Care Management. At home, the patient with a leg amputation needs to have enough room to use a wheelchair if the prosthesis is not yet available. He or she must be able to use toileting facilities and have access to areas necessary for self-management, such as the kitchen. Structural home modifications may be required before the patient goes home.

Self-Management Education. After the sutures or staples are removed, the patient begins residual limb care. A home care nurse may be needed to teach the patient and/or family how to care for the limb and the prosthesis if it is available (see the Home Care Considerations: The Patient With a Lower-Extremity Amputation in the Home box).

HOME CARE CONSIDERATIONS

The Patient With a Lower-Extremity Amputation in the Home

Assess the residual limb for:
- Adequate circulation
- **Infection**
- Healing
- Flexion contracture
- Dressing/elastic wrap

Assess the patient's ability to perform ADLs in the home.
- Evaluate the patient's ability to use ambulatory aids and care for the prosthetic device (if available).
- Assess the patient's pain level (intensity and quality).
- Assess the patient's nutritional status.
- Assess the patient's ability to cope with body image change.

The limb should be rewrapped several times a day with an elastic bandage applied in a figure-eight manner. For many patients, a shrinker stocking or sock is easier to apply. After the limb is healed, it is cleaned each day with the rest of the body during bathing with soap and water. Teach the patient and/or family to inspect it every day for signs of inflammation or skin breakdown.

! NURSING SAFETY PRIORITY (QSEN)

Action Alert

Collaborate with the prosthetist to teach the patient about prosthesis care after amputation to ensure its reliability and proper function. These devices are custom made, taking into account the patient's level of amputation, lifestyle, and occupation. Proper teaching regarding correct cleansing of the socket and inserts, wearing the correct liners, and assessing shoe wear and a schedule of follow-up care are essential before discharge. This information may need to be reviewed by the home care nurse.

Health Care Resources. A patient who seems to adjust to the amputation during hospitalization may realize that it is difficult to cope with the loss after discharge from the hospital. Teach the patient and family about available resources and support from organizations such as the Amputee Coalition of America (ACA) (www.amputee-coalition.org) and the National Amputation Foundation (NAF) (www.nationalamputation.org). The NAF was originally started for veterans but has since expanded to offer services to civilians.

PATIENT-CENTERED CARE: VETERANS HEALTH CONSIDERATIONS (QSEN)

Teach patients who are veterans about the many resources that can help them adjust to one or more amputations. In addition to specialty clinics and other services offered by the Veterans Administration in the United States, many other community and military services exist to help veterans adapt their lifestyle and remain active. Many of these services also assist families of veterans who have been injured (Table 47.2).

◆ **Evaluation: Evaluate Outcomes.** Evaluate the care of the patient with one or more amputations based on the identified priority patient problems. The expected outcomes include that the patient:
- Have adequate **perfusion** to the residual limb
- State that **pain** is controlled to between a 2 and 3 or as acceptable to the patient on a 0 to 10 pain intensity assessment scale
- Perform **mobility** skills independently and not experience complications of decreased mobility
- Be free of surgical site **infection**
- Have a positive self-esteem and lifestyle adaptation to live a productive, high-quality life

CARPAL TUNNEL SYNDROME

Pathophysiology Review

Carpal tunnel syndrome (CTS) is a common condition in which the median nerve in the wrist becomes compressed, causing pain and numbness (Durham & VanRavenstein, 2017). The carpal tunnel is a rigid canal that lies between the carpal bones and a fibrous tissue sheet. A group of tendons surround the synovium and share space with the median nerve in the carpal tunnel. When the synovium becomes swollen or thickened, this nerve is compressed.

The median nerve supplies motor, sensory, and autonomic function for the first three fingers of the hand and the palmar aspect of the fourth (ring) finger. Because the median nerve is close to other structures, wrist flexion causes nerve impingement and extension causes increased pressure in the lower portion of the carpal tunnel.

CTS is the most common type of repetitive stress injury (RSI). RSIs are the fastest-growing type of occupational injury. People whose jobs require repetitive hand activities, such as pinching or grasping during wrist flexion (e.g., factory workers, computer operators, jackhammer operators), are predisposed to CTS. In more recent years, young adults have an increased incidence of CTS due to texting and other cell phone use. It can also result from overuse in sports activities such as golf, tennis, or racquetball.

CTS usually presents as a chronic problem. Acute cases are rare. Excessive hand exercise, edema or hemorrhage into the carpal tunnel, or thrombosis of the median artery can lead to acute CTS. *Patients with hand burns or a Colles fracture of the wrist are particularly at risk for this problem.* In most cases, the cause may not result in nerve deficit for years.

TABLE 47.2 **Examples of Military and Community Resources for Veterans With Amputations in the United States**

Resource	Website Address
Hope for the Warriors™	www.hopeforthewarriors.org
Military OneSource	www.militaryonesource.com
U.S. Army Wounded Warrior Program	www.aw2.army.mil
Veterans Administration	www.va.gov
Amputee Coalition of America	www.amputee-coalition.org
Wounded Warrior Project	www.woundedwarriorproject.org
American Amputee Foundation	www.americanamputee.org
Amputee Resources for Canada	www.amputee.ca

CTS is also a common complication of certain metabolic and connective tissue diseases. For example, synovitis (inflammation of the synovium) occurs in patients with rheumatoid arthritis (RA). The hypertrophied synovium compresses the median nerve. In other chronic disorders such as diabetes mellitus, inadequate blood supply can cause median nerve neuropathy or dysfunction, resulting in CTS.

In a few cases, CTS may be a familial or congenital problem that manifests in adulthood. Space-occupying growths such as ganglia, tophi, and lipomas can also result in nerve compression.

PATIENT-CENTERED CARE: GENDER HEALTH CONSIDERATIONS (QSEN)

Women, especially those older than 50 years, are much more likely than men to experience CTS, probably due to the higher prevalence of diseases such as RA in women. The problem usually affects the dominant hand but can occur in both hands simultaneously. CTS is beginning to be found in children and adolescents as a result of the increased use of cell phones and other handheld mobile devices (Durham & VanRavenstein, 2017).

Health Promotion and Maintenance

Most businesses recognize the hazards of repetitive motion as a primary cause of occupational injury and disability. Both men and women in the labor force are experiencing increasing numbers of RSIs. Occupational health nurses have played an important role in ergonomics and in the development of ergonomically designed furniture and various aids to decrease CTS and other musculoskeletal injuries. Ergonomics is the study of how equipment and furniture can be arranged so that people can do work or other activities more efficiently and comfortably without injury.

U.S. federal and state legislation has been passed to ensure that all businesses, including health care organizations (HCOs), provide *ergonomically appropriate workstations* for their employees (Occupational Safety and Health Administration [OSHA]). The Joint Commission also requires that hospitals and other HCOs provide a safe work environment for all staff. In Canada, each province requires the work setting to have joint health and safety committees in which employees are actively involved in setting safety standards (Canadian Centre for Occupational Health and Safety). The Best Practice for Patient Safety & Quality Care: Health Promotion Activities to Prevent Carpal Tunnel Syndrome box lists best practices for preventing CTS in the health care setting.

❖ Interprofessional Collaborative Care

◆ **Assessment: Recognize Cues.** A diagnosis is often made based on the patient's history and report of hand pain and numbness and without further assessment. Ask about the nature, intensity, and location of the pain. Patients often state that the pain is worse at night as a result of flexion or direct pressure during sleep. The pain may radiate to the arm, shoulder and neck, or chest.

In addition to reports of numbness, patients with carpal tunnel syndrome (CTS) may also have paresthesia (painful numbness and tingling). *Sensory* changes usually occur weeks or months before *motor* manifestations.

BEST PRACTICE FOR PATIENT SAFETY & QUALITY CARE (QSEN)

Health Promotion Activities to Prevent Carpal Tunnel Syndrome

- Become familiar with federal and state laws regarding workplace requirements to prevent repetitive stress injuries such as carpal tunnel syndrome (CTS).
- When using equipment or computer workstations that can contribute to developing CTS, assess that they are ergonomically appropriate, including:
  - Specially designed wrist rest devices
  - Geometrically designed computer keyboards
  - Chair height that allows good posture
- Take regular short breaks away from activities that cause repetitive stress, such as working at computers and using cell phones and other handheld devices.
- Stretch fingers and wrists frequently during work hours.
- Stay as relaxed as possible when using equipment that causes repetitive stress.

The primary health care provider performs several tests for abnormal sensory findings. The Phalen wrist test, sometimes called **Phalen maneuver,** produces paresthesia in the median nerve distribution (palmar side of the thumb, index and middle fingers, and half of the ring finger) within 60 seconds as a result of increased internal carpal pressure. The patient is asked to relax the wrist into flexion or to place the back of the hands together and flex both wrists at the same time. The Phalen test is positive in most patients with CTS (Jarvis, 2018).

Motor changes in CTS begin with a weak pinch, clumsiness, and difficulty with fine movements. These changes progress to muscle weakness and wasting, which can impair self-management. If desired, test for pinching ability and ask the patient to perform a fine-movement task, such as threading a needle. Strenuous hand activity worsens the pain and numbness (McCance et al., 2019).

In addition to inspecting for muscle atrophy and task performance, observe the wrist for swelling. Gently palpate the area and note any unusual findings. Autonomic changes may be evidenced by skin discoloration, nail changes (e.g., brittleness), and increased or decreased hand sweating.

◆ **Interventions: Take Action.** The primary health care provider uses conservative measures before surgical intervention. However, CTS can recur with either type of treatment. Management depends on the patient, but established best practices have not been determined.

Nonsurgical Management. Aggressive drug therapy and immobilization of the wrist are the major components of nonsurgical management. Teach the patient the importance of these modalities in the hope of preventing surgical intervention.

NSAIDs are the most commonly prescribed drugs for the relief of *pain* and inflammation, if present, but they do not slow the progression of CTS (Blevins, 2020). In addition to or instead of systemic medications, the primary health care provider may inject corticosteroids directly into the carpal tunnel. If the patient responds to the injection, several additional weekly or monthly injections are given. Teach him or her to take NSAIDs with or after meals to reduce gastric irritation.

A splint or hand brace may be used to immobilize the wrist during the day, during the night, or both. Many patients experience temporary relief with these devices. The occupational therapist places the wrist in the neutral position or in slight extension.

Laser or ultrasound therapy may also be helpful. Some patients report fewer symptoms after beginning yoga or another exercise routine. For some patients, wrist-stretching exercises are recommended, including wrist extension and flexion stretches (Blevins, 2020).

Surgical Management. Surgery can relieve the pressure on the median nerve by providing nerve decompression to prevent irreversible damage for patients with extended cases of CTS. Major surgical complications are rare after CTS surgery.

The nurse in the surgeon's office or same-day surgical center reinforces the teaching provided by the surgeon regarding the nature of the surgery. Postoperative care is reviewed so that the patient knows what to expect. Chapter 9 describes general preoperative care in detail.

Whatever the cause of nerve compression, the surgeon removes it by either cutting or laser. The most common surgery is the endoscopic carpal tunnel release (ECTR). In this procedure, the surgeon makes a very small incision (less than ½ inch [1.2 cm]) through which the endoscope is inserted. He or she then uses special instruments to free the trapped median nerve. Although ECTR is less invasive and costs less than the open procedure, the patient may have a longer period of postoperative pain and numbness compared with recovery from open carpal tunnel release (OCTR). Surgical treatment seems to be more effective than conservative measures over the long term. However, there is no evidence that one type of procedure, open or endoscopic, is more effective than the other; it is basically surgeon preference (Durham & VanRavenstein, 2017).

After surgery, monitor vital signs and check the dressing carefully for drainage and tightness. If ECTR has been performed, the dressing is very small. The surgeon may require that the patient's affected hand and arm be elevated above heart level for several days to reduce postoperative swelling. Check the neurovascular status of the fingers every hour during the immediate postoperative period and encourage the patient to move them frequently. Offer pain medication and assure him or her that a prescription for analgesics will be provided before discharge. Discomfort should not last more than 24 to 72 hours (Blevins, 2020).

Hand movements, including lifting heavy objects, may be restricted for 4 to 6 weeks after surgery. The patient can expect weakness for weeks or perhaps months. Teach him or her to report any changes in neurovascular status, including increased pain, bleeding, or infection, to the surgeon's office immediately.

Remind the patient and family that the surgical procedure might not be a cure. For example, synovitis may recur with rheumatoid arthritis and may recompress the median nerve. Multiple surgeries and other treatments are common with CTS.

The patient may need help with self-management activities during recovery. Ensure that assistance in the home is available before discharge; this is usually provided by the family or significant others.

BEST PRACTICE FOR PATIENT SAFETY & QUALITY CARE (QSEN)

Emergency Care of Patients With Sports-Related Injuries

- Do not move the victim until spinal cord injury is ascertained (see Chapter 40 for assessment of spinal cord injury).
- Use RICE:
  - **Rest** the injured part; immobilize the joint above and below the injury by applying a splint if needed.
  - Apply **ice** intermittently for the first 24 to 48 hours (heat may be used thereafter).
  - Use **compression** for the first 24 to 48 hours (e.g., elastic wrap).
  - **Elevate** the affected limb to decrease swelling.
- Always assume that the area is fractured until x-ray studies are done.
- Assess neurovascular status in the area distal to the injury.

NCLEX EXAMINATION CHALLENGE 47.4

Safe and Effective Care Environment

What is the nurse's **priority** when doing an admission for a client who returned directly from the operating suite after a carpal tunnel repair?
A. Monitor vital signs, including pulse oximetry.
B. Check the surgical dressing to ensure that it is intact.
C. Assess neurovascular assessment in the affected arm.
D. Monitor intake and output.

KNEE INJURIES

In addition to the bone and muscle problems already discussed, trauma can cause cartilage, ligament, and tendon injury. Many musculoskeletal injuries are the result of playing sports (professional and recreational) or doing other strenuous physical activities. The popularity of all-terrain vehicles (ATVs) and skateboarding has increased injuries in younger patients. Sports injuries have become so common that large metropolitan hospitals have sports medicine clinics and physicians who specialize in this field.

The principles of injury to one part of the body are similar to those of other sports injuries and accidents. For example, a tendon rupture in a knee is cared for in the same manner as a tendon rupture in the wrist. The Best Practice for Patient Safety & Quality Care box lists general emergency measures for sports-related injuries.

Because the knee is most often injured, it is discussed as a typical example of other areas of the body. Trauma to the knee results in *internal derangement,* a broad term for disturbances of an injured knee joint. When surgery is required to resolve the problem, most surgeons prefer to perform the procedure through an arthroscope when possible. A description of arthroscopy is presented in Chapter 44. Postoperative care for knee surgeries generally includes analgesics, physical therapy, and bracing or splinting, often using a knee immobilizer (Fig. 47.11). All patients require frequent neurovascular monitoring. Table 47.3 lists examples of common knee injuries and their interprofessional management.

ROTATOR CUFF INJURIES

The musculotendinous, or rotator, cuff of the shoulder functions to stabilize the head of the humerus in the glenoid cavity during shoulder abduction. Young adults usually sustain a tear of the cuff by substantial trauma, such as may occur during a fall, while throwing a ball, or with heavy lifting. Older adults tend to have small tears related to aging, repetitive motions, or falls, and the tears are usually painless.

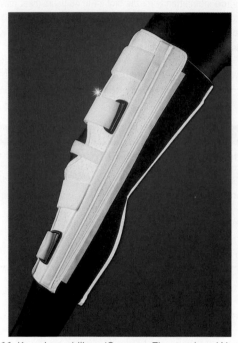

FIG. 47.11 Knee immobilizer. (Courtesy Zimmer, Inc., Warsaw, IN.)

The patient with a torn rotator cuff has shoulder *pain* and cannot easily abduct the arm at the shoulder. When the arm is abducted, he or she usually drops it because abduction cannot be maintained (drop arm test). Pain is more intense at night and with overhead activities. Partial-thickness tears are more painful than full-thickness tears, but full-thickness tears result in more weakness and loss of function. Muscle atrophy is commonly seen, and *mobility* is reduced. Diagnosis is confirmed with x-rays, MRI, ultrasonography, and/or CT scans.

The primary health care provider usually treats the patient with partial-thickness tears conservatively with NSAIDs, intermittent steroid injections, physical therapy, and activity limitations while the tear heals. Physical therapy treatments may include ultrasound, electrical stimulation, ice, and heat.

For patients who do not respond to conservative treatment in 3 to 6 months or for those who have a complete (full-thickness) tear, the surgeon repairs the cuff using mini-open or arthroscopic procedures. An interscalene nerve block may be used to extend analgesia for an open repair. If a peripheral nerve block is used, remind the patient that the arm will feel numb and cannot be moved for up to 20 or more hours after surgery. Observe, report, and document complications of respiratory distress and neurovascular compromise.

After surgery, the affected arm is usually immobilized for several weeks. Pendulum exercises are started on the third or fourth postoperative day and progress to active exercises in about 2 weeks. Patients then begin rehabilitation in the ambulatory-care occupational therapy department. Teach them that they may not have full function for several months.

TABLE 47.3	Examples of Acute Soft-Tissue Musculoskeletal Injuries
Acute Injury/Description	**Management**
Sprain: excessive stretching of a ligament	Immobilization, RICE, possible surgery if severe
Strain: excessive stretching of a muscle or tendon	Heat/cold, activity limitations, NSAIDs, muscle relaxants, possible tendon repair
Ligament tear (such as anterior cruciate ligament in knee): damage to ligament most often caused by sports or vehicular crash	RICE, surgery if does not heal or is severe (usually arthroscopic)
Meniscus tear: damage to knee cartilage caused by sports or other trauma	RICE, bracing, splinting, NSAIDs, surgery (usually arthroscopic)
Tendon rupture (such as the Achilles tendon in heel): often caused by sports or wearing high-heeled shoes; in some cases can occur after taking fluoroquinolones such as ciprofloxacin (Cipro)	RICE, NSAIDs, orthotic devices, ultrasound, surgery if severe or does not heal
Patellofemoral pain syndrome (PFPS): knee pain caused by overuse of the knee joint; also called *runner's knee*	Rest, splinting, bracing, NSAIDs, possibly surgery as last resort
Joint dislocation: displacement of a bone from its usual position in a synovial joint	Manual joint relocation; possible surgery

GET READY FOR THE NEXT-GENERATION NCLEX® EXAMINATION!

Key Points

Review these Key Points for each NCLEX Examination Client Needs Category.

Safe and Effective Care Environment

- Collaborate with physical and occupational therapists for care of patients with fractures to improve *mobility* and muscle strength. **QSEN: Teamwork and Collaboration**
- Remember that the priority care for patients with fractures and amputations is to maintain perfusion, reduce *pain,* and prevent decreased *mobility*. **QSEN: Evidence-Based Practice**
- Monitor for potentially life-threatening complications of fractures, including hemorrhage, venous thromboembolism, fat embolism syndrome, acute compartment syndrome, and *infection*. **Clinical Judgment**

Health Promotion and Maintenance

- Teach people to avoid musculoskeletal injury by treating or preventing osteoporosis (see Chapter 45), being cautious when walking to prevent a fall, wearing supportive shoes, avoiding dangerous sports or activities, and decreasing time spent doing repetitive stress activities, such as using a computer keyboard or cell phone. **QSEN: Safety**
- Several community organizations, such as the Amputee Coalition of America, are available to help patients and their families cope with the loss of a body part. **QSEN: Patient-Centered Care**
- Teach patients and their family members and significant others how to care for casts or other orthopedic devices at home. **QSEN: Safety**
- In collaboration with the interprofessional health team, reinforce teaching for ambulating with crutches, walkers, or canes and teach exercises to patients with leg amputation to prevent hip flexion contractures. **QSEN: Teamwork and Collaboration**
- Provide special care for older adults with hip fractures, including preventing heel pressure injuries and promoting early ambulation to prevent complications of immobility. **QSEN: Patient-Centered Care**

Psychosocial Integrity

- For patients with severe trauma or amputation, assess coping skills and encourage verbalization. **QSEN: Patient-Centered Care**
- Recognize that the patient having an amputation may need to adjust to an altered lifestyle but can be active and productive. **QSEN: Patient-Centered Care**

Physiological Integrity

- Be aware that open fractures cause a higher risk for infection than do closed fractures; use strict aseptic technique when providing wound management. **QSEN: Evidence-Based Care**
- Recognize that fat embolism syndrome is different from pulmonary (blood clot) embolism. **Clinical Judgment**
- Provide emergency care of the patient with a fracture. **Clinical Judgment**
- Identify the patient at risk for acute compartment syndrome; loosen bandages or request that the patient's cast be cut if neurovascular compromise is assessed; notify the health care provider immediately. **QSEN: Evidence-Based Practice**
- As a priority, document neurovascular status frequently in patients with musculoskeletal injury, traction, or cast and manage *pain* adequately. **QSEN: Informatics**
- Provide evidence-based appropriate cast care, depending on the type of cast (plaster or synthetic); check for pressure necrosis under the cast by feeling for heat, assessing the patient's pain level, and smelling the cast for an unpleasant odor. **QSEN: Evidence-Based Practice**
- Provide pin care for patients with skeletal traction or external fixation; assess for signs and symptoms of infection at the pin sites. **QSEN: Evidence-Based Practice**
- Provide postoperative care for the patient having a fracture repair, including promoting *mobility* and monitoring for complications of immobility. **QSEN: Safety**
- Provide emergency care for a patient having a traumatic amputation in the community. Call 911, assess the patient for ABCs, apply direct pressure on the amputation site, and elevate the extremity above the patient's heart to decrease bleeding. For finger parts, wrap the amputated part with a clean cloth and place in a sealed bag, which is lowered into ice water. **QSEN: Evidence-Based Practice**
- After surgery, assess for and promptly manage phantom limb *pain* in the patient who has an amputation; collaborate with specialists to incorporate complementary and integrative therapies and drug therapy into the patient's plan of care. **QSEN: Patient-Centered Care**
- Assess and document neurovascular status frequently after an endoscopic carpal tunnel release. **QSEN: Safety**
- Provide emergency care for patients with a sports-related injury using RICE (Rest, Ice, Compression, Elevation). **QSEN: Evidence-Based Practice**
- Recall that carpal tunnel syndrome (CTS) is the most common type of repetitive stress injury (RSI) caused by certain occupations such as computer operators and factory workers. **QSEN: Evidence-Based Practice**
- Many acute musculoskeletal injuries are initially treated by RICE: *rest, ice, compression,* and *elevation*. **QSEN: Evidence-Based Practice**

MASTERY QUESTIONS

1. The nurse is assigned to care for a postoperative client who had an open reduction, internal fixation of the right tibia yesterday. The client reports increased right leg pain, numbness, and tingling. What would be the nurse's **first** action at this time?
   A. Elevate the surgical leg on a pillow.
   B. Perform a neurovascular assessment.
   C. Administer pain medication.
   D. Call the primary health care provider.

2. The nurse teaches assistive personnel (AP) how to position a client who had an above-the-knee amputation (AKA) last week. Which statement by the AP indicates **understanding** of the teaching?
   A. "We should keep the surgical leg elevated on two pillows at all times."
   B. "We should keep the client in a sitting position as long as possible."
   C. "We should keep the surgical leg as flat on the bed as possible."
   D. "We should keep the client in a prone position most of the day."

3. The nurse is caring for a client who was admitted to the emergency department (ED) with report of left knee pain and swelling after playing baseball with friends. Which nursing actions are appropriate when caring for the client? **Select all that apply.**
   A. Apply heat to the affected area.
   B. Assess the severity and quality of pain.
   C. Perform a neurovascular assessment.
   D. Elevate the affected extremity.
   E. Immobilize the injured knee joint.

REFERENCES

Blevins, S. (2020). Carpal tunnel syndrome. *Medsurg Nursing, 29*(1), 53–55.

Conley, R.B., Adib, G., Adler, R.A., Akesson, K.E., Alexander, I.M., Amenta, K.C., et al. (2020). Secondary fracture prevention: Consensus clinical recommendations from a multistakeholder coalition. *Orthopaedic Nursing, 39*(3), 145-161.

Duperouzel, W., Gray, B., & Santy-Tomlinson, J. (2018). The principles of traction and the application of lower limb skin traction. *International Journal of Orthopaedic and Trauma Nursing, 29*, 54–57.

Durham, C. O., & VanRavenstein, K. (2017). It's all in the wrist: Diagnosis and management of carpal tunnel syndrome. *Orthopaedic Nursing, 36*(5), 323–327.

Freysteinson, W., Thomas, L., Sebastian-Deutsch, A., Douglas, D., Meltom, D., Celia, T., et al. (2016). A study of the amputee experience of viewing self in the mirror. *Rehabilitation Nursing.* https://doi.org/10.1002/mj.256. [Epub ahead of print].

Georgiades, D. S. (2018). A systematic integrative review of pin site crusts. *Orthopaedic Nursing, 37*(1), 36–42.

Hohler, S. E. (2018). Providing evidence-based practices for patients with hip fractures. *Nursing, 48*(6), 52–57.

Jarvis, C. (2018). *Physical examination & health assessment* (8th ed.). St. Louis: Elsevier Saunders.

MacDonald, V., Maher, A. B., Mainz, H., Meehan, A. J., Brent, L., Hommel, A., et al. (2018). Developing and testing an international audit of quality indicators for older adults with fragility fractures. *Orthopaedic Nursing, 37*(2), 115–121.

McCance, K., Huether, S., Brashers, V., & Rote, N. (2019). *Pathophysiology: The biologic basis for disease in adults and children* (8th ed.). St. Louis: Mosby.

Schreiber, M. L. (2017). Lower limb amputation: Postoperative nursing care and considerations. *Medsurg Nursing, 26*(4), 274–279.

Slusser, M. M., Garcia, L. I., Reed, C.-R., & McGinnis, P. Q. (2019). *Foundations of interprofessional collaborative practice in health care.* St. Louis: Elsevier.

Thurlow, G., & Gray, B. (2018). Complex regional pain syndrome. *International Journal of Orthopaedic and Trauma Nursing, 30*, 44–47.

Turkowski, B. B. (2018). "I can't poop": Medication-induced constipation. *Orthopaedic Nursing, 37*(3), 192–196.

Wennberg, P., Andersson, H., & Sundstrom, B. W. (2018). Patients with suspected hip fractures in the chain of emergency care: An integrative review of the literature. *International Journal of Orthopaedic and Trauma Nursing, 29*, 16–31.

Williams, M. G., Jeffery, Z., Corner, H. W., Charity, J., Quantick, M., & Sartin, N. (2019). A robust approach to implementing fascia iliaca compartment nerve blocks in hip fracture patients. *Orthopaedic Nursing, 37*(3), 185–189.

Yildirim, M., & Sen, S. (2020). Mirror therapy in the management of phantom limb pain. *AJN, 120*(3), 41–46.

48

Assessment of the Gastrointestinal System

Charity Hacker

http://evolve.elsevier.com/Iggy/

LEARNING OUTCOMES

1. Collaborate with the interprofessional team to perform a gastrointestinal (GI) assessment.
2. Prioritize evidence-based care for patients having invasive diagnostic testing affecting *nutrition, elimination,* and GI *pain.*
3. Teach evidence-based ways for adults to prevent GI problems.
4. Explain how physiologic aging changes of the gastrointestinal system affect *nutrition* and *elimination.*
5. Implement nursing interventions to decrease the psychosocial impact caused by GI problems.
6. Apply knowledge of anatomy and physiology, genetic risk, and principles of aging to perform a focused GI assessment.
7. Use clinical judgment to document the GI assessment in the electronic health record.
8. Interpret assessment findings for patients with a suspected or actual GI problem.

KEY TERMS

amylase An enzyme that converts starch and glycogen into simple sugars; found most commonly in saliva and pancreatic fluids.

borborygmus High-pitched bowel sounds that are proximal (above) an obstruction.

bruit An audible swishing sound produced when the volume of blood or the diameter of the blood vessel changes.

colonoscopy An endoscopic examination of the entire large bowel.

digestion The mechanical and chemical process in which complex foodstuffs are broken down into simpler forms that can be used by the body.

dyspepsia An epigastric burning sensation, often referred to as "heartburn."

endoscope A tube that allows viewing and manipulation of internal body areas.

endoscopic retrograde cholangiopancreatography (ERCP) A procedure in which the bile ducts, pancreatic duct, and gallbladder are visualized through endoscopy.

endoscopy The direct visualization of the gastrointestinal tract by means of a flexible fiberoptic endoscope.

enteroscopy Visualization of the small intestine.

esophageal stricture Narrowing of the esophageal opening.

esophagogastroduodenoscopy (EGD) The visual examination of the esophagus, stomach, and duodenum by means of a fiberoptic endoscope.

flatulence Gas in the lower gastrointestinal tract.

guaiac-based fecal occult blood test (gFOBT) A diagnostic test that measures the presence of blood in the stool from gastrointestinal bleeding—a common finding associated with colorectal cancer.

lipase An enzyme secreted by the pancreas that facilitates the breakdown of triglycerides into fatty acids.

NPO (nothing by mouth) No eating, drinking (including water), or smoking.

PQRST A mnemonic (memory device) that may help in the assessment of abdominal pain. The letters represent these areas: P, precipitating or palliative (What brings it on? What makes it better or worse?); Q, quality or quantity (How does it look, feel, or sound?); R, region or radiation (Where is it? Does it spread anywhere?); S, severity scale (How bad is it [on a scale of 0 to 10]? Is it getting better, worse, or staying the same?); T, timing (Onset, duration, and frequency?).

reflux Reverse or backward flow.

sigmoidoscopy An endoscopic examination of the rectum and sigmoid colon using a flexible scope.

steatorrhea Fatty stools.

virtual colonoscopy Three-dimensional images of the colon and rectum created by use of an abdominal and pelvic CT scan.

The *alimentary canal,* known as the GI tract, consists of the mouth, esophagus, stomach, small and large intestines, and rectum. The GI system is formed when the salivary glands, liver, gallbladder, and pancreas secrete substances into this tract (Fig. 48.1). The main functions of the GI tract, with the aid of organs such as the pancreas and the liver, are the digestion of food to adequately meet the body's *nutrition* needs, and the *elimination* of waste resulting from digestion. The GI tract is susceptible to numerous health problems, including structural or mechanical alterations, impaired motility, infection, inflammation or autoimmune disease, and cancer.

ANATOMY AND PHYSIOLOGY REVIEW

Structure

The lumen, or inner wall, of the GI tract consists of four layers: mucosa, submucosa, muscularis, and serosa. The *mucosa,* the innermost layer, includes a thin layer of smooth muscle and specialized exocrine gland cells. It is surrounded by the *submucosa,* which is made up of connective tissue. The *submucosa* layer is surrounded by the muscularis. The *muscularis* is composed of both circular and longitudinal smooth muscles, which work to keep contents moving through the tract. The outermost layer, the *serosa,* is composed of connective tissue. Although the GI tract is continuous from the mouth to the anus, it is divided into specialized regions. The mouth, pharynx, esophagus, stomach, and small and large intestines each perform a specific function. In addition, the secretions of the salivary, gastric, and intestinal glands; liver; and pancreas empty into the GI tract to aid digestion.

Function

The functions of the GI tract include secretion, digestion, absorption, motility, and *elimination.* Food and fluids are ingested, swallowed, and propelled along the lumen of the GI tract to the anus for elimination. The smooth muscles contract to move food from the mouth to the anus. Before food can be absorbed, it must be broken down to a liquid, called *chyme.* Digestion is the mechanical and chemical process in which complex foodstuffs are broken down into simpler forms that can be used by the body. During digestion, the stomach secretes hydrochloric acid, the liver secretes bile, and digestive enzymes are released from accessory organs, aiding in food breakdown. After the digestive process is complete, absorption takes place. *Absorption* is carried out as the nutrients produced by digestion move from the lumen of the GI tract into the body's circulatory system for uptake by individual cells (McCance & Huether, 2019).

Oral Cavity. The oral cavity (mouth) includes the buccal mucosa, lips, tongue, hard palate, soft palate, teeth, and salivary glands. The buccal mucosa is the mucous membrane lining the inside of the mouth. The tongue is involved in speech, taste, and *mastication* (chewing). Small projections called *papillae* cover the tongue and provide a roughened surface, permitting the movement of food in the mouth during chewing. The hard palate and the soft palate together form the roof of the mouth.

Adults have 32 permanent teeth: 16 each in upper and lower arches. The different types of teeth function to prepare food for digestion by cutting, tearing, crushing, or grinding the food. Swallowing begins after food is taken into the mouth and chewed. Saliva is secreted in response to the presence of food in the mouth and begins to soften the food. Saliva contains mucin and an enzyme called *salivary alpha-amylase* (McCance & Huether, 2019) (also known as *ptyalin*), which begins the breakdown of carbohydrates.

Esophagus. The *esophagus* is a muscular canal that extends from the pharynx (throat) to the stomach and passes through the center of the diaphragm. Its primary function is to move food and fluids from the pharynx to the stomach. At the upper end of the esophagus is a sphincter referred to as the upper esophageal sphincter (UES). When at rest, the UES is closed to prevent air into the esophagus during respiration. The portion of the esophagus just above the gastroesophageal (GE) junction is referred to as the lower esophageal sphincter (LES). When at rest, the LES is normally closed to prevent reflux of gastric contents into the esophagus. If the LES does not work properly, gastroesophageal reflux disease (GERD) can develop.

Stomach. The *stomach* is located in the midline and left upper quadrant (LUQ) of the abdomen and has three functional regions: the fundus, body, and antrum (McCance & Huether, 2019). Anatomically, the *cardia* is the narrow portion of the stomach that is below the gastroesophageal (GE) junction. The *fundus* is the area nearest to the cardia. The main area of the stomach is referred to as the *body* or *corpus.* The *antrum* (pylorus) is the distal (lower) portion of the stomach and is separated from the duodenum by the pyloric sphincter. Both ends of the stomach are guarded by sphincters (cardiac [LES] and pyloric), which aid in the transport of food through the GI tract and prevent backflow.

Smooth muscle cells that line the stomach are responsible for gastric motility. The stomach is also richly innervated with intrinsic and extrinsic nerves. Parietal cells lining the wall of the stomach secrete hydrochloric acid, whereas chief cells secrete pepsinogen (a precursor to pepsin, a digestive enzyme). Parietal cells also produce intrinsic factor, a substance that aids in the absorption of vitamin B_{12}. Absence of intrinsic factor causes pernicious anemia.

After ingestion of food, the stomach functions as a food reservoir where the digestive process begins, using mechanical movements and chemical secretions. The stomach mixes or churns the food, breaking apart the large food molecules and mixing them with gastric secretions to form chyme, which then empties into the duodenum. The *intestinal phase* begins as the chyme passes from the stomach into the duodenum, causing distention. It is assisted by secretin and cholecystokinin,

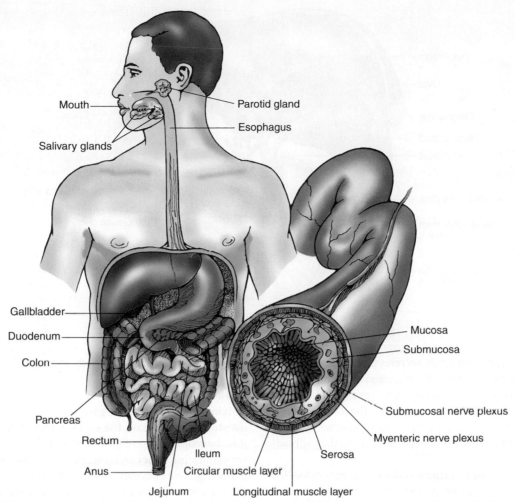

FIG. 48.1 The GI system (GI tract) can be thought of as a tube (with necessary structures) extending from the mouth to the anus for a 25-foot length. The structure of this tube *(shown enlarged)* is basically the same throughout its length.

hormones that inhibit further acid production and decrease gastric motility (Peate & Nair, 2016).

Pancreas. The *pancreas* is a fish-shaped gland that lies behind the stomach and extends horizontally from the duodenal C-loop to the spleen (McCance & Huether, 2019). The pancreas is divided into portions known as the head, the body, and the tail (Fig. 48.2).

Two major cellular bodies (exocrine and endocrine) within the pancreas have separate functions. The exocrine part consists of cells that secrete enzymes needed for digestion of carbohydrates, fats, and proteins (proteases, amylase, and lipase). The endocrine part of the pancreas is made up of the *islets of Langerhans,* with alpha cells producing glucagon and beta cells producing insulin, as well as delta and f (or PP) cells (McCance & Huether, 2019). The hormones produced are essential in the regulation of metabolism.

Liver and Gallbladder. The liver is the largest organ in the body (other than skin) and is located mainly in the right upper quadrant (RUQ) of the abdomen. The right and left hepatic ducts transport bile from the liver. It receives its blood supply from

the hepatic artery and portal vein, resulting in approximately 1200 mL of blood flow through the liver every minute.

The liver performs more than 400 functions in three major categories: storage, protection, and metabolism. It stores many minerals and vitamins, such as iron; magnesium; fat-soluble vitamins A, D, E, and K; and water-soluble vitamin B_{12} (McCance & Huether, 2019).

The protective function of the liver involves phagocytic *Kupffer cells,* which are part of the body's reticuloendothelial system. They engulf harmful bacteria and anemic red blood cells. The liver also detoxifies potentially harmful compounds (e.g., drugs, chemicals, alcohol). Therefore the risk for drug toxicity increases with aging because of decreased liver function.

The liver functions in the metabolism of proteins that are vital for survival. It breaks down amino acids to remove ammonia, which is then converted to urea and is excreted via the kidneys as urine (McCance & Huether, 2019). It synthesizes several plasma proteins, including albumin, prothrombin, and fibrinogen. The liver's role in carbohydrate metabolism involves storing and releasing glycogen as the body's energy requirements change. The organ also synthesizes, breaks down, and temporarily stores fatty acids and triglycerides.

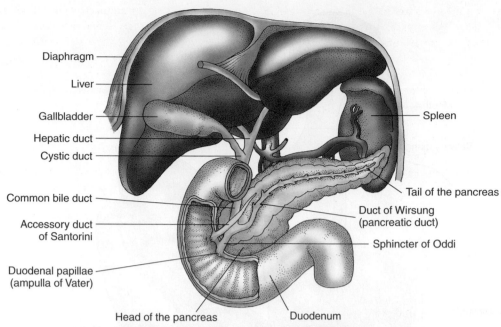

FIG. 48.2 Anatomy of the pancreas, liver, and gallbladder.

The liver forms and continually secretes bile, which is essential for the breakdown of fat. The secretion of bile increases in response to gastrin, secretin, and cholecystokinin. Bile is secreted into small ducts that empty into the common bile duct (CBD) and into the duodenum at the *sphincter of Oddi.* However, if the sphincter is closed, the bile goes to the gallbladder for storage.

The *gallbladder* is a pear-shaped, bulbous sac that is located underneath the liver. It is drained by the cystic duct, which joins with the hepatic duct from the liver to form the CBD. The gallbladder collects, concentrates, and stores the bile that has come from the liver. It releases the bile into the duodenum via the CBD when fat is present.

Small Intestine. The small intestine is the longest and most convoluted portion of the digestive tract, measuring an average of 9 to 16 feet (3 to 5 m) in length in an adult (Collins & Badireddy, 2020). It is composed of three different regions: duodenum, jejunum, and ileum. The *duodenum* is the first 8 to 10 inches (20 to 25 cm) of the small intestine and is attached to the distal end of the pylorus (Collins & Badireddy, 2020). The common bile duct and pancreatic duct join to form the ampulla of Vater, emptying into the duodenum at the duodenal papilla. This papillary opening is surrounded by muscle known as the sphincter of Oddi. The 8-foot (2.5-m) portion of the small intestine that follows the sphincter of Oddi is the *jejunum.* The last 10 feet (3 m) of the small intestine is called the *ileum* (Collins & Badireddy, 2020). The ileocecal valve separates the entrance of the ileum from the cecum of the large intestine (Peate & Nair, 2016).

The inner surface of the small intestine has a velvety appearance because of numerous mucous membrane finger-like projections. These projections are called *intestinal villi.* In addition to the intestinal villi, the small intestine has circular folds of mucosa and submucosa, which increase the surface area for digestion and absorption.

The small intestine has three main *functions*: movement (mixing and peristalsis), digestion, and absorption. Because the intestinal villi increase the surface area of the small intestine, it is the major organ of absorption of the digestive system. The small intestine mixes and transports the chyme to combine with many digestive enzymes. It takes an average of 3 to 6 hours for the contents to be passed by peristalsis through the small intestine (Peate & Nair, 2016). Intestinal enzymes aid the body in the digestion of proteins, carbohydrates, and lipids.

Large Intestine. The large intestine extends about 5 to 6 feet in length from the ileocecal valve to the anus and is lined with columnar epithelium that has absorptive and mucous cells. It begins with the *cecum,* a dilated, pouchlike structure that is inferior to the ileocecal opening. At the base of the cecum is the vermiform appendix, which has been discovered to play a role in intestinal immunity (Girard-Madoux et al., 2018). The large intestine then extends upward from the cecum as the colon. The colon consists of four divisions: ascending colon, transverse colon, descending colon, and sigmoid colon (McCance & Huether, 2019). The sigmoid colon empties into the rectum.

Beyond the sigmoid colon, the large intestine bends downward to form the rectum. The last 1 to 1½ inches (3 to 4 cm) of the large intestine are called the *anal canal,* which opens to the exterior of the body through the anus. The internal and external sphincter muscles surround the anal canal and control defecation.

The large intestine's *functions* are movement, absorption, and ***elimination.*** Movement in the large intestine consists mainly of segmental contractions, such as those in the small intestine, to allow enough time for the absorption of water and electrolytes. In addition, peristaltic contractions are triggered by colonic distention to move the contents toward the rectum, where the material is stored until the urge to defecate occurs. Absorption of water and some electrolytes occurs in the large intestine to reduce the fluid volume of the chyme. This process creates a more solid material, the feces, for *elimination.*

Gastrointestinal Changes Associated With Aging

As people age, and especially after 65 years of age, physiologic changes occur in the GI system. Common digestive and *elimination* changes can affect *nutrition* (Terrery & Nicoteri, 2016). The Patient-Centered Care: Older Adult Considerations: Changes in the Gastrointestinal System Associated With Aging box lists common GI changes in older adults.

PATIENT-CENTERED CARE: OLDER ADULT CONSIDERATIONS (QSEN)

Changes in the Gastrointestinal System Associated With Aging

Physiologic Change	Disorders Related to Change
Atrophy of the gastric mucosa leads to decreased hydrochloric acid levels (hypochlorhydria).	Decreased absorption of iron and vitamin B_{12} and proliferation of bacteria. Atrophic gastritis occurs as a consequence of bacterial overgrowth.
Peristalsis decreases, and nerve impulses are dulled.	Decreased sensation to defecate can result in postponement of bowel movements, which leads to constipation and impaction.
Distention and dilation of pancreatic ducts change. Calcification of pancreatic vessels occurs with a decrease in lipase production.	Decreased lipase level results in decreased fat absorption and digestion. Steatorrhea (fatty stool) occurs because of decreased fat digestion.
A decrease in the number and size of hepatic cells leads to decreased liver weight and mass. This change and an increase in fibrous tissue lead to decreased protein synthesis and changes in liver enzymes. Enzyme activity and cholesterol synthesis are diminished.	Decreased enzyme activity depresses drug metabolism, which leads to accumulation of drugs—possibly to toxic levels.
The delicate microbial balance of good anaerobic and aerobic flora is disrupted over time, negatively affecting the immune response (Vemuri et al., 2018).	Dysfunctional microbial activity contributes to obesity, inflammatory disease, and reduced immunity.

ASSESSMENT: RECOGNIZE CUES

Patient History

The purpose of the health history is to determine the events related to the current health problem (see the Best Practice for Patient Safety & Quality Care: Questions for Gastrointestinal Health History box). Ask questions about changes in appetite, weight, and stool. Determine the patient's experience with *pain,* if that is one of his or her concerns.

Collect data about the patient's age, gender, and culture. This information can be helpful in assessing who is likely to have particular GI system disorders. For instance, older adults

are more at risk for stomach cancer than are younger adults. Younger adults are at higher risk for inflammatory bowel disease (IBD). The exact reasons for these differences continue to be studied. Colon cancer, once a disease that affected older adults, has become more common among young people with obesity (Colorectal Cancer Alliance, 2019).

NCLEX EXAMINATION CHALLENGE 48.1

Physiological Integrity

Which daily behavior of a client with GI problems requires **further** nursing assessment? **Select all that apply.**
A. Smokes a pack of cigarettes
B. Uses Fleet enemas frequently to assist with bowel movements
C. Practices intentional relaxation
D. Eats multiple servings of fruits
E. Takes 325 mg of aspirin at night for arthritic pain
F. Exercises for 30 minutes three times weekly
G. Travels extensively across the world

Finally, investigate the patient's travel history. Ask whether he or she has traveled outside of the country recently or has been camping near lakes and streams in his or her country of residence. This information may provide clues about the cause of symptoms such as diarrhea.

BEST PRACTICE FOR PATIENT SAFETY & QUALITY CARE (QSEN)

Questions for Gastrointestinal Health History

- What is your typical daily food intake?
- What medications are you taking? (Obtain name, dose, and frequency)
- Do you take any vitamins, minerals, or herbal supplements? If so, what are they?
- How is your appetite? Has there been a recent change?
- Have you lost or gained weight recently? If so, was the weight loss or gain intentional?
- Are you on a special diet? If so, what kind, and for what purpose?
- Do you have difficulty chewing or swallowing?
- Do you wear dentures? If so, how well do they fit?
- Do you experience indigestion or "heartburn"? If so, how often? What seems to cause it? What helps it?
- Have you had GI disorders or surgeries in the past? If so, what are they and when did they occur?
- Is there a family history of GI health problems?
- Do you smoke (or vape), or have you ever smoked (vaped) in the past?
- Do you chew or have you ever chewed tobacco?
- Do you drink alcoholic beverages? If so, what kind, how much, and how many each week?
- Do you have pain, diarrhea, constipation, or gas? Do any specific foods accompany the problem?
- Have you traveled out of the country recently? If so, where and when?
- What is your usual bowel *elimination* pattern? Frequency? Character?
- Do you use laxatives to produce a bowel movement? If so, how frequently?
- Do you have any pain or bleeding associated with bowel movements?
- Have you experienced changes in your usual bowel pattern or stool?
- Have you ever had an endoscopy or a colonoscopy? If so, which one, and when?

Nutrition History. A *nutrition* history is important when assessing GI system function. Many conditions arise as a result of alterations in intake and absorption of nutrients. The purpose of a nutrition assessment is to gather information about how well the patient's needs are being met. Inquire about any special diet and whether there are any known food allergies. Ask the patient to describe the usual foods that are eaten daily and the times that meals are taken.

> ### 👤 PATIENT-CENTERED CARE: CULTURAL/SPIRITUAL CONSIDERATIONS (QSEN)
>
> Cultural and spiritual patterns are important in obtaining a complete *nutrition* history. Ask if certain foods pose a problem for the patient. For example, spices or hot pepper used in cooking can aggravate or precipitate GI tract symptoms such as indigestion. Note spiritual observations such as fasting or abstinence.
>
> Many non-white Americans and those of Asian and South American heritage are lactose intolerant as a result of having insufficient amounts of the enzyme *lactase* or producing a less active form of the enzyme (Bass, 2017). A much smaller percentage of Caucasian people also have this problem. Lactase is needed to convert lactose in milk and other dairy products to glucose and galactose. Lactose intolerance causes bloating, cramping, and diarrhea as a result of lack of lactase.

Health problems can also affect *nutrition*; therefore explore changes that have occurred in eating habits as a result of illness. Assess for *anorexia* (loss of appetite for food), changes in taste, and any difficulty or *pain* with swallowing (dysphagia) that could be associated with esophageal disorders. Also ask if abdominal *pain* or discomfort occurs with eating and whether the patient has experienced nausea, vomiting, or dyspepsia (an epigastric burning sensation, often referred to as "heartburn"). Unknown food allergies may be a cause of these symptoms. Inquire about unintentional weight loss because some GI cancers may present in this manner. Assess for alcohol and caffeine consumption because both substances are associated with many GI disorders, such as gastritis and peptic ulcer disease.

The patient's socioeconomic status may have a profound impact on *nutrition.* People who have limited budgets, such as some older adults or the unemployed, may not be able to purchase foods required for a balanced diet. They may substitute less expensive and less effective OTC medications or herbs for prescription drugs. People who live in "food deserts" (i.e., places with little access to fresh fruits and vegetables [U.S. Department of Agriculture, 2019] and other healthy foods) may also be affected by lack of *nutrition.* Necessary medical care may be delayed, and patients may not seek health care until conditions are well advanced.

Family History and Genetic Risk. Ask about a family history of GI disorders. Some GI health problems have a genetic predisposition. For example, familial adenomatous polyposis (FAP) is an inherited autosomal dominant disorder that predisposes the patient to colon cancer (Simonson, 2018). Pertinent genetic risks are discussed with the GI problems in later chapters.

Current Health Problems. Because GI signs and symptoms are often vague and difficult for the patient to describe, it is important to obtain a chronologic account of the current problem, symptoms, and any treatments taken. If a patient has kept a diary of dates, symptoms, and treatments used, this can be helpful to establish patterns. Ask about the location, quality, quantity, and timing of each symptom (onset, duration), and factors that may aggravate or alleviate it (see the Best Practice for Patient Safety and Quality Care: Questions for Gastrointestinal Health History box).

Changes in bowel habits are common assessment findings. Obtain this information from the patient:
- Pattern of bowel movements
- Color and consistency of the feces
- Occurrence of diarrhea or constipation
- Effective action taken to relieve diarrhea or constipation
- Presence of frank blood or tarry stools
- Presence of abdominal distention or gas
- Weight gain or loss that has been unintentional

Assess the patient's:
- Normal weight
- Weight gain or loss
- Period of time for weight change
- Changes in appetite or oral intake

Pain is a common concern of patients with GI tract disorders. Abdominal pain is often vague and difficult to evaluate. The mnemonic **PQRST** may be helpful in conducting a pain assessment (Jarvis, 2020):

P: Provocation or palliation
- What were you doing when the pain started?
- What caused it?
- What makes it better or worse?
- What seems to trigger it (e.g., stress, position, certain activities)?

Q: Quality or quantity
- Describe the feeling (e.g., sharp, dull, stabbing, burning, crushing, throbbing, nauseating, shooting, twisting, or stretching).

R: Region or radiation
- Where is the pain located?
- Does it radiate? (Where?)
- Does it feel as if it travels or moves around?
- Did it start elsewhere and is now localized to one spot?

S: Severity scale
- How severe is the pain on a scale of 0 to 10, with 0 being no pain and 10 being the worst pain ever?
- Does it interfere with activities?
- How bad is it at its worst?
- Does it force you to sit down, lie down, slow down?
- How long does an episode last?

T: Timing
- When or at what time did the pain start?
- How long did it last?
- How often does it occur (e.g., hourly, daily, weekly, monthly)?
- Is it sudden or gradual?

- What were you doing when you first experienced it?
- When do you usually experience it (e.g., daytime, night, early morning)?
- Are you ever awakened by it?
- Does it lead to anything else?
- Is it accompanied by other signs and symptoms?
- Does it ever occur before, during, or after meals?
- Does it occur seasonally?

Skin changes may result from GI tract disorders such as liver and biliary system *obstruction*. Ask whether these clinical signs and symptoms have occurred in the past or are currently present:

- Skin discolorations or rashes
- Itching
- *Jaundice* (yellowing of skin caused by bilirubin pigments)
- Increased bruising or tendency to bleed

Physical Assessment

Physical assessment involves a comprehensive examination of the patient's **nutrition** status, mouth, and abdomen. Nutrition assessment is discussed in detail in Chapter 55. Oral assessment is described in Chapter 49.

In preparation for assessment of the abdomen, ask the patient to empty his or her bladder and then to lie in a supine position with knees bent, keeping the arms at the sides to prevent tensing of the abdominal muscles.

The abdomen is assessed by using the four techniques of examination in a specific order. Nurse generalists perform inspection, auscultation, and light palpation. Health care providers perform inspection, auscultation, percussion, and deep palpation. These sequences are preferred so percussion and palpation do not increase intestinal activity and bowel sounds. If appendicitis or an abdominal aneurysm is suspected, palpation is not done.

Inspection. The abdominal examination usually begins with inspection of the patient's right side and proceeds in a systematic fashion (Fig. 48.3):

- Right upper quadrant (RUQ)
- Left upper quadrant (LUQ)
- Left lower quadrant (LLQ)
- Right lower quadrant (RLQ)

Table 48.1 lists the organs that lie in each of these areas.

If areas of *pain* or discomfort are noted from the history, they are cautiously assessed last in the examination sequence. This sequence should prevent the patient from tensing abdominal muscles because of the pain, which can make the examination difficult.

Inspect the skin and note any of these findings:

- Overall asymmetry of the abdomen
- Discoloration or scarring
- Abdominal distention
- Bulging flanks
- Taut, glistening skin
- Skin folds
- Subcutaneous fat noted
- Location, size, and description of any pressure injuries

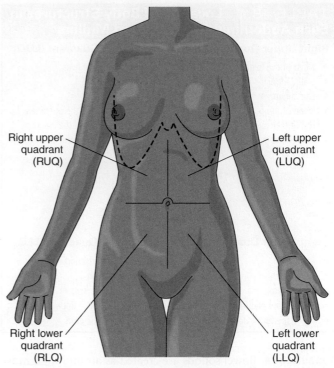

Right upper quadrant (RUQ)
Left upper quadrant (LUQ)
Right lower quadrant (RLQ)
Left lower quadrant (LLQ)

FIG. 48.3 Topographic division of the abdomen into quadrants.

Observe the contour and symmetry of the abdomen, which can be rounded, flat, concave, or distended. It is best determined when standing at the side of the bed or treatment table and looking down on the abdomen. View the abdomen at eye level from the side. Asymmetry of the abdomen can indicate problems affecting the underlying body structures (see Table 48.1). Note the shape and position of the umbilicus for any deviations.

> **! NURSING SAFETY PRIORITY** (QSEN)
> **Action Alert**
>
> Peristaltic movements are rarely seen unless the patient is thin and has increased peristalsis. If these movements are observed, note the quadrant of origin and the direction of peristaltic flow. Report this finding to the health care provider because it may indicate an intestinal obstruction.

Finally, observe abdominal movements, including the normal rising and falling with inspiration and expiration, and note any distress during movement. Occasionally pulsations may be visible, particularly in the area of the abdominal aorta.

> **! NURSING SAFETY PRIORITY** (QSEN)
> **Action Alert**
>
> If a bulging, pulsating mass is present during assessment of the abdomen, **do not touch** the area because the patient may have an abdominal aortic aneurysm, a life-threatening problem. Notify the health care provider of this finding immediately!

TABLE 48.1 Location of Body Structures in Each Abdominal Quadrant and Midline

Right Upper Quadrant (RUQ)	Left Upper Quadrant (LUQ)
• Most of the liver	• Left lobe of the liver
• Gallbladder	• Stomach
• Duodenum	• Spleen
• Head of the pancreas	• Body and tail of the pancreas
• Hepatic flexure of the colon	• Splenic flexure of the colon
• Part of the ascending and transverse colon	• Part of the transverse and descending colon

Midline

- Abdominal aorta
- Uterus (if enlarged)
- Bladder (if distended)

Right Lower Quadrant (RLQ)	Left Lower Quadrant (LLQ)
• Cecum	• Part of the descending colon
• Appendix	• Sigmoid colon
• Right ureter	• Left ureter
• Right ovary and fallopian tube	• Left ovary and fallopian tube
• Right spermatic cord	• Left spermatic cord

Auscultation. Bowel sounds are created as air and fluid move through the GI tract. They are normally heard as relatively high-pitched, irregular gurgles with a normal frequency range of 5 to 30 per minute (Jarvis, 2020). They are characterized as normal, hypoactive, or hyperactive. They are diminished or absent after abdominal surgery or in the patient with peritonitis or paralytic ileus. The most reliable method for assessing the return of peristalsis after abdominal surgery is to ask the patient if he or she has passed flatus within the past 8 hours or had a stool within the past 12 to 24 hours.

Increased high-pitched bowel sounds, especially loud, gurgling sounds, result from increased motility of the bowel (**borborygmus**). These sounds are usually heard in the patient with diarrhea or gastroenteritis or are heard above a complete intestinal obstruction.

Auscultation of the abdomen is performed with the diaphragm of the stethoscope because bowel sounds are usually high pitched. Place the stethoscope lightly on the abdominal wall, beginning in the RLQ in the area of the ileocecal valve, where bowel sounds are normally present (Jarvis, 2020). Proceed with listening to other quadrants.

During auscultation, also listen for vascular sounds or **bruits** ("swooshing" sounds) over the abdominal aorta, the renal arteries, and the iliac arteries. A bruit heard over the aorta usually indicates the presence of an aneurysm. *If this sound is heard, do not percuss or palpate the abdomen. Notify the health care provider immediately of your findings!*

Percussion. Percussion may be done by the **health care provider** to determine the size of solid organs; to detect the presence of masses, fluid, and air; and to estimate the size of the liver and spleen. The percussion notes heard in the abdomen are termed *tympanic* (the high-pitched, loud, musical sound of an air-filled intestine) or *dull* (the medium-pitched, softer, thudlike sound over a solid organ, such as the liver).

The liver and spleen can be percussed. An enlarged liver is called *hepatomegaly*. Dullness heard in the left anterior axillary line indicates enlargement of the spleen (*splenomegaly*). Mild-to-moderate splenomegaly can be detected by percussion before the spleen becomes palpable.

Palpation. The purpose of palpation is to determine the size and location of abdominal organs and to assess for the presence of masses or tenderness. Palpation of the abdomen consists of two types: light and deep. Nurse generalists perform light palpation. The technique of *light palpation* is used to detect large masses and areas of tenderness. Place the first four fingers of the palpating hand close together and then place them lightly on the abdomen and proceed smoothly and systematically from quadrant to quadrant. Depress the abdomen to a depth of ½ to 1 inch (1.25 to 2.5 cm). Proceed with a rotational movement of the palpating hand. Note any areas of tenderness or guarding because these areas will be examined last and cautiously during deep palpation. While performing light palpation, note signs of rigidity, which, unlike voluntary guarding, is a sign of peritoneal inflammation. Only health care providers, such as physicians, physician assistants, and advance practice nurses, should perform deep palpation. Deep palpation is used to further determine the size and shape of abdominal organs and masses.

NCLEX EXAMINATION CHALLENGE 48.2
Physiological Integrity

While performing an abdominal assessment on a client, the nurse notes a bruit over the aorta. What is the appropriate nursing action?

A. Consult another nurse to verify the bruit.
B. Auscultate each quadrant for 5 minutes each.
C. Notify the health care provider of the findings.
D. Perform light palpation to further assess the pulsation.

Psychosocial Assessment

Psychosocial assessment focuses on how the GI health problem affects the patient's life and lifestyle. Remember that patients are often reluctant to discuss **elimination** problems, which may be very personal and embarrassing. The interview focus is on whether usual daily activities and/or employment have been interrupted or disturbed. Ask about recent stressful events, as stress has been associated with the development or exacerbation (flare-up) of irritable bowel syndrome (IBS) and other GI disorders. If the patient is diagnosed with cancer, he or she is likely to experience the stages of the grieving process. Patients may be depressed, angry, or in denial.

Diagnostic Assessment

Laboratory Assessment. To make an accurate assessment of the many possible causes of GI system abnormalities, laboratory testing of blood, urine, and stool specimens may be performed.

Serum Tests. A *complete blood count (CBC)* aids in the diagnosis of anemia and infection. It also detects changes in the blood's formed elements. In adults, GI bleeding is the most frequent cause of anemia. It is associated with GI cancer, peptic ulcer disease, diverticulitis, and inflammatory bowel disease.

Prothrombin time (PT) is useful in evaluating levels of clotting factors. PT measures the rate at which prothrombin is converted to thrombin, a process that depends on vitamin K–associated clotting factors. Hepatocellular liver disease leads to a prolonged PT secondary to impaired synthesis of clotting proteins (Pagana & Pagana, 2018).

Many *electrolytes* are altered in GI tract dysfunction. For example, calcium is absorbed in the GI tract and may be measured to detect malabsorption. Excessive vomiting or diarrhea causes sodium or potassium depletion, thus requiring replacement.

Assays of serum enzymes are important in the evaluation of liver damage. *Aspartate aminotransferase (AST)* and *alanine aminotransferase (ALT)* are two enzymes found in the liver and other organs. These enzymes are elevated in most liver disorders, but they are highest in conditions that cause necrosis, such as hepatitis and cirrhosis.

Elevations in serum amylase and lipase may indicate acute pancreatitis, a serious inflammation of the pancreas characterized by a sudden onset of abdominal pain, nausea, and vomiting. In this disease, serum amylase levels begin to elevate within 24 hours of onset and remain elevated for up to 5 days. Serum amylase and lipase are not elevated when extensive pancreatic necrosis is present because there are few pancreatic cells manufacturing the enzymes.

Bilirubin is the primary pigment in bile, which is normally conjugated and excreted by the liver and biliary system. It is measured as total serum bilirubin, conjugated (direct) bilirubin, and unconjugated (indirect) bilirubin. These measurements are important in the evaluation of jaundice and liver and biliary tract functioning. Elevations in direct and indirect bilirubin levels and/or gamma-glutamyl transferase (GGT) can indicate impaired excretion.

The serum level of *ammonia* may also be measured to evaluate hepatic function. Ammonia is normally used to rebuild amino acids or is converted to urea for excretion. Elevated levels are seen in conditions that cause hepatocellular injury, such as pancreatitis, cholecystitis, and gastrointestinal disease (Pagana & Pagana, 2018).

Two primary *oncofetal antigens—CA19-9* and *CEA—*are evaluated to monitor the efficacy of cancer therapy and assess for the recurrence of cancer in the GI tract. These antigens may also be increased in benign GI conditions. The Laboratory Profile: Gastrointestinal Assessment box lists blood tests commonly used by the health care provider in the diagnosis of GI disorders. Additional serum tests are described in other GI chapters within this text.

Urine Tests. Amylase can be detected in the urine. In acute pancreatitis, renal clearance of amylase is increased. Amylase levels in the urine remain elevated 5 to 7 days after onset of disease processes, even after serum levels return to normal within 1 to 2 days (Pagana & Pagana, 2018). This becomes an important finding in patients who are symptomatic for several days or longer.

Urine *urobilinogen* is a form of bilirubin that is converted by the intestinal flora and excreted in the urine. Its measurement is useful in the evaluation of hepatic and biliary obstruction, because the presence of bilirubin in the urine often occurs before jaundice is seen.

Stool Tests. The American Cancer Society (ACS) recommends regular screening to detect colorectal cancer early when it can most effectively be treated (ACS, 2018). Options include an annual high-sensitivity fecal immunochemical test (FIT), an annual guaiac-based fecal occult blood test (gFOBT) (such as the Hemoccult II Sensa), or a FIT-DNA test performed every 3 years. These tests use a take-home, multisample method rather than having the test done during a digital rectal examination. These tests use a take-home, multisample method rather than having the test done during a digital rectal examination.

The traditionally used gFOBT (e.g., Hemoccult II Sensa) requires an active component of guaiac and is therefore more likely than the FIT (e.g., HemeSelect) to yield false-positive results. In addition, patients having the guaiac-based test must avoid NSAIDs for 7 days prior to and during the collection period, as well as red meat, citrus fruits and juices, and vitamin C in excess of 250 mg/day for 3 days prior to and during the test period (CliaWaived, 2019). Patient adherence is likely to be higher with the FIT method because drugs and food do not interfere with the test results.

As an alternate to the gFOBT or FIT, a stool DNA test (sDNA) can be completed every 3 years (American Cancer Society [ACS], 2018). Available only by prescription, this type of at-home diagnostic kit (such as Cologuard) is shipped directly to the patient after the health care provider has ordered the testing. Although less specific in detection than a colonoscopy, this type of testing can be encouraging to patients who may be fearful of undergoing a traditional colonoscopy or have concerns about financial coverage.

The cost for Cologuard testing is covered by Medicare and Medicare Advantage, with no additional cost to the patient (Exact Sciences Corporation, 2020). It also should be covered, based on the Affordable Care Act, by most private insurances; Cologuard reports that 94% of users have no out-of-pocket expenditures for this type of screening (Exact Sciences Corporation, 2020).

Once received in the mail, the test is easy to complete. The patient does not have to undergo any special preparation, such as the bowel cleansing that is required prior to a traditional colonoscopy. The patient collects one stool sample and returns it via a prepaid postage container. Although false-negative or false-positive results are possible, Cologuard reports identifying 92% of colon cancers and 42% of high-risk precancers per 10,000 samples (Imperiale et al., 2014).

Teach patients to talk openly with their health care provider to determine if a home screening test is appropriate. People who have a personal or family history of colon cancer, who have a condition that places them at risk (such as inflammatory bowel disease or Crohn's disease), or who have had previous positive results from another type of colon cancer screening test should be taught that a traditional colonoscopy is preferred over a home test. Emphasize the need to promptly follow up with the health care provider after the test to discuss results and possible subsequent actions that need to be taken.

LABORATORY PROFILE

Gastrointestinal Assessment

Test (Serum)	Normal Range for Adults	Significance of Abnormal Findings
Alanine aminotransferase (ALT)	4-36 units/L (may be slightly higher in older adults) Canadian: 5-35 mU/mL	*Increased* values indicate possible: • Liver disease • Hepatitis • Cirrhosis
Albumin	3.5-5.0 g/dL Canadian: 3.5-5.5 g/L	*Decreased* values indicate possible: • Hepatic disease • Undernutrition
Alkaline phosphatase	30-120 units/L (may be slightly higher in older adults) Canadian: 40-160 units/L	*Increased* values indicate possible: • Cirrhosis • Biliary obstruction • Liver tumor
Ammonia	10-80 mg/dL Canadian: 6-47 mcmol/L (10-80 mcg/dL)	*Increased* values indicate possible: • Hepatic disease such as cirrhosis
Aspartate aminotransferase (AST)	0-35 units/L (may be slightly higher in older adults; women may have slightly lower levels than men) Canadian: 7-40 units/L (may be slightly higher in older adults; women may have slightly lower levels than men)	*Increased* values indicate possible: • Liver disease • Hepatitis • Cirrhosis
Bilirubin (total)	0.3-1.0 mg/dL Canadian: 3-22 mcmol/L (0.2-1.3 mg/dL)	*Increased* values indicate possible: • Hemolysis • Biliary obstruction • Hepatic damage
Calcium (total)	9.0-10.5 mg/dL (values decrease in older adults) Canadian: 8.4-10.6 mg/dL	*Decreased* values indicate possible: • Malabsorption • Kidney failure • Acute pancreatitis
Cancer antigen 19-9 (CA19-9)	<37 units/mL Canadian: <37 kU/L	*Increased* values indicate possible: • Cancer of the pancreas, stomach, colon, gallbladder • Acute pancreatitis • Inflammatory bowel disease
Carcinoembryonic antigen (CEA)	<5 ng/mL Canadian: <5 mcg/L (<5 ng/mL)	*Increased* values indicate possible: • Colorectal, stomach, pancreatic cancer • Ulcerative colitis • Crohn's disease • Hepatitis • Cirrhosis
Cholesterol	<200 mg/dL Canadian: Same	*Increased* values indicate possible: • Pancreatitis • Biliary obstruction *Decreased* values indicate possible: • Liver cell damage
Conjugated (direct) bilirubin	0.1-0.3 mg/dL Canadian: 1.7-5.1 mcmol/L (0.1-0.3 mg/dL)	*Increased* values indicate possible: • Biliary obstruction
Potassium	3.5-5.0 mEq/L or 3.5-5.0 mmol/L Canadian: 3.5-5.1 mmol/L	*Decreased* values indicate possible: • Vomiting • Gastric suctioning • Diarrhea • Drainage from intestinal fistulas
Serum amylase	30-220 units/L Canadian: 25-125 units/L	*Increased* values indicate possible: • Acute pancreatitis
Serum lipase	0-160 units/L Canadian: Same	*Increased* values indicate possible: • Acute pancreatitis
Unconjugated (indirect) bilirubin	0.2-0.8 mg/dL Canadian: 3.4-12.0 mcmol/L (0.2-0.8 mg/dL)	*Increased* values indicate possible: • Hemolysis • Hepatic damage

LABORATORY PROFILE—cont'd

Gastrointestinal Assessment

Test (Serum)	Normal Range for Adults	Significance of Abnormal Findings
Xylose absorption	20-57 mg/dL (60-min plasma) 30-58 mg/dL (120-min plasma) Canadian: >1.3 mmol/L (>20 mg/dL) (60-min plasma) >1.6 mmol/L (>25 mg/dL) (120-min plasma)	*Decreased* values in blood and urine indicate possible: • Malabsorption in the small intestine

Data from Pagana, K., & Pagana, T. (2018). *Mosby's manual of diagnostic and laboratory tests* (6th ed.). St. Louis: Mosby; and Pagana, K., Pagana, T., & Pike-MacDonald, S. (2019). *Mosby's Canadian manual of diagnostic and laboratory tests* (2nd ed.). St. Louis: Mosby.

Stool samples may also be collected to test for *ova and parasites* to aid in the diagnosis of parasitic infection. They may also be tested for *fecal fats* when steatorrhea (fatty stools) or malabsorption is suspected. Fat is normally absorbed in the small intestine in the presence of biliary and pancreatic secretions; in malabsorption, fat is abnormally excreted in the stool. Stool samples can also be tested to detect the presence of infectious agents, such as *Clostridium difficile*, a common cause of diarrhea in older adults and patients on prolonged antibiotic therapy.

Imaging Assessment. Radiographic examinations and similar diagnostic procedures are useful in detecting structural and functional disorders of the GI system. Provide information about preparation for the examination, provide an explanation of the procedure, and teach the required postprocedure care.

A *plain film of the abdomen* may be the first x-ray study that the health care provider requests when diagnosing a GI problem. This film can reveal masses, tumors, and strictures or obstructions. Patterns of bowel gas appear light on the abdominal film and can be useful in detecting an obstruction (ileus). No preparation is required except to wear a hospital gown and remove any jewelry or belts, which may interfere with the film.

When abdominal *pain* is severe or bowel perforation is suspected, an *acute abdomen series* may be requested. This procedure consists of a chest x-ray, a supine abdomen film, and an upright abdomen film. The chest x-ray may reveal a hiatal hernia, and an upright abdomen film may show air in the peritoneum from a bowel perforation. Although x-rays are helpful, CT, MRI, and ultrasound scans are used more often (Gangadhar et al., 2016).

The 2019 American Cancer Society screening guidelines include the following tests as options to determine the presence of colorectal cancer and polyps in adults older than 45 years (ACS, 2019):

• Flexible sigmoidoscopy every 5 years, *or*
• CT colonography (virtual colonoscopy) every 5 years, *or*
• Colonoscopy every 10 years

CT, also referred to as a *CT scan,* provides a noninvasive cross-sectional x-ray view that can detect tissue densities and abnormalities in the abdomen, including the liver, pancreas, spleen, and biliary tract. It may be performed with or without contrast medium. If contrast medium is to be used, ask about allergies to seafood and iodine. The patient is to remain NPO, which means "nothing by mouth," for at least 4 hours before the test if a contrast medium is to be used. IV access is required for injection of the contrast medium. Advise the patient that on injection he or she may feel warm and flushed or experience a metallic taste. The patient who has claustrophobia may require a mild sedative to tolerate the study. The radiologic technician instructs the patient to lie still and to hold his or her breath when asked, as a series of images are taken. The test takes about 10 minutes.

Like other parts of the body, the abdomen and its organs may also be evaluated by *MRI,* such as *magnetic resonance cholangiopancreatography (MRCP).* Because of the use of powerful magnets, a special questionnaire is used and special precautions are taken to ensure that the patient meets requirements for this type of testing. Although this type of imaging takes longer than a CT scan, it does not expose patients to radiation.

NCLEX EXAMINATION CHALLENGE 48.3

Health Promotion and Maintenance

Which teaching will the nurse provide to a community group about early detection of colorectal cancer? **Select all that apply.**

A. Home testing kits are available with a prescription.
B. Sigmoidoscopy should be performed every 10 years.
C. People over 40 years old should be tested for colon cancer.
D. Bowel preparation is necessary prior to performance of a colonoscopy.
E. Virtual colonoscopies (CT colonography) can be performed every 5 years.

Other Diagnostic Assessment

Endoscopy. Endoscopy is direct visualization of the GI tract using a flexible fiberoptic endoscope, a tube that allows viewing and manipulation of internal body areas. It is commonly prescribed to evaluate bleeding, ulceration, inflammation, tumors, and cancer of the esophagus, stomach, biliary system, or bowel. Specimens for biopsy and cell studies (e.g., *Helicobacter pylori*) can be obtained through the endoscope. There are several types of endoscopic examinations, and the patient must sign an informed consent form before having any of these invasive studies performed.

Esophagogastroduodenoscopy. Esophagogastroduodenoscopy (EGD) is a visual examination of the esophagus, stomach, and duodenum by means of a fiberoptic endoscope. If GI bleeding is found during an EGD, the health care provider can use clips, thermocoagulation, injection therapy, or a topical hemostatic agent (National Institute of Diabetes and Digestive and Kidney Diseases [NIDDK], 2017). If the patient has an **esophageal stricture**, a narrowing of the esophageal opening, it can be dilated during EGD. Gastric lesions can be visualized using this procedure, and suspicion for celiac disease can be affirmed.

Usually patients are asked to avoid anticoagulants, aspirin, or other NSAIDs for several days before EGD unless it is absolutely necessary. The patient can take regularly prescribed medications the morning of the test unless otherwise instructed by the health care provider. Patients with diabetes should consult their primary health care provider for special instructions. Teach the patient to remain NPO for 6 to 8 hours before the procedure. If the patient has dentures, they are removed. Tell the patient that a flexible tube will be passed down the esophagus while he or she is under moderate sedation. Midazolam, fentanyl, or propofol is commonly used for sedation (Cohen, 2020). *These drugs can depress the rate and depth of the patient's respirations.* Atropine may be administered to dry secretions. A local anesthetic is sprayed to inactivate the gag reflex and facilitate passage of the tube. Explain that this anesthetic will depress the gag reflex and that swallowing will be difficult.

After the drugs are given, the patient is placed in a position with the head of the bed elevated. A bite block is inserted to prevent biting down on the endoscope and to protect the teeth. The health care provider passes the tube through the mouth and into the esophagus (Fig. 48.4). The procedure takes about 20 to 30 minutes.

During the test, the endoscopy nurse monitors the patient's respirations for rate and depth. Oxygenation saturation level is measured via pulse oximetry and ventilation is measured via capnography, capnometry, or mass spectroscopy (American Society of Anesthesiologists, 2015). Shallow respirations decrease the amount of carbon dioxide that the patient exhales. *If the patient's respiratory rate is below 10 breaths/min or the exhaled carbon dioxide level falls below 20%, the nurse typically uses a stimulus such as a sternal rub to encourage deeper and faster respirations.*

After the test, check vital signs frequently (usually every 15 to 30 minutes) until the sedation begins to wear off. The side rails of the bed are raised during this time. Keep the patient NPO until the gag reflex returns (usually in 30 to 60 minutes). IV fluids that were started before the procedure can be discontinued when the patient is able to tolerate oral fluids without nausea or vomiting.

> ### ! NURSING SAFETY PRIORITY (QSEN)
> **Action Alert**
>
> The priority for care to promote patient safety after esophagogastroduodenoscopy is to prevent aspiration. Do not offer fluids or food by mouth until you are sure that the gag reflex is intact! Monitor for signs of perforation, such as **pain,** bleeding, or fever.

Because EGD is most often performed as an ambulatory care (outpatient) procedure requiring moderate sedation, be sure that the patient has someone to drive him or her home. Remind the patient to not drive for at least 12 to 18 hours after the procedure because of sedation. Teach him or her that a hoarse voice or sore throat may persist for several days after the test. Throat lozenges can be used to relieve throat discomfort.

Endoscopic Retrograde Cholangiopancreatography. Endoscopic retrograde cholangiopancreatography (ERCP) includes visual and radiographic examination of the liver, gallbladder, bile ducts, and pancreas to identify the cause and location of obstruction. It is commonly used today for therapeutic purposes rather than for diagnosis. After a cannula is inserted into the common bile duct, a radiopaque dye is instilled, and several x-ray images are obtained. The health care provider may perform a *papillotomy* (a small incision in the sphincter around the ampulla of Vater) to remove gallstones. If a biliary duct stricture is found, plastic or metal stents may be inserted to keep the ducts open. Biopsy samples of tissue are also frequently taken during this test.

The patient prepares for this test in the same manner as for an EGD. Perform medication reconciliation to determine if the patient is taking anticoagulants, NSAIDs, antiplatelet drugs, or antihyperglycemic agents. The health care provider will determine whether drugs are safe to take and whether any will need to be stopped before the test.

The patient must be NPO for 6 to 8 hours before the test. If the patient has dentures, they are removed. Ask about prior exposure to x-ray contrast media and any sensitivities or allergies. IV access is required to administer drugs that cause moderate sedation. Ask the patient about any implantable medical devices, such as a cardiac pacemaker. Modern pacemakers generally are not affected by electrocautery; however, it is recommended that implantable defibrillators be deactivated, if possible, when electrocautery is used (Association of periOperative Registered Nurses [AORN], 2017).

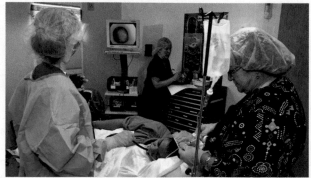

FIG. 48.4 Esophagogastroduodenoscopy allows visualization of the esophagus, the stomach, and the duodenum. If the esophagus is the focus of the examination, the procedure is called *esophagoscopy.* If the stomach is the focus, the procedure is called *gastroscopy.*

The endoscopic procedure and nursing care for a patient having an ERCP are similar to those for the EGD procedure, except that the endoscope is advanced farther into the duodenum and into the biliary tract. Once the cannula is in the common duct, contrast medium is injected, and x-rays are taken to view the biliary tract. A tilt table assists in distributing the contrast medium to all areas to be assessed. The patient is placed in a left lateral position for viewing the common bile duct. Once the cannula is placed, he or she is put in a prone position. After examination of the biliary tree, the cannula is directed into the pancreatic duct for examination. The ERCP lasts from 30 minutes to 2 hours, depending on the treatment that may be done.

After the test, assess vital signs frequently, usually every 15 minutes, until the patient is stable. To prevent aspiration, check to ensure that the gag reflex has returned before offering fluids or food. Discontinue IV fluids that were started before the procedure when the patient is able to tolerate oral fluids without nausea or vomiting.

> ### ! NURSING SAFETY PRIORITY (QSEN)
> #### Action Alert
>
> Teach the patient and family to monitor for severe postprocedure complications at home, including cholecystitis or cholangitis (gallbladder inflammation or infection), bleeding, perforation, sepsis, and pancreatitis (Lee et al., 2018). The patient has severe *pain* if any of these complications occur. Fever is present in sepsis. These problems do not occur immediately after the procedure; they may take several hours to 2 days to develop.

Colicky abdominal *pain* and flatulence can result from air instilled during the procedure. Instruct the patient to report abdominal pain, fever, nausea, or vomiting that fails to resolve after returning home. Be sure that the patient has someone to drive him or her home if the test was done on an ambulatory care basis. Remind the patient to not drive for at least 12 to 18 hours after the procedure because of sedation.

Small Bowel Capsule Endoscopy. Small bowel endoscopy, or enteroscopy, provides a view of the small intestine. Video capsule endoscopy (VCE) is a procedure that uses a small-bowel enteroscopy device to visualize the entire small bowel (Keuchel et al., 2015), including the distal ileum. These devices are used to evaluate and locate the source of GI bleeding. Before the development of the VCE capsule endoscopes, viewing the small intestine was inadequate. The capsule battery lasts around 10 hours, so it is not used to view the colon.

Prepare the patient by explaining the procedure, the purpose, and what to expect during the testing. The patient must not eat or drink, including water, for 12 hours before the test and be NPO for the first 2 hours of the testing. The patient may drink clear liquids after 2 hours and have a light lunch after 4 hours (American Society for Gastrointestinal Endoscopy, 2020).

At the time of the procedure, the patient's abdomen is marked for the location of the sensors, and the sensors are applied. The patient wears an abdominal belt that houses a data recorder to capture the transmitted images. After the capsule is swallowed with a glass of water, the patient may return to normal activity, but should try to avoid vigorous activity and remain calm for the remainder of the study. At the end of the procedure, the patient returns the capsule equipment to the facility for downloading to a central computer. The procedure lasts about 8 hours or until the capsule is passed from the body.

Because the capsule endoscope is a single-use device that moves through the GI tract by peristalsis and is excreted naturally, explain to the patient that the capsule will be seen in the stool and is discarded after *elimination.* No other follow-up is necessary. The patient should report to the health care provider any signs or symptoms of GI obstruction, fever, chest pain, or difficulty breathing or if the capsule is not passed within 2 weeks.

Colonoscopy. Colonoscopy is an endoscopic examination of the entire large bowel. Be sure to fully assess all patients who may need a colonoscopy. The American Cancer Society recommends that beginning at age 45 years all healthy men and women should have a colonoscopy every 10 years or choose another equally effective recommended screening option (ACS, 2018). Evidence currently shows that younger adults with obesity are developing colon cancer, possibly due to chronic low-level inflammation that leads to cancer over a period of time (National Cancer Institute, 2017). Those at high risk for cancer (e.g., family history) or those who had polyps removed should have the test more often.

The health care provider can obtain tissue biopsy specimens or remove polyps through the colonoscope during this procedure. A colonoscopy can also evaluate the cause of chronic diarrhea or locate the source of GI bleeding. Topical hemostatic agents or other methods may be used to manage the bleeding.

Patient Preparation. Patients who have their first colonoscopy are often very anxious. Provide information about the procedure, level of sedation, and possibility of *pain* (Kartin et al., 2017). Reassure them that pain will be controlled with medication as needed.

Remind patients to avoid aspirin, anticoagulants, and antiplatelet drugs for several days before the procedure. Patients with diabetes should check with their primary health care provider about drug therapy requirements on the day of the test because they are NPO.

The health care provider will prescribe the specific method of preparation of the bowel, which begins the night before the procedure. Drinkable solutions can be chilled to improve taste. Teach the patient to partake of a clear liquid diet the day before the scheduled colonoscopy. Gatorade or other sports drinks will be recommended by the health care provider to replace electrolytes that are lost during bowel preparation. Instruct him or her to avoid red, orange, or purple (grape) beverages or gelatin. The patient should be NPO for several hours before the procedure, based on the health care provider's instructions.

Watery diarrhea usually begins in about an hour after starting the bowel preparation process. In some cases, the patient may also require laxatives, suppositories (e.g., bisacodyl), or one or more small-volume cleansing enemas (e.g., Fleet).

The failure to achieve adequate bowel preparation prior to this procedure can lead to decreased visualization of adenoma or unsuccessful colonoscopy. Patient education and type of bowel preparation solution are critical to a successful procedure (Writers, 2018).

Procedure. IV access is necessary for the administration of moderate sedation. The health care provider prescribes drugs to aid in relaxation, usually IV midazolam, fentanyl, or propofol (Cohen, 2020). Alternate therapies, such as using music, can improve the person's experience with a colposcopy, although it is not a substitute for sedation or pain medication (Kartin et al., 2017).

Initially the patient is placed on the left side with the knees drawn up while the endoscope is placed into the rectum and moved to the cecum. Air or carbon dioxide may be instilled for better visualization. Research indicates that the use of carbon dioxide is associated with decreased patient *pain* and distention (Lee & Salzman, 2020). The entire procedure lasts about 30 to 60 minutes. Atropine sulfate is kept available in case of bradycardia resulting from vasovagal response.

During the test, monitor the patient's respirations for rate and depth, and the oxygen saturation level via pulse oximetry. Shallow respirations decrease the amount of carbon dioxide that the patient exhales. If the patient's respiratory rate is below 10 breaths/min or the exhaled carbon dioxide level falls below 20%, use a stimulus such as a sternal rub to encourage deeper and faster respirations.

Follow-up Care. Check vital signs every 15 minutes until the patient is stable. Keep the side rails up until the patient is fully alert, and maintain NPO status. Ask the patient to lie on his or her left side to promote comfort and encourage passing flatus. Observe for signs of perforation (severe *pain*) and hemorrhage, such as a rapid drop in blood pressure. Reassure the patient that a feeling of fullness, cramping, and passage of flatus is expected for several hours after the test. Fluids are permitted after the patient passes flatus to indicate that peristalsis has returned. Discontinue IV fluids that were started before the procedure when the patient is able to tolerate oral fluids without nausea or vomiting.

If a polypectomy or tissue biopsy was performed, there may be a small amount of blood in the first stool after the colonoscopy. Complications of colonoscopy are not common. *Report excessive bleeding or severe **pain** to the health care provider immediately* (see the Best Practice for Patient Safety & Quality Care: Care of the Patient After a Colonoscopy box).

As with other endoscopic procedures, the patient will need someone to provide transportation home if the procedure was done in an ambulatory care setting. Remind the patient to avoid driving and making important or legal decisions for the rest of the day after the procedure because of the effects of sedation.

Virtual Colonoscopy. A noninvasive imaging procedure to obtain multidimensional views of the entire colon is the *CT colonography,* known as **virtual colonoscopy** (Fig. 48.5). The bowel preparation and dietary restrictions are similar to those for traditional colonoscopy. However, if a polyp is detected during a virtual colonoscopy or bleeding is found, the patient must have

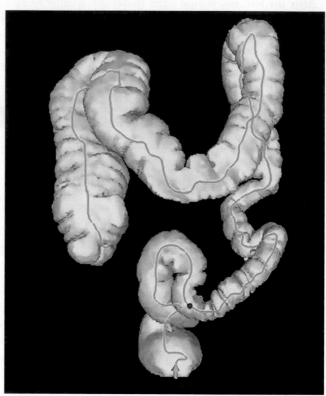

FIG. 48.5 Virtual colonoscopy. (From Pickhardt, P. J., & Kim, D. H. [2007]. CT colonography (virtual colonoscopy): A practical approach for population screening. *Radiologic Clinics of North America, 45*[2], 361-375.)

BEST PRACTICE FOR PATIENT SAFETY & QUALITY CARE (QSEN)

Care of the Patient After a Colonoscopy

- Do not allow the patient to take anything by mouth until sedation wears off
- Take vital signs every 15 to 30 minutes until the patient is alert.
- Keep patient in left lateral position to promote passing of flatus.
- Keep the top side rails up until the patient is alert.
- Assess for rectal bleeding or severe pain.
- Remind the patient that fullness and mild abdominal cramping are expected for several hours.
- Assess for signs and symptoms of bowel perforation, including severe abdominal pain and guarding. Fever may occur later.
- Assess for signs and symptoms of hypovolemic shock, including dizziness, light-headedness, decreased blood pressure, tachycardia, pallor, and altered mental status (this may be the first sign in older adults).
- If the procedure is performed in an ambulatory care setting, arrange for another person to drive the patient home.
- Teach the patient to refrain from driving, making legal decisions, or carrying out other work that requires focus for the rest of the day.

CLINICAL JUDGMENT CHALLENGE 48.1

Safety; Evidence-Based Practice

The nurse is providing preprocedure education to a 55-year-old client who is scheduled for an initial screening colonoscopy in 1 week. The electronic health record indicates a personal history of Crohn's disease and a family history of colon cancer. The client does not wish to go through the preparation process for a traditional colonoscopy, and voices a preference to have a home screening test performed.

1. **Recognize Cues:** What assessment information in this client situation is the most important and immediate concern for the nurse? (Hint: Identify the **relevant** information *first* to determine what is most important.)
2. **Analyze Cues:** What client conditions are consistent with the **most relevant** information? (Hint: Think about priority collaborative problems that support and contradict the information presented in this situation.)

a follow-up invasive colonoscopy for treatment. Therefore the advantage of the traditional colonoscopy is that both diagnostic testing and minor surgical procedures can be done at the same time.

Sigmoidoscopy. Proctosigmoidoscopy, referred to as a sigmoidoscopy, is an endoscopic examination of the rectum and sigmoid colon using a flexible scope. This procedures screens for colon cancer, investigates the source of GI bleeding, and can be used to diagnose or monitor inflammatory bowel disease. If sigmoidoscopy is used as an alternative to colonoscopy for colorectal cancer screening, it is recommended that screening begin at 45 years of age and be done every 5 years thereafter (ACS, 2018). Patients at high risk for cancer may require more frequent screening.

As with similar tests, the health care provider will determine which medicines, such as NSAIDs and anticoagulants, should be discontinued prior to the procedure. Teach the patient to consume a clear liquid diet for a period of time determined by the health care provider before the test. A laxative may be prescribed for the night before the test. A cleansing enema or sodium biphosphate (Fleet) enema is usually required the morning of the procedure.

The patient is placed on the left side in the knee-chest position. Moderate sedation is not required. The endoscope is lubricated and inserted into the anus to the required depth for viewing. Tissue biopsy may be performed during this procedure, but the patient cannot feel it. The examination usually lasts between 5 and 15 minutes.

Inform the patient that mild gas ***pain*** and flatulence may be experienced from air instilled into the rectum during the examination. If a biopsy specimen was obtained, a small amount of bleeding may be observed. Instruct the patient that excessive bleeding should be reported immediately to the health care provider.

Ultrasonography. Ultrasonography is a technique in which high-frequency, inaudible vibratory sound waves are passed through the body via a transducer. The echoes created by the sound waves are then recorded and converted into images for analysis. Ultrasonography is commonly used to view soft tissues, such as the liver, spleen, pancreas, and biliary system.

The advantages of this test are that it is painless, is noninvasive, requires no radiation, and requires no specific preparation.

The patient may be fasting, depending on the abdominal organs to be examined. Inform him or her that it will be necessary to lie still during the study.

The patient is usually placed in a supine position. The technician applies insulating gel to the end of the transducer and on the area of the abdomen under study. This gel allows airtight contact of the transducer with the skin. The technician moves the transducer back and forth over the skin until the desired images are obtained. The study takes about 15 to 30 minutes. No follow-up care is necessary.

Endoscopic Ultrasonography. Endoscopic ultrasonography (EUS) provides images of the GI wall and high-resolution images of the digestive organs. The ultrasonography is performed through the endoscope. This procedure is useful in diagnosing the presence of lymph node tumors; mucosal tumors; and tumors of the pancreas, stomach, and rectum. The patient preparation and follow-up care are similar to those for both endoscopy and ultrasonography.

Liver-Spleen Scan. A liver-spleen scan uses IV injection of a radioactive material that is taken up primarily by the liver and secondarily by the spleen. The scan evaluates the liver and spleen for tumors or abscesses, organ size and location, and blood flow.

Teach the patient about the need to lie still during the scanning. Assure him or her that the injection has only small amounts of radioactivity and is not dangerous. Ask female patients of childbearing age if they may be pregnant or are currently breast-feeding. The radionuclide can be found in breast milk, and radiation from x-rays or scans should be avoided in pregnancy.

The technician or the health care provider gives the radioactive injection through an IV line, and a wait of about 15 minutes is necessary for uptake. The patient is placed in many different positions while the scanning takes place. Tell the patient that the radionuclide is eliminated from the body through the urine in 24 hours. Careful handwashing after toileting decreases the exposure to any radiation present in the urine.

GET READY FOR THE NEXT-GENERATION NCLEX® EXAMINATION!

Key Points
Review these Key Points for each NCLEX Examination Client Needs Category.

Safe and Effective Care Environment
- Remind the patient to have someone available to drive him or her home after an endoscopic procedure because of the effects of moderate sedation. **QSEN: Safety**
- Check for the return of the gag reflex after an upper endoscopic procedure before offering fluids or food; aspiration may occur if the gag reflex is not intact. **QSEN: Safety**

Health Promotion and Maintenance
- Teach patients to carefully follow instructions for bowel preparation before diagnostic testing; the bowel must be clear to visualize the colon. **QSEN: Evidence-Based Practice**

- Instruct the patient to avoid vigorous activity, and follow the health care provider's instructions for eating, following a video capsule endoscopy. **QSEN: Evidence-Based Practice**

Psychosocial Integrity
- Remember that GI health problems markedly affect lifestyle and may cause anger, denial, and depression. **QSEN: Patient-Centered Care**
- Recall that GI testing may cause anxiety, fear, and/or embarrassment. **QSEN: Patient-Centered Care**

Physiological Integrity
- Recognize age-related changes in the GI system. **QSEN: Patient-Centered Care**
- Perform a focused abdominal assessment using inspection, auscultation, and light palpation. **QSEN: Evidence-Based Practice**

- Do not palpate or auscultate any abdominal pulsating mass because it could be a life-threatening aortic aneurysm. **QSEN: Safety**
- Assess and report major complications of GI testing to the health care provider. **QSEN: Safety**
- Review and interpret laboratory results and report abnormal findings to the health care provider. **Clinical Judgment**

- Monitor vital signs, and assess for bleeding, fever, and pain, for the patient having an endoscopic procedure. **QSEN: Safety**
- Do not allow foods or fluids for the patient who has had a colonoscopy until sedation wears off. **QSEN: Safety**

■ MASTERY QUESTIONS

1. Immediately following a colonoscopy, which client behavior will the nurse report to the health care provider? **Select all that apply.**
   A. Passing of flatus
   B. Blood pressure 128/80 mm Hg
   C. Abdominal guarding
   D. Change in mental status
   E. Report of mild abdominal cramping

2. Which teaching will the nurse include when educating a client who is scheduled to have an esophagogastroduodenoscopy (EGD)? **Select all that apply.**
   A. "Anesthesia will be used for sedation."
   B. "The procedure takes about 20 to 30 minutes to complete."
   C. "Informed consent will be needed prior to the procedure."
   D. "A separate test will be required to obtain any needed biopsies."
   E. "You will need to refrain from eating for at least 6 to 8 hours before the EGD."

REFERENCES

American Cancer Society (ACS). (2018). *Colorectal cancer screening test*. www.cancer.org/cancer/colon-rectal-cancer/detection-diagnosis-staging/screening-tests-used.html.

American Cancer Society (ACS). (2019). *American Cancer Society guidelines for the early detection of cancer*. https://www.cancer.org/healthy/find-cancer-early/cancer-screening-guidelines/american-cancer-society-guidelines-for-the-early-detection-of-cancer.html.

American Society of Anesthesiologists (ASA). (2015). *Standards for basic anesthetic monitoring*. www.asahq.org/quality-and-practice-management/standards-guidelines-and-related-resources/standards-for-basic-anesthetic-monitoring.

American Society for Gastrointestinal Endoscopy. (2020). *Understanding capsule endoscopy*. www.asge.org/home/for-patients/patient-information/understanding-capsule-endoscopy.

Association of periOperative Registered Nurses. (2017). Guideline summary: Energy-generating devices, Part 1--electrosurgery. (2017). *AORN Journal, 105*(3), 311–315. https://doi.org/10.1016/j.aorn.2016.12.021.

Bass, P. F., III. (2017). Lactose intolerance diagnosis and diet strategies. *Contemporary Pediatrics, 34*(6), 17–20.

CliaWaived. (2019). *Hemoccult II sensitive (fecal occult blood) tests*. https://www.cliawaived.com/hemoccult-ii-sensa-fecal-occult-blood-tests.html.

Cohen, J. (2020). Gastrointestinal endoscopy in adults: Procedural sedation administered by endoscopists. In Salzman, J., & Joshi, G. (Eds.), *UpToDate*, Waltham, MA.

Collins, J., & Badireddy, M. (2020). *StatPearls:Anatomy, abdomen and Pelvis, small intestine*. Treasure Island, FL: StatPearls Publishing.

Colorectal Cancer Alliance. (2019). Young onset. https://www.ccalliance.org/colorectal-cancer-information/young-onset.

Exact Sciences Corporation. (2020). *The easy Cologuard experience*. https://www.cologuardtest.com/meet-cologuard/easy-cologuard-experience.

Gangadhar, K., Kielar, A., Dighe, M. K., O'malley, R., Wang, C., Gross, J. A., et al, (2016). Multimodality approach for imaging of non-traumatic acute abdominal emergencies. *Abdominal Radiology, 41*(1), 136–148. https://doi.org/10.1007/s00261-015-0586-6.

Girard-Madoux, M., Gomez de Aguero, M., Ganal-Vonarburg, S., Mooser, C., Belz, G., Macpherson, A., et al. (2018). The immunological functions of the Appendix: An example of redundancy? *Seminars in Immunology, 36*, 31–44. https://doi.org/10.1016/j.smim.2018.02.005.

Imperiale, T. F., Ransohoff, D. F., Itzkowitz, S. H., et al. (2014). Multitarget stool DNA testing for colorectal-cancer screening. *New England Journal of Medicine, 370*(14), 1287–1297.

Jarvis, C. (2020). *Physical examination & health assessment* (8th ed.). St. Louis: Saunders.

Kartin, P., Bulut, F., Ceyhan, O., Tasci, S., Gursoy, S., & Isik, N. (2017). The effect of meditation and music listening on the anxiety level, operation tolerance and pain perception in people who were performed colonoscopy. *International Journal of Caring Sciences, 10*(3), 1587–1594.

Keuchel, M., Kurniawan, N., Baltes, P., Bandorski, D., & Koulaouzidis, A. (2015). Quantitative measurements in capsule endoscopy. *Computers in Biology and Medicine, 65*, 333–347.

Lee, H. S., Moon, J. C., Park, J. Y., Bang, S., Seung, W. P., Si, Y. S., et al. (2018). Urgent endoscopic retrograde cholangiopancreatography is not superior to early ERCP in acute biliary pancreatitis with biliary obstruction without cholangitis. *PLoS One, 13*(2). https://doi.org/10.1371/journal.pone.0190835.

Lee, L., & Salzman, J. (2020). Overview of colonoscopy in adults. In Howell, D. (Ed.), *UpToDate*, Waltham, MA.

McCance, K. L., & Huether, S. E. (2019). *Pathophysiology: The biologic basis for disease in adults and children* (8th ed.). St. Louis: Elsevier.

National Cancer Institute at the National Institutes of Health. (2017). *Obesity and cancer*. www.cancer.gov/about-cancer/causes-prevention/risk/obesity/obesity-fact-sheet#q4.

National Institute of Diabetes and Digestive and Kidney Diseases (NIDDK). (2017). *Upper GI endoscopy*. www.niddk.nih.gov/health-information/diagnostic-tests/upper-gi-endoscopy.

Pagana, K., & Pagana, T. (2018). *Mosby's manual of diagnostic and laboratory tests* (6th ed.). St. Louis: Mosby.

Peate, I., & Nair, M. (2016). *Fundamentals of anatomy and physiology: For nursing and healthcare students* (2nd ed.). Hoboken, NJ: John Wiley & Sons.

Simonson, C. (2018). Colorectal cancer—an update for primary care nurse practitioners. *The Journal for Nurse Practitioners, 14*(4), 344–350. https://doi.org/10.1016/j.nurpra.2017.12.030.

Terrery, C. L., & Nicoteri, J. A. L. (2016). The 2015 American Geriatric Society beers criteria: Implications for nurse practitioners. *The Journal for Nurse Practitioners, 12*(3), 192–200. https://doi.org/10.1016/j.nurpra.2015.11.027.

U.S. Department of Agriculture. (2019). *Food access research atlas*. https://www.ers.usda.gov/data-products/food-access-research-atlas/documentation/.

Vemuri, R., Gundamaraju, R., Shastri, M. D., Shukla, S. D., Kalpurath, K., Ball, M., et al. (2018). Gut microbial changes, interactions, and their implications on human lifecycle: An ageing perspective. *BioMed Research International*, 1–13. https://doi.org/10.1155/2018/4178607.

Writers, A. M. (2018). Rates of adequate bowel preparation for colonoscopy may be improved by individualized treatment, education and support. *Drugs & Therapy Perspectives, 34*(1), 29–33. https://doi.org/10.1007/s40267-017-0454-2.

49

Concepts of Care for Patients With Oral Cavity and Esophageal Problems

Keelin C. Cromar, Cherie R. Rebar

http://evolve.elsevier.com/Iggy/

LEARNING OUTCOMES

1. Collaborate with the interprofessional team to coordinate high-quality care for patients with oral cavity or esophageal problems.
2. Describe factors that place a patient at high risk for oral cavity or esophageal problems and refer to the health care provider.
3. Implement patient-centered nursing interventions to decrease the psychosocial impact of living with an oral cavity or esophageal problem.
4. Apply knowledge of anatomy, physiology, and pathophysiology to assess patients with an oral cavity or esophageal problem.
5. Use clinical judgment to analyze assessment findings and diagnostic data in the care of patients with an oral cavity or esophageal problem.
6. Prioritize evidence-based care for patients with an oral cavity or esophageal problem affecting *tissue integrity*, *nutrition*, or *gas exchange* or that induces *pain*.
7. Plan care coordination and transition management for patients with an oral cavity or esophageal problem.

KEY TERMS

aphthous stomatitis Noninfectious stomatitis.

Barrett epithelium Columnar epithelium (instead of the normal squamous cell epithelium) that develops in the lower esophagus during the process of healing from gastroesophageal reflux disease. It is considered premalignant and is associated with an increased risk of cancer in patients with prolonged disease.

candidiasis An infection caused by the fungus *Candida albicans*.

dysphagia Difficulty swallowing.

erythroplakia A velvety red mucosal lesion, most often occurring in the oral cavity.

esophageal stricture Narrowing of the esophageal opening.

esophagogastroduodenoscopy (EGD) The visual examination of the esophagus, stomach, and duodenum by means of a fiberoptic endoscope.

gastroesophageal reflux (GER) Condition that occurs as a result of backward flow of stomach contents into the esophagus.

gastroesophageal reflux disease (GERD) An upper gastrointestinal disease caused by the backward flow (reflux) of gastrointestinal contents into the esophagus.

hiatal hernia A condition, also called a diaphragmatic hernia, that involves the protrusion of the stomach through the esophageal hiatus of the diaphragm into the chest.

leukoplakia White, patchy lesions on a mucous membrane.

minimally invasive esophagectomy (MIE) A laparoscopic surgical procedure to remove part of the esophagus; may be performed in patients with early-stage cancer.

reflux esophagitis Damage to the esophageal mucosa, often with erosion and ulceration, in patients with gastroesophageal reflux disease.

regurgitation Backward flow of stomach contents into the esophagus.

sialadenitis Inflammation of a salivary gland.

stomatitis Inflammation of the oral mucosa; characterized by painful single or multiple ulcerations that impair the protective lining of the mouth. The ulcerations are commonly referred to as "canker sores."

upper endoscopy See *esophagogastroduodenoscopy*.

volvulus Obstruction of the bowel caused by twisting of the bowel.

xerostomia Very dry mouth caused by a severe reduction in saliva flow.

✴ PRIORITY AND INTERRELATED CONCEPTS

The priority concepts for this chapter are:
- *Tissue Integrity*
- *Nutrition*

    The *Tissue Integrity* concept exemplar for this chapter is Stomatitis.

    The *Nutrition* concept exemplar for this chapter is Gastroesophageal Reflux Disease (GERD).

The interrelated concepts for this chapter are:
- *Gas Exchange*
- *Pain*

A HEALTHY ORAL CAVITY

Oral and esophageal problems can compromise *tissue integrity,* impair *nutrition* status and *gas exchange,* and induce *pain.* This chapter discusses the most common oral and esophageal health problems. The nurse plays an important role in maintaining and restoring oral and esophageal health through nursing interventions, including provision of patient and family education to restore optimal *nutrition* comfort.

Inside the mouth, teeth tear, grind, and crush food into small particles to promote swallowing, beginning the process of digestion. Saliva enzymes begin carbohydrate breakdown. The esophagus moves partially digested food from the mouth to the stomach. Oral cavity disorders can severely affect physiologic well-being, speech, body image, and self-esteem. Those at highest risk include people who (Fischer et al., 2017):

- Have developmental delays or mental health disorders
- Have limited access to care due to homelessness or health disparities
- Reside in institutions
- Use tobacco and/or alcohol
- Consume an unhealthy diet
- Have a type of oral cancer
- Consume dietary excess

✴ TISSUE INTEGRITY CONCEPT EXEMPLAR: STOMATITIS

Pathophysiology Review

Stomatitis is a broad term that refers to inflammation within the oral cavity. Painful, inflamed ulcerations (called *aphthous ulcers* or *canker sores*) (Fig. 49.1) that erode *tissue integrity* of the mouth are one of the most common forms of stomatitis. The sores cause *pain* and place the patient at risk for bleeding and infection. Treatment ranges from topical applicants to opioid analgesics and/or antifungal medication, depending on the source and degree of inflammation. Stomatitis is classified according to the cause of the inflammation.

Etiology and Genetic Risk. *Primary stomatitis,* the most common type, includes aphthous stomatitis (noninfectious stomatitis), herpes simplex stomatitis, and traumatic ulcers. *Secondary stomatitis* generally results from infection by opportunistic viruses,

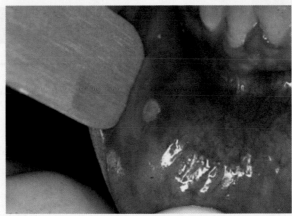

FIG. 49.1 Aphthous ulcer. (From Auerbach, P.S., Cushing, T.A., & Stuart H.N. [2017]. *Auerbach's wilderness medicine* [7th ed.]. Philadelphia: Elsevier.)

fungi, or bacteria in patients who are immunocompromised or as a result of chemotherapy, radiation, or steroid drug therapy.

A common type of secondary stomatitis is caused by *Candida albicans,* which is sometimes present in small amounts in the mouth, especially in older adults. Long-term antibiotic therapy can destroy normal flora, which allows *Candida* to overgrow. The result can be candidiasis, *(moniliasis),* a painful fungal infection.

👤 PATIENT-CENTERED CARE: OLDER ADULT CONSIDERATIONS (QSEN)

Older adults are at high risk for candidiasis because the immune system naturally declines during aging. The risk increases for those with diabetes or malnourishment, or those under great stress. Taking multiple medications can contribute to oral dryness and decreased salivation. Teach proper mouth care to preserve *tissue integrity*, as prevention is much easier than treatment of this painful kind of stomatitis.

Stomatitis can result from infection, allergy, vitamin or mineral deficiency (complex B vitamins, folate, zinc, iron), systemic disease, and irritants such as tobacco and alcohol. Certain foods such as coffee, potatoes, cheese, nuts, citrus fruits, and gluten may trigger allergic responses that cause aphthous ulcers. Evidence suggests that activation of the cell-mediated immune system in some patients may be related to a genetic predisposition (Plewa & Chatterjee, 2020).

Incidence and Prevalence. The most common type of stomatitis, recurrent aphthous stomatitis (RAS), affects approximately 20% of the general population and is more commonly found in females (Plewa & Chatterjee, 2020).

Health Promotion and Maintenance. Proper oral hygiene can decrease the frequency and severity of stomatitis. The Patient and Family Education: Preparing for Self-Management: Maintaining a Healthy Oral Cavity box contains important teaching points to provide to all adults, which will also help them to improve and maintain oral health.

PATIENT AND FAMILY EDUCATION: PREPARING FOR SELF-MANAGEMENT

Maintaining a Healthy Oral Cavity

- Eat a well-balanced diet and stay hydrated by drinking water.
- Manage stress by using healthy coping mechanisms; stress can increase inflammation.
- Perform a weekly self-examination of your mouth; report changes or unusual findings to the primary health care provider or dentist.
- Report occlusion of teeth, mouth *pain*, or swelling to the primary health care provider.
- If you wear dentures, make sure that they are in good repair and fit properly.
- Thoroughly brush and floss your teeth (or brush dentures) consistently twice daily.
- Avoid mouthwashes that contain alcohol, which can damage *tissue integrity.*
- Avoid drugs that increase inflammation of the mouth or reduce saliva flow.
- See your dentist regularly; have dental problems addressed as soon as they are noted.

❖ Interprofessional Collaborative Care

Care for the patient with stomatitis usually takes place in the community setting. The interprofessional team that collaborates to care for this patient includes the primary health care provider and nurse; a dentist and dental hygienist to provide care for the teeth, gums, and oral cavity; and an ear, nose, and throat specialist if needed.

◆ Assessment: Recognize Cues

History. Ask about a history of recent infections, *nutrition* changes, oral hygiene habits, oral trauma, and stress. Also collect a drug history, including over-the-counter (OTC) drugs and nutrition and herbal supplements. Document the course of the current symptoms, and determine if stomatitis has occurred in the past. Ask if the lesions interfere with swallowing, eating, or communicating. Severe stomatitis and edema have the potential to obstruct the airway. In cases of oral candidiasis, white plaquelike lesions appear on the tongue, palate, pharynx (throat), and buccal mucosa (inside the cheeks) (Fig. 49.2). When these patches are wiped away, the underlying surface is red, sore, and painful, and *tissue integrity* is compromised.

Physical Assessment/Signs and Symptoms. Assess for lesions, coating, and cracking. Document characteristics of the lesions, including location, size, shape, odor, color, and drainage. If lesions are seen along the pharynx and the patient reports dysphagia (difficulty with swallowing) or throat *pain*, they might extend down the esophagus. To establish a definitive diagnosis, the primary health care provider may prescribe additional swallowing studies.

Psychosocial Assessment. Severe stomatitis can be very painful, which can cause distress. Assess the patient's ability to cope with pain. Also determine if the presence of stomatitis has an effect on the patient's body image or self-image.

◆ Analysis: Analyze Cues and Prioritize Hypotheses. The priority collaborative problems for the patient with stomatitis include:

1. Impaired *tissue integrity* due to oral and/or esophageal lesions
2. *Pain* due to oral and/or esophageal lesions

❗ NURSING SAFETY PRIORITY (QSEN)

Action Alert

Airway obstruction, aspiration pneumonia, and malnutrition can result from dysphagia. Assess for signs and symptoms such as coughing or choking when swallowing, a sensation of food "sticking" in the pharynx, or difficulty swallowing. If dysphagia is suspected, use the PASS acronym for quick assessment: Is it **P**robable that the patient will have swallowing difficulty? **A**ccount for previous swallowing problems. **S**creen for signs and symptoms. Obtain a **S**peech-language pathologist (SLP) referral (Mountain & Golles, 2017). Report signs and symptoms to the primary health care provider, and institute aspiration prevention interventions.

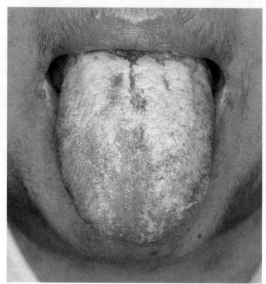

FIG. 49.2 Oral candidiasis. (From Millsop, J.W., & Fazel, N. [2016]. Oral candidiasis. *Clinics in Dermatology, 34*[4], 487–494. https://doi.org/10.1016/j.clindermatol.2016.02.022.)

◆ Planning and Implementation: Generate Solutions and Take Action

Preserving Tissue Integrity

Planning: Expected Outcomes. The patient with stomatitis is expected to regain a healthy oral cavity with intact *tissue integrity.*

Interventions. Interventions for stomatitis are targeted toward health promotion and reduced risk for infection through careful *oral hygiene* and food selection. Delegate oral care to assistive personnel (AP), as this task falls within an AP's skill set, and inspect the patient's oral cavity when the AP is done. Follow the procedures described in the Best Practice for Patient Safety & Quality Care: Care of the Patient With Problems of the Oral Cavity box for best oral care.

Drug therapy used for stomatitis includes solutions to address pain and infection. Commonly used drugs to address infection include (Brice, 2019):

- Clotrimazole troches
- Nystatin suspension (swish and spit)
- Chlorhexidine (swish and spit)

BEST PRACTICE FOR PATIENT SAFETY & QUALITY CARE (QSEN)

Care of the Patient With Problems of the Oral Cavity

- Remove dentures if the patient has severe stomatitis or oral *pain*.
- Encourage the patient who is able to do so to perform oral hygiene twice daily, after meals, and as often as needed. If the patient is unable, provide mouth care.
- Increase oral care frequency to every 2 hours or more if stomatitis is not controlled.
- Teach patient to use a soft toothbrush or gauze, to use toothpaste free of sodium lauryl sulfate (SLS), and to avoid commercial mouthwashes and lemon-glycerin swabs, which can irritate mucosa.
- Encourage frequent rinsing of the mouth with warm saline, sodium bicarbonate (baking soda) solution, or a combination of these solutions.
- Help the patient select soft, bland, and nonacidic foods.
- Apply topical analgesics or anesthetics as prescribed by the primary health care provider and document effectiveness.

Minimizing Pain

Planning: Expected Outcomes. The patient with stomatitis is expected to experience minimized discomfort or absence of *pain*.

Interventions. Dietary changes may help decrease discomfort. Cool or cold liquids can be very soothing, whereas hard, spicy, salty, and acidic foods or fluids can further irritate the ulcers. Include foods high in protein to promote healing. Vitamin C may be recommended as a supplement; eating citrus fruits rich in vitamin C may be painful.

Over-the-counter (OTC) oral anesthetics can be recommended. Prescription drugs used as "swish and spit" agents for pain management include (Brice, 2019):

- Viscous lidocaine
- Diphenhydramine liquid
- Aluminum hydroxide, magnesium hydroxide, and simethicone suspension

! NURSING SAFETY PRIORITY (QSEN)

Drug Alert

Teach patients to use viscous lidocaine with extreme caution. Lidocaine causes a topical anesthetic effect, so patients may not easily feel burns from hot liquids. As sensation in the mouth and throat decreases, the risk for aspiration raises.

NCLEX EXAMINATION CHALLENGE 49.1

Physiological Integrity

A nurse is caring for a client with recurrent aphthous stomatitis (RAS) who asks about food choices while healing. Which food will the nurse suggest?

A. Half of an orange
B. Chocolate pudding
C. Chips with hummus
D. Glass of tomato juice

Care Coordination and Transition Management

Home Care Management. Remind the patient to take all medications as prescribed, especially antibiotics, even if he or she begins to feel better. If the patient has been prescribed medication for *pain*, teach about possible side effects and discourage driving and activities that require concentration. Teach which drugs should be used to swish and swallow, which are to be used only as a rinse, and which are taken orally.

Self-Management Education. Teach about dietary choices that will not irritate the oral cavity and how to gently brush to promote good oral hygiene while preserving *tissue integrity* and minimizing *pain*.

Health Care Resources. Although most cases of stomatitis are self-limiting, some patients may experience persistent pain (e.g., for stomatitis related to ongoing treatment with chemotherapy and/or radiation). These patients may benefit from a support group related to their underlying illness or a group designated for those who are coping with persistent pain.

◆ **Evaluation: Evaluate Outcomes.** Evaluate the care of the patient with stomatitis based on the identified priority patient problems. The expected outcomes include that the patient will:

1. Have healthy oral mucosa without inflammation or infection
2. Experience minimized discomfort or absence of *pain*

ORAL CAVITY DISORDERS

ORAL TUMORS: PREMALIGNANT LESIONS

Tumors of the mouth, whether benign, precancerous, or cancerous, can affect swallowing, chewing, and speaking. *Pain* can also limit daily activities and self-care. Oral tumors affect body image, especially if treatment involves removal of the tongue or part of the mandible (jaw) or requires a tracheostomy.

ERYTHROPLAKIA

Erythroplakia, which is considered precancerous, appears as red, velvety mucosal lesions on the floor of the mouth, tongue, palate, and mandibular mucosa. It can be difficult to distinguish from inflammatory or immune reactions.

LEUKOPLAKIA

Leukoplakia causes thickened, white, firmly attached patches on the oral mucosa that cannot easily be scraped off. These common oral lesions appear slightly raised and sharply rounded. Most of these lesions are benign; however, lesions on the lips or tongue can progress to cancer. Tobacco use increases the chance of development of leukoplakia.

! CORE MEASURES

Always ask patients about current or historical tobacco use. The Joint Commission's Tobacco Treatment Measures (TOB) (2020b) requires offering practical counseling and treatment to people who use tobacco.

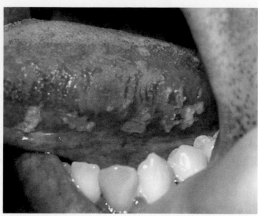

FIG. 49.3 Hairy leukoplakia. (From Sapp, J.P., Eversole, L.R., & Wysocki, G.P. [2004]. *Contemporary oral and maxillofacial pathology* [2nd ed.]. St. Louis: Elsevier.)

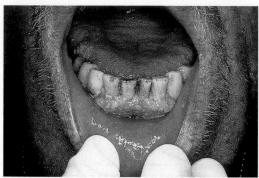

FIG. 49.4 Oral cancer. (From Salvo, S.G. [2014]. *Mosby's pathology for massage therapists* [3rd ed.]. St. Louis: Mosby.)

Long-term oral mucous membrane irritation (poorly fitting dentures, cheek chewing, broken teeth) can precede development of leukoplakia.

Oral hairy leukoplakia (Fig. 49.3) develops in people with immune compromise. It is often found in those with human immune deficiency virus (HIV) (as an early symptom) or Epstein-Barr virus (EBV).

ORAL CANCER

Teach adults to visit a dentist at least twice a year for professional dental hygiene and an oral cancer screening, which includes inspecting and palpating the mouth for lesions (Fig. 49.4). Prevention strategies including stopping use of tobacco and alcohol, avoiding sun exposure to lips, and avoiding exposure to human papillomavirus (HPV), a sexually transmitted infection (see Chapter 69).

Textile workers, plumbers, and coal and metal workers, who have prolonged exposure to polycyclic aromatic hydrocarbons (PAHs), are at high risk for development of oral cancer, particularly if they have exposure to HPV (Zhang et al., 2019). People with *periodontal disease* (gum disease) (Fig. 49.5) in which mandibular (jaw) bone loss has occurred are also at risk.

Teach adults to follow the guidelines in the Patient and Family Education: Preparing for Self-Management: Maintaining a Healthy Oral Cavity box to maintain oral health.

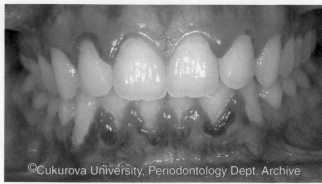

©Cukurova University, Periodontology Dept. Archive

FIG. 49.5 Periodontal (gum) disease. (From Newman, M.G., Takei, H., Klokkevold, P.R., & Carranza, F.A. [2019]. *Newman and Carranza's Clinical Periodontology* [13th ed.]. Philadelphia: Elsevier.)

Pathophysiology Review

Most oral cancers are squamous cell carcinomas that begin on the lips, tongue, buccal mucosa, and oropharynx in people over the age of 40. Oral lesions that are red, raised, and eroded are suspicious for cancer. A lesion that does not heal within 2 weeks or a lump or thickening in the cheek warrants further assessment (Oral Cancer Foundation [OCF], 2019a).

Basal cell carcinoma of the mouth occurs primarily on the lips and is related most closely to sunlight exposure. The lesion is asymptomatic and resembles a raised scab. With time, it evolves into a characteristic ulcer with a raised, pearly border. Basal cell carcinomas do not metastasize but can aggressively involve the skin of the face.

Kaposi sarcoma is a vascular tumor, appearing as a raised, purple, reddish, or brownish nodule or plaque, which is usually painless. It can be found on the hard palate, gums, tongue, or tonsils. It is most often associated with acquired immune deficiency syndrome (AIDS [HIV-III]) (see Chapter 17).

PATIENT-CENTERED CARE: GENETIC/GENOMIC CONSIDERATIONS QSEN

Ask about history of any cancer in patients who are at risk for, or may have, oral cancer. Genetic variations in patients with oral cancer have been found, especially the mutation of the *TP53* gene (McCance et al., 2019). The tumor protein p53 is essential for cell division regulation and prevention of tumor formation (National Institutes of Health, 2020).

NCLEX EXAMINATION CHALLENGE 49.2
Health Promotion and Maintenance

A nurse is caring for four clients. Which individual does the nurse identify as being at the **highest** risk for development of oral cancer?
A. 28-year-old with human papillomavirus (HPV) infection
B. 30-year-old with recurrent aphthous stomatitis (RAS)
C. 55-year-old who quit chewing tobacco 5 years ago
D. 76-year-old who is sometimes negligent in denture care

⟫ KEY FEATURES

Oral Cancer

- Bleeding from the mouth
- Poor appetite, compromised **nutrition** status
- Difficulty chewing or swallowing
- Unplanned weight loss
- Thick or absent saliva
- Painless oral lesion that is red, raised, or eroded
- Thickening or lump in cheek

❖ Interprofessional Collaborative Care

Care of the patient with oral cancer takes place in a variety of settings from the hospital to the community, depending on the degree of treatment needed. The interprofessional team that treats and cares for a patient with oral cancer may include the primary health care provider, dentist, surgeon, oncologist, nurse, speech therapist, registered dietitian nutritionist, social worker, and spiritual leader of the patient's choosing.

◆ **Assessment: Recognize Cues.** Assess the patient's oral hygiene regimen and use of dentures or oral appliances. Ask about oral bleeding; alcohol or tobacco use; difficulty eating, chewing, or swallowing; and whether there has been unplanned recent weight loss (see the Key Features: Oral Cancer box). Assess for educational, cultural, and/or spiritual needs that might affect health teaching or treatment, as well as the patient's self-image. Evaluate for presence of a support system.

Thoroughly inspect the oral cavity for any lesions, **pain,** or restriction of movement; using gloves, a tongue blade, and penlight, examine all areas of the mouth. The primary health care provider will palpate for cervical nodes (Fig. 49.6).

A needle biopsy or an incisional biopsy of the abnormal tissue will be performed by the provider to assess for malignant or premalignant changes. In very small lesions, an excisional biopsy can permit complete tumor removal (OCF, 2019a). CT or MRI may be performed to determine if there is metastasis (or if staging is needed), and MRI is useful in detecting perineural involvement and evaluating thickness in cancers of the tongue.

◆ **Interventions: Take Action.** Oral cavity lesions can be treated by surgical excision; radiation and surgery; or radiation, surgery, and chemotherapy. Multimodal therapy is most effective for more major oral cancers (OCF, 2019a). Airway maintenance to facilitate **gas exchange** is the priority of care for patients with oral cancer. Other nursing interventions focus on restoring and maintaining oral health to the best degree possible.

Nonsurgical Management. Implement interventions targeted to promote **gas exchange,** remove secretions, and prevent aspiration. Assess for dyspnea resulting from obstruction or excessive secretions. Assess the quality, rate, and depth of respirations. Auscultate the lungs for adventitious sounds, such as wheezes caused by aspiration. Listen for stridor caused by partial airway obstruction. Promote deep breathing to help produce an effective cough to mobilize secretions.

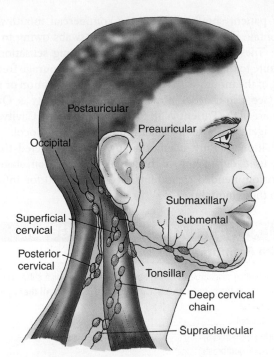

FIG. 49.6 The lymph nodes of the cervical region.

Place the patient in semi-Fowler or high-Fowler position. If the patient is able to swallow and the gag reflex is intact, it is beneficial to encourage fluids to liquefy secretions for easier removal. Chest physiotherapy, often performed by the respiratory therapist, can be helpful. If needed, use oral suction equipment with a dental tip or a tonsil tip (Yankauer) to remove secretions. Teach the patient and family to use suction catheters as appropriate.

Steroids, which reduce inflammation, may be prescribed for edema associated with oral cavity lesions. Antibiotics may be prescribed for infection. A cool mist supplied by a face tent may help with oxygen transport and edema control.

! NURSING SAFETY PRIORITY (QSEN)

Action Alert

Aspiration precautions must be instituted for patients with oral cancer. Assess the patient's level of consciousness (LOC), gag reflex (especially before giving fluids), and ability to swallow. Place the patient in a semi-Fowler or high-Fowler position and keep suction equipment nearby. Remind assistive personnel to feed patients at risk for aspiration in small amounts. All family and visitors should be instructed to speak with the nurse before offering any type of food or drink to the patient. Thickened liquids may be needed; collaborate with the speech-language pathologist, who may recommend a swallow study.

Perform oral hygiene every 2 hours. Use a soft-bristle toothbrush or an ultrasoft "chemobrush," especially for patients with a low platelet count. Do not use oral swabs or disposable foam brushes, which do not adequately control bacteremia-promoting plaque and may further dry the oral mucosa. Water-based lubricant can be applied to moisten the lips and oral mucosa as needed.

The patient should avoid using commercial mouthwashes that contain alcohol and lemon-glycerin swabs owing to their acidity. These substances can cause a burning sensation and contribute to dry oral mucous membranes. Encourage frequent rinsing of the mouth with sodium bicarbonate solution or warm saline (see also the Best Practice for Patient Safety & Quality Care: Care of the Patient With Problems of the Oral Cavity box). Follow agency or primary health care provider protocol.

Radiation therapy, chemotherapy, and/or targeted therapy may be used, depending on the tumor type, location, stage, and other recommended treatments. See Chapter 20 for information on these modalities.

NCLEX EXAMINATION CHALLENGE 49.3
Health Promotion and Maintenance

When providing discharge teaching about mouth care, which substance will the nurse teach the client with oral cancer to avoid? **Select all that apply.**
A. Mouthwash
B. Lip lubricant
C. Warm saline rinses
D. Ultrasoft toothbrush
E. Disposable foam brushes
F. Bicarbonate mouth rinse

Surgical Management. Depending on the type and stage of cancer, a different surgery may be recommended. Common surgeries for oral cancer include (Cancer Treatment Centers of America, 2020):

- Scalpel, laser, or cryoprobe removal (of erythroplakia or leukoplakia, depending on type)
- Glossectomy—removal of the tongue
- Laryngectomy—removal of the larynx and tumor
- Mandible resection (full or partial)—removal of part or all of the mandible
- Maxillectomy—removal of part or all of the hard palate
- Microsurgery—reconstruction of the mouth, throat, or mandible with body tissue from the patient (e.g., from the intestine, arm, abdomen)
- Mohs micrographic surgery—removal of cancer on the lip by taking of thin slices until no cancer is left
- Neck dissection (partial, modified radical, or radical)—removal of lymph nodes in the neck, with or without muscle, nerve tissue, and veins
- Pedicle or free flap reconstruction—repair of the mouth, throat, or neck after a tumor is removed (often with the use of a skin graft)
- Tumor resection—removal of an entire oral tumor, with some surrounding normal tissue

Preoperative Care. Preoperative care for patients undergoing significant head and neck cancer is discussed in Chapter 26. For patients undergoing same-day procedures on an ambulatory basis, such as the scalpel, laser, or cryoprobe removal of erythroplakia or leukoplakia, document the patient's level of understanding of the disease process, the rationale for the procedure, and the planned intervention. Evidence shows that preoperative oral health reduces postoperative inflammation

---

PATIENT AND FAMILY EDUCATION: PREPARING FOR SELF-MANAGEMENT
Care of the Patient With Oral Cancer at Home

- Inspect the mouth daily for changes, such as redness or lesions, or signs of infection.
- Continue meticulous oral hygiene at home.
- Use an ultrasoft toothbrush or chemobrush; clean brush after every use.
- Keep all follow-up appointments.
- Use a thickening agent for liquids if dysphagia is present.
- Eat soft foods if stomatitis occurs.
- Use saliva substitute as prescribed, if needed.

---

and complications, so provide teaching and encourage starting proper oral care before any procedure takes place.

Operative Procedures. The procedure chosen for isolated tumors is dependent on size, stage, and location. Removal may be done by scalpel, laser, or cryoprobe. Operative procedures for patients undergoing significant head and neck cancer are described in Chapter 26.

Postoperative Care. For small, local excisions, postoperative teaching includes planning for liquid diet for a day, and then advancing as tolerated. Activity can resume as tolerated, and *pain* is managed on a case-by-case basis. Remind the patient to keep any follow-up appointments, and to continue meticulous oral care. Postoperative care for patients undergoing significant head and neck cancer is located in Chapter 26.

Care Coordination and Transition Management. Continuing care for the patient with an oral tumor depends on the severity of the tumor and the degree of treatment. Teach the patient who underwent a minor procedure for localized oral cancer about *nutrition* therapies to best restore oral and systemic health, drug therapy (if prescribed), and symptoms of infection to report. See the Patient and Family Education: Preparing for Self-Management: Care of the Patient With Oral Cancer at Home box for more information. Also see Chapter 26 for care of the patient who underwent significant head and neck cancer surgery.

SIALADENITIS

Pathophysiology Review

Acute sialadenitis, inflammation of a salivary gland, can be associated with:

- Bacteria or viruses (commonly associated with cytomegalovirus)
- •Immunologic compromise (e.g., HIV infection, Sjögren syndrome)
- Decrease in saliva production (especially in patients undergoing radiation for head and neck, or thyroid, cancer)
- Systemic drugs (phenothiazines, tetracyclines)

Acute sialadenitis most commonly affects the parotid or submandibular gland in adults. Although there is not a defining timeline to mark the transition, sialadenitis can become chronic if swelling persists over weeks to months (Hoffman, 2019).

Untreated infections of the salivary glands can evolve into an abscess, which can rupture and spread infection into the tissues of the neck and the mediastinum. The best prevention for acute sialadenitis is adherence to routine oral hygiene, which prevents infection from ascending to the salivary glands.

❖ Interprofessional Collaborative Care

Assess for any predisposing factors for sialadenitis, such as ionizing radiation to the head or neck area. Collect a thorough drug history and ask about systemic illnesses, especially ones where immunity is compromised.

Assess the oral cavity for dryness, *pain,* and swelling of the face in the area of the affected gland. Purulent drainage can sometimes be massaged from the affected area. Assess facial function, as the branches of cranial nerve VII (the facial nerve) are near the salivary glands. The patient may also report fever and general malaise.

Conservative care is directed at treating the underlying cause and increasing the flow of saliva. Teach the patient to stay hydrated, apply moist heat, and massage the gland by sweeping the fingers along the course of the gland with gentle pressure. *Pain* and inflammation can be managed with NSAIDs, and antibiotics will be prescribed if infection is suspected. *Sialagogues* (substances that stimulate the flow of saliva) may be recommended if saliva production has decreased.

The salivary glands are sensitive to ionizing radiation, such as from radiation therapy or radioactive iodine treatment of thyroid cancers. Radiation of the salivary glands can cause *pain* and edema, which generally subside after several days. Exposure of the glands to radiation produces a type of sialadenitis known as xerostomia (very dry mouth caused by a severe reduction in the flow of saliva) within 24 hours.

Xerostomia may be temporary or permanent, depending on the radiation dose and percentage of total salivary gland tissue irradiated. Frequent sips of water and frequent mouth care, especially before meals, are the most effective interventions to address xerostomia. After the course of radiation therapy has been completed, saliva substitutes may provide moisture for short periods of time. Over-the-counter solutions are available.

✴ NUTRITION CONCEPT EXEMPLAR: GASTROESOPHAGEAL REFLUX DISEASE (GERD)

Pathophysiology Review

Gastroesophageal reflux disease (GERD), the most common upper gastrointestinal disorder in the United States, occurs most often in middle-age and older adults. Gastroesophageal reflux (GER) occurs as a result of backward flow of stomach contents into the esophagus, known as regurgitation. GERD is the chronic and more serious condition that arises from persistent GER.

Patients who are overweight or have obesity are at highest risk for GERD because increased weight increases intra-abdominal pressure, which contributes to reflux. *Helicobacter pylori* may contribute to reflux (McCance et al., 2019) by causing gastritis and thus poor gastric emptying. This increases frequency of GER events and acid exposure to the esophagus.

TABLE 49.1 Factors Contributing to Decreased Lower Esophageal Sphincter Pressure	
• Caffeinated beverages	• Smoking and use of other tobacco products
• Coffee, tea, and cola	
• Chocolate	• Calcium channel blockers
• Nitrates	• Anticholinergic drugs
• Citrus fruits	• High levels of estrogen and progesterone
• Tomatoes and tomato products	
• Alcohol	• Nasogastric tube placement
• Peppermint, spearmint	

Etiology and Genetic Risk. There is not a single causative agent for GERD. Reflux produces symptoms by exposing the esophageal mucosa to the irritating effects of gastric or duodenal contents, resulting in inflammation. A patient with acute symptoms of inflammation is often described as having mild or severe reflux esophagitis (McCance et al., 2019). When the lower esophageal sphincter (LES) is compromised (relaxed), gastric contents reflux into the esophagus. Eating large meals or certain foods, taking certain drugs, smoking, and using alcohol influence the tone function of the LES (Table 49.1). Reflux is generally sour or bitter. Although rare, a reflex salivary hypersecretion known as *water brash* can occur in response to reflux. Water brash is different from regurgitation. The patient reports a sensation of fluid in the throat, but unlike with regurgitation, there is no bitter or sour taste.

Patients who have a nasogastric (NG) tube have decreased esophageal sphincter function. The tube keeps the cardiac sphincter open and allows acidic contents from the stomach to enter the esophagus. Other factors that increase intra-abdominal and intragastric pressure (e.g., pregnancy, wearing tight belts or abdominal binders, bending over, ascites) overcome the gastroesophageal pressure gradient maintained by the LES and allow reflux to occur. Many patients with obstructive sleep apnea report frequent episodes of GERD. Nighttime reflux causes prolonged exposure of the esophagus to acid because the patient is usually in supine position, and secretions do not drain back down with gravity.

Twin and family studies have demonstrated an approximate 31% heritability of GERD (Argyrou et al., 2018). As with many disorders, lifestyle choices contribute very significantly to this condition.

During the process of healing, the body may substitute Barrett epithelium (columnar epithelium) for the normal squamous cell epithelium of the lower esophagus; this becomes known as Barrett esophagus. Although this new tissue is more resistant to acid and supports esophageal healing, it is premalignant and is associated with an increased risk for cancer in patients with prolonged GERD. The fibrosis and scarring that accompany the healing process can produce esophageal stricture (narrowing of the esophageal opening), which leads to progressive difficulty swallowing. Uncontrolled esophageal reflux also increases the risk for other complications such as asthma, laryngitis, dental decay, and cardiac disease, as well as serious concerns for hemorrhage and aspiration pneumonia.

Incidence and Prevalence. The population affected by GERD continues to get younger. The greatest recent rise in proportion of people with GERD, as well as those using proton pump inhibitor (PPI) therapy, is seen in the 30- to 39-year-old demographic (Yamasaki et al., 2018). Prevalence in North America is 18.1% to 27.8% (Yamasaki et al., 2018).

Health Promotion and Maintenance. Adults with gastroesophageal reflux (GER) may initially be asymptomatic. Teach patients to engage in healthy eating habits that include consuming small, frequent meals and limiting intake of fried, fatty, and spicy foods, and caffeine. Sitting upright for at least 1 hour after eating can promote proper digestion and reduce the risk for reflux.

NCLEX EXAMINATION CHALLENGE 49.4
Health Promotion and Maintenance

Which client statement about GERD triggers requires further nursing teaching? **Select all that apply.**
A. "I will decrease my alcohol intake."
B. "Smoking one or two cigarettes a day won't hurt."
C. "My plan is to eat six small meals daily."
D. "Tomato-based foods should be avoided.'"
E. "I love soda but I'm going to stop drinking it."
F. "Our family eats tacos and burritos several times weekly."

❖ Interprofessional Collaborative Care

Care for the patient with GERD usually takes place in the community setting. Seldom is surgery needed to correct the problem. The interprofessional team that collaborates to care for this patient typically includes the primary health care provider, nurse, and registered dietitian nutritionist (RDN).

◆ Assessment: Recognize Cues

History. Ask the patient about a history of heartburn or atypical chest pain associated with the reflux of GI contents. Ask whether he or she has been newly diagnosed with asthma, has experienced morning hoarseness, or has coughing or wheezing, especially at night. These symptoms may indicate severe reflux reaching the pharynx or mouth or pulmonary aspiration.

Ask about dysphagia and *odynophagia* (painful swallowing), which can accompany chronic GERD.

Physical Assessment/Signs and Symptoms. Dyspepsia, also known as *indigestion,* and regurgitation are the main symptoms of GERD, although symptoms may vary in severity (see the Key Features: Gastroesophageal Reflux Disease box). With severe GERD, this sensation generally occurs after each meal and lasts for 20 minutes to 2 hours. Discomfort may worsen when the patient lies down. Drinking fluids, taking antacids, or maintaining an upright posture usually provides prompt relief.

Other symptoms may include abdominal discomfort, feeling uncomfortably full, nausea, flatulence, eructation (belching), and bloating. Because indigestion might not be viewed as a serious concern, patients often delay seeking treatment. The symptoms

---

⏩ KEY FEATURES
Gastroesophageal Reflux Disease

- Dyspepsia (indigestion)
- Regurgitation (may lead to aspiration or bronchitis)
- Water brash (hypersalivation)
- Dental caries (severe cases)
- Dysphagia
- Odynophagia (painful swallowing)
- Globus (feeling of something in back of throat)
- Pharyngitis
- Coughing, hoarseness, or wheezing at night
- Chest pain
- Pyrosis (heartburn)
- Epigastric *pain*
- Generalized abdominal *pain*
- Belching
- Flatulence
- Nausea

---

typically worsen when the patient bends over, strains, or lies down. If the indigestion is severe, the *pain* may be felt in the chest and may radiate to the neck, jaw, or back, mimicking cardiac pain.

In addition to performing a gastrointestinal assessment, auscultate the patient's lung fields, assessing for crackles, which can be an indication of associated aspiration.

Psychosocial Assessment. Patients may come to the emergency department (ED) fearing that they are having a myocardial infarction. Stay with the patient as much as possible until a diagnosis is made, as worrying can create intense anxiety. Assess the client's ability to cope with stress and fear, and provide referrals as necessary.

👤 PATIENT-CENTERED CARE: OLDER ADULT CONSIDERATIONS QSEN

Older adults are at risk for developing severe complications associated with GERD caused by age-related physiologic changes, comorbidities, increased prevalence of obesity, and polypharmacy (Commisso & Fidelindo, 2019). Instead of the typical symptoms related to GERD, this population experiences more severe complications of the disease such as atypical chest pain; ear, nose, and throat infections; and pulmonary problems, such as aspiration pneumonia, sleep apnea, and asthma. Barrett esophagus and esophageal erosions are also more common in older adults.

Diagnostic Assessment. A definitive diagnostic test for GERD does not exist; however, the primary health care provider may use a clinical history and diagnostic tests to establish a diagnosis when GERD is suspected (Gyawali et al., 2018). Usually, patients with classic GERD symptoms are diagnosed on the basis of clinical symptoms and history alone (Kahrilas, 2020). Those with atypical symptoms may benefit from an upper endoscopy (also called esophagogastroduodenoscopy [EGD]). This procedure involves insertion of an endoscope (a flexible plastic tube equipped with a light and lens) down the throat, which shows the esophagus and any associated abnormalities. A biopsy can be performed at the same time (see Chapter 48) (Gyawali et al., 2018). This test requires the use of moderate sedation during the procedure, and patients must have someone drive them home after recovery.

Ambulatory esophageal pH monitoring is the most accurate method of diagnosing GERD. In this procedure, a transnasally placed catheter or wireless, capsule-like device is affixed to the distal esophageal mucosa (Kahrilas, 2020). The patient is asked to keep a diary of activities and symptoms over 24 to 48 hours (depending on diagnostic method), and the pH is continuously monitored and recorded.

Although not as common, *esophageal manometry*, or motility testing, may be performed. Water-filled catheters are inserted in the patient's nose or mouth and slowly withdrawn while measurements of LES pressure and peristalsis are recorded. When used alone, manometry cannot establish a diagnosis of GERD (Gyawali et al., 2018); it is used to rule out an esophageal motility disorder before considering surgery for GERD (Kahrilas, 2020).

◆ Analysis: Analyze Cues and Prioritize Hypotheses

The priority collaborative problems for the patient with gastroesophageal reflux disease (GERD) include:

1. Potential for compromised *nutrition* status due to dietary selection
2. Acute *pain* due to reflux of gastric contents

◆ Planning and Implementation: Generate Solutions and Take Action

Balancing Nutrition

Planning: Expected Outcomes. The patient with imbalanced *nutrition* is expected to have improvement in nutrition status while esophagitis heals.

Interventions. Interventions are designed to optimize *nutrition* status, decrease symptoms experienced with GERD, and prevent complications. Nursing care priorities focus on teaching the patient about proper dietary selections that provide optimum nutrients and that do not contribute to reflux.

Nonsurgical Management. For most patients, GERD can be controlled with *nutrition* therapy, lifestyle changes, and drug therapy. The most important role of the nurse is patient and caregiver education. Teach the patient that GERD is a chronic disorder that requires ongoing management. The disease should be treated more aggressively in older adults.

Ask about the patient's basic meal patterns and food preferences. Coordinate with the registered dietitian nutritionist (RDN), patient, and caregiver to adopt changes in eating that may decrease reflux symptoms.

Teach the patient to limit or eliminate foods that decrease LES pressure. Foods that irritate inflamed tissue and cause heartburn, such as peppermint, chocolate, fatty foods (especially fried), caffeine, and carbonated beverages, should be avoided. The patient should also restrict spicy and acidic foods (e.g., orange juice, tomatoes) until esophageal healing occurs. Recommend applications ("apps") that can help the patient follow a healthier diet, such as MyFitnessPal (www.myfitnesspal.com) or MyPlate (www.livestrong.com).

Explain that large meals increase volume and pressure within the stomach and delay gastric emptying. Recommend eating four to six small meals each day rather than three large ones. Advise the patient to eat slowly and chew thoroughly to facilitate digestion and prevent eructation (belching). Teach to avoid eating at least 3 hours before going to bed, because reflux episodes are most damaging at night. The risk for aspiration is increased if regurgitation occurs when the patient is lying down. Remind the patient to sleep propped up to promote **gas exchange**. This can be done by placing blocks under the head of the bed or by using a large, wedge-style pillow instead of a standard pillow.

Teach that alcohol and tobacco should be avoided, and make referrals to cessation groups and programs if needed. If weight management is needed, refer to the appropriate resources and community support groups.

Minimizing Pain

Planning: Expected Outcomes. The patient is expected to have relief of *pain* associated with GERD.

Interventions. Interventions are designed to minimize the patient's *pain*. Nursing care priorities focus on teaching the patient about lifestyle modifications that will improve comfort.

Nonsurgical Management. In addition to appropriate dietary selections that promote *nutrition* and allow esophageal tissues to heal, the patient should be encouraged to adhere to other methods of controlling symptoms to minimize *pain.*

Lifestyle changes. In addition to nutrition modifications, teach the patient about other lifestyle changes that decrease symptoms of GERD. Discourage heavy lifting, straining, and working in a position in which the patient bends at the abdomen. Encourage comfortable, nonrestrictive clothing.

Emphasize that these general adaptations are an essential and effective part of disease management and can produce prompt results in uncomplicated cases.

Patients with obesity often have obstructive sleep apnea in addition to GERD. Those who receive continuous positive airway pressure (CPAP) treatment report improved sleeping and decreased episodes of reflux at night. See Chapter 26 for a discussion of CPAP.

Drug therapy. Some drugs lower LES pressure and cause reflux; these include oral contraceptives, anticholinergic agents, sedatives, NSAIDs (e.g., ibuprofen), nitrates, and calcium channel blockers. Although not always possible, the elimination of drugs causing reflux should be explored with the primary health care provider.

Drug therapy for GERD management includes three major types: antacids, histamine blockers, and proton pump inhibitors (PPIs). These drugs, which are also used for peptic ulcer disease, have one or more of these functions:

- Inhibit gastric acid secretion
- Accelerate gastric emptying
- Protect the gastric mucosa

The stomach responds to these actions, and the *pain* that a patient experiences should decrease. See Table 50.1 in Chapter 50 for drug therapy used for GERD management.

Some PPIs, such as esomeprazole and pantoprazole, may be administered in IV form for short-term use to treat or prevent stress ulcers that can result from surgery. PPIs promote rapid tissue healing, but recurrence is common when the drug is stopped. Long-term use may mask reflux symptoms, and stopping the drug determines if reflux has been resolved. Recent research has linked long-term PPI use to community-acquired pneumonia, *Clostridium difficile*, bone fractures, chronic kidney injury, and vitamin and mineral deficiencies. Evidence is still being gathered regarding several of these adverse effects, but it is important to acknowledge the need for monitoring during extended PPI use (Nehra et al., 2018).

PATIENT-CENTERED CARE: OLDER ADULT CONSIDERATIONS (QSEN)

Research has found that long-term use of proton pump inhibitors (PPIs) may increase the risk for hip fracture, especially in older adults. PPIs can interfere with calcium absorption and protein digestion and therefore reduce available calcium to bone tissue. Decreased calcium makes bones more brittle and likely to fracture, especially as adults get older (Maes et al., 2017).

Endoscopic therapies. The Stretta procedure, a nonsurgical method, can replace surgery for GERD when other measures are not effective. In the Stretta procedure, the health care provider applies radiofrequency (RF) energy through the endoscope using needles placed near the gastroesophageal junction. The RF energy decreases vagus nerve activity, thus reducing discomfort for the patient. Patients with obesity or those who have severe symptoms may not be candidates for this procedure. Postoperative instructions for patients who have undergone the Stretta procedure can be found in the Patient and Family Education: Preparing for Self-Management box.

Surgical Management. A very small percentage of patients with GERD require antireflux surgery. It is usually indicated for patients who have not responded to medical treatment, have high-volume reflux, and have severe esophagitis; in some cases, it is also beneficial for patients with upper respiratory symptoms associated with GERD (Schwaitzberg, 2019). Various surgical procedures may be used through conventional open or laparoscopic techniques.

PATIENT AND FAMILY EDUCATION: PREPARING FOR SELF-MANAGEMENT

Postoperative Instructions for Patients Having the Stretta Procedure

- Remain on clear liquids for 24 hours after the procedure.
- After the first day, consume a soft diet, such as custard, pureed vegetables, mashed potatoes, and applesauce.
- Avoid NSAIDs and aspirin for 10 days.
- Continue drug therapy as prescribed, usually proton pump inhibitors.
- Use liquid medications whenever possible.
- Do not allow nasogastric tubes to be inserted for at least 1 month because the esophagus could be perforated.
- Contact the primary health care provider immediately if these problems occur:
  - Abdominal *pain*
  - Bleeding
  - Chest *pain*
  - Dysphagia
  - Nausea or vomiting
  - Shortness of breath

Laparoscopic Nissen fundoplication (LNF) is minimally invasive surgery (MIS) and is the standard surgical approach for treatment of severe GERD (Mermelstein et al., 2018). Information about this procedure can be found in the next section (Hiatal Hernias) in the Surgical Management discussion. Patients who have surgery are encouraged to continue following the basic antireflux regimen of antacids and *nutrition* therapy because the rate of recurrence is high.

The LINX Reflux Management System is a device that augments the LES with a ring composed of rare earth magnets (Schwaitzberg, 2020). The magnets attract to increase the closure pressure of the LES, yet still allow food passage with swallowing. The LINX can be effective for patients with typical GERD symptoms who have an abnormal pH study, only partially respond to daily PPI therapy, and do not have a hiatal hernia or severe esophagitis (Schwaitzberg, 2020). *Teach patients who have had LINX to talk with all health care providers before having an MRI.* Older LINX devices should *never* be in the presence of MRI, as serious injury could occur; newer devices, called MR Conditional, can undergo scanning under *certain* conditions (Schwaitzberg, 2020).

For patients having surgery for GERD, follow preoperative and postoperative interventions presented in Chapter 9.

! NURSING SAFETY PRIORITY (QSEN)
Safety Alert

When caring for a patient who has had LINX device insertion, emphasize the importance of telling each health care provider about this procedure. If an MRI is recommended, only certain patients with more recent LINX devices *may* be eligible to undergo scanning. Patients with older LINX devices (which contain magnets) should *never* undergo MRI scanning. The health care provider can determine whether MRI is acceptable for the patient, given the date of LINX device insertion.

Care Coordination and Transition Management. Patients with GERD that does not require surgical intervention are usually managed in the community setting. Nursing interventions focus on helping the patient and family with current treatment and reducing risk for continuing symptoms and complications.

Home Care Management. Remind the patient to make appropriate dietary selections that enhance *nutrition* and decrease symptoms associated with GERD. Teach how to properly adhere to drug therapy to minimize GERD-related *pain.*

Self-Management Education. For patients with nonsurgical GERD, teach about signs and symptoms of more serious complications such as esophageal stricture and Barrett esophagus.

Health Care Resources. Patients may find it helpful to work with a registered dietitian nutritionist (RDN) or a support group for meal-planning purposes. Give the patient information about local support groups for people with GERD and direct toward online communities that provide credible information and discussion for ongoing management of this condition.

◆ **Evaluation: Evaluate Outcomes.** Evaluate the care of the patient with GERD based on the identified priority patient problem. The expected outcomes include that the patient will:

- Adhere to appropriate dietary selections, medication therapy, and lifestyle modifications, which decrease signs and symptoms of GERD
- Experience minimized or absence of *pain*

HIATAL HERNIAS

Hiatal hernias, also called *diaphragmatic hernias,* involve the protrusion of the stomach through the esophageal hiatus of the diaphragm into the chest. The esophageal hiatus is the opening in the diaphragm through which the esophagus passes from the thorax to the abdomen.

CLINICAL JUDGMENT CHALLENGE 49.1
Patient-Centered Care; Evidence-Based Practice

The nurse is caring for a 33-year-old male client who is seeing the primary health care provider for several months of "heartburn" after lunch and dinner. He reports that these episodes last about an hour after eating, and are much worse if he lays down for sleep after a meal. Most of the time, he also experiences belching and bloating with the "heartburn". He has been taking over-the-counter antacids with minimal relief. He says that his wife sent him today because she was getting concerned about the amount of antacids he has been using. Reading in the electronic health record, the nurse notes a medical history of mild hypertension controlled with amlodipine, and a social history of smoking a pack of cigarettes daily and drinking 4 to 5 alcoholic beverages weekly. Further data collected today include: height 5'9" tall, weight 203 lb. The patient confirms that this information is still current.

1. **Recognize Cues:** What assessment information in this client situation is the most important and immediate concern for the nurse? (Hint: Identify the **relevant** information *first* to determine what is most important.)
2. **Analyze Cues:** What client conditions are consistent with the **most relevant** information? (Hint: Think about priority collaborative problems that support and contradict the information presented in this situation.)
3. **Prioritize Hypotheses:** Which possibilities or explanations are **most likely** to be present in this client situation? Which possibilities or explanations are the most serious? (Hint: Consider all possibilities and determine their urgency and risk for this client.)
4. **Generate Solutions:** What actions would most likely achieve the desired outcomes for this client? Which actions should be **avoided** or are **potentially harmful**? (Hint: Determine the desired outcomes first to decide which interventions are appropriate and those that should be avoided.)
5. **Take Action:** Which actions are the most appropriate and how should they be implemented? In what **priority order** should they be implemented? (Hint: Consider health teaching, documentation, requested health care provider orders or prescriptions, nursing skills, collaboration with or referral to health team members, etc.)
6. **Evaluate Outcomes:** What client assessment would indicate that the nurse's actions were **effective**? (Hint: Think about signs that would indicate an improvement, decline, or unchanged client condition.)

Pathophysiology Review

Hiatal hernias are classified as type I (*sliding* hernias, which are most common) or types II through IV (paraesophageal, or *rolling,* hernias). In a type I (sliding) hernia, the esophagogastric junction and a portion of the fundus of the stomach slide upward through the esophageal hiatus into the chest, usually as a result of weakening of the diaphragm (Fig. 49.7). The hernia generally moves freely and slides into and out of the chest during changes in position or intra-abdominal pressure. Although **volvulus** (twisting of a GI structure) and obstruction do occur rarely, the major concern for a sliding hernia is the development of esophageal reflux and associated complications (see the section Nutrition Concept Exemplar: Gastroesophageal Reflux Disease [GERD]earlier in this chapter).

Types II through IV (paraesophageal) hernias are characterized as follows (Kahrilas, 2019):

- Type II—The gastroesophageal junction remains in its normal intra-abdominal location, but the fundus (and possibly portions of the stomach's greater curvature) rolls through the esophageal hiatus and into the chest beside the esophagus (see Fig. 49.7).
- Type III—The gastroesophageal junction and the fundus both herniate through the hiatus, with the fundus lying above the gastroesophageal junction.
- Type IV—The colon, spleen, pancreas, or small intestine is found in the hernia sac (instead of the stomach).

The risks for volvulus (twisting of a GI structure), obstruction (blockage), and strangulation (stricture) are high. The development of iron deficiency anemia is common because slow bleeding from venous obstruction causes the gastric mucosa to become engorged and ooze. Significant bleeding or hemorrhage is rare.

❖ Interprofessional Collaborative Care

Care for the patient with a hiatal hernia usually takes place in the community setting, unless surgery is needed to correct the problem. The interprofessional health care team includes the primary health care provider, nurse, surgeon, registered dietitian nutritionist, and spiritual leader of the patient's choice.

◆ **Assessment: Recognize Cues.** Most patients with hiatal hernias are asymptomatic, but some experience symptoms similar to those with GERD (McCance et al., 2019) as listed in the Key Features: Hiatal Hernias box. Symptoms usually worsen after a meal or when the patient is supine. Obtain a history and perform a physical assessment as you would for a patient with GERD (covered earlier in this chapter).

The *barium swallow study with fluoroscopy* is the most specific diagnostic test for identifying hiatal hernia. Rolling hernias are usually clearly visible, and sliding hernias can often be observed when the patient moves through a series of positions that increase intra-abdominal pressure. To visualize sliding hernias, an esophagogastroduodenoscopy (EGD) may be performed to view both the esophagus and gastric lining (see Chapter 48). High-resolution manometry (HRM) with esophageal pressure topography (EPT) is used to identify larger sliding hiatal hernias (Kahrilas, 2020).

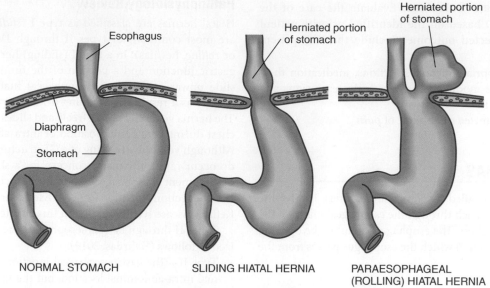

FIG. 49.7 Comparison of the normal stomach and sliding and paraesophageal (rolling) hiatal hernias.

<table>
<tr><td colspan="2"></td></tr>
</table>

▶▶ KEY FEATURES
Hiatal Hernias

Sliding Hiatal Hernias	**Paraesophageal Hernias**
• Heartburn	• Feeling of fullness (after eating)
• Regurgitation	• Breathlessness (after eating)
• Chest pain	• Feeling of suffocation (after eating)
• Dysphagia	• Chest pain that mimics angina
• Belching	• Worsening of symptoms in a recumbent position

◆ **Interventions: Take Action.** Type I (sliding) hiatal hernias are usually treated medically. Treatment of types II through IV (paraesophageal) hiatal hernias are treated based on type, the severity of symptoms, and the risk for serious complications. When possible, medical management is favored. For patients at risk for, or who experience, volvulus, bleeding, obstruction, strangulation, perforation, or airway obstruction, surgery is performed (Kahrilas, 2020).

Nonsurgical Management. Interventions for patients with a type I (sliding) hiatal hernia are similar to those for GERD. These include drug therapy, *nutrition* therapy, and lifestyle changes. The primary health care provider typically recommends antacids or a proton-pump inhibitor in an attempt to control reflux and its symptoms. *Nutrition* therapy is also important and follows the guidelines discussed earlier for GERD.

❗ NURSING SAFETY PRIORITY (QSEN)
Action Alert

When caring for a patient with hiatal hernia, education is one of the most important parts of nursing care. Follow health teaching as described for patients with GERD.

Surgical Management. Surgery may be required when the risk for complications is high or when damage from chronic reflux becomes severe.

Preoperative Care. If the surgery is not urgent, the surgeon may instruct a patient who is overweight to lose weight before surgery. Any patient who is to undergo surgery for hiatal hernia is advised to quit smoking. As part of preoperative teaching, reinforce the surgeon's instructions and prepare the patient for what to expect after surgery. See Chapter 9 for preoperative intervention.

Operative Procedures. Surgical repair can be done transabdominally or transthoracically. The transabdominal approach can be done as an open procedure or laparoscopically (Rosen & Blatnik, 2019). Surgery involves fundoplication, in which the stomach fundus is wrapped around the distal esophagus. The wrap is then closed with sutures to anchor the lower esophagus below the diaphragm (Fig. 49.8).

Laparoscopic Nissen fundoplication (LNF) is a minimally invasive surgical procedure commonly used for hiatal hernia repair. Complications after LNF occur less frequently compared with those seen in patients having the more traditional open surgical approach. A small percentage of patients are not candidates for LNF and therefore require a conventional open fundoplication.

Prepare the patient undergoing a transthoracic approach for a chest tube and a nasogastric tube, which will be present after surgery. These will be inserted during surgery and remain in place for several days.

Postoperative Care. Patients having the *LNF procedure* or paraesophageal repair via laparoscope are at risk for bleeding and infection, although these problems are not common. The nursing care priority is to observe for these complications and provide health teaching. See specific education in the Patient and Family Education: Preparing for Self-Management: Postoperative Instructions for Patients Having Laparoscopic

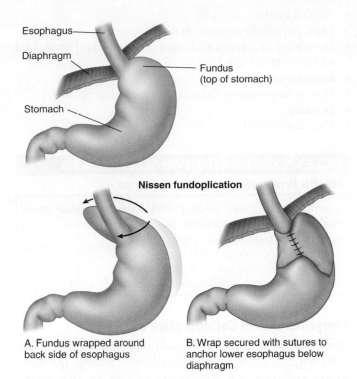

Esophagus

Diaphragm

Fundus (top of stomach)

Stomach

Nissen fundoplication

A. Fundus wrapped around back side of esophagus

B. Wrap secured with sutures to anchor lower esophagus below diaphragm

FIG. 49.8 Open surgical approach for Nissen fundoplication for gastro-esophageal reflux disease or hiatal hernia repair.

Nissen Fundoplication (LNF) or Paraesophageal Repair via Laparoscope box.

Postoperative care after *open repair* closely follows that required after any esophageal surgery. Carefully assess for complications of open surgery as shown in the Best Practice for Patient Safety & Quality Care: Assessment of Postoperative Complications Related to Fundoplication Procedures box. Report any unusual assessment findings to the surgeon.

! NURSING SAFETY PRIORITY (QSEN)

Action Alert

The primary focus of care after conventional surgery for a hiatal hernia repair is the prevention of respiratory complications. Elevate the head of the patient's bed at least 30 degrees to lower the diaphragm and promote lung expansion. Help the patient out of bed and begin ambulation as soon as possible. Be sure to support the incision during coughing to reduce *pain* and prevent excessive strain on the suture line, especially in patients with obesity.

For the patient who has undergone an open procedure, provide postoperative interventions presented in Chapter 9 regarding incentive spirometry, deep breathing, and prevention of venous thromboembolism. Patients with large hiatal hernias are at the highest risk for developing respiratory complications. The patient will have a large-bore (diameter) nasogastric (NG) tube to prevent the fundoplication wrap from becoming too tight around the esophagus. Initially the NG drainage should be dark brown with old blood. The drainage should become normal yellowish green within the first 8 hours after surgery. Check the

PATIENT AND FAMILY EDUCATION: PREPARING FOR SELF-MANAGEMENT

Postoperative Instructions for Patients Having Laparoscopic Nissen Fundoplication (LNF) or Paraesophageal Repair via Laparoscope

- Consume a soft diet for about a week; avoid carbonated beverages, tough foods, and raw vegetables that are difficult to swallow.
- Remain on antireflux medications as prescribed for at least a month or per your health care provider's recommendation.
- Do not drive for a week after surgery; do not drive if taking opioid pain medication.
- Walk every day but do not do any heavy lifting.
- Remove small dressings 2 days after surgery and shower; do not remove wound closure strips until 10 days after surgery.
- Wash incisions with soap and water, rinse well, and pat dry; report any redness or drainage from the incisions to your surgeon.
- Report fever above 101°F (38.3°C), nausea, vomiting, or uncontrollable bloating or *pain.* For patients older than 65 years, report temperature elevations above 100°F (37.8°C).
- Keep your follow-up appointment with your surgeon, usually 3 to 4 weeks after surgery.

BEST PRACTICE FOR PATIENT SAFETY & QUALITY CARE (QSEN)

Assessment of Postoperative Complications Related to Fundoplication Procedures

Complication	Assessment Findings
Temporary dysphagia	Difficulty swallowing when oral feeding begins
Gas bloat syndrome	Difficulty belching to relieve distention
Atelectasis, pneumonia	Dyspnea, chest pain, or fever
Obstructed nasogastric tube	Nausea, vomiting, or abdominal distention, and/or a nondraining nasogastric tube

NG tube every 4 to 8 hours for proper placement in the stomach. It should be properly anchored so it does not become displaced, because reinsertion could perforate the fundoplication. Follow the surgeon's recommendations for care of the patient with an NG tube.

Monitor patency of the NG tube to keep the stomach decompressed. This prevents retching or vomiting, which can strain or rupture the stomach sutures. The NG tube is irritating, so provide frequent oral hygiene to minimize *pain.* Assess hydration status regularly, and document accurate measures of intake and output. Adequate fluid replacement helps thin respiratory secretions.

Beginning with clear fluids, the patient gradually progresses to a near-normal diet during the first 4 to 6 weeks. Some foods, especially caffeinated or carbonated beverages and alcohol, are either restricted or eliminated. The food storage area of the stomach is reduced by the surgery, and meals need to be smaller and more frequent. *Carefully supervise the first oral feedings because temporary dysphagia is common.* Continuous dysphagia usually indicates that the fundoplication is too tight, and dilation may be required.

Other patients have *aerophagia* (air swallowing) from attempting to reverse or clear acid reflux. Teach them to relax consciously before and after meals, to eat and drink slowly, and to chew all food thoroughly. Air in the stomach that cannot be removed by belching can be extremely uncomfortable.

Some patients develop *gas bloat syndrome,* in which patients cannot voluntarily eructate (belch). The syndrome is usually temporary but may persist. Teach the patient to avoid drinking carbonated beverages and eating gas-producing foods (especially high-fat foods), chewing gum, and drinking with a straw. Frequent position changes and ambulation are often effective interventions for eliminating air from the GI tract. If gas *pain* is still present, it may be recommended that patients take simethicone, which relieves gas pressure.

Care Coordination and Transition Management. Patients undergoing open surgical repair require activity restrictions for 3 to 6 weeks postoperatively. For those who have undergone laparoscopic surgery, activity is typically restricted for a shorter time, and the patient can return to his or her usual lifestyle more quickly, usually in about a week.

For long-term management, educate the patient on:
- Appropriate *nutrition* modifications
- Use of stool softeners or bulk laxatives to prevent constipation and straining
- Daily incisional inspection
- Conditions that require notification of the health care provider, including swelling, redness, tenderness, discharge, or fever
- Avoidance of people with a respiratory infections; development of a respiratory infection with coughing can cause the incision or the fundoplication to dehisce

ESOPHAGEAL TUMORS

Pathophysiology Review

Although esophageal tumors can be benign, most are malignant (cancerous), and the majority develop from the epithelium. Squamous cell carcinomas of the esophagus are located in the upper two-thirds of the esophagus. Adenocarcinomas are more commonly found in the distal third and at the gastroesophageal junction and are now the most common type of esophageal cancer (McCance et al., 2019). Esophageal tumors grow rapidly because there is no serosal layer to limit their extension. Because the esophageal mucosa is richly supplied with lymph tissue, there is typically early spread of tumors to lymph nodes. Esophageal tumors can protrude into the esophageal lumen and can cause thickening or invade deeply into surrounding tissue. In rare cases, the lesion may be confined to the epithelial layer (in situ). In most cases, the tumor is large and well established at diagnosis. More than half of esophageal cancers metastasize throughout the body.

Primary risk factors associated with the development of esophageal cancer include:

- Alcohol intake
- Diets chronically deficient in fresh fruits and vegetables
- Diets high in nitrates and nitrosamines (found in pickled and fermented foods)
- Malnutrition
- Obesity (especially with increased abdominal pressure)
- Smoking
- Untreated GERD

NCLEX EXAMINATION CHALLENGE 49.5
Health Promotion and Maintenance

A community health nurse is screening clients for esophageal cancer. Which client is identified as being at **highest** risk?
A. 22-year-old who drinks a glass of beer weekly
B. 44-year-old who smokes a pack of cigarettes daily
C. 50-year-old who takes over-the-counter omeprazole
D. 63-year-old who uses protein supplements regularly

❖ Interprofessional Collaborative Care

Care of the patient with esophageal tumors usually takes place in the hospital, followed by the community setting. The interprofessional team that collaborates to care for this patient generally includes the primary health care provider, nurse, surgeon, registered dietitian nutritionist (RDN), respiratory therapist, social worker, and spiritual leader of the patient's choice.

◆ **Assessment: Recognize Cues.** Assess for risk factors related to the development or symptoms of esophageal cancer. Men, regardless of race or ethnicity, have higher incidence and mortality rates associated with esophageal cancer (American Cancer Society [ACS], 2020a).

Cancer of the esophagus is a silent tumor in its early stages, with few observable signs. By the time the tumor causes symptoms, it usually has spread extensively. One of the most common symptoms of esophageal cancer is dysphagia. This symptom may not be present until the esophageal opening has narrowed. Weight loss often accompanies progressive dysphagia and can exceed 20 lb over several months. See the Key Features: Esophageal Tumors box for more common clinical symptoms of esophageal tumors.

▶ **KEY FEATURES**
Esophageal Tumors

- Persistent and progressive dysphagia (most common feature)
- Feeling of food sticking in the throat
- Odynophagia (painful swallowing)
- Halitosis
- Chronic hiccups
- Chronic cough with increasing secretions
- Hoarseness
- Severe, persistent chest or abdominal pain or discomfort
- Anorexia
- Regurgitation
- Nausea and vomiting
- Weight loss (often more than 20 lb)
- Changes in bowel habits (diarrhea, constipation, bleeding)

The diagnosis of esophageal cancer may cause significant anxiety. The disease is accompanied by distressing symptoms and is often terminal. The fear of choking can create unusual stress, especially at mealtimes. The loss of pleasure and social aspects of eating may affect relationships. Assess the patient's response to the diagnosis and prognosis. Ask about usual coping strengths and resources. Determine the availability of support systems and the potential impact of the disease and its treatment. Refer to psychological counseling, pastoral care, and/or the social worker or case manager as needed. Chapter 8 describes end-of-life care for patients in the terminal stage of the disease.

NCLEX EXAMINATION CHALLENGE 49.6
Psychosocial Integrity

The nurse is caring for a client with esophageal cancer who is scheduled for surgery. When the client asks, "Is this treatment going to cure me?" which nursing response is appropriate? **Select all that apply.**

A. "The surgery has been useful for many patients so it should work for you."

B. "You can beat this disease if you just put your mind to it and do not give up."

C. "Yes, and you have the best surgeon around who specializes in cancer treatment."

D. "Your surgeon can give more information about the effectiveness of this treatment."

E. "It sounds like you are concerned about surgical outcomes; let's talk about your feelings."

Diagnostic Assessment. An esophagogastroduodenoscopy (EGD) with biopsy is performed to inspect the esophagus and obtain tissue specimens for cell studies and disease staging. A complete cancer staging workup is performed, often by endoscopic ultrasound, to determine the extent of the disease and plan appropriate therapy.

Positron emission tomography (PET) may identify metastatic disease with more accuracy than a CT scan. PET can also help evaluate response to chemotherapy to treat the cancer.

◆ **Interventions: Take Action.** Treatment of patients with esophageal cancer depends on staging at diagnosis. Multimodal therapy is often necessary to treat esophageal cancer, as it is often advanced at diagnosis. Along with treatment of the cancer itself, patients with cancer of the esophagus experience many physical problems, and symptom management becomes essential.

Nonsurgical Management. Nonsurgical treatment options for cancer of the esophagus that can assist in disease and ***nutrition*** management may include:

- Nutrition and swallowing therapy
- Chemotherapy, radiation, and chemoradiation
- Photodynamic therapy and porfimer sodium
- Other therapies

Nutrition and Swallowing Therapy. Conduct a screening assessment to provide information about the patient's ***nutrition*** status. The registered dietitian nutritionist (RDN) determines the caloric needs of the patient to meet daily requirements. Perform weights daily before breakfast on the same scale each day. To keep the esophagus patent, position the patient upright for several hours after meals, and avoid allowing the patient to lay completely flat. Remind assistive personnel (AP) and other health care team members to keep the head of the bed elevated to a 30-degree angle or more to prevent reflux.

Semisoft foods and thickened liquids are preferred because they are easier to swallow. Document the amount of food and fluid intake every day to monitor progress in meeting desired ***nutrition*** outcomes. Liquid supplements are used between feedings to increase caloric intake. Ongoing efforts are made to preserve the ability to swallow, but enteral feedings (tube feedings) may be needed temporarily when dysphagia is severe. In patients with complete esophageal obstruction or life-threatening fistulas, the surgeon may create a gastrostomy or jejunostomy for feeding. Chapter 55 describes care for patients receiving enteral feeding.

Collaborate with the speech-language pathologist (SLP) to help the patient with oral exercises to improve swallowing (*swallowing therapy*) and with the occupational therapist (OT) for feeding techniques.

⚠ NURSING SAFETY PRIORITY (QSEN)
Critical Rescue

When the patient with an esophageal tumor is eating or drinking, recognize that you must monitor for signs and symptoms of aspiration, which can cause airway obstruction, pneumonia, or both, especially in older adults. In coordination with the SLP, respond by teaching caregivers how to feed the patient, how to monitor for aspiration, and how to respond quickly if choking occurs.

Chemotherapy and Radiation. *Chemotherapy* may be given preoperatively or in concurrence with other treatments. *Radiation therapy* can also be used alone but is used most frequently in combination with other treatments. *Chemoradiation* is a treatment for esophageal cancer that involves the use of chemotherapy at the same time as radiation therapy.

Photodynamic Therapy and Porfimer Sodium. *Photodynamic therapy (PDT)* is used as palliative treatment for patients with advanced esophageal cancer; it can relieve pain or make swallowing somewhat easier. PDT is sometimes used with *porfimer sodium* (Photofrin), a light-sensitive drug that collects in cancer cells, for palliation. Chapter 20 describes these approaches to care in detail.

Other Therapies. *Esophageal dilation* may be performed as necessary throughout the course of the disease to achieve temporary but immediate relief of dysphagia. It is usually performed in an ambulatory care setting. Dilators are used to tear soft tissue, thereby widening the esophageal lumen (opening). In most cases, malignant tumors can be dilated safely, but perforation remains a significant risk. Large metal stents may be used to keep the esophagus open for longer periods. A stent covered with graft material can be used to seal a perforation. Bacteremia may also occur. To reduce the risk for sepsis and endocarditis, antibiotics are given. The treatment is repeated as often as needed to preserve the patient's ability to swallow. Prolonged stent embedment into benign esophageal tissue can cause ulceration, bleeding, fistula, dysphagia, and formation of a new stricture if the stent is not removed (Vermeulen & Siersema, 2018).

Endoscopic therapies like stenting can be offered as palliative care for patients who are not surgical candidates. Stenting can be performed with metal, plastic, or biodegradable mechanisms that are intended to relieve obstruction.

Targeted therapies such as trastuzumab, which targets the HER2 protein, may be given IV every 3 weeks; at this time the optimal length of treatment is not known (ACS, 2020b). This treatment can be used with chemotherapy, or alone if chemotherapy has not been effective.

Surgical Management. The purposes of different types of surgical resection vary from cure to palliation. *Esophagectomy* is the removal of all or part of the esophagus, and is usually selected as the initial surgical approach to esophageal cancer (Swanson, 2020). For patients with early-stage cancer, a laparoscopic-assisted minimally invasive esophagectomy (MIE) may be performed. However, most patients require conventional open surgery because of tumor size and metastasis by the time they are diagnosed with the disease.

Preoperative Care. Preoperative preparation for patients undergoing esophagectomy can be quite extensive. Advise the patient to stop smoking 2 to 4 weeks before surgery to enhance pulmonary function. Intensive preoperative respiratory rehabilitation may be prescribed to strengthen the pulmonary system, which has been shown to decrease postoperative pulmonary complications (Swanson, 2020). Patient preparation may include lengthy **nutrition** support to decrease the risk for postoperative complications. Ideally this supplementation is given orally, but some patients require tube feeding or parenteral nutrition. Teach the patient and caregiver to monitor the patient's weight and intake and output. A preoperative evaluation may be required to treat dental disease. Instruct the patient to practice meticulous oral care four times daily to decrease the risk for postoperative infection.

Preoperative nursing care focuses on teaching and psychological support regarding the surgical procedure and preoperative and postoperative instructions. See Chapter 9 for specific preoperative teaching. On the day of surgery, the surgeon usually prescribes prophylactic antibiotics and supplemental oxygen.

Operative Procedures. There are numerous types of esophagectomies that can be performed based on the tumor location, length, extension, and protrusion into surrounding structures (Swanson, 2020). The extent of lymphadenectomy needed and the surgeon's preferences also influence surgical approach. Surgery may be minimally invasive, or open. Carefully review the specific type of procedure performed in order to optimize postprocedure nursing care.

Postoperative Care. Intensive postoperative care is necessary for the patient who has had an esophagectomy, because of the risk for multiple serious complications. Follow postoperative care as outlined in Chapter 9.

Remind all staff to keep the patient in a semi-Fowler or high-Fowler position to support ventilation and prevent reflux. *Ensure the patency of the chest tube drainage system and monitor for changes in the volume or color of the drainage.*

> **! NURSING SAFETY PRIORITY** QSEN
> *Action Alert*
>
> Respiratory care is the highest postoperative priority for patients having an esophagectomy. For those who had traditional surgery, intubation with mechanical ventilation is necessary for at least the first 16 to 24 hours. Pulmonary complications include atelectasis and pneumonia. The risk for postoperative pulmonary complications is increased in the patient who has received preoperative radiation. Once the patient is extubated, support deep breathing, turning, and coughing every 1 to 2 hours. Assess the patient for decreased breath sounds and shortness of breath every 1 to 2 hours. Provide incisional support and adequate analgesia to enhance effective coughing.

Cardiovascular complications, particularly hypotension during surgery, can occur as a result of pressure placed on the posterior heart. Carefully monitor cardiovascular and pulmonary statuses in the postoperative period. See the Nursing Safety Priority box.

> **! NURSING SAFETY PRIORITY** QSEN
> *Action Alert*
>
> Monitor for symptoms of fluid volume overload, particularly in older patients and those who have undergone lymph node dissection. Assess for edema, crackles in the lungs, and increased jugular venous pressure. In the immediate postoperative phase, the patient is often admitted to the intensive care unit. Critical care nurses assess hemodynamic parameters such as cardiac output, cardiac index, and systemic vascular resistance every 2 hours to monitor for myocardial ischemia. Observe for atrial fibrillation, which can result from irritation of the vagus nerve during surgery, and manage according to agency protocol.

Wound management is a major postoperative concern with conventional surgery because the patient typically has multiple incisions and drains. *Provide direct support to the incision during turning and coughing to prevent dehiscence.* Wound infection can occur 4 to 5 days after surgery. Leakage from the site of anastomosis is a dreaded complication that can appear 2 to 10 days after surgery. If an anastomotic leak occurs, all oral intake is discontinued and does not resume until the site of the leak has healed. *Mediastinitis* (inflammation of the mediastinum) resulting from an anastomotic leak can lead to fatal sepsis.

> **! NURSING SAFETY PRIORITY** QSEN
> *Critical Rescue*
>
> After esophageal surgery, recognize fever, fluid accumulation, signs of inflammation, and symptoms of early shock (e.g., tachycardia, tachypnea). Respond immediately by reporting any of these findings to the surgeon *and* the Rapid Response Team!

A nasogastric (NG) tube is placed intraoperatively to decompress the stomach to prevent tension on the suture line. Monitor the NG tube for patency and carefully secure the tube to prevent dislodgment, which can disrupt the sutures at the anastomosis. *Do not irrigate or reposition the NG tube in patients who have undergone esophageal surgery unless prescribed by the surgeon.* See the Best Practice for Patient Safety & Quality Care:

BEST PRACTICE FOR PATIENT SAFETY & QUALITY CARE (QSEN)

Managing the Patient With a Nasogastric Tube After Esophageal Surgery

- Check for tube placement every 4 to 8 hours.
- Ensure that the tube is patent (open) and draining; drainage should turn from bloody to yellowish green by the end of the first postoperative day.
- Secure the tube well to prevent dislodgment.
- Do not irrigate or reposition the tube without a health care provider's order.
- Provide meticulous oral and nasal hygiene every 2 to 4 hours.
- Keep the head of the bed elevated to at least 30 degrees.
- When the patient is permitted to have a small amount of water, place him or her in an upright position and observe for dysphagia (difficulty swallowing).
- Observe for leakage from the anastomosis site (indicated by fever, fluid accumulation, and symptoms of early shock [tachycardia, tachypnea, altered mental status]).

Managing the Patient With a Nasogastric Tube After Esophageal Surgery box for specific interventions.

Nutrition management of the patient who has undergone esophageal surgery is an early postoperative concern. After conventional surgery, on the second postoperative day, initial feedings usually begin through the jejunostomy tube (J tube). Do not aspirate for residual because this increases the risk for mucosal tearing. Feedings are slowly increased over the next several days through the fifth postoperative day. A barium swallow is performed on the seventh postoperative day; if no anastomotic leaks are seen, the NG tube is discontinued (Swanson, 2020). A minimal liquid diet should be continued for the following 2 weeks. Further oral intake should be prescribed by the surgeon at the time of follow-up.

Care Coordination and Transition Management.
Patients with esophageal cancer have many challenges to face once they are discharged home. Treatment regimens cause long-lasting side effects, such as fatigue and weakness. These complex treatments also require the patient and caregiver to be knowledgeable about symptom management and to know when to report concerns.

Once the patient is discharged to home, ongoing respiratory care remains a priority. Give the patient and caregiver instructions for ambulation and incentive spirometer use. Encourage the patient to be as active as possible and avoid excessive bed rest because this can lead to complications of immobility.

Nutrition support is important. Encourage the patient to continue increasing oral feedings as prescribed by the surgeon. Remind him or her to eat small, frequent meals containing high-calorie, high-protein foods that are soft and easily swallowed. Teach the

⚠ NATIONAL PATIENT SAFETY GOALS

In accordance with The Joint Commission National Patient Safety Goals for 2020 (The Joint Commission, 2020a), teach the family to protect the patient from infection by following the World Health Organization (WHO) or the Centers for Disease Control and Prevention (CDC) handwashing guidelines and to contact the health care provider immediately if signs of respiratory infection develop. Patients should stay away from people with infections and avoid large crowds.

value of using supplemental shakes. Emphasize the importance of sitting upright to eat, and remaining upright after meals. Patients who have undergone esophageal resection can lose up to 10% of their body weight. Teach the patient to monitor his or her weight at home and to report a weight loss of 5 lb or more in 1 month. If sufficient oral intake is not possible, tube feedings or parenteral nutrition at home at home may be needed.

Teach the patient that dysphagia or odynophagia may recur because of stricture, reflux, or cancer recurrence. These symptoms should be reported to the health care provider promptly.

Despite radical surgery, the patient with cancer of the esophagus often still has a terminal illness and a relatively short life expectancy. This can cause significant anxiety and depression in some patients (see the Evidence-Based Practice box). Emphasis is placed on maximizing quality of life. Realistic planning is important. Help family members in exploring sources of support and in arranging for hospice care when it becomes necessary. Chapter 8 describes end-of-life care.

EVIDENCE-BASED PRACTICE (QSEN)

Anxiety and Depression Among Esophageal Cancer Patients

Hellstadius, Y., Lagergren, J., Zylstra, J., Gossage, J., Davies, A., Hultman, C.M., et al. (2017). Prevalence and predictors of anxiety and depression among esophageal cancer patients prior to surgery. *Diseases of the Esophagus, 30*(8), 1-7.

This study aimed to establish the prevalence and predictors of anxiety and depression in 106 esophageal cancer patients after diagnosis but before surgical intervention. The researchers collected information about prevalence and predictor variables in hospital records and self-report questionnaires from patients with esophageal cancer at one hospital in London, England from 2011 to 2014. The research focused on clinical and sociodemographic characteristics and how they related to each patient's results on the Hospital Anxiety and Depression Scale (HADS). The study found that a significant number of patients reported anxiety and depression following an esophageal cancer diagnosis. The two groups that reported anxiety and depression most often were women and those who had limitations to their physical activity. Overall, they found that 40% of all patients in this study reported anxiety or depression immediately on being diagnosed with esophageal cancer.

Level of Evidence: 4
The research design was a cross-sectional study.

Commentary: Implications for Practice and Research
The observations made by this study have important implications for those caring for patients who have an esophageal cancer diagnosis. Due to the poor prognosis in patients with esophageal cancer, emotional assessment and supportive care are imperative. This study also helps health care providers to identify specific sociodemographic groups that are at higher risk for anxiety and depression during treatment. This information can assist the interprofessional health care team in providing patient-centered mental health interventions throughout esophageal cancer treatment. Because this study is of a cross-sectional design, no direct correlations can be made, but it does present significant trends that can guide future research and aid in improving care of those diagnosed with esophageal cancer.

Refer patients to community or home care organizations for in-home care. Teach about services available through the American Cancer Society (www.cancer.org), including support groups and transportation. Coordinate resource referrals with the case manager or home care agency as needed.

ESOPHAGEAL TRAUMA

Trauma to the esophagus can result from blunt injuries, chemical burns, surgery or endoscopy (although rare), or the stress of continuous severe vomiting. Trauma may affect the esophagus directly or it may create problems in the lungs or mediastinum. When excessive force is exerted on the esophageal mucosa, it may perforate or rupture, allowing the caustic acid secretions to enter the mediastinal cavity. These tears are associated with a high mortality rate related to shock, respiratory impairment, or sepsis.

Common causes of esophageal perforation include:

- Straining
- Seizures
- Trauma
- Foreign objects
- Instruments or tubes
- Chemical injury
- Complications of esophageal surgery
- Ulcers

Chemical injury is usually a result of the accidental or intentional ingestion of caustic substances. The damage to the mouth and esophagus is rapid and severe. Acid burns tend to affect the superficial mucosal lining, whereas alkaline substances cause deeper penetrating injuries. Strong alkalis can cause full perforation of the esophagus within 1 minute. Additional complications may include aspiration pneumonia and hemorrhage. Esophageal strictures may develop as scar tissue forms.

Patients with esophageal trauma are initially evaluated and treated in the emergency department. Assessment focuses on the nature of the injury and the circumstances surrounding it. *Assess for airway patency, breathing, chest pain, dysphagia, vomiting, and bleeding as the priorities for patient care.* If the risk for extending the damage is not excessive, an endoscopic study may be requested to evaluate tears or perforation. A CT scan of the chest can be done to assess for the presence of mediastinal air.

After the injury, keep the patient NPO to prevent further leakage of esophageal secretions. Esophageal and gastric suction can be used for drainage and to rest the esophagus. Esophageal rest is maintained for more than a week after injury to allow for initial healing of the mucosa. Total parenteral nutrition (TPN) is prescribed to provide calories and protein for wound healing while the patient is not eating.

To prevent sepsis, the health care provider prescribes broad-spectrum antibiotics. High-dose corticosteroids may be administered to suppress inflammation and prevent strictures (esophageal narrowing). Opioid and nonopioid analgesics may be prescribed for *pain* management. When caustic burns involve the mouth, topical agents such as viscous lidocaine may be used.

If nonsurgical management is not effective in healing injured esophageal tissue, the patient may need surgery to remove the damaged tissue. Those with severe injuries may require resection of part of the esophagus with a gastric pull-through and repositioning or replacement by a bowel segment. A gastrostomy tube (G-tube) placement may be needed to meet *nutrition* needs while healing.

GET READY FOR THE NEXT-GENERATION NCLEX® EXAMINATION!

Key Points

Review these key points for each NCLEX Examination Client Needs Category.

Safe and Effective Care Environment

- Check the gag reflex and implement airway management interventions for patients having oral or esophageal surgery. **QSEN: Safety**
- Collaborate with the registered dietitian nutritionist (RDN) to plan *nutrition* modifications for patients with GERD. **QSEN: Teamwork and Collaboration**
- Assess for complications and provide postoperative care for patients having surgical procedures for oral and esophageal problems. **QSEN: Safety**
- Teach the patient and caregiver to recognize dysphagia symptoms. **QSEN: Safety**

Health Promotion and Maintenance

- Teach oral hygiene techniques and remind adults to visit their dentist twice a year. **QSEN: Patient-Centered Care**
- Teach patients with nonhealing oral wounds to contact their primary health care provider or dentist. **QSEN: Safety**
- Teach adults to avoid tobacco, alcohol, and sun exposure to decrease risk for oral cancer. **QSEN: Evidence-Based Practice**

Psychosocial Integrity

- Assess the patient's response to an oral or esophageal cancer diagnosis, and refer to psychological and community resources as needed. **QSEN: Patient-Centered Care**
- Explain all procedures, restrictions, drug therapy, and follow-up care. **Ethics**

Physiological Integrity

- Assess all patients for oral lesions or tumors. **Clinical Judgment**
- Provide gentle oral care for patients with oral lesions to preserve *tissue integrity*. **QSEN: Safety**
- Monitor the *nutrition* status of patients with GERD, hiatal hernia, and oral or esophageal cancer. **Clinical Judgment**
- Stress the importance of controlling reflux through *nutrition* and drug therapy. **QSEN: Evidence-Based Practice**
- Teach the patient with GERD to elevate the head of the bed or sleep propped up. **QSEN: Evidence-Based Practice**
- Teach the patient with esophageal cancer to report weight loss. **QSEN: Patient-Centered Care**
- Collaborate with the interprofessional team to design a plan of care for the patient with impaired swallowing and/or impaired *nutrition*. **QSEN: Teamwork and Collaboration**

MASTERY QUESTIONS

1. A nurse is caring for a 34-year-old client newly diagnosed with GERD. Which lifestyle change will the nurse suggest? **Select all that apply.**
   A. Lose weight if needed.
   B. Do not eat before bed.
   C. Elevate the foot of your bed by 6 to 12 inches.
   D. Avoid pants with a tight waistband or belt.
   E. Eat fatty foods to minimize ongoing hunger.
2. A client who had the Stretta procedure to treat severe GERD is being discharged. Which client statement requires further nursing teaching? **Select all that apply.**
   A. "Dysphagia after this procedure is normal."
   B. "It's important to stop my proton pump inhibitor."
   C. "I will not take NSAIDs and aspirin for at least 10 days."
   D. "I might cough up some blood following this procedure."
   E. "Today I will drink clear liquids and tomorrow I can eat soft food."
3. A public health nurse is assessing community clients for oral health disorders. Which client is identified at highest risk?
   A. 23-year-old with three dental fillings
   B. 34-year-old with schizophrenia
   C. 55-year-old with stable angina
   D. 62-year-old with irritable bowel syndrome

REFERENCES

American Cancer Society (ACS). (2020a). *Esophageal cancer risk factors.* https://www.cancer.org/cancer/esophagus-cancer/causes-risks-prevention/risk-factors.html.

American Cancer Society (ACS). (2020b). *Targeted therapy for esophageal cancer.* https://www.cancer.org/cancer/esophagus-cancer/treating/targeted-therapy.html.

Argyrou, A., Legaki, E., et al. (2018). Rick factors for gastroesophageal reflux disease and analysis of genetic contributors. *World Journal of Clinical Cases, 6*(8), 176–182.

Brice, S. (2019). Recurrent aphthous stomatitis. In Dellavalle, R. (Ed.), *UpToDate.* Waltham, MA.

Cancer Treatment Centers of America. (2020). *Surgery for oral cancer.* https://www.cancercenter.com/cancer-types/oral-cancer/treatments/surgery.

Commisso, A., & Fidelindo, L. (2019). Lifestyle modifications in adults and older adults with chronic gastroesophageal reflux disease (GERD). *Critical Care Nursing Quarterly, 42*(1), 64–74. https://doi.org/10.1097/CNQ.0000000000000239.

Fischer, D. J., O'Hayre, M., Kusiak, J. W., Somerman, M. J., & Hill, C. V. (2017). Oral health disparities: A perspective from the national institute of dental and craniofacial research. *American Journal of Public Health, 107*(S1), S36–S38. https://doi.org/10.2105/AJPH.2016.303622.

Gyawali, C. P., Kahrilas, P. J., Savarino, E., Zerbib, F., Mion, F., Smout, A., et al. (2018). Modern diagnosis of GERD: The lyon consensus. *Gut, 67,* 1351–1362. https://doi.org/10.1136/gutjnl-2017-314722.

Hellstadius, Y., Lagergren, J., Zylstra, J., Gossage, J., Davies, A., Hultman, C. M., et al. (2017). Prevalence and predictors of anxiety and depression among esophageal cancer patients prior to surgery. *Diseases of the Esophagus, 30*(8), 1–7. https://doi.org/10.1111/dote.12437.

Hoffman, H. (2019). Salivary gland swelling: Evaluation and diagnostic approach. In Deschler, D. (Ed.), *UpToDate.* Waltham, MA.

Kahrilas, P. (2020). Clinical manifestations and diagnosis of gastroesophageal reflux in adults. In Talley, N. (Ed.), *UpToDate.* Waltham, MA.

Kahrilas, P. (2019). Hiatus hernia. In Talley, N. (Ed.), *UpToDate.* Waltham, MA.

Maes, M., Fixen, D., & Linnebur, S. (2017). Adverse effects of proton-pump inhibitor use in older adults: A review of the evidence. *Therapeutic Advances in Drug Safety, 8*(9), 273–297.

McCance, K., Huether, S., Brashers, V., & Rote, N. (2019). *Pathophysiology: The biologic basis for disease in adults and children* (8th ed.). St. Louis: Elsevier.

Mermelstein, J., Chait-Mermelstein, A., & Chait, M. M. (2018). Proton pump inhibitor-refractory gastroesophageal reflux disease: Challenges and solutions. *Clinical and Experimental Gastroenterology, 11,* 119–134. https://doi.org/10.2147/CEG.S121056.

Mountain, C., & Golles, K. (2017). Detecting dysphagia. *American Nurse Today, 12*(5). https://www.americannursetoday.com/detecting-dysphagia/.

National Institutes of Health. (2020). *Genetics home reference: TP53.* www.ghr.nlm.nih.gov/gene/TP53.

Nehra, A. K., Alexander, J. A., Loftus, C. G., & Nehra, V. (2018). Proton pump inhibitors: Review of emerging concerns. *Mayo Clinic Proceedings, 93*(2), 240–246. https://doi.org/10.1016/j.mayocp.2017.10.022.

Oral Cancer Foundation (OCF). (2020). *April is oral cancer awareness month.* https://oralcancerfoundation.org/april-is-oral-cancer-awareness-month/.

Plewa, M. C., & Chatterjee, K. (2020). *Aphthous stomatitis. StatPearls. Treasure island (FL).* StatPearls Publishing. https://www.ncbi.nlm.nih.gov/books/NBK431059/.

Rosen, M., & Blatnik, J. (2019). Surgical management of paraesophageal hernia. In Friedberg, J., & Talley, N. (Eds.), *UpToDate.* Waltham, MA.

Schwaitzberg, S. (2020). Surgical management of gastroesophageal reflux in adults. In Friedberg, J., & Talley, N. (Eds.), *UpToDate.* Waltham, MA.

Swanson, S. (2020). Surgical management of resectable esophageal and esophagogastric junction cancers. In Tanabe, K. (Ed.), *UpToDate.* Waltham, MA.

The Joint Commission. (2020a). *National patient safety Goals, 2020.* https://www.jointcommission.org/standards/national-patient-safety-goals/.

The Joint Commission. (2020b). *Core measures.* https://www.jointcommission.org/measurement/measures/.

Vermeulen, B. D., & Siersema, P. D. (2018). Esophageal stenting in clinical practice: An overview. *Current Treatment Options in Gastroenterology, 16*(2), 260–273. https://doi.org/10.1007/s11938-018-0181-3.

Yamasaki, T., et al. (2018). The changing epidemiology of gastroesophageal reflux disease: Are patients getting younger? *Journal of Neurogastroenterology and Motility, 24*(4), 559–569.

Zhang, C., et al. (2019). Role of polycyclic aromatic hydrocarbons as a co-factor in human papillomavirus–mediated carcinogenesis. *BMC Cancer, 19,* 138.

50

Concepts of Care for Patients With Stomach Disorders

Lara Carver, Jennifer Powers, Donna D. Ignatavicius

http://evolve.elsevier.com/Iggy/

LEARNING OUTCOMES

1. Collaborate with the interprofessional team to manage quality care for patients with *inflammation* and *pain* caused by caused by stomach disorders.
2. Identify community resources for families and patients recovering from stomach disorders.
3. Apply knowledge of pathophysiology of stomach disorders to identify common assessment findings, including actual or risk for impaired *nutrition.*
4. Prioritize evidence-based nursing interventions for patients with stomach disorders to promote *nutrition* and manage *infection.*
5. Plan transition management and care coordination for the patient who has stomach disorders, including health teaching.

KEY TERMS

dumping syndrome A postgastrectomy condition that refers to a group of vasomotor symptoms that occur after eating.

dyspepsia An epigastric burning sensation, often referred to as "heartburn."

gastrectomy Surgical removal of all (total gastrectomy) or part (subtotal gastrectomy) of the stomach.

gastritis The *inflammation* of gastric mucosa (stomach lining).

hematemesis Vomiting bright red or coffee-ground blood.

melena Dark, "tarry" (sticky) stool, indicating occult blood caused by digestion of blood within the small intestine.

peptic ulcer disease A condition that results when GI mucosal defenses become impaired and no longer protect the epithelium from the effects of acid and pepsin.

peritonitis An abdominal *infection* in which the abdomen is tender, rigid, and boardlike.

stress ulcer Acute gastric mucosal lesion occurring after an acute medical crisis or trauma, such as sepsis or a head injury, or surgery.

✳ PRIORITY AND INTERRELATED CONCEPTS

The priority concept for this chapter is:

- *Infection*

  The *Infection* concept exemplar for this chapter is Peptic Ulcer Disease (PUD).

The interrelated concepts for this chapter are:

- *Inflammation*
- *Nutrition*
- *Pain*

The stomach is part of the upper GI system that is responsible for a large part of the digestive process. It is affected by only a few diseases, including gastritis, peptic ulcer disease (PUD), and cancer, yet these conditions can be very serious and sometimes life threatening. Each of these health problems can result in impaired or altered *nutrition. Inflammation* and *infection* can cause *pain* and discomfort. Chapter 3 briefly reviews each of these health concepts.

GASTRITIS

Gastritis is the *inflammation* of gastric mucosa (stomach lining) (see complete discussion of inflammation in Chapter 16). It can be classified according to cause, cellular changes, or distribution of the lesions, and can be erosive (causing ulcers) or nonerosive. Although the mucosal changes that result from *acute* gastritis typically heal after several months, this is not true for *chronic* gastritis.

Pathophysiology Review

Prostaglandins provide a protective mucosal barrier that prevents the stomach from digesting itself. If there is a break in the protective barrier, mucosal injury can occur. The resulting injury is worsened by histamine release and vagal nerve stimulation. Hydrochloric acid can then diffuse back into the mucosa and injure small vessels. This back-diffusion can cause edema, bleeding, and erosion of the stomach's lining.

Inflammation of the gastric mucosa or submucosa after exposure to local irritants or other causes can result in *acute gastritis*. The early pathologic manifestation of gastritis is a thickened, reddened mucous membrane with prominent rugae, or folds. Various degrees of mucosal necrosis and inflammation occur in acute disease. The diagnosis cannot be based solely on clinical symptoms. If the stomach muscle is not involved, complete recovery usually occurs in a few days with no residual evidence of gastric *inflammation*. If the muscle is affected, bleeding or hemorrhage may occur during an episode of acute gastritis.

Long-term NSAID use creates a high risk for acute gastritis. NSAIDs inhibit prostaglandin production in the mucosal barrier. Other risk factors include use of alcohol, coffee, and caffeine. Stress and cigarette smoking are considered risk factors for the development of acute gastritis (Ankita et al., 2017). Local irritation from radiation therapy and accidental or intentional ingestion of corrosive substances, including acids or alkalis (e.g., lye and drain cleaners), can also cause acute gastritis. Use of drugs such as steroids, aldosterone antagonists, and selective serotonin reuptake inhibitors can contribute to gastroduodenal *inflammation* and ulceration.

Chronic gastritis appears as a patchy, diffuse (spread out) *inflammation* of the mucosal lining of the stomach. As the disease progresses, the walls and lining of the stomach thin and atrophy. With progressive gastric atrophy from chronic mucosal injury, the function of the parietal (acid-secreting) cells decreases, and the source of intrinsic factor is lost. Intrinsic factor is critical for absorption of vitamin B_{12}. When body stores of vitamin B_{12} are eventually depleted, pernicious anemia results. The amount and concentration of acid in stomach secretions gradually decrease until the secretions consist of only mucus and water.

The most common form of chronic gastritis is type B gastritis, caused by *Helicobacter pylori* **infection**. A direct correlation exists between the number of organisms and the degree of cellular abnormality present. The host response to the *H. pylori* infection is activation of lymphocytes and neutrophils. Release of inflammatory cytokines, such as interleukin (IL)-1, IL-8, and tumor necrosis factor–alpha (TNF-α), damages the gastric mucosa (McCance et al., 2019).

Chronic gastritis is associated with an increased risk for gastric cancer. The persistent **inflammation** extends deep into the mucosa, causing gastric gland destruction and cellular changes (McCance et al., 2019). Chronic local irritation and toxic effects caused by alcohol ingestion, radiation therapy, and smoking have been linked to chronic gastritis. Surgical procedures that involve the pyloric sphincter, such as pyloroplasty, can lead to gastritis by causing reflux of alkaline secretions into the stomach. Other systemic disorders such as Crohn's disease, graft-versus-host disease, and uremia can also precipitate the development of chronic gastritis (McCance et al., 2019).

Health Promotion and Maintenance

Gastritis is a very common health problem in the United States. A balanced diet, regular exercise, and stress-reduction techniques can help prevent it (see the Patient and Family Education: Preparing for Self-Management: Gastritis Prevention box).

PATIENT AND FAMILY EDUCATION: PREPARING FOR SELF-MANAGEMENT

Gastritis Prevention

- Eat a well-balanced diet and exercise regularly.
- Avoid drinking excessive amounts of alcoholic beverages.
- Do not take large doses of aspirin, other NSAIDs (e.g., ibuprofen), or corticosteroids.
- Avoid excessive intake of coffee (even decaffeinated).
- Be sure that foods and water are safe to avoid contamination.
- Manage stress levels using complementary and integrative therapies such as relaxation and meditation techniques.
- Stop smoking and/or using other forms of tobacco.
- Protect yourself against exposure to toxic substances in the workplace such as lead and nickel.
- Seek medical treatment if you are experiencing symptoms of gastroesophageal reflux (see Chapter 49).

A balanced diet includes following the recommendations of the U.S. Department of Agriculture (USDA) and limiting intake of foods and spices that can cause gastric distress, such as caffeine, chocolate, mustard, pepper, and other strong or hot spices. Alcohol and tobacco should also be avoided. Regular exercise maintains peristalsis, which helps prevent gastric contents from irritating the gastric mucosa. Stress-reduction techniques can include aerobic exercise, meditation, and/or yoga, depending on individual preferences.

❖ Interprofessional Collaborative Care

Care of the patient with gastritis usually takes place in the community setting. However, if symptoms are severe, the patient may be hospitalized.

◆ **Assessment: Recognize Cues.** Symptoms of *acute gastritis* range from mild to severe. Clients typically report a rapid onset of epigastric **pain** and dyspepsia (an epigastric burning sensation, often referred to as "heartburn"). In some cases, gastric bleeding may occur and manifest as hematemesis (vomiting bright red or coffee-ground blood), or melena (dark, "tarry" [sticky] stool, indicating occult blood caused by digestion of blood within the small intestine).

Gastritis or food poisoning caused by endotoxins, such as staphylococcal endotoxin, has an abrupt onset. Severe nausea and vomiting often occur within 5 hours of ingestion of the contaminated food. *In some cases gastric hemorrhage is the presenting symptom, which is a life-threatening emergency.*

Chronic gastritis causes few symptoms unless ulceration occurs. Patients may report nausea, vomiting, or upper abdominal discomfort. Periodic epigastric **pain** may occur after a meal. Some patients have anorexia.

Esophagogastroduodenoscopy (EGD) via an endoscope with biopsy is the gold standard for diagnosing gastritis. (See Chapter 48 for discussion of nursing care associated with this diagnostic procedure.) The primary health care provider performs a biopsy to establish a definitive diagnosis of the type of gastritis. If lesions are patchy and diffuse, biopsy of several suspicious areas may be necessary to avoid misdiagnosis. A *cytologic examination* of the biopsy specimen is performed to confirm or rule out gastric cancer. Tissue samples can also be taken to detect *H. pylori infection* using *rapid urease testing.* The results of these tests are more reliable if the patient has discontinued taking antacids and proton pump inhibitors (PPIs) for at least a week (Pagana & Pagana, 2018; Pagana et al., 2019).

◆ **Interventions: Take Action.** Patients with gastritis are not often seen in the acute care setting unless they have an exacerbation ("flare-up") of acute or chronic gastritis that results in fluid and electrolyte imbalance, bleeding, or increased *pain.* Collaborative care is directed toward supportive care for relieving the symptoms and removing or reducing the cause of discomfort.

Acute gastritis is treated symptomatically and supportively because the healing process is spontaneous, usually occurring within a few days. When the cause is removed, *pain* and discomfort usually subside. If bleeding occurs, a blood transfusion and fluid replacement may be given. Surgery, such as partial gastrectomy, pyloroplasty, and/or vagotomy, may be needed for patients with major bleeding or ulceration. (See discussion of gastric surgery procedures in this chapter later under Gastric Cancer.)

Eliminating the causative factor(s) is the primary treatment approach for *acute* gastritis. *Nutrition* and drug therapy may also be used. Teach the patient to limit intake of any foods and spices that cause distress, such as those that contain caffeine or high acid content (e.g., tomato products, citrus juices) or those that are heavily seasoned with strong or hot spices. Bell peppers and onions are also commonly irritating foods. Most patients seem to progress better with a bland, nonspicy diet and smaller, more frequent meals. Alcohol and tobacco should also be avoided.

The primary health care provider often prescribes drugs that block and buffer gastric acid secretions to relieve *pain.* H_2-*receptor antagonists,* such as famotidine and nizatidine, are typically used to block gastric secretions. Sucralfate, a *mucosal barrier fortifier,* may also be prescribed. Antisecretory agents *(proton pump inhibitors [PPIs]),* such as omeprazole or pantoprazole, may be prescribed to suppress gastric acid. *Antacids* used as buffering agents include aluminum hydroxide combined with magnesium hydroxide and aluminum hydroxide combined with simethicone and magnesium hydroxide (see the Common Examples of Drug Therapy: Gastritis and Peptic Ulcer Disease box). Calcium carbonate (chewable or liquid) is also a potent antacid, but it triggers gastrin release, causing rebound acid secretion.

Teach the patient about various techniques that reduce stress and *pain,* such as progressive relaxation, cutaneous stimulation, guided imagery, and distraction. Table 50.1 lists commonly used complementary and integrative therapies for gastritis and peptic ulcer disease.

Treatment of *chronic* gastritis varies with the cause. The approach to management includes the elimination of causative agents, treatment of any underlying disease (e.g., chronic kidney disease, Crohn's disease), avoidance of toxic substances (e.g., alcohol, tobacco), and health teaching.

Patients with *chronic* gastritis may require vitamin B_{12} for prevention or treatment of pernicious anemia. If *H. pylori* is found, the primary health care provider treats the *infection.* Current practice for infection treatment is described in the Drug Therapy discussion in the Peptic Ulcer Disease section.

TABLE 50.1   Commonly Used Complementary and Integrative Therapies for Gastritis and Peptic Ulcer Disease (PUD)

Herbs and Vitamins	Homeopathy
• Cranberry	• Carbo vegetabilis
• Deglycyrrhizinated licorice (DGL)	• Ipecacuanha
• Zinc	• Nux vomica
• Ginger	• Pulsatilla
• Glutamine	
• Acidophilus	
• Probiotics	
• Slippery elm	
• Vitamin A	
• Vitamin C	

✴ INFECTION CONCEPT EXEMPLAR: PEPTIC ULCER DISEASE (PUD)

Peptic ulcer disease (PUD) results when GI mucosal defenses become impaired and no longer protect the epithelium from the effects of acid and pepsin.

Pathophysiology Review

Types of Ulcers. Three types of peptic ulcers may occur: duodenal ulcers, gastric ulcers, and stress ulcers (less common). Many ulcers are caused by *H. pylori infection* (National Institute of Diabetes and Digestive and Kidney Diseases, 2020). The most common route of *H. pylori* infection transmission is either oral-to-oral (stomach contents are transmitted from mouth to mouth) or fecal-to-oral (from stool to mouth) contact.

As a response to the bacteria, cytokines, neutrophils, and other substances are activated and cause epithelial cell necrosis. Urease produced by *H. pylori* breaks down urea into ammonia, which neutralizes the acidity of the stomach. In addition, the helical shape of *H. pylori* allows the bacterium to burrow into the mucus layer of the stomach and become undetectable by the body's immune cells. Although this bacterium does not cause illness in most people, it is a major risk factor for peptic ulcers and gastric cancer (McCance et al., 2019).

Duodenal ulcers occur more often than other types. Most duodenal ulcers present in the upper portion of the duodenum. They are deep, sharply demarcated lesions that penetrate through the mucosa and submucosa into the muscularis propria (muscle layer). The floor of the ulcer consists of a necrotic area residing on granulation tissue and surrounded by areas of fibrosis (McCance et al., 2019) (Fig. 50.1).

The main feature of a duodenal ulcer is high gastric acid secretion, although a wide range of secretory levels are found. In patients with duodenal ulcers, pH levels are low (excess acid) in the duodenum for long periods. Protein-rich meals, calcium, and vagus nerve excitation stimulate acid secretion. Combined with hypersecretion, a rapid emptying of food from the stomach reduces the buffering effect of food and delivers a large acid bolus to the duodenum. Inhibitory secretory mechanisms and pancreatic secretion may be insufficient to control the acid load.

⬭ COMMON EXAMPLES OF DRUG THERAPY

Gastritis and Peptic Ulcer Disease

Class and Common Examples	Selected Nursing Implications
Antacids	
Increase pH of gastric contents by deactivating pepsin	
Magnesium hydroxide with aluminum hydroxide	Give 2 hr after meals and at bedtime. *Hydrogen ion load is high after ingestion of foods.*
	Use liquid rather than tablets. *Suspensions are more effective than chewable tablets.*
	Do not give other drugs within 1-2 hr of antacids. *Antacids interfere with absorption of other drugs.*
	Assess patients for a history of chronic kidney disease. *Hypermagnesemia may result, especially in patients with poorly functioning kidneys, thus causing toxicity.*
	Assess the patient for a history of heart failure. *Inadequate renal perfusion from heart failure decreases the ability of the kidneys to excrete magnesium, thus causing toxicity.*
	Observe the patient for the side effect of diarrhea. *Magnesium often causes diarrhea.*
Aluminum hydroxide	Give 1 hr after meals and at bedtime. *Hydrogen ion load is high after ingestion of food.*
	Use liquid rather than tablets if palatable. *Suspensions are more effective than chewable tablets.*
	Do not give other drugs within 1-2 hr of antacids. *Antacids interfere with absorption of other drugs.*
	Observe patients for the side effect of constipation. If constipation occurs, consider alternating with magnesium antacid. *Aluminum causes constipation, and magnesium has a laxative effect.*
	Use for patients with chronic kidney disease. *Aluminum binds with phosphates in the GI tract. This antacid does not contain magnesium.*
H₂ Antagonists (Blockers)	
Decrease gastric acid secretions by blocking histamine receptors in parietal cells	
Famotidine	Give single dose at bedtime for treatment of heartburn and PUD. *Bedtime administration suppresses nocturnal acid production.*
Nizatidine	
NOTE: IV famotidine may also be given to prevent surgical stress ulcers.	
Mucosal Barrier Fortifiers	
Protect stomach mucosa	
Sucralfate	Give 1 hr before and 2 hr after meals and at bedtime. *Food may interfere with drug's adherence to mucosa.*
	Do not give within 30 min of giving antacids or other drugs. *Antacids may interfere with effect*
Bismuth subsalicylate	Remind patient to refrain from taking aspirin while on this drug. *Aspirin is a salicylic acid and can lead to overdose.*
Proton Pump Inhibitors	
Suppress HK–ATPase enzyme system of gastric acid secretion to suppress acid	
Omeprazole	Have patients take capsule whole; do not crush. *Delayed-release capsules allow absorption after granules leave the stomach.*
	Give 30 min before the main meal of the day. *The proton pump is activated by the presence of food. Therefore the drug needs a chance to work before the patient eats.*
Lansoprazole	Give 30 min before the main meal of the day. *The proton pump is activated by the presence of food. Therefore the drug needs a chance to work before the patient eats.*
Rabeprazole	Take after the morning meal. *This drug promotes healing and symptom relief of duodenal ulcers.*
	Do not crush capsule. *This drug is a sustained-release capsule.*
Pantoprazole	Do not crush. *This drug is enteric coated.*
	IV form must be given on a pump with a filter and in a separate line. *Given IV, this drug precipitates easily.*
	Do not give IV pantoprazole with other IV drugs.
	Monitor for adverse drug interactions if patient is on other medications. *The IV form is not compatible with most other drugs. This drug will alter how other drugs are metabolized, either increasing or decreasing their effectiveness.*
Esomeprazole	Assess for hepatic impairment. *Patients with severe hepatic problems need a low dose.*
	Do not give Nexium IV with other IV drugs. *The IV form is not compatible with most other drugs.*
	Monitor for adverse drug interactions if patient is on other medications. *This drug will alter how other drugs are metabolized, either increasing or decreasing the effectiveness.*

Continued

💊 COMMON EXAMPLES OF DRUG THERAPY—cont'd

Gastritis and Peptic Ulcer Disease

Class and Common Examples	Selected Nursing Implications
Prostaglandin Analogs Stimulate mucosal protection and decrease gastric acid secretions	
Misoprostol	Not commonly given, but used for clients receiving NSAIDs to *protect the stomach mucosa.* Avoid magnesium-containing antacids. *Misoprostol and magnesium-containing antacids can cause diarrhea.* Do not administer to pregnant women. *This drug can cause abortion, premature birth, or birth defects.*
Antimicrobials Treat *H. pylori* infection	
Clarithromycin	Give with caution to patients with renal impairment; monitor renal function laboratory values. *This drug can increase the patient's BUN level and should be monitored.*
Amoxicillin	Teach patients to take the drug with food or immediately after a meal. *This drug can cause GI disturbances, including nausea, vomiting, and diarrhea.*
Tetracycline	Teach patients to take the drug at least 1 hr before meals or 2 hr after meals. *Dairy products and other foods may interfere with drug absorption.* Teach patients to avoid direct sunlight and wear sunscreen when outdoors. *This drug can cause the skin to burn as a result of photosensitivity.*
Metronidazole	Teach patients to take the drug with food. *This drug can cause GI disturbances, especially nausea.* Teach patients to avoid alcohol during drug therapy and for at least 3 days after therapy is completed. *The patient can experience a drug-alcohol reaction, including severe nausea, vomiting, and headache.*

BUN, Blood urea nitrogen; *PUD,* peptic ulcer disease.

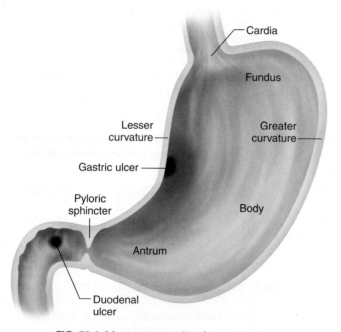

FIG. 50.1 Most common sites for peptic ulcers.

Gastric ulcers usually develop in the antrum of the stomach near acid-secreting mucosa (see Fig. 50.1). When a break in the mucosal barrier occurs (such as that caused by *H. pylori infection*), hydrochloric acid injures the epithelium. Gastric ulcers may then result from back-diffusion of acid or dysfunction of the pyloric sphincter. Without normal functioning of the pyloric sphincter, bile refluxes (backs up) into the stomach. This reflux of bile acids may break the integrity of the mucosal barrier, which leads to mucosal **inflammation.** Toxic agents and bile then destroy the membrane of the gastric mucosa.

Gastric emptying is often delayed in patients with gastric ulceration. This causes regurgitation of duodenal contents, which worsens the gastric mucosal injury. Decreased blood flow to the gastric mucosa may also alter the defense barrier and thereby allow ulceration to occur.

Stress ulcers are acute gastric mucosal lesions occurring after an acute medical crisis or trauma, such as sepsis or a head injury. In the patient who is NPO for major surgery, gastritis may lead to stress ulcers. Patients who are critically ill, especially those with extensive burns (Curling ulcer), sepsis (ischemic ulcer), or increased intracranial pressure (Cushing ulcer), are also susceptible to these ulcers. Stress ulcers are associated with lengthened hospital stay and increased mortality rates. Therefore most patients who have major trauma or surgery receive IV drug therapy (e.g., PPIs) to prevent stress ulcer development.

Bleeding caused by gastric erosion is the main manifestation of acute stress ulcers. Multifocal lesions associated with stress ulcers occur in the stomach and proximal duodenum. These lesions begin as areas of ischemia and evolve into erosions and ulcerations that may progress to massive hemorrhage.

Complications of Ulcers. The most common complications of PUD are hemorrhage, perforation, pyloric obstruction, and intractable disease. *Hemorrhage is the most serious complication.* It tends to occur more often in patients with *gastric* ulcers and in older adults. Many patients have a second episode of bleeding if underlying **infection** with *H. pylori* remains untreated

KEY FEATURES

Upper GI Bleeding

- Bright red or coffee-ground vomitus (hematemesis)
- Melena (tarry or dark sticky stools)
- Decreased hemoglobin and hematocrit
- Decreased blood pressure
- Increased heart rate
- Weak peripheral pulses
- Acute confusion (in older adults)
- Vertigo
- Dizziness or light-headedness
- Syncope (loss of consciousness)

or if therapy does not include an H_2 antagonist. With massive bleeding the patient vomits bright red or coffee-ground blood (**hematemesis**). Gastric acid digestion of blood typically results in the coffee-ground appearance. Hematemesis usually indicates bleeding at or above the duodenojejunal junction (upper GI bleeding). Other signs and symptoms are listed in the Key Features: Upper GI Bleeding box.

Minimal bleeding from ulcers manifests with occult blood in a dark, "tarry" stool (**melena**). Melena may occur in patients with gastric ulcers but is more common in those with duodenal ulcers.

Gastric and duodenal ulcers can perforate and bleed (Fig. 50.2). *Perforation* occurs when the ulcer becomes so deep that the entire thickness of the stomach or duodenum is worn away. The stomach or duodenal contents can then leak into the peritoneal cavity. Sudden, sharp **pain** begins in the mid-epigastric region and spreads over the entire abdomen. The amount of pain correlates with the amount and type of GI contents spilled. The classic pain causes the patient to be apprehensive. The abdomen is tender, rigid, and boardlike as a result of this **infection** (**peritonitis**). The patient often assumes a "fetal" position to decrease the tension on the abdominal muscles. He or she can become severely ill within hours. Bacterial septicemia and hypovolemic shock can follow. Peristalsis diminishes, and paralytic ileus develops. *Peptic ulcer perforation is a surgical emergency and can be life threatening!*

NCLEX EXAMINATION CHALLENGE 50.1

Safe and Effective Care Environment

The nurse is caring for a client diagnosed with peptic ulcer disease (PUD). For which potential complications will the nurse monitor? **Select all that apply.**
A. Pneumonia
B. Peritonitis
C. Anemia
D. Stroke
E. Hypotension
F. Cirrhosis

Pyloric (gastric outlet) obstruction (blockage) occurs in a small percentage of patients and manifests with vomiting caused by stasis and gastric dilation. Obstruction occurs at the pylorus (the gastric outlet) and is caused by scarring, edema, inflammation, or a combination of these factors. Symptoms of obstruction include abdominal bloating, nausea, and vomiting. When vomiting persists, the

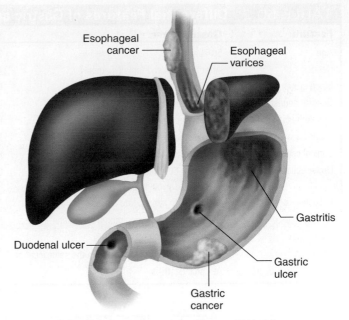

FIG. 50.2 Common causes of upper GI bleeding.

patient may have *metabolic alkalosis* from loss of large quantities of acid gastric juice (hydrogen and chloride ions) in the vomitus. *Hypokalemia* may also result from the vomiting or metabolic alkalosis.

Many patients with ulcers have a single episode with no recurrence. However, *intractability* may develop from complications of ulcers, excessive stressors in the patient's life, or an inability to adhere to long-term therapy. He or she no longer responds to conservative management, or recurrences of symptoms interfere with ADLs. In general, the patient continues to have recurrent pain despite treatment. Those who fail to respond to traditional treatments or who have a relapse after discontinuation of therapy are referred to a gastroenterology practitioner.

Etiology and Genetic Risk. Peptic ulcer disease is caused most often by bacterial **infection** with *H. pylori* and long-term use of NSAIDs such as ibuprofen. NSAIDs break down the mucosal barrier and disrupt the mucosal protection mediated systemically by cyclooxygenase (COX) inhibition. Other risk factors for PUD are the same as for gastritis (see discussion earlier in this chapter). Patients with duodenal ulcers often have a positive family history of the disease.

Incidence and Prevalence. PUD affects millions of adults across the world. In the United States, the prevalence of PUD is over 15 million (McCance et al., 2019). However, primary health care provider visits, hospitalizations, and the mortality rate for PUD have decreased in the past few decades, in part because of the use of proton pump inhibitors and earlier treatment for *H. pylori*.

❖ Interprofessional Collaborative Care

Care of the patient with PUD generally takes place in the community setting, unless the patient develops a more serious condition such as upper GI bleeding, which requires acute management.

TABLE 50.2   Differential Features of Gastric and Duodenal Ulcers

Feature	Gastric Ulcer	Duodenal Ulcer
Age	50-70 yr	20-50 yr
Gender	Affects males and females equally	Affects males and females equally
Blood group	No differentiation	Most often type O
General nourishment	May be malnourished	Usually well nourished
Stomach acid production	Normal secretion or hyposecretion	Hypersecretion
Occurrence	Mucosa exposed to acid-pepsin secretion	Mucosa exposed to acid-pepsin secretion; positive family history
Clinical course	Healing and recurrence	Healing and recurrence
Upper abdominal pain	Occurs 30-60 min after a meal; at night, rarely Worsened by ingestion of food	Occurs 1½-3 hr after a meal; at night: often awakens patient between 1 and 2 a.m. Relieved by ingestion of food
Response to treatment	Healing with appropriate therapy	Remissions and exacerbations
Hemorrhage	Hematemesis more common than melena	Melena more common than hematemesis
Cancer risk	Increased, but in less than 10%	Not increased
Recurrence	Tends to heal and recurs often in the same location	60% recur within 1 yr; 90% recur within 2 yr
Surrounding mucosa	Atrophic gastritis	No gastritis

◆ Assessment: Recognize Cues

History. A history of current or past medical conditions focuses on GI problems, particularly any history of diagnosis or treatment for *H. pylori* **infection.** Review all prescription and OTC drugs the patient is taking. Specifically inquire whether the patient is taking corticosteroids, chemotherapy, or NSAIDs. Also ask whether he or she has ever undergone radiation treatments. Assess whether the patient has had any GI surgeries, especially a partial gastrectomy, which can cause chronic gastritis.

Collect data related to the causes and risk factors for peptic ulcer disease (PUD). Question the patient about factors that can influence the development of PUD, including alcohol intake and tobacco use. Note if certain foods such as tomatoes or caffeinated beverages precipitate or worsen symptoms. Information regarding actual or perceived daily stressors should also be obtained.

A history of GI upset, pain and its relationship to eating and sleep patterns, and actions taken to relieve pain are also important. Inquire about any changes in the character of the pain because this may signal the development of complications. For example, if ***pain*** that was once intermittent and relieved by food and antacids becomes constant and radiates to the back or upper quadrant, the patient may have ulcer perforation. However, many adults with active duodenal or gastric ulcers report having no ulcer symptoms.

Physical Assessment/Signs and Symptoms. Physical assessment findings may reveal epigastric tenderness and ***pain***, usually located at the midline between the umbilicus and the xiphoid process. *If perforation into the peritoneal cavity is present, the patient typically has a rigid, boardlike abdomen accompanied by rebound tenderness and intense pain* (**peritonitis**). Initially, auscultation of the abdomen may reveal hyperactive bowel sounds, but these may diminish with progression of the **infection.** Perform a comprehensive pain assessment. **Dyspepsia** is the most commonly reported symptom associated with PUD. It is typically described as sharp, burning, or gnawing pain. Some patients may perceive discomfort as a sensation of abdominal pressure or of fullness or hunger. Specific differences between gastric and duodenal ulcers are listed in Table 50.2 (McCance et al., 2019).

To assess for fluid volume deficit that may occur from a bleeding ulcer, take orthostatic blood pressures and monitor for signs and symptoms of dehydration. Also assess for dizziness, especially when the patient is upright, because this is a symptom of fluid volume deficit. *Older adults often experience dizziness when they get out of bed and are at risk for falls.*

Psychosocial Assessment. Assess the impact of ulcer disease on the patient's lifestyle, occupation, family, and social and leisure activities. Evaluate the impact that lifestyle changes will have on the patient and family. This assessment may reveal information about the patient's ability to adhere to the prescribed treatment regimen and obtain the needed social support to alter his or her lifestyle.

Laboratory Assessment. There are three simple, noninvasive tests to detect *H. pylori* in the patient's blood, breath, or stool. Although the breath and stool tests are considered more accurate, *serologic testing* for *H. pylori* antibodies is the most common method to confirm *H. pylori* infection. The *urea breath test* involves swallowing a capsule, liquid, or pudding that contains urea with a special carbon atom. After a few minutes the patient exhales; and, if the special carbon atom is found, the bacterium is present. The *stool antigen test* is performed on a stool sample provided by the patient, which is tested for *H. pylori* antigens. Patients who have bleeding from a peptic ulcer may have *decreased hemoglobin and hematocrit* values. The *stool* may also be positive for occult (not seen) blood if bleeding is present (Pagana & Pagana, 2018; Pagana et al., 2019).

Other Diagnostic Assessment. *The major diagnostic test for PUD is esophagogastroduodenoscopy (EGD), which is the most accurate means of establishing a diagnosis.* Direct visualization of the ulcer crater by EGD allows the primary health care provider to take specimens for *H. pylori* testing and biopsy and cytologic studies for ruling out gastric cancer. The *rapid urease test* can confirm a quick diagnosis because urease is produced by the bacteria in the gastric mucosa. EGD may be repeated at 4- to 6-week intervals while the primary health care provider evaluates the progress of healing in response to therapy. Chapter 48 describes this test in more detail.

GI bleeding may be tested using a *nuclear medicine scan.* No special preparation is required for this scan. The patient is injected with a contrast medium (usually technetium [^{99m}Tc]), and the GI system is scanned for the presence of bleeding after a waiting period. A second scan may be done 1 to 2 days after treatment for the bleeding to determine if the interventions were effective.

◆ **Analysis: Analyze Cues and Prioritize Hypotheses.** The priority collaborative problems for patients with peptic ulcer disease (PUD) include:

1. Acute or persistent *pain* due to gastric and/or duodenal ulceration
2. Potential for upper GI bleeding due to gastric and/or duodenal ulceration or perforation

◆ **Planning and Implementation: Generate Solutions and Take Action**

Managing Acute or Persistent Pain

Planning: Expected Outcomes. The patient with PUD is expected to report pain control as evidenced by no more than a 3 on a 0 to 10 pain intensity scale.

Interventions. PUD causes significant discomfort that affects many aspects of daily living. Interventions to manage pain focus on drug therapy and dietary changes.

Drug Therapy. The primary purposes of drug therapy in the treatment of PUD are to (1) provide *pain* relief, (2) eliminate *H. pylori infection,* (3) heal ulcerations, and (4) prevent recurrence. Several different regimens can be used. Although numerous drugs have been evaluated for the treatment of *H. pylori* infection, no single agent has been used successfully against the organism. A common drug regimen for *H. pylori* infection is PPI–triple therapy, which includes a proton pump inhibitor (PPI), such as lansoprazole, plus two antibiotics such as metronidazole and tetracycline or clarithromycin and amoxicillin for 10 to 14 days. Some primary health care providers may prefer to use quadruple therapy, which contains a combination of a proton pump inhibitor (PPI), any two commonly used antibiotics as described previously, and the addition of bismuth. Bismuth therapy is often used in patients who are allergic to penicillin-based medications.

Bismuth subsalicylate inhibits *H. pylori* from binding to the mucosal lining and stimulates mucosal protection and prostaglandin production. Teach patients that they cannot take aspirin while on this drug because aspirin is a salicylic acid and could cause an overdose of salicylates. Patients should also be taught that bismuth may cause the stools and/or tongue to be discolored black. This discoloration is temporary and harmless.

> ### 👤 PATIENT-CENTERED CARE: OLDER ADULT CONSIDERATIONS (QSEN)
>
> Many older adults have *H. pylori* infection that is undiagnosed because of vague symptoms associated with physiologic changes of aging and comorbidities that mask **dyspepsia**. Because the average age of gastric cancer diagnosis is 70 years, it is important to teach older adults about the symptoms of PUD and to consider *H. pylori* screening. Early detection and aggressive treatment can prevent PUD and gastric cancer.

Hyposecretory drugs reduce gastric acid secretions and are therefore used for both peptic ulcer disease (PUD) and gastritis management. The primary prescribed drugs include proton pump inhibitors and H₂-receptor antagonists (see the Common Examples of Drug Therapy: Gastritis and Peptic Ulcer Disease box).

A *proton pump inhibitor (PPI) is the drug class of choice for treating patients with acid-related disorders.* Omeprazole, lansoprazole, and esomeprazole are each available as delayed-release capsules designed to release their contents after they pass through the stomach. Omeprazole and lansoprazole may be dissolved in a sodium bicarbonate solution and given through any feeding tube. Bicarbonate protects the dissolved omeprazole and lansoprazole granules in gastric acid. Therefore the drugs are still absorbed correctly. These capsules can also be opened. The enteric-coated capsules can be put in apple juice or orange juice and given through a large-bore feeding tube. Rabeprazole and pantoprazole are enteric-coated tablets that quickly dissolve after the tablet has moved through the stomach and should not be crushed before they are taken. Several of the PPIs, such as pantoprazole, are also available in an IV form, which is useful for patients who are NPO (Burchum & Rosenthal, 2019).

Some patients use PPIs for years and perhaps a lifetime; these patients should be assessed periodically to determine the necessity of PPI use. Some studies have suggested there may be an increased risk of osteoporotic fractures related to long-term PPI use, yet current research is ongoing to determine if there is a definitive link (Burchum & Rosenthal, 2019). Omeprazole reduces the effect of clopidogrel, an antiplatelet drug. Teach patients to tell their primary health care provider if they are taking clopidogrel. PPIs should not be discontinued abruptly, to prevent rebound activation of the proton pump; a step-down approach over several days is recommended (Burchum & Rosenthal, 2019).

Nutrition Therapy. The role of diet in the management of ulcer disease is controversial. There is no evidence that dietary restriction reduces gastric acid secretion or promotes tissue healing, although a bland diet may assist in relieving symptoms. Food itself acts as an antacid by neutralizing gastric acid for 30 to 60 minutes. An increased rate of gastric acid secretion, called *rebound,* may follow.

> ### ❗ NURSING SAFETY PRIORITY (QSEN)
> #### *Action Alert*
>
> Teach the patient with peptic ulcer disease to follow healthy *nutrition* habits and avoid substances that increase gastric acid secretion. This includes caffeine-containing beverages (coffee, tea, cola). Both caffeinated and decaffeinated coffees should be avoided because coffee contains peptides that stimulate gastrin release (Priyanka et al., 2016).

Teach the patient to exclude any foods that cause discomfort. A bland, nonirritating diet is recommended during the acute symptomatic phase. Bedtime snacks are avoided because they may stimulate gastric acid secretion. Eating six smaller meals daily may help, but this regimen is no longer a regular part of therapy. No evidence supports the theory that eating six meals daily promotes healing of the ulcer. This practice may actually stimulate gastric acid secretion. Patients should avoid alcohol and tobacco because of their stimulatory effects on gastric acid secretion.

Complementary and Integrative Health. Teach patients about complementary and integrative therapies that can reduce stress, including hypnosis and imagery. For example, the use of yoga and meditation techniques has demonstrated a beneficial effect on anxiety disorders. Many have suggested that GI disorders result from the dysfunction of both the GI tract itself and the brain. This means that emotional stress is thought to worsen GI disorders such as peptic ulcer disease. Yoga may alter the activities of the central and autonomic nervous systems.

Herbs and other supplements may be used by some patients as discussed earlier in this chapter under Gastritis.

Managing Upper GI Bleeding

Planning: Expected Outcomes. The patient with upper GI bleeding (often called *upper GI hemorrhage* or *UGH*) is expected to have bleeding promptly and effectively controlled and vital signs within normal limits.

Interventions. Blood loss from PUD results in high morbidity and mortality. Fluid volume loss secondary to vomiting can lead to dehydration and electrolyte imbalances. Interventions aimed at managing complications associated with PUD include prevention and/or management of bleeding, perforation, and gastric outlet obstruction. In some cases surgical treatment of complications becomes necessary.

Nonsurgical Management. Because prevention or early detection of complications is needed to obtain a positive clinical outcome, monitor the patient carefully and immediately report changes to the Rapid Response Team or primary health care provider.

Emergency: upper GI bleeding. The patient who is actively bleeding has a life-threatening emergency and needs supportive therapy to prevent hypovolemic shock and possible death (Farrar, 2018).

! NURSING SAFETY PRIORITY (QSEN)

Critical Rescue

> Recognize that your priority for care of the patient with upper GI bleeding is to maintain **a**irway, **b**reathing, and **c**irculation (ABCs). Respond to these needs by providing oxygen and other ventilatory support as needed, starting two large-bore IV lines for replacing fluids and blood, and monitoring vital signs, hematocrit, and oxygen saturation.

The purpose of managing hypovolemia is to expand intravascular fluid in a patient who is volume depleted. Carefully monitor the patient's fluid status, including intake and output. *Fluid replacement in older adults should be closely monitored to prevent fluid overload.* Serum electrolytes are also assessed because depletions from vomiting or nasogastric suctioning must be replaced. Volume replacement with isotonic solutions (e.g., 0.9% normal saline solution, lactated Ringer's solution) should be started immediately. The primary health care provider may prescribe blood products such as packed red blood cells (PRBCs) to expand volume and correct a low hemoglobin and hematocrit. For patients with active bleeding, fresh frozen plasma may be given if the prothrombin time is 1.5 times higher than the midrange control value (Farrar, 2018).

Continue to monitor the patient's hematocrit, hemoglobin, and coagulation studies for changes from the baseline measurements. With mild bleeding (less than 500 mL), slight feelings of weakness and mild perspiration may be present. When blood loss exceeds 1 L/24 hr, manifestations of hypovolemic shock may occur, such as hypotension, chills, palpitations, diaphoresis, and a weak, thready pulse (see Chapter 34 for management of shock).

A combination of several different treatments, including nasogastric tube (NGT) placement and lavage, endoscopic therapy, interventional radiologic procedures, and acid suppression, can be used to control acute bleeding and prevent rebleeding. If the patient is actively bleeding at home, he or she is usually admitted to the emergency department. After the bleeding has stopped, H_2-receptor antagonists and proton pump inhibitors are the primary drugs used.

Nasogastric tube placement and lavage. Upper GI bleeding or obstruction often requires the primary health care provider or nurse to insert a large-bore NGT to:
- Determine the presence or absence of blood in the stomach
- Assess the rate of bleeding
- Prevent gastric dilation
- Administer lavage

Although not performed as commonly today, *gastric lavage* requires the insertion of a large-bore NGT with instillation of a room-temperature solution in volumes of 200 to 300 mL. There is no evidence that sterile saline or sterile water is better than tap water for this procedure. Follow agency protocol for the solution that is required. The solution and blood are repeatedly withdrawn manually until returns are clear or light pink and without clots. Instruct the patient to lie on the left side during this procedure. The NGT may remain in place for a few days or be removed after lavage.

Treatment of pyloric obstruction is directed toward restoring fluid and electrolyte balance and decompressing the dilated stomach. Obstruction related to edema and spasm generally responds to medical therapy. First, the stomach must be decompressed with nasogastric suction. Next, interventions are directed at correcting metabolic alkalosis and dehydration. The NGT is typically clamped after about 72 hours. Check the patient for retention of gastric contents. If the amount retained is not more than 50 mL in 30 minutes or other prescribed parameters, the primary health care provider may allow oral fluids. In some cases, surgical intervention may be required to treat PUD.

Endoscopic therapy. Endoscopic therapy via an esophagogastroduodenoscopy (EGD) can assist in achieving homeostasis during an acute hemorrhage by isolating the bleeding artery to embolize (clot) it. The endoscopist can insert instruments through the endoscope during the procedure to stop bleeding in three different ways: (1) inject chemicals into the bleeding site; (2) treat the bleeding area with heat, electric current, or laser; or (3) close the affected blood vessels with a band or clip. During the EGD, a specialized endoscopy nurse and technician assist the physician with the procedure.

Pre-EGD nursing care involves inserting one or two large-bore IV catheters if they are not in place. A large catheter allows the patient to receive IV moderate sedation (e.g., midazolam [Versed] and an opioid) and possibly a blood transfusion. Keep the patient NPO for 4 to 6 hours before the procedure. This prevents the risk for aspiration and allows the endoscopist to view and treat the ulcer. A patient must sign a consent form before the EGD *after* the primary health care provider informs him or her about the procedure.

! NURSING SAFETY PRIORITY (QSEN)

Action Alert

> After esophagogastroduodenoscopy (EGD), monitor vital signs, heart rhythm, and oxygen saturation frequently per agency protocol until they return to baseline. In addition, frequently assess the patient's ability to swallow saliva. The patient's gag reflex may initially be absent after EGD because of anesthetizing (numbing) of the throat with a spray before the procedure. *After the procedure, do not allow the patient to have food or liquids until the gag reflex has returned!*

Endoscopic therapy is beneficial for most patients with active bleeding. However, ulcers that continue to bleed or continue to rebleed despite endoscopic therapy may require an interventional radiologic procedure or surgical repair.

Interventional radiologic procedures. For patients with persistent, massive upper GI bleeding or those who are not surgical candidates, catheter-directed embolization may be performed. This endovascular procedure is usually done if endoscopic procedures are not successful or available. A femoral approach is most often used, but brachial access may be used. An arteriogram is performed to identify the arterial anatomy and find the exact location of the bleeding. The radiologist injects medication or other material into the blood vessels to stop the bleeding. Care of the patient following an arteriogram is similar to care following a percutaneous vascular intervention, which is described in Chapters 30 and 33. Postarteriogram nursing care should be provided after the procedure.

❓ CLINICAL JUDGMENT CHALLENGE 50.1

Safety; Teamwork and Collaboration

A 52-year-old woman was admitted after vomiting bright red blood last night. She states that she has a history of gastritis and hypertension and takes medication for both. She cannot provide the names of the medications she is taking. This morning's nursing assessment findings include:

- States that she has been taking ibuprofen 1600 mg every day for over a year for osteoarthritis in her hands and feet
- Blood pressure = 112/68 mm Hg (down from 150/90 mm Hg last night)
- Apical pulse = 108 beats/min
- Respirations = 22 breaths/min
- Has dry, pale skin
- Has a slightly distended abdomen with mid-epigastric moderate pain (5 out of 10)
- Is alert and oriented × 3
- Has adequate bowel sounds × 4

1. **Recognize Cues:** What assessment information in this client situation is the most important and immediate concern for the nurse? (Hint: Identify the **relevant** information *first* to determine what is most important.)
2. **Analyze Cues:** What client conditions are consistent with the **most relevant** information? (Hint: Think about priority collaborative problems that support and contradict the information presented in this situation.)
3. **Prioritize Hypotheses:** Which possibilities or explanations are **most likely** to be present in this client situation? Which possibilities or explanations are the most serious? (Hint: Consider all possibilities and determine their urgency and risk for this client.)
4. **Generate Solutions:** What actions would most likely achieve the desired outcomes for this client? Which actions should be **avoided** or are **potentially harmful**? (Hint: Determine the desired outcomes first to decide which interventions are appropriate and those that should be avoided.)
5. **Take Action:** Which actions are the most appropriate and how should they be implemented? In what **priority order** should they be implemented? (Hint: Consider health teaching, documentation, requested health care provider orders or prescriptions, nursing skills, collaboration with or referral to health team members, etc.)
6. **Evaluate Outcomes:** What client assessment would indicate that the nurse's actions were **effective**? (Hint: Think about signs that would indicate an improvement, decline, or unchanged client condition.)

Drug therapy. *Aggressive acid suppression is used to prevent rebleeding.* When acute bleeding is stopped and clot formation has taken place within the ulcer crater, the clot remains in contact with gastric contents. Acid-suppressive agents are used to stabilize the clot by raising the pH level of gastric contents. Several types of drugs are used. H_2-receptor antagonists prevent acid from being produced by parietal cells. Proton pump inhibitors prevent the transport of acid across the parietal cell membrane (Burchum & Rosenthal, 2019).

Surgical Management. Evidence-based guidelines for the treatment of PUD that include *H. pylori* treatment and the development of nonsurgical means of controlling bleeding have led to a decline in the need for surgical intervention. In PUD, surgical intervention may be used to:

- Treat patients who do not respond to medical therapy or other nonsurgical procedures
- Treat a surgical emergency that develops as a complication of PUD, such as perforation

Two general surgical approaches are available for PUD: minimally invasive surgery and conventional open surgery.

Minimally invasive surgery (MIS) via laparoscopy may be used to remove a chronic gastric ulcer or treat hemorrhage from perforation. Several small incisions allow access to the stomach and duodenum. The patient may have partial stomach removal (subtotal gastrectomy), pyloroplasty (to open the pylorus), and/or a vagotomy (vagus nerve cutting) to control acid secretion. Acid-reduction surgery may not be necessary because of the increased use of PPIs and endoscopic procedures in the treatment of PUD. The advantages of MIS over traditional open surgical procedures include a shorter hospital stay, fewer complications, less pain, and better, quicker recovery. Care of patients having gastric surgery is discussed later in this chapter under Gastric Cancer.

Care Coordination and Transition Management. Patients may be discharged from the hospital if there is no evidence of ongoing bleeding, orthostatic changes, or cardiopulmonary distress or compromise. Those discharged after treatment for peptic ulcer disease (PUD) and/or complications secondary to the disease face several challenges to manage the disease successfully. Long-term adherence to drug therapy may require the patient to take several drugs each day. Permanent lifestyle alterations in **nutrition** habits must also be made.

Home Care Management. Most patients are discharged to home to continue their recovery. Those who have had major surgery or complications, such as hemorrhage, may require one or two visits from a home care nurse to assess clinical progress, especially if the patient is an older adult (see the Home Care Considerations: The Patient with Peptic Ulcer Disease box).

Self-Management Education. The primary focus of home care preparation is patient and family teaching regarding risk factors for the recurrence of PUD. Teach them how to recognize new complications and what to do if they occur.

Help the patient plan ways to make needed lifestyle changes. For postsurgical patients, especially those who have undergone partial stomach removal, smaller meals may be required. Other postoperative **nutrition** changes are described in the Self-Management Education discussion in the Gastric Cancer section.

🏠 **HOME CARE CONSIDERATIONS**

The Patient With Peptic Ulcer Disease

Assess gastrointestinal and cardiovascular status, including:
- Vital signs, including orthostatic vital signs
- Skin color
- Presence of abdominal pain (location, severity, character, duration, precipitating factors, and relief measures)
- Character, color, and consistency of stools
- Changes in bowel elimination pattern
- Hemoglobin and hematocrit
- Bowel sounds; palpate for areas of tenderness

Assess nutritional status, including:
- Dietary patterns and habits
- Intake of coffee and alcohol
- Relationship of food ingestion to symptoms

Assess medication history:
- Use of steroids
- Use of NSAIDs
- Use of over-the-counter medications

Assess patient's coping style:
- Recent stressors
- Past coping style

Assess patient's understanding of illness and ability to adhere to the therapeutic regimen:
- Symptoms to report to the primary health care provider
- Expected and side effects of medications
- Food and drug interactions
- Need for smoking cessation

⚠️ **NURSING SAFETY PRIORITY** (QSEN)

Action Alert

Teach the patient who has peptic ulcer disease to seek immediate medical attention if experiencing any of these symptoms:
- Sharp, sudden, persistent, and severe epigastric or abdominal pain
- Bloody or black stools
- Bloody vomit or vomit that looks like coffee grounds

⚠️ **NURSING SAFETY PRIORITY** (QSEN)

Action Alert

Teach the patient who has had surgery for PUD to avoid any OTC product containing aspirin or other NSAIDs. Emphasize the importance of following the treatment regimen for *H. pylori* infection and healing the ulcer and of keeping all follow-up appointments. Help the patient identify situations that cause stress, describe feelings during stressful situations, and develop a plan for coping with stressors.

Health Care Resources. If needed, refer the patient and family to the National Institute of Diabetes and Digestive and Kidney Diseases Health Information Center (www.digestive. niddk.nih.gov/) in the United States or to the Canadian Digestive Health Foundation (https://cdhf.ca/). These groups provide information and support to patients who have digestive disorders.

◆ **Evaluation: Evaluate Outcomes.** Evaluate the care of the patient with peptic ulcer disease (PUD) based on the identified priority patient problems. The expected outcomes are that the patient:

- Does not have active PUD or *H. pylori* **infection**
- Verbalizes relief or control of **pain**
- Adheres to the drug regimen and lifestyle changes to prevent recurrence and heal the ulcer
- Does not experience upper GI bleeding; if bleeding occurs, it will be promptly and effectively managed

GASTRIC CANCER

Most cancers of the stomach are adenocarcinomas. This type of cancer develops in the mucosal cells that form the innermost lining of any portion or all of the stomach. In general, gastric cancer is more common in males than in females, and there is a sharp increase in adults over 50 years of age (American Cancer Society, 2020). *Often there are no symptoms in the early stages, and the disease is advanced when detected.*

Pathophysiology Review

Gastric cancer usually begins in the glands of the stomach mucosa. Atrophic gastritis and intestinal metaplasia (abnormal tissue development) are precancerous conditions. Inadequate acid secretion in patients with atrophic gastritis creates an alkaline environment that allows bacteria (especially *H. pylori*) to multiply. This ***infection*** causes mucosa-associated lymphoid tissue (MALT) lymphoma, which starts in the stomach (McCance et al., 2019).

Gastric cancers spread by direct extension through the gastric wall and into regional lymphatics, which carry tumor deposits to lymph nodes. Direct invasion of and adherence to adjacent organs (e.g., the liver, pancreas, and transverse colon) may also result. Hematogenous spread via the portal vein to the liver and via the systemic circulation to the lungs and bones is the most common mode of metastasis. Peritoneal seeding of cancer cells from the tumor areas to the omentum, peritoneum, ovary, and pelvic cul-de-sac can also occur.

In adults with *advanced* gastric cancer, there is invasion of the muscularis (stomach muscle) or beyond. These lesions are not cured by surgical resection. The overall 5-year survival rate of adults with stomach cancer in the United States is poor because most patients have no symptoms until the disease advances.

Infection with *H. pylori* is the largest risk factor for gastric cancer because it carries the cytotoxin-associated gene A (*CagA*) gene. Patients with pernicious anemia, gastric polyps, chronic atrophic gastritis, and achlorhydria (absence of secretion of hydrochloric acid) are two to three times more likely to develop gastric cancer.

The disease also seems to be positively correlated with eating excessive pickled foods, nitrates from processed foods, and salt added to food. The ingestion of these foods over a long period can lead to atrophic gastritis, a precancerous condition. A low intake of fruits and vegetables is also a risk factor for cancer (McCance et al., 2019).

Gastric surgery seems to increase the risk for gastric cancer because of the possible development of atrophic gastritis, which results in changes to the mucosa. Patients with Barrett esophagus from prolonged or severe gastroesophageal reflux disease (GERD) have an increased risk for cancer in the cardia (at the point where the stomach connects to the esophagus). Chapter 49 discusses GERD and esophageal cancer in detail.

❖ Interprofessional Collaborative Care

Care of the patient with gastric cancer takes place in all settings, ranging from the home and community environment to the inpatient setting, depending on the stage of disease and the immediate course of treatment.

◆ Assessment: Recognize Cues.

Although patients with *early* gastric cancer may be asymptomatic, dyspepsia and abdominal discomfort are the *most* common symptoms. However, these symptoms are often ignored, or a change in diet or use of antacids relieves them. As the tumor grows, these symptoms become more severe and do not respond to *nutrition* changes or drug therapy (see the Key Features: Early versus Advanced Gastric Cancer box).

In patients with advanced disease, anemia is evidenced by *low hematocrit* and hemoglobin values. Patients may have macrocytic or microcytic anemia associated with decreased iron or vitamin B$_{12}$ absorption. *The stool may be positive for occult blood.* Hypoalbuminemia and *abnormal results of liver tests* (e.g., bilirubin and alkaline phosphatase) occur with advanced disease and hepatic metastasis. The level of carcinoembryonic antigen (CEA) is elevated in advanced cancer of the stomach (Pagana & Pagana, 2018; Pagana et al., 2019).

The primary health care provider uses esophagogastroduodenoscopy (EGD) with biopsy for definitive diagnosis of gastric cancer. (See Chapter 48 for a discussion of nursing care associated with this diagnostic test.) The lesion can be viewed directly, and biopsies of all visible lesions can be performed to determine the presence of cancer cells. During the endoscopy, an endoscopic (endoluminal) ultrasound (EUS) of the gastric mucosa can also be performed. This technology allows the primary health care provider to evaluate the depth of the tumor and the presence of lymph node involvement, which permits more accurate staging of the disease. CT, positron emission tomography (PET), and MRI scans of the chest, abdomen, and pelvis are used in determining the extent of the disease and planning therapy.

▶▶ KEY FEATURES

Early Versus Advanced Gastric Cancer

Early Gastric Cancer
- Dyspepsia
- Abdominal discomfort initially relieved with antacids
- Feeling of fullness
- Epigastric, back, or retrosternal pain

Advanced Gastric Cancer
- Nausea and vomiting
- Iron deficiency anemia
- Palpable epigastric mass
- Enlarged lymph nodes
- Weakness and fatigue
- Progressive weight loss

◆ Interventions: Take Action.

Management of gastric cancer includes drug therapy, radiation, and/or surgery. Drug therapy and radiation may be used instead of surgery or as an adjunct before and/or after surgery.

Nonsurgical Management. The treatment of gastric cancer depends highly on the stage of the disease. Radiation and chemotherapy commonly prolong survival of patients with advanced gastric disease.

Combination *chemotherapy* with multiple cycles of drugs such as cisplatin and epirubicin before and after surgery may be given. Bone marrow suppression, nausea, and vomiting are common adverse drug effects. Chapter 20 discusses the general nursing care of patients receiving chemotherapy.

Although gastric cancers are somewhat sensitive to the effects of radiation, the use of this treatment is limited because the disease is often widely spread to other abdominal organs at diagnosis. Organs such as the liver, kidneys, and spinal cord can endure only a limited amount of radiation. Intraoperative radiotherapy (IORT) is available in large tertiary care health care systems.

Surgical Management. Surgical resection by removing the tumor is the preferred method for treating gastric cancer. The primary surgical procedures for the treatment of gastric cancer are total and subtotal (partial) gastrectomy. In early stages, laparoscopic surgery (minimally invasive surgery [MIS]) plus adjuvant chemotherapy or radiation may be curative. Patients having MIS have less pain, shorter hospital stays, rare postoperative complications, and quicker recovery. However, MIS is performed less often in the United States than in Europe because very few patients are diagnosed in the early stage of the disease. A recent study in a U.S. cancer center examined outcomes of MIS and an Enhanced Recovery After Surgery protocol. In addition to expected outcomes associated with laparoscopic surgery, patients in the study advanced their diets more quickly, experienced less weight loss, and increased their physical activity more quickly within the first week after the procedure when compared with patients having open traditional surgery (Desiderio et al., 2018).

Most patients with advanced disease are candidates for palliative surgical treatment. Metastasis in the supraclavicular lymph nodes, inguinal lymph nodes, liver, umbilicus, or perirectal wall indicates that the opportunity for cure by resection has been lost. Palliative resection may significantly improve the quality of life for a patient with obstruction, hemorrhage, or pain.

Preoperative Care. Before conventional open-approach surgery, a nasogastric tube (NGT) is often inserted and connected to suction to remove secretions and empty the stomach. This allows surgery to take place without contamination of the peritoneal cavity by gastric secretions. The NGT remains in place for a few days *after surgery* to prevent the accumulation of secretions, which may lead to vomiting or GI distention and pressure on the incision. Patients having laparoscopic surgery (minimally invasive surgery [MIS]) do not require an NGT.

Because weight loss is problematic for patients with gastric cancer, **nutrition** therapy is a vital aspect of preoperative and postoperative management. Before surgery, compression by the tumor can prevent adequate nutritional intake. To correct malnutrition before surgery, if present, the primary health care provider may prescribe enteral supplements to the diet and/or total parenteral nutrition (TPN). Vitamin, mineral, iron, and protein supplements are essential to correct nutritional deficits.

Other preoperative nursing measures for the patient undergoing open gastric surgery are the same as those for any patient undergoing abdominal surgery and general anesthesia (see Chapter 9).

Operative Procedures. The surgeon usually removes part or all of the stomach to take out the tumor. When the tumor is located in the mid-portion or distal (lower) portion of the stomach, a subtotal (partial) gastrectomy is typically performed. The omentum and relevant lymph nodes are also removed. The surgery may be performed as an MIS procedure or as an open conventional surgical technique, with or without robotic assistance.

For the patient with a removable growth in the proximal (upper) third of the stomach, a total gastrectomy is typically performed (Fig. 50.3). In this procedure the surgeon removes the entire stomach along with the lymph nodes and omentum. The surgeon sutures the esophagus to the duodenum or jejunum to reestablish continuity of the GI tract. More radical surgery involving removal of the spleen and distal pancreas is controversial, although the Whipple procedure may be used to prolong life. The complications of this drastic surgery are very serious and common (see Chapter 54). For patients with advanced disease, total gastrectomy is performed when gastric bleeding or obstruction is present.

Patients with tumors at the gastric outlet who are not candidates for subtotal or total gastrectomy may undergo gastroenterostomy for palliation. The surgeon creates a passage between the body of the stomach and the small bowel, often the duodenum.

Postoperative Care. Provide evidence-based postoperative care for patients who have had general anesthesia to prevent atelectasis, paralytic ileus, wound *infection,* and peritonitis (see Chapter 9). Document and report any signs and symptoms of these complications immediately to the surgeon.

Auscultate the lungs for adventitious sounds (crackles or reduced breath sounds) and monitor for the return of bowel sounds. Take vital signs as appropriate to detect signs of infection or bleeding. Aggressive pulmonary exercises and early ambulation can help prevent respiratory complications and deep vein thrombosis. Also inspect the operative site every 8 to 12 hours for the presence of redness, swelling, or drainage, which indicate wound infection. Keep the head of the bed elevated to prevent aspiration from reflux.

Decreased patency caused by a clogged NGT can result in *acute gastric dilation* after surgery. This problem is characterized by epigastric pain and a feeling of fullness, hiccups, tachycardia, and hypotension. Notify the surgeon to obtain an order for irrigation or replacement of the NGT to relieve these symptoms.

Dumping syndrome is a term that refers to a group of vasomotor symptoms that occur after eating in patients who have had a gastrectomy. This syndrome is believed to occur as a result of the rapid emptying of food contents into the small intestine, which shifts fluid into the gut, causing abdominal distention. Observe for *early* manifestations of this syndrome, which typically occur within 30 minutes of eating. Symptoms include vertigo, tachycardia, syncope, sweating, pallor, palpitations, and the desire to lie down. Report these manifestations to the surgeon, and encourage the patient to lie down. Monitor the patient for late symptoms.

Late dumping syndrome, which occurs 90 minutes to 3 hours after eating, is caused by a release of an excessive amount of insulin. The insulin release follows a rapid rise in the blood glucose level that results from the rapid entry of high-carbohydrate food into the jejunum. Observe for manifestations, including dizziness, light-headedness, palpitations, diaphoresis, and confusion.

Dumping syndrome is managed by *nutrition* changes that include decreasing the amount of food taken at one time and eliminating liquids ingested with meals. In collaboration with the registered dietitian nutritionist, teach the patient to eat a high-protein, high-fat, low- to moderate-carbohydrate diet (Table 50.3). Acarbose may be used to decrease carbohydrate absorption. A somatostatin analog, octreotide, 50 mcg subcutaneously two or three times daily 30 minutes before meals, may be prescribed in severe cases. This drug decreases gastric and intestinal hormone secretion and slows stomach and intestinal transit time.

Delayed gastric emptying is often present after gastric surgery and usually resolves within 1 week. Edema at the anastomosis (surgical connection areas) or adhesions (scar tissue) obstructing the distal loop may cause mechanical blockage. Metabolic causes (e.g., hypokalemia, hypoproteinemia, or hyponatremia) should be considered. The edema usually resolves with nasogastric suction, maintenance of fluid and electrolyte balance, and proper *nutrition.*

Several problems related to *nutrition* develop as a result of partial removal of the stomach, including deficiencies of vitamin B_{12}, folic acid, and iron; impaired calcium metabolism; and reduced absorption of calcium and vitamin D. These problems are caused by a reduction of intrinsic factor. The decrease results from the resection and from inadequate absorption because of rapid entry of food into the bowel. In the absence of intrinsic

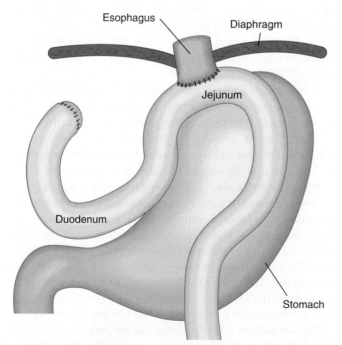

FIG. 50.3 Total gastrectomy with anastomosis of the esophagus to the jejunum (esophagojejunostomy) is the principal surgical intervention for extensive gastric cancer.

TABLE 50.3 Diet for Dumping Syndrome

Food Group	Foods Allowed or Encouraged	Foods to Use With Caution	Foods That Must Be Excluded
Soups		Fluids 1 hr before and after meals	Spicy soups
Meat and meat substitutes	8 ounces or more per day: fish, poultry, beef, pork, veal, lamb, eggs, cheese, peanut butter		Spicy meats or meat substitutes
Potatoes	Potato, rice, pasta, starchy vegetables (small amount)		Highly spiced potatoes or potato substitutes
Bread and cereal	White bread, rolls, muffins, crackers, and cereals (small amount)	Whole-grain bread, rolls, crackers, and cereals	Breads with frosting or jelly, sweet rolls, and coffee cake
Vegetables	Two or more cooked vegetables	Gas-producing vegetables, such as cabbage, onions, broccoli, or raw vegetables	
Fruits	Limit three per day: unsweetened cooked or canned fruits	Unsweetened juice or fruit drinks 30-45 min after meals; fresh fruit	Sweetened fruit or juice
Beverages	Dietetic drinks	Limit to 1 hr after meals; caffeine-containing beverages, such as coffee, tea, and cola; if tolerated, diet carbonated beverages	Milk shakes, malts, and other sweet drinks; regular carbonated beverages and alcohol
Fats	Margarine, oils, shortening, butter, bacon, and salad dressings	Mayonnaise	Any milk products with fat
Desserts	Fruit (see Fruits)	Sugar-free gelatin, pudding, and custard	All sweets, cakes, pies, cookies, candy, ice cream, and sherbet
Seasonings and miscellaneous	Diet jelly, diet syrups, sugar substitutes	Excessive amounts of salt	Excessive amounts of spices, sugar, jelly, honey, syrup, or molasses

General Principles for Patients to Follow
- Several small meals daily
- Relatively high fat and protein content
- Low roughage
- Relatively low carbohydrate content
- No milk, sweets, or sugars
- Liquid between meals *only*

factor, signs and symptoms of pernicious anemia may occur. Assess for the development of atrophic glossitis secondary to vitamin B_{12} deficiency. In atrophic glossitis, the tongue takes on a shiny, smooth, and "beefy" appearance. The patient may also have signs of anemia secondary to folic acid and iron deficiency. Monitor the complete blood count (CBC) for signs of megaloblastic anemia (low red blood cell [RBC] level) and leukopenia (low white blood cell [WBC] level). These manifestations are corrected by the administration of vitamin B_{12}. The primary health care provider may also prescribe folic acid or iron preparations. Anemias are discussed elsewhere in this textbook.

Care Coordination and Transition Management. Patients who have undergone total gastrectomy and those who are debilitated with advanced gastric cancer are discharged to home with maximal assistance and support or to a transitional care unit or skilled nursing facility. Patients who have undergone subtotal gastrectomy and are not debilitated may be discharged to home with partial assistance for ADLs. Recurrence of cancer is common, and patients need regular follow-up examinations and imaging assessments. Collaborate with the case manager to ensure continuity of care and thorough follow-up with diagnostic testing.

Home Care Management. Gastric cancer is a life-threatening illness. Therefore the patient and family members require physical and emotional care. Assess their ability to cope with

the disease and the possible need for end-of-life care. The adverse effects of gastric cancer treatment can be debilitating, and patients need to learn symptom-management strategies. Hospice programs can help both the patient and the family cope with these physical and emotional needs.

Patients may fear returning home because of their inability for self-management. Enlisting family and health care resources for the patient may ease some of this anxiety. Provide the family with adequate information about community support systems to make the transition to home care easier. If the prognosis is poor, they need continued professional support from case managers, social workers, and/or nurses to cope with death and dying. (See Chapter 8 for a discussion of end-of-life care.)

Self-Management Education. Educate the patient and family about any continuing needs, drug therapy, and nutrition therapy. If patients are discharged to home with surgical dressings, teach the patient and family how to change them. Review the manifestations of incisional infection (e.g., fever, redness, and drainage) that they should report to their surgeon.

Patients who will be receiving radiation therapy or chemotherapy require instructions related to the side effects of these treatments. Nausea and vomiting are common side effects of chemotherapy, and instruction in the use of prescribed antiemetics may be needed. (See Chapter 20 for health teaching for patients receiving chemotherapy or radiation therapy.)

In collaboration with the registered dietitian nutritionist, teach the patient and family about the type and quantity of foods that will provide optimal nutritional value. Interventions to minimize dumping syndrome and decrease gastric stimulants are also emphasized (see Table 50.3). Remind the patient to:

- Eat small, frequent meals
- Avoid drinking liquids with meals
- Avoid foods that cause discomfort
- Eliminate caffeine and alcohol consumption
- Begin a smoking-cessation program, if needed
- Receive B_{12} injections, as prescribed
- Lie flat for a short time after eating

Health Care Resources. A home care referral provides continued assessment, assistance, and encouragement to the patient and family. A home care nurse can help with care procedures and provide valuable psychological support. Additional referrals to a registered dietitian nutritionist, professional counselor, or clergy/spiritual leader may be necessary. Referral to a hospice agency can be of great assistance for the patient with advanced disease. Hospice care may be delivered in the home or in an institutional setting. Appropriate support groups (e.g., I Can Cope, provided by the American Cancer Society [http://www.cancer.org/treatment/index]) can be a major resource.

NCLEX EXAMINATION CHALLENGE 50.2
Psychosocial Integrity

Which client statement regarding diet and nutrition after a total gastrectomy requires **further teaching** by the nurse?
A. "I should stay sitting up for an hour after I eat."
B. "I will avoid liquids with my meals."
C. "I need to eat small frequent meals."
D. "I need to stay away from concentrated sweets."

GET READY FOR THE NEXT-GENERATION NCLEX® EXAMINATION!

Key Points
Review these Key Points for each NCLEX Examination Client Needs Category.

Safe and Effective Care Environment

- When caring for patients with gastric health problems, collaborate with the members of the interprofessional team, including the pharmacist, registered dietitian nutritionist, health care provider, and/or case manager. **QSEN: Teamwork and Collaboration**

Health Promotion and Maintenance

- Refer the patient with gastric cancer to the American Cancer Society. **QSEN: Patient-Centered Care**
- Identify patients at risk for gastritis and PUD, especially those with *H. pylori* and older adults who take large amounts of NSAIDs. **QSEN: Safety**
- Teach adults to prevent PUD by avoiding excess consumption of caffeine, alcohol, coffee, aspirin, NSAIDs, and contaminated food and water and by avoiding smoking. **QSEN: Evidence-Based Practice**
- Teach patients the importance of adhering to *H. pylori* treatment to prevent development of gastric cancer. **QSEN: Evidence-Based Practice**

Psychosocial Integrity

- Allow patients with gastric cancer to express feelings of grief, fear, and anxiety. **QSEN: Patient-Centered Care**
- For patients with advanced gastric cancer, identify end-of-life care needs, including referral to hospice care. **Ethics**

Physiological Integrity

- Recall that *acute* gastritis causes a rapid onset of epigastric pain and dyspepsia; *chronic* gastritis causes vague epigastric pain (usually relieved with food) and intolerance to fatty and spicy foods. **QSEN: Patient-Centered Care**
- Remember that patients with gastric ulcers may be malnourished and have pain that is worsened by ingestion of food; patients with duodenal ulcers are usually well nourished, have pain that is relieved by ingestion of food, and awaken with pain during the night. **QSEN: Patient-Centered Care**
- For patients who have undergone a gastrectomy, collaborate with the registered dietitian nutritionist and instruct the patient regarding diet changes to avoid abdominal distention and dumping syndrome. **QSEN: Teamwork and Collaboration**
- Teach patients with abnormal abdominal symptoms to consult with their health care provider immediately. **QSEN: Safety**
- Teach that hematemesis is a medical emergency and refer to the emergency department for prompt treatment. **QSEN: Safety**
- Teach the proper administration of antacids (one or two after meals), reminding patients that antacids can interfere with the effectiveness of certain drugs, such as phenytoin (Dilantin). **QSEN: Evidence-Based Practice**
- Teach the proper administration of H_2 antagonists and explain that they should be taken at bedtime (see the Common Examples of Drug Therapy: Gastritis and Peptic Ulcer Disease box.). **QSEN: Evidence-Based Practice**
- Teach the proper administration of antisecretory agents, noting that most cannot be crushed because they are sustained-release or enteric-coated tablets. **QSEN: Evidence-Based Practice**
- Monitor patients with ulcers for signs and symptoms of upper GI bleeding, such as hematemesis, melena, and low blood pressure. Report any of these symptoms to the primary health care provider immediately. **QSEN: Safety; Clinical Judgment**
- After EGD, monitor vital signs, heart rhythm, and oxygen saturation frequently until they return to baseline. To prevent aspiration, assess the gag reflex and ensure that it is intact before giving the patient food or fluids. **QSEN: Safety; Clinical Judgment**
- Observe for signs and symptoms of dumping syndrome after gastric surgery; teach characteristics and management of this syndrome. **QSEN: Evidence-Based Practice**

■ MASTERY QUESTIONS

1. The primary health care provider prescribes bismuth subsalicylate for a client as part of treating *H. pylori* infection. What health teaching will the nurse include for the client about this drug?
   A. "Do not crush this drug before taking."
   B. "The drug may cause your tongue and stool to turn black."
   C. "Take the drug at night only."
   D. "The drug may cause you to have diarrhea."

2. What health teaching will the nurse include to promote gastric health for an adult client? **Select all that apply.**
   A. "Stop smoking or using tobacco of any form."
   B. "Do not drink excessive amounts of alcohol."
   C. "Consume high-fat foods and decrease carbohydrates."
   D. "Avoid excessive amounts of pickled or smoked food."
   E. "Avoid taking large amounts of NSAIDs."

REFERENCES

American Cancer Society. (2020). *Stomach cancer.* http://www.cancer.org/cancer/stomachcancer/detailedguide/stomach-cancer-key-statistics.

Ankita, C., Nehal, G., Komal, K., Lambole, V., & Shah, D. P. (2017). A review: Peptic ulcer disease. *Pharma Science Monitor: An International Journal of Pharmaceutical Sciences, 8*(2), 210–218.

Benmassaoud, A., McDonald, E. G., & Lee, T. C. (2016). Potential harms of proton pump inhibitor therapy: Rare adverse effects of commonly used drugs. *Canadian Medical Association Journal, 188*(9), 657–662.

Burchum, J. L. R., & Rosenthal, L. D. (2019). *Lehne's pharmacology for nursing care* (10th ed.). St. Louis: Elsevier.

Desiderio, J., Stewart, C. L., Sun, V., Melstrom, L., Warner, S., Lee, B., et al. (2018). Enhanced recovery after surgery for gastric cancer improves clinical outcomes at a U.S. cancer center. *Journal of Gastric Cancer, 18*(3), 230–241.

Farrar, F. C. (2018). Management of acute gastrointestinal bleeding. *Critical Care Nursing Clinics of North America, 30*(1), 55–66.

McCance, K., Huether, S., Brashers, V., & Rote, N. (2019). *Pathophysiology: The biologic basis for disease in adults and children* (8th ed.). St. Louis: Mosby.

National Institute of Diabetes and Digestive and Kidney Diseases. (2020). *Definitions and facts for peptic ulcers (stomach ulcers).* https://www.niddk.nih.gov/health-information/health-topics/digestive-diseases/peptic-ulcer/pages/definition-facts.aspx.

Pagana, K. D., & Pagana, T. J. (2018). *Manual of diagnostic and laboratory tests* (6th ed.). St. Louis: Mosby.

Pagana, K. D., Pagana, T. J., & Pike-MacDonald, S. A. (2019). *Mosby's Canadian manual of diagnostic and laboratory tests* (2nd ed.). Toronto, ON: Elsevier.

Priyanka, C., Jenish, R., Gajera, V., Lambole, V., & Shah, D. P. (2016). Peptic ulcer: A review on epidemiology, etiology, pathogenesis and management strategies. *Pharma Science Monitor: An International Journal of Pharmaceutical Sciences, 7*(2), 139–147.

51

Concepts of Care for Patients With Noninflammatory Intestinal Disorders

Keelin Cromar

http://evolve.elsevier.com/Iggy/

LEARNING OUTCOMES

1. Collaborate with the interprofessional team to manage quality care for patients with impaired *elimination* caused by noninflammatory bowel disorders.
2. Identify community resources for families and patients recovering from noninflammatory bowel disorders.
3. Apply knowledge of pathophysiology of noninflammatory bowel disorders to identify common assessment findings, including actual or risk for impaired *nutrition* and *fluid and electrolyte balance.*
4. Prioritize evidence-based nursing interventions for patients with noninflammatory bowel disorders to promote *nutrition,* maintain *fluid and electrolyte balance,* and manage *pain.*
5. Plan transition management and care coordination for the patient who has a colostomy, including health teaching.

KEY TERMS

abdominoperineal (AP) resection Surgical removal of the sigmoid colon, rectum, and anus through combined abdominal and perineal incisions.

borborygmi High-pitched bowel sounds that are proximal (above) an obstruction.

colectomy Surgical removal of the entire colon.

colon resection Surgical removal of part of the colon and regional lymph nodes.

colostomy The surgical creation of an opening of the colon (stoma) onto the surface of the abdomen to allow passage of stool.

exploratory laparotomy A surgical opening of the abdominal cavity.

fecal occult blood test [FOBT] A laboratory test to determine the presence of occult (microscopic) blood in the stool.

flatulence Excessive gas (flatus) in the intestines.

hemorrhoidectomy Surgical removal of hemorrhoids.

hemorrhoids Unnaturally swollen or distended veins in the anorectal region.

hernia A weakness in the abdominal muscle wall through which a segment of the bowel or other abdominal structure protrudes.

hernioplasty A surgical hernia repair procedure performed to reinforce the weakened outside abdominal muscle wall with a mesh patch.

herniorrhaphy Surgical repair of a hernia.

intussusception Telescoping of a segment of the intestine within itself.

irreducible (incarcerated) hernia A hernia that cannot be reduced or placed back into the abdominal cavity. Any hernia that is not reducible requires immediate surgical evaluation.

irritable bowel syndrome A functional GI disorder that causes chronic or recurrent diarrhea, constipation, and/or abdominal pain and bloating.

mechanical obstruction A condition in which the bowel is physically blocked by problems outside the intestine (e.g., adhesions), in the bowel wall (e.g., Crohn's disease), or in the intestinal lumen (e.g., tumors).

minimally invasive inguinal hernia repair (MIIHR) Surgical hernia repair through a laparoscope.

nonmechanical obstruction A condition in which peristalsis is decreased or absent because of neuromuscular disturbance, resulting in a slowing of the movement or a backup of intestinal contents; also known as *paralytic ileus.*

obstipation No passage of stool.

polyps In the intestinal tract, small growths covered with mucosa and attached to the surface of the intestine; although most are benign, they are significant because some have the potential to become malignant.

reducible hernia A hernia that can be reduced or placed back into the abdominal cavity.

strangulated obstruction Bowel obstruction or hernia that has compromised blood flow (can be life-threatening).

volvulus Twisting of the intestine.

If not diagnosed and managed early, some intestinal problems can lead to inadequate absorption of vital nutrients and affect *nutrition* and *elimination.* If these disorders become severe or progress, *pain* and problems with *fluid and electrolyte balance* may occur. Chapter 3 briefly reviews each of these health concepts. Intestinal health problems may be classified as inflammatory or noninflammatory; this chapter focuses on disorders that are noninflammatory in origin.

✳ ELIMINATION CONCEPT EXEMPLAR: INTESTINAL OBSTRUCTION

Pathophysiology Review

Intestinal obstructions can be partial or complete and are classified as mechanical or nonmechanical. With either condition, *elimination* is compromised by this common and serious disorder.

Types of Intestinal Obstructions. In mechanical obstruction, the bowel is physically blocked by problems outside the intestine (e.g., adhesions), in the bowel wall (e.g., Crohn's disease), or in the intestinal lumen (e.g., tumors). Nonmechanical obstruction (also known as paralytic ileus or *functional obstruction*) does not involve a physical obstruction in or outside the intestine. Instead, peristalsis is decreased or absent because of neuromuscular disturbance, resulting in a slowing of the movement or a backup of intestinal contents (McCance et al., 2019).

Intestinal contents are composed of ingested fluid, food, and saliva; gastric, pancreatic, and biliary secretions; digestive enzymes; and swallowed air. In both mechanical and nonmechanical obstructions, the intestinal contents accumulate at and above the area of obstruction. Abdominal distention results from the intestine's inability to absorb the contents and move the waste down through the intestinal tract. To compensate for the delay, peristalsis increases in an effort to move the intestinal contents forward. This increase stimulates more secretions, which then leads to additional distention. The bowel then becomes edematous and increased capillary permeability results. Plasma leaking into the peritoneal cavity and fluid trapped in the intestinal lumen decrease the absorption of fluid and electrolytes into the vascular space. Reduced circulatory blood volume (hypovolemia) and electrolyte imbalances typically occur. Hypovolemia ranges from mild to extreme (hypovolemic shock).

Complications of Intestinal Obstruction. Specific problems related to *fluid and electrolyte balance* and acid-base balance

result, depending on the part of the intestine that is blocked. An obstruction high in the small intestine causes a loss of gastric hydrochloric acid, which can lead to *metabolic alkalosis.* Obstruction below the duodenum but above the large bowel results in a loss of both acids and bases, so acid-base balance is usually not compromised. Obstruction at the end of the small intestine and lower in the intestinal tract causes loss of alkaline fluids, which can lead to *metabolic acidosis* (McCance et al., 2019).

If hypovolemia is severe, acute kidney injury or even death can occur. Bacterial peritonitis with or without actual perforation can also result. Bacteria in the intestinal contents lie stagnant in the obstructed intestine. This is not a problem unless the blood flow to the intestine is compromised. However, with *closed-loop obstruction* (blockage in two different areas) or a strangulated obstruction (obstruction with compromised blood flow that can be life threatening), the risk for peritonitis (infection) is greatly increased. Bacteria without blood supply can form and release endotoxins into the peritoneal or systemic circulation and cause septic shock. The same process occurs when gangrene results from intestinal ischemia caused by mesenteric arterial occlusion.

With a strangulated obstruction, major blood loss into the intestine and the peritoneum can occur. Sepsis and bleeding can result in an increased intra-abdominal pressure (IAP) or acute compartment syndrome.

Etiology. Intestinal obstruction is caused by a variety of conditions and is associated with significant morbidity. It can occur anywhere in the intestinal tract, although the ileum in the small intestine (the narrowest part of the intestinal tract) is the most common site.

Mechanical obstruction can result from:
- Adhesions (scar tissue from surgeries or pathology)
- Benign or malignant tumor
- Complications of appendicitis
- Hernias
- Fecal impactions (especially in older adults)
- Strictures due to Crohn's disease (a chronic inflammatory bowel disease) or previous radiation therapy
- Intussusception (telescoping of a segment of the intestine within itself) (Fig. 51.1)
- Volvulus (twisting of the intestine) (see Fig. 51.1)
- Fibrosis due to disorders such as endometriosis

In people ages 60 years or older, diverticulitis, tumors, and fecal impaction are the most common causes of obstruction (McCance et al., 2019).

Postoperative ileus (POI) (paralytic ileus), or *nonmechanical* obstruction, is most commonly caused by handling of the intestines during abdominal surgery. In patients with POI, intestinal function is lost for a few hours to several days. Electrolyte disturbances, especially hypokalemia, predispose the patient to this problem. The ileus can also be a consequence of peritonitis because leakage of colonic contents causes severe irritation and triggers an inflammatory response and infection (see Peritonitis in Chapter 52). Vascular insufficiency to the bowel, also referred to as *intestinal ischemia,* is another potential cause of an ileus.

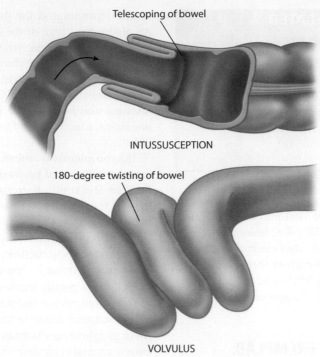

Telescoping of bowel

INTUSSUSCEPTION

180-degree twisting of bowel

VOLVULUS

Fig. 51.1 Two major types of mechanical obstruction.

It results when arterial or venous thrombosis or an embolus decreases blood flow to or in the mesenteric blood vessels surrounding the intestines. Severe insufficiency of blood supply can result in infarction of surrounding organs (e.g., bowel infarction), gangrene, and eventually sepsis and septic shock.

Incidence and Prevalence. Because there are many causes of intestinal obstruction, the incidence and prevalence is not well known. However, it occurs much more commonly in patients who have had bowel surgery and those with intestinal tumors. Older adults are the most likely group to have a bowel obstruction.

❖ Interprofessional Collaborative Care

Care for the patient with an intestinal obstruction takes place in the hospital setting. The interprofessional team that primarily collaborates to care for this patient generally includes the primary health care provider, nurse, and registered dietitian nutritionist.

◆ Assessment: Recognize Cues

History. Collect information about a history of GI disorders, surgeries, and treatments. Question the patient about recent nausea and vomiting and the color of emesis, noting if vomitus is described as greenish-yellow, bilious, or hematemesis. Perform a thorough pain assessment with particular attention to the onset, aggravating factors, alleviating factors, and patterns or rhythms of the *pain.* Severe pain that then stops and changes to tenderness on palpation may indicate perforation; this finding should be reported promptly to the primary health care provider. Ask about *elimination* patterns, including the passage of flatus and the time, character, and consistency of the last bowel movement. Singultus (hiccups) is common with all types

of intestinal obstruction. When an obstruction is suspected, keep the patient NPO and contact the primary health care provider promptly for further direction.

Assess for a family history of colorectal cancer (CRC) and ask about blood in the stool or a change in bowel pattern. Body temperature with uncomplicated obstruction is rarely higher than 100°F (37.8°C). A temperature higher than this, with or without guarding and tenderness, and a sustained elevation in pulse could indicate a strangulated obstruction, peritonitis, or intestinal ischemia. A fever, tachycardia, hypotension, increasing abdominal pain, abdominal rigidity, or change in color of skin overlying the abdomen should be reported to the health primary health care provider immediately.

Physical Assessment/Signs and Symptoms. The patient with *mechanical* obstruction in the *small intestine* often has mid-abdominal *pain* or cramping. The pain can be sporadic, and the patient may feel comfortable between episodes. If strangulation is present, the pain becomes more localized and steady. Vomiting often accompanies obstruction and is more profuse with obstructions in the proximal small intestine. The vomitus may contain bile and mucus or be orange-brown and foul smelling because of bacterial overgrowth with low ileal obstruction. Prolonged vomiting can result in a disruption in *fluid and electrolyte balance.* Obstipation (no passage of stool) and failure to pass flatus are associated with complete obstruction; diarrhea may be present in partial obstruction.

Mechanical colonic obstruction causes a milder, more intermittent colicky abdominal *pain* than is seen with small-bowel obstruction. Lower abdominal distention and obstipation may be present, or the patient may have ribbon-like stools if obstruction is partial. Alterations in bowel patterns and blood in the stools may accompany the obstruction if colorectal cancer or diverticulitis is the cause.

KEY FEATURES
Small-Bowel and Large-Bowel Obstructions

Small-Bowel Obstructions	Large-Bowel Obstructions
Abdominal discomfort or pain possibly accompanied by visible peristaltic waves in upper and middle abdomen	Intermittent lower abdominal cramping
Upper or epigastric abdominal distention	Lower abdominal distention
Nausea and early, profuse vomiting (may contain fecal material)	Minimal or no vomiting
Obstipation	Obstipation or ribbon-like stools
Severe fluid and electrolyte imbalances	No major fluid and electrolyte imbalances
Metabolic alkalosis (not always present)	Metabolic acidosis (not always present)

On examination of the abdomen, observe for abdominal distention, which is common in all forms of intestinal obstruction. Peristaltic waves may also be visible. Auscultate for proximal (above the obstruction) high-pitched bowel sounds (**borborygmi**), which are associated with cramping early in the obstructive process as the intestine tries to push the mechanical obstruction forward. In later stages of mechanical obstruction, bowel sounds are absent, especially distal to the obstruction. Abdominal tenderness and rigidity are usually minimal. The presence of a tense, fluid-filled bowel loop mimicking a palpable abdominal mass may signal a closed-loop, strangulating small-bowel obstruction.

In most types of *nonmechanical* obstruction, the pain is described as a constant, diffuse discomfort. Colicky cramping is not characteristic of this type of obstruction. *Pain* associated with obstruction caused by vascular insufficiency or infarction is usually severe and constant. On inspection, abdominal distention is typically present. On auscultation of the abdomen, note and document decreased bowel sounds in early obstruction and absent bowel sounds in later stages. Vomiting of gastric contents and bile is frequent, but the vomitus rarely has a foul odor and is rarely profuse. Obstipation may or may not be present. A comparison of small- and large-bowel obstructions is outlined in the Key Features: Small-Bowel and Large-Bowel Obstructions box.

Laboratory Assessment. There is no definitive laboratory test to confirm a diagnosis of mechanical or nonmechanical obstruction. *White blood cell (WBC) counts* are normal unless there is a strangulated obstruction, infarction, and/or gangrene. *Hemoglobin, hematocrit,* and *blood urea nitrogen (BUN)* values are often elevated, indicating dehydration. Serum sodium, chloride, and potassium are decreased. Elevations in serum amylase levels may occur with strangulating obstructions, which can damage the pancreas (Pagana & Pagana, 2018).

Other Diagnostic Assessment. The primary health care provider obtains imaging information from an *abdominal CT scan* or MRI as soon as an obstruction is suspected. Distention with fluid and gas in the small intestine with the absence of gas in the colon indicates an obstruction in the small intestine.

The diagnostic examination chosen depends on the suspected location of the obstruction. As an initial assessment, the primary health care provider may request an *abdominal ultrasound* to evaluate the potential cause of the obstruction. An endoscopy (sigmoidoscopy or colonoscopy) may also be performed to determine the cause of the obstruction, except when perforation or complete obstruction is suspected.

◆ **Analysis: Analyze Cues and Prioritize Hypotheses.** The priority collaborative problem for patients with intestinal obstruction is *Potential for life-threatening complications due to reduced flow or blocked flow of intestinal contents.*

◆ **Planning and Implementation: Generate Solutions and Take Action.** Interventions are aimed at uncovering the cause and relieving the obstruction. Relieving the obstruction decreases the potential for medical complications and reduces *pain.* Intestinal obstructions can be relieved by nonsurgical or surgical means.

Reducing the Risk of Life-Threatening Complications

Planning: Expected Outcomes. The expected outcome is that the patient's obstruction will resolve to restore normal bowel *elimination,* prevent potentially life-threatening complications, and relieve *pain.*

Interventions. Collaborative and nursing interventions depend on the location, cause, type, and severity of the bowel obstruction. Therefore a nonsurgical or surgical approach may be used.

Nonsurgical Management. If the obstruction is partial and there is no evidence of strangulation or ischemia, nonsurgical management may be the treatment of choice, as summarized in the Best Practice for Patient Safety & Quality Care: Nursing Care of Patients Who Have an Intestinal Obstruction box. Once the obstruction has been addressed effectively, *elimination* patterns are expected to resume.

BEST PRACTICE FOR PATIENT SAFETY & QUALITY CARE (QSEN)

Nursing Care of Patients Who Have an Intestinal Obstruction

- Monitor vital signs, especially blood pressure and pulse, for indications of fluid balance.
- Assess the patient's abdomen at least twice a day for bowel sounds, distention, and passage of flatus.
- Monitor *fluid and electrolyte balance* status, including laboratory values.
- Manage the patient who has a nasogastric tube (NGT):
  - Monitor drainage.
  - Ensure tube patency.
  - Check tube placement.
  - Irrigate tube as prescribed.
  - Maintain the patient on NPO status.
  - Provide frequent mouth and nares care.
  - Maintain the patient in a semi-Fowler position.
- Give analgesics for *pain* as prescribed.
- Maintain IV therapy for fluid and electrolyte replacement.
- Give alvimopan as prescribed for patients with a postoperative ileus.
- Maintain parenteral *nutrition* if prescribed.

Paralytic ileus responds very well to nonsurgical methods of relieving obstruction. Nonsurgical approaches are also preferred in the treatment of patients with terminal disease associated with bowel obstruction. In addition to being NPO, patients typically have a nasogastric tube (NGT) inserted to decompress the bowel by draining fluid and air. The tube is attached to suction.

Nasogastric tubes. Most patients with an obstruction have an NGT unless the obstruction is mild. A Salem sump tube is inserted through the nose and placed into the stomach. It is attached to low *continuous* suction. This tube has a vent ("pigtail") that prevents the stomach mucosa from being pulled away during suctioning. Levin tubes do not have a vent and therefore should be connected only to low *intermittent* suction. They are used far less often than the Salem sump tubes.

! NURSING SAFETY PRIORITY (QSEN)

Action Alert

At least every 4 hours, assess the patient with an NGT for proper placement of the tube, tube patency, and output (quality and quantity). Monitor the nasal skin around the tube for irritation. Use an approved device that secures the tube to the nose to prevent accidental removal. Assess for peristalsis by auscultating for bowel sounds with the suction disconnected (suction masks peristaltic sounds).

Monitor any NGT for proper functioning. Occasionally, NGTs move out of optimal drainage position or become plugged. In this case, note a decrease in gastric output or stasis of the tube's contents. Assess the patient for nausea, vomiting, increased abdominal distention, and placement of the tube. If the NGT is repositioned or replaced, confirmation of proper placement may be obtained by x-ray before use. After appropriate placement is established, aspirate the contents and irrigate the tube with 30 mL of normal saline every 4 hours or as requested by the primary health care provider.

Other nonsurgical interventions. Most types of nonmechanical obstruction respond to nasogastric decompression with medical treatment of the primary disorder. Incomplete mechanical obstruction can sometimes be treated successfully without surgery. Obstruction caused by lower fecal impaction usually resolves after disimpaction and enema administration. Intussusception may respond to hydrostatic pressure changes during a barium enema.

For patients with a postoperative ileus (POI), alvimopan may be given for short-term use. This drug is an oral, peripherally acting mu opioid receptor antagonist that increases GI motility (Al-Mazrou et al., 2017).

IV fluid replacement and maintenance are indicated for all patients with intestinal obstruction because the patient is NPO and *fluid and electrolyte balance* is altered (particularly potassium and sodium) as a result of vomiting and nasogastric suction. On the basis of serum electrolytes and blood urea nitrogen (BUN) levels, the primary health care provider prescribes aggressive fluid replacement with 2 to 4 L of an isotonic solution (normal saline or lactated Ringer's solution) with potassium added. Use care with patients who are susceptible to fluid overload (e.g., older adults with a history of heart or chronic kidney disease). Monitor lung sounds, weight, and intake and output daily. *Weight is the most reliable indicator of fluid balance!* Blood replacement may be indicated in strangulated obstruction because of blood loss into the bowel or peritoneal cavity.

Monitor vital signs and other measures of fluid status (e.g., urine output, skin turgor, mucous membranes) every 2 to 4 hours, depending on the severity of the patient's symptoms. In collaboration with the registered dietitian nutritionist, the primary health care provider may prescribe parenteral **nutrition** (PN), especially if the patient has had chronic nutritional problems and has been NPO for an extended period. Chapter 55 discusses the nursing care of patients receiving PN.

The patient with intestinal obstruction is usually thirsty, although some older adults have a decreased thirst response. Remind assistive personnel (AP) to provide frequent mouth care to help maintain moist mucous membranes. A few ice chips may be allowed if the patient is not having surgery. Follow agency protocol or the primary health care provider's request regarding ice chips.

Abdominal distention can cause severe **pain.** The colicky, crampy pain that comes and goes with mechanical obstruction, as well as the nausea, vomiting, dry mucous membranes, and thirst, contribute to the patient's discomfort. Continually assess the character and location of the pain and immediately report any **pain** that significantly increases or changes from colicky and intermittent to a constant discomfort. These changes can indicate perforation of the intestine or peritonitis.

Analgesics may be temporarily withheld in the diagnostic workup period so that signs and symptoms of perforation or peritonitis are not masked. Explain to the patient and family the rationale for not giving analgesics. In addition, if analgesics such as morphine are given, they may slow intestinal motility and can cause vomiting. Be alert to this side effect because nausea and vomiting are also signs of NGT obstruction or worsening bowel obstruction. Consider the importance of nonpharmacologic pain control measures when withdrawing this type of medication (see Chapter 5 for detailed description of pain management).

Help the patient achieve a position of comfort, with frequent position changes to promote increased peristalsis. A semi-Fowler position helps alleviate the pressure of abdominal distention on the chest and promotes thoracic excursion to facilitate breathing.

Pain is generally less with nonmechanical obstruction than with mechanical obstruction. With both types of obstruction, food or oral fluids aggravate the GI tract and increase pain (McCance et al., 2019).

If strangulation is thought to be likely, the primary health care provider prescribes IV broad-spectrum antibiotics. In addition, in cases of partial obstruction or paralytic ileus, drugs that enhance gastric motility (prokinetic agents) such as metoclopramide may be used.

Surgical Management. In patients with complete mechanical obstruction and in some cases of incomplete mechanical obstruction, surgical intervention is necessary to relieve the obstruction. A strangulated obstruction is complete, and surgical intervention is always required. If surgery is needed, an exploratory laparotomy (a surgical opening of the abdominal cavity) to investigate the cause of the obstruction is performed. More specific surgical procedures depend on the cause of the obstruction.

Provide general preoperative teaching for both the patient and family as discussed in Chapter 9. In cases of complete obstruction, the patient may feel too ill to understand the information. In this case, reinforce the information with the family or other caregiver. Depending on the cause and severity of the obstruction and the expertise of the surgeon, patients have either minimally invasive surgery (MIS) via laparoscopy or a conventional open approach.

In the *conventional open surgical approach,* the surgeon makes a large incision, enters the abdominal cavity, and explores for obstruction and its cause, if possible (exploratory laparotomy). If adhesions are found, they are lysed (cut and released). Obstruction caused by a tumor or diverticulitis requires a colon resection with primary anastomosis or a temporary or permanent colostomy. If obstruction is caused by intestinal infarction, an embolectomy, thrombectomy, or resection of the gangrenous small or large bowel may be necessary. In severe cases a colectomy (surgical removal of the entire colon) may be needed.

Most patients today have laparoscopic surgery (MIS) for mechanical intestinal obstructions and do *not* have an NGT. For the *MIS* approach, the specially trained surgeon makes several small incisions in the abdomen and places a video camera to view the abdominal contents to determine the extent of the obstruction. This procedure takes longer than the open approach, but blood loss is less, and healing is faster. Robotic assistance may be used, depending on the experience of the surgeon and available equipment.

General postoperative care for the patient undergoing an *exploratory laparotomy* is similar to that described in Chapter 9. In addition, patients who had an open surgical approach have an NGT in place until peristalsis resumes. A clear liquid diet may be prescribed to encourage return of peristalsis. As liquids are started, the NGT can be disconnected from suction and capped for 1 to 2 hours after the patient has taken clear liquids to determine if he or she is able to tolerate them. If the patient vomits after liquids, the suction is resumed. When the patient has return of peristalsis, the NGT suction is discontinued, and the tube is clamped for a scheduled amount of time. If the patient does *not* experience nausea while the NGT is clamped, the tube is removed.

The hospital stay for a patient having MIS to remove tumors, adhesions, and other obstructions may be as short as 1 to 2 days compared with 3 days or longer for the patients undergoing the conventional open surgical approach. Recovery is much quicker because there is less *pain* and there are fewer postoperative complications among those who had laparoscopic surgery.

Care Coordination and Transition Management. All patients with intestinal obstruction are hospitalized for monitoring and treatment. The length of stay varies according to the type of

CLINICAL JUDGMENT CHALLENGE 51.1

Patient-Centered Care; Teamwork and Collaboration; Informatics

A 45-year-old woman is transferred to a medical-surgical unit after having been admitted from the emergency department for a bowel obstruction. She has a history of Crohn's disease and a bowel resection for this disease. When the client arrives, she has a Salem sump nasogastric tube (NGT) in place that is attached to NGT suction and draining greenish drainage. She also has IV normal saline running at 150 mL/hr. The client's vital signs are stable, except for her blood pressure, which remains low at 95/50 mm Hg. She reports a pain score of 5/10 in her upper abdomen.

Additional nursing assessment data include:

- Abdominal distention present
- Reports mild nausea
- No bowel sounds in lower quadrants
- Distant bowel sounds in upper quadrants
- Apical pulse = 96 beats/min
- Oxygen saturation = 95% (on room air)

Lab results include:

- Serum sodium = 129 mEq/L (129 mmol/L)
- Serum chloride – 92 mEq/L (92 mmol/L)
- Serum potassium = 3.3 mEq/L (3.3 mmol/L)

1. **Recognize Cues:** What assessment information in this client situation is the most important and immediate concern for the nurse? (Hint: Identify the **relevant** information *first* to determine what is most important.)
2. **Analyze Cues:** What client conditions are consistent with the **most relevant** information? (Hint: Think about priority collaborative problems that support and contradict the information presented in this situation.)
3. **Prioritize Hypotheses:** Which possibilities or explanations are **most likely** to be present in this client situation? Which possibilities or explanations are the most serious? (Hint: Consider all possibilities and determine their urgency and risk for this client.)
4. **Generate Solutions:** What actions would most likely achieve the desired outcomes for this client? Which actions should be **avoided** or are **potentially harmful**? (Hint: Determine the desired outcomes first to decide which interventions are appropriate and those that should be avoided.)
5. **Take Action:** Which actions are the most appropriate and how should they be implemented? In what **priority order** should they be implemented? (Hint: Consider health teaching, documentation, requested health care provider orders or prescriptions, nursing skills, collaboration with or referral to health team members, etc.)
6. **Evaluate Outcomes:** What client assessment would indicate that the nurse's actions were **effective**? (Hint: Think about signs that would indicate an improvement, decline, or unchanged client condition.)

obstruction, the treatment, and the presence of complications. Patients who have complicated obstruction, such as strangulation or incarceration, are at greater risk for peritonitis, sepsis, and shock.

Patients with nonmechanical (functional) intestinal obstruction are less likely to require a lengthy hospitalization because of the obstruction alone. Nonmechanical obstruction generally responds to nasogastric suction and possible drug therapy within a few days. However, if an ileus occurs as a complication of an abdominal surgery, the hospital stay could be lengthy.

Home Care Management. Preparation for home care depends on the cause of the obstruction and the treatment required. Those who have resolution of obstruction without surgical intervention are assessed for their knowledge of strategies to avoid recurrent obstruction. For example, if fecal impaction in an older adult was the cause of the obstruction, assess the patient's ability to carry out a bowel regimen independently (see the Patient-Centered Care: Older Adult Considerations box).

For those who have had surgery, evaluate their ability to function at home with the added tasks of incision care and possibly colostomy care (see later discussion of colostomy care in the Colorectal Cancer section).

Self-Management Education. Instruct the patient to report any abdominal *pain* or distention, nausea, or vomiting, with or without constipation, because these symptoms might indicate recurrent obstruction. However, the patient should be reassured that recurrent paralytic ileus is not common.

Teach the patient who has had surgery about incision care, drug therapy, and activity limitations. Drug therapy consists of an oral opioid analgesic, such as oxycodone hydrochloride with acetaminophen, to be taken as needed for incisional discomfort. As with any opioid therapy, an over-the-counter laxative with a softener (e.g., docusate with senna) may be added to prevent constipation and possible recurrent obstruction.

Health Care Resources. The need for follow-up appointments depends on the cause of the obstruction and the treatment required. In collaboration with the case manager, make arrangements for a home care nurse if the patient needs help with incision or colostomy care, discussed later in this chapter.

◆ **Evaluation: Evaluate Outcomes.** Evaluate the care of the patient with intestinal obstruction based on the identified priority patient problems. The expected outcomes are that the patient will:
- Have relief from the obstruction and no evidence of life-threatening complications.
- Report that he or she has returned to having usual bowel *elimination*.

COLORECTAL CANCER

Pathophysiology Review

Colorectal refers to the colon and rectum, which together make up the large intestine, also known as the *large bowel*. Colorectal cancer (CRC) is cancer of the colon or rectum. In the United States, it is the third most common malignancy among adults (American Cancer Society [ACS], 2019a). Patients often consider a diagnosis of cancer as a "death sentence," but colon cancer is highly curable for many patients, especially if diagnosed early.

Tumors occur in different areas of the colon, with about two-thirds occurring within the rectosigmoid region as shown in Fig. 51.2. Most CRCs are adenocarcinomas, which are tumors that arise from the glandular epithelial tissue of the colon. Abnormal cellular regulation develops as a multistep process affecting immunity, resulting in a number of molecular changes. These changes include loss of key tumor suppressor genes and activation of certain oncogenes that alter colonic mucosa cell division. The increased proliferation of the colonic mucosa forms polyps that can transform into malignant tumors. Most CRCs are believed to arise from adenomatous **polyps** that present as small growths covered with mucosa and attached to the surface of the intestine (McCance et al., 2019).

CRC can metastasize by direct extension or by spreading through the blood or lymph. The tumor may spread locally into the four layers of the bowel wall and into neighboring organs. It may enlarge into the lumen of the bowel or spread through the lymphatics or the circulatory system. CRC enters the circulatory system directly from the primary tumor through blood vessels in the bowel or via the lymphatic system. The liver is the most common site of metastasis from circulatory spread. Metastasis to the lungs, brain, bones, and adrenal glands may also occur. Colon tumors can also spread by peritoneal seeding during surgical resection of the tumor. Seeding may occur when a tumor is excised and cancer

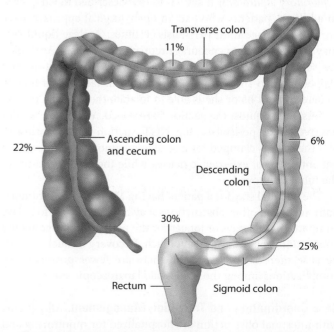

Fig. 51.2 Incidence of cancer in relation to colorectal anatomy.

cells break off from the tumor into the peritoneal cavity. Chapter 19 discusses cancer pathophysiology in more detail.

The major risk factors for the development of colorectal cancer (CRC) include age older than 50 years, genetic predisposition, and/or personal or family history of cancer. However, increasing numbers of adults under 45 years of age are being diagnosed with CRC. Some diseases also predispose the patient to cancer, such as familial adenomatous polyposis (FAP), Crohn's disease, and ulcerative colitis (McCance et al., 2019).

PATIENT-CENTERED CARE: GENETIC/ GENOMIC CONSIDERATIONS (QSEN)

People with a first-degree relative (parent, sibling, or child) diagnosed with colorectal cancer (CRC) have three to four times the risk for developing the disease. Many genes are associated with CRC. An autosomal dominant inherited genetic disorder known as *familial adenomatous polyposis (FAP)* accounts for 1% of CRCs. FAP is the result of one or more mutations in the adenomatous polyposis coli *(APC)* gene. In very young patients, thousands of adenomatous polyps develop over the course of 10 to 15 years and have nearly a 100% chance of becoming malignant (McCance, et al., 2019). By 20 years of age, most patients require surgical intervention, usually a colectomy with ileostomy or ileoanal pull-through, to prevent cancer.

Lynch syndrome, also known as hereditary nonpolyposis colorectal cancer (HNPCC), is another autosomal dominant disorder and accounts for approximately 3% of all CRCs. Lynch syndrome is also caused by gene mutations, including mutations in *MLH1* and *MLH2*. People with these mutations have an 80% chance of developing CRC at an average of 45 years of age. They also tend to have a higher incidence of endometrial, ovarian, stomach, small bowel, brain, and ureteral cancers (McCance et al., 2019). Genetic testing is available for both of these familial CRC syndromes. Refer patients for genetic counseling and testing if the patient prefers.

The role of infectious agents in the development of colorectal and anal cancer continues to be investigated. Some lower GI cancers are related to *Helicobacter pylori, Streptococcus bovis,* and human papillomavirus (HPV) infections.

There is also strong evidence that long-term smoking, obesity, physical inactivity, and heavy alcohol consumption are risk factors for CRC (ACS, 2019b). A high-fat diet, particularly animal fat from red meats, increases bile acid secretion and anaerobic bacteria, which are thought to be carcinogenic for the bowel. Diets with large amounts of refined carbohydrates that lack fiber decrease bowel transit time.

NCLEX EXAMINATION CHALLENGE 51.1

Health Promotion and Maintenance

The nurse is talking with a group of older clients about colorectal cancer (CRC) risk factors. Which of the following factors are considered to be common CRC risk factors? **Select all that apply.**

A. High-fat diet
B. Crohn's disease
C. Smoking
D. Alcoholism
E. Family history of cancer
F. Obesity

Health Promotion and Maintenance. People at risk can take action to decrease their chance of getting CRC and/or increase their chance of surviving it. For example, those whose family members have had hereditary CRC should be genetically tested for FAP and Lynch syndrome. If gene mutations are present, the person at risk can collaborate with the health care team to decide which prevention or treatment plan to implement.

Teach adults about the need for diagnostic screening. When an adult turns 40 years of age, he or she should discuss with the primary health care provider the need for colon cancer screening. The interval depends on level of risk. Adults of average risk who are 45 years of age and older and without a family history should undergo regular CRC screening as recommended by the American Cancer Society (ACS). The ACS screening options include fecal occult blood testing (FOBT) every year, colonoscopy every 10 years, or flexible sigmoidoscopy or CT colonography every 5 years. Adults who have a personal or family history of the disease should begin screening earlier and more frequently.

Teach adults, regardless of risk, to modify their diets as needed to decrease fat, refined carbohydrates, and low-fiber foods. Obesity is a major risk factor for most types of cancer. Encourage baked or broiled foods, especially those high in fiber and low in animal fat. Remind adults to eat increased amounts of brassica vegetables, including broccoli, cabbage, cauliflower, and sprouts.

Educate about the hazards of smoking, excessive alcohol, and physical inactivity. Refer patients as needed for smoking- or alcohol-cessation programs and recommend ways to increase regular physical exercise.

❖ Interprofessional Collaborative Care

Care for the patient with CRC usually takes place in a variety of health care settings. The interprofessional team that collaborates to care for this patient generally includes the surgeon, oncologist, and nurse and may include the registered dietitian nutritionist, psychologist, social worker, and spiritual leader of the patient's choice.

◆ Assessment: Recognize Cues

Physical Assessment/Signs and Symptoms. Ask whether vomiting and changes in bowel *elimination* habits, such as constipation or change in shape of stool with or without blood, have been noted. The patient may also report fatigue (related to anemias), abdominal fullness, vague abdominal pain, or unintentional weight loss. These symptoms suggest advanced disease.

Additional signs and symptoms of CRC depend on the location of the tumor. *However, the most common signs are rectal bleeding, anemia, and a change in stool consistency or shape.* Stools may contain microscopic amounts of blood that are occult (hidden), or the patient may have mahogany (dark)-colored or bright red stools (Fig. 51.3). Gross blood is not usually detected with tumors of the right side of the colon, but it is common (but not massive) with tumors of the left side of the colon and the rectum.

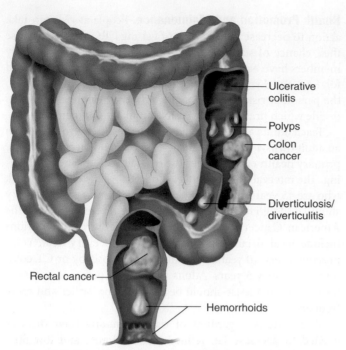

Fig. 51.3 Common causes of lower gastrointestinal bleeding.

Tumors in the transverse and descending colon result in symptoms of obstruction as growth of the tumor blocks the passage of stool. The patient may report "gas pains," cramping, or incomplete evacuation. Tumors in the rectosigmoid colon are associated with hematochezia (the passage of red blood via the rectum), straining to pass stools, and narrowing of stools. Patients may report dull pain. Right-sided tumors can grow quite large without disrupting bowel patterns or appearance because the stool consistency is more liquid in this part of the colon. These tumors ulcerate and bleed intermittently; consequently stools can contain mahogany (dark)-colored blood. A mass may be palpated in the lower right quadrant, and the patient often has anemia secondary to blood loss (McCance et al., 2019).

Laboratory Assessment. A positive test result for occult (microscopic) blood in the stool (**fecal occult blood test [FOBT]** or fecal immunochemical test [FIT]) indicates bleeding in the GI tract. These tests can yield false-positive results if certain vitamins or drugs are taken before the test. Depending on the type of test being used, the patient may need to avoid aspirin, vitamin C, iron, and red meat for 48 hours before giving a stool specimen. Also assess whether the patient is taking anti-inflammatory drugs (e.g., ibuprofen, corticosteroids, or salicylates). These drugs should be discontinued for a designated period before the test. For the FOBT two or three separate stool samples should be tested on 3 consecutive days. Negative results do not completely rule out the possibility of CRC; for this reason additional testing may be suggested (Pagana & Pagana, 2018).

Carcinoembryonic antigen (CEA), an oncofetal antigen, is elevated in many people with CRC. The normal value is less than 5 ng/mL (Pagana & Pagana, 2018). This protein is not specifically associated with the CRC, and it may be elevated in the presence of other benign or malignant diseases and in smokers.

CEA is often used to monitor the effectiveness of treatment and to identify disease recurrence.

Other Diagnostic Assessment. *CT-guided virtual colonoscopy* is growing in popularity. This test is noninvasive and includes a CT scan of the rectum and colon. It is thought to be more thorough than traditional invasive colonoscopy. However, treatments, biopsies, or surgeries cannot be performed when a virtual colonoscopy is used.

A *sigmoidoscopy* provides visualization of the lower colon using a fiberoptic scope. Polyps can be visualized, and tissue samples can be taken for biopsy. Polyps are usually removed during the procedure. A *colonoscopy* provides views of the entire large bowel from the rectum to the ileocecal valve. As with sigmoidoscopy, polyps can be seen and removed, and tissue samples can be taken for biopsy. *Colonoscopy is the definitive test for the diagnosis of colorectal cancer.* These procedures and associated nursing care are discussed in Chapter 48.

◆ **Interventions: Take Action.** The primary approach to treating CRC is to remove the entire tumor or as much of the tumor as possible to prevent or slow metastatic spread of the disease. A patient-centered collaborative care approach is essential to meet the desired outcomes.

Although surgical resection is the primary method used to control the disease, several adjuvant (additional) therapies are used. Adjuvant therapies are administered before or after surgery to achieve a cure and prevent recurrence, if possible.

Nonsurgical Management. The type of therapy used is based on the pathologic staging of the disease. The staging system used most often in colorectal cancer is the TNM (tumor, nodes, metastasis) classification; more information on the use of this system can be found in Chapter 19.

The administration of preoperative *radiation therapy* has not improved overall survival rates for colon cancer, but it has been effective in providing local or regional control of the disease. Postoperative radiation has not demonstrated any consistent improvement in survival or recurrence. However, as a palliative measure, radiation therapy may be used to control pain, hemorrhage, bowel obstruction, or metastasis to the lung in advanced disease. For rectal cancer, unlike colon cancer, radiation therapy is often a part of the treatment plan. Reinforce information about the radiation therapy procedure to the patient and family and monitor for possible side effects (e.g., diarrhea, fatigue). Chapter 20 describes the general nursing care of patients undergoing radiation therapy.

Adjuvant *chemotherapy* after primary surgery is recommended for patients with stage II or stage III disease to interrupt the DNA production of cells and destroy them. The drugs of choice are IV 5-fluorouracil with leucovorin (5-FU/LV), capecitabine, and irinotecan hydrochloride (Burchum & Rosenthal, 2019). These drugs can be used individually but are generally used in combination for the greatest treatment benefit. As with other chemotherapeutic drugs, these agents cannot discriminate between cancer and healthy cells. Therefore, common side effects are diarrhea, mucositis, leukopenia, mouth ulcers, and peripheral neuropathy (Benson et al., 2017).

Bevacizumab is an antiangiogenesis drug, also known as a *vascular endothelial growth factor (VEGF) inhibitor,* approved for metastatic CRC. This drug reduces blood flow to the growing tumor cells, thereby depriving them of necessary nutrients needed to grow (Seow et al., 2016). A VEGF inhibitor is usually given in combination with other chemotherapeutic agents.

Cetuximab and panitumumab are monoclonal antibodies known as *epidermal growth factor receptor (EGFR) inhibitors (EGFRIs),* and may also be given in combination with other drugs for metastatic disease (Seow et al., 2016). These drugs work by blocking factors that promote cancer cell growth.

Intrahepatic arterial chemotherapy, often with 5-FU, may be administered to patients with liver metastasis. Patients with CRC also receive drugs for relief of symptoms, such as opioid analgesics and antiemetics. Chapter 20 describes care of patients receiving chemotherapy in detail.

Surgical Management. Surgical removal of the tumor with margins free of disease is the best method of ensuring removal of CRC. The size of the tumor, its location, the extent of metastasis, the integrity of the bowel, and the condition of the patient determine which surgical procedure is performed for colorectal cancer. Many regional lymph nodes are removed and examined for presence of cancer. The number of lymph nodes that contain cancer is a strong predictor of prognosis. The most common surgeries performed are colon resection (removal of the part of the colon and regional lymph nodes) with reanastomosis, partial colectomy with a *colostomy (temporary or permanent)* or total colectomy with an *ileostomy/ileoanal pull-through,* and *abdominoperineal resection.* A colostomy is the surgical creation of an opening (stoma) of the colon onto the surface of the abdomen to allow passage of stool. An abdominoperineal (AP) resection is performed when rectal tumors are present. In this procedure, the surgeon removes the sigmoid colon, rectum, and anus through combined abdominal and perineal incisions.

For patients having a colon resection, minimally invasive surgery (MIS) via laparoscopy is commonly performed today. This procedure results in shorter hospital stays, less pain, fewer complications, and quicker recovery compared with the conventional open surgical approach (Papageorge et al., 2016).

Preoperative Care. Reinforce the surgeon's explanation of the planned procedure. The patient is told as accurately as possible what anatomic and physiologic changes will occur with surgery. The location and number of incision sites and drains are also discussed.

Before evaluating the tumor and colon during surgery, the surgeon may not be able to determine whether a colostomy (or less commonly, an ileostomy) will be necessary. The patient is told that a colostomy is a possibility. If a colostomy is planned, the surgeon consults a certified wound, ostomy, and continence nurse (CWOCN, sometimes referred to as the WOC nurse) to recommend optimal placement of the ostomy. The CWOCN teaches the patient about the rationale and general principles of ostomy care. In many settings, the CWOCN marks the patient's abdomen to indicate a potential ostomy site that will decrease the risk for complications such as interference from undergarments or a prosthesis with the ostomy appliance. Table 51.1 describes the preoperative role of the CWOCN.

TABLE 51.1   **Preoperative Assessment by the CWOCN Before Ostomy Surgery**
Key Points of Psychosocial Assessment
• Patient's and family's level of knowledge of disease and ostomy care
• Patient's educational level
• Patient's physical limitations (particularly sensory)
• Support available to patient
• Patient's type of employment
• Patient's involvement in activities such as hobbies
• Financial concerns regarding purchase of ostomy supplies
Key Points of Physical Assessment
Before marking the placement for the ostomy, the nurse specialist considers:
• Contour of the abdomen in lying, sitting, and standing positions
• Presence of skinfolds, creases, bony prominences, and scars
• Location of belt line
• Location that is easily visible to the patient
• Possible location in the rectus muscle

CWOCN, Certified wound, ostomy, and continence nurse.

The patient who requires low rectal surgery (e.g., abdominoperineal resection) is faced with the risk for postoperative sexual dysfunction and urinary incontinence after surgery as a result of nerve damage during surgery. The surgeon discusses the risk for these problems with the patient before surgery and allows him or her to verbalize concerns and questions related to this risk before he or she gives informed consent. Reinforce teaching about abdominal surgery performed for the patient under general anesthesia and review the routines for turning and deep breathing (see Chapter 9). Teach the patient about the method of *pain* management to be used after surgery such as IV patient-controlled analgesia (PCA), epidural analgesia, or other method.

If the bowel is not obstructed or perforated, elective surgery is planned. The patient may be instructed to thoroughly clean the bowel, or perform "bowel prep," to minimize bacterial growth and prevent complications. Mechanical cleaning is accomplished with laxatives and enemas or with "whole-gut lavage." The use of bowel preps is controversial, and some surgeons do not recommend it. For example, older adults may become dehydrated from this process.

To reduce the risk for infection, the surgeon may prescribe one dose of oral or IV antibiotics to be given before the surgical incision is made. Teach patients that a nasogastric tube (NGT) may be placed for decompression of the stomach after conventional open surgery. A peripheral IV or central venous catheter is also placed for fluid and electrolyte replacement while the patient is NPO after surgery. Patients having minimally invasive surgeries do not need an NGT.

The patient with colorectal cancer faces a serious illness with long-term consequences of the disease and treatment. A case manager or social worker can be very helpful in identifying patient and family needs and ensuring continuity of care and support.

Operative Procedures. For the conventional open surgical approach, the surgeon makes a large incision in the abdomen and explores the abdominal cavity to determine whether the tumor can be removed. For a colon resection, the portion of the colon with the tumor is excised, and the two open ends of

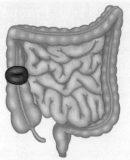

The **ascending colostomy** is done for right-sided tumors.

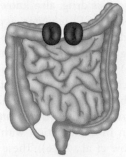

The **transverse (double-barrel) colostomy** is often used in such emergencies as intestinal obstruction or perforation because it can be created quickly. There are two stomas. The proximal one, closest to the small intestine, drains feces. The distal stoma drains mucus.

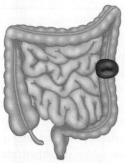

The **descending colostomy** is done for left-sided tumors.

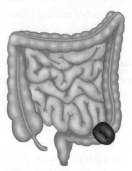

The **sigmoid colostomy** is done for rectal tumors.

Fig. 51.4 Different locations of colostomies in the colon.

the bowel are irrigated before anastomosis (reattachment) of the colon. If an anastomosis is not feasible because of the location of the tumor or inflammation of the bowel, a colostomy is created.

A temporary or permanent colostomy may be created in the ascending, transverse, descending, or sigmoid colon (Fig. 51.4). One of several techniques is used to construct a colostomy. A loop stoma (surgical opening) is made by bringing a loop of colon to the skin surface, severing and everting the anterior wall, and suturing it to the abdominal wall. Loop colostomies are usually performed in the transverse colon and are usually temporary. An external rod may be used to support the loop until the intestinal tissue adheres to the abdominal wall. Care must be taken to avoid displacing the rod, especially during appliance changes.

An end stoma is often constructed, usually in the descending or sigmoid colon, when a colostomy is intended to be permanent. It may also be done when the surgeon oversews the distal stump of the colon and places it in the abdominal cavity, preserving it for future reattachment. An end stoma is constructed by severing the end of the proximal portion of the bowel and bringing it out through the abdominal wall.

The least common colostomy is the *double-barrel stoma,* which is created by dividing the bowel and bringing both the proximal and distal portions to the abdominal surface to create two stomas. The proximal stoma (closest to the patient's

head) is the functioning stoma and eliminates stool. The distal stoma (farthest from the head) is considered nonfunctioning, although it may secrete some mucus. The distal stoma is sometimes referred to as a *mucous fistula.*

Laparoscopic (MIS) colon resection or total colectomy allows complete tumor removal with an adequate surgical margin and removal of associated lymph nodes. Several small incisions are made, and a miniature video camera is placed within the abdomen to help see the area that is involved. This technique takes longer than the conventional procedure and requires specialized training. However, blood loss and postoperative pain are reduced.

Postoperative Care. Patients who have an *open colon resection* without a colostomy receive care similar to that of those having any abdominal surgery (see Chapter 9). Other patients have surgeries that also require colostomy management. They typically have a nasogastric tube (NGT) after open surgery and receive IV PCA for the first 24 to 36 hours. After NGT removal, the diet is slowly progressed from liquids to solid foods as tolerated. The care of patients with an NGT is found in the Interventions discussion in the Intestinal Obstruction section earlier in this chapter.

By contrast, patients who have *laparoscopic surgery* (MIS) can eat solid foods very soon after the procedure. Because they usually have less **pain** and are at risk for fewer postoperative complications, they are able to ambulate and heal earlier than those who have the conventional approach. The hospital stay is usually shorter for the patient with MIS—typically 1 to 2 days, depending on the patient's age and general condition.

Colostomy Management. The patient who has a colostomy may return from surgery with a clear ostomy pouch system in place. A clear pouch allows the health care team to observe the stoma. If no pouch system is in place, a petrolatum gauze dressing is usually placed over the stoma to keep it moist. This is covered with a dry, sterile dressing. In collaboration with the CWOCN, place a pouch system as soon as possible. The colostomy pouch system, also called an *appliance,* allows more convenient and suitable collection of stool than a dressing does. Pouches are available in both one and two-piece systems and ae held in place by adhesive barriers or wafers.

Assess the color and integrity of the stoma frequently. *A healthy stoma should be reddish pink (or dark red to pink) and moist and protrude about 1 to 3 cm from the abdominal wall but most commonly about ¾ inch (2 cm)* (Fig. 51.5). During the initial postoperative period, the stoma may be slightly edematous. A small amount of bleeding at the stoma is common. These minor problems tend to resolve within 6 to 8 weeks (Stelton, 2019).

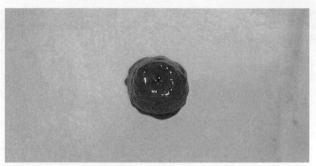

Fig. 51.5 Mature colostomy. (From Evans, S. [2009]. *Surgical pitfalls.* Philadelphia: Saunders.)

! NURSING SAFETY PRIORITY (QSEN)

Action Alert

Report any of these early postoperative stoma problems to the surgeon:
- Stoma ischemia and necrosis (dark red, purplish, or black color; dry)
- Continuous heavy bleeding
- Mucocutaneous separation (breakdown of the suture line securing the stoma to the abdominal wall)

Also assess the condition of the peristomal skin (skin around the stoma) and frequently check the pouch system for proper fit and signs of leakage. The skin should be intact, smooth, and without redness or excoriation. The most common peristomal skin complications are irritant dermatitis (from fecal content), skin stripping (from the adhesive barrier or wafer), and candidiasis (fungal infection under the barrier or wafer) (Stelton, 2019).

The colostomy should start functioning 2 to 3 days after surgery. When it begins to function, the pouch may need to be emptied frequently because of excess gas collection. It should be emptied when it is one-third to one-half full of stool. Stool is liquid immediately after surgery but becomes more solid, depending on where in the colon the stoma was placed. For example, stool from an ascending colon colostomy continues to be liquid, stool from a transverse colon colostomy becomes pasty, and stool from a descending colon colostomy becomes more solid (similar to stool expelled from the rectum).

Wound Management. For an AP resection, the perineal wound is generally surgically closed, and two bulb suction drains such as Jackson-Pratt drains are typically placed in the wound or through stab wounds near the wound. The drains help prevent drainage from collecting within the wound and are usually left in place for several days, depending on the character and amount of drainage. These drains are described in more detail in Chapter 9.

Monitoring drainage from the perineal wound and cavity is important because of the possibility of infection and abscess formation. Serosanguineous drainage from the perineal wound may be observed for 1 to 2 months after surgery. Complete healing of the perineal wound may take 6 to 8 months. This wound can be a greater source of *pain* than the abdominal incision and ostomy, and more care may be required. The patient may experience phantom rectal sensations because sympathetic innervation for rectal control has not been interrupted. Rectal pain and itching may occasionally occur after healing. Interventions may include use of antipruritic drugs, such as benzocaine, and warm compresses. Continually assess for signs of infection, abscess, or other complications and implement methods for promoting wound drainage and comfort (see the Best Practice for Patient Safety & Quality Care: Perineal Wound Care box).

BEST PRACTICE FOR PATIENT SAFETY & QUALITY CARE (QSEN)

Perineal Wound Care

Wound Care
- Place an absorbent dressing (e.g., abdominal pad) over the wound.
- Instruct the patient that he or she may:
  - Use a feminine napkin as a dressing
  - Wear jockey-type shorts rather than boxers

Comfort Measures
- If prescribed, soak the wound area in a sitz bath for 10 to 20 minutes three or four times per day or use warm/hot compresses or packs.
- Administer an analgesic as prescribed and assess its effectiveness.
- Instruct the patient about permissible activities. The patient should:
  - Assume a side-lying position in bed; avoid sitting for long periods
  - Use foam pads or a soft pillow on which to sit whenever in a sitting position
  - Avoid the use of air rings or rubber donut devices

Prevention of Complications
- Maintain ***fluid and electrolyte balance*** by monitoring intake and output and output from the perineal wound.
- Observe incision integrity and monitor wound drains; watch for erythema, edema, bleeding, drainage, unusual odor, and excessive or constant ***pain.***

NCLEX EXAMINATION CHALLENGE 51.2

Physiological Integrity

A client had an open partial colectomy and colostomy placement 6 hours ago. Which assessment would **concern** the nurse?

A. Purple, moist stoma
B. Stoma edema
C. Liquid stool collecting in the drainage bag
D. Serosanguineous fluid draining from the drain(s)

Care Coordination and Transition Management. The patient and family are faced with a possible alteration in body functions. Medical and surgical interventions for the treatment of colorectal cancer may result in cure, disease control, or palliation. Nursing interventions are designed to help the patient and family plan effective strategies for expressing feelings of grief and developing coping skills.

Collaborate with the case manager to help patients and their families cope with the immediate postoperative phase of recovery. After hospitalization for surgery, the patient is usually managed at home. Radiation therapy or chemotherapy is typically administered on an ambulatory care basis. For the patient with advanced cancer, hospice care may be an option (see Chapter 8).

Home Care Management. Assess all patients for their ability for self-management within limitations. For those requiring assistance with care, home care visits by nurses or assistive nursing personnel can be provided.

For the patient who has undergone a colostomy, review the home situation to help the patient arrange for care. Ostomy products should be kept in an area (preferably the bathroom) where the temperature is neither hot nor cold (skin barriers may become stiff or melt in extreme temperatures) to ensure proper functioning.

Self-Management Education. Before discharge, teach the patient to avoid lifting heavy objects or straining on defecation to prevent tension on the anastomosis site. If he or she had the open surgical approach, the patient should avoid driving and vigorous physical activity for 4 to 6 weeks while the incision heals. Patients who have had laparoscopy can usually return to all usual activities in 1 to 2 weeks.

! NURSING SAFETY PRIORITY (QSEN)

Action Alert

A stool softener may be prescribed to keep stools soft in consistency for ease of passage. Teach patients to note the frequency, amount, and character of the stools. In addition to this information, teach those with colon resections to watch for and report signs and symptoms of intestinal obstruction and perforation (e.g., cramping, abdominal pain, nausea, vomiting). Advise the patient to avoid gas-producing foods and carbonated beverages. The patient may require 4 to 6 weeks to establish the effects of certain foods on bowel patterns.

Ongoing Colostomy Care. Rehabilitation after surgery requires that patients and family members or other caregivers learn how to perform colostomy care. Provide adequate opportunity before discharge for patients to learn the psychomotor skills involved in this care. Plan sufficient practice time for learning how to handle, assemble, and apply all ostomy equipment. Teach patients and families or other caregivers about:

- Appearance of a normal stoma
- Signs and symptoms of complications
- Measurement of the stoma
- Choice, use, care, and application of the appropriate appliance to cover the stoma
- Measures to protect the skin adjacent to the stoma
- *Nutrition* changes to control gas and odor
- What to expect in terms of stool consistency
- Resumption of normal activities, including work, travel, and sexual intercourse

The appropriate pouch system must be selected and fitted to the stoma. Patients with flat, firm abdomens may use either flexible (bordered with paper tape) or nonflexible (full skin barrier wafer) pouch systems. A firm abdomen with lateral creases or folds requires a flexible system. Patients with deep creases, flabby abdomens, a retracted stoma, or a stoma that is flush or concave to the abdominal surface can benefit from a convex appliance with a stoma belt. This type of system presses into the skin around the stoma, causing the stoma to protrude. This protrusion helps tighten the skin and prevents leaks around the stoma opening onto the peristomal skin.

Measurement of the stoma is necessary to determine the correct size of the stoma opening on the appliance. The opening should be large enough not only to cover the peristomal skin but also to avoid stoma trauma. The stoma shrinks within 6 to 8 weeks after surgery. Therefore it needs to be measured at least once weekly during this time to gauge appliance fit and comfort. Measurements are also necessary if the patient gains or loses weight. Teach the patient and family caregiver to trace the pattern of the stoma area on the wafer portion of the appliance and to cut an opening about 1/8 to 1/16 inch larger than the stoma pattern to ensure that stoma tissue will not be constricted.

Skin preparation may include clipping peristomal hair or shaving the area (moving from the stoma outward) to achieve a smooth surface, prevent unnecessary discomfort when the wafer is removed, and minimize the risk for infected hair follicles. Advise the patient to clean around the stoma with mild soap and water before putting on an appliance. He or she should avoid using moisturizing soaps to clean the area because the lubricants can interfere with adhesion of the appliance.

! NURSING SAFETY PRIORITY (QSEN)

Action Alert

Teach the patient and family to apply a skin sealant (preferably without alcohol) and allow it to dry before application of the appliance (colostomy pouch) to facilitate less painful removal of the tape or adhesive. If peristomal skin becomes raw (skin stripping), stoma powder or paste or a combination may also be applied. The paste or other filler cream is also used to fill in crevices and creases to create a flat surface for the flange of the colostomy bag. If the patient develops a fungal rash (candidiasis), an antifungal cream or powder should be used.

Control of gas and odor from the colostomy is often an important outcome for patients with new ostomies. Although a leaking or inadequately closed pouch is the usual cause of odor, flatus can also contribute to it. Remind the patient with an ostomy that although, in general, no foods are forbidden, certain foods (such as vegetables) can cause flatus or contribute to odor when the pouch is open. Charcoal filters, pouch deodorizers, or placement of a breath mint in the pouch helps eliminate odors. The patient should be cautioned to not put aspirin tablets in the pouch because they may cause ulceration of the stoma. Vents that allow release of gas from the ostomy bag through a deodorizing filter are available and may decrease the patient's level of self-consciousness about odor.

The patient with a sigmoid colostomy may benefit from colostomy irrigation to regulate *elimination.* However, most patients with a sigmoid colostomy can become regulated through diet. Irrigation is similar to an enema but is administered through the stoma rather than the rectum.

In addition to teaching the patient about the signs and symptoms of obstruction and perforation, ask him or her to report any fever or sudden onset of pain or swelling around the stoma. Other home care assessment is listed in the Home Care Considerations: The Patient With A Colostomy box.

Psychosocial Concerns. The diagnosis of cancer can be emotionally immobilizing for the patient and family or significant others, but treatment may be welcomed because it may provide hope for control of the disease. Explore reactions to the illness and perceptions of planned interventions.

The patient's reaction to ostomy surgery may include:

- Fear of not being accepted by others
- Feelings of grief related to disturbance in body image
- Concerns about sexuality

🏠 **HOME CARE CONSIDERATIONS**

The Patient With a Colostomy

Assess gastrointestinal status, including:
- Dietary and fluid intake and habits
- Presence or absence of nausea and vomiting
- Weight gain or loss
- Bowel *elimination* pattern and characteristics and amount of effluent stool
- Bowel sounds

Assess condition of stoma at least weekly, including:
- Location, size, protrusion, color, and integrity (check for stoma retraction, prolapse or stenosis)
- Presence of peristomal hernia
- Signs of ischemia, such as dull coloring or dark or purplish bruising

Assess peristomal skin for:
- Presence or absence of excoriated skin, leakage underneath drainage system
- Presence of folliculitis (inflammation of hair follicles) or dermatitis (inflammation of skin)
- Fit of appliance and effectiveness of skin barrier and appliance

Assess the patient's and family's coping skills, including:
- Self-care abilities in the home
- Acknowledgment of changes in body image and function
- Sense of loss

Encourage the patient and family to verbalize their feelings. Education about how to physically manage the ostomy will empower both the family and patient to begin restoration of self-esteem and improvement of body image. Inclusion of family and significant others in the rehabilitation process may help preserve relationships and raise self-esteem. Anticipatory instruction includes information on leakage accidents, odor control measures, and adjustments to resuming sexual relationships.

Health Care Resources. Several resources are available to maintain continuity of care in the home environment and provide for patient needs that the nurse is not able to meet. Make referrals to community-based case managers or social workers who can provide further emotional counseling, aid in managing financial concerns, or arrange for services in the home or long-term care facility as needed.

Provide information about the United Ostomy Associations of America (www.ostomy.org), a self-help group of people with ostomies. This group has literature, online resources, and information about local chapters. The organization conducts a visitor program that sends specially trained visitors (who have an ostomy ["ostomate"]) to talk with patients. After obtaining consent, make a referral to the visitor program so the volunteer ostomate can see the patient both before and after surgery. A primary health care provider's consent for visitation may be necessary.

The local division or unit of the American Cancer Society (ACS) (www.cancer.org) can help provide necessary medical equipment and supplies, home care services, travel accommodations, and other resources for the patient who is having cancer treatment or surgery. Inform the patient and family of the programs available through the local division or unit. Other excellent Internet resources include Cancer Care (www.cancercare.org), the Colorectal Cancer Alliance (www.ccalliance.org), and the National Cancer Institute (www.cancer.gov). The Canadian Cancer Society (www.cancer.ca) is an excellent resource for patients who live in Canada.

Because of short hospital stays, patients with new ostomies receive much health teaching from nurses working for home health care agencies. This resource also helps provide physical care needs, medication management, and emotional support. If the patient has advanced colorectal cancer, a referral for hospice services in the home, nursing home, or other long-term care setting may be appropriate. The home health care nurse informs the patient and family about which ostomy supplies are needed and where they can be purchased. Price and location are considered before recommendations are made.

IRRITABLE BOWEL SYNDROME

Pathophysiology Review

Irritable bowel syndrome (IBS) is a functional GI disorder that causes chronic or recurrent diarrhea, constipation, and/or abdominal *pain* and bloating. It is sometimes referred to as *spastic colon, mucous colon,* or *nervous colon.* IBS is the most common digestive disorder seen in clinical practice and may affect as many as one in five people in the United States (McCance et al., 2019).

In patients with IBS, GI motility changes, and increased or decreased bowel transit times result in changes in the normal *elimination* pattern to one of these classifications: diarrhea (IBS-D), constipation (IBS-C), alternating diarrhea and constipation (IBS-A), or a mix of diarrhea and constipation (IBS-M). Symptoms of the disease typically begin to appear in young adulthood and continue throughout the patient's life.

The etiology of IBS remains unclear. Research suggests that a combination of environmental, immunologic, genetic, hormonal, and stress factors play a role in the development and course of the disorder. Examples of environmental factors include foods and fluids such as caffeinated or carbonated beverages and dairy products. Infectious agents have also been identified. Several studies have found that patients with IBS often have small-bowel bacterial overgrowth, which causes bloating and abdominal distention. Multiple normal flora and pathogenic agents have been identified, including *Pseudomonas aeruginosa*. Researchers believe that these agents are less causative and serve as measurable biomarkers for the disease (Derkacz et al., 2018).

Immunologic and genetic factors have also been associated with IBS, especially cytokine genes, including proinflammatory interleukins (ILs), such as IL-6 and IL-8, and tumor necrosis factor–alpha (TNF-α). These findings may provide the basis of targeted drug therapy for the disease (McCance et al., 2019).

In the United States, women are two times more likely to have IBS than are men. This difference may be the result of hormonal differences. However, in other areas of the world, this distribution pattern may not occur.

Considerable evidence relates the role of stress and mental or behavioral illness, especially anxiety and depression, to IBS. Many patients diagnosed with IBS meet the criteria for at least one primary mental health disorder. However, the *pain* and other chronic symptoms of the disease may lead to secondary mental health disorders. For example, when diarrhea is predominant, patients fear that there will be no bathroom facilities available and can become very anxious. As a result, they may not want to leave their homes or travel on trips where bathrooms are not available at all times. The long-term nature of dealing with a chronic disease for which there is no cure can lead to secondary depression in some patients (McCance et al., 2019).

❖ Interprofessional Collaborative Care

Care for the patient with IBS usually takes place in the outpatient setting, although patients with severe cases of IBS may be hospitalized for a period of time.

◆ **Assessment: Recognize Cues.** Ask the patient about a history of fatigue, malaise, abdominal *pain,* changes in the bowel pattern (constipation, diarrhea, or an alternating pattern of both) or consistency of stools, and the passage of mucus. Patients with IBS do not usually lose weight. Ask whether the patient has had any GI infections. Collect information on all drugs that the patient is taking because some can cause symptoms similar to those of IBS. Ask about the *nutrition* history, including the use of caffeinated drinks or beverages sweetened with sorbitol or fructose, which can cause bloating or diarrhea.

The course of the illness is specific to each patient. Most patients can identify factors that cause exacerbations, such as diet, stress, or anxiety. Food intolerance may be associated with IBS. Dairy products (e.g., for those with lactose intolerance or milk protein), raw fruits, and grains can contribute to bloating, flatulence (excessive gas [flatus] in the intestines), and abdominal distention. Patients may keep a food diary to record possible triggers for IBS symptoms.

A flare-up of worsening cramps, abdominal *pain,* and diarrhea and/or constipation may bring the patient to the primary health care provider. One of the *most common concerns of patients with IBS is pain in the left lower quadrant of the abdomen, although it is not always present.* Assess the location, intensity, and quality of the *pain.* Some patients have internal visceral (organ) hypersensitivity that can cause or contribute to it. Nausea may be associated with mealtime and defecation. The constipated stools are small and hard and are generally followed by several softer stools. The diarrheal stools are soft and watery, and mucus is often present. Patients with IBS often report belching, gas, anorexia, and bloating.

The patient generally appears well, with a stable weight, and nutritional and fluid status is within normal ranges. Inspect and auscultate the abdomen. Bowel sounds vary but are generally within normal range. With constipation, bowel sounds may be hypoactive; with severe diarrhea, they may be hyperactive.

Routine laboratory values (including a complete blood count [CBC], serum albumin, erythrocyte sedimentation rate [ESR], and stools for occult blood) remain normal in IBS. Some health care providers request a *hydrogen breath test* or small-bowel bacterial overgrowth breath test (Ghoshal et al., 2017). When small-intestinal bacterial overgrowth or malabsorption of nutrients is present, an excess of hydrogen is produced. Some of this hydrogen is absorbed into the bloodstream and travels to the lungs, where it is exhaled. Patients with IBS often exhale an increased amount of hydrogen.

Teach the patient that he or she will need to be NPO (may have water) for at least 12 hours before the hydrogen breath test. At the beginning of the test, the patient blows into a hydrogen analyzer. Then, small amounts of test sugar are ingested, depending on the purpose of the test, and additional breath samples are taken every 15 minutes for 1 to 5 hours (Pagana & Pagana, 2018).

◆ **Interventions: Take Action.** The patient with IBS is usually managed on an ambulatory care basis and learns self-management strategies. Interventions include health teaching, drug therapy, and stress reduction. Some patients also use complementary and integrative therapies. A holistic approach to patient care is essential for positive outcomes (Sultan & Malhotra, 2017).

Dietary fiber and bulk help produce bulky, soft stools and establish regular bowel *elimination* habits. The patient should ingest about 30 to 40 g of fiber each day. Eating regular meals, drinking 8 to 10 glasses of water each day, and chewing food slowly help promote normal bowel function.

Drug therapy depends on the main symptom of IBS. The primary health care provider may prescribe bulk-forming or antidiarrheal agents and/or newer drugs to control symptoms.

For the treatment of *constipation-predominant IBS (IBS-C)*, bulk-forming laxatives, such as psyllium hydrophilic mucilloid, are generally taken at mealtimes with a glass of water. The hydrophilic properties of these drugs help prevent dry, hard, or liquid stools. Lubiprostone is an oral laxative approved for women with IBS-C, which increases fluid in the intestines to promote bowel *elimination.* Teach the patient to take the drug with food and water. Linaclotide is the newest drug for IBS-C, which works by simulating receptors in the intestines to increase fluid and promote bowel transit time. The drug also helps relieve *pain* and cramping that are associated with IBS. Teach patients to take this drug once a day about 30 minutes before breakfast.

Diarrhea-predominant IBS (IBS-D) may be treated with antidiarrheal agents, such as loperamide and psyllium (a bulk-forming agent). Alosetron, a selective serotonin (5-HT3) receptor antagonist, may be used with caution in *women* with IBS-D as a last resort when they have not responded to conventional therapy (Lacy et al., 2018). Patients taking this drug must agree to report symptoms of colitis or constipation early because it is associated with potentially life-threatening bowel complications, including ischemic colitis (lack of blood flow to the colon).

! NURSING SAFETY PRIORITY (QSEN)

Drug Alert

Before the patient begins alosetron, take a thorough drug history (including alternative treatments), both prescribed and over the counter, because it interacts with many drugs in a variety of classes. Remind patients that they should not take psychoactive drugs and antihistamines while taking alosetron. Teach patients to report severe constipation, fever, increasing abdominal *pain,* increasing fatigue, darkened urine, bloody diarrhea, or rectal bleeding as soon as it occurs and to stop the drug immediately (Burchum & Rosenthal, 2019).

Many patients with IBS who have bloating and abdominal distention *without constipation* have success with rifaximin, an antibiotic that works locally with little systemic absorption. The U.S. Food and Drug Administration (FDA) originally approved this drug for "traveler's diarrhea," and it now has been approved for use in IBS-D (Lembo et al., 2016).

For IBS in which *pain* is the predominant symptom, tricyclic antidepressants such as amitriptyline have also been used successfully. It is unclear whether their effectiveness is the result of the antidepressant or anticholinergic effects of the drugs. If patients have postprandial (after eating) *pain,* they should take these drugs 30 to 45 minutes before mealtime.

Complementary and Integrative Health. For patients with increased intestinal bacterial overgrowth, recommend daily probiotic supplements. *Probiotics* have been shown to be effective for reducing bacteria and successfully alleviating GI symptoms of IBS. There is also evidence that peppermint oil

capsules may be effective in reducing symptoms for patients with IBS (Currò et al., 2017).

Stress management is also an important part of holistic care. Relaxation techniques, meditation, and/or yoga may help the patient decrease GI symptoms. If the patient has a stressful work or family situation, personal counseling may be helpful. Based on patient preference, make appropriate referrals or assist in making appointments if needed. The opportunity to discuss problems and attempt creative problem solving is often helpful. Teach the patient that regular exercise is important for managing stress and promoting regular bowel *elimination.*

HERNIATION

Pathophysiology Review

A hernia is a weakness in the abdominal muscle wall through which a segment of the bowel or other abdominal structure protrudes. Hernias can also penetrate through any other defect in the abdominal wall, through the diaphragm, or through other structures in the abdominal cavity.

The most important elements in the development of a hernia are congenital or acquired muscle weakness and increased intra-abdominal pressure. The most significant factors contributing to increased intra-abdominal pressure are obesity, pregnancy, and lifting heavy objects.

The most common types of abdominal hernias are indirect, direct, femoral, umbilical, and incisional (McCance et al., 2019).

- An *indirect inguinal hernia* is a sac formed from the peritoneum that contains a portion of the intestine or omentum. The hernia pushes downward at an angle into the inguinal canal. In males, indirect inguinal hernias can become large and often descend into the scrotum.
- *Direct inguinal hernias,* in contrast, pass through a weak point in the abdominal wall.
- *Femoral hernias* protrude through the femoral ring. A plug of fat in the femoral canal enlarges and eventually pulls the peritoneum and often the urinary bladder into the sac.
- *Umbilical hernias* are congenital or acquired. Congenital umbilical hernias appear in infancy. Acquired umbilical hernias directly result from increased intra-abdominal pressure. They are most commonly seen in people who are obese.
- *Incisional,* or *ventral, hernias* occur at the site of a previous surgical incision. These hernias result from inadequate healing of the incision, which is usually caused by postoperative wound infections, inadequate *nutrition,* and obesity.

Hernias may also be classified as reducible, irreducible (incarcerated), or strangulated. A reducible hernia is one in which the contents of the hernial sac can be placed back into the abdominal cavity by application of gentle pressure. An irreducible (incarcerated) hernia cannot be reduced or placed back into the abdominal cavity. *Any hernia that is not reducible requires immediate surgical evaluation.*

A hernia is strangulated when the blood supply to the herniated segment of the bowel is cut off by pressure from the hernial ring (the band of muscle around the hernia). If a hernia is strangulated, there is ischemia and obstruction of the bowel loop. *This can lead to necrosis of the bowel, sepsis, and possibly bowel perforation. Signs of strangulation are abdominal distention, nausea, vomiting, pain, fever, and tachycardia.*

Indirect inguinal hernias, the most common type, occur mostly in men because they follow the tract that develops when the testes descend into the scrotum before birth. Direct hernias occur more often in older adults. Femoral and adult umbilical hernias are most common in pregnant women or those with obesity. Incisional hernias can occur in people who have undergone abdominal surgery.

❖ Interprofessional Collaborative Care

Care for the patient with a hernia usually takes place in the ambulatory outpatient setting. Patients with inguinal hernias often need surgery in a same-day surgical facility.

◆ Assessment: Recognize Cues.
The patient with a hernia typically comes to the primary health care provider's office, clinic, or the emergency department with a report of a "lump" or protrusion felt at the involved site. The development of the hernia may be associated with straining or lifting.

Perform an abdominal assessment, inspecting the abdomen when the patient is lying and again when he or she is standing. If the hernia is reducible, it may disappear when the patient is lying flat. The primary health care provider asks the patient to strain or perform the Valsalva maneuver and observes for bulging. Auscultate for active bowel sounds. *Absent bowel sounds may indicate obstruction and strangulation, which are considered medical emergencies.*

To palpate an inguinal hernia, the primary health care provider gently examines the ring and its contents by inserting a finger in the ring and noting any changes when the patient coughs. *The hernia is never forcibly reduced; this maneuver could cause strangulated intestine to rupture.*

If a male patient suspects a hernia in his groin, the primary health care provider has him stand for the examination. Using the right hand for the patient's right side and the left hand for the patient's left side, the examiner pushes in the loose scrotal skin with the index finger, following the spermatic cord upward to the external inguinal cord. At this point, the patient is asked to cough, and any palpable herniation is noted.

◆ Interventions: Take Action.
The type of treatment selected depends on patient factors such as age and the type and severity of the hernia.

Nonsurgical Management. If the patient is not a surgical candidate (often an older man with multiple health problems), the primary health care provider may prescribe a truss for an inguinal hernia, usually for men. A truss is a pad made with firm material. It is held in place over the hernia with a belt to help keep the abdominal contents from protruding into the hernial sac. If a truss is used, it is applied only after the primary health care provider has reduced the hernia if it is not incarcerated. The patient usually applies the truss on awakening. Teach him to assess the skin under the truss daily and to protect it with a light layer of powder.

Surgical Management. Most hernias are inguinal, and surgical repair is the treatment of choice. Surgery is usually performed on an ambulatory care basis for patients who have

no pre-existing health conditions that would complicate the operative course. In same-day surgery centers, anesthesia may be regional or general, and the procedure is typically laparoscopic. If bowel strangulation and tissue death occur, more extensive surgery, such as a bowel resection or temporary colostomy, may be necessary. Patients undergoing this extensive surgery are hospitalized for a longer period.

Surgical repair of a hernia is called **herniorrhaphy**. A **minimally invasive inguinal hernia repair (MIIHR)** through a laparoscope is the surgery of choice. A conventional open herniorrhaphy may be performed when laparoscopy is not appropriate. Patients having minimally invasive surgery (MIS) recover more quickly, have less pain, and develop fewer postoperative complications compared with those having a conventional open surgery.

In addition to patient education about the procedure, the most important preoperative preparation is to teach the patient to remain NPO for the number of hours before surgery that the surgeon specifies. If same-day surgery is planned, remind the patient to arrange for someone to take him or her home and for that adult to be available for the rest of the day at home. For patients having a conventional open approach, provide general preoperative care as described in Chapter 9.

During an MIIHR, the surgeon makes several small incisions, identifies the defect, and places the intestinal contents back into the abdomen. During a conventional open herniorrhaphy, the surgeon makes an abdominal incision to perform this procedure. When a **hernioplasty** is also performed, the surgeon reinforces the weakened outside abdominal muscle wall with a mesh patch.

The patient who has had MIIHR is discharged from the surgical center in 3 to 5 hours, depending on recovery from anesthesia. Teach the patient to avoid strenuous activity for several days before returning to work and a normal routine. A stool softener may be needed to prevent constipation. Caution patients who are taking oral opioids for pain management to not drive or operate heavy machinery. Teach them to observe incisions for redness, swelling, heat, drainage, and increased pain and promptly report their occurrence to the surgeon. Remind patients that soreness and discomfort (rather than severe, acute pain) are common after MIIHR. Be sure to make a follow-up telephone call on the day after surgery to check on the patient's status.

General postoperative care of patients having a hernia repair is the same as that described in Chapter 9 *except that they should avoid coughing.* To promote lung expansion, encourage deep breathing and ambulation. With repair of an indirect inguinal hernia, the primary health care provider may suggest a scrotal support and ice bags applied to the scrotum to prevent swelling, which often contributes to pain. Elevation of the scrotum with a soft pillow helps prevent and control swelling.

In the immediate postoperative period, male patients who have had an inguinal hernia repair may experience difficulty voiding. Encourage them to stand to allow a more natural position for gravity to facilitate voiding and bladder emptying. Urine output of less than 30 mL/hr should be reported to the surgeon. Techniques to stimulate voiding such as allowing water to run may also be used. A fluid intake of at least 1500 to 2500 mL daily prevents dehydration, maintains urinary function, and minimizes constipation. A "straight" or intermittent ("in and out") catheterization is required if the patient cannot void. The Best Practice for Patient Safety & Quality Care: Nursing Care of the Postoperative Patient Having a Minimally Invasive Inguinal Hernia Repair (MIIHR) box summarizes best nursing practices for postoperative care after an MIIHR.

Most patients have uneventful recoveries after a hernia repair. Surgeons generally allow them to return to their usual activities after surgery, with avoidance of straining and lifting for several weeks while subcutaneous tissues heal and strengthen.

On discharge, provide oral instructions and a written list of symptoms to be reported, including fever, chills, wound drainage, redness or separation of the incision, and increasing incisional pain. Teach the patient to keep the wound dry and clean with antibacterial soap and water. Showering is usually permitted in a few days.

NCLEX EXAMINATION CHALLENGE 51.3

Physiological Integrity

A nurse provides discharge teaching for a male client who had a minimally invasive hernia repair this morning. Which statement by the client indicates a need for **further** teaching?

A. "I should avoid coughing if at all possible."

B. "I can shower in a day or two after I remove my surgical bandage."

C. "I can't go back to work for at least 6 weeks."

D. "I should use an ice pack to help relieve my pain."

HEMORRHOIDS

Pathophysiology Review

Hemorrhoids are unnaturally swollen or distended veins in the anorectal region. The veins involved in the development of hemorrhoids are part of the normal structure of the anal region. With limited distention, the veins function as a valve overlying the anal sphincter that assists in continence. Increased intra-abdominal pressure causes elevated systemic and portal venous pressure, which is transmitted to the anorectal veins. Arterioles in the anorectal region shunt blood directly to the distended anorectal veins, which increases the pressure. With repeated elevations in pressure from increased intra-abdominal pressure and engorgement from arteriolar shunting of blood, the distended veins eventually separate from the smooth muscle surrounding them. The result is prolapse of the hemorrhoidal vessels.

Hemorrhoids can be internal or external (Fig. 51.6). *Internal hemorrhoids,* which cannot be seen on inspection of the perineal area, are above the anal sphincter. *External hemorrhoids* lie below the anal sphincter and can be seen on inspection of the anal region. *Prolapsed hemorrhoids* can become thrombosed or inflamed, or they can bleed (McCance et al., 2019).

Hemorrhoids are common and not significant unless they cause prolonged *pain* or bleeding. Because of the increase in

---

BEST PRACTICE FOR PATIENT SAFETY & QUALITY CARE (QSEN)

Nursing Care of the Postoperative Patient Having a Minimally Invasive Inguinal Hernia Repair (MIIHR)

- Monitor vital signs, especially blood pressure and pulse, for indications of internal bleeding.
- Assess and manage incisional pain with oral analgesics; report and document severe *pain* that does not respond to drug therapy immediately.
- Encourage deep breathing and use of incentive spirometry after surgery; *teach the patient to avoid excessive coughing!*
- Encourage ambulation with assistance as soon as possible after surgery (within the first few hours).
- Apply ice packs as prescribed to the surgical area.
- Help the patient to void by standing the first time after surgery.
- Teach patients at discharge to:
  - Rest for several days after surgery.
  - Observe the incision sites for redness or drainage and report these findings to the surgeon.
  - Shower after 24 to 36 hours after removing any bandage, but do not remove wound closure strips; be aware that the strips will fall off in about a week.
  - Monitor temperature for the first few days and report the occurrence of a fever.
  - Do not lift more than 10 lb (4.5 kg) until allowed by the surgeon.
  - Avoid constipation by eating high fiber foods and drinking extra fluids.
  - Return to work when allowed by the surgeon, usually in 1 to 2 weeks, depending on the patient's work responsibilities.

---

abdominal pressure, the condition worsens during pregnancy, or with constipation with straining, obesity, heart failure, prolonged sitting or standing, and strenuous exercise and weight lifting. Decreased fluid intake can also cause hemorrhoids because of the development of hard stool and subsequent constipation. Straining while evacuating stool causes hemorrhoids to enlarge.

Health Promotion and Maintenance. Prevention of constipation is the most essential measure to prevent hemorrhoids. Constipation can be prevented by increasing fiber in the diet, such as eating more whole grains and raw vegetables and fruits. Encourage patients to drink plenty of water unless otherwise contraindicated (e.g., kidney disease, heart disease). Remind the patient to avoid straining at stool. Remind him or her to exercise regularly with a gradual buildup in intensity. Maintaining a healthy weight also helps prevent hemorrhoids.

❖ Interprofessional Collaborative Care

Care of the patient with hemorrhoids usually takes place in the ambulatory care setting and is provided by the primary health care provider and nurse. If surgery is required, the patient will be admitted to a same-day surgical center.

The most common symptoms of hemorrhoids are bleeding, swelling, and prolapse (bulging). Blood is characteristically bright red and is present on toilet tissue or streaked in the stool. *Pain* is a common symptom and is often associated with

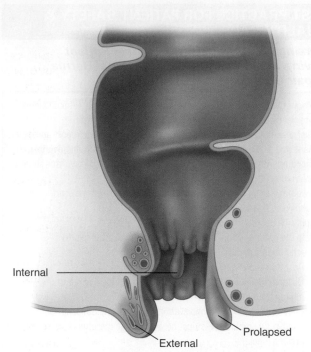

Internal

External

Prolapsed

Fig. 51.6 Internal, external, and prolapsed hemorrhoids. *Internal hemorrhoids* lie above the anal sphincter and cannot be seen on inspection of the anal area. *External hemorrhoids* lie below the anal sphincter and can be seen on inspection of the anal region. Hemorrhoids that enlarge, fall down, and protrude through the anus are called *prolapsed hemorrhoids.*

thrombosis, especially if thrombosis occurs suddenly. Other symptoms include itching and a mucous discharge. Diagnosis is usually made by inspection and digital examination.

Interventions are typically conservative and are aimed at reducing symptoms with minimal discomfort, cost, and time lost from usual activities. Cold packs applied to the anorectal region for a few minutes at a time beginning with the onset of pain and tepid sitz baths three or four times per day are often enough to relieve discomfort, even if the hemorrhoids are thrombosed.

Topical anesthetics, such as lidocaine, are useful for severe pain. Dibucaine ointment and similar products are available over the counter and may be applied for mild-to-moderate *pain* and itching. However, this ointment should be used only temporarily, because it can mask worsening symptoms and delay diagnosis of a severe disorder. If itching or inflammation is present, the primary health care provider may prescribe a steroid preparation, such as hydrocortisone. Cleansing the anal area with moistened cleansing tissues rather than standard toilet tissue helps avoid irritation. The

anal area should be cleansed gently by dabbing rather than wiping.

Diets high in fiber and fluids are recommended to promote regular bowel movements without straining. Stool softeners, such as docusate sodium, can be used temporarily. Irritating laxatives are avoided, as are foods and beverages that can make hemorrhoids worse. Spicy foods, nuts, coffee, and alcohol can be irritating. Remind patients to avoid sitting for long periods. The primary health care provider may prescribe mild oral analgesics for pain if the hemorrhoids are thrombosed.

Conservative treatment should alleviate symptoms in 3 to 5 days. If symptoms continue or recur frequently, the patient may require surgical intervention.

The surgeon can perform several procedures in an ambulatory care setting to remove symptomatic hemorrhoids (**hemorrhoidectomy**). The type of surgery (e.g., ultrasound or laser removal) depends on the degree of prolapse, whether there is thrombosis, and the overall condition of the patient. Complications of these procedures include *pain,* thrombosis of other hemorrhoids, infection, bleeding, and abscess formation. If the hemorrhoid is prolapsed, a circular stapling device may be used to excise a band of mucosa above the prolapse and restore the hemorrhoidal tissue back into the anal canal.

Teach patients with hemorrhoids about the need to eat high-fiber, high-fluid diets to promote regular bowel patterns before and after surgery. Advise them to avoid stimulant laxatives, which can be habit forming.

For patients who undergo any type of surgical intervention, monitor for bleeding and *pain* after surgery and teach them to report these problems to their health care provider. Using moist heat (e.g., sitz baths or warm compresses) three or four times per day can help promote comfort.

> **⚠ NURSING SAFETY PRIORITY** (QSEN)
> ### *Action Alert*
>
> Tell the patient who has had surgical intervention for hemorrhoids that the first postoperative bowel movement may be very painful. Be sure that someone is with or near the patient when this happens. Some patients become lightheaded and diaphoretic and may have syncope (temporary loss of consciousness) related to a vasovagal response.

The primary health care provider usually prescribes stool softeners such as docusate sodium to begin before surgery and continue after surgery. Analgesics and anti-inflammatory drugs are prescribed. A mild laxative should be administered if the patient has not had a bowel movement by the third postoperative day.

GET READY FOR THE NEXT-GENERATION NCLEX® EXAMINATION!

Key Points

Review these Key Points for each NCLEX Examination Client Needs Category.

Safe and Effective Care Environment

- Collaborate with the certified wound, ostomy, and continence nurse (CWOCN) when a patient is scheduled for or has a new colostomy. **QSEN: Teamwork and Collaboration**
- Collaborate with the case manager/discharge planner, health care provider, and CWOCN to plan care for the patient with colorectal cancer (CRC). **QSEN: Teamwork and Collaboration**

Health Promotion and Maintenance

- Refer patients with familial CRC syndromes for genetic counseling and testing. **QSEN: Evidence-Based Practice**
- Refer ostomy patients to the United Ostomy Associations of America and the American Cancer Society for additional information and support groups. **QSEN: Patient-Centered Care**
- Teach patients with irritable bowel syndrome (IBS) to avoid GI stimulants, such as caffeine, alcohol, and milk and milk products, and to manage stress. **QSEN: Evidence-Based Practice**
- Instruct patients on dietary modifications to decrease the occurrence of CRC, such as eating a diet high in fiber and avoiding red meat. **QSEN: Evidence-Based Practice**
- Teach adults age 45 years and older to have routine screening for CRC; people with genetic predispositions should have earlier and more frequent screening. **QSEN: Evidence-Based Practice**
- Teach patients to prevent or manage constipation to help avoid hemorrhoids; teach patients the importance of maintaining a healthy weight to decrease the risk for hemorrhoids. **QSEN: Evidence-Based Practice**
- Teach patients and caregivers how to provide colostomy care, including dietary measures, skin care, and ostomy products. **QSEN: Patient-Centered Care**

Psychosocial Integrity

- Assist the patient with CRC with the grieving process. **QSEN: Patient-Centered Care**
- Be aware that having a colostomy is a life-altering event that can severely impact one's body image; issues related to sexuality and fear of acceptance should be discussed. **QSEN: Patient-Centered Care**

Physiological Integrity

- Be aware that minimally invasive inguinal hernia repair is an ambulatory care procedure done via laparoscopy; postoperative management requires health teaching regarding rest for a few days and inspection of incisions for signs of infection. **QSEN: Evidence-Based Practice**
- Be aware that a strangulated hernia can cause ischemia and bowel obstruction, requiring immediate intervention. **QSEN: Safety**
- Monitor patients who have conventional open herniorrhaphy for ability to void. **QSEN: Safety**
- Recall that changes in bowel habits or stool characteristics and/or rectal bleeding are often associated with a diagnosis of CRC. **QSEN: Safety**
- Keep the peristomal skin clean and dry; observe for leakage around the pouch seal. **QSEN: Evidence-Based Practice**
- Provide meticulous perineal wound care for patients having an abdominoperineal resection. **QSEN: Safety**
- Recognize characteristics of the colostomy stoma, which should be reddish pink and moist; report abnormalities such as ischemia and necrosis (purplish or black) or unusual bleeding to the surgeon. **Clinical Judgment**
- Recall that bowel sounds are altered in patients with obstruction; absent bowel sounds imply total obstruction. **QSEN: Safety**
- Assess the patient's nasogastric tube (NGT) for proper placement, patency, and output at least every 4 hours. **QSEN: Safety**
- Monitor patients with bowel obstruction for signs and symptoms of fluid, electrolyte, and acid-base imbalances; patients with small bowel obstruction are at greater risk for problems with *fluid and electrolyte balance.* **QSEN: Safety**
- Teach patients having hemorrhoid surgery to take stool softeners before and after surgery to decrease discomfort during *elimination.* **QSEN: Evidence-Based Practice**
- Provide comfort measures for the patient who has chronic diarrhea associated with malabsorption. **QSEN: Patient-Centered Care**
- Reinforce teaching regarding supplements or dietary restrictions needed for malabsorption management. **QSEN: Evidence-Based Practice**

MASTERY QUESTIONS

1. The nurse is caring for a client with a complete large bowel obstruction. What assessment findings would the nurse expect? **Select all that apply.**
   A. Obstipation
   B. Dehydration
   C. Metabolic alkalosis
   D. Abdominal distention
   E. Abdominal pain
   F. Profuse vomiting

2. A client has a new diagnosis of irritable bowel syndrome (IBS) with diarrhea. What health teaching by the nurse is **appropriate** for this client?
   A. "Take a stool softener every day to ease defecation."
   B. "Avoid high-fiber foods in your diet."
   C. "Avoid dairy products and caffeinated beverages."
   D. "Ask your primary health care provider for an antidepressant."

REFERENCES

Al-Mazrou, A. M., Baser, O., & Pokala, R. K. (2017). Alvimopan, regardless of ileus risk, significantly impacts ileus, length of stay, and Readmission after intestinal surgery. *Journal of the American College of Surgeons*, 225(4), S37.

American Cancer Society (ACS). (2019a). *Cancer facts and figures.* Atlanta: ACS.

American Cancer Society (ACS). (2019b). *Colorectal cancer risk factors.* Atlanta: ACS.

Benson, A. B., Venook, A. P., Cederquist, L., Chan, E., Chen, Y., Cooper, H. S., et al. (2017). Colon cancer: Clinical practice guidelines in oncology. *Journal of the National Comprehensive Cancer Network*, 15(3), 370–398.

Burchum, J. L. R., & Rosenthal, L. D. (2019). *Lehne's pharmacology for nursing care* (10th ed.). St. Louis: Elsevier.

Currò, D., Ianiro, G., Pecere, S., Bibbò, S., & Cammarota, G. (2017). Probiotics, fibre and herbal medicinal products for functional and inflammatory bowel disorders. *British Journal of Pharmacology*, 174(11), 1426–1449. https://doi.org/10.1111/bph.13632.

Derkacz, A., Olczyk, P., & Komosinska-Vassev, K. (2018). Diagnostic markers for Nonspecific inflammatory bowel diseases. *Disease Markers*, 2018, 7451946. https://doi.org/10.1155/2018/7451946.

Ghoshal, U. C., Shukla, R., & Ghoshal, U. (2017). Small intestinal bacterial overgrowth and irritable bowel syndrome: A Bridge between functional organic Dichotomy. *Gut and Liver*, 11(2), 196–208. https://doi.org/10.5009/gnl16126.

Lacy, B. E., Nicandro, J. P., Chuang, E., & Earnest, D. L. (2018). Alosetron use in clinical practice: Significant improvement in irritable bowel syndrome symptoms evaluated using the US food and drug administration composite endpoint. *Therapeutic Advances in Gastroenterology*, 111756284818771674. https://doi.org/10.1177/1756284818771674.

Lembo, A., Pimentel, M., Rao, S. S., Schoenfeld, P., Cash, B., Weinstock, L. B., et al. (2016). Repeat treatment with rifaximin is Safe and effective in patients with diarrhea-predominant irritable bowel syndrome. *Gastroenterology*, 151(6), 1113–1121. https://doi.org/10.1053/j.gastro.2016.08.003.

McCance, K., Huether, S., Brashers, V., & Rote, N. (2019). *Pathophysiology: The biologic basis for disease in adults and children* (8th ed.). St. Louis: Elsevier.

Pagana, K. D., & Pagana, T. J. (2018). *Mosby's manual of diagnostic and laboratory tests* (6th ed.). St. Louis: Mosby.

Papageorge, C. M., Zhao, Q., Foley, E. F., Harms, B., Heise, C. P., Carchman, E. H., et al. (2016). Short-term outcomes of minimally invasive versus open colectomy for colon cancer. *Journal of Surgical Research*, 204(1), 89–93.

Seow, H. F., Yip, W. K., & Fifis, T. (2016). Advances in targeted and immunobased therapies for colorectal cancer in the genomic era. *OncoTargets and Therapy*, 9, 1899–1920.

Stelton, S. (2019). Stoma and peristomal skin care: A clinical review. *AJN*, 119(6), 38–45.

Sultan, S., & Malhotra, A. (2017). Irritable bowel syndrome. *Annals of Internal Medicine*, 166(11), ITC81–ITC96. https://doi.org/10.7326/AITC201706060.

52

Concepts of Care for Patients With Inflammatory Intestinal Disorders

Keelin Cromar

http://evolve.elsevier.com/Iggy/

LEARNING OUTCOMES

1. Collaborate with the interprofessional team to manage quality care for patients with impaired *elimination* caused by chronic inflammatory bowel disorders.
2. Identify community resources for families and patients recovering from inflammatory bowel disorders.
3. Apply knowledge of pathophysiology of inflammatory bowel disorders to identify common assessment findings, including actual or risk for impaired *nutrition* and *fluid and electrolyte balance.*
4. Prioritize evidence-based nursing interventions for patients with inflammatory bowel disorders to promote *nutrition,* maintain *fluid and electrolyte balance,* and manage *pain, infection,* and/or *inflammation.*
5. Plan transition management and care coordination for the patient who has an ileostomy, including health teaching.

KEY TERMS

abscess A localized infection in which there is a collection of pus.

appendectomy The removal of the inflamed appendix by one of several surgical approaches.

appendicitis An acute inflammation of the vermiform appendix that occurs most often among young adults.

celiac disease A chronic inflammation of the small intestinal mucosa that can cause bowel wall atrophy, malabsorption, and diarrhea.

Crohn's disease (CD) A chronic inflammatory disease of the small intestine (most often), the colon, or both; the terminal ileum is most often affected.

diverticulitis The inflammation or infection of diverticula.

diverticulosis The presence of many abnormal pouchlike herniations (diverticula) in the wall of the intestine.

effluent Drainage.

fissure A tear, crack, or split in skin and underlying tissue.

fistula Abnormal opening (tract) between two organs or structures.

gastroenteritis A very common health problem worldwide that causes diarrhea and/or vomiting related to inflammation of the mucous membranes of the stomach and intestinal tract.

ileostomy A procedure in which a loop of the ileum is placed through an opening in the abdominal wall (stoma) for drainage of fecal material into a pouching system worn on the abdomen.

intestinal malabsorption (malabsorption syndrome) The inability of essential nutrients to be absorbed through a diseased intestinal wall, causing anemia and malnutrition (most common in Crohn's disease).

laparoscopy A minimally invasive surgery (MIS) with one or more small incisions near the umbilicus through which a small endoscope and tools are placed.

laparotomy An open surgical approach requiring a large abdominal incision.

ostomate A person who has an ostomy.

peritonitis A life-threatening, acute inflammation and infection of the visceral/parietal peritoneum and endothelial lining of the abdominal cavity.

progressive multifocal leukoencephalopathy (PML) A deadly infection that affects the brain.

steatorrhea Fatty diarrheal stools.

tenesmus An unpleasant and urgent sensation to defecate.

toxic megacolon Massive dilation of the colon and subsequent colonic ileus that can lead to gangrene and peritonitis.

ulcerative colitis (UC) A disease that creates widespread chronic inflammation of the rectum and rectosigmoid colon but can extend to the entire colon when the disease is extensive.

PRIORITY AND INTERRELATED CONCEPTS

The priority concepts for this chapter are:
- **Infection**
- **Inflammation**

The **Infection** concept exemplar for this chapter is Peritonitis.
The **Inflammation** concept exemplar for this chapter is Ulcerative Colitis.

The interrelated concepts for this chapter are:
- **Nutrition**
- **Elimination**
- **Pain**
- **Fluid and Electrolyte Balance**

The *intestinal tract* is made up of the small intestine and large intestine (colon). Continued digestion of food and absorption of nutrients occurs primarily in the small intestine to meet the body's needs for energy. Water is reabsorbed in the large intestine to help maintain a fluid balance and promote the passage of waste products. When the intestinal tract and its nearby structures become acutely inflamed, *pain* and *infection* can occur. Chronic bowel *inflammation* can affect *nutrition*, *elimination*, and *fluid and electrolyte balance.* Chapter 3 briefly reviews each of these health concepts.

Appendicitis, gastroenteritis, and peritonitis are the most common *acute* inflammatory bowel disorders (IBDs). These disorders can be potentially life threatening and can have major systemic complications if not treated promptly. Ulcerative colitis and Crohn's disease are the two most common *chronic* IBDs that affect adults.

INFECTION CONCEPT EXEMPLAR: PERITONITIS

Pathophysiology Review

Peritonitis is a life-threatening, acute *inflammation* and *infection* of the visceral/parietal peritoneum and endothelial lining of the abdominal cavity. The peritoneal cavity normally contains about 50 mL of sterile fluid (transudate), which prevents friction in the abdominal cavity during peristalsis. When the peritoneal cavity is contaminated by bacteria, the body begins an inflammatory reaction, walling off a localized area to fight the infection. Vascular dilation and increased capillary permeability occur, allowing transport of leukocytes and subsequent phagocytosis of the offending organisms. If the process of walling off fails, the *inflammation* spreads and contamination becomes massive, resulting in diffuse (widespread) *infection.*

Peritonitis is most often caused by contamination of the peritoneal cavity by bacteria or chemicals. Bacteria gain entry into the peritoneum by perforation (from appendicitis, diverticulitis, peptic ulcer disease) or from an external penetrating wound, a gangrenous gallbladder or bowel segment, bowel obstruction, or ascending infection through the genital tract. Less common causes include invasive tumors, leakage or contamination during surgery, or *infection* by skin pathogens in patients undergoing continuous ambulatory peritoneal dialysis (CAPD) (McCance et al., 2019).

When diagnosis and treatment of peritonitis are delayed, blood vessel dilation continues. The body responds to the continuing infectious process by shunting extra blood to the area of inflammation (hyperemia). Fluid is shifted from the extracellular fluid compartment into the peritoneal cavity, connective tissues, and GI tract *("third spacing").* This shift of fluid can result in a significant decrease in circulatory volume and *hypovolemic shock.* Severely decreased circulatory volume can result in insufficient perfusion of the kidneys, leading to acute kidney injury with impaired *fluid and electrolyte balance* (McCance et al., 2019).

Peristalsis slows or *stops* in response to severe peritoneal *inflammation* and *infection,* and the lumen of the bowel becomes distended with gas and fluid. Fluid that normally flows to the small bowel and the colon for reabsorption accumulates in the intestine in volumes of 7 to 8 L daily. The toxins or bacteria responsible for the peritonitis can also enter the bloodstream from the peritoneal area and lead to bacteremia, or septicemia (bacterial invasion of the blood), a life-threatening condition that can lead to systemic sepsis and septic shock (see Chapter 34 on *infection.*)

Respiratory problems can occur as a result of increased abdominal pressure against the diaphragm from intestinal distention and fluid shifts to the peritoneal cavity. Also, *pain* can interfere with respirations at a time when the patient has an increased oxygen demand because of the infectious process.

Etiology. Common bacteria responsible for peritonitis include *Escherichia coli, Streptococcus, Staphylococcus, Pneumococcus,* and *Gonococcus.* Chemical peritonitis results from leakage of bile, pancreatic enzymes, and gastric acid (McCance et al., 2019).

Incidence and Prevalence. Peritonitis is the dominant cause of death from surgical infections, with a mortality rate of up to 20% (Ross et al., 2018). It occurs most commonly in young adults who have appendicitis and older adults whose immunity is often decreased.

❖ Interprofessional Collaborative Care

Patients with peritonitis are hospitalized because of the severe nature of the illness. If complications are extensive, the patients are often admitted to a critical care unit.

◆ Assessment: Recognize Cues

History. Ask the patient about abdominal *pain* and determine the character of the pain (e.g., cramping, sharp, aching), location of the pain, and whether the pain is localized or generalized. Ask about a history of a low-grade fever or recent spikes in temperature.

Physical Assessment/Signs and Symptoms. Physical findings of peritonitis depend on several factors: the stage of the disease, the ability of the body to localize the process by walling off the *infection,* and whether the *inflammation* has progressed to generalized peritonitis (see the Key Features: Peritonitis box).

The patient most often appears acutely ill, lying still, possibly with the knees flexed. Movement is guarded, and he or she may report and show signs of *pain* (e.g., facial grimacing) with coughing or movement of any type. During inspection, observe for progressive abdominal distention, often seen when the

» KEY FEATURES

Peritonitis

- Rigid, board-like abdomen (classic)
- Abdominal *pain* (localized, poorly localized, or referred to the shoulder or chest)
- Distended abdomen
- Nausea, anorexia, vomiting
- Diminishing bowel sounds
- Inability to pass flatus or feces
- Rebound tenderness in the abdomen
- High fever
- Tachycardia
- Dehydration from high fever (poor skin turgor)
- Decreased urine output
- Hiccups
- Possible compromise in respiratory status

inflammation and *infection* markedly reduce intestinal motility. Auscultate for bowel sounds, which usually disappear with progression of the inflammation.

*The cardinal signs of peritonitis are abdominal **pain**, tenderness, and distention.* In the patient with *localized* peritonitis, the abdomen is tender on palpation in a well-defined area with rebound tenderness in this area. With *generalized* peritonitis, tenderness is widespread.

Psychosocial Assessment. The patient with peritonitis may be very fearful and anxious about the implications of a diagnosis of peritonitis and may be distressed regarding the physical *pain* that he or she feels. Provide a calm, nonanxious presence and reassure the patient that you will be there (presence) to help him or her during this time. Allow the patient to express feelings of fear and anxiety, and provide nonjudgmental listening and presence.

Laboratory Assessment. *White blood cell (WBC) counts* are often elevated to 20,000/mm^3 with a high neutrophil count (*leukocytosis*). *Blood culture* studies may be done to determine whether septicemia has occurred and to identify the causative organism to determine appropriate antibiotic therapy. The primary health care provider may request laboratory tests to assess *fluid and electrolyte balance* and renal status, including blood urea nitrogen (BUN), creatinine, hemoglobin, and hematocrit. Oxygen saturation and arterial blood gases may be obtained to assess respiratory function and acid-base balance.

Imaging Assessment. *Abdominal x-rays* can assess for free air or fluid in the abdominal cavity, indicating perforation. The x-rays may also show dilation, edema, and *inflammation* of the small and large intestines. An *abdominal ultrasound* or *computerized tomography (CT) scan* may also be performed.

◆ **Analysis: Analyze Cues and Prioritize Hypotheses.** The priority collaborative problems for patients with peritonitis include:
1. Acute *pain* due to abdominal *inflammation* and *infection*
2. Potential for fluid volume shift due to fluid moving into interstitial or peritoneal space

◆ **Planning and Implementation: Generate Solutions and Take Action.** The collaborative plan of care for the patient diagnosed with peritonitis focuses on treating the cause of the infection and managing the infectious process. Nonsurgical and/or surgical modalities may be required to resolve the *infection*.

Managing Pain

Planning: Expected Outcomes. The patient is expected to report pain of 2 to 3 on a 0 to 10 pain intensity scale as the *inflammation* and *infection* resolve.

Interventions. Interventions for peritonitis are usually nonsurgical, but surgery may be required to remove abscesses or other infectious material.

Nonsurgical Management. Assess vital signs frequently, noting any change that may indicate septic shock, such as unresolved or progressive hypotension, decreased pulse pressure, tachycardia, fever, skin changes, and/or tachypnea. Monitor mental status changes for any sign of confusion or altered level of consciousness. Practice proper handwashing and maintain strict asepsis when caring for wounds, drains, and dressings to decrease chance of superimposed *infection*. If the patient has or requires a urinary catheter, maintain strict sterile technique and provide appropriate catheter care. Observe and document wound drainage; report any changes immediately to the primary health care provider. Administer broad-spectrum antibiotics as prescribed to treat known or potential pathogens. Provide oxygen as prescribed and according to the patient's respiratory status and oxygen saturation via pulse oximetry.

Surgical Management. Abdominal surgery may be needed to identify and repair the cause of the peritonitis. If the patient is critically ill and surgery could be life threatening, it may be delayed. Surgery focuses on controlling the contamination, removing foreign material from the peritoneal cavity, and draining collected fluid.

An *exploratory laparotomy* (an open surgical approach requiring a large abdominal incision) or laparoscopy is used to remove or repair an inflamed or perforated organ (e.g., appendectomy for an inflamed appendix; a colon resection, with or without a colostomy, for a perforated diverticulum). Before the incision(s) is closed, the surgeon irrigates the peritoneum with antibiotic solutions. Several catheters may be inserted to drain the cavity and provide a route for irrigation after surgery.

If an *open* conventional surgical procedure is needed, the *infection* may slow healing of an incision or the incision may be partially open to heal by second or third intention. These wounds require special care involving manual irrigation or packing as prescribed by the surgeon. If the surgeon requests peritoneal irrigation through a drain, *maintain sterile technique during manual irrigation* to prevent further risk for infection. Chapter 9 describes general preoperative and postoperative care.

⚠ NURSING SAFETY PRIORITY (QSEN)

Action Alert

Monitor the patient's level of consciousness, vital signs, respiratory status (respiratory rate and breath sounds), and intake and output at least hourly immediately after abdominal surgery. Maintain the patient in a semi-Fowler position to promote drainage of peritoneal contents into the lower region of the abdominal cavity. This position also helps increase lung expansion.

Restoring Fluid Volume Balance

Planning: Expected Outcomes. The patient will experience restoration of fluid volume balance.

Interventions. The primary health care provider prescribes hypertonic IV fluids and broad-spectrum antibiotics immediately after establishing the diagnosis of peritonitis. Remind assistive personnel to take a daily weight using the same scale each morning, and record intake and output carefully. A nasogastric tube (NGT) is inserted to decompress the stomach and the intestine if a laparotomy is anticipated.

Multisystem complications can occur with peritonitis. Loss of fluids and electrolytes from the extracellular space to the peritoneal cavity, NGT suctioning, and NPO status require that the patient receives IV fluid replacement. Fluid rates may be changed frequently on the basis of laboratory values, assessment findings, and patient condition.

Assess whether the patient retains fluid used for irrigation by comparing and recording the amount of fluid returned with the amount of fluid instilled. Fluid retention could cause abdominal distention or pain.

Care Coordination and Transition Management

Home Care Management. The length of hospitalization for a patient with peritonitis depends on the extent and severity of the infectious process. Patients who have a localized **abscess** (a localized *infection* in which there is a collection of pus) drained and who respond to antibiotics and IV fluids without multisystem complications are discharged in several days. Others may require mechanical ventilation or hemodialysis with longer hospital stays. Some patients may be transferred to a transitional care unit to complete their antibiotic therapy and recovery. Convalescence is often longer than other surgeries because of multisystem involvement.

Self-Management Education. Before being discharged home, assess the patient's ability for self-management. Provide the patient and family with written and oral instructions to report the following problems to the primary health care provider immediately:

- Unusual or foul-smelling drainage
- Swelling, redness, or warmth or bleeding from the incision site
- A temperature higher than 101°F (38.3°C)
- Abdominal *pain*
- Signs of wound dehiscence or ileus

Patients with large incisions that are left open heal by secondary or tertiary intention and require dressings, solution, and catheter-tipped syringes to irrigate the wound. A home care nurse may be needed to assess, irrigate, or pack the wound and change the dressing as needed until the patient and family feel comfortable with the procedure. If the patient needs assistance with ADLs, a home care aide or temporary placement in a skilled care facility may be indicated.

Review information about antibiotics and analgesics. For patients taking short-term oral opioid analgesics such as oxycodone with acetaminophen, a stool softener such as docusate sodium may be prescribed with a laxative. Older adults are especially at risk for constipation from codeine-based drugs. Remind patients to avoid taking additional acetaminophen to prevent liver toxicity.

Teach patients to refrain from any lifting for *at least* 6 weeks after an open surgical procedure. Other activity limitations are based on individual need and the primary health care provider's recommendation. Patients who have laparoscopic surgery can resume activities within a week or two and may not have any major restrictions.

NCLEX EXAMINATION CHALLENGE 52.1

Safe and Effective Care Environment

A client had an exploratory laparotomy to treat the cause of peritonitis and has a large incision that is closed with staples and two abdominal drains. Which finding(s) would the nurse report **immediately** to the surgeon? **Select all that apply.**

A. Serosanguineous drainage
B. Increased abdominal distention
C. Fever and chills
D. Pain level 2 on a scale of 0 to 10
E. Passing flatus

Health Care Resources. Patients with peritonitis may benefit from a social services consultation. Social workers can help patients locate the most appropriate and affordable supplies that will be needed for ongoing care. Collaborate with the case manager to determine the appropriate setting for seamless continuing care in the community.

◆ **Evaluation: Evaluate Outcomes.** Evaluate the care of the patient with peritonitis based on the identified priority patient problems. The expected outcomes are that the patient:

- Verbalizes relief or control of pain as *infection* resolves
- Experiences *fluid and electrolyte balance*

APPENDICITIS

Pathophysiology Review

Appendicitis is an acute *inflammation* of the vermiform appendix that occurs most often among young adults. It is the most common cause of right lower quadrant (RLQ) pain. The appendix usually extends off the proximal cecum of the colon just below the ileocecal valve. Inflammation occurs when the lumen (opening) of the appendix is obstructed (blocked), leading to *infection* as bacteria invade the wall of the appendix. The initial obstruction is usually a result of fecaliths (very hard pieces of feces) composed of calcium phosphate–rich mucus and inorganic salts (McCance et al., 2019).

When the lumen is blocked, the mucosa secretes fluid, increasing the internal pressure and restricting blood flow, which results in *pain.* If the process occurs slowly, an **abscess** may develop, but a rapid process may result in **peritonitis**. *All complications of peritonitis are serious. Gangrene and sepsis can occur within 24 to 36 hours, are life threatening, and are some of the most common indications for emergency surgery. Perforation may develop within*

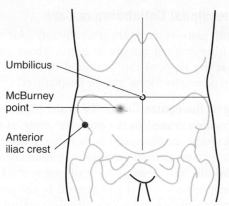

Fig. 52.1 The McBurney point is located midway between the anterior iliac crest and the umbilicus in the right lower quadrant. This is the classic area for localized tenderness during the later stages of appendicitis.

24 hours, but the risk rises rapidly after 48 hours. Perforation of the appendix results in peritonitis with a temperature of greater than 101°F (38.3°C) and a rise in pulse rate.

❖ Interprofessional Collaborative Care

◆ Assessment: Recognize Cues. History taking and tracking the sequence of symptoms are important because nausea or vomiting before abdominal pain can indicate gastroenteritis. Abdominal pain followed by nausea and vomiting can indicate appendicitis. Classically, patients with appendicitis have cramping *pain* in the epigastric or periumbilical area. Anorexia is also a frequent symptom.

Perform a complete *pain* assessment. Initially pain can present anywhere in the abdomen or flank area. As the *inflammation* and *infection* progress, the pain becomes more severe and shifts to the RLQ between the anterior iliac crest and the umbilicus. This area is referred to as the *McBurney point* (Fig. 52.1). *Abdominal pain that increases with cough or movement and is relieved by bending the right hip or the knees suggests perforation and peritonitis.* The primary health care provider assesses for muscle rigidity and guarding on palpation of the abdomen. The patient may report pain after release of pressure. This sensation is referred to as *rebound* tenderness.

Laboratory findings do not establish the diagnosis, but often there is a moderate elevation of the *white blood cell (WBC) count* (leukocytosis) to 10,000 to 18,000/mm³ with a "shift to the left" (an increased number of immature WBCs). A WBC elevation to greater than 20,000/mm³ may indicate a perforated appendix. An *ultrasound* study may show the presence of an enlarged appendix. If symptoms are recurrent or prolonged, a CT scan can be used to diagnose and may reveal the presence of a fecaloma (a small "stone" of feces) (Pagana & Pagana, 2018).

◆ Interventions: Take Action. All patients with suspected or confirmed appendicitis are hospitalized, and most have surgery to remove the inflamed appendix.

Nonsurgical Management. Keep the patient with suspected or known appendicitis NPO to prepare for the probability of surgery and to avoid making the *inflammation* worse. Be sure that the patient's *pain* is adequately managed before surgical intervention.

> ## ❗ NURSING SAFETY PRIORITY (QSEN)
> ### Action Alert
>
> For the patient with suspected appendicitis, administer IV fluids as prescribed to maintain **fluid and electrolyte balance** and replace fluid volume. If tolerated, advise the patient to maintain a semi-Fowler position so that abdominal drainage can be contained in the lower abdomen. Once the diagnosis of appendicitis is confirmed and surgery is scheduled, administer opioid analgesics and antibiotics as prescribed. *The patient with suspected or confirmed appendicitis should not receive laxatives or enemas, which can cause perforation of the appendix. Do not apply heat to the abdomen because this may increase circulation to the appendix and result in increased **inflammation** and perforation!*

Surgical Management. Surgery is required as soon as possible for most patients. An **appendectomy** is the removal of the inflamed appendix by one of several surgical approaches. Uncomplicated appendectomy procedures are done via laparoscopy. A **laparoscopy** is a minimally invasive surgery (MIS) with one or more small incisions near the umbilicus, through which a small endoscope and tools are inserted. Patients having this type of surgery for appendix removal have few postoperative complications (see Chapter 9). A procedure known as *natural orifice transluminal endoscopic surgery (NOTES)* (e.g., transvaginal endoscopic appendectomy) does not require an external skin incision. During this procedure, the surgeon places the endoscope into the vagina or other orifice and makes a small incision to enter the peritoneal space. Patients having any type of laparoscopic procedure are typically discharged the same day of surgery with less pain and few complications after discharge. Most patients can return to usual activities in 1 to 2 weeks.

If the diagnosis is not definitive but the patient is at high risk for complications from suspected appendicitis, the surgeon may perform an exploratory laparotomy. A **laparotomy** is an open surgical approach with a large abdominal incision.

Preoperative teaching is often limited because the patient is in *pain* or may be admitted quickly for emergency surgery. The patient is prepared for general anesthesia. After surgery, care of the patient who has undergone an appendectomy is the same as that required for anyone who has received general anesthesia (see Chapter 9).

If complications such as peritonitis or abscesses are found during *open* traditional surgery, wound drains are inserted and a nasogastric tube may be placed to decompress the stomach and prevent abdominal distention. Administer IV antibiotics and opioid analgesics as prescribed. Help the patient out of bed on the evening of surgery to help prevent respiratory complications, such as atelectasis. He or she may be hospitalized for as long as 3 to 5 days and return to usual activity in 4 to 6 weeks.

GASTROENTERITIS

Pathophysiology Review

Gastroenteritis is a very common health problem worldwide that causes diarrhea and/or vomiting related to *inflammation* of the mucous membranes of the stomach and intestinal tract. The small

TABLE 52.1 Common Types of Gastroenteritis and Their Characteristics

Type	Characteristics
Viral Gastroenteritis	
Epidemic viral	Caused by many parvovirus-type organisms Transmitted by the fecal-oral route in food and water Incubation period 10-51 hr Communicable during acute illness
Norovirus (Norwalk viruses)	Transmitted by the fecal-oral route and possibly the respiratory route (vomitus) Incubation in 48 hr Affects adults of all ages Older adults can become hypovolemic and experience electrolyte imbalances
Bacterial Gastroenteritis	
Campylobacter enteritis	Transmitted by the fecal-oral route or contact with infected animals or infants Incubation period 1-10 days Communicable for 2-7 wk
Escherichia coli diarrhea	Transmitted by fecal contamination of food, water, or fomites
Shigellosis	Transmitted by direct and indirect fecal-oral routes Incubation period 1-7 days Communicable during the acute illness to 4 wk after the illness Humans possibly carriers for months

bowel is most commonly affected and can be caused by either viral (more common) or bacterial *infection*. Table 52.1 lists common types of gastroenteritis and their primary characteristics.

Norovirus (also known as a *Norwalk-like virus*) is the leading foodborne disease that causes gastroenteritis. It occurs most often between November and April because it is resistant to low temperatures and has a long viral shedding before and after the illness. Norovirus is transmitted (spread) through the fecal-oral route from person to person and from contaminated food and water. Infected individuals can also contaminate surfaces and objects in the environment. Vomiting may cause the virus to become airborne. The incubation time is 1 to 2 days (McCance et al., 2019).

In most cases of gastroenteritis, the illness is self-limiting and lasts about 3 days. However, in those who are immunosuppressed or in older adults, dehydration and hypovolemia can occur as complications requiring medical attention and possibly hospitalization.

Health Promotion and Maintenance. Outbreaks of norovirus have occurred in prisons, on cruise ships, and in nursing homes, college dormitories, and other places where large groups of people are in close proximity. Teach individuals that handwashing and sanitizing surfaces and other environmental items help prevent the spread of the illness. Hand sanitizers are often placed in public areas so that hands can be cleaned when washing with soap and water is inconvenient. Proper food and beverage preparation is also important to prevent contamination.

❖ Interprofessional Collaborative Care

Patients with gastroenteritis are generally cared for in the community setting and self-manage at home. Those who develop the more severe types of this condition or become extremely dehydrated during its course may be hospitalized.

◆ **Assessment: Recognize Cues.** The patient history can provide information related to the potential cause of the illness. Ask about recent travel, especially to tropical regions of Asia, Africa, Mexico, or Central or South America, because these areas historically have been a source of gastroenteritis. Inquire if the patient has eaten at any restaurant in the past 24 to 36 hours. Some people acquire gastroenteritis from eating in "fast-food" restaurants or from food items purchased at a farmer's market or grocery store. Bacterial infections have caused large outbreaks that resulted from contaminated spinach and lettuce in the United States. Raw or undercooked food such as oysters, sushi, and rare meat can also cause GI infections.

The patient who has gastroenteritis usually looks ill. Nausea and vomiting typically occur first, followed by abdominal cramping and diarrhea. For patients who are older or for those who have inadequate immune systems, weakness and cardiac dysrhythmias may occur from loss of potassium (hypokalemia) from diarrhea. Monitor for and document manifestations of hypokalemia and hypovolemia (dehydration).

> **⚠ NURSING SAFETY PRIORITY** (QSEN)
> ***Action Alert***
>
> For patients with gastroenteritis, note any abdominal distention and listen for hyperactive bowel sounds. Depending on the amount of fluids and electrolytes lost through diarrhea and vomiting, patients may have varying degrees of dehydration manifested by:
> - Weight loss (unintentional)
> - Poor skin turgor
> - Fever (not common in older adults)
> - Dry mucous membranes
> - Orthostatic blood pressure changes (which can cause a fall, especially for older adults)
> - Hypotension
> - Oliguria (decreased or absent urinary output)
>
> In some cases, dehydration may be severe. It can occur very rapidly in older adults. Monitor mental status changes, such as acute confusion, that result from hypoxia due to dehydration in the older adult. These changes may be the only initial signs and symptoms of dehydration in older adults.

◆ **Interventions: Take Action.** For any type of gastroenteritis, encourage fluid replacement. The amount and route of fluid administration are determined by the patient's hydration status and overall health condition. Teach patients to drink extra fluids to replace fluid lost through vomiting and diarrhea. Oral rehydration therapy (ORT) may be needed for some patients to replace fluids and electrolytes. Examples of ORT solutions include sports drinks and Pedialyte. Depending on the patient's age and severity of dehydration, he or she may be treated in the hospital with IV fluids to restore hydration.

Drugs that suppress intestinal motility may not be given for bacterial or viral gastroenteritis. *Use of these drugs can prevent the infecting organisms from being eliminated from the body.* If the primary health care provider determines that antiperistaltic/antidiarrheal agents are necessary, loperamide may be recommended.

! NURSING SAFETY PRIORITY (QSEN)

Drug Alert

Diphenoxylate hydrochloride with atropine sulfate reduces GI motility but is used sparingly because of its habit-forming ability. *The drug should not be used for older adults because it also causes drowsiness and could contribute to falls.*

Treatment with antibiotics may be needed if the gastroenteritis is caused by bacterial **infection** with fever and severe diarrhea. Depending on the type and severity of the illness, examples of drugs that may be prescribed include ciprofloxacin or azithromycin. If the gastroenteritis is caused by shigellosis, anti-infective agents such as ciprofloxacin, ceftriaxone, or azithromycin are prescribed (Burchum & Rosenthal, 2019).

Frequent stools that are rich in electrolytes and enzymes and frequent wiping and washing of the anal region can irritate the skin. Teach the patient to avoid toilet paper and harsh soaps. Ideally, he or she can gently clean the area with warm water or an absorbent material, followed by thorough but gentle drying. Cream, oil, or gel can be applied to a damp, warm washcloth to remove stool that sticks to open skin. Special prepared skin wipes can also be used. Protective barrier cream can be applied to the skin between stools. Sitz baths for 10 minutes two or three times daily can also relieve discomfort.

If leakage of stool is a problem, the patient can use an absorbent cotton or panty liner and keep it in place with snug underwear. For patients who are incontinent, the use of incontinent pads at night instead of briefs allows air to circulate to the skin and prevents irritation. Remind assistive personnel to keep the perineal and buttock areas clean and dry and that frequent changes will be necessary.

During the acute phase of the illness, teach the patient and family about the importance of fluid replacement. Patient and family education regarding risk for transmission of gastroenteritis is also important (see the Patient and Family Education: Preparing for Self-Management: Preventing Transmission of Gastroenteritis box).

PATIENT AND FAMILY EDUCATION: PREPARING FOR SELF-MANAGEMENT

Preventing Transmission of Gastroenteritis

Advise the patient to:
- Wash hands well for at least 30 seconds with an antibacterial soap, especially after a bowel movement, and maintain good personal hygiene.
- Restrict the use of glasses, dishes, eating utensils, and tubes of toothpaste for his or her own use. In severe cases, disposable utensils may be used.
- Maintain clean bathroom facilities to avoid exposure to stool.
- Inform the primary health care provider if symptoms persist beyond 3 days.
- Do not prepare or handle food that will be consumed by others. If you (the patient) are employed as a food handler, the public health department should be consulted for recommendations about the return to work.

TABLE 52.2 Differential Features of Ulcerative Colitis and Crohn's Disease

Feature	Ulcerative Colitis	Crohn's Disease
Location	Begins in the rectum and proceeds in a continuous manner toward the cecum	Most often in the terminal ileum, with patchy involvement through all layers of the bowel
Etiology	Unknown	Unknown
Peak incidence at age	15-25 yr and 55-65 yr	15-40 yr
Number of stools	10-20 liquid, bloody stools per day	5-6 soft, loose stools per day, nonbloody
Complications	Hemorrhage Nutritional deficiencies	Fistulas (common) Nutritional deficiencies
Client need for surgery	20%-40%	75%

Preparing for Self-Management: Preventing Transmission of Gastroenteritis box).

✳ INFLAMMATION CONCEPT EXEMPLAR: ULCERATIVE COLITIS

Pathophysiology Review

Ulcerative colitis (UC) is a disease that creates widespread chronic **inflammation** of the rectum and rectosigmoid colon but can extend to the entire colon when the disease is extensive. Distribution of the disease can remain constant for years. UC is a disease that is associated with periodic remissions and exacerbations (flare-ups) and is often confused with Crohn's disease. Comparisons and differences are listed in Table 52.2.

Many factors can cause exacerbations, including intestinal **infection**. Most patients who are affected have mild-to-moderate disease, but a small percentage of patients present with severe symptoms. Older adults with UC are at high risk for impaired **fluid and electrolyte balance** as a result of diarrhea, including dehydration and hypokalemia (McCance et al., 2019).

The intestinal mucosa becomes hyperemic (has increased blood flow), edematous, and reddened. In more severe inflammation, the lining can bleed and small erosions, or ulcers, occur. Abscesses can form in these ulcerative areas and result in tissue necrosis (cell death). Continued edema and mucosal thickening can lead to a narrowed colon and possibly a partial bowel obstruction. Table 52.3 lists the categories of the severity of UC.

The patient's stool typically contains blood and mucus. Patients report tenesmus (an unpleasant and urgent sensation to defecate) and lower abdominal colicky pain relieved with defecation. Malaise, anorexia, anemia, dehydration, fever, and weight loss are common. Extraintestinal manifestations such as migratory polyarthritis, ankylosing spondylitis, and erythema nodosum are present in a large number of patients. The common and extraintestinal complications of UC are listed in Table 52.4.

Etiology and Genetic Risk. The exact cause of UC is unknown, but a combination of genetic, immunologic, and environmental factors likely contributes to disease development. A genetic

TABLE 52.3 American College of Gastroenterologists Classification of Ulcerative Colitis Severity

Severity	Stool Frequency	Signs/Symptoms
Mild	<4 stools/day with/without blood	Asymptomatic Laboratory values usually normal
Moderate	>4 stools/day with/without blood	Minimal symptoms Mild abdominal pain Mild intermittent nausea Possible increased C-reactive protein[a] or ESR[b]
Severe	>6 bloody stools/day	Fever Tachycardia Anemia Abdominal pain Elevated C-reactive protein[a] and/or ESR[b]
Fulminant	>10 bloody stools/day	Increasing symptoms Anemia may require transfusion Colonic distention on x-ray

UC, Ulcerative colitis.

[a]C-reactive protein is a sensitive acute-phase serum marker that is evident in the first 6 hours of an inflammatory process.

[b]ESR, erythrocyte sedimentation rate; may be helpful but is less sensitive than C-reactive protein.

TABLE 52.4 Complications of Ulcerative Colitis and Crohn's Disease

Complication	Description
Hemorrhage/perforation	Lower GI bleeding results from erosion of the bowel wall.
Abscess formation	Localized pockets of **infection** develop in the ulcerated bowel lining.
Toxic megacolon	Massive dilation of the colon and subsequent colonic ileus that can lead to gangrene and peritonitis.
Intestinal malabsorption	Essential nutrients cannot be absorbed through the diseased intestinal wall, causing anemia and malnutrition (most common in Crohn's disease).
Nonmechanical bowel obstruction	Obstruction results from toxic megacolon or cancer.
Fistulas	In Crohn's disease in which the **inflammation** is transmural, fistulas can occur anywhere but usually track between the bowel and bladder, resulting in pyuria and fecaluria.
Colorectal cancer	Patients with ulcerative colitis with a history longer than 10 years have a high risk for colorectal cancer. This complication accounts for about one-third of all deaths related to ulcerative colitis.
Extraintestinal complications	Complications include arthritis, hepatic and biliary disease (especially cholelithiasis), oral and skin lesions, and ocular disorders, such as iritis. The cause is unknown.
Osteoporosis	Osteoporosis occurs, especially in patients with Crohn's disease.

basis of the disease has been supported because it is often found in families and twins. Immunologic causes, including autoimmune dysfunction, are likely the etiology of extraintestinal manifestations of the disease. Epithelial antibodies in the immunoglobulin G (IgG) class have been identified in the blood of some patients with UC (McCance et al., 2019).

With long-term disease, cellular changes can occur that increase the risk for colon cancer. Damage from proinflammatory cytokines, such as specific interleukins (ILs) (e.g., IL-1, IL-6, IL-8) and tumor necrosis factor (TNF)–alpha, have cytotoxic effects on the colonic mucosa (McCance et al., 2019).

PATIENT-CENTERED CARE: CULTURAL/SPIRITUAL CONSIDERATIONS (QSEN)

Ulcerative colitis is more common among Askenazki Jewish individuals than among those who are not Jewish and among whites more than non-whites (McCance et al., 2019). The reasons for these cultural differences are not known.

Incidence and Prevalence. In the United States, 1.6 million individuals are affected by chronic inflammatory bowel disease (IBD). Between the two primary types of IBD, ulcerative colitis (UC) and Crohn's disease (discussed later), the incidence is split almost equally. Although diagnosis can occur at any age, most people are diagnosed between 15 and 35 years of age (Crohn's & Colitis Foundation, 2020). Women are more often affected than men in their younger years, but men have the disease more often as middle-age and older adults (McCance et al., 2019).

❖ Interprofessional Collaborative Care

Patients with UC may be self-managed at home, cared for in the community setting, or hospitalized, depending on their immediate condition related to this chronic bowel disease.

◆ Assessment: Recognize Cues

History. Collect data on family history of IBD, previous and current therapy for the illness, and dates and types of surgery. Obtain a *nutrition* history, including intolerance of milk and milk products and fried, spicy, or hot foods. Ask about usual bowel *elimination* pattern (color, number, consistency, and character of stools); abdominal pain; tenesmus; anorexia; and fatigue. Note any relationship between diarrhea, timing of meals, emotional distress, and activity. Inquire about recent (past 2 to 3 months) exposure to antibiotics to rule out a *Clostridium difficile* infection. Has the patient traveled to or emigrated from tropical areas? Ask about recent use of NSAIDs because these can cause a flare-up of the disease. Inquire about any extraintestinal symptoms, such as arthritis, mouth sores, vision problems, and skin disorders.

Physical Assessment/Signs and Symptoms. Symptoms vary with an acuteness of onset. Vital signs are usually within normal limits in mild disease. In more severe cases, the patient may have a low-grade fever (99° to 100° F [37.2° to 37.8° C]). The physical assessment findings are usually nonspecific, and in milder cases the physical examination may be normal. Viral and bacterial infections can cause symptoms similar to those of UC.

Note any abdominal distention along the colon. Fever associated with tachycardia may indicate dehydration, peritonitis, and bowel perforation. Assess for signs and symptoms associated with extraintestinal complications, such as inflamed joints and lesions inside the mouth.

Psychosocial Assessment. Many patients are very concerned about the frequency of stools and the presence of blood. *The inability to control the disease symptoms, particularly diarrhea, can be disruptive and anxiety producing.* Severe illness may limit the patient's activities outside the home with fear of fecal incontinence resulting in feeling "tied to the toilet." Severe anxiety and depression may result. Eating may be associated with pain and cramping and an increased frequency of stools. This can make mealtimes an unpleasant experience. Frequent visits to primary health care providers and close monitoring of the colon mucosa for abnormal cell changes can be anxiety provoking.

Assess the patient's understanding of the illness and its impact on his or her lifestyle. Encourage and support the patient while exploring:

- The relationship of life events to disease exacerbations
- Stress factors that produce symptoms
- Family and social support systems
- Concerns regarding the possible genetic basis and associated cancer risks of the disease
- Internet access for reliable education information

Laboratory Assessment. Hematocrit and hemoglobin levels may be low related to chronic blood loss, which indicates anemia and a chronic disease state. *An increased WBC count, C-reactive protein, or erythrocyte sedimentation rate (ESR) is consistent with inflammatory disease.* Blood levels of sodium, potassium, and chloride may be *low* as a result of frequent diarrheal stools and malabsorption through the diseased bowel (Pagana & Pagana, 2018). Hypoalbuminemia (decreased serum albumin) is found in patients with extensive disease from losing protein in the stool.

Other Diagnostic Assessment. *Magnetic resonance enterography (MRE)* is the main examination used to study the bowel in patients who have chronic IBD. An MRE allows the primary health care provider to visualize the bowel lumen and wall, mesentery, and surrounding abdominal organs. Teach the patient that he or she will need to fast for 4 to 6 hours before the test. As part of the test the patient drinks a large amount of contrast medium; this can cause abdominal discomfort and diarrhea. Be sure that the patient has the opportunity to go to the restroom before positioning on the MRI table. The patient then lies prone while the first of two doses of glucagon are given subcutaneously. This substance helps to slow the bowel's activity and motility (Khatri et al., 2018).

An upper endoscopy and/or *colonoscopy* may be done to aid in diagnosis, but the bowel preparation ("prep") can be especially uncomfortable for patients with inflammatory bowel disease (IBD). Frequent colonoscopies are recommended when patients have longer than a 10-year history of UC involving the entire colon because they are at high risk for colorectal cancer. In some cases, a *CT scan* may be done to confirm the disease or its complications. *Barium enemas* with air contrast can show differences between UC and Crohn's disease and identify complications, mucosal patterns, and

the distribution and depth of disease involvement. In early disease, the barium enema may show incomplete filling as a result of *inflammation* and fine ulcerations along the bowel contour, which appear deeper in more advanced disease.

◆ **Analysis: Analyze Cues and Prioritize Hypotheses.** The priority collaborative problems for patients with UC include:

1. Diarrhea due to *inflammation* of the bowel mucosa
2. Acute or persistent *pain* due to *inflammation* and ulceration of the bowel mucosa and skin irritation
3. Potential for lower GI bleeding and resulting anemia due to UC

◆ **Planning and Implementation: Generate Solutions and Take Action**

Managing Diarrhea

Planning: Expected Outcomes. The major concern for a patient with ulcerative colitis is the occurrence of frequent, bloody diarrhea and fecal incontinence from tenesmus. Therefore the expected outcome of treatment is for the patient to have decreased diarrhea, formed stools, and control of bowel movements, which allow for mucosal healing.

Interventions. Many measures are used to relieve symptoms and reduce intestinal motility, decrease *inflammation,* and promote intestinal healing. Nonsurgical and/or surgical management may be needed.

Nonsurgical Management. Nonsurgical management includes drug and *nutrition* therapy. The use of physical and emotional rest is also an important consideration. Teach the patient to record color, volume, frequency, and consistency of stools, either on paper or via an electronic app, to determine severity of the problem.

Monitor the skin in the perianal area for irritation and ulceration resulting from loose, frequent stools. Stool cultures may be sent for analysis if diarrhea continues. Have the patient record their weight one or two times per week. If the patient is hospitalized, remind assistive personnel to weigh him or her on admission and daily in the morning using the same scale before breakfast and document all weights.

NCLEX EXAMINATION CHALLENGE 52.2

Physiological Integrity

The nurse is caring for an older adult client who experiences an exacerbation of ulcerative colitis with severe diarrhea and rectal bleeding that have lasted a week. For which complication(s) will the nurse assess? **Select all that apply.**

A. Increased BUN

B. Hypokalemia

C. Leukocytosis

D. Anemia

E. Hyponatremia

Drug therapy. Common drug therapy for UC includes aminosalicylates, glucocorticoids, antidiarrheal drugs, and immunomodulators. Teach patients about side effects and adverse drug events (ADEs) and when to call their primary health care provider.

The *aminosalicylates* are drugs commonly used to treat mild-to-moderate UC and/or maintain remission. Several aminosalicylic acid compounds are available. These drugs, also called *5-ASAs,* are thought to have an anti-inflammatory effect on the lining of the intestine by inhibiting prostaglandins and are usually effective in 2 to 4 weeks.

Sulfasalazine, the first aminosalicylate approved for UC, is metabolized by the intestinal bacteria into 5-ASA, which delivers the beneficial effects of the drug, and sulfapyridine, which is responsible for unwanted side effects. Teach patients to take a folic acid supplement because sulfasalazine decreases its absorption (Burchum & Rosenthal, 2019).

! NURSING SAFETY PRIORITY (QSEN)

Drug Alert

Teach patients taking sulfasalazine to report nausea, vomiting, anorexia, rash, and headache to the health care provider. With higher doses, hemolytic anemia, hepatitis, male infertility, or agranulocytosis can occur. This drug is in the same family as sulfonamide antibiotics. *Therefore, assess the patient for an allergy to sulfonamide or other drugs that contain sulfa before the patient takes the drug.* The use of a thiazide diuretic may be a contraindication for sulfasalazine (Burchum & Rosenthal, 2019).

Mesalamine is better tolerated than sulfasalazine because none of its preparations contain sulfapyridine. It may be given as a delayed-release drug in the terminal ileum and beyond within the colon, or as an extended-release drug that works throughout the colon and rectum. Mesalamine can also be given as an enema or a suppository. These preparations have minimal systemic absorption and therefore have fewer side effects (Crohn's and Colitis Foundation, 2020).

Glucocorticoids, such as prednisone and prednisolone, are corticosteroid therapies that may be prescribed during exacerbations of the disease. Prednisone is typically prescribed, and the dose may be increased as acute flare-ups occur. Once clinical improvement occurs, the corticosteroids are tapered because of the adverse effects that commonly occur with long-term steroid therapy (e.g., hyperglycemia, osteoporosis, peptic ulcer disease, increased potential for infection, adrenal insufficiency). For patients with rectal *inflammation,* topical steroids in the form of small retention enemas or suppositories may be prescribed. Medications such as budesonide, steroids that are thought to work mostly in the bowel, produce fewer systemic side effects (Burchum & Rosenthal, 2019).

To provide symptomatic management of diarrhea, *antidiarrheal drugs* may be prescribed. However, these drugs are given very cautiously because they can cause colon dilation and toxic megacolon (massive dilation of the colon and subsequent colonic ileus that can lead to gangrene and peritonitis). Common antidiarrheal drugs include diphenoxylate hydrochloride and atropine sulfate and loperamide.

Immunomodulators are drugs that alter an individual's immune response. Alone, they are often not effective in the treatment of UC. However, in combination with steroids, they may offer a synergistic effect to a quicker response, thereby decreasing the amount of steroids needed. Biologic response modifiers (BRMs) used for UC (and Crohn's disease, discussed later in this chapter) include infliximab and adalimumab (Humira). Although not approved as a first-line therapy for UC, infliximab may be used for refractory disease or for severe complications, such as toxic megacolon and extraintestinal manifestations. Infliximab is an immunoglobulin G (IgG) monoclonal antibody that reduces the activity of tumor necrosis factor (TNF) to decrease *inflammation.* Adalimumab is another monoclonal antibody approved for refractory (not responsive to other therapies) cases. BRMs are used more commonly in management of Crohn's disease. These drugs cause immunosuppression and should be used with caution. Teach the patient to report any signs of a beginning *infection,* including a cold, and to avoid large crowds or others who are sick.

Several newer monoclonal antibodies have recently been approved by the U.S. Food and Drug Administration (FDA) for use in patients with chronic IBD. One of these drugs, vedolizumab, is an intestinal-specific leukocyte traffic inhibitor in that it prevents white blood cells from migrating to inflamed bowel tissue (Engel et al., 2018)).

Nutrition therapy and rest. Patients with severe symptoms who are hospitalized are kept NPO to ensure bowel rest. The primary health care provider may prescribe total parenteral *nutrition* (TPN) for severely ill and malnourished patients during severe exacerbations. Chapter 55 describes this therapy in detail. Patients with less severe symptoms may drink elemental formulas, which have components that are absorbed in the small bowel and reduce bowel stimulation.

Diet is not a major factor in the inflammatory process, but some patients with ulcerative colitis (UC) find that caffeine and alcohol increase diarrhea and cramping. For some patients, raw vegetables and other high-fiber foods can cause GI symptoms. Lactose-containing foods may be poorly tolerated and should be reduced or eliminated. Teach patients that carbonated beverages, pepper, nuts and corn, dried fruits, and smoking are common GI stimulants that could cause discomfort. Each patient differs in his or her food and fluid tolerances.

During an exacerbation of the disease, patient activity is generally restricted because rest can reduce intestinal activity, provide comfort, and promote healing. Ensure that the patient has easy access to a bedpan, bedside commode, or bathroom in case of urgency or tenesmus.

Complementary and integrative health. In addition to dietary changes, complementary and integrative therapies may be used to supplement traditional management of UC. Examples include herbs (e.g., flaxseed), selenium, and vitamin C. Biofeedback, hypnosis, yoga, acupuncture, and ayurveda (a combination of diet, yoga, herbs, and breathing exercises) may be helpful. These therapies need further study to validate their effectiveness, but some patients find them helpful.

Surgical Management. Some patients with UC require surgery to help manage their disease when medical therapies alone are not effective. In some cases, surgery is performed for complications of UC such as toxic megacolon, hemorrhage, bowel perforation, dysplastic biopsy results, and colon cancer.

Preoperative care. General preoperative teaching related to abdominal surgery is described in Chapter 9. If a temporary or permanent ileostomy is planned, provide an in-depth explanation to the patient and family. An ileostomy is a procedure in which a loop of the ileum is placed through an opening in the abdominal wall (stoma) for drainage of fecal material into a pouching system worn on the abdomen. This *external* pouching system consists of a solid skin barrier (wafer) to protect the skin and a fecal collection device (pouch), similar to the system used for patients with colostomies (discussed in Chapter 51).

If an ileostomy is planned, the surgeon consults with a certified wound, ostomy, continence nurse (CWOCN) before surgery for recommendations on the best location of the stoma. A visit before surgery from an ostomate (a patient with an ostomy) may be helpful.

Operative procedures. Any one of several surgical approaches may be used for the patient with UC. Minimally invasive procedures, such as laparoscopic, laparoscopic-assisted, hand-assisted, and robotic-assisted surgery, are common for patients with UC in large tertiary care centers (Valente & Hull, 2018). Laparoscopic surgery usually involves one or several small incisions but often takes longer to perform than the open surgical approach. The natural orifice transluminal endoscopic surgery (NOTES) procedure can be performed via the anus or vagina for certain patients. The availability of this type of procedure depends greatly on the training of the surgeon. Patients may have moderate sedation or general anesthesia for minimally invasive surgical procedures. These patients are *not* typically admitted to critical care units for continuing postoperative care.

Patients who are obese, have had previous abdominal surgeries, or have dense scar tissue (adhesions) may not be candidates for laparoscopic procedures. A conventional open surgical approach involves general anesthesia and an abdominal incision. Patients with open procedures are initially admitted to critical care units for short-term stabilization.

Restorative proctocolectomy with ileo pouch–anal anastomosis (RPC-IPAA). This procedure has become the gold standard for patients with UC. In some centers, the surgery is performed via laparoscopy (laparoscopic RPC-IPAA). Typically, it is a two-stage procedure that includes the removal of the colon and most of the rectum (Fig. 52.2); the anus and anal sphincter remain intact. The surgeon then surgically creates an *internal* pouch (reservoir) using the last 1½ feet of the small intestine. The ileo-anal pouch, sometimes called a *J-pouch, S-pouch,* or *pelvic pouch,* is then connected to the anus. A *temporary* ileostomy through the abdominal skin is created to allow healing of the internal pouch and all anastomosis sites. It also allows for an increase in the capacity of the internal pouch. In the *second* surgical stage, the temporary loop ileostomy is closed. The time interval between the first and second stages varies, but many patients have the second surgical stage to close the ileostomy within 1 to 2 months of the first surgery.

Usually bowel continence is excellent after this procedure, but some patients report leakage of stool during sleep. They may take antidiarrheal drugs to help control this problem. Reassure the patient that they might have frequent stools and urgency after this procedure.

Total proctocolectomy with a permanent ileostomy. Total proctocolectomy with a *permanent* ileostomy is done for patients who are not candidates for or do not want the ileo-anal pouch. The procedure involves the removal of the colon, rectum, and anus with surgical closure of the anus (Fig. 52.3A). The surgeon brings the end of the ileum out through the abdominal wall and forms a stoma, or permanent ostomy.

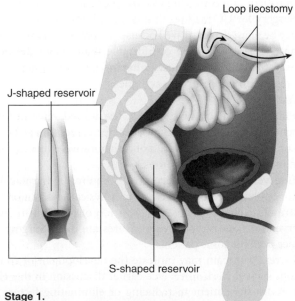

Stage 1.
After removal of the colon, a temporary loop ileostomy is created, and an ileo-anal reservoir is formed. The reservoir is created in an S-shaped reservoir (using three loops of ileum) or a J-shaped reservoir (suturing a portion of ileum to the rectal cuff, with an upward loop).

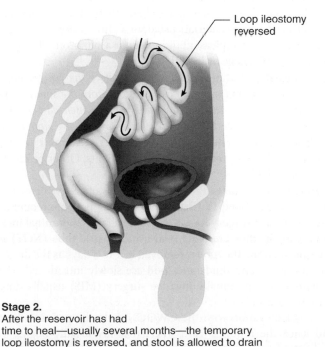

Stage 2.
After the reservoir has had time to heal—usually several months—the temporary loop ileostomy is reversed, and stool is allowed to drain into the reservoir.

Fig. 52.2 Creation of an ileo-anal reservoir.

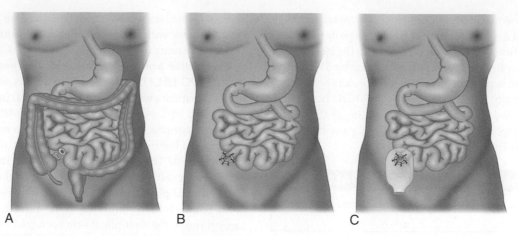

Fig 52.3 (A) Total proctocolectomy with a permanent ileostomy. This involved removal of the colon, the rectum, and the anus with closure of the anus. (B) Ileostomy surgical stoma placement. (C) Ileostomy with ostomy appliance attached.

> ## ⚠ NURSING SAFETY PRIORITY (QSEN)
> ### *Critical Rescue*
>
> The ileostomy stoma (Fig. 52.3B) is usually placed in the right lower quadrant of the abdomen below the belt line. It should not be prolapsed or retract into the abdominal wall. *Assess the stoma frequently after stoma placement. Recognize that it should be pinkish to cherry red to ensure an adequate blood supply. If the stoma looks pale, bluish, or dark, respond by reporting these findings to the surgeon immediately (Stelton, 2019)!*

Initially after surgery, the output from an ileostomy is a loose, dark green liquid that may contain some blood. Over time, a process called *ileostomy adaptation* occurs. The small intestine begins to perform some of the functions that had previously been done by the colon, including the absorption of increased amounts of sodium and water. Stool volume decreases, becomes thicker (paste-like), and turns yellow-green or yellow-brown. The **effluent** (fluid material) usually has little odor or a sweet odor. Any foul or unpleasant odor may be a symptom of a problem such as blockage or infection.

The ileostomy drains frequently. *Therefore the patient must wear a pouch system at all times. The stool from the small intestine contains many enzymes and bile salts, which can quickly irritate and excoriate the skin. Skin care around the stoma is a priority!* A pouch system with a skin barrier (gelatin or pectin) provides sufficient protection for most patients. Other products are also available.

Postoperative care. Provide general postoperative care after surgery, as described in Chapter 9. The few patients requiring open-approach surgery for UC will have a large abdominal incision. Initially, they are NPO, and a nasogastric tube (NGT) is used for suction. The tube is removed in 1 to 2 days as the drainage decreases, and fluids and food are slowly introduced. The patient having minimally invasive surgery (MIS) usually does *not* have an NGT.

In collaboration with the CWOCN, help the patient adjust and learn the required care. The ileostomy usually begins to drain stool within 24 hours after surgery at more than 1 L/day. Be sure that fluids are replaced by adding 500 mL or more each day to prevent dehydration. After about a week of high-volume output, the stool drainage slows and becomes thicker. During this period, some patients need antidiarrheal drugs.

The hospital stay is usually from 1 to 4 days, depending on whether the patient has laparoscopic or conventional open surgery. Patients having MIS have less pain from surgery, fewer complications, and faster restoration of bowel function when compared with other surgical patients (Valente & Hull, 2018).

For those who have the RPC-IPAA procedure, remind them that the internal pouch can become inflamed (pouchitis). This problem is usually treated effectively with metronidazole for 7 to 10 days. Teach patients that, after the second stage of surgery, they might have burning during bowel *elimination* because gastric acid cannot be absorbed well by the ileum. Also, instruct them to omit foods that can cause odors or gas, such as cabbage, asparagus, brussels sprouts, and beans. Teach patients to eliminate foods that cannot be digested well, such as nuts and corn. Each patient differs in which foods he or she can tolerate.

Surgery for UC may result in altered body image. However, it may be viewed as positive because the patient will have fewer symptoms and feel more comfortable than before the procedure. Patients have to adjust to having an ostomy before they can resume their presurgery activities.

Managing Pain

Planning: Expected Outcomes. The desired outcome for the patient is that he or she will verbalize decreased *pain* at 2 to 3 or less on a 0 to 10 scale as a result of collaborative, evidence-based pain management interventions.

Interventions. *Pain* control requires pharmacologic and nonpharmacologic measures. Physical discomfort can contribute to emotional distress. A variety of symptom-reducing interventions and supportive measures are used. Surgery may reduce *pain* for some patients.

Increases in pain may indicate the development of complications such as peritonitis (see earlier discussion in this chapter). Assist the patient in reducing or eliminating factors that can cause or increase the *pain* experience. For example, he or she may benefit from *nutrition* changes to decrease abdominal discomfort such as cramping and bloating.

Antidiarrheal drugs may be needed to control diarrhea, thus reducing the discomfort. However, they must be used with caution and for a short time because toxic megacolon can develop.

Perineal skin can be irritated by contact with loose stools and frequent cleaning. Explain special measures for skin care. Use of medicated wipes is soothing if the rectal area is tender or sensitive from the use of toilet tissue. A number of ostomy manufacturers (e.g., Hollister, ConvaTec) produce a system for skin care that may help prevent and heal perineal skin irritation. These systems usually include a skin-cleaning solution, a moisturizing and healing cream, and a petroleum jelly–like barrier that prevents contact of moisture and stool with the skin.

Preventing or Monitoring for Lower GI Bleeding

Planning: Expected Outcomes. If possible, patients are expected to remain free of complications that can cause bleeding, such as perforation or anemia. For the patient experiencing lower GI bleeding, he or she is expected to have a cessation of bleeding with prompt collaborative care.

Interventions. The nursing priority is to monitor the patient closely for signs and symptoms of GI bleeding resulting from the disease or its complications. If the patient has lower GI bleeding of more than 0.5 mL/min, a *GI bleeding scan* may be useful to localize the site of the bleeding (Pagana & Pagana, 2018). However, this test cannot indicate the cause of the bleeding and may take several hours to administer. Patients in the critical care unit are not candidates for the test because they must leave the unit for it. *Keep in mind that GI bleeding is considered a medical emergency; therefore the patient should be monitored closely to prevent complications!*

⚠ NURSING SAFETY PRIORITY (QSEN)

Critical Rescue

Recognize that it is important to monitor stools for blood loss for the patient with ulcerative colitis. The blood may be bright red (frank bleeding) or black and tarry (melena). Monitor hematocrit, hemoglobin, and electrolyte values and assess vital signs. Prolonged slow bleeding can lead to anemia. Observe for fever, tachycardia, and signs of fluid volume depletion. Changes in mental status may occur, especially among older adults, and may be the first indication of dehydration or anemia.

If symptoms of GI bleeding begin, respond by notifying the Rapid Response Team or primary health care provider immediately. Blood products are often prescribed for patients with severe anemia. Prepare for the blood transfusion by inserting a large-bore IV catheter if it is not already in place. Chapter 37 outlines nursing actions during blood transfusion.

Care Coordination and Transition Management

Home Care Management. The patient with ulcerative colitis provides self-management at home but may require hospitalization during severe exacerbations or after surgical intervention. In addition, those who have extraintestinal problems often need ongoing collaborative care for joint and/or skin problems.

Home care management focuses on controlling signs and symptoms and monitoring for complications. For patients returning home or transferring to nursing home or transitional care after surgery, ongoing respiratory care, incision care

(if applicable), ostomy care, and pain management should be continued.

Self-Management Education. Teach the patient about the nature of ulcerative colitis, including its acute episodes, remissions, and symptom management. Stress that even though the cause is unknown, relapses can be prevented with proper health care. Teach patients taking immunosuppressive drugs, such as corticosteroids and biologic response modifiers—more commonly known as *biologics* (monoclonal antibodies), to report signs of possible **infection** to the primary health care provider. Remind them to avoid crowds and anyone who has an infection. Review the purpose of drug therapy, when drugs should be taken, side effects, and adverse drug events.

Instruct the patient about measures to reduce or control abdominal *pain,* cramping, and diarrhea. Also teach the patient and family about symptoms associated with disease exacerbation that should be reported to the primary health care provider, such as fever higher than 101°F (38.3°C), tachycardia, palpitations, and an increase in diarrhea, severe abdominal *pain,* or nausea/vomiting. Provide written information and contact numbers for the primary health care provider.

There is no special diet for a patient with an ileostomy. However, teach the patient to avoid any foods that cause gas. Examples include high-fiber foods such as nuts, raw cabbage, corn, celery, and popcorn. The patient needs to learn which foods he or she tolerates best and adjust the diet accordingly.

If the patient has undergone a temporary or permanent surgical diversion, collaborate with the CWOCN to explain and demonstrate required care so that the patient can self-manage or the family/caregiver can assist. Teach the importance of including adequate amounts of salt and water in the diet because the diversion can increase the loss of these substances. Urge the patient to be cautious in situations that lead to heavy sweating or fluid loss, such as strenuous physical activity, high environmental heat, and episodes of diarrhea and vomiting.

Finding the best ostomy pouching system is a major issue for many patients with an ileostomy. An effective system is one that:

- Protects the skin
- Contains the effluent (drainage) and reduces odor, if any
- Remains securely attached to the skin for a dependable period of time

Most patients desire an adhesive barrier that will last for 3 to 7 days. The barrier must create a solid seal to prevent the enzymes in the drainage from irritating the skin. Solid barriers are classified as "regular wear" or "extended wear." An adult with a high output may want an extended-wear barrier. A special cream can be used to help fill any uneven skin surfaces and provide a consistent seal. Pouches can also be individualized by the patient. Large pouches can hold more but are heavy when full. Patients also have to consider the costs of the various systems and if or how much their insurance will help pay for them. The Patient and Family Education: Preparing for Self-Management: Ileostomy Care box describes the main aspects of ileostomy care, including skin care.

A patient with an ileostomy may have many concerns about management at home and about sexual and social adjustments. Considering possible sexual issues helps the patient

PATIENT AND FAMILY EDUCATION: PREPARING FOR SELF-MANAGEMENT
Ileostomy Care

Skin Protection
- Use a skin barrier to protect your skin from contact with contents from the ostomy.
- Use skin-care products, such as skin sealants and ostomy skin creams. If your skin continues to be exposed to ostomy contents, select a product to fill in problem areas and provide an even skin surface.
- Watch your skin for any irritation or redness.

Pouch Care
- Empty your pouch when it is one-third to one-half full.
- Change the pouch during inactive times, such as before meals, before retiring at night, on waking in the morning, and 2 to 4 hours after eating.
- Change the entire pouch system every 3 to 7 days.

Nutrition
- Chew food thoroughly.
- Be cautious about high-fiber and high-cellulose foods. You may need to eliminate these from the diet if they cause severe problems (diarrhea, constipation, or blockage). Examples include coconut, popcorn, tough-fiber meats, rice, cabbage, and vegetables with skins (tomatoes, corn, and peas).

Drug Therapy
- Avoid taking enteric-coated and capsule medications.
- Inform any primary health care provider who is prescribing medications for you that you have an ostomy. Before having prescriptions filled, inform your pharmacist that you have an ostomy.
- Do not take any laxative or enemas. You should usually have loose stool and should contact your primary health care provider if no stool has passed in 6 to 12 hours.

Symptoms to Watch
- Report any drastic increase or decrease in drainage to your primary health care provider.
- If stomal swelling, abdominal cramping, or distention occurs or if ileostomy contents stop draining:
  - Remove the pouch with faceplate.
  - Lie down, assuming a knee-chest position.
  - Begin abdominal massage.
  - Apply moist towels to the abdomen.
  - Drink hot tea.
- If none of these maneuvers is effective in resuming ileostomy flow or if abdominal pain is severe, call your primary health care provider right away.

🏠 HOME CARE CONSIDERATIONS
The Patient With Inflammatory Bowel Disease

Assess gastrointestinal function and nutritional status, including:
- Abdominal cramping or *pain*
- Bowel *elimination* pattern, specifically frequency, characteristics, and amount of stools and presence or absence of blood in stools
- Food and fluid intake (include relationship of specific foods to cramping and stools)
- Weight gain or loss
- Signs and symptoms of dehydration
- Presence or absence of fever, rectal tenesmus, or urgency
- Bowel sounds
- Condition of perianal skin, including presence or absence of perianal **fistula, fissure,** or **abscess**

Assess patient's and family's coping skills, including:
- Current and ongoing stress level and coping style
- Availability of support system

Assess home environment, including:
- Adequacy and availability of bathroom facilities
- Opportunity for rest and relaxation

Assess ability to self-manage therapeutic regimen, including:
- Drug therapy
- Signs and symptoms to report
- Nutrition therapy
- Availability of community resources
- Importance of follow-up care

Health Care Resources. If the patient needs assistance with self-management at home, collaborate with the case manager or social worker to arrange the services of a home care aide or nurse. A home care nurse can provide assessment and guidance in integrating ostomy care into the patient's lifestyle. The nurse may also teach about wound care, including monitoring wound healing, if needed (see the Home Care Considerations: The Patient With Inflammatory Bowel Disease box).

The patient and family need to know where to purchase ostomy supplies, along with the name, size, and manufacturer's order number.

For patients with a permanent ileostomy, locate a community ostomy support group by contacting the United Ostomy Associations of America (www.ostomy.org). The United Ostomy Association of Canada serves the needs of Canadian patients (www.ostomycanada.ca). A local support group or the Crohn's and Colitis Foundation of America (www.ccfa.org) may be helpful in obtaining supplies and providing education for ostomates. Inform the patient and family members of available ostomy ambulatory care clinics and ostomy specialists. If the patient agrees, a visit from an ostomate can be continued after discharge to home.

◆ **Evaluation: Evaluate Outcomes.** Evaluate the care of the patient with ulcerative colitis based on the identified priority patient problems. Expected outcomes may include that the patient will:
- Experience no diarrhea or a decrease in diarrheal episodes
- Verbalize decreased pain
- Have absence of lower GI bleeding
- Self-manage the ileostomy or ileo-anal pouch (temporary or permanent)

identify and discuss these concerns with the sex partner. For example, a change in positioning during intercourse may alleviate apprehension. Social situations may cause anxiety related to decreased self-esteem and a disturbance in body image. Encourage the patient to discuss possible concerns in addressing and resolving these potentially stressful events. Clinical depression is common among patients with ulcerative colitis. Refer patients to appropriate mental health resources if depression is suspected.

Some hospitals provide community support groups for their patients with inflammatory bowel disease (IBD). These groups help patients and their families cope with the psychological impact of IBD and educate them about *nutrition* and complementary and integrative therapies.

CROHN'S DISEASE

Pathophysiology Review

Crohn's disease (CD) is a chronic inflammatory disease of the small intestine (most often), the colon, or both. It can affect the GI tract from the mouth to the anus but most commonly affects the terminal ileum. CD is a slowly progressive and unpredictable disease with involvement of multiple regions of the intestine with normal sections in between (called *skip lesions* on x-rays). Like ulcerative colitis (UC), this disease is recurrent, with remissions and exacerbations.

CD presents as **inflammation** that causes a thickened bowel wall. Strictures and deep ulcerations (cobblestone appearance) also occur, which put the patient at risk for developing a bowel fistula (abnormal opening [tract] between two organs or structures). The result is severe diarrhea and malabsorption of vital nutrients. Anemia is common, usually from iron deficiency or malabsorption issues (McCance et al., 2019).

The complications associated with CD are similar to those of UC (see Table 52.4). Hemorrhage is more common in UC, but it can occur in CD as well. Severe malabsorption by the small intestine is more common in patients with CD versus UC that may not involve the small bowel to any significant extent. Patients with CD can become very malnourished and debilitated due to intestinal malabsorption of dietary nutrients.

Rarely, cancer of the small bowel and colon develop but can occur after the disease has been present for 15 to 20 years. Fistula formation is a common complication of CD but is rare in UC. Fistulas can occur between segments of the intestine or manifest as cutaneous fistulas (opening to the skin) or perirectal abscesses. They can also extend from the bowel to other organs and body cavities, such as the bladder or vagina (Fig. 52.4). Some patients develop intestinal obstruction, which at first is secondary to **inflammation** and edema. Over time, fibrosis and scar tissue develop and obstruction results from a narrowing of the bowel. Most patients with CD require surgery at some point. Chapter 51 ok discusses surgical procedures for intestinal obstruction.

Almost a million individuals in the United States have Crohn's disease, and Canada has one of the highest incidences of Crohn's disease and colitis worldwide (Crohn's and Colitis Canada, 2020). Most patients experience symptoms and are

PATIENT-CENTERED CARE: GENETIC/ GENOMIC CONSIDERATIONS (QSEN)

The exact cause of CD is unknown. A combination of genetic, immune, and environmental factors may contribute to its development. About 20% of patients have a positive family history for the disease (Cleynen et al., 2016). The discovery of a mutation in the *NOD2/CARD15* gene on chromosome 16 seems to be associated with some patients who have CD. This gene is found in monocytes that normally recognize and destroy bacteria.

Proinflammatory cytokines, such as tumor necrosis factor–alpha (TNF-alpha) and interleukins (ILs) (e.g., IL-6 and IL-8), are immunologic factors that contribute to the etiology of CD (McCance et al., 2019). Many of the drugs used for the disease inhibit or block one or more of these factors.

Other risk factors include tobacco use, Jewish ethnicity, and living in urban areas (McCance et al., 2019). CD is more common in individuals of Ashkenazi Jewish background than in any other group. Current research has found genetic markers in this population that contribute to higher rates of CD (Santos et al., 2018). It was once thought that stress and nutrition play a role in the development of CD, but these factors have not been proven. However, inadequate **nutrition** can exacerbate the patient's symptoms.

diagnosed as adolescents or young adults between 15 and 35 years of age (Crohn's and Colitis Foundation, 2020).

❖ Interprofessional Collaborative Care

Similar to patients with ulcerative colitis, patients with Crohn's disease may be self-managed at home, cared for in the community setting, or hospitalized depending on their immediate condition related to this chronic bowel disease.

◆ **Assessment: Recognize Cues.** Crohn's disease can be exacerbated by bacterial infection. A detailed history is needed to identify manifestations specific to the disease. Ask about recent unintentional weight loss, the frequency and consistency of stools, the presence of blood in the stool, fever, and abdominal pain.

Perform a thorough abdominal assessment. Assess for manifestations of the disease, and evaluate the patient's **nutrition** and hydration status.

When inspecting the abdomen, assess for distention, masses, or visible peristalsis. Inspection of the perianal area may reveal ulcerations, fissures, or fistulas. During auscultation, bowel sounds may be decreased or absent with severe **inflammation** or obstruction. An increase in high-pitched or rushing sounds

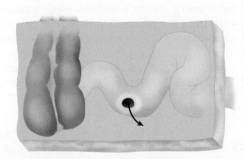

External enterocutaneous
(between skin and intestine)

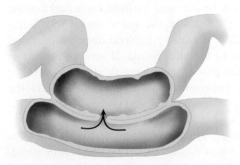

Enteroenteric
(between intestine and intestine)

Fig. 52.4 Types of fistulas that are complications of Crohn's disease.

may be present over areas of narrowed bowel loops. Muscle guarding, masses, rigidity, or tenderness may be noted on palpation by the primary health care provider.

The signs and symptoms associated with Crohn's disease vary greatly from person to person. Most patients report diarrhea, abdominal *pain,* and low-grade fever. Fever is common with fistulas, abscesses, and severe inflammation. If the disease occurs in only the ileum, diarrhea occurs five or six times per day, often with a soft, loose stool. Steatorrhea (fatty diarrheal stools) is common. Stools may contain bright red blood (McCance et al., 2019).

Abdominal pain from **inflammation** is usually constant and often located in the right lower quadrant. The patient also may have pain around the umbilicus before and after bowel movements. If the lower colon is diseased, pain is common in both lower abdominal quadrants.

Most patients with Crohn's disease have *weight loss.* Nutritional problems are the result of increased catabolism from chronic inflammation, anorexia, malabsorption, or self-imposed dietary restrictions. These problems result in impaired **fluid and electrolyte balance** and vital nutrient deficiencies (see Chapter 13 for more information on fluids and electrolytes).

The patient who has Crohn's disease (CD) needs a complete psychosocial assessment. The chronic nature of the problem and the associated complications can greatly affect patients and their families. Lifestyle changes are necessary to cope with such a disruptive and painful chronic illness. Assess the patient's coping

---

> ### ! NURSING SAFETY PRIORITY (QSEN)
> #### Action Alert
>
> For the patient with Crohn's disease, be especially alert for signs and symptoms of **peritonitis** (discussed earlier in this chapter), small-bowel obstruction, and nutritional and fluid imbalances. Early detection of a change in the patient's status helps reduce these life-threatening complications.

---

skill and help identify support systems. Similar to problems associated with other chronic diseases, clinical depression and severe anxiety disorders are common among patients with CD.

Anemia is common as a result of slow bleeding and poor nutrition. Serum levels of folic acid and vitamin B_{12} are generally low because of malabsorption, further contributing to anemia. Amino acid malabsorption and protein-losing enteropathy may result in *decreased albumin* levels. C-reactive protein and ESR may be elevated to indicate inflammation. White blood cells (WBCs) in the urine may show **infection** (pyuria), which is caused by ureteral obstruction or an enterovesical (bowel to bladder) fistula. If severe diarrhea or fistula is present, the patient may have fluid and electrolyte losses, particularly potassium and magnesium. Assess the patient for signs and symptoms that can occur related to electrolyte losses (see Chapter 13).

X-rays show the narrowing, ulcerations, strictures, and fistulas common with Crohn's disease. *Magnetic resonance enterography (MRE)* is performed to determine bowel activity and motility as discussed under the Other Diagnostic Assessment in the Ulcerative Colitis concept exemplar.

◆ **Interventions: Take Action.** Collaborative care for patients with Crohn's disease is similar to that described in the Nonsurgical Management discussion in the Ulcerative Colitis section. Specific interventions vary with the severity of disease and the complications that are present.

Nonsurgical Management

Drug Therapy. Drugs used to manage Crohn's disease (CD) are similar to those used in the treatment of ulcerative colitis (UC). For mild-to-moderate disease, 5-ASA drugs may be effective, although research shows that their usage for CD has produced mixed results (see the Drug Therapy discussion in the Ulcerative Colitis section).

Most patients have moderate-to-severe disease and need stronger drug therapy to control their symptoms. Two agents that may be prescribed for CD are azathioprine and mercaptopurine. These drugs suppress the immune system and can lead to serious infections. Methotrexate may also be given to suppress immune activity of the disease.

A group of biologic response modifiers (BRMs), also known as *monoclonal antibody drugs,* have been approved for use in CD when other drugs have been ineffective. These drugs inhibit tumor necrosis factor (TNF)–alpha, which decreases the inflammatory response. Examples of commonly used drugs for patients with CD include infliximab, adalimumab, natalizumab, and certolizumab pegol. These agents are not given to patients with a history of cancer, heart disease, or multiple sclerosis (Winter & Burakoff, 2017).

> ### ! NURSING SAFETY PRIORITY (QSEN)
> #### Drug Alert
>
> Both infliximab and certolizumab pegol must be given in a health care setting, such as a medical office, via parenteral routes. Teach patients how to give themselves a subcutaneous injection for those drugs that come in that form. Teach them to report injection site reactions, including redness and swelling. Remind patients that headache, abdominal pain, and nausea and vomiting are common side effects. Teach them to avoid crowds and people with infection. Reinforce the need to report any **infection,** including a cold or sore throat, to the primary health care provider immediately (Burchum & Rosenthal, 2019).
>
> Natalizumab is given IV under medical supervision every 4 weeks for moderate-to-severe CD and when other drugs are not effective. Natalizumab can cause **progressive multifocal leukoencephalopathy** (PML), a deadly infection that affects the brain. Before giving the drug, be sure that the patient is free of all infections. Teach patients the importance of reporting any cognitive, motor, or sensory changes immediately to the primary health care provider. Vedolizumab is used for treatment of moderate-to-severe CD. This drug is administered IV at weeks 0, 2, and 6, and then the first maintenance dose is given at 8 weeks. The maintenance doses continue every 8 weeks after that (Engel et al., 2018). Clinical trials verify that vedolizumab does not increase the risk for PML, but because of its mechanism of action, the FDA strongly encourages education regarding this possible complication (Card et al., 2018).

Although glucocorticoids can be effective for patients with CD, sepsis can result from abscesses or fistulas that may be present. These drugs mask the symptoms of **infection.** Therefore they must be used with caution and only on a short-term basis. Monitor the patient closely for signs of infection. Teach the patient not to stop the steroids abruptly because of the potential for adrenal insufficiency. Ciprofloxacin and metronidazole have been helpful in patients with fistulas, anorectal abscesses, and *infection* related to CD.

Nutrition Therapy. Long-standing nutritional deficits can have severe consequences for the patient with Crohn's disease. Poor *nutrition* can lead to inadequate fistula and wound healing, loss of lean muscle mass, decreased immune responses, and increased morbidity and mortality. During severe exacerbations of the disease, the patient may be hospitalized to provide bowel rest and nutritional support with total parenteral nutrition (TPN). Nutritional supplements such as Ensure or Sustacal can be given to provide nutrients and more calories. Teach the patient to avoid GI stimulants, such as caffeinated beverages and alcohol.

Fistula Management. Fistulas are common with acute exacerbations of Crohn's disease. They can be between the bowel and bladder (enterovesical), between two segments of bowel (enteroenteric), between the skin and bowel (enterocutaneous), or between the bowel and vagina (enterovaginal) (see Fig. 52.4). The patient with multiple fistulas often has complications such as systemic infections, skin problems (including abscesses and fissures), and malnutrition. Treatment of the patient with an abscess (a localized infection in which there is a collection of pus) requires an incision and drainage (I & D) local procedure. Management of the patient with a fistula is more complicated and includes *nutrition* and electrolyte therapy, skin care, and prevention of infection.

❗ NURSING SAFETY PRIORITY (QSEN)

Action Alert

Adequate *nutrition* and ***fluid and electrolyte balance*** are priorities in the care of the patient with a fistula. GI secretions are high in volume and rich in electrolytes and enzymes. The patient is at high risk for malnutrition, dehydration, and hypokalemia (decreased serum potassium). Assess for these complications and collaborate with the health care team to manage them. Carefully monitor urinary output and daily weights. A decrease in either measurement indicates possible dehydration, which should be treated immediately by providing additional fluids.

The patient requires at least 3000 calories daily to promote healing of the fistula. If he or she cannot take adequate oral fluids and nutrients, total enteral nutrition (TEN) or TPN may be prescribed. For patients who do not require TEN or TPN, collaborate with the registered dietitian nutritionist to:

- Carefully monitor the patient's tolerance of the prescribed diet
- Help the patient select high-calorie, high-protein, high-vitamin, low-fiber meals
- Offer enteral supplements
- Record food intake for accurate calorie counts

Remind assistive personnel to provide enteral supplements, record accurate intake and output, and take daily weights while the patient is in the hospital. Collaborate with the certified wound, ostomy, and continence nurse (CWOCN) to select the most appropriate wound management for each patient.

❗ NURSING SAFETY PRIORITY (QSEN)

Action Alert

For patients with fistulas, preserving and protecting the skin are the nursing priorities. Be sure that wound drainage is not in direct contact with skin because intestinal fluid enzymes are caustic! Clean the skin promptly to prevent skin breakdown or fungal infection, which can cause major discomfort for the patient.

Enzymes and bile in the stool contribute to the problem of skin irritation and excoriation. Skin irritation needs to be prevented. This may be accomplished by using skin barriers, pouching systems, and insertion of drains (Fig. 52.5). Skin barriers or dressings are used when the fistula drainage is less than 100 mL in 24 hours. A pouch is used for heavily draining fistulas to reduce the risk for skin breakdown and measure the **effluent**. However, they are very challenging because of location and drainage amount. Treatment with an antifungal powder applied to the skin around the fistula is often very helpful to prevent or treat *Candida* infection.

For some fistulas, pouching may not be possible because of their location. Drainage may need to be managed using regulated wall suction or a negative-pressure wound therapy device. Continuous low wall suction is attached to a suction catheter in the wound bed of the fistula, not into the fistula tract. These systems are not meant for long-term management.

Negative-pressure wound therapy (e.g., vacuum-assisted closure, or wound VAC therapy) promotes wound healing by secondary intention as it prepares the wound bed for closure, reduces edema, promotes granulation and perfusion, and removes exudate and infectious material. It should not be used for patients who are at risk for bleeding or only for the purpose of drainage containment.

Patients with fistulas are also at high risk for intra-abdominal abscesses and sepsis. Antibiotic therapy is commonly prescribed. Observe for signs of sepsis (systemic infection), such as fever, abdominal pain, or a change in mental status. Monitor for increased WBC levels that could indicate a systemic infection (McCance et al., 2019).

Other helpful interventions for the patient with CD are those that relax the patient and soothe the GI tract. Such therapies may include naturopathy, herbs (e.g., ginger), acupuncture, hypnotherapy, and ayurveda (a combination of diet, herbs, yoga, and breathing exercises). The evidence supporting the use of these substances for CD is lacking, but many patients find them helpful for overall physical and emotional health. Teach patients about the availability of these therapies and recommend that they include them in their collaborative plan of care.

Surgical Management. Surgery for Crohn's disease may be performed for patients who have not improved with medical management or for those who have complications from the disease. Surgery to manage Crohn's disease is not as successful as that for ulcerative colitis because of the extent of the disease. The patient with a fistula may undergo resection of the diseased area. Other indications for surgical treatment include perforation, massive hemorrhage, intestinal obstruction or strictures, abscesses, or cancer.

🔳 CLINICAL JUDGMENT CHALLENGE 52.1

Patient-Centered Care; Evidence-Based Practice; Teamwork and Collaboration

A 28-year-old woman has had Crohn's disease for over 5 years. She is admitted today to the hospital for severe diarrhea and abdominal pain and is receiving IV fluids. The primary health care provider suspects that she has a small enteroenteric (between two segments of bowel) fistula. This client reports that she is newly married and is worried about the impacts this complication may have on her life as they are trying to get pregnant with their first child. She was taking prednisone to control her exacerbation, but now it has been discontinued. This evening, the nurse notes these assessment findings:

- Hyperactive bowel sounds × 4
- Reports abdominal pain and cramping as a 7 on a 0-10 pain intensity scale
- Severe abdominal distention
- Temperature = 101° F (38.3° C)
- Apical pulse = 88 beats/min
- Blood pressure = 124/76 mm Hg
- Respirations = 24 breaths/min
- Na = 136 mEq/L (136 mmol/L)
- K = 3.3 mEq/L (3.3 mmol/L)

1. **Recognize Cues:** What assessment information in this client situation is the most important and immediate concern for the nurse? (Hint: Identify the **relevant** information *first* to determine what is most important.)
2. **Analyze Cues:** What client conditions are consistent with the **most relevant** information? (Hint: Think about priority collaborative problems that support and contradict the information presented in this situation.)
3. **Prioritize Hypotheses:** Which possibilities or explanations are **most likely** to be present in this client situation? Which possibilities or explanations are the most serious? (Hint: Consider all possibilities and determine their urgency and risk for this client.)
4. **Generate Solutions:** What actions would most likely achieve the desired outcomes for this client? Which actions should be **avoided** or are **potentially harmful**? (Hint: Determine the desired outcomes first to decide which interventions are appropriate and those that should be avoided.)
5. **Take Action:** Which actions are the most appropriate and how should they be implemented? In what **priority order** should they be implemented? (Hint: Consider health teaching, documentation, requested health care provider orders or prescriptions, nursing skills, collaboration with or referral to health team members, etc.)
6. **Evaluate Outcomes:** What client assessment would indicate that the nurse's actions were **effective**? (Hint: Think about signs that would indicate an improvement, decline, or unchanged client condition.)

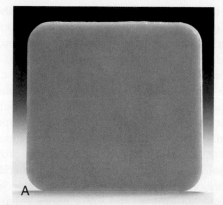

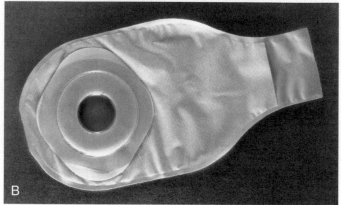

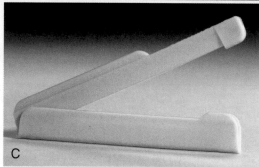

Fig. 52.5 Skin barriers, such as wafers **(A)**, are cut to fit ⅛ inch around the fistula. A drainable pouch **(B)** is applied over the wafer and clamped **(C)** until the pouch is to be emptied. Effluent should drain into the bag and not contact the skin. (Courtesy ConvaTec, a Bristol-Myers Squibb Company, Princeton, NJ.)

In some cases, a resection (removal of part of the small bowel) can be performed via minimally invasive surgery (MIS) via laparoscopy. This surgery involves one or more small incisions, less pain, and a quicker surgical recovery when compared with traditional open surgery. Both small-bowel resection (usually the ileum) and ileocecal resection can be done using this procedure. For other patients, an open surgical approach is used to allow for better visual access to the bowel.

Stricturoplasty may be performed for bowel strictures related to Crohn's disease. This procedure increases the bowel diameter. Care before and after each of these surgical procedures is similar to care for patients undergoing other types of abdominal surgery (see Chapter 9).

Care Coordination and Transition Management

Home Care Management. The discharge care plan for the patient with Crohn's disease is similar to that for the patient with ulcerative colitis (see the Care Coordination and Transition Management discussion in the Ulcerative Colitis section). Collaborate with the case manager and CWOCN or wound nurse to help the patient plan self-management.

Self-Management Education. Reinforce measures to control the disease and related symptoms and manage *nutrition*. Teach the patient and family to make arrangements for the patient to have easy access to the bathroom and privacy to perform fistula care, if needed.

The health teaching plan for Crohn's disease is similar to that for the patient with ulcerative colitis. Teach the patient about the usual course of the disease, symptoms of complications, and when to notify the health care provider. Provide health teaching for drug therapy, including purpose, dose, and side effects. In addition to other drugs, vitamin supplements, including monthly vitamin B_{12} injections, may be needed because of the inability of the ileum to absorb certain nutrients. In collaboration with the dietitian, instruct the patient to follow a low-residue, high-calorie diet and to avoid foods that cause discomfort, such as milk, gluten (wheat products), and other GI stimulants like caffeine.

Remind the patient to take rest periods, especially during exacerbations of the disease. If stress appears to increase symptoms of the disease, recommend stress-management techniques, counseling, and/or physical activity to improve quality of life. For long-term teaching, inform the patient about the increased risk for bowel cancer and the importance of frequent colorectal cancer screening (see Chapter 51).

If a patient has a fistula, explain and demonstrate wound care. Provide the opportunity for the patient to practice this care in the hospital. Ideally, he or she should be independent in fistula care before leaving the hospital. However, because of location of the fistula (perirectal or vaginal) or a large abdomen, assistance may be needed. If this is the case, teach a family member or other caregiver how to manage the wound. Patients may be transferred to a transitional or skilled nursing unit for collaborative care.

Health Care Resources. Patients who are discharged to home after undergoing resection and anastomosis may require visits from a home care nurse to assess the surgical wound and monitor for complications. Assess the patient's and family's ability to monitor the progress of fistula healing and to watch for indications of infection and sepsis. A home care aide or other service might be helpful for the patient who cannot meet nutritional needs or who needs help with grocery shopping and meal preparation.

In collaboration with the case manager, assist with obtaining the equipment and supplies for fistula care, such as skin barriers and wound drainage bags. A support group sponsored by the United Ostomy Associations of America (www.ostomy.org) or a local hospital in the community may also be available to help with meeting physical and psychosocial needs.

DIVERTICULAR DISEASE

Diverticula are pouchlike herniations of the mucosa through the muscular wall of any part of the gut, but most commonly the colon. **Diverticulosis** is the presence of many abnormal pouchlike herniations (diverticula) in the wall of the intestine. Acute **diverticulitis** is the inflammation or infection of diverticula.

Pathophysiology Review

Diverticula can occur in any part of the small or large intestine, but they usually occur in the sigmoid colon (Fig. 52.6). The muscle of the colon hypertrophies, thickens, and becomes rigid, and herniation of the mucosa and submucosa through the colon wall is seen. Diverticula seem to occur at points of weakness in the intestinal wall, often at areas where blood vessels interrupt

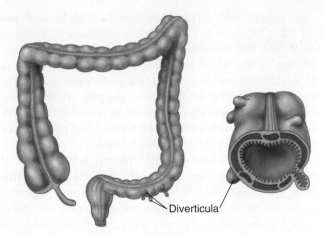

Fig. 52.6 Several abnormal outpouchings, or herniations, in the wall of the intestine, which are diverticula. These can occur anywhere in the small or large intestine but are found most often in the colon. Diverticulitis is the inflammation of a diverticulum that occurs when undigested food or bacteria become trapped in the diverticulum.

the muscle layer. Muscle weakness develops as part of the aging process or because of a lack of fiber in the diet.

Diverticula *without* **inflammation** cause few problems. However, if undigested food or bacteria become trapped in a diverticulum, blood supply to that area is reduced. Bacteria invade the diverticulum, resulting in diverticulitis, which then can perforate and develop a local **abscess**. A perforated diverticulum can progress to an intra-abdominal perforation with **peritonitis**. Lower GI bleeding may also occur (see earlier discussion in this chapter under Ulcerative Colitis).

High intraluminal pressure forces the formation of a pouch in the weakened area of the mucosa. Diets low in fiber that cause less bulky stool and constipation have been implicated in the formation of diverticula. Retained undigested food in diverticula is suggested to be one cause of diverticulitis. The retained food reduces blood flow to that area and makes bacterial invasion of the sac easier (McCance et al., 2019).

The exact incidence of diverticulosis is unknown, but millions are affected by the problem. It is found in two thirds of adults older than 80 years, with more men than women affected.

❖ Interprofessional Collaborative Care

Patients with diverticular disease are self-managed at home, cared for in the community setting, or hospitalized if surgery is needed to correct a concern.

◆ **Assessment: Recognize Cues.** The patient with *diverticulosis* usually has no symptoms. Unless pain or bleeding develops, the condition may go undiagnosed. Diverticula are most often diagnosed during routine colonoscopy. Occasionally diverticulosis will cause symptoms. For the patient with uncomplicated diverticulosis, ask about intermittent **pain** in the left lower quadrant and a history of constipation. If diverticulitis is suspected, ask about a history of low-grade fever, nausea, and abdominal pain. Inquire about recent bowel **elimination** patterns because constipation may develop as a result of intestinal inflammation. Also, ask about any bleeding from the rectum.

The patient with *diverticulitis* may have abdominal *pain,* most often localized to the left lower quadrant. It is intermittent at first but becomes progressively steady. Occasionally, pain may be just above the pubic bone or may occur on one side. Abdominal pain is generalized if peritonitis has occurred. Nausea and vomiting are common. The patient's temperature is elevated, ranging from a low-grade fever to 101°F (38.3°C). Chills may be present. Often an increased heart rate (tachycardia) occurs with fever (Elisei & Tursi, 2016).

On examination of the abdomen, observe for distention. The patient may report tenderness over the involved area. Localized muscle spasm, guarded movement, and rebound tenderness may be present with peritoneal irritation. If generalized peritonitis is present, profound guarding occurs; rebound tenderness is more widespread; and sepsis, hypotension, or hypovolemic shock can occur. If the perforated diverticulum is close to the rectum, the health care provider may palpate a tender mass during the rectal examination. Blood pressure checks may show orthostatic changes. *If bleeding is massive, the patient may have hypovolemia and hypotension that result in shock.*

For the patient with uncomplicated diverticulosis, laboratory studies are not indicated. However, the patient with diverticulitis has an *elevated white blood cell (WBC) count. Decreased hematocrit and hemoglobin* values are common if chronic or severe bleeding occurs. Stool tests for occult blood, if requested, are sometimes positive. Abdominal x-rays may be done to evaluate for free air and fluid indicating perforation. A CT scan may be performed to diagnose an abscess or thickening of the bowel related to diverticulitis.

Abdominal ultrasonography, a noninvasive test, may also reveal bowel thickening or an abscess. The primary health care provider may recommend a colonoscopy 4 to 8 weeks *after the acute phase* of the illness to rule out a tumor in the large intestine, particularly if the patient has rectal bleeding.

◆ **Interventions: Take Action.** Patients are managed on an ambulatory care basis if the symptoms are mild. Monitor the patient for any prolonged or increased fever, abdominal *pain,* or blood in the stool. The patient with moderate-to-severe diverticulitis may be hospitalized, especially if he or she is older or has complications. Manifestations suggesting the need for admission are a temperature higher than 101°F (38.3°C), persistent and severe abdominal pain for more than 3 days, and/or lower GI bleeding.

Nonsurgical Management. A combination of drug and *nutrition* therapy with rest is used to decrease the *inflammation* associated with diverticular disease. Broad-spectrum antimicrobial drugs, such as metronidazole in conjunction with trimethoprim/sulfamethoxazole (TMZ) or ciprofloxacin, are often prescribed. A mild analgesic may be given for pain. The Patient-Centered Care: Older Adult Considerations: Diverticulitis box lists nursing interventions needed for care of older adults with diverticulitis.

The patient with more severe *pain* may be admitted to the hospital for IV fluids to correct dehydration and IV drug therapy. For patients with moderate-to-severe diverticulitis, an opioid analgesic may alleviate pain.

👤 PATIENT-CENTERED CARE: OLDER ADULT CONSIDERATIONS (QSEN)

Diverticulitis

- Provide antibiotics and analgesics as prescribed. Observe older patients carefully for side effects of these drugs, especially confusion (or increased confusion), and orthostatic hypotension.
- Do not give laxatives or enemas. Teach the patient and family about the importance of avoiding these measures.
- Encourage the patient to rest and to avoid activities that may increase intra-abdominal pressure, such as straining and bending.
- While diverticulitis is active, provide a *low*-fiber diet. When the *inflammation* resolves, provide a *high*-fiber diet. Teach the patient and family about these diets and when they are appropriate.
- Because older patients do not always experience the typical *pain* or fever expected, observe carefully for other signs of active disease, such as a sudden change in mental status.
- Perform frequent abdominal assessments to determine distention and tenderness on palpation.
- Check stools for occult or frank bleeding.

Laxatives and enemas are avoided because they increase intestinal motility. Assess the patient on an ongoing basis for manifestations of impaired *fluid and electrolyte balance.*

Teach the patient to rest during the acute phase of illness. Remind him or her to refrain from lifting, straining, coughing, or bending to avoid an increase in intra-abdominal pressure, which can result in perforation of the diverticulum. *Nutrition* therapy should be restricted to low fiber or clear liquids based on symptoms. The patient with more severe symptoms is NPO. A nasogastric tube (NGT) is inserted if nausea, vomiting, or abdominal distention is severe. Infuse IV fluids as prescribed for hydration. In collaboration with a dietitian, the patient increases dietary intake slowly as symptoms subside. When *inflammation* has resolved and bowel function returns to normal, a fiber-containing diet is introduced gradually.

Surgical Management. Diverticulitis can result in rupture of the diverticulum with peritonitis, pelvic abscess, bowel obstruction, fistula, persistent fever or *pain,* or uncontrolled bleeding. The surgeon performs emergency surgery if peritonitis, bowel obstruction, or pelvic abscess is present. Colon resection, with or without a colostomy, is the most common surgical procedure for patients with diverticular disease. Chapter 51 discusses the nursing care for patients with this procedure.

Care Coordination and Transition Management. Discharge plans vary according to the treatment. The patient who has surgical intervention has the added responsibilities of incision care and possibly colostomy care with temporary limitations placed on activities.

Patients with diverticular disease need education regarding a high-fiber diet. Encourage the patient with *diverticulosis* to eat a diet high in cellulose and hemicellulose types of fiber. These substances can be found in wheat bran, whole-grain breads, and cereals. Teach the patient to eat at least 25 to 35 g of fiber per day. Fresh fruits and vegetables with high fiber content are added to provide bulk to stools.

If not accustomed to eating high-fiber foods, teach the patient to add them to the diet gradually to avoid flatulence and abdominal cramping. If he or she cannot tolerate the recommended fiber requirement, a bulk-forming laxative, such as psyllium hydrophilic mucilloid, can be taken to increase fecal size and consistency. Teach the patient to drink plenty of fluids to help prevent bloating that may occur with a high-fiber diet. Alcohol should be avoided because it irritates the bowel. Foods containing seeds or indigestible material that may block a diverticulum, such as nuts, corn, popcorn, cucumbers, tomatoes, and figs, may need to be eliminated. Teach the patient that dietary fat intake should not exceed 30% of the total daily caloric intake.

The patient should be instructed to avoid all fiber when symptoms of *diverticulitis* are present, because high-fiber foods can be irritating. As *inflammation* resolves, fiber can gradually be added until progression to a high-fiber diet is established. The patient who has undergone surgery is usually taking solid food by the time of discharge from the hospital.

Provide oral and written instructions on incision care and the signs and symptoms to report to the health care provider for the patient who had abdominal surgery. If a colostomy was created, reinforce ostomy care as needed. Encourage the patient to express concerns about body image. Allow time and address sexual concerns regarding the changed body image.

Instruct the patient with any type of diverticular disease about the manifestations of acute diverticulitis, including fever, abdominal pain, and bloody, mahogany, or tarry stools. Instruct patients to avoid the use of laxatives (other than bulk-forming types) and enemas. Reassure them that this disorder should not cause problems if a proper diet is followed.

In collaboration with the case manager, arrange for a home care nurse, if needed, to assess wound healing and proper functioning of the ostomy and the appliance. If the patient is interested, arrange for a visit from an ostomy volunteer (**ostomate**) or an ostomy nurse. For information about other community resources, remind the patient to contact the United Ostomy Associations of America (www.ostomy.org).

NCLEX EXAMINATION CHALLENGE 52.3
Physiological Integrity

The nurse is teaching a client about nutrition and diverticulosis. Which food will the nurse teach the client to avoid?
A. Cucumber
B. Beans
C. Carrot
D. Radish

CELIAC DISEASE

Celiac disease was once thought to be a rare disease but, because of improved diagnostic testing, many cases have been diagnosed in the past 10 to 15 years. Celiac disease is a multisystem autoimmune disease with an estimated incidence as high as 1 in 250

of the world's population (McCance et al., 2019). Patients who have other autoimmune diseases, such as rheumatoid arthritis and diabetes mellitus type 1, are at the highest risk for the disease.

Celiac disease is a chronic *inflammation* of the small intestinal mucosa that can cause bowel wall atrophy, malabsorption, and diarrhea. Like many inflammatory disorders, it is thought to be caused by a combination of genetic, immunologic, and environmental factors. The primary complication of celiac disease is cancer, specifically non-Hodgkin lymphoma or GI cancers and *nutrition* deficiencies.

Patients with celiac disease have varying signs and symptoms with cycles of remission and exacerbation (flare-up), usually related to how well they monitor their diet. Classic symptoms include anorexia, diarrhea and/or constipation, steatorrhea (fatty stools), abdominal pain, abdominal bloating and distention, and weight loss. Some patients have no symptoms. Still others have atypical symptoms that affect every body system, as listed in the Key Features: Celiac Disease box. Diagnosis is usually made by obtaining a screening blood test and endoscopy.

Dietary management is the only available treatment for achieving disease remission. In most cases, a gluten-free diet (GFD) results in healing the intestinal mucosa after about 2 years. Gluten is the primary substance in wheat and wheat-based products. Teach patients to carefully check for hidden sources of gluten that are in foods, food additives, drugs, and cosmetics. Patients often take vitamin and mineral supplements to replace those lost in avoiding gluten foods. A registered dietitian nutritionist should be included in the patient's long-term planning and overall treatment.

▶▶ KEY FEATURES
Celiac Disease

Classic Symptoms
- Weight loss
- Anorexia
- Diarrhea and/or constipation
- Steatorrhea
- Abdominal pain and distention
- Vomiting

Atypical Symptoms
- Osteoporosis
- Joint *pain* and *inflammation*
- Lactose intolerance
- Iron deficiency anemia
- Depression
- Migraines
- Epilepsy
- Autoimmune disorders
- Stomatitis
- Early menopause
- Protein-calorie malnutrition
- Infertility

TABLE 52.5   Comparison of Common Parasitic Infections

	Giardiasis *(Giardia lamblia)*	Amebiasis *(Entamoeba histolytica)*	*Cryptosporidium*
Description	Occurs in cysts and trophozoites Causes superficial invasion, destruction, and *inflammation* of small intestine mucosa	Occurs most commonly in crowded areas with poor sanitation Invades and ulcerates large intestinal mucosa	Occurs most commonly in immunosuppressed individuals Source is often contaminated swimming pools
Common assessment findings	Diarrhea Malabsorption syndrome Weight loss Nutrient deficiencies Acute phase is self-limiting Chronic phase can last for years	Can occur without symptoms May be mild or severe symptoms if they occur, including foul-smelling stools, abdominal cramping, and weight loss Can have extraintestinal symptoms	Primarily diarrhea Self-limiting health problem in individuals with normal immune system

PARASITIC INFECTION

Pathophysiology Review

Parasites can enter and invade the gastrointestinal tract and cause *infection*. They commonly enter through the mouth (oral-fecal transmission) from contaminated food or water, oral-anal sexual practices, or contact with feces from a contaminated person. Common parasites that cause infection in humans are *Giardia lamblia*, which causes giardiasis; *Entamoeba histolytica*, which causes amebiasis (amoebic dysentery); and *Cryptosporidium*. The primary method for determining which parasitic infection is present is through stool analysis. The white blood cell (WBC) count can be very high when severe diarrhea (dysentery) is present. Table 52.5 differentiates these three common types of parasites.

A less common parasitic infection is increasing in the United States. Chagas disease is caused by the *Trypanosoma cruzi* parasite, which is most commonly transmitted in impoverished areas of Latin America by the triatomine (kissing) bug. Patients first develop an acute *infection,* followed by an intermediate asymptomatic period and a chronic infection. Patients with chronic Chagas disease often develop cardiac dysrhythmias or heart failure and colon or esophagus dilation, causing impaired digestion and bowel *elimination*. An estimated 300,000 individuals in the United States have the disease (most in the southern areas of the United States), which can be transmitted through blood transfusions and organ transplantations. The Centers for Disease Control and Prevention (CDC) has targeted Chagas disease as one of five neglected parasitic infections that require public health action as the number of cases is expected to increase (CDC, 2019).

❖ Interprofessional Collaborative Care

◆ **Assessment: Recognize Cues.** A thorough history can help determine potential sources of exposure to parasitic infection. A history of travel to parts of the world where such infections are prevalent increases suspicion for infection with parasites. GI symptoms related to travel might be delayed as long as 1 to 2 weeks after the return home. Immigrants (newcomers) may have the *infection* on entering a new country. A *nutrition* history is especially helpful if several people in a group become ill. Common water supplies or bodies of water may be infected with *Giardia* or *Cryptosporidium*. Trichinosis should be considered if the patient has eaten pork products.

Mild-to-moderate *E. histolytica* infestation causes the daily passage of several strongly foul-smelling stools, possibly with mucus but without blood, accompanied by abdominal cramping, flatulence (gas), fatigue, and weight loss.

The infected patient usually experiences remissions and recurrences. Severe amoebic dysentery is manifested by frequent, liquid, and foul-smelling stools with mucus *and* blood. Fever up to 104° F (40° C), tenesmus, generalized abdominal tenderness, and vomiting can also occur. The ulcerations of invading amebiasis that occur in the colon can cause pain, bleeding, and obstruction. Ulcerations can also occur in the rectum, resulting in formed stool with blood. Complications are rare but include appendicitis and bowel perforation.

Extraintestinal amebiasis can occur without symptoms of intestinal infection. The most common form is amoebic liver abscess, which causes symptoms of fever, pain, and an enlarged liver. The abscess can rupture, and death can result if the infection and complications are not treated.

◆ **Interventions: Take Action.** *Handwashing is the best way to prevent the spread of parasitic infections.* Treatment for all types of *amebiasis* involves the use of amebicide drugs. Metronidazole followed by a luminal agent such as paromomycin, is commonly prescribed (Houpt et al., 2016). The patient with severe amoebic dysentery requires IV fluid replacement and possibly an opiate-like drug, such as diphenoxylate hydrochloride and atropine sulfate, to control bowel motility. The patient with extraintestinal amebiasis or severe dehydration, especially the older adult, is hospitalized. The patient with asymptomatic, mild, or moderate disease is treated with drug therapy on an ambulatory care basis. Therapy effectiveness is based on the examination of at least three stools at 2- to 3-day intervals, starting 2 to 4 weeks after drug therapy has been completed. *Teach patients* the importance of keeping their follow-up appointments and taking all drugs as prescribed.

Treatment for *giardiasis* is drug therapy. Metronidazole is the drug of choice. Tinidazole can be used as an alternative. Stools are examined 2 weeks after treatment to assess for drug effectiveness.

Infection with *Cryptosporidium* is usually self-limiting in adults who have normal immune function. Drug therapy for patients who are immunosuppressed may include paromomycin, an aminoglycoside antibiotic. Teach patients that this drug can cause dizziness.

> **! NURSING SAFETY PRIORITY (QSEN)**
> **Action Alert**
>
> Explain modes of transmission of parasitic infections and means to avoid the spread of infection and recurrent contact with parasitic organisms. *Inform the patient that the infection can be transmitted to others until amebicides effectively kill the parasites. Teach the patient to:*
> - Avoid contact with stool
> - Keep toilet areas clean
> - Wash hands meticulously with an antimicrobial soap after bowel movements
> - Maintain good personal hygiene by bathing or showering daily
> - Avoid stool from dogs and beavers
>
> Advise the patient to avoid sexual practices that allow rectal contact until drug therapy is completed. *All household and sexual partners should have stool examinations for parasites.* If the water supply is suspected as the source, a sample is obtained and sent for analysis. Multiple infections are common in households, often as a result of contaminated shared water supplies. Well water and water from areas with inadequate or no filtration equipment can be sources of contamination.

GET READY FOR THE NEXT-GENERATION NCLEX® EXAMINATION!

Key Points

Review these Key Points for each NCLEX Examination Client Needs Category.

Safe and Effective Care Environment

- Collaborate with a CWOCN, health care provider, and case manager to plan care for patients with IBD. **QSEN: Teamwork and Collaboration**
- When transitioning care, remind patients and families about community resources for IBD, including the United Ostomy Associations of America and the Crohn's and Colitis Foundation of America. **QSEN: Teamwork and Collaboration**

Health Promotion and Maintenance

- Teach patients to use *infection* control measures to prevent transmission of gastroenteritis. **QSEN: Safety**
- Teach patients how to self-manage an ileostomy or other surgical diversion, including skin care, pouch management, and stoma assessment. **QSEN: Patient-Centered Care**

Psychosocial Integrity

- Be aware that all IBDs (acute and chronic) are very disruptive to one's daily routine; living with IBD requires a lifetime of modifications. **QSEN: Patient-Centered Care**
- Recognize that having a chronic bowel disease or an ileostomy impacts the patient's body image and self-esteem; assess for coping strategies that the patient has previously used, and identify personal support systems, such as family members, to assist in coping. **QSEN: Patient-Centered Care**

Physiological Integrity

- Assess for the classic signs and symptoms of appendicitis, which can include abdominal pain, nausea and vomiting, and abdominal tenderness on palpation (McBurney point); some patients also have leukocytosis. **QSEN: Safety**
- Recognize that perforation (rupture) of the appendix requires prompt intervention and can result in peritonitis. **QSEN: Safety**
- Assess for signs and symptoms of dehydration and blood loss in patients who have acute and chronic inflammatory bowel disorders, such as anemia and hypotension. **QSEN: Safety**
- Administer antidiarrheal medications as prescribed to decrease stools and therefore prevent dehydration in patients with acute and chronic inflammatory bowel disorders. **QSEN: Evidence-Based Practice**
- Be alert for GI bleeding in the patient with chronic IBD. **QSEN: Safety**
- Be aware that patients with Crohn's disease are at high risk for malnutrition as a result of an inability to absorb nutrients via the small intestine. **Clinical Judgment**
- Priority problems for patients with UC include diarrhea, pain, and potential for lower GI bleeding. **Clinical Judgment**
- Teach patients with IBD to avoid GI stimulants, such as alcohol and caffeine. **QSEN: Evidence-Based Practice**
- Administer infliximab or other monoclonal antibody agent as prescribed for patients with Crohn's disease; these drugs may also be useful for those with UC in selected cases but can cause secondary *infection.*
- Observe for signs and symptoms of lower GI bleeding in patients with chronic inflammatory and diverticular disease. **QSEN: Safety**
- Teach patients with diverticulosis to eat a high-fiber diet; diverticulitis requires a low-fiber diet. **QSEN: Evidence-Based Practice**
- Instruct patients with diverticulosis about nutrition modifications, such as avoiding nuts, foods with seeds, and GI stimulants. **QSEN: Evidence-Based Practice**
- Be aware that patients with celiac disease have various signs and symptoms; some have no symptoms, some have

classic symptoms, and some have atypical symptoms. **QSEN: Patient-Centered Care**
- Teach patients with celiac disease about the need to consume a strict gluten-free diet, which avoids wheat and wheat-based products. **QSEN: Evidence-Based Practice**

- Be aware that GI problems, including diarrhea, may be caused by parasites and contaminated or undercooked food. **QSEN: Safety**

▮ MASTERY QUESTIONS

1. The nurse is caring for a client with peritonitis from a perforated appendix. Which abdominal assessment finding will the nurse most likely expect?
   A. Soft abdomen
   B. Board-like abdomen
   C. Slightly distended abdomen
   D. Absent bowel sounds

2. A client had a colectomy with creation of an ileo-anal pouch and temporary ileostomy yesterday morning. The nurse assesses the ostomy and its functioning. Which assessment finding will the nurse report to the primary health care provider?
   A. Client's report of abdominal pain of 3 on a 0 to 10 pain intensity scale
   B. Slight abdominal distention
   C. No drainage from the ileostomy
   D. Serosanguinous effluent from the drain

REFERENCES

Burchum, J. L. R., & Rosenthal, L. D. (2019). *Lehne's pharmacology for nursing care* (10th ed.). St. Louis: Elsevier.

Card, T., Xu, J., Liang, H., & Bhayat, F. (2018). What is the risk of progressive multifocal leukoencephalopathy in patients with ulcerative colitis or Crohn's disease treated with vedolizumab? *Inflammatory Bowel Diseases, 24*(5), 953–959.

Centers for Disease Control and Prevention (CDC). (2019). Parasites-American trypanosomiasis. http://www.cdc.gov/parasites/chagas.

Cleynen, I., Boucher, G., Jostins, L., Schumm, L. P., Zeissig, S., Ahmad, T., et al. (2016). Inherited determinants of Crohn's disease and ulcerative colitis phenotypes: A genetic association study. *Lancet, 387*, 156–167.

Crohn's and Colitis Foundation. (2020). *Crohn's disease & colitis.* http://www.crohnscolitisfoundation.org.

Crohn's and Colitis Canada. (2020). *Canada leads the fight against IBD.* http://www.crohnsandcolitis.ca.

Elisei, W., & Tursi, A. (2016). Recent advances in the treatment of colonic diverticular disease and prevention of acute diverticulitis. *Annals of Gastroenterology: Quarterly Publication of the Hellenic Society of Gastroenterology, 29*(1), 24–32.

Engel, T., Ungar, B., Yung, D. E., Ben-Horin, S., Eliakim, R., & Kopylov, U. (2018). Vedolizumab in IBD: Lessons from real-world experience; A systematic review and pooled analysis. *Journal of Crohn's and Colitis, 12*(2), 245–257.

Houpt, E., Hung, C. C., & Petri, W. (2016). *Entamoeba histolytica (Amebiasis). Infectious disease and antimicrobial agents.* http://antimicrobe.org/new/b137.asp.

Khatri, G., Coleman, J., & Levendecker, J. R. (2018). Magnetic resonance enterography for inflammatory and noninflammatory conditions of the small bowel. *Radiologic Clinics of North America, 56*(5), 671–689.

McCance, K., Huether, S., Brashers, V., & Rote, N. (2019). *Pathophysiology: The biologic basis for disease in adults and children* (8th ed.). St. Louis: Elsevier.

Pagana, K. D., & Pagana, T. J. (2018). *Manual of diagnostic and laboratory tests* (6th ed.). St. Louis: Mosby.

Ross, J. T., Matthay, M. A., & Harris, H. W. (2018). Secondary peritonitis: Principles of diagnosis and intervention. *British Medical Journal, 361*, k1407.

Santos, M. P. C., Gomes, C., & Torres, J. (2018). Familial and ethnic risk in inflammatory bowel disease. *Annals of Gastroenterology, 31*(1), 14–23.

Stelton, S. (2019). Stoma and peristomal skin care: A clinical review. *AJN, 119*(6), 38–45.

Valente, M. A., & Hull, T. L. (2018). Minimally invasive techniques for inflammatory bowel disease. In A. Pigazzi (Ed.), *Techniques in minimally invasive rectal surgery.* New York, NY: Springer Publishing.

Winter, R. W., & Burakoff, R. (2017). How should we treat mild and moderate-severe Crohn's disease in 2017? A brief overview of available therapies. *Expert Review of Gastroenterology & Hepatology, 11*(2), 95–97.

53

Concepts of Care for Patients With Liver Problems

Lara Carver, Jennifer Powers

http://evolve.elsevier.com/Iggy/

LEARNING OUTCOMES

1. Collaborate with the interprofessional team to manage quality care for patients with liver problems caused by impaired **cellular regulation** and **infection**.
2. Identify community resources for families and patients recovering from liver problems.
3. Apply knowledge of pathophysiology of liver problems to identify common assessment findings, including actual or risk for impaired **nutrition** and **fluid and electrolyte balance.**
4. Prioritize nursing and collaborative care for patients with common liver problems to manage **pain**, control **inflammation**, and promote **nutrition.**
5. Plan transition management and care coordination for the patient who has a liver problem, including health teaching.

KEY TERMS

alcohol withdrawal A condition that occurs after stopping heavy and prolonged alcohol intake, which often results in tremors, acute confusion, psychotic behaviors (such as delusions and hallucinations), and autonomic symptoms including tachycardia, elevated blood pressure, and diaphoresis.

ascites The collection of free fluid within the peritoneal cavity caused by increased hydrostatic pressure from portal hypertension.

asterixis A coarse tremor characterized by rapid, nonrhythmic extensions and flexions in the wrists and fingers (hand flapping).

cirrhosis A disease characterized by widespread fibrotic (scarred) bands of connective tissue that change the liver's anatomy and physiology.

ecchymoses Large purple, blue, or yellow bruises.

esophageal varices A complication of cirrhosis in which fragile, thin-walled esophageal veins become distended and tortuous from increased pressure (portal hypertension).

fetor hepaticus The distinctive breath odor of chronic liver disease and hepatic encephalopathy that is characterized by a fruity or musty odor.

hepatic encephalopathy (also called *portal-systemic encephalopathy [PSE]*) is a complex cognitive syndrome that results from liver failure and cirrhosis.

hepatitis Widespread inflammation and infection of liver cells.

hepatomegaly Liver enlargement that commonly occurs in patients with early cirrhosis.

hepatopulmonary syndrome A complication of cirrhosis caused by excessive ascitic volume and manifested by dyspnea as a result of intraabdominal pressure, which limits thoracic expansion and diaphragmatic excursion.

hepatorenal syndrome A late complication of cirrhosis affecting the kidneys and manifested by oliguria, elevated blood urea nitrogen (BUN) and creatinine levels, and increased urine osmolarity.

icterus Yellow coloration of the eye sclerae.

jaundice Yellowish coloration of the skin caused by increased serum bilirubin.

nonalcoholic fatty liver disease (NAFLD) A rapidly growing liver disease that is associated with obesity, diabetes mellitus type 2, and metabolic syndrome.

paracentesis An invasive procedure performed to remove abdominal fluid in patients who have massive ascites.

petechiae Round, pinpoint, red-purple hemorrhagic lesions.

portal hypertension A major complication of cirrhosis resulting in persistent increase in pressure within the portal vein >5 mm Hg.

splenomegaly Spleen enlargement.

spontaneous bacterial peritonitis (SBP) An infection that results from bacteria collected in ascitic fluid.

transjugular intrahepatic portal-systemic shunt (TIPS) An interventional radiologic procedure performed for patients who have not responded to other modalities to manage hemorrhage or long-term ascites.

ultrasound transient elastography A noninvasive imaging test that measures liver stiffness, which helps the primary health care provider determine the amount of liver disease present.

PRIORITY AND INTERRELATED CONCEPTS

The priority concepts for this chapter are:
- *Cellular Regulation*
- *Infection*

The **Cellular Regulation** concept exemplar for this chapter is Cirrhosis.
The **Infection** concept exemplar for this chapter is Hepatitis.

The interrelated concepts for this chapter are:
- *Fluid and Electrolyte Balance*
- *Inflammation*
- *Pain*
- *Nutrition*

As the largest and one of the most vital internal organs, the liver performs more than 400 functions and affects every body system. Common problems of the liver affect *cellular regulation, nutrition,* and *fluid and electrolyte balance.* Liver diseases range in severity from mild hepatic *inflammation* and *infection* to chronic end-stage cirrhosis. Many of these problems can cause *pain* or discomfort. Chapter 3 briefly reviews these concepts.

CELLULAR REGULATION CONCEPT EXEMPLAR: CIRRHOSIS

Cirrhosis is extensive, irreversible scarring of the liver, usually caused by a chronic reaction to hepatic *inflammation* and necrosis. This scarring process directly impairs *cellular regulation.* The disease typically develops slowly and has a progressive, prolonged, destructive course resulting in end-stage liver disease.

Pathophysiology Review

Cirrhosis is characterized by widespread fibrotic (scarred) bands of connective tissue that change the liver's anatomy and physiology. *Inflammation* caused by either toxins or disease results in extensive degeneration and destruction of hepatocytes (liver cells). As cirrhosis develops, the tissue becomes nodular. These nodules can block bile ducts and normal blood flow throughout the liver. Impairments in blood and lymph flow result from compression caused by excessive fibrous tissue. In early disease, the liver is usually enlarged and firm. As the pathologic process continues, the liver shrinks in size and becomes harder, resulting in decreased liver function over weeks to years. Some patients with cirrhosis have no symptoms until serious complications occur. The impaired liver function results in elevated serum liver enzymes.

Cirrhosis of the liver can be divided into several common types, depending on the cause of the disease (McCance et al., 2019):
- Postnecrotic cirrhosis (caused by viral hepatitis [especially hepatitis C] and certain drugs or other toxins)
- Laennec's or alcoholic cirrhosis (caused by chronic alcoholism)
- Biliary cirrhosis (also called *cholestatic;* caused by chronic biliary obstruction or autoimmune disease)

Complications of Cirrhosis. Common problems and complications associated with hepatic cirrhosis depend on the amount of damage sustained by the liver. In *compensated* cirrhosis, the liver is scarred and ***cellular regulation*** is impaired, but the organ can still perform essential functions without causing major symptoms. In *decompensated* cirrhosis, liver function is impaired with obvious signs and symptoms of liver failure.

The loss of hepatic function contributes to the development of metabolic abnormalities. Hepatic cell damage may lead to these common complications:
- Portal hypertension
- Ascites and esophageal varices
- Biliary obstruction
- Hepatic encephalopathy

Portal Hypertension. Portal hypertension, a persistent increase in pressure within the portal vein greater than 5 mm Hg, is a major complication of cirrhosis. It results from increased resistance to or obstruction (blockage) of the flow of blood through the portal vein and its branches. The blood meets resistance to flow and seeks collateral (alternative) venous channels around the high-pressure area.

Blood flow backs into the spleen, causing splenomegaly (spleen enlargement). Veins in the esophagus, stomach, intestines, abdomen, and rectum become dilated. Portal hypertension can result in ascites (excessive abdominal [peritoneal] fluid), esophageal varices (distended veins), prominent abdominal veins (caput medusae), and hemorrhoids.

Ascites and Gastroesophageal Varices. Ascites is the collection of free fluid within the peritoneal cavity caused by increased hydrostatic pressure from portal hypertension (McCance et al., 2019). The collection of plasma protein in the peritoneal fluid reduces the amount of circulating plasma protein in the blood. When this decrease is combined with the inability of the liver to produce albumin because of impaired liver cell functioning, the serum colloid osmotic pressure is decreased in the circulatory system. The result is a fluid shift from the vascular system into the abdomen, a form of "third spacing." As a result, the patient may have hypovolemia and edema at the same time.

Massive ascites may cause renal vasoconstriction, triggering the renin-angiotensin system. This results in sodium and water retention, which increases hydrostatic pressure and the vascular volume and leads to more ascites.

As a result of portal hypertension, the blood backs up from the liver and enters the esophageal and gastric veins. Esophageal varices occur when fragile, thin-walled esophageal veins become distended and tortuous from increased pressure. The potential for varices to bleed depends on their size; size is determined by direct endoscopic observation. Varices occur most often in the distal esophagus but can be present also in the stomach and rectum.

Decreased prothrombin production places the patient with cirrhosis at risk for bleeding. Bleeding esophageal varices are a life-threatening medical emergency. Severe blood loss may occur, resulting in shock from hypovolemia. The bleeding may present as either hematemesis (vomiting blood) or melena (black, tarry stools). Loss of consciousness may occur before

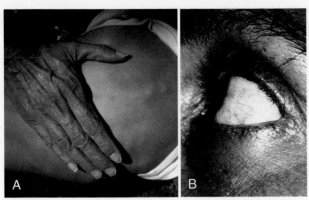

FIG. 53.1 (A and B) Jaundice as a result of liver dysfunction such as cirrhosis and hepatitis. (From Leonard PC. [2020]. *Quick & easy medical terminology* [9th ed.]. St. Louis: Elsevier.)

TABLE 53.1   Stages of Hepatic Encephalopathy
Stage I
• Subtle manifestations that may not be recognized immediately
• Personality changes
• Behavior changes (agitation, belligerence)
• Emotional lability (euphoria, depression)
• Impaired thinking
• Inability to concentrate
• Fatigue, drowsiness
• Slurred or slowed speech
• Sleep pattern disturbances
Stage II
• Continuing mental changes
• Mental confusion
• Disorientation to time, place, or person
• Asterixis (hand flapping)
Stage III
• Progressive deterioration
• Marked mental confusion
• Stuporous, drowsy but arousable
• Abnormal electroencephalogram tracing
• Muscle twitching
• Hyperreflexia
• Asterixis (hand flapping)
Stage IV
• Unresponsiveness, leading to death in most patients progressing to this stage
• Unarousable, obtunded
• Usually no response to painful stimulus
• No asterixis
• Positive Babinski sign
• Muscle rigidity
• Fetor hepaticus (characteristic liver breath—musty, sweet odor)
• Seizures

any observed bleeding. Variceal bleeding can occur spontaneously with no precipitating factors. However, any activity that increases abdominal pressure may increase the likelihood of a variceal bleed, including heavy lifting or vigorous physical exercise. In addition, chest trauma or dry, hard food in the esophagus can cause bleeding.

Patients with portal hypertension may also have portal hypertensive gastropathy. This complication can occur with or without esophageal varices. Slow gastric mucosal bleeding occurs, which may result in chronic slow blood loss, occult-positive stools, and anemia.

Splenomegaly results from the backup of blood into the spleen. The enlarged spleen destroys platelets, causing thrombocytopenia (low serum platelet count) and increased risk for bleeding. Thrombocytopenia is often the first clinical sign that a patient has liver dysfunction.

Biliary Obstruction. In patients with cirrhosis, the production of bile in the liver is decreased. This prevents the absorption of fat-soluble vitamins (e.g., vitamin K). Without vitamin K, clotting factors II, VII, IX, and X are not produced in sufficient quantities, and the patient is susceptible to bleeding and easy bruising. These abnormalities are confirmed by coagulation studies. Some patients have a genetic predisposition to obstruction of the bile duct that leads to biliary cirrhosis—usually from gallbladder disease or an autoimmune form of the disease called *primary biliary cirrhosis (PBC)*.

Jaundice (yellowish coloration of the skin) in patients with cirrhosis is caused by one of two mechanisms: hepatocellular disease or intrahepatic obstruction (Fig. 53.1). *Hepatocellular* jaundice develops because the liver cells cannot effectively excrete bilirubin. This decreased excretion results in excessive circulating bilirubin levels. *Intrahepatic obstructive* jaundice results from edema, fibrosis, or scarring of the hepatic bile channels and bile ducts, which interferes with normal bile and bilirubin excretion. Patients with jaundice often report pruritus (itching).

Hepatic Encephalopathy. Hepatic encephalopathy (also called **portal-systemic encephalopathy [PSE]**) is a complex cognitive syndrome that results from liver failure and cirrhosis. Patients report sleep disturbance, mood disturbance, mental status changes, and speech problems early as this complication begins. Hepatic

encephalopathy may be reversible with early intervention. Later neurologic symptoms include an altered level of consciousness, impaired thinking processes, and neuromuscular problems.

Hepatic encephalopathy may develop slowly in patients with chronic liver disease and go undetected until the late stages. Symptoms develop rapidly in acute liver dysfunction. Four stages of development have been identified (Table 53.1). The patient's symptoms may gradually progress to coma or fluctuate among the four stages.

The exact mechanisms causing hepatic encephalopathy are not clearly understood but probably are the result of the shunting of portal venous blood into the central circulation, so the liver is bypassed. As a result, substances absorbed by the intestine are not broken down or detoxified and may lead to metabolic abnormalities, such as elevated serum ammonia and gamma-aminobutyric acid (GABA). Elevated serum ammonia results from the inability of the liver to detoxify protein by-products and is common in patients with hepatic encephalopathy. However, it is not a clear indicator of the presence of encephalopathy. Some patients may have major impairment without high elevations of serum ammonia, and elevations of ammonia can occur without evidence of encephalopathy.

Factors that may contribute to or worsen hepatic encephalopathy in patients with cirrhosis include:

- High-protein diet
- Infection
- Hypovolemia (decreased fluid volume)
- Hypokalemia (decreased serum potassium)
- Constipation
- GI bleeding (causes a large protein load in the intestines)
- Drugs (e.g., hypnotics, opioids, sedatives, analgesics, diuretics, illicit drugs)

The prognosis depends on the severity of the underlying cause, precipitating factors, and degree of liver dysfunction (McCance et al., 2019).

Other Complications. The development of hepatorenal syndrome indicates a poor prognosis for the patient with liver failure. It is often the cause of death in these patients. This syndrome is manifested by:

- A sudden decrease in urinary flow (<500 mL/24 hr) (oliguria)
- Elevated blood urea nitrogen (BUN) and creatinine levels with abnormally decreased urine sodium excretion
- Increased urine osmolarity

Hepatorenal syndrome often occurs after clinical deterioration from GI bleeding or the onset of hepatic encephalopathy. It may also complicate other liver diseases, including acute hepatitis and fulminant liver failure.

Patients with cirrhosis and ascites may develop acute spontaneous bacterial peritonitis (SBP). Those who are particularly susceptible are patients with very advanced liver disease. This may be the result of low concentrations of proteins; proteins normally provide some protection against bacteria.

The bacteria responsible for SBP are typically from the bowel and reach the ascitic fluid after migrating through the bowel wall and transversing the lymphatics. Symptoms vary but may include fever, chills, *pain* (especially in the abdomen), and tenderness. However, indications can also be minimal with only mild symptoms in the absence of fever. Worsening encephalopathy and increased jaundice may also be present without abdominal symptoms (McCance et al., 2019).

The diagnosis of SBP is made when a sample of ascitic fluid is obtained by paracentesis for cell counts and culture. An ascitic fluid leukocyte count of more than 250 polymorphonuclear (PMN) leukocytes may indicate the need for treatment (McCance et al., 2019).

Another major complication of cirrhosis is hepatopulmonary syndrome caused by excessive ascitic volume. The client experiences dyspnea as a result of intra-abdominal pressure, which limits thoracic expansion and diaphragmatic excursion.

Etiology and Genetic Risk. The most common causes for cirrhosis in the United States are chronic alcoholism, chronic viral hepatitis, and bile duct disease (Table 53.2). Hepatitis C is a leading cause of cirrhosis and liver cancer in the United States (Centers for Disease Control and Prevention, 2020b). It is an infectious bloodborne illness that usually causes chronic disease

TABLE 53.2	Common Causes of Cirrhosis
• Alcoholic liver disease	• Drugs and chemical toxins
• Viral hepatitis	• Gallbladder disease
• Autoimmune hepatitis	• Metabolic/genetic causes
• Steatohepatitis (from fatty liver)	• Cardiovascular disease

and compromises the body's immunity. *Inflammation* caused by *infection* over time leads to progressive scarring of the liver. It usually takes decades for cirrhosis to develop, although alcohol use in combination with hepatitis C may speed the process.

Hepatitis B and hepatitis D are the most common causes of cirrhosis worldwide. Hepatitis B also causes *inflammation* and low-grade damage over decades that can ultimately lead to cirrhosis. Hepatitis D virus can infect the liver but only in people who already have hepatitis B (see discussion in **Infection Concept Exemplar: Hepatitis**).

Cirrhosis may also occur as a result of nonalcoholic fatty liver disease (NAFLD), a rapidly growing health care concern. NAFLD is associated with aging, obesity, diabetes mellitus type 2, and metabolic syndrome (Vacca, 2020). This disease can progress to liver cancer, cirrhosis, or failure, causing premature death. Up to 30% of Americans may have NAFLD (American Liver Foundation, 2020a). The Patatin-like phospholipase domain-containing 3 gene *(PNPLA3)* has been identified as a risk gene for the disease. Latinos have this gene more often than other ethnic groups and therefore are at the highest risk for NAFLD (McCance et al., 2019).

Another common cause of cirrhosis is excessive and prolonged alcohol use. Alcohol has a direct toxic effect on the hepatocytes and causes liver *inflammation* (alcoholic hepatitis). The liver becomes enlarged, with cellular degeneration and infiltration by fat, leukocytes, and lymphocytes. Over time, the inflammatory process decreases and the destructive phase increases. Early scar formation is caused by fibroblast infiltration and collagen formation. Damage to the liver tissue progresses as malnutrition and repeated exposure to the alcohol continue. If alcohol is withheld, the fatty infiltration and *inflammation* are reversible. If alcohol use continues, widespread scar tissue formation and fibrosis infiltrate the liver as a result of cellular necrosis. The long-term use of illicit drugs, such as cocaine, has similar effects on the liver.

PATIENT-CENTERED CARE: GENDER HEALTH CONSIDERATIONS (QSEN)

The amount of alcohol necessary to cause cirrhosis varies widely from individual to individual, and there are gender differences. In women, it may take as few as two or three drinks per day over a minimum of 10 years. In men, perhaps six drinks per day over the same time period may be needed to cause disease. However, a smaller amount of alcohol over a long period of time can increase memory loss from alcohol toxicity of the cerebral cortex. Binge drinking can increase risk for hepatitis and fatty liver (McCance et al., 2019).

Incidence and Prevalence. Approximately 3.2 million Americans have hepatitis C (American Liver Foundation, 2020b), and 1 in 7 Americans have hepatitis B, which can particularly affect Asian American and Pacific Islander-born individuals (Immunization Action Coalition, 2020).

Combined, the incidence of chronic liver disease and cirrhosis is a major common cause of death in the United States. The national prevalence of hepatitis B in Canada is 270,000 individuals (Canadian Digestive Health Association, 2020). It is more challenging to quantify the exact number of Canadians with liver disease, since these statistics are grouped with other digestive disorders; however, it is known that approximately 7000 Canadians die annually after being affected with a liver disorder (Canadian Digestive Health Association, 2020.)

❖ Interprofessional Collaborative Care

Care for the patient with cirrhosis can take place in various settings by many members of the interprofessional health care team. These patients may, at different times, self-manage at home, be hospitalized for immediate concerns, need rehabilitative care, or be cared for in the community setting, including possible hospice care.

◆ Assessment: Recognize Cues

History. Obtain data from patients with suspected cirrhosis, including age, gender, and employment history, especially history of exposure to alcohol, drugs (prescribed and illicit), use of herbal preparations, and chemical toxins. Keep in mind that all exposures are important, regardless of how long ago they occurred. Determine whether there has ever been a needlestick injury. Sexual history and orientation may be important in determining an infectious cause for liver disease, because men having sex with men (MSM) are at high risk for hepatitis A, hepatitis B, and hepatitis C. People with hepatitis can develop cirrhosis (McCance et al., 2019).

Inquire about whether there is a family history of alcoholism and/or liver disease. Ask the patient to describe his or her alcohol intake, including the amount consumed during a given period. Is there a history of illicit drug use, including oral, IV, and intranasal forms? Is there a history of obtaining tattoos? If so, when and where were they done? Has the patient been in the military or in prison? Is the patient a health care worker, firefighter, or police officer? For patients previously or currently in an alcohol or drug recovery program, how long have they been sober? This information is sensitive and often difficult for the patient to answer. Be sure to establish why you are asking these questions and accept answers in a nonjudgmental manner. Provide privacy during the interview. For many people, the behaviors causing the liver disease occurred years before the onset of their current illness, and they are regretful and often embarrassed.

Ask the patient about previous medical conditions, such as an episode of jaundice or acute viral hepatitis, biliary tract disorders (such as cholecystitis [gallbladder *inflammation*]), viral *infection,* surgery, blood transfusions, autoimmune disorders, obesity, altered lipid profile, heart failure, respiratory disorders, or liver injury.

Physical Assessment/Signs and Symptoms. Because cirrhosis has a slow onset, many of the *early* signs and symptoms are vague and nonspecific. Assess for:

- Fatigue
- Significant change in weight
- GI symptoms, such as anorexia and vomiting
- *Pain* in the abdominal area and liver tenderness (both of which may be ignored by the patient)

Liver function problems are often found during a routine physical examination or when laboratory tests are completed for an unrelated illness or problem. The patient with *compensated cirrhosis* may be completely unaware that there is a liver problem. The first sign may present before the onset of symptoms when routine laboratory tests, presurgical evaluations, or life and health insurance assessments show abnormalities. These tests could indicate abnormal liver function or thrombocytopenia (decreased serum platelet count), requiring a more thorough diagnostic workup.

The development of late signs of *advanced cirrhosis* (also called *end-stage liver failure*) usually causes the patient to seek medical treatment. GI bleeding, jaundice, ascites, and spontaneous bruising indicate poor liver function and complications of cirrhosis.

Thoroughly assess the patient with liver dysfunction or failure because it affects every body system. The clinical picture and course vary from patient to patient, depending on the severity of the disease. Assess for the common late disease signs and symptoms outlined in the Key Features: Late-Stage Cirrhosis box.

Abdominal Assessment. *Massive* ascites can be detected as a distended abdomen with bulging flanks (Fig. 53.2). The umbilicus may protrude, and dilated abdominal veins (caput medusae) may radiate from the umbilicus. Ascites can cause physical problems. For example, orthopnea and dyspnea from increased abdominal distention can interfere with lung expansion. The patient may have difficulty maintaining an erect body posture, and problems with balance may affect walking. Inspect and palpate for the presence of inguinal or umbilical hernias, which are likely to develop because of increased intra-abdominal pressure. *Minimal* ascites is often more difficult to detect, especially in the obese patient.

When performing an assessment of the abdomen, keep in mind that **hepatomegaly** (liver enlargement) occurs in many cases of early cirrhosis. **Splenomegaly** is common in

---

▶ KEY FEATURES

Late-Stage Cirrhosis

- **Jaundice** and **icterus** (yellow coloration of the eye sclerae)
- Dry skin
- Pruritus (itchy skin)
- Rashes
- Purpuric lesions, such as **petechiae** (round, pinpoint, red-purple hemorrhagic lesions) or **ecchymoses** (large purple, blue, or yellow bruises)
- Warm and bright red palms of the hands (palmar erythema)
- Vascular lesions with a red center and radiating branches, known as spider angiomas (also called telangiectases, spider nevi, or vascular spiders), on the nose, cheeks, upper thorax, and shoulders
- **Ascites**
- Peripheral dependent edema of the extremities and sacrum
- Vitamin deficiency (especially fat-soluble vitamins A, D, E, and K)

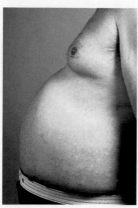

FIG. 53.2 Patient with abdominal ascites in late-stage cirrhosis. (From Leonard PC. [2020]. *Quick & easy medical terminology* [9th ed.]. St. Louis: Elsevier.)

nonalcoholic causes of cirrhosis. As the liver deteriorates, it may become hard and small.

Measure the patient's abdominal girth to evaluate the progression of ascites (see Fig. 53.2). To measure abdominal girth, the patient lies flat while the nurse or other examiner pulls a tape measure around the largest diameter (usually over the umbilicus) of the abdomen. The girth is measured at the end of exhalation. Mark the abdominal skin and flanks to ensure the same tape measure placement on subsequent readings. *However, taking daily weights is the most reliable indicator of fluid retention.*

Other Physical Assessment. Observe vomitus and stool for blood. This may be indicated by frank blood in the excrement or by a positive fecal occult blood test (FOBT). Gastritis, stomach ulceration, or oozing esophageal varices may be responsible for the blood in the stool. Note the presence of **fetor hepaticus,** which is the distinctive breath odor of chronic liver disease and hepatic encephalopathy and is characterized by a fruity or musty odor. Amenorrhea (no menstrual period) may occur in women, and men may exhibit testicular atrophy, gynecomastia (enlarged breasts), and impotence as a result of inactive hormones.

Continually assess the patient's neurologic function; it may also be helpful to include family members in conversations about the patient's baseline mental status if the patient is unable to effectively communicate. Subtle changes in mental status and personality often progress to coma—a late complication of hepatic encephalopathy. Monitor for **asterixis**—a coarse tremor characterized by rapid, nonrhythmic extensions and flexions in the wrists and fingers (hand flapping).

Psychosocial Assessment. The patient with hepatic cirrhosis may undergo subtle or obvious personality, cognitive, and behavior changes, such as agitation. He or she may experience sleep pattern disturbances or exhibit signs of emotional lability (fluctuations in emotions), euphoria (a very elevated mood), or depression. A psychosocial assessment identifies needs and helps guide care.

Repeated hospitalizations are common for patients with cirrhosis. It is a life-altering chronic disease, impacting not only the patient but also the immediate and extended family members and significant others. There are significant emotional, physical, and financial changes. Substance use may continue

even as health worsens. It is important, whenever possible, to use resources available to these patients and their families. Collaborate with social workers, substance use counselors, and mental health/behavioral health care professionals as needed for patient assessment and management.

Part of the psychosocial assessment is determining if the patient is alcohol dependent. If this is the case, observe and prepare for alcohol withdrawal. **Alcohol withdrawal** occurs after stopping alcohol intake after heavy and prolonged use. Monitor for tremors, sometimes called the "jitters," which can begin as early as 6 to 8 hours after alcohol cessation. Cognitive and neurologic changes associated with delirium tremens (DTs) may include acute confusion, anxiety, and psychotic behaviors, such as delusions and hallucinations. Autonomic changes may include tachycardia, elevated blood pressure, and diaphoresis (Halter, 2018). Care of the patient experiencing withdrawal can be a medical emergency. Consult mental health textbooks for more information about caring for the alcohol-dependent patient.

Laboratory Assessment. Laboratory study abnormalities are common in patients with liver disease (Table 53.3). Serum levels of *aspartate aminotransferase* (AST), *alanine aminotransferase* (ALT), and *lactate dehydrogenase* (LDH) typically are elevated because these enzymes are released into the blood during hepatic **inflammation.** However, as the liver deteriorates, the hepatocytes may be unable to create an inflammatory response, and the AST and ALT may be normal. ALT levels are more specific to the liver, whereas AST can be found in muscle, kidney, brain, and heart. An AST/ALT ratio greater than 1.0 is usually found in alcoholic liver disease (Pagana & Pagana, 2018).

Increased *alkaline phosphatase* and gamma-glutamyl transpeptidase (GGT) levels are caused by biliary obstruction and therefore may increase in patients with cirrhosis. Alkaline phosphatase is a nonspecific bone, intestinal, and liver enzyme. However, alkaline phosphatase also increases when bone disease, such as osteoporosis, is present. Total serum *bilirubin* levels also rise. Indirect bilirubin levels increase in patients with cirrhosis because of the inability of the failing liver to excrete bilirubin. Therefore bilirubin is present in the urine (urobilinogen) in increased amounts. Fecal urobilinogen concentration is decreased in patients with biliary tract obstruction. These patients have light- or clay-colored stools.

Total serum *albumin* levels are decreased in patients with severe or chronic liver disease as a result of decreased synthesis by the liver (Pagana & Pagana, 2018). Loss of osmotic "pull" proteins such as albumin promotes the movement of intravascular fluid into the interstitial tissues (e.g., ascites). Prothrombin time/*international normalized ratio* (PT/INR) is prolonged because the liver decreases the production of prothrombin. The platelet count is low, resulting in a characteristic thrombocytopenia of cirrhosis. Anemia may be reflected by decreased red blood cell (RBC), hemoglobin, and hematocrit values. The white blood cell (WBC) count may also be decreased. *Ammonia* levels are usually elevated in patients with advanced liver disease. Serum creatinine may be elevated in patients with deteriorating kidney function. Dilutional hyponatremia (low serum sodium) may occur in patients with ascites.

TABLE 53.3 Assessment of Abnormal Laboratory Findings in Liver Disease

Abnormal Finding	Significance
Serum Enzymes	
Elevated serum aspartate aminotransferase (AST)	Hepatic cell destruction, hepatitis
Elevated serum alanine aminotransferase (ALT)	Hepatic cell destruction, hepatitis (most specific indicator)
Elevated lactate dehydrogenase (LDH)	Hepatic cell destruction
Elevated serum alkaline phosphatase	Obstructive jaundice, hepatic metastasis
Elevated gamma-glutamyl transpeptidase (GGT)	Biliary obstruction, cirrhosis
Bilirubin	
Elevated serum total bilirubin	Hepatic cell disease
Elevated serum direct conjugated bilirubin	Hepatitis, liver metastasis
Elevated serum indirect unconjugated bilirubin	Cirrhosis
Elevated urine bilirubin	Hepatocellular obstruction, viral or toxic liver disease
Elevated urine urobilinogen	Hepatic dysfunction
Decreased fecal urobilinogen	Obstructive liver disease
Serum Proteins	
Increased serum total protein	Acute liver disease
Decreased serum total protein	Chronic liver disease
Decreased serum albumin	Severe liver disease
Elevated serum globulin	Immune response to liver disease
Other Tests	
Elevated serum ammonia	Advanced liver disease or portal-systemic encephalopathy (PSE)
Prolonged prothrombin time (PT) or international normalized ratio (INR)	Hepatic cell damage and decreased synthesis of prothrombin

NCLEX EXAMINATION CHALLENGE 53.1

Physiological Integrity

The nurse is caring for a client who is diagnosed with cirrhosis. Which serum laboratory value(s) will the nurse expect to be abnormal? **Select all that apply.**
A. Prothrombin time
B. Serum bilirubin
C. Albumin
D. Aspartate aminotransferase (AST)
E. Lactate dehydrogenase (LDH)
F. Acid phosphatase

Imaging Assessment. Plain x-rays of the abdomen may show hepatomegaly, splenomegaly, or massive ascites. A CT scan may be requested.

MRI is another test used to diagnose the patient with liver disease. It can reveal mass lesions, giving additional specific information. This information is helpful in determining whether the condition is malignant or benign.

Other Diagnostic Assessment. Ultrasound (US) of the liver is often the first assessment for an adult with suspected liver disease to detect ascites, hepatomegaly, and splenomegaly. It can also determine the presence of biliary stones or biliary duct obstruction. Liver US with Doppler is useful in detecting portal vein thrombosis and evaluating whether the direction of portal blood flow is normal. Ultrasound transient elastography is a noninvasive test that measures liver stiffness, which helps the primary health care provider determine the amount of liver disease present. The normal amount of stiffness is 5.0 kilopascals (kPa). Higher degrees of stiffness indicate liver fibrosis. More than 11 kPa indicates that the client has cirrhosis. The imaging study may not be as reliable for patients who have excessive ascites or obesity (Chancy, 2019).

Some patients being assessed for liver disease require biopsies to determine the exact pathology and the extent of disease progression. This procedure can be problematic because a large number of patients are at risk for bleeding. Even a percutaneous (through the skin) biopsy can pose a significant risk to the patient. To minimize this risk, an interventional radiologist can perform a liver biopsy using a long sheath through a jugular vein that then is threaded into the hepatic vein and liver. A tissue sample is obtained for microscopic evaluation. If a biopsy procedure is not possible, a radioisotope liver scan may be used to identify cirrhosis or other diffuse disease.

The primary health care provider may request *arteriography* if US is not conclusive in finding portal vein thrombosis. To evaluate the portal vein and its branches, a portal venogram may be performed instead, by passing a catheter into the liver and portal vein. This procedure is described in the Transjugular Intrahepatic Portal-Systemic Shunt (TIPS) section.

The primary health care provider may perform an *esophago-gastroduodenoscopy (EGD)* to directly visualize the upper GI tract to detect complications of liver failure. These complications may include bleeding or oozing esophageal varices, stomach irritation and ulceration, or duodenal ulceration and bleeding. EGD is performed by introducing a flexible fiberoptic endoscope into the mouth, esophagus, and stomach while the patient is under moderate sedation. A camera attached to the scope permits direct visualization of the mucosal lining of the upper GI tract. An *endoscopic retrograde cholangiopancreatography (ERCP)* uses the endoscope to inject contrast material via the sphincter of Oddi to view the biliary tract and allow for stone removals, sphincterotomies, biopsies, and stent placements if required. These procedures are described in more detail in Chapter 48.

◆ **Analysis: Analyze Cues and Prioritize Hypotheses.** The priority collaborative problems for patients with cirrhosis include:
1. Fluid overload due to third spacing of abdominal and peripheral fluid (ascites)
2. Potential for hemorrhage due to portal hypertension and subsequent GI varices
3. Acute confusion and other cognitive changes due to increased serum ammonia levels and/or alcohol withdrawal
4. Pruritus due to increased serum bilirubin and jaundice

◆ **Planning and Implementation: Generate Solutions and Take Action**

Managing Fluid Volume

Planning: Expected Outcomes. The patient with cirrhosis is expected to have less excess fluid volume as evidenced by decreased ascites and peripheral edema, as well as adequate circulatory volume.

Interventions. Fluid accumulations are minimal during the early stages of cirrhosis. Therefore nursing and interprofessional interventions are aimed at preventing the accumulation of additional fluid and decreasing any existing fluid collection. Nonsurgical treatment measures are used to treat ascites in most cases.

Supportive measures to control abdominal ascites include *nutrition* therapy, drug therapy, paracentesis, and respiratory support. The patient's *fluid and electrolyte balance* is carefully monitored during the treatment period.

Nutrition Therapy. The primary health care provider usually places the patient with early abdominal ascites on a low-sodium diet as an initial means of controlling fluid accumulation. The amount of daily sodium (Na^+) intake restriction varies, but a 1- to 2-g (2000 mg) Na^+ restriction may be tried first. In collaboration with the registered dietitian nutritionist, explain the purpose of the restriction and advise the patient and family to read the sodium content labels on all food and beverages. Table salt should be completely excluded. Low-sodium diets may be distasteful, so suggest alternative flavoring additives such as lemon, vinegar, parsley, oregano, and pepper. Remind the patient that seasoned and salty food is an acquired taste; in time, he or she will become used to the decrease in dietary sodium.

In general, patients with *late-stage* cirrhosis are malnourished and have multiple dietary deficiencies. IV vitamin supplements such as thiamine, folate, and multivitamin preparations are typically given because the liver cannot store vitamins. For patients with biliary cirrhosis, bile may not be available for fat-soluble vitamin transport and absorption. Oral vitamins are prescribed when IV fluid administration is discontinued.

Drug Therapy. The primary health care provider usually prescribes a *diuretic* to reduce fluid accumulation and prevent cardiac and respiratory problems. Monitor the effect of diuretic therapy by weighing the patient daily, measuring daily intake and output, measuring abdominal girth, documenting peripheral edema, and assessing electrolyte levels. Serious fluid and electrolyte imbalances, such as dehydration, hypokalemia (decreased potassium), and hyponatremia (decreased sodium), may occur with loop diuretic therapy. Depending on the diuretic selected, the provider may prescribe an oral or IV potassium supplement. Some clinicians prescribe furosemide and spironolactone as a combination diuretic therapy for the treatment of ascites. Because these drugs work differently, they are used for maintenance of sodium and potassium balance. For example, furosemide causes potassium loss, whereas spironolactone conserves it in the body.

All patients with ascites have the potential to develop spontaneous bacterial peritonitis (SBP) from bacteria in the collected ascitic fluid. In some patients, mild symptoms such as low-grade fever and loss of appetite occur. In others, there may be abdominal pain, fever, and change in mental status. When performing an abdominal assessment, listen for bowel sounds and assess for abdominal wall rigidity. Treatment involves IV cefotaxime or other third-generation cephalosporins or fluroquinolones.

Paracentesis. For some patients, abdominal paracentesis may be needed if ascites affects respiratory effort. A paracentesis is an invasive procedure performed to remove abdominal fluid. The procedure is performed at the bedside, in an interventional radiology department, or in an ambulatory care setting. The primary health care provider inserts a trocar catheter or drain into the abdomen to remove the ascitic fluid from the peritoneal cavity. This procedure is done using ultrasound for added safety. In some situations, a short-term ascites drain catheter may be placed while the patient is awaiting surgical intervention, or tunneled ascites drains can allow a patient or family caregiver to drain ascitic fluid at home. Nursing implications associated with this procedure are described in the Best Practice for Patient Safety & Quality Care box: The Patient Having a Paracentesis.

BEST PRACTICE FOR PATIENT SAFETY & QUALITY CARE (QSEN)

The Patient Having a Paracentesis

- Explain the procedure and answer patient questions.
- Obtain vital signs, including weight, before the procedure.
- Ask the patient to void before the procedure to prevent injury to the bladder!
- Position the patient in bed with the head of the bed elevated.
- Monitor vital signs per protocol or primary health care provider request during the procedure.
- Measure the drainage and record accurately.
- Document the characteristics of the collected fluid.
- Label and send the fluid for laboratory analysis; document in the patient health record that specimens were sent.
- After the catheter is removed, apply a dressing to the site; assess for leakage.
- Maintain bedrest per protocol.
- Take vital signs and weigh the patient after the paracentesis; document in the patient record weight both before and after paracentesis. (The patient should experience a weight loss due to fluid removal.)

If SBP is suspected, a sample of fluid is withdrawn and sent for cell count and culture. If the patient has symptoms of *infection,* the primary health care provider may prescribe antibiotics while awaiting the culture results.

Respiratory Support. Excessive ascitic fluid volume may cause the patient to have respiratory problems. He or she may develop *hepatopulmonary syndrome.* Dyspnea develops as a result of increased intra-abdominal pressure, which limits thoracic expansion and diaphragmatic excursion. Auscultate lungs every 4 to 8 hours for crackles that could indicate pulmonary complications, depending on the patient's overall condition.

> ### ! NURSING SAFETY PRIORITY (QSEN)
> #### *Action Alert*
>
> For the patient with hepatopulmonary syndrome, monitor his or her oxygen saturation with pulse oximetry. If needed, apply oxygen therapy to ease breathing. Elevate the head of the bed to at least 30 degrees or as high as the patient wants to improve breathing. This position, with his or her feet elevated to decrease dependent ankle edema, often relieves dyspnea. Remind assistive personnel to weigh the patient daily every morning before breakfast using the same scale.

Fluid and electrolyte balance problems are common as a result of the disease or treatment. Laboratory tests, such as blood urea nitrogen (BUN), serum protein, hematocrit, and electrolytes, help determine fluid and electrolyte status. An elevated BUN, decreased serum proteins, and increased hematocrit may indicate hypovolemia.

If medical management fails to control ascites, the primary health care provider may choose to divert ascites into the venous system by creating a shunt. Patients with ascites are poor surgical risks. The transjugular intrahepatic portal-systemic shunt (TIPS) is a nonsurgical procedure that is used to control long-term ascites and reduce variceal bleeding. This procedure is described in the discussion of Interventions in the Preventing or Managing Hemorrhage section that follows.

Preventing or Managing Hemorrhage

Planning: Expected Outcomes. The patient is expected to be free of bleeding episodes. However, if he or she has a hemorrhage, it is expected to be controlled by prompt, evidence-based professional interventions. Esophageal variceal bleeds are the most common cause of upper GI bleeding (also see Chapter 50 on management of upper GI bleeding).

Interventions. All patients with cirrhosis should be screened for esophageal varices by endoscopy to detect them early *before they bleed.* If patients have varices, they are placed on preventive therapy. If acute bleeding occurs, early interventions are used to manage it. *Because massive esophageal bleeding can cause rapid blood loss, emergency interventions are needed.*

The role of early drug therapy is to *prevent* bleeding and infection in patients who have varices. A nonselective *beta-blocking agent* such as propranolol is usually prescribed to prevent bleeding. By decreasing heart rate and the hepatic venous pressure gradient, the chance of bleeding may be reduced.

Up to 20% of cirrhotic patients who are admitted to the hospital as a result of upper GI bleeding have bacterial *infection,* and even more patients develop health care–associated infection, usually cellulitis, urinary tract infections, or pneumonia (McCance et al., 2019). Infection is one of the most common indicators that patients will have an acute variceal bleed (AVB). Therefore cirrhotic patients with GI bleeding should receive *antibiotics* when admitted to the hospital.

If bleeding occurs, the health care team intervenes quickly to control it by combining vasoactive drugs with endoscopic therapies. *Vasoactive* drugs, such as octreotide acetate and vasopressin, reduce blood flow through vasoconstriction to decrease portal pressure. Octreotide also suppresses secretion of gastrin, serotonin, and intestinal peptides, which decreases GI blood flow to help with pressure reduction within the varices (Burchum & Rosenthal, 2019). Vasopressin is used less commonly because it is a very potent drug (Pezzotti, 2020).

Endoscopic therapies include ligation of the bleeding veins or sclerotherapy. Both procedures are very effective in controlling bleeding and improving patient survival rates. Esophageal varices may be managed with *endoscopic variceal ligation (EVL) (banding).* This procedure involves the application of small "O" bands around the base of the varices to decrease their blood supply. The patient is unaware of the bands, and they cause no discomfort.

Endoscopic sclerotherapy (EST), also called *injection sclerotherapy,* may be done to stop bleeding. The varices are injected with a sclerosing agent via a catheter. This procedure is associated with complications such as mucosal ulceration, which could result in further bleeding.

If rebleeding occurs, rescue therapies are used. These procedures include a second endoscopic procedure, balloon tamponade and esophageal stents, and shunting procedures. Short-term esophagogastric balloon tamponade with esophageal stents is a very effective way to control bleeding. However, the procedure can cause potentially life-threatening complications, such as aspiration, asphyxia, and esophageal perforation. Similar to a nasogastric tube, the tube is placed through the nose and into the stomach. An attached balloon is inflated to apply pressure to the bleeding variceal area. Before this tamponade, the patient is usually intubated and placed on a mechanical ventilator to protect the airway. This therapy is used if the patient is not able to have a second endoscopy or TIPS procedure.

The **transjugular intrahepatic portal-systemic shunt (TIPS)** is a nonsurgical procedure performed in interventional radiology departments. This procedure is used for patients who have not responded to other modalities for hemorrhage or long-term ascites. If time permits, patients have a Doppler ultrasound to assess jugular vein anatomy and patency. The patient receives heavy IV sedation or general anesthesia for this procedure. The radiologist places a large sheath through the jugular vein. A needle is guided through the sheath and pushed through the liver into the portal vein. A balloon enlarges this tract, and a stent keeps it open. Most patients also have a Doppler ultrasound study of the liver after the TIPS procedure to record the blood flow through the shunt. Treating patients with TIPS who have esophageal/gastric varix hemorrhage problems may also require esophageal/gastric vein embolization as a part of the procedure. Patients with a highly cirrhotic liver usually have little flow through the liver parenchyma. These patients develop large portal-esophageal (or portal-gastric) veins diverting blood away from the diseased liver. Even after a successful TIPS, the diverting veins may persist and must be embolized (intentionally blocked) so they will not rebleed.

Serious complications of TIPS are not common. Patients are usually discharged in 1 or 2 days and are followed up with ultrasounds for the first year after the shunt is placed to ensure continued patency. Patients must also be monitored for hepatic encephalopathy, which can be caused by a TIPS. After creation of the TIPS, blood now bypasses most of the liver's filtration processes, allowing toxins to circulate throughout the body. For some patients, this can cause disturbances in consciousness and behavior. Lactulose or other medications may be given to counteract this effect, and dietary modification may also be helpful. In some cases, a TIPS may have to have the flow reduced or closed completely to reverse the encephalopathy. This is done by deploying a smaller stent or occluding device inside the original TIPS. This is a delicate decision for the health care provider to make, because reduction of flow through the shunt will likely cause the initial esophageal hemorrhaging to recur.

Patients receiving TIPS can also have significant elevation of their pulmonary artery pressure. This is a result of the sudden increase of blood flow to the right heart. Diuretics may help to treat this problem. For this reason, patients must be carefully evaluated for right heart failure before TIPS placement.

Depending on the procedure done to control esophageal bleeding, patients usually have a nasogastric tube (NGT) inserted to detect any new bleeding episodes. They often receive packed red blood cells, fresh frozen plasma, dextran, albumin, and platelets through large-bore IV catheters. Monitor vital signs every hour and check coagulation studies, including prothrombin time (PT), partial thromboplastin time (PTT), platelet count, and international normalized ratio (INR).

Preventing or Managing Confusion

Planning: Expected Outcomes. The patient is expected to be free of acute or chronic confusion. However, if it occurs, it is expected that the interprofessional health care team will intervene early to maintain patient safety and prevent further health problems or death from encephalopathy.

Interventions. Collaborative interventions are planned around the management of slowing or stopping the accumulation of ammonia in the body to improve mental status and orientation. Assess the patient's neurologic status and monitor during treatment.

Because ammonia is formed in the GI tract by the action of bacteria on protein, nonsurgical treatment measures to decrease ammonia production include dietary limitations and drug therapy to reduce bacterial breakdown. Patients with cirrhosis have increased nutritional requirements—high-carbohydrate, moderate-fat, and high-protein foods. However, the diet may be changed for those who have elevated serum ammonia levels with signs of encephalopathy. Patients should have a moderate amount of protein and fat foods and simple carbohydrates. Strict protein restrictions are not required because patients need protein for healing. In collaboration with the registered dietitian nutritionist, be sure to include family members or significant others in **nutrition** counseling. The patient is often weak and unable to remember complicated guidelines. Brief, simple directions regarding dietary dos and don'ts are recommended. Keep in mind any financial, cultural, or personal implications and the patient's food allergies when discussing food choices to provide optimal patient-centered care.

Drugs are used sparingly because they are difficult for the failing liver to metabolize. In particular, opioid analgesics, sedatives, and barbiturates should be restricted, especially for the patient with a history of encephalopathy.

However, several types of drugs may eliminate or reduce ammonia levels in the body. These include lactulose or lactitol and nonabsorbable antibiotics. The primary health care provider may prescribe *lactulose* (or lactitol) to promote the excretion of ammonia in the stool. This drug is a viscous, sticky, sweet-tasting liquid that is given either orally or by NG tube. The purpose is to obtain a laxative effect. Cleansing the bowels may rid the intestinal tract of the toxins that contribute to encephalopathy. It works by increasing osmotic pressure to draw fluid into the colon and prevents absorption of ammonia in the colon. The drug may be prescribed to the patient who has manifested signs of encephalopathy, regardless of the stage (Burchum & Rosenthal, 2019). The desired effect of the drug is production of two or three soft stools per day and a decrease in patient confusion caused by this complication.

Observe for response to lactulose. The patient may report intestinal bloating and cramping. Serum ammonia levels may be monitored but do not always correlate with symptoms. Hypokalemia and dehydration may result from excessive stools. Remind assistive personnel to help the patient with skin care if needed to prevent breakdown caused by excessive stools.

Several *nonabsorbable antibiotics* may be given if lactulose does not help the patient meet the desired outcome or if he or she cannot tolerate the drug. These drugs should not be given together. Older adults can become weak and dehydrated from having multiple stools. Neomycin sulfate or rifaximin, both broad-spectrum antibiotics, may be given to act as intestinal antiseptics. These drugs destroy the normal flora in the bowel, diminishing protein breakdown and decreasing the rate of ammonia production. Maintenance doses of neomycin are given orally but may also be administered as a retention enema. Long-term use has the potential for kidney toxicity and therefore is not commonly used for an extended period of time. It cannot be used for patients with existing kidney disease (Burchum & Rosenthal, 2019).

Frequently assess for changes in level of consciousness and orientation. Check for **asterixis** and **fetor hepaticus**. These signs suggest worsening encephalopathy. Thiamine supplements and benzodiazepines may be needed if the patient is at risk for alcohol withdrawal.

Physiological Integrity

The nurse is caring for a client in end-stage liver failure. Which interventions should be implemented when observing for hepatic encephalopathy? **Select all that apply.**

A. Assess the client's neurologic status as prescribed.
B. Monitor the client's hemoglobin and hematocrit levels.
C. Monitor the client's serum ammonia level.
D. Monitor the client's electrolyte values daily.
E. Prepare to insert an esophageal balloon tamponade tube.
F. Make sure the client's fingernails are short.

Managing Pruritus

Planning: Expected Outcomes. The patient is expected to experience less discomfort from pruritus as a result of comfort measures and possibly drug therapy.

Interventions. Patients frequently report pruritus and dry skin as a result of jaundice from increased levels of serum bilirubin as cirrhosis progresses. Pruritus tends to increase in warmer conditions and in the early evening and at night. Therefore comfort measures include avoiding being too warm, moisturizing the skin, and avoiding irritants to the skin. Some patients find that cool compresses and/or corticosteroids creams provide temporary relief. If these measures are not effective, drug therapy, including selective serotonin reuptake inhibitors like sertraline, may be helpful.

Care Coordination and Transition Management.
If the patient with late-stage cirrhosis survives life-threatening complications, he or she is usually discharged to home or to a long-term care facility after treatment measures have managed the acute medical problems. A home care referral may be needed if the patient is discharged to home. These chronically ill patients are often readmitted multiple times, and community-based care is aimed at optimizing comfort, promoting independence, supporting caregivers, and preventing rehospitalization.

INTERPROFESSIONAL COLLABORATION
Care of Patients with Cirrhosis

For patients with moderate-to-late-stage liver disease, collaborate with the case manager (CM) or other discharge planner to coordinate interprofessional continuing care. According to the Interprofessional Education Collaborative (IPEC) Expert Panel's Competency of Roles and Responsibilities, using the unique and complementary abilities of other team members optimizes health and patient care (IPEC Expert Panel, 2016; Slusser et al., 2019). Collaborate with health care team members to help the client be as ADL independent as possible, including physical and occupational therapists. Patients with end-stage disease may benefit from hospice care.

Home Care Management. In collaboration with the patient, family, and case manager, assess physical adaptations needed to prepare the patient's home for recovery. His or her rest area needs to be close to a bathroom because diuretic and/or lactulose therapy increases the frequency of urination and stools. If the patient has difficulty reaching the toilet, additional equipment (e.g., bedside commode) is necessary. Special adult-size incontinence pads or briefs may be helpful if the patient has an altered mental status and incontinence. If the patient has shortness of breath from massive ascites, elevating the head of the bed and maintaining him or her in a semi-Fowler to high-Fowler position may help alleviate respiratory distress. Alternatively, a reclining chair with an elevated foot rest may be used.

Self-Management Education. The patient is discharged to the home setting with an individualized teaching plan that includes **nutrition** therapy, drug therapy, and alcohol abstinence. The patient who has a tunneled ascites drain will need to be taught how to access the drain and remove excess fluid. *Review the home care instructions that are provided with the drainage system with both the patient and family/caregiver. Remind them not to remove more than 2000 mL from the abdomen at one time to prevent hypovolemic shock.*

The patient with encephalopathy often finds that small, frequent meals are best tolerated. If his or her nutritional intake or albumin/prealbumin is decreased after discharge, multivitamin and oral nutritional supplements are usually needed. Teach patients to avoid excessive vitamins and minerals that can be toxic to the liver, such as fat-soluble vitamins, excessive iron supplements, and niacin. Remind patients to check with their primary health care provider before taking any vitamin supplement.

The patient is often discharged while receiving diuretics. Provide instructions regarding the primary health care provider's prescription for the diuretic. Teach about side effects of therapy, such as hypokalemia. The patient may need to take a potassium supplement if he or she is taking a diuretic that is not potassium sparing.

If the patient has had problems with bleeding from gastric ulcers, the primary health care provider may prescribe an H_2-receptor antagonist agent or proton pump inhibitor to reduce acid reflux (see Chapter 50). Patients who have had episodes of spontaneous bacterial peritonitis (SBP) may be on a daily low-dose maintenance antibiotic.

Teach family members how to recognize signs of encephalopathy and to contact the primary health care provider if these signs develop. Reinforce that constipation, bleeding, and **infection** can increase the risk for encephalopathy.

Advise the patient to avoid all over-the-counter drugs, especially NSAIDs and hepatic toxic herbs, vitamins, and minerals. Reinforce the need to keep appointments for follow-up medical care. Remind the patient and family to notify the primary health care provider immediately if any GI bleeding (overt bleeding or melena) is noted so that re-evaluation can begin quickly.

! NURSING SAFETY PRIORITY (QSEN)
Action Alert

One of the most important aspects of ongoing care for the patient with cirrhosis is health teaching about the need for the client to avoid acetaminophen, alcohol, smoking, and illicit drugs. By avoiding these substances, the patient may:
- Prevent further fibrosis of the liver from scarring
- Allow the liver to heal and regenerate
- Prevent gastric and esophageal irritation
- Reduce the incidence of bleeding
- Prevent other life-threatening complications

Health Care Resources. The patient with chronic cirrhosis may require a home care nurse for several visits after hospital discharge. The home care nurse can monitor the effectiveness of treatment in controlling ascites. The encephalopathic patient may need to be monitored for adherence to drug therapy and alcohol abstinence, if appropriate. Individual and group therapy sessions may be arranged to help patients deal with alcohol abstinence if they are too ill to attend a formal treatment program. Because some patients may have alienated relatives over the years because of substance use, it may be necessary to help them identify a friend, neighbor, or adult in their recovery group for support. If needed, refer the patient and family to self-help groups, such as Alcoholics Anonymous and Al-Anon. In Canada, SMART Recovery offers similar support, as well as additional services to control addictions.

The patient with cirrhosis may also desire spiritual or other psychosocial support. Finances are frequently a problem for the chronically ill patient and family; social support and community services need to be identified. The American Liver Foundation (www.liverfoundation.org) and American Gastroenterological Association (www.gastro.org) are excellent sources for more information about liver disease.

For patients who are not candidates for liver transplantation, address end-of-life issues. Discuss options such as hospice care with patients and their families (see Chapter 8). Be aware that they will go through a grieving process and will perhaps be in denial or very angry.

◆ **Evaluation: Evaluate Outcomes.** Evaluate the care of the patient with cirrhosis based on the identified priority patient problems. The expected outcomes include that the patient will:
- Have a decrease in or have no ascites
- Achieve *fluid and electrolyte balance*
- Not have hemorrhage or will be managed immediately if bleeding occurs
- Not develop encephalopathy or will be managed immediately if it occurs
- Successfully abstain from alcohol or drugs (if disease is caused by one or more of these substances) and have adequate *nutrition*

✳ INFECTION CONCEPT EXEMPLAR: HEPATITIS

Pathophysiology Review

Hepatitis is the widespread *inflammation* and *infection* of liver cells. *Viral* hepatitis, which can be acute or chronic, is the most common type. Less common types of hepatitis are caused by chemicals, drugs, and some herbs. This section discusses hepatitis caused by a virus. Viral hepatitis results from an infection caused by one of five categories of viruses:
- Hepatitis A virus (HAV)
- Hepatitis B virus (HBV)
- Hepatitis C virus (HCV)
- Hepatitis D virus (HDV)
- Hepatitis E virus (HEV)

Some cases of viral hepatitis are not caused by any of these viruses. These patients have non–A-E hepatitis. This section focuses on the most common viral types.

Liver injury with *inflammation* can develop after exposure to a number of drugs and chemicals by inhalation, ingestion, or parenteral (IV) administration. *Toxic and drug-induced hepatitis* can result from exposure to hepatotoxins (e.g., industrial toxins, alcohol, and drugs). Hepatitis may also occur as a secondary *infection* during the course of infections with other viruses, such as Epstein-Barr, herpes simplex, varicella-zoster, and cytomegalovirus.

After the liver has been exposed to any causative agent (e.g., a virus), it becomes enlarged and congested with inflammatory cells, lymphocytes, and fluid, resulting in right upper quadrant pain and discomfort. As the disease progresses, the liver's normal lobular pattern becomes distorted as *cellular regulation* is compromised as a result of widespread *inflammation,* necrosis, and hepatocellular regeneration. This distortion increases pressure within the portal circulation, interfering with the blood flow into the hepatic lobules. Edema of the liver's bile channels results in obstructive jaundice.

Etiology. The five major types of acute viral hepatitis vary by etiology, mode of transmission, manner of onset, and incubation periods. Hepatitis cases must be reported to the local public health department, which then notifies the Centers for Disease Control and Prevention (CDC).

Hepatitis A. The causative agent of hepatitis A, hepatitis A virus (HAV), is a ribonucleic acid (RNA) virus of the enterovirus family. *It is a hardy virus and survives on human hands.* The virus is resistant to detergents and acids but is destroyed by chlorine (bleach) and extremely high temperatures.

Hepatitis A usually has a mild course similar to that of a typical flulike infection and often goes unrecognized. It is spread most often by the fecal-oral route by fecal contamination either from person-to-person contact (e.g., oral-anal sexual activity) or by consuming contaminated food or water. Common sources of *infection* include shellfish caught in contaminated water and food contaminated by food handlers infected with HAV. The incubation period of hepatitis A is usually 15 to 50 days, with a peak of 25 to 30 days. The disease is usually not life threatening, but its course may be more severe in adults older than 40 years and those with pre-existing liver disease such as hepatitis C (McCance et al., 2019).

In a small percentage of hepatitis A cases, severe illness with extrahepatic signs and symptoms can occur. Advanced age and conditions such as chronic liver disease may cause widespread damage that requires a liver transplant. In some cases when the patient's immunity is decreased, death may occur. The incidence of hepatitis A is particularly high in nonaffluent countries in which sanitation is poor; however, cases are diagnosed internationally across the globe (World Health Organization, 2017). Some adults have hepatitis A and do not know it. The course is similar to that of a GI illness, and the disease and recovery are usually uneventful.

Hepatitis B. The hepatitis B virus (HBV) is not transmitted like HAV. It is a double-shelled particle containing DNA composed of a core antigen (HBcAg), a surface antigen (HBsAg), and another antigen found within the core (HBeAg) that circulates in the blood. HBV may be spread through these common modes of transmission (CDC, 2020a):

- Unprotected sexual intercourse with an infected partner
- Sharing needles, syringes, or other drug-injection equipment
- Sharing razors or toothbrushes with an infected individual
- Accidental needlesticks or injuries from sharp instruments primarily in health care workers (low incidence)
- Blood transfusions (that have not been screened for the virus, before 1992)
- Hemodialysis
- Direct contact with the blood or open sores of an infected individual
- Birth (spread from an infected mother to baby during birth)

In addition, patients whose immunity is compromised by either disease or drug therapy are more likely to develop hepatitis B. The clinical course of hepatitis B may be varied. Symptoms usually occur within 25 to 180 days of exposure.

Blood tests confirm the disease, although many individuals with hepatitis B have no symptoms. Most adults who get hepatitis B recover and clear the virus from their body and develop immunity. However, a small percentage of people do not develop immunity and become carriers. Hepatitis carriers can infect others even though they are not sick and have no obvious signs of hepatitis B. Chronic carriers are at high risk for cirrhosis and liver cancer. Because of the high number of newcomers from endemic areas, the incidence of hepatitis B has increased in the United States.

Hepatitis C. Hepatitis C (HCV) is the leading cause of end-stage liver disease in the world (Chaney, 2019). The causative virus of hepatitis C is an enveloped, single-stranded RNA virus, which is genetically unstable and has at least six known major genotypes. Transmission is blood to blood. The rate of sexual transmission is very low in a single-couple relationship but increases with multiple sex partners or in men who have unprotected sex with men. HCV is spread most commonly by (Chaney, 2019):

- Illicit IV drug needle sharing (highest incidence)
- Blood, blood products, or organ transplants received before 1992
- Baby boomers (those adults born between 1945 and 1965)

- Needlestick injury with HCV-contaminated blood (health care workers at high risk)
- Hemodialysis
- Health care workers
- People who are incarcerated (prisoners)
- Sharing of drug paraphernalia

The disease is *not* transmitted by casual contact or intimate household contact. However, those infected are advised not to share razors, toothbrushes, or pierced earrings because microscopic blood may be on these items.

The incubation period ranges from 2 weeks to 6 months. Acute infection and illness are not common. Most people are completely unaware that they have been infected. They may be asymptomatic and not diagnosed until many months or years after the initial exposure when an abnormality is detected during a routine laboratory evaluation or when liver problems occur. Unlike with hepatitis B, most people infected with hepatitis C do not clear the virus, and a chronic infection develops.

HCV usually does its damage to the body's immunity over decades by causing a chronic **inflammation** in the liver that eventually causes the liver cells to scar. Scarring from chronic **infection** with either HBV and HCV frequently leads to cirrhosis, which is a risk factor for developing primary liver cancer (McCance et al., 2019). Patients who develop liver cancer may have interventional radiologic procedures (such as transarterial chemoembolization [TACE]), cryotherapy, ablation, traditional chemotherapy, or selective radiation therapy (SIRT) (see Chapter 20 for more information on cancer management modalities and associated nursing care). Liver cancer can also occur as a metastatic disease process and is not associated with hepatitis or cirrhosis.

Hepatitis D. Hepatitis D (delta hepatitis) is caused by a defective RNA virus that needs the helper function of HBV. It occurs only with HBV to cause viral replication. This usually develops into chronic disease. The incubation period is about 14 to 56 days. As with hepatitis B, the disease is transmitted primarily by parenteral routes, especially in patients who are IV drug users. Having sexual contact with someone with HDV is also a high-risk factor (McCance et al., 2019).

Hepatitis E. The hepatitis E virus (HEV) causes a waterborne infection associated with epidemics in the Indian subcontinent, Asia, Africa, the Middle East, Mexico, and Central and South America. Many large outbreaks have occurred after heavy rains and flooding. Like hepatitis A, hepatitis E is caused by fecal contamination of food and water.

In the United States, hepatitis E has been found only in international travelers. It is transmitted via the fecal-oral route, and the clinical course resembles that of hepatitis A. Hepatitis E has an incubation period of 15 to 64 days. There is no evidence at this time of a chronic form of the disease. The disease tends to be self-limiting and resolves on its own (McCance et al., 2019).

Complications of Hepatitis. Failure of the liver cells to regenerate, with progression of the necrotic process, results in a severe acute and often fatal form of hepatitis known as *fulminant hepatitis.* Hepatitis is considered to be chronic when liver *inflammation* lasts longer than 6 months. *Chronic hepatitis* usually occurs as a result of hepatitis B or hepatitis C. Superimposed infection with hepatitis D virus (HDV) in patients with chronic hepatitis B may also result in chronic hepatitis. Chronic hepatitis can lead to cirrhosis and liver cancer. Many patients have multiple infections, especially a combination of HBV with HCV, HDV, or HIV infections (McCance et al., 2019).

Incidence and Prevalence. The incidence of hepatitis A and hepatitis B is declining as a result of CDC recommendations for vaccination. However, hepatitis B and hepatitis C are a concern because of their association with cirrhosis and liver cancer. Although exact numbers are not known, it is estimated that over 170 million people worldwide have the hepatitis C virus (HCV) with 3 to 4 million new cases occurring every year. It is the most common chronic bloodborne infection in the United States (Chaney, 2019; Horsley-Silva & Vargas, 2017). Most hepatitis A (HAV) infections in the United States today occur in patients who have drug abuse or those who are homeless (Heavey, 2020).

Currently there is no vaccine for HCV; however, patients may be treated with antiviral drug therapies. The desired outcome of treatment of HCV-infected patients is to reduce mortality and liver-related health adverse consequences, including end-stage liver disease and liver cancer. It is expected that the cases of HCV may rise over the next several decades as a result of increasing illicit drug use.

Health Promotion and Maintenance. Hepatitis vaccines for infants, children, and adolescents have helped to decrease the incidence of hepatitis A and hepatitis B. Teach adults the importance of obtaining immunizations for their children. These vaccines are safe and not associated with major complications. Some adults are also advised to receive these immunizations.

Measures for preventing hepatitis A in adults include:
- Proper handwashing, especially after handling shellfish
- Avoiding contaminated food or water (including tap water in countries with high incidence)
- Receiving immunoglobulin within 14 days if exposed to the virus
- Receiving the HAV vaccine before traveling to areas where the disease is common (e.g., Mexico, Caribbean)
- Receiving the vaccine if living or working in enclosed areas with others, such as college dormitories, correctional institutions, day-care centers, and long-term care facilities

Several HAV vaccines are made of inactivated hepatitis A virus and are given in the deltoid muscle. Several vaccines can also provide protection against hepatitis B virus (HBV) infection. A combination HAV and HBV vaccine is also available for adults. Examples of groups for whom immunization against HBV should be used include:
- People who have sexual intercourse with more than one partner
- People with sexually transmitted infection (STI) or a history of STI
- Men having unprotected sex with men (MSM)

BEST PRACTICE FOR PATIENT SAFETY & QUALITY CARE (QSEN)

Prevention of Viral Hepatitis in Health Care Workers

- Use Standard Precautions to prevent the transmission of disease between patients or between patients and health care staff (see Chapter 21).
- Eliminate needles and other sharp instruments by substituting needleless systems. (Needlesticks are the major source of hepatitis B transmission in health care workers.)
- Take the hepatitis B vaccine, which is given in a series of three injections. This vaccine also prevents hepatitis D by preventing hepatitis B.
- For postexposure prevention of hepatitis A, seek medical attention immediately for immunoglobulin (Ig) administration.
- Report all cases of hepatitis to the local health department.

- People with any chronic liver disease (such as hepatitis C or cirrhosis)
- Patients with human immune deficiency virus (HIV) infection
- People who are exposed to blood or body fluids in the workplace, including health care workers, firefighters, and police
- People in correctional facilities (prisoners)
- Patients needing immunosuppressant drugs
- Family members, household members, and sexual contacts of people with HBV infection

Multiple HCV genotypes have made it difficult to develop an effective vaccine against hepatitis C. Teach baby boomer adults to have a one-time screening test for HCV due to the high risk of this infection in this population (Chaney, 2019).

Additional measures to prevent viral hepatitis for health care workers and others in contact with infected patients are listed in the Best Practice for Patient Safety & Quality Care: Prevention of Viral Hepatitis in Health Care Workers box.

❖ Interprofessional Collaborative Care

Care for the patient with hepatitis can take place in various settings. These patients may, at different times, self-manage at home, be hospitalized for immediate concerns, or be cared for in the community setting.

◆ Assessment: Recognize Cues

History. Begin by asking the patient whether or not he or she has had known exposure to a person with hepatitis. For the patient who presents with few or no symptoms of liver disease but has abnormal laboratory tests (e.g., elevated alanine aminotransferase [ALT] or aspartate aminotransferase [AST] level), the history may need to include additional questions regarding risk factors.

Physical Assessment/Signs and Symptoms. Assess whether the patient has any of the signs and symptoms associated with most types of vital hepatitis as listed in the Key Features: Viral Hepatitis box. Although HCV may be asymptomatic for most adults, some patients with a new HCV *infection* can experience some of these signs and symptoms.

⟫ KEY FEATURES
Viral Hepatitis

- Abdominal pain
- Yellowish sclera (**icterus**)
- Arthralgia (joint pain) or myalgia (muscle pain)
- Diarrhea/constipation
- Light clay-colored stools
- Dark yellow to brownish urine
- **Jaundice**
- Fever
- Fatigue
- Malaise
- Anorexia
- Nausea and vomiting
- Dry skin
- Pruritus (itching)

Lightly palpate the right upper abdominal quadrant to assess for liver tenderness. The patient may report right upper quadrant pain with jarring movements. Inspect the skin, sclerae, and mucous membranes for **jaundice**. He or she may present for medical treatment only after jaundice appears, believing that other vague symptoms are related to a flulike syndrome.

Jaundice in hepatitis results from intrahepatic obstruction and is caused by edema of the liver's bile channels. Dark urine and clay-colored stools are often reported by the patient. If possible, obtain a urine and stool specimen for visual inspection and laboratory analysis. The patient may also have skin abrasions from scratching because of pruritus (itching).

Patients with chronic HCV infection often have extrahepatic complications. Examples include:

- Depression
- Polyarthritis
- Myalgia
- Renal insufficiency
- Cognitive impairment
- Cardiovascular problems such as vasculitis and heart disease

Psychosocial Assessment. Viral hepatitis has various presentations, but for most infected people the initial course is mild with few or no symptoms. The long-term complications of fibrosis and cirrhosis cause the more serious problem. This is especially true for patients who have chronic HBV and HCV infection.

Emotional problems for affected patients may center on their feeling sick and fatigued. General malaise, inactivity, and vague symptoms contribute to depression. Some patients often feel guilty and are remorseful about decisions made that caused the disease. These feelings are most likely to occur when the source of infection is from drug use.

Infectious diseases such as hepatitis continue to have a social stigma. (See the Evidence-Based Practice box.) The patient may feel embarrassed by the precautions that are imposed in the hospital and continue to be necessary at home. This embarrassment may cause the patient to limit social interactions. Patients may be afraid that they will spread the virus to family and friends.

EVIDENCE-BASED PRACTICE (QSEN)
Caring for Military Veterans With Hepatitis C

Phillips, F., & Barnes, D. (2016). Social support and adherence for military veterans with hepatitis C. *Clinical Nurse Specialist, 30*(1), 38–44.

This qualitative study's aim was to describe military veterans' experience of support after diagnosis of hepatitis C and how support impacted their adherence to treatment.

A convenience sample of 21 veterans was used for this phenomenological study. Inclusion criteria were composed of veterans who were older than 18 years of age; were receiving standard care for hepatitis C; and could read, write, and communicate in English. In keeping with a phenomenological design, researchers collected data during a one-time, in-depth interview with each participant. Follow-up phone calls were used to verify that the themes identified were congruent with the lived experience of subjects.

Results indicated that veterans selectively tell only certain individuals about their diagnosis due to fear of stigma. In turn, this limits the amount of people in their circle of support. Veterans found some level of support, yet some level of burden, when disclosing their status to family members, friends, and health care providers.

Level of Evidence: 3
This qualitative research was designed as a phenomenological study.

Commentary: Implications for Practice and Research
Nurses must use empathy and concern while assessing availability of support systems for patients. In absence of a personal support network, or in addition to an existing support system, nurses should recommend support groups or counseling to help the patient adhere to treatment and management of hepatitis C.

Family members are sometimes afraid of getting the disease and may distance themselves from the patient. Allow them to verbalize these feelings and explore the reasons for these fears. Educate the patient and family members about modes of transmission, and clarify information as needed.

Patients may be unable to return to work for several weeks during the acute phases of illness. The loss of wages and the cost of hospitalization for a patient without insurance coverage may produce great anxiety and financial burden. This situation may last for months or years if hepatitis becomes chronic.

Laboratory Assessment. Hepatitis A, hepatitis B, and hepatitis C are usually confirmed by acute elevations in levels of liver enzymes, indicating liver cellular damage, and by specific serologic markers.

Levels of ALT and AST may possibly rise into the thousands in acute or fulminant cases of hepatitis. Alkaline phosphatase levels may be normal or elevated. Serum total bilirubin levels are elevated and are consistent with the clinical appearance of jaundice.

The presence of *hepatitis A* is established when hepatitis A virus (HAV) antibodies (anti-HAV) are found in the blood. Ongoing **inflammation** of the liver by HAV is indicated by the presence of immunoglobulin M (IgM) antibodies, which persist in the blood for 4 to 6 weeks. Previous infection is identified by the presence of immunoglobulin G (IgG) antibodies. These antibodies persist in the serum and provide permanent immunity to HAV (Pagana & Pagana, 2018).

The presence of the *hepatitis B* virus (HBV) is established when serologic testing confirms the presence of hepatitis B antigen-antibody systems in the blood and a detectable viral count (HBV polymerase chain reaction [PCR] DNA). Antigens located on the surface (shell) of the virus (HBsAg) and IgM antibodies to hepatitis B core antigen (anti-HBcAg IgM) are the most significant serologic markers. The presence of these markers establishes the diagnosis of hepatitis B. *The patient is infectious as long as hepatitis B surface antigen (HBsAg) is present in the blood.* Persistence of this serologic marker after 6 months or longer indicates a carrier state or chronic hepatitis. HBsAg levels normally decline and disappear after the acute hepatitis B episode. The presence of antibodies to HBsAg in the blood indicates recovery and immunity to hepatitis B. *People who have been vaccinated against HBV have a positive HBsAg because they also have immunity to the disease (Pagana & Pagana, 2018).*

To detect HCV infection, blood is tested for anti-HCV antibodies to HCV recombinant core antigen, *NS3 gene*, NS4 antigen, and NS5 antibody. The antibodies can be detected within 4 weeks of the infection (Pagana & Pagana, 2018). To identify the actual circulating virus, the HCV RNA test is used. This confirms active virus and can measure the viral load. A diagnostic tool called the *OraQuick HCV Rapid Antibody Test* has the advantage of providing a quick diagnosis of the disease as a point-of-care test.

The presence of *hepatitis D* virus (HDV) can be confirmed by the identification of intrahepatic delta antigen or, more often, by a rise in the hepatitis D virus antibodies (anti-HDV) titer. This increase can be seen within a few days of **infection** (Pagana & Pagana, 2018).

Hepatitis E virus (HEV) testing is usually reserved for travelers in whom hepatitis is present but the virus cannot be detected. Hepatitis E antibodies (anti-HEV) are found in people infected with the virus.

Other Diagnostic Assessment. *Liver biopsy* may be used to confirm the diagnosis of hepatitis and establish the stage and grade of liver damage or cancer. Characteristic changes help the pathologist distinguish among a virus, drug, toxin, fatty liver, iron, and other disease. It is usually performed in an ambulatory care setting as a percutaneous procedure (through the skin) after a local anesthetic is given. However, if coagulation is abnormal, it may be done using either a CT-guided or transjugular route to reduce the risk for pneumothorax or hemothorax. *Ultrasound* also may be used.

◆ **Analysis: Analyze Cues and Prioritize Hypotheses.** The priority collaborative problems for patients with hepatitis include:
1. Weight loss due to complications associated with **inflammation** of the liver
2. Fatigue due to **infection** and decreased metabolic energy production

◆ **Planning and Implementation: Generate Solutions and Take Action.** The patient with viral hepatitis can be mildly or acutely ill, depending on the severity of the **inflammation** and **infection**. Most patients are not hospitalized, although older adults and those with dehydration may be admitted

for a short-term stay. The plan of care for all patients with viral hepatitis is based on measures to rest the liver, promote hepatic regeneration, strengthen immunity, and prevent complications, if possible.

Promoting Nutrition
Planning: Expected Outcomes. The patient will maintain appropriate weight and **nutrition** status.

Interventions. The patient with hepatitis, especially hepatitis A, may decline food because of general malaise, anorexia, abdominal discomfort, or nausea. The patient's diet should be high in carbohydrates and calories with moderate amounts of fat and protein added after nausea and anorexia subside. Small, frequent meals are often preferable to three standard meals daily. Ask the patient about appealing food preferences because favorite foods are tolerated better than randomly selected foods. High-calorie snacks may be needed. Supplemental vitamins are often prescribed.

Managing Fatigue
Planning: Expected Outcomes. The patient will progressively exhibit increasing energy as evidenced by participation in ADLs and self-reported decrease in level of fatigue.

Interventions. During the acute stage of viral hepatitis, interventions are aimed at resting the inflamed liver to promote hepatic cell regeneration. *Rest* is an essential intervention to reduce the liver's metabolic demands and increase its blood supply. Collaborative care is generally supportive. The patient is usually tired and expresses feelings of general malaise. Complete bedrest is usually not required, but rest periods alternating with periods of activity are indicated and are often enough to promote hepatic healing. Individualize the patient's plan of care and change it as needed to reflect the severity of symptoms, fatigue, and results of liver function tests and enzyme determinations. Activities such as self-care and ambulating are gradually added to the activity schedule as tolerated.

Drugs of any kind are used sparingly for patients with hepatitis to allow the liver to rest. An antiemetic to relieve nausea may be prescribed. However, because of the life-threatening nature of chronic hepatitis B and hepatitis C, a number of drugs are given, including antiviral and immunomodulating drugs.

Two groups of drugs are approved for management of Hepatitis B—*interferon alfa preparations* and *nucleoside analogs*. Examples of interferon alfa drugs include interferon alfa-2b and Peginterferon alfa-2a. These drugs are not used as often today because newer, more effective medications are available. Examples of nucleoside analogs include lamivudine and adefovir (see the Common Examples of Drug Therapy: Chronic Hepatitis B and Hepatitis C box).

For a number of years, the standard of care for hepatitis C was pegylated (PEG) interferon alfa plus ribavirin (Burchum & Rosenthal, 2019). In the past decade, new direct-acting antiviral (DAA) drugs that target specific steps in HCV replication have been used with much more success and fewer side or adverse effects. In 2011, the U.S. Food and Drug Administration approved the first two first-generation *protease inhibitors (PIs)*. These drugs have been taken off the market in favor of better second-generation PIs (Chaney, 2019). The current standard of

COMMON EXAMPLES OF DRUG THERAPY

Chronic Hepatitis B and Hepatitis C

Drug	Nursing Implications
Chronic Hepatitis B	
Tenofovir	Monitor kidney function. *Drug is excreted through kidneys; monitoring for renal impairment is important.*
	Teach risk for falls to prevent fractures. *Can cause bone demineralization.*
Adefovir	Monitor kidney function. *Drug is excreted through kidneys; monitoring for renal impairment is important.*
Lamivudine	Monitor kidney function. *Drug is excreted through kidneys; monitoring for renal impairment is important.*
	Remind patient to not discontinue drug without consulting with primary health care provider. *Discontinuation of drug can cause flareup of HBV.*
Entecavir	Monitor kidney function. Teach the patient to avoid alcohol to prevent serious interaction. *Drug is excreted through kidneys; monitoring for renal impairment is important.*
Chronic Hepatitis C	
Second-generation protease inhibitors:	Monitor CBC and chemistry panel.
• Grazoprevir	Instruct the patient on common reactions, such as rash, itching, nausea, and headache.
• Simprevir	*Kidney and liver function may become impaired, and electrolyte imbalances may occur when taking this drug.*
• Paritaprevir	
NS5A inhibitors:	
• Elbasvir (also available in combination with grazoprevir)	Ask the patient if he or she has a history of or current hepatitis B. *The combination drug can reactivate hepatitis B and cause liver failure.*
	Teach patients that their liver enzymes must be monitored, especially ALT elevation. *The combination drug can cause liver toxicity, including an increase in liver enzymes.*
• Ledipasvir/Sofosbuvir (for hepatitis C genotype 1 only)	Ask if the patient has had any other type of hepatitis or cirrhosis. *This combination drug can reactivate hepatitis B and cause liver failure.*
	Do not give this drug to patients receiving amiodarone. *If this drug combination is taken with amiodarone, the patient may experience severe symptomatic bradycardia and other cardiac problems, including chest pain.*
NS5A-NS5B polymerase inhibitor:	
• Sofosbuvir/velpatasvir (for almost all main types of hepatitis C)	Ask the patient if he or she has a history of or current hepatitis B. *The combination drug can reactivate hepatitis B and cause liver failure.*
	Teach patients that their liver enzymes must be monitored, especially ALT elevation.

HBV, Hepatitis B virus; *HIV,* human immune deficiency virus.

practice for hepatitis C treatment is that a patient's drug regimen is determined by HCV viral genotype (AASLD, 2018). Examples of newer single and combination PIs are presented in the Common Examples of Drug Therapy: Chronic Hepatitis B and Hepatitis C box. All of these drugs can affect the immune system and make patients susceptible to *infection. Teach patients to avoid crowds and people who are infected!*

Similar to patients with other chronic diseases, patients with hepatitis often use complementary and integrative therapies to promote general well-being and improve quality of life. Examples include herbs and vitamin supplements including silymarin (milk thistle plant), green tea, and vitamin E. The effectiveness of these substances has not been well researched.

Care Coordination and Transition Management. Home care management varies according to the type of hepatitis and whether the disease is acute or chronic. A primary focus in any case is preventing the spread of the infection. For hepatitis transmitted by the fecal-oral route, careful handwashing and sanitary disposal of feces are important. Therefore education is very important.

! NURSING SAFETY PRIORITY (QSEN)

Action Alert

Teach the patient with viral hepatitis and the family to use measures to prevent infection transmission. In addition, instruct the patient to avoid alcohol and check with the primary health care provider before taking any medication or vitamin, supplement, or herbal preparation.

Encourage the patient to increase activity gradually to prevent fatigue. Suggest that the patient eat small, frequent meals of high-carbohydrate foods and plan frequent rest periods.

Collaborate with the certified infection control practitioner and infectious disease specialist if needed in caring for these patients. These experts can suggest appropriate resources for the patient and family.

◆ **Evaluation: Evaluate Outcomes.** Evaluate the care of the patient with hepatitis based on the identified priority patient problems. The expected outcomes include that the patient will:
• Maintain adequate *nutrition* for body requirements
• Report increasing energy levels as the liver rests
• Achieve appropriate management of *infection* and *inflammation*

? CLINICAL JUDGMENT CHALLENGE 53.1

Patient-Centered Care; Safety

A 19-year-old woman presents at the college health clinic 3 weeks after a spring break trip to Las Vegas. She tells the nurse that the highlight of the trip was an "all-you-can-eat" seafood buffet. Since that time, she reports that she has been experiencing periodic fevers, abdominal pain, loss of appetite, nausea, vomiting, and fatigue. At first, she states that she thought she had the flu, but she now thinks that something else "must be terribly wrong" because her eyes and skin are turning yellow. She confirms that she is a nonsmoker and only drinks one to two alcoholic drinks per month.

1. **Recognize Cues:** What assessment information in this client situation is the most important and immediate concern for the nurse? (Hint: Identify the **relevant** information *first* to determine what is most important.)
2. **Analyze Cues:** What client conditions are consistent with the **most relevant** information? (Hint: Think about priority collaborative problems that support and contradict the information presented in this situation.)
3. **Prioritize Hypotheses:** Which possibilities or explanations are **most likely** to be present in this client situation? Which possibilities or explanations are the most serious? (Hint: Consider all possibilities and determine their urgency and risk for this client.)
4. **Generate Solutions:** What actions would most likely achieve the desired outcomes for this client? Which actions should be **avoided** or are **potentially harmful**? (Hint: Determine the desired outcomes first to decide which interventions are appropriate and those that should be avoided.)
5. **Take Action:** Which actions are the most appropriate and how should they be implemented? In what **priority order** should they be implemented? (Hint: Consider health teaching, documentation, requested health care providsser orders or prescriptions, nursing skills, collaboration with or referral to health team members, etc.)
6. **Evaluate Outcomes:** What client assessment would indicate that the nurse's actions were **effective**? (Hint: Think about signs that would indicate an improvement, decline, or unchanged client condition.)

LIVER TRANSPLANTATION

Pathophysiology Review

Liver transplantation has become a common procedure worldwide. The patient with end-stage liver disease or acute liver failure who has not responded to conventional medical or surgical intervention is a potential candidate for liver transplantation. Many diseases can cause liver failure. Cirrhosis (scarring of the liver) is the most common reason for liver transplants. Other common reasons are chronic hepatitis B and hepatitis C, bile duct diseases, autoimmune liver disease, alcoholic liver disease, and fatty liver disease.

Transplantation Considerations. The patient for potential transplantation has extensive physiologic and psychological assessment and evaluation by primary health care providers and transplant coordinators. Alternative treatment should be extensively explored before committing a patient for a liver transplant. Patients who are *not* considered candidates for transplantation are those with:

• Severe cardiovascular instability with advanced cardiac disease
• Severe respiratory disease
• Metastatic tumors
• Inability to follow instructions regarding drug therapy and self-management

Liver transplantation has become the most effective treatment for an increasing number of patients with acute and chronic liver diseases. Inclusion and exclusion criteria vary among transplantation centers and are continually revised as treatment options change and surgical techniques improve.

Donor livers are obtained primarily from trauma victims who have not had liver damage. They are distributed through a nationwide program, the United Network of Organ Sharing (UNOS). This system distributes donor livers based on regional considerations and patient acuity. Candidates with the highest level of acuity receive highest priority.

The donor liver is transported to the surgery center in a solution that preserves the organ for up to 8 hours. The diseased liver is removed through an incision made in the upper abdomen. The new liver is carefully put in its place and attached to the patient's blood vessels and bile ducts. The procedure can take many hours to complete and requires a highly specialized team and large volumes of fluid and blood replacement.

Living donors have also been used and are usually close family members or a spouse. This is done on a voluntary basis after careful psychological and physiologic preparation and testing. The donor's liver is resected (usually removal of one lobe) and implanted into the recipient after removal of the diseased liver. In both the donor and the recipient, the liver regenerates and grows in size to meet the demands of the body.

Transplantation Complications. Although liver transplantations are commonly performed, complications can occur. Some problems can be managed medically, whereas others require hospitalizations or removal of the transplant. The most common complications are acute graft rejection, infection, and bleeding (Lynn, 2016; McCance et al., 2019).

The success rate for transplantations has greatly improved since the introduction many years ago of cyclosporine (cyclosporin A), an immunosuppressant drug. Today, many other antirejection drugs are used. (See Chapter 18 for a discussion of rejection and preventive drug therapy for organ transplantation.)

! NURSING SAFETY PRIORITY QSEN

Action Alert

For the patient who has undergone liver transplantation, monitor for clinical signs and symptoms of rejection, which may include tachycardia, fever, *pain* in the right upper quadrant or flank, decreased bile pigment and volume, and increasing jaundice. Laboratory findings include elevated serum bilirubin, rising ALT and AST levels, elevated alkaline phosphatase levels, and increased prothrombin time/international normalized ratio (PT/INR) (Pagana & Pagana, 2018).

Transplant rejection is treated aggressively with immunosuppressive drugs. As with all rejection treatments, the patient is at a greater risk for infection. If therapy is not effective, liver function rapidly deteriorates. Multisystem organ failure, including respiratory and renal involvement, develops along with diffuse coagulopathies and portal-systemic encephalopathy (PSE). The only alternative for treatment is emergency retransplantation.

Infection is another potential threat to the transplanted graft and the patient's survival. Vaccinations and prophylactic antibiotics are helpful in prevention. Immunosuppressant therapy, which must be used to prevent and treat organ rejection, significantly increases the patient's risk for infection. Other risk factors include the presence of multiple tubes and intravascular lines, immobility, and prolonged anesthesia.

In the early posttransplantation period, common infections include pneumonia, wound infections, and urinary tract infections. Opportunistic *infections* usually develop after the first postoperative month and include cytomegalovirus, mycobacterial infections, and parasitic infections. Latent infections such as tuberculosis and herpes simplex may be reactivated. Women, Hispanics, and patients with less than a high school education are most likely to be readmitted with transplant complications, although the cause is not known (Dols et al., 2020).

The primary health care provider prescribes broad-spectrum antibiotics for prophylaxis during and after surgery. Obtain culture specimens from all lines and tubes and collect specimens for culture at predetermined time intervals as dictated by the agency's policy. If an *infection* is detected, the primary health care provider prescribes organism-specific anti-infective agents. The patient should be taught to contact the primary health care provider at any time that signs of *infection* are present.

The biliary anastomosis is susceptible to breakdown, obstruction, and infection. If leakage occurs or if the site becomes necrotic or obstructed, an abscess can form; or peritonitis, bacteremia, and cirrhosis may develop. Observe for potential complications, which are listed in Table 53.4.

> **! NURSING SAFETY PRIORITY** (QSEN)
> **Action Alert**
>
> For the patient who has had a liver transplantation, monitor the temperature frequently per hospital protocol and report elevations, increased abdominal pain, distention, and rigidity, which are indicators of peritonitis. Nursing assessment also includes monitoring for a change in neurologic status that could indicate encephalopathy from a nonfunctioning liver. Report signs of clotting problems (e.g., bloody oozing from a catheter, petechiae, ecchymosis) to the surgeon immediately because they may indicate impaired function of the transplanted liver.

❖ Interprofessional Collaborative Care

Care of the patient undergoing liver transplantation requires an interprofessional team approach. Receiving a transplant has a major psychosocial impact. Transplant complications cause patients to be very anxious. In collaboration with the members of the interprofessional health care team, assure them and their families that these problems are common and usually treated successfully.

After the patient is identified as a candidate and a donor organ is procured, the actual liver transplantation surgical procedure usually takes many hours. The length of the procedure can vary greatly.

In the immediate postoperative period, the patient is managed in the critical care unit and requires aggressive monitoring and

TABLE 53.4 Assessment and Prevention of Common Postoperative Complications Associated With Liver Transplantation

Assessment	Prevention
Acute Graft Rejection	
Occurs from the 4th to 10th postoperative day	Prophylaxis with immunosuppressant agents, such as cyclosporine
Manifested by tachycardia, fever, right upper quadrant (RUQ) or flank pain, diminished bile drainage or change in bile color, or increased jaundice	Early diagnosis to treat with more potent antirejection drugs
Laboratory changes: (1) increased levels of serum bilirubin, transaminases, and alkaline phosphatase; (2) prolonged prothrombin time	
Infection	
Can occur at any time during recovery	Antibiotic prophylaxis; vaccinations
Manifested by fever or excessive, foul-smelling drainage (urine, wound, or bile); other indicators depend on location and type of infection	Frequent cultures of tubes, lines, and drainage
	Early removal of invasive lines
	Good handwashing
	Early diagnosis and treatment with organism-specific anti-infective agents
Hepatic Complications (Bile Leakage, Abscess Formation, Hepatic Thrombosis)	
Manifested by decreased bile drainage, increased RUQ abdominal pain with distention and guarding, nausea or vomiting, increased jaundice, and clay-colored stools	If present, keep T-tube in dependent position and secure to patient; empty frequently, recording quality and quantity of drainage
Laboratory changes: increased levels of serum bilirubin and transaminases	Report signs and symptoms to surgeon immediately
	May need surgical intervention
Acute Kidney Injury	
Caused by hypotension, antibiotics, cyclosporine, acute liver failure, or hypothermia	Monitor all drug levels with nephrotoxic side effects
Indicators of hypothermia: shivering, hyperventilation, increased cardiac output, vasoconstriction, and alkalemia	Prevent hypotension
Early indicators of acute kidney injury: changes in urine output, increased blood urea nitrogen (BUN) and creatinine levels, and electrolyte imbalance	Observe for early signs of acute kidney injury and report them immediately to the surgeon

care. Monitor for signs and symptoms of complications of surgery and immediately report them to the surgeon (see Table 53.4).

Post–liver transplant patients are living longer today than ever. Teach patients to be aware of side effects of immunosuppressive drugs, such as hypertension, nephrotoxicity, drug-induced *infection,* and gastrointestinal disturbances. Remind them that long-term management of care includes surveillance for malignancy, metabolic syndrome, and diabetes. Teaching the patient self-examination for skin, breast, and testicular malignancies and reminders for annual Papanicolaou (Pap) smears and other cancer screening tests are important. Posttransplant patients need to maintain lifestyle changes to increase their longevity after surgery.

GET READY FOR THE NEXT-GENERATION NCLEX® EXAMINATION!

Key Points

Review these Key Points for each NCLEX Examination Client Needs Category.

Safe and Effective Care Environment

- Refer patients with liver disorders to the American Liver Foundation; refer dying patients to hospice and other community resources as needed. **QSEN: Patient-Centered Care**

Health Promotion and Maintenance

- Teach patients to take precautions to prevent viral hepatitis in the community. **QSEN: Evidence-Based Practice**
- Teach patients to avoid alcohol and illicit drugs to prevent or slow the progression of alcohol-induced cirrhosis; remind them not to take any medication (including over-the-counter drugs) without checking with their primary health care provider. **QSEN: Safety**

Psychosocial Integrity

- Recognize that patients with cirrhosis have mental and emotional changes (including confusion) due to hepatic encephalopathy. **QSEN: Patient-Centered Care**
- Be aware that patients with cirrhosis and/or chronic hepatitis may feel guilty about their disease because of past habits such as drug and alcohol use. Allow patients to express feelings openly. **Ethics**
- Be aware that patients having liver transplantation have major concerns about the possibility of complications, such as organ rejection. **QSEN: Patient-Centered Care**

Physiological Integrity

- Be aware that cirrhosis has many causes other than alcohol use.
- Observe for clinical signs and symptoms of hepatic encephalopathy (PSE) as listed in Table 53.2. **QSEN: Safety**
- Monitor laboratory values of patients suspected of or diagnosed with cirrhosis of the liver as listed in Table 53.3. **Clinical Judgment**
- Monitor the patient with cirrhosis for bleeding and neurologic changes. **QSEN: Safety**
- Administer drug therapy to decrease ammonia levels (that cause PSE) in patients with cirrhosis, such as lactulose and nonabsorbable antibiotics. **QSEN: Safety**
- Differentiate the five major types of hepatitis: A, B, C, D, and E. Hepatitis D occurs only with hepatitis B and is transmitted most commonly by blood and body fluid exposure. Hepatitis A is transmitted via the fecal-oral route. Hepatitis C is the most common type and is also transmitted via blood and body fluids. **QSEN: Evidence-Based Practice**
- Be aware that patients with chronic viral hepatitis often develop cirrhosis and cancer of the liver. **QSEN: Evidence-Based Practice**
- Recognize that potent immunomodulators and antivirals are given to treat hepatitis B and hepatitis C; teach patients on immunomodulators to avoid large crowds and people who have infections. **QSEN: Safety**
- Monitor the patient having a liver transplantation for complications, such as those described in Table 53.4. **QSEN: Safety**
- Report and document elevated temperature, increased abdominal pain and rigidity, bleeding, and/or neurologic status changes as possible indicators of liver transplantation complications. **QSEN: Safety**

MASTERY QUESTIONS

1. A client is receiving adefovir for management of hepatitis B. What health teaching will the nurse provide for the client about this drug? **Select all that apply.**
   A. "Avoid places with crowds and individuals who have infection."
   B. "Report increased bruising to your doctor because the drug can cause bleeding."
   C. "Get your lab work done regularly because the drug can affect your kidneys."
   D. "Be careful and avoid falls because the drug can cause fractures."
   E. "Follow up with the dietitian to ensure that you adhere to your special diet."

2. The nurse is caring for a patient with cirrhosis who has hepatic encephalopathy. Which assessment finding should the nurse report to the primary health care provider?
   A. Fatigue
   B. Difficulty sleeping
   C. Seizure
   D. Disorientation

REFERENCES

American Association for the Study of Liver Diseases (AASLD). (2018). *Recommendations for testing, managing and treating hepatitis C.* http://hcvguidelines.org/sites/default/files/HCV-Guidance_February_2016_a1.pdf.

American Liver Foundation. (2020a). *Non-alcoholic fatty liver disease.* http://www.liverfoundation.org/abouttheliver/info/nafld/.

American Liver Foundation. (2020b). *Hepatitis C.* http://hepc.liver-foundation.org/.

Burchum, J. L. R., & Rosenthal, L. D. (2019). *Lehne's pharmacology for nursing care* (10th ed.). St. Louis: Elsevier.

Centers for Disease Control and Prevention (CDC). (2020a). *Hepatitis B FAQs for the public.* http://www.cdc.gov/hepatitis/hbv/bfaq.htm#bFAQ10.

Centers for Disease Control and Prevention (CDC). (2020b). *Liver cancer.* https://www.cdc.gov/cancer/liver/index.htm.

Chaney, A. (2019). Caring for patients with chronic hepatitis C infection. *Nursing 2019, 49*(3), 36–42.

Digestive Health Association, C. (2020). *Statistics.* http://www.cdhf.ca/en/statistics#19.

Dols, J. D., Mendoza, A., Pomerleau, T., Purcell, C. V., Gonzalez, M., et al. (2020). Causation and risk factors for 30-day readmission of patients post-liver transplant: A descriptive study. *MEDSURG Nursing, 29*(1), 27–33.

Halter, M. J. (2018). *Varcarolis' foundations of psychiatric-mental health nursing* (8th ed.). St. Louis: Elsevier.

Heavey, E. (2020). Hepatitis A takes hold in the community. *Nursing 2020, 50*(7), 24–28.

Horsley-Silva, J. L., & Vargas, H. E. (2017). New therapies for hepatitis C virus infection. *Gastroenterology and Hepatology, 13*(3), 22–31.

Immunization Action Coalition. (2020). *Hepatitis B information for Asian Americans and Pacific Islanders.* http://www.immunize.org/catg.d/p4190.pdf.

Interprofessional Education Collaborative Expert Panel. (2016). *Core competencies for interprofessional collaborative practice: Report of an expert panel* (2nd ed.). Washington, D.C: Interprofessional Education Collaborative.

Lynn, S. (2016). How to help patients with liver failure. *American Nurse Today, 11*(9), 26–29.

McCance, K., Huether, S., Brashers, V., & Rote, N. (2019). *Pathophysiology: The biologic basis for disease in adults and children* (8th ed.). St. Louis: Mosby.

Pagana, K. D., & Pagana, T. J. (2018). *Manual of diagnostic and laboratory tests* (6th ed.). St. Louis: Mosby.

Pezzotti, W. (2020). Understanding acute upper gastrointestinal bleeding in adults. *Nursing2020, 50*(5), 25–29.

Saab, S., Manne, V., Neito, J., Schwimmer, J. B., & Chalasani, N. P. (2016). Perspectives in clinical gastroenterology and hepatology: Nonalcoholic fatty liver disease in Latinos. *Clinical Gastroenterology and Hepatology, 14*, 5–12.

Slusser, M. M., Garcia, L. I., Reed, C.-R., & McGinnis, P. Q. (2019). *Foundations of interprofessional collaborative practice in health care.* St. Louis: Elsevier.

Vacca, V.M. (2020). Nonalcoholic fatty liver disease: What nurses need to know. *Nursing 2020, 50*(3), 32–39.

World Health Organization. (2017). *Global hepatitis report 2017.* http://apps.who.int/iris/bitstream/10665/255016/1/9789241565455-eng.pdf?ua=1.

54

Concepts of Care for Patients With Problems of the Biliary System and Pancreas

Lara Carver, Jennifer Powers

http://evolve.elsevier.com/Iggy/

LEARNING OUTCOMES

1. Collaborate with the interprofessional team to manage quality care for patients with biliary and pancreatic problems caused by *inflammation.*
2. Identify community resources for families and patients recovering from biliary and pancreatic problems.
3. Apply knowledge of pathophysiology of liver problems to identify common assessment findings, including actual or risk for impaired *nutrition* and *pain*.
4. Prioritize nursing and collaborative care for patients with common gallbladder or pancreatic disorders.
5. Plan transition management and care coordination for the patient who has a biliary or pancreatic problem, including health teaching.

KEY TERMS

acute pancreatitis A serious, and at times life-threatening, *inflammation* of the pancreas.

biliary colic Severe right upper abdominal pain caused by obstruction of the cystic duct or movement of one or more gallstones.

cholecystectomy The surgical removal of the gallbladder.

cholecystitis An *inflammation* of the gallbladder that may be acute or chronic.

cholelithiasis Gallstones (also known as *calculi*).

chronic pancreatitis A progressive, destructive disease of the pancreas that has remissions and exacerbations ("flare-ups").

dyspepsia An epigastric burning sensation, often referred to as "heartburn."

eructation Belching.

flatulence Gas (flatus) in the lower GI tract.

icterus Yellow coloration of the eye sclera.

jaundice Yellow coloration of the skin and mucous membranes.

pancreatic abscess Suppuration (pus formation) of pancreatic tissue caused by secondary bacterial invasion; often occurs in patients with acute or chronic pancreatitis.

pancreatic pseudocyst A condition in which infected pancreatic fluid becomes walled off by fibrous tissue.

partial pancreatectomy Surgical removal of part of the pancreas.

postcholecystectomy syndrome (PCS) A complication of cholecystectomy that causes increased abdominal or epigastric *pain* and vomiting and/or diarrhea weeks to months after surgery.

splenectomy Surgical removal of the spleen.

steatorrhea Fatty stools.

Whipple procedure (radical pancreaticoduodenectomy) Extensive surgical procedure used most often to treat cancer of the head of the pancreas; entails removal of the proximal head of the pancreas, the duodenum, a portion of the jejunum, the stomach (partial or total gastrectomy), and the gallbladder, with anastomosis of the pancreatic duct (pancreaticojejunostomy), the common bile duct (choledochojejunostomy), and the stomach (gastrojejunostomy) to the jejunum.

The liver, gallbladder, and pancreas make up the biliary system. This chapter focuses on common problems of the gallbladder and pancreas. Liver disorders are described in Chapter 53. The biliary system secretes enzymes and other substances that promote food digestion in the stomach and small intestine. When these organs do not work properly, adults may experience impaired *digestion*, which can result in inadequate **nutrition**.

Disorders of the gallbladder and pancreas may extend to other organs because of the close anatomic location of these organs, if the primary health problem is not treated early. *Inflammation* and obstruction (blockage) can occur in the biliary system from gallstones, edema, stricture, or tumors. These problems frequently cause the patient to have moderate-to-severe acute or persistent abdominal **pain**. These concepts are briefly reviewed in Chapter 3.

✴ INFLAMMATION CONCEPT EXEMPLAR: CHOLECYSTITIS

Pathophysiology Review

Cholecystitis is an *inflammation* of the gallbladder that affects many adults, very commonly in affluent countries. It may be either acute or chronic, although most patients have the acute type. The inflammatory process often affects the client's **nutrition** status.

Acute Cholecystitis. Two types of acute cholecystitis can occur: calculous and acalculous cholecystitis. The most common type is calculous cholecystitis, in which chemical irritation and inflammation result from gallstones, or calculi (cholelithiasis), that obstruct the cystic duct (most often), gallbladder neck, or common bile duct (choledocholithiasis) (Fig. 54.1). When the gallbladder is inflamed, trapped bile is reabsorbed and acts as a chemical irritant to the gallbladder wall. Reabsorbed bile, in combination with impaired circulation, edema, and distention of the gallbladder, causes ischemia and infection. The result is tissue sloughing with necrosis and gangrene within the gallbladder itself. The gallbladder wall may eventually perforate (rupture). If the perforation is small and localized, an abscess may form. Peritonitis (infection of the peritoneum) may result if the perforation is large.

The exact mechanism of gallstone formation is not clearly understood, but abnormal metabolism of cholesterol and bile salts plays an important role. The gallbladder provides an excellent environment for the production of stones because it only occasionally mixes its normally abundant mucus with its highly viscous, concentrated bile. Impaired gallbladder motility can

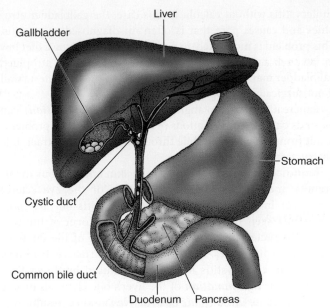

FIG. 54.1 Gallstones within the gallbladder and obstructing the common bile and cystic ducts.

lead to stone formation by delaying bile emptying and causing biliary stasis.

Gallstones are composed of substances normally found in bile, such as cholesterol, bilirubin, bile salts, calcium, and various proteins. They are classified as either cholesterol stones or pigment stones. Cholesterol calculi form as a result of metabolic imbalances of cholesterol and bile salts. They are the most common type found in adults in the United States (McCance et al., 2019).

Bacteria can collect around the stones in the biliary system. Severe bacterial invasion can lead to life-threatening *suppurative* cholangitis when symptoms are not recognized quickly and pus accumulates in the ductal system.

Acalculous cholecystitis (*inflammation* occurring without gallstones) is typically associated with biliary stasis caused by any condition that affects the regular filling or emptying of the gallbladder. For example, a decrease in blood flow to the gallbladder or anatomic problems such as twisting or kinking of the gallbladder neck or cystic duct can result in pancreatic enzyme reflux into the gallbladder, causing *inflammation*. Sphincter of Oddi dysfunction (SOD) can also occur to cause reflux and inflammation. Most cases of this type of cholecystitis occur in patients with:
- Sepsis
- Severe trauma or burns
- Long-term total parenteral **nutrition** (TPN)
- Multiple organ dysfunction syndrome (MODS)
- Major abdominal surgery
- Hypovolemia

Chronic Cholecystitis. Chronic cholecystitis most often results when repeated episodes of cystic duct obstruction cause chronic inflammation. Calculi are almost always present. The gallbladder becomes fibrotic and atrophied, which results in decreased motility and deficient absorption. Young thin women, especially those who are athletic (e.g., gymnasts), may experience chronic cholecystitis without calculi. In this case, the gallbladder atrophies and causes pain that is often misdiagnosed as gastritis. This problem is most likely to occur when consuming a diet low in fat, such as a vegetarian diet. In some cases, the atrophied gallbladder may adhere to nearby organs or the mesenteric wall if not surgically removed.

Pancreatitis and cholangitis (bile duct *inflammation*) can occur as chronic complications of cholecystitis. These problems result from the backup of bile throughout the biliary tract. Bile obstruction leads to jaundice.

Jaundice (yellow coloration of the skin and mucous membranes) and icterus (yellow coloration of the eye sclera) can occur in patients with acute cholecystitis but are most commonly seen in those with the *chronic* form of the disease. Obstructed bile flow caused by edema of the ducts or gallstones contributes to *extrahepatic* obstructive jaundice. Jaundice in cholecystitis may also be caused by direct liver involvement. *Inflammation* of the liver's bile channels or bile ducts may cause *intrahepatic* obstructive jaundice, resulting in an increase in circulating levels of bilirubin, the major pigment of bile.

In an adult with obstructive jaundice, the normal flow of bile into the duodenum is blocked, and excessive bile salts accumulate in the skin. This accumulation of bile salts leads to pruritus (itching) or a burning sensation. The bile flow blockage also prevents bilirubin from reaching the large intestine, where it is converted to urobilinogen. Because urobilinogen accounts for the normal brown color of feces, clay-colored stools result. Water-soluble bilirubin is normally excreted by the kidneys in the urine. When an excess of circulating bilirubin occurs, the urine becomes dark because of the kidneys' effort to clear the bilirubin.

Etiology and Genetic Risk. A familial or genetic tendency appears to contribute to the development of cholelithiasis, but this may be partially related to familial *nutrition* habits (excessive dietary cholesterol intake) and sedentary lifestyles. Gene-environment interactions may contribute to gallstone production. For example, some gene variations program some people to make and secrete more cholesterol into bile, leading to the increase in cholesterol-containing gallstones. The highest frequency of gallstone production occurs among the American Indian and Mexican-American populations (McCance et al., 2019). Other risk factors for cholecystitis are listed in Table 54.1.

PATIENT-CENTERED CARE: GENDER HEALTH CONSIDERATIONS (QSEN)

Obesity is a major risk factor for gallstone formation, especially in women. Pregnancy and drugs such as hormone replacements and birth control pills alter hormone levels and delay muscular contraction of the gallbladder, decreasing the rate of bile emptying. The incidence is higher in women who have had multiple pregnancies. Therefore some clinicians continue to refer to the patient *most* at risk for acute cholecystitis and gallstones by the four *F*s: *F*emale, *F*orty, *F*at, and *F*ertile. However, cholecystitis often occurs in younger and older women and in those who are thin.

TABLE 54.1 Risk Factors for Cholecystitis

- Women of all ages (risk of calculi increases with aging)
- American Indian, Mexican American, or Caucasian
- Obesity
- Rapid weight loss or prolonged fasting; low-fat diet
- Increased serum cholesterol and lipids
- Women on hormone replacement therapy (HRT)
- Cholesterol-lowering drugs
- Family history of gallstones
- Prolonged total parenteral nutrition
- Crohn's disease
- Gastric bypass surgery
- Sickle cell disease
- Glucose intolerance/diabetes mellitus type 2
- Pregnancy
- Genetic factors

Incidence and Prevalence. Cholecystitis and cholelithiasis most often occur in affluent countries throughout the world. The incidence is 60% to 70% in American Indians and 15% in Caucasian adults (McCance et al., 2019).

❖ Interprofessional Collaborative Care

Care of the patient with cholecystitis primarily takes place by self-management at home, in the community, or within the same-day surgical center or hospital if surgery is required.

◆ Assessment: Recognize Cues

History. Obtain the patient's height, weight, and vital signs; or ask that these activities be performed by assistive personnel (AP) with appropriate supervision. Ask about food preferences and determine whether excessive fat and cholesterol are part of the diet. Typically, diets high in fat, high in calories, low in fiber, and high in refined white carbohydrates place patients at high risk for developing gallstones. Consuming low-fat diets can contribute to chronic cholecystitis in young thin women.

Inquire if intake of certain foods causes pain. Question whether any GI symptoms occur when fatty food is eaten, such as flatulence (gas [flatus]in the lower GI tract), dyspepsia (an epigastric burning sensation, often referred to as "heartburn"), indigestion, eructation (belching), anorexia, nausea, vomiting, and abdominal *pain.*

Ask patients to describe their daily activity or exercise routines to determine whether they are sedentary, a risk factor for developing gallstones. Question whether there is a family history of gallbladder disease. Ask the patient about taking current or previous hormone replacement therapy (HRT). If the patient is female, ask if she is taking or has recently been on oral contraceptives (birth control pills).

Physical Assessment/Signs and Symptoms. Patients with cholecystitis have abdominal *pain*, although symptoms vary in intensity and frequency. Ask the patient to describe the pain, including its intensity and duration, precipitating factors, and any measures that relieve it. Pain may be described as indigestion of varying intensity, ranging from a mild, persistent ache to a steady, constant pain in the right upper abdominal quadrant. It may radiate to the right shoulder or scapula. In some cases the abdominal *pain* of chronic cholecystitis may be vague and nonspecific. The usual pattern is episodic. Patients often refer to acute pain episodes as "gallbladder attacks."

PATIENT-CENTERED CARE: OLDER ADULT CONSIDERATIONS (QSEN)

Older adults and patients with diabetes mellitus may have atypical symptoms of cholecystitis, including the absence of *pain* and fever. Localized tenderness may be the only presenting sign. The older patient may become acutely confused (delirium) as the first symptom of gallbladder disease.

! **NURSING SAFETY PRIORITY** (QSEN)

Critical Rescue

The severe pain of **biliary colic** is produced by obstruction of the cystic duct of the gallbladder or movement of one or more gallstones. When a stone is moving through or is lodged within the duct, tissue spasm occurs in an effort to get the stone through the small duct. Biliary colic may be so severe that it occurs with tachycardia, pallor, diaphoresis, and prostration (extreme exhaustion). Assess the patient for possible shock caused by biliary colic. *Notify the health care provider or Rapid Response Team if these symptoms occur.* Stay with the patient and keep the head of the bed flat if shock occurs.

Advanced physical assessment for rebound tenderness (Blumberg sign) and deep palpation is performed only by a primary health care provider (Jarvis, 2020). To elicit rebound tenderness, the primary health care provider pushes his or her fingers deeply and steadily into the patient's abdomen and then quickly releases the pressure. Pain that results from the rebound of the palpated tissue may indicate peritoneal *inflammation.* Deep palpation below the liver border in the right upper quadrant may reveal a sausage-shaped mass, representing the distended, inflamed gallbladder. Percussion over the posterior rib cage worsens localized abdominal *pain.*

In *chronic* cholecystitis, patients may have slowly developing symptoms and may not seek medical treatment until late symptoms such as **jaundice**, clay-colored stools, and dark urine occur from biliary obstruction. **Icterus** may also be present. **Steatorrhea** (fatty stools) occurs because fat absorption is decreased as a result of the lack of bile. Bile is needed for the absorption of fats and fat-soluble vitamins in the intestine. As with any inflammatory process, the patient may have an elevated temperature of 99°F to 102°F (37.2°C to 38.9°C), tachycardia, and dehydration from fever and vomiting. He or she often will decline food intake because of the resulting *pain* or other

▶ **KEY FEATURES**

Cholecystitis

- Episodic or vague upper abdominal *pain* or discomfort that can radiate to the right shoulder
- Pain triggered by a high-fat or high-volume meal
- Anorexia
- Nausea and/or vomiting
- **Dyspepsia**
- **Eructation**
- **Flatulence**
- Feeling of abdominal fullness
- Rebound tenderness (Blumberg sign)
- Fever
- Jaundice, clay-colored stools, dark urine
- **Steatorrhea** (most common with chronic cholecystitis)

 PATIENT-CENTERED CARE: OLDER ADULT CONSIDERATIONS (QSEN)

Older adults become dehydrated much more quickly than other age-groups, and they may not present with a fever. Monitor for a new onset of disorientation or acute confusion due to decreased blood volume available to oxygenate the cells of the brain (hypoxia).

symptoms that may occur. The Key Features: Cholecystitis box lists the most common signs and symptoms of cholecystitis.

Laboratory Assessment. A differential diagnosis rules out other diseases that may cause similar symptoms, such as peptic ulcer disease, hepatitis, and pancreatitis. An increased *white blood cell (WBC)* count indicates **inflammation**. Serum levels of *alkaline phosphatase, aspartate aminotransferase (AST),* and *lactate dehydrogenase (LDH)* may be elevated, indicating abnormalities in liver function in patients with severe biliary obstruction. The direct (conjugated) and indirect (unconjugated) *serum bilirubin levels* are also elevated. If the pancreas is involved, serum amylase and lipase levels are elevated.

Other Diagnostic Assessment. Calcified gallstones are easily viewed on abdominal x-ray. Stones that are not calcified cannot be seen. *Ultrasonography (US) of the right upper quadrant is the best initial diagnostic test for cholecystitis.* It is safe, accurate, and painless. Acute cholecystitis is seen as edema of the gallbladder wall and pericholecystic fluid.

A hepatobiliary scan (sometimes called a *hepatobiliary iminodiacetic acid [HIDA] scan*) can be performed to visualize the gallbladder and determine patency of the biliary system. In this nuclear medicine test, a radioactive tracer or chemical is injected IV. About 20 minutes after the injection, a gamma camera tracks the flow of the tracer from the gallbladder to determine the ejection rate of bile into the biliary duct. A decreased bile flow indicates gallbladder disease with obstruction. Teach patients having this test to have nothing by mouth before the procedure. Remind the patient that the camera is large and close to the body for most of the procedure.

When the cause of cholecystitis or cholelithiasis is not known or the patient has symptoms of biliary obstruction (e.g., jaundice), an *endoscopic retrograde cholangiopancreatography (ERCP)* may be performed. Some patients have the less invasive and safer *magnetic resonance cholangiopancreatography (MRCP),* which can be performed by an interventional radiologist. For this procedure, the patient is given oral or IV contrast material (gadolinium) before having an MRI scan. Before the test, ask the patient about any history of urticaria (hives) or other allergy. MRI is also contraindicated in patients with a pacemaker or other incompatible devices. Gadolinium does not contain iodine, which decreases the risk for an allergic response. Chapter 48 discusses these tests in more detail.

◆ **Analysis: Analyze Cues and Prioritize Hypotheses.** The priority collaborative problems for patients with cholecystitis include:

1. Acute or persistent *pain* due to gallbladder *inflammation* and/or gallstones
2. Weight loss due to decreased intake because of pain, nausea, and anorexia

◆ **Planning and Implementation: Generate Solutions and Take Action.** If cholecystitis and its associated pain cannot be managed medically, a laparoscopic cholecystectomy is the treatment of choice for patients with acute or long-term chronic cholecystitis. *Nutrition* status and *pain* control must be addressed before and after surgery.

Managing Acute Pain

Planning: Expected Outcomes. The patient with cholecystitis is expected to report a decrease in abdominal *pain* as evidenced by self-report of a level of 2 or 3 level on a 0 to10 pain intensity scale.

Interventions. The priorities for patient care include providing supportive care by relieving symptoms and decreasing *inflammation*. *Pain* assessment to measure the effectiveness of these interventions is an essential part of nursing care.

NCLEX Examination Challenge 54.1
Physiologic Integrity

A young adult client admitted with a diagnosis of cholecystitis from cholelithiasis has severe abdominal pain, nausea, and vomiting. Based on these assessment findings, which client problem is the **highest priority** for nursing intervention at this time?

A. Anxiety
B. Risk for dehydration
C. Acute pain
D. Malnutrition

Nonsurgical Management. Many patients with acute cholecystitis, with or without gallstones, have no symptoms. Acute *pain* usually occurs when gallstones partially or totally obstruct the cystic or common bile duct. Most patients find that they need to avoid fatty foods to prevent further episodes of biliary colic. Withhold food and fluids if nausea and vomiting occur. IV therapy is used to prevent dehydration. Persistent pain may occur in patients with chronic cholecystitis without gallstones, and may be misdiagnosed as gastritis.

Acute biliary pain requires opioid analgesia, such as morphine or hydromorphone (Dilaudid). All opioids may cause some degree of sphincter of Oddi spasm.

Ketorolac, a potent NSAID, may be used for mild-to-moderate *pain*. Be sure to monitor the patient for increased pain, tachycardia, and hypotension because the drug can cause GI bleeding. The primary health care provider prescribes antiemetics to control nausea and vomiting. IV antibiotic therapy may also be given, depending on the cause of cholecystitis or as a one-time dose for surgery.

An option for a small number of patients with cholelithiasis (gallstones) is the use of oral bile acid dissolution or gallstone-stabilizing agents. Drugs such as ursodiol and chenodiol may be given as long-term therapy to dissolve or stabilize gallstones (Burchum & Rosenthal, 2019). A gallbladder ultrasound is required every 6 months for the first year of therapy to determine the effectiveness of the drug. Teach patients on this type of drug therapy to report diarrhea, vomiting, or severe abdominal pain, especially if it radiates to the shoulders, to their primary health care provider immediately. Remind them to take the medication with food and milk.

For some patients with small stones or for those who are not good surgical candidates, a treatment that is commonly used for kidney stones can be used to break up gallstones—*extracorporeal shock wave lithotripsy (ESWL)*. This procedure can be used only for patients who have a normal weight, cholesterol-based stones, and good gallbladder function. The patient lies on a water-filled pad, and shock waves break up the large stones into smaller ones that can be passed through the digestive system. During the procedure, the patient might have *pain* resulting from the movement of the stones or duct or gallbladder spasms. A therapeutic bile acid, such as ursodeoxycholic acid (UDCA), may be used after the procedure to help dissolve the remaining stone fragments.

Another treatment option for patients who cannot have surgery is the insertion of a *percutaneous transhepatic biliary catheter* (drain) using CT or ultrasound guidance to open the blocked duct(s) so bile can flow (cholecystostomy). Catheters can be placed several ways, depending on the condition of the biliary ducts, in an internal, external, or internal/external drain. Biliary catheters usually divert bile from the liver into the duodenum to bypass a stricture. When all of the bile enters the duodenum, it is called an *internal* drain. However, in some cases a patient has an *internal/external* drain in which part of the bile empties into a drainage bag. Patients who need this drain for an extended period may have the external drain capped. If jaundice or leakage around the catheter site occurs, teach the patient to reconnect the catheter to a drainage bag and have a follow-up cholangiogram injection done by an interventional radiologist. An *external*-only catheter is connected either temporarily or permanently to a drainage bag that should be *positioned lower than the catheter insertion site* to drain by gravity. A reduction in bile drainage indicates that the drain is no longer working.

Surgical Management. Cholecystectomy is the surgical removal of the gallbladder. One of two procedures is performed: the laparoscopic cholecystectomy or, in rare cases, the traditional open-approach cholecystectomy.

Laparoscopic cholecystectomy. Laparoscopic cholecystectomy, a minimally invasive surgery (MIS), is the "gold standard" and is performed far more often than the traditional open approach. The advantages of MIS when compared with the open approach include:

- Complications are not common.
- The death rate is very low.
- Bile duct injuries are rare.
- Patient recovery is quicker.
- Postoperative pain is less severe.

The laparoscopic procedure (often called a "lap chole") is commonly performed on an ambulatory care basis in a same-day surgery suite or agency. The surgeon explains the procedure, and the nurse answers questions and reinforces the instructions. Reinforce what to expect after surgery and review *pain* management, deep-breathing exercises, incisional care, and leg exercises to prevent deep vein thrombosis. There is no special preoperative preparation other than the routine preparation for surgery under general anesthesia described in Chapter 9.

During the surgery the surgeon makes a very small midline puncture at the umbilicus. Additional small incisions may be needed, although *single-incision laparoscopic cholecystectomy (SILC)* using a flexible endoscope is often done. The abdominal cavity is insufflated with 3 to 4 L of carbon dioxide. Gasless laparoscopic cholecystectomy using abdominal wall–lifting devices are used in some centers. This technique results in improved pulmonary and cardiac function. A trocar catheter is inserted, through which a laparoscope is introduced. The laparoscope is attached to a video camera, and the abdominal organs are viewed on a monitor. The gallbladder is dissected from the liver bed, and the cystic artery and duct are closed. The surgeon aspirates the bile and crushes any large stones, if present, and then extracts the gallbladder through the umbilical puncture site.

Removing the gallbladder with the laparoscopic technique reduces the risk for wound complications. Some patients have mild-to-severe discomfort from carbon dioxide retention in the abdomen, which may be felt throughout the thorax and shoulders.

> ### ⚠ NURSING SAFETY PRIORITY (QSEN)
> #### *Action Alert*
>
> After a laparoscopic cholecystectomy, assess the patient's oxygen saturation level using pulse oximetry frequently until the effects of the anesthesia have passed. Remind the patient to perform deep-breathing exercises every hour.

Other postoperative care for the patient after a laparoscopic procedure is similar to that for any patient having minimally invasive endoscopic surgery (see Chapter 9). Offer the patient food and water when he or she is fully awake, and monitor for the nausea and/or vomiting that often results from anesthesia. If needed, administer an antiemetic drug such as ondansetron hydrochloride either IV push or as a disintegrating tablet. Several drug doses may be needed. Maintain an IV line to administer fluids until nausea and vomiting subside. Be sure to have the head of the bed elevated in the same-day surgery unit to prevent aspiration from vomiting. After nausea subsides, assist the patient to the bathroom to void. Early ambulation also promotes absorption of the carbon dioxide, which can decrease postoperative discomfort.

Administer an oral or IV push opioid and anti-inflammatory drug as needed immediately after surgery. Continuous IV pain control is usually not required because there is only one or a few small incisions, which are covered with wound closure strips (e.g., Steri-Strips) and small adhesive bandages or are surgically glued. The glue or closure strips lose their adhesiveness in about a week to 10 days and can be removed or fall off as the incision heals.

The patient is usually discharged from the hospital or surgery center the same day, although older and obese patients may stay overnight. Provide postoperative teaching regarding *pain* management, incision care, and follow-up appointments. Teach the patient to use ice and oral opioids for incisional pain, if needed, for a few days. For abdominal or thoracic discomfort from carbon dioxide retention, many patients report that heat application is helpful. The patient is typically allowed to bathe or shower the day after surgery.

After laparoscopic surgery the patient can return to usual activities much sooner than those having an open cholecystectomy. Instruct the patient to rest for the first 24 hours and then begin to resume usual activities Most patients are able to resume usual activities within a week.

Some patients are able to return to their usual diet after surgery, whereas others must carefully avoid high-fat foods. A large intake of fatty foods may result in abdominal *pain* and diarrhea, which could result in a *mild* **postcholecystectomy syndrome (PCS)** (see later discussion of PCS in the Traditional Cholecystectomy section). Teach patients to introduce foods high in fat one at a time to determine which foods are best tolerated.

A newer minimally invasive surgical procedure is *natural orifice transluminal endoscopic surgery (NOTES)* for removal or repair of organs. Surgery can be performed on many body organs through the mouth, vagina, and rectum. For removal of the gallbladder, the vagina is used most often in women because it can be easily decontaminated with an antiseptic and allows easy access into the peritoneal cavity. The surgeon makes a small internal incision through the cul-de-sac of Douglas between the rectum and uterine wall to access the gallbladder. The main advantages of this procedure are the lack of visible incisions and minimal, if any, postoperative complications (Roberts & Kate, 2016).

> ### ❓ CLINICAL JUDGMENT CHALLENGE 54.1
> #### *Patient-Centered Care; Evidence-Based Practice*
>
> Today a 28-year-old woman had a scheduled laparoscopic cholecystectomy in the same-day surgical center as a result of ongoing pain intolerance to fatty foods, spices, and caffeine. Over the past few months, she has had multiple tests to rule out gastritis, peptic ulcer disease, and other GI disorders. She is currently completing graduate studies and has been on a vegetarian diet for 10 years. Her height is 5 feet 7 inches (1.7 m) and her current weight is 115 lb (52.16 kg). She has been on oral contraceptives since she turned 18 and has never been pregnant. Her immediate postoperative assessment reveals the following:
>
> - Temperature = 98°F (36.7°C)
> - Pulse = 88 beats/min
> - Respirations = 22 breaths/min
> - Blood pressure = 138/78 mm Hg
> - Pain level = 7/10 on a 0-to-10 pain intensity scale
> - Crying and states she is very nauseated
> - Drowsy but easily aroused
> - Wound closures intact
>
> 1. **Recognize Cues:** What assessment information in this client situation is the most important and immediate concern for the nurse? (Hint: Identify the **relevant** information *first* to determine what is most important.)
> 2. **Analyze Cues:** What client conditions are consistent with the **most relevant** information? (Hint: Think about priority collaborative problems that support and contradict the information presented in this situation.)
> 3. **Prioritize Hypotheses:** Which possibilities or explanations are **most likely** to be present in this client situation? Which possibilities or explanations are the most serious? (Hint: Consider all possibilities and determine their urgency and risk for this client.)
> 4. **Generate Solutions:** What actions would most likely achieve the desired outcomes for this client? Which actions should be **avoided** or are **potentially harmful**? (Hint: Determine the desired outcomes first to decide which interventions are appropriate and those that should be avoided.)
> 5. **Take Action:** Which actions are the most appropriate and how should they be implemented? In what **priority order** should they be implemented? (Hint: Consider health teaching, documentation, requested health care provider orders or prescriptions, nursing skills, collaboration with or referral to health team members, etc.)
> 6. **Evaluate Outcomes:** What client assessment would indicate that the nurse's actions were **effective**? (Hint: Think about signs that would indicate an improvement, decline, or unchanged client condition.)

Traditional cholecystectomy. Use of the open surgical approach (abdominal laparotomy) has greatly declined during the past several decades. The few patients who have this type of surgical approach usually have severe biliary obstruction, and the ducts need to be explored to ensure patency.

The nurse provides the usual preoperative care and teaching in the operating suite on the day of surgery (see Chapter 9). The surgeon removes the gallbladder through a right upper quadrant incision and explores the biliary ducts for the presence of stones or other cause of obstruction. The surgeon usually inserts a drainage tube such as a Jackson-Pratt (JP) drain. This tube is placed in the gallbladder bed to prevent fluid accumulation. The drainage is usually serosanguineous (serous fluid mixed with blood) and is stained with bile in the first 24 hours after surgery. A one-dose IV antibiotic may be given to prevent infection before or during surgery.

Nursing care for a patient who has had a traditional open cholecystectomy is similar to the care for any patient who has had abdominal surgery under general anesthesia as described in Chapter 9. Postoperative incisional *pain* after a traditional cholecystectomy is controlled with opioids, IV acetaminophen, and/or IV anti-inflammatory drug. Encourage the patient to use coughing and deep-breathing exercises when pain is controlled and the incision is splinted.

Antiemetics may be necessary for episodes of postoperative nausea and vomiting. Administer the antiemetic early, as prescribed, to prevent retching associated with vomiting and increased incisional *pain.*

Provide care for the incision and the surgical drain. The surgeon typically removes the surgical dressing and drain within 24 hours after surgery.

The patient is NPO until fully awake after surgery. Document his or her level of consciousness, vital signs, and pain level. Assess the surgical incision for signs of infection, such as excessive redness or purulent drainage. Report changes to the surgeon immediately. Begin ambulation as soon as possible to prevent deep vein thrombosis and promote peristalsis.

Advance the diet from clear liquids to solid foods as peristalsis returns. The patient usually resumes solid foods and is discharged to home 1 to 2 days after surgery, depending on any complications and the patient's general condition. In the early postoperative period, if bile flow is reduced, a low-fat diet may reduce discomfort and prevent nausea.

Promoting Nutrition

Planning: Expected Outcomes. The patient will not lose weight or will regain usual weight if indicated to meet metabolic needs.

Interventions. The patient with cholecystitis may decline food because of abdominal discomfort, nausea, and anorexia. The patient's diet should be high in fiber and low in fat. Teach patients to avoid gas-producing foods. Small, frequent meals are often preferable to three standard meals daily. Ask the patient about appealing food preferences because favorite foods are tolerated more readily than randomly selected foods. Teach the patient to weigh regularly to assess for stabilization of weight or report concerns associated with weight loss. If needed, monitor laboratory results such as blood urea nitrogen (BUN), prealbumin, albumin, and total protein and transferrin levels to assess ongoing *nutrition* status.

TABLE 54.2 Common Causes of Postcholecystectomy Syndrome	
Biliary	**Nonbiliary**
• Pseudocyst	• Coronary artery disease
• Common bile duct (CBD) leak	• Intercostal neuritis
• CBD or pancreatic duct stricture or obstruction	• Unexplained pain syndrome
• Sphincter of Oddi dysfunction	• Psychiatric or neurologic disorder
• Retained or new CBD gallstone	
• Pancreatic or liver mass	
• Primary sclerosing cholangitis	
• Diverticular compression	

Care Coordination and Transition Management. Some patients with cholecystitis may have mild-to-moderate discomfort that can be managed by nutrition intervention; others may require surgery and subsequent hospitalization. Home care preparation is individual, based on each patient's circumstances.

Education needs to be started as soon as a patient has an initial experience with cholecystitis and has appropriate pain relief. Assess the patient's and family's knowledge of the disease and provide teaching as needed. The desired outcomes for discharge planning and education are to avoid further episodes of cholecystitis.

For most patients, a special diet is not required. Advise them to eat nutritious meals and avoid excessive intake of fatty foods, especially fried food, butter, and "fast food." If the patient is obese, recommend a weight-reduction program.

Remind the patient to report repeated abdominal or epigastric pain with vomiting and/or diarrhea that may occur several weeks to months after surgery. These symptoms indicate possible **postcholecystectomy syndrome (PCS)**. There are multiple causes of PCS, some of which are related to the biliary system, and others are not. Common causes of PCS are listed in Table 54.2.

Management depends on the exact cause but usually involves the use of endoscopic retrograde cholangiopancreatography (ERCP) to find the cause of the problem and repair it. This procedure and related nursing care are described in Chapter 48. Collaborative care includes *pain* management, antibiotics, *nutrition* and hydration therapy (possibly short-term parenteral nutrition), and control of nausea and vomiting.

◆ **Evaluation: Evaluate Outcomes.** Evaluate the care of the patient with cholecystitis based on the identified priority patient problems. The expected outcomes include that the patient will:
- Report control of abdominal pain, as indicated by self-report and pain scale measurement
- Have adequate *nutrition* available to meet metabolic needs

✳ INFLAMMATION CONCEPT EXEMPLAR: ACUTE PANCREATITIS

Pathophysiology Review

Acute pancreatitis is a serious and at times life-threatening *inflammation* of the pancreas. This inflammatory process is caused by a premature activation of excessive pancreatic enzymes that destroy ductal tissue and pancreatic cells, resulting in autodigestion and fibrosis of the pancreas. The pathologic changes occur in different degrees. The severity of pancreatitis depends on the extent of *inflammation* and tissue damage. Pancreatitis can range from mild involvement evidenced by edema and inflammation to *necrotizing hemorrhagic pancreatitis (NHP)*. NHP is diffuse bleeding pancreatic tissue with fibrosis and tissue death.

The pancreas is unusual in that it functions as both an exocrine gland and an endocrine gland. The primary *endocrine* disorder is diabetes mellitus and is discussed in Chapter 59. The *exocrine* function of the pancreas is responsible for secreting enzymes that assist in the breakdown of starches, proteins, and fats. These enzymes are normally secreted in the inactive form and become activated once they enter the small intestine. Early activation (i.e., activation within the pancreas rather than the intestinal lumen) results in the inflammatory process of pancreatitis. Direct toxic injury to the pancreatic cells and the production and release of pancreatic enzymes (e.g., trypsin, lipase, elastase) result from the obstructive damage. After pancreatic duct obstruction, increased pressure may contribute to ductal rupture, allowing spillage of trypsin and other enzymes into the pancreatic parenchymal tissue. *Autodigestion* of the pancreas occurs as a result (Fig. 54.2). In *acute* pancreatitis, four major pathophysiologic processes occur: lipolysis, proteolysis, necrosis of blood vessels, and *inflammation*.

The hallmark of pancreatic necrosis is enzymatic fat necrosis of the endocrine and exocrine cells of the pancreas caused by the enzyme *lipase*. Fatty acids are released during this *lipolytic process* and combine with ionized calcium to form a soaplike

product. The initial rapid lowering of serum calcium levels is not readily compensated for by the parathyroid gland. Because the body needs ionized calcium and cannot use bound calcium, hypocalcemia occurs (McCance et al., 2019).

Proteolysis involves the splitting of proteins by hydrolysis of the peptide bonds, resulting in the formation of smaller polypeptides. Proteolytic activity may lead to thrombosis and gangrene of the pancreas. Pancreatic destruction may be localized and confined to one area or may involve the entire organ.

Elastase is activated by trypsin and causes elastic fibers of the blood vessels and ducts to dissolve. The *necrosis of blood vessels* results in bleeding, ranging from minor bleeding to massive hemorrhage of pancreatic tissue. Another pancreatic enzyme, kallikrein, causes the release of vasoactive peptides, bradykinin, and a plasma kinin known as kallidin. These substances contribute to vasodilation and increased vascular permeability, further compounding the hemorrhagic process. This massive destruction of blood vessels by necrosis may lead to generalized hemorrhage, with blood escaping into the retroperitoneal tissues. *Many deaths in patients with acute pancreatitis result from irreversible hypovolemic shock due to hemorrhage.*

The *inflammatory stage* occurs when leukocytes cluster around the hemorrhagic and necrotic areas of the pancreas. A secondary bacterial invasion may lead to suppuration (pus formation) of the pancreatic tissue called a **pancreatic abscess**. Pancreatic abscesses must be drained promptly to prevent sepsis. Mild infected lesions may be absorbed. When infected lesions are severe, calcification and fibrosis occur. If the infected

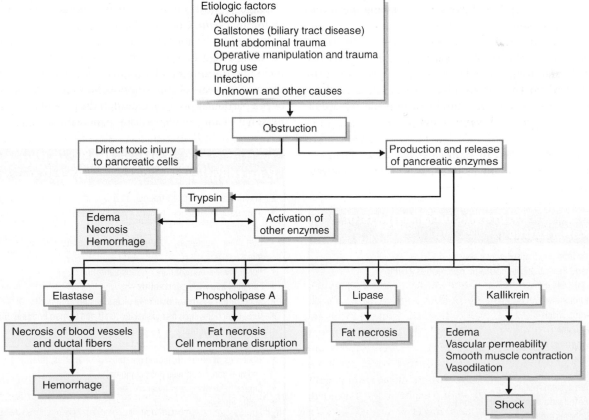

FIG. 54.2 The process of autodigestion in acute pancreatitis.

fluid becomes walled off by fibrous tissue, a **pancreatic pseudo-cyst** forms. Pseudocysts often rupture spontaneously but may require surgical removal.

Complications of Acute Pancreatitis.
Acute pancreatitis may result in severe, life-threatening complications (Table 54.3). **Jaundice** occurs from swelling of the head of the pancreas, which slows bile flow through the common bile duct. The bile duct may also be compressed by calculi (stones) or a **pancreatic pseudocyst**. The resulting total bile flow obstruction causes severe jaundice. Intermittent hyperglycemia occurs from the release of glucagon, as well as the decreased release of insulin due to damage to the pancreatic islet cells. Total destruction of the pancreas may occur, leading to type 1 diabetes mellitus (McCance et al., 2019).

Left lung pleural effusions frequently develop in the patient with acute pancreatitis. *Atelectasis and pneumonia may occur also, especially in older patients.*

Multisystem organ failure is caused by necrotizing hemorrhagic pancreatitis (NHP). The patient is at risk for acute respiratory distress syndrome (ARDS). This severe form of pulmonary edema is caused by disruption of the alveolar-capillary membrane and is a serious complication of acute pancreatitis. (See Chapter 29 for a discussion of ARDS.) In acute pancreatitis, pulmonary failure accounts for more than half of all deaths that occur in the first week of the disease.

Coagulation defects are another major potential complication and may result in death. Complex physiologic changes in the pancreas cause the release of necrotic tissue and enzymes into the bloodstream, resulting in altered coagulation. Disseminated intravascular coagulation (DIC) involves hypercoagulation of the blood, with consumption of clotting factors and the development of microthrombi.

Shock in acute pancreatitis results from peripheral vasodilation from the released vasoactive substances and the retroperitoneal loss of protein-rich fluid from proteolytic digestion. Hypovolemia may result in decreased renal perfusion and acute renal failure. Paralytic (adynamic) ileus results from peritoneal irritation and seepage of pancreatic enzymes into the abdominal cavity.

Etiology and Genetic Risk.
In many cases the cause of pancreatitis is not known, but many factors can injure the pancreas.

The most common cause is biliary tract disease, with gallstones accounting for almost half of the cases of obstructive pancreatitis (McCance et al., 2019). Acute pancreatitis may occur as a result of trauma from surgical manipulation after biliary tract, pancreatic, gastric, and duodenal procedures, such as cholecystectomy, the Whipple procedure, and partial gastrectomy. The trauma may also occur as a complication of the diagnostic procedure *endoscopic retrograde cholangiopancreatography (ERCP)*, although this rarely occurs. Additional factors that can cause acute pancreatitis are listed in Table 54.4.

Incidence and Prevalence.
Pancreatic "attacks" are especially common during holidays and vacations when alcohol consumption may be high, especially in men. Women are affected most often after having cholelithiasis and biliary tract problems. They are also most at risk for pancreatitis within several months after childbirth (McCance et al., 2019).

Death occurs in a small percentage of patients with acute pancreatitis, but with early diagnosis and treatment, mortality can be reduced. It occurs at a higher rate in *older adults* and in patients with postoperative pancreatitis. The prognosis for recovery is usually good for pancreatitis associated with biliary tract disease and poor if pancreatitis accompanies alcoholism.

❖ Interprofessional Collaborative Care

Care for the patient with acute pancreatitis usually takes place in the hospital setting for **pain** control and possible surgical intervention.

◆ Assessment: Recognize Cues

History. Most often the patient reports severe and constant abdominal **pain**. Conduct the interview *after pain is controlled.* Ask whether the abdominal pain occurs when drinking alcohol or eating a high-fat meal. Obtain information about alcohol use, including the amount of alcohol consumed during what period of time (i.e., years of consumption, how much usually consumed over a particular period). Question the patient about a family or personal history of alcoholism, pancreatitis, trauma, or biliary

---

TABLE 54.3   Potential Complications of Acute Pancreatitis

- Pancreatic infection (causes septic shock)
- Hemorrhage (necrotizing hemorrhagic pancreatitis [NHP])
- Acute kidney failure
- Paralytic ileus
- Hypovolemic shock
- Pleural effusion
- Acute respiratory distress syndrome (ARDS)
- Atelectasis
- Pneumonia
- Multiorgan system failure
- Disseminated intravascular coagulation (DIC)
- Type 2 diabetes mellitus

TABLE 54.4   Factors That Can Cause Acute Pancreatitis

- Trauma: external (blunt trauma, stab wounds, gunshot wounds [GSWs])
- Pancreatic obstruction: tumors, cysts, or abscesses; abnormal organ structure
- Metabolic problems: hyperlipidemia, hyperparathyroidism, or hypercalcemia
- Renal involvement: failure or transplantation
- Familial, inherited pancreatitis
- Penetrating gastric or duodenal ulcers, resulting in peritonitis
- Viral infections such as coxsackievirus B and human immune deficiency virus (HIV) infection
- Alcoholism
- Toxicities of drugs, including opiates, sulfonamides, thiazides, steroids, and oral contraceptives (less common)
- Cigarette smoking and tobacco use
- Cystic fibrosis
- Gallstones

tract disease. Ask whether any abdominal surgical interventions such as cholecystectomy, or diagnostic procedures such as ERCP, have been performed recently.

Ask about other medical problems known to cause pancreatitis. Inquire about recent viral infections. Ask the patient or family member to list all prescription and over-the-counter (OTC) drugs taken recently, including nutritional and herbal supplements.

Physical Assessment/Signs and Symptoms. The diagnosis of acute pancreatitis is made based on the clinical presentation combined with the results of diagnostic studies, both laboratory and imaging assessments. Symptoms of acute pancreatitis vary widely and depend on the severity of the *inflammation.* Typically, a patient is diagnosed after presenting with severe abdominal *pain* in the mid-epigastric area or left upper quadrant. Assess the intensity and quality of pain. The patient often states that the pain had a sudden onset and radiates to the back, left flank, or left shoulder. The pain is described as intense, *boring* (feeling that it is going through the body), and continuous, and is worsened by lying in the supine position. Often the patient finds relief by assuming the fetal position (with the knees drawn up to the chest and the spine flexed) or by sitting upright and bending forward. He or she may report weight loss resulting from nausea and vomiting. Obtain the patient's weight.

When performing an abdominal assessment, inspect for:

- Generalized jaundice
- Gray-blue discoloration of the abdomen and periumbilical area
- Gray-blue discoloration of the flanks, caused by pancreatic enzyme leakage to cutaneous tissue from the peritoneal cavity

Listen for bowel sounds; absent or decreased bowel sounds usually indicate paralytic (adynamic) ileus. On light palpation, note abdominal tenderness, rigidity, and guarding as a result of peritonitis. Pancreatic ascites creates a dull sound on percussion.

Monitor and record vital signs frequently to assess for elevated temperature, tachycardia, and decreased blood pressure, or assign and closely supervise this activity. Auscultate the lung fields for adventitious sounds or diminished breath sounds and observe for dyspnea or orthopnea.

! NURSING SAFETY PRIORITY (QSEN)

Critical Rescue

For the patient with acute pancreatitis, monitor for significant changes in vital signs that may indicate the life-threatening complication of shock. Hypotension and tachycardia may result from pancreatic hemorrhage, excessive fluid volume shifting, or the toxic effects of abdominal sepsis from enzyme damage. Observe for changes in behavior and level of consciousness (LOC) that may be related to alcohol withdrawal, hypoxia, or impending sepsis with shock.

Psychosocial Assessment. If excessive alcohol is a causative factor, tactfully explore the patient's alcohol intake history after the patient has adequate pain control. Provide patient privacy and establish a trusting relationship. Discuss the intake of alcohol and the reasons for overindulging. Using the CAGE questionnaire to assist with determining alcohol use may be beneficial. Ask the

TABLE 54.5 Causes of Serum Laboratory Abnormalities in Acute Pancreatitis

Abnormal Finding	Cause
Increased amylase	Pancreatic cell injury
Elevated lipase	Pancreatic cell injury
Elevated trypsin	Pancreatic cell injury
Elevated elastase	Pancreatic cell injury
Other Diagnostic Tests	
Elevated glucose	Pancreatic cell injury resulting in impaired carbohydrate metabolism; decreased insulin release
Decreased calcium and magnesium	Fatty acids combined with calcium; seen in fat necrosis
Elevated bilirubin	Hepatobiliary obstructive process
Elevated alanine aminotransferase (ALT)	Hepatobiliary involvement/obstruction
Elevated aspartate aminotransferase (AST)	Hepatobiliary involvement
Elevated leukocyte count and presence of C-reactive protein	Inflammatory response

patient when increased drinking episodes occur and, in particular, whether binges occur during holidays, vacations, or weekends or revolve around particular activities, such as television viewing. Question him or her about any recent traumatic or stressful event that may have contributed to increased alcohol consumption, such as the death of a family member or a job loss.

Laboratory Assessment. Diagnostic laboratory abnormalities are typical in patients with acute pancreatitis (Table 54.5). A variety of pancreatic and nonpancreatic disorders can cause increased serum amylase levels. In patients with pancreatitis, *amylase* levels usually increase within 12 to 24 hours and remain elevated for 2 to 3 days. Persistent elevations may be an indicator of duct obstruction or pancreatic duct leak (Pagana & Pagana, 2018).

Lipase also helps determine the presence of acute pancreatitis. Serum levels may rise later than amylase and remain elevated for up to 2 weeks. Because these levels stay elevated for such a long time, the primary health care provider may find this test useful in diagnosing patients who are not examined until several days after the initial onset of symptoms. An increase in lipase and amylase in the urine is also expected (Pagana & Pagana, 2018).

If pancreatitis is accompanied by biliary dysfunction (biliary pancreatitis), serum *bilirubin* and *alkaline phosphatase* levels are usually elevated. A sensitive indicator of biliary obstruction in acute pancreatitis is serum *alanine aminotransferase (ALT)*. A threefold or greater rise in concentration indicates that the diagnosis of acute biliary pancreatitis is valid. Elevated *white blood cell (WBC) count and differential, erythrocyte sedimentation rate (ESR),* and serum *glucose* levels are also common in acute pancreatitis. The levels often correlate with disease severity.

Decreased serum *calcium* and *magnesium* levels are seen with fat necrosis. Calcium levels may fall and remain decreased for 7 to 10 days. Those that consistently remain below 8 mg/dL are associated with a poor prognosis. Other tests include the basic metabolic panel (BMP), complete blood count (CBC), triglycerides, serum total protein, and albumin. The blood urea nitrogen (BUN), serum glucose, and triglycerides are usually elevated. Hemoconcentration is common as a result of third-space fluid loss. Leukocytosis (elevated WBCs) and thrombocytopenia (decreased platelets) are common. Albumin levels are decreased because cytokines (e.g., tumor necrosis factor [TNF]) released as part of the inflammatory response allow it to move from the bloodstream into the extravascular space. The presence of C-reactive protein suggests possible pancreatic *inflammation* and necrosis (Pagana & Pagana, 2018).

Imaging Assessment. Abdominal ultrasound is the most sensitive test to diagnose causes of pancreatitis, such as gallstones, and can be performed at the bedside. However, it is not helpful in viewing the pancreas because of overlying bowel gas. Therefore *contrast-enhanced CT* provides a more reliable image and diagnosis of acute pancreatitis. This noninvasive technique may also be used to rule out **pancreatic pseudocyst** or ductal calculi.

An abdominal x-ray may also reveal gallstones. A chest x-ray may show elevation of the left side of the diaphragm or pleural effusion. Pancreatic stones are best diagnosed through ERCP.

◆ **Analysis: Analyze Cues and Prioritize Hypotheses.** The priority collaborative problems for patients with acute pancreatitis include:

1. Severe acute *pain* due to pancreatic *inflammation* and enzyme leakage
2. Weight loss due to inability to ingest food and absorb nutrients

NCLEX Examination Challenge 54.2
Physiologic Integrity

A client was admitted to the hospital yesterday with a diagnosis of acute pancreatitis. What assessment findings will the nurse expect for this client? **Select all that apply.**

A. Severe boring abdominal pain
B. Jaundice
C. Nausea and/or vomiting
D. Decreased serum amylase level
E. Leukocytosis
F. Dyspnea

◆ **Planning and Implementation: Generate Solutions and Take Action**

Managing Acute Pain

Planning: Expected Outcomes. The patient with acute pancreatitis is expected to state that he or she has a decrease in or absence of abdominal *pain,* as evidenced by self-report of a level of 2 or 3 on a 0 to 10 pain intensity scale.

Interventions. The priorities for care for the patient with acute pancreatitis are to provide supportive care by relieving symptoms, to decrease *inflammation,* and to anticipate or treat complications. *As for any patient, continually assess for and support the ABCs (airway, breathing, and circulation).*

In collaboration with the respiratory therapist, if available, provide oxygen and other respiratory support as needed. The collaborative plan of care depends on the severity of the illness.

Severe continuous "boring" abdominal pain is the most common symptom of pancreatitis! The main focus of nursing care is aimed at controlling **pain** by interventions that decrease GI tract activity, thus decreasing pancreatic stimulation. Pain assessment to measure the effectiveness of these interventions is an essential part of nursing care.

Nonsurgical Management. *Mild* pancreatitis requires hydration with IV fluids, *pain* control, and drug therapy. The interprofessional health care team initially attempts to relieve pain with nonsurgical interventions, which include fasting and rest, drug therapy, and comfort measures. If the patient has a life-threatening complication or requires frequent assessment, he or she is admitted to a critical care unit for invasive hemodynamic monitoring.

To rest the pancreas and reduce pancreatic enzyme secretion, withhold food and fluids (NPO) during the acute period. The primary health care provider prescribes IV isotonic fluid administration to maintain hydration. IV replacement of calcium and magnesium may also be needed. Measure and document intake and output. Some patients have an indwelling urinary catheter to obtain accurate measurements.

Nasogastric drainage and suction are reserved for more *severely ill* patients who have continuous vomiting or biliary obstruction. Gastric decompression using a nasogastric tube (NGT) prevents gastric juices from flowing into the duodenum.

> ### ! NURSING SAFETY PRIORITY QSEN
> #### Action Alert
>
> Because paralytic (adynamic) ileus is a common complication of acute pancreatitis, prolonged nasogastric intubation may be necessary. Assess frequently for the return of peristalsis by asking the patient if he or she has passed flatus or had a stool. The return of bowel sounds is not reliable as an indicator of peristalsis return; passage of flatus or a bowel movement is the most reliable indicator. See the discussion of intestinal obstruction in Chapter 51.

Pain management for acute pancreatitis typically begins with the administration of opioids by patient-controlled analgesia (PCA). Drugs such as morphine or hydromorphone are typically given. Other options that have been used successfully to manage acute pain include IV or transdermal fentanyl and epidural analgesia (Burchum & Rosenthal, 2019).

In *mild* pancreatitis, the pain usually subsides in 2 to 3 days. However, with *severe* acute pancreatitis, the abdominal pain and tenderness may persist for up to 2 weeks. Drug dosages and intervals are individualized according to the severity of the disease and the symptoms.

Histamine receptor antagonists (e.g., famotidine) and proton pump inhibitors (e.g., pantoprazole) help decrease gastric acid secretion. Antibiotics may be prescribed, but they are indicated primarily for patients with acute necrotizing pancreatitis or pancreatic abscess.

Helping the patient assume a side-lying position (with the legs drawn up to the chest) may help decrease the abdominal *pain* of pancreatitis ("fetal position"). Sitting with the knees flexed toward the chest is also helpful.

If the patient is NPO or has an NGT, remind assistive personnel to implement frequent oral and nares hygiene measures to keep mucous membranes moist and free of inflammation or crusting. Because of the drying effect of drugs and the absence of oral fluids, the mouth and oral cavity may be extremely dry, resulting in considerable discomfort and possibly parotitis (inflammation of the parotid [salivary] glands).

> ### ! NURSING SAFETY PRIORITY (QSEN)
> #### *Action Alert*
>
> For the patient with acute pancreatitis, monitor his or her respiratory status every 4 to 8 hours or more often as needed and provide oxygen to promote comfort in breathing. Respiratory complications such as pleural effusions increase patient discomfort. Fluid overload can be detected by assessing for weight gain, listening for crackles, and observing for dyspnea. Carefully monitor for signs of respiratory failure.

Observe for signs and symptoms of hypocalcemia, such as muscle twitching, numbness, and irritability. Chapter 13 discusses assessment and care of patients with hypocalcemia in more detail.

Lowering the patient's anxiety level may also reduce pain. Explain all procedures and other aspects of patient care thoroughly. Provide reassurance, offer diversional activities such as music and reading material, and encourage visitors to direct attention away from the pain.

If pancreatitis was caused by gallstones, an ERCP with a sphincterotomy (opening of the sphincter of Oddi) may be performed on an urgent or emergent basis. If this procedure is not successful, surgery is required. ERCP is described in detail in Chapter 48.

Surgical Management. Surgical intervention for acute pancreatitis is usually not indicated. However, if an ERCP is not successful in removing gallstones, a laparoscopic cholecystectomy may be performed as described in the Surgical Management discussion in the section Inflammation Concept Exemplar: Cholecystitis.

Complications of pancreatitis, such as pancreatic pseudocyst and abscess, may also require surgical intervention. Laparoscopy (minimally invasive surgery [MIS]) may be done to drain an abscess or pseudocyst. For patients who are at high surgical risk, pseudocysts or abscesses can be treated by percutaneous drainage under CT guidance.

Promoting Nutrition

Planning: Expected Outcomes. The patient with acute pancreatitis is expected to have adequate *nutrition* to meet his or her metabolic needs.

Interventions. The patient is maintained on NPO status in the early stages of pancreatitis. Antiemetics for nausea and vomiting are prescribed as needed. Patients who have severe pancreatitis and are unable to eat for 24 to 48 hours after illness onset may begin jejunal tube feeding unless paralytic ileus is present. *Early nutrition* intervention enhances immune system functioning and may prevent complications and worsening *inflammation*. Enteral feeding is preferred over total parenteral nutrition (TPN) because it causes fewer episodes of glucose elevation and other complications

associated with TPN. Be sure that the patient is weighed every day. Collaborate with the primary health care provider, registered dietitian nutritionist, and pharmacist to plan and implement the most appropriate nutrition intervention. Chapter 55 describes collaborative care of patients receiving enteral feeding and TPN.

When food is tolerated during the healing phase, the primary health care provider prescribes small, frequent, moderate- to high-carbohydrate, high-protein, low-fat meals. Food should be bland with little spice. GI stimulants such as caffeine-containing food (tea, coffee, cola, and chocolate), as well as alcohol, should be avoided. Monitor the patient beginning to resume oral food intake for nausea, vomiting, and diarrhea. *If any of these symptoms occur, notify the primary health care provider immediately.*

To boost caloric intake, commercial liquid nutritional preparations supplement the diet. The health care provider may also prescribe fat-soluble and other vitamin and mineral replacement supplements. Glutamine, omega-3 fatty acids, fiber, antioxidants, and/or nucleotides may be added to the patient's nutrition plan.

Care Coordination and Transition Management

Home Care Management. Home care preparation is individualized for each patient's circumstances. Some patients may be severely weakened from their acute illness and need to confine activity to one floor, limiting stair climbing and other strenuous activities until they regain their strength. Collaborate with the case manager (CM) to plan the best place for the patient to recover and resources that may be needed.

Self-Management Education. Education needs to be started early in the hospitalization period—as soon as the acute episodes of pain have subsided. Assess the patient's and family's knowledge of the disease.

The desired outcomes for discharge planning and education are to avoid further episodes of pancreatitis and prevent progression to a chronic disease. If the patient uses alcohol, instruct him or her to abstain from drinking to prevent further pain attacks and extension of *inflammation* and pancreatic insufficiency. Tell the patient that if alcohol is consumed, acute *pain* will return, and further autodigestion of the pancreas may lead to chronic pancreatitis.

Teach the patient to notify the primary health care provider after discharge to home if acute abdominal pain or biliary tract disease (as evidenced by jaundice, clay-colored stools, or darkened urine) occurs. These signs and symptoms are possible indicators of complications or disease progression.

Health Care Resources. Patients with acute pancreatitis may require several visits by a home care nurse if the hospital course was complicated. In these cases, home care may be needed for wound care and assistance with ADLs. The patient requires medical follow-up with the primary care provider to monitor the disease process. For those with alcoholism, provide information about groups such as Alcoholics Anonymous (AA). Family members may attend support groups such as Al-Anon and Alateen.

◆ **Evaluation: Evaluate Outcomes.** Evaluate the care of the patient with acute pancreatitis based on the identified priority patient problems. The expected outcomes include that the patient will:

- Have control of abdominal *pain,* as indicated by self-report and pain scale measurement
- Have adequate *nutrition* available to meet metabolic needs

CHRONIC PANCREATITIS

Pathophysiology Review

Chronic pancreatitis is a progressive, destructive disease of the pancreas that has remissions and exacerbations ("flare-ups"). *Inflammation* and fibrosis of the tissue contribute to pancreatic insufficiency and diminished function of the organ.

Chronic pancreatitis can be classified into several categories. Alcoholism is the primary risk factor for *chronic calcifying pancreatitis (CCP)*, the most common type. In the early stages of the disease, pancreatic secretions precipitate as insoluble proteins that plug the pancreatic ducts and flow of pancreatic juices. As the protein plugs become more widespread, the cellular lining of the ducts changes and ulcerates. This inflammatory process causes fibrosis of the pancreatic tissue. Intraductal calcification and marked pancreatic tissue destruction (necrosis) develop in the late stages. The organ becomes hard and firm as a result of cell atrophy and pancreatic insufficiency (McCance et al., 2019).

CCP is found predominantly in men, but the incidence in women is increasing. In women, chronic pancreatitis occurs more commonly among those with biliary tract disease (cholecystitis and cholelithiasis).

Chronic obstructive pancreatitis develops from **inflammation,** spasm, and obstruction of the sphincter of Oddi, often from cholelithiasis (gallstones). Inflammatory and sclerotic lesions occur in the head of the pancreas and around the ducts, causing an obstruction and backflow of pancreatic secretions. (See the Complications of Acute Pancreatitis section.)

Autoimmune pancreatitis is a chronic inflammatory process in which immunoglobulins invade the pancreas. Other organs may also be infiltrated, including the lungs and liver. There is evidence to show that autoimmune pancreatitis puts the patient at risk for pancreatic cancer (Lew et al., 2017).

Idiopathic and *hereditary chronic pancreatitis* may be associated with *SPINK1* and *CFTR* gene mutations and with mutations in the *BRCA2* gene. People with hereditary pancreatitis have been shown to have a 53-fold increased risk of pancreatic cancer (Lew et al., 2017). The protein encoded by the *SPINK1* gene is a trypsin inhibitor. The *CFTR* gene is associated with cystic fibrosis. Research on these gene mutations can help in developing targeted drug therapy for treatment of these diseases.

Pancreatic insufficiency in any type of chronic pancreatitis causes loss of *exocrine* function. Most patients with chronic pancreatitis have decreased pancreatic secretions and bicarbonate. Pancreatic enzyme secretion must be greatly reduced to produce steatorrhea resulting from severe malabsorption of fats. These characteristic stools are pale, bulky, and frothy and have an offensive odor. The action of colonic bacteria on unabsorbed lipids and proteins is responsible for the extremely foul odor. On inspection of the stools, the fat content is visible.

Fat malabsorption also contributes to weight loss and muscle wasting (a decrease in muscle mass) and leads to general debilitation. Protein malabsorption results in a "starvation" edema of the feet, legs, and hands caused by decreased levels of circulating albumin.

The loss of pancreatic *endocrine* function is responsible for the development of diabetes mellitus in patients with chronic pancreatic insufficiency. (See Chapter 59 for a complete discussion of diabetes mellitus.)

The patient with chronic pancreatitis may have pulmonary complications, such as pleuritic pain, pleural effusions, and pulmonary infiltrates. Pancreatic ascites may decrease diaphragmatic excursion and lung expansion, resulting in impaired ventilation. In the ill patient with chronic pancreatitis, acute respiratory distress syndrome (ARDS) may develop.

❖ Interprofessional Collaborative Care

Care for the patient with chronic pancreatitis takes place in the home or community setting but moves to the hospital setting for *pain* control and possible surgical intervention.

◆ **Assessment: Recognize Cues.** Many symptoms of chronic pancreatitis differ from those of an acute **inflammation**. Abdominal pain is the major symptom for most types of pancreatitis. For those with chronic pancreatitis, pain is typically described as a continuous burning or gnawing dullness with periods of acute exacerbation (flare-ups). The pain is very intense and relentless. The frequency of acute exacerbations may increase as the pancreatic fibrosis develops. Key features of chronic pancreatitis are listed in the Key Features: Chronic Pancreatitis box.

Perform an abdominal assessment. Abdominal tenderness is less intense in patients with chronic pancreatitis than in those with acute pancreatitis. Massive pancreatic ascites may be present, producing dullness on abdominal percussion. Because respiratory complications can occur, auscultate the lung fields for adventitious sounds or decreased aeration and observe for dyspnea or orthopnea.

Ask the patient to collect a random stool specimen if able or ask him or her to describe the stools. The specimen may show **steatorrhea**. Assess for unintentional weight loss; muscle wasting; **jaundice**; dark urine; and the symptoms of diabetes mellitus, such as polyuria (increased urinary output), polydipsia (excessive thirst), and polyphagia (increased appetite).

Diagnosis is based on the patient's symptoms and laboratory and imaging assessment. *Endoscopic retrograde cholangiopancreatography* (ERCP) is done to visualize the pancreatic and common bile ducts. *Imaging studies* such as CT scanning, contrast-enhanced MRI, abdominal ultrasound (US), and endoscopic ultrasound (EUS) are also useful in making the diagnosis. In chronic pancreatitis, laboratory findings include normal or moderately elevated serum *amylase* and *lipase* levels. Obstruction of the intrahepatic bile duct can cause elevated

---

▶▶ KEY FEATURES

Chronic Pancreatitis

- Intense abdominal *pain,* a major symptom, that is continuous and burning or gnawing
- Abdominal tenderness
- Ascites
- Possible left upper quadrant mass (if pancreatic pseudocyst or abscess is present)
- Respiratory compromise manifesting with adventitious or diminished breath sounds, dyspnea, or orthopnea
- **Steatorrhea**; clay-colored stools
- Weight loss
- **Jaundice**
- Dark urine
- Polyuria, polydipsia, polyphagia (diabetes mellitus)

serum *bilirubin* and *alkaline phosphatase* levels. Intermittent elevations in serum *glucose* levels are common and can be detected by blood glucose monitoring, both fasting and nonfasting.

◆ **Interventions: Take Action.** The focus of caring for the patient with chronic pancreatitis is to manage acute or persistent *pain,* maintain adequate *nutrition,* and prevent disease recurrence.

Nonsurgical Management. The primary nonsurgical interventions include drug and *nutrition* therapy. The major intervention for the pain of chronic pancreatitis is drug therapy. Medicate the patient as prescribed according to the assessment of the intensity of pain. Evaluate the effectiveness of the drug intervention. Initially opioid analgesia is used most frequently, but dependency may occur. Nonopioid analgesics may be tried to relieve pain. (See Chapter 5 for other interventions for acute and persistent pain.)

Pancreatic enzyme replacement therapy (PERT) is the standard of care to prevent malnutrition, malabsorption, and excessive weight loss. Pancreatic enzymes are usually prescribed in the form of capsules or tablets that contain varying amounts of amylase, lipase, and protease. Teach patients not to chew or crush pancreatic enzyme replacements that are available as delayed-release capsules or enteric tablets. Teach them to take the enzymes with all meals and snacks (Burchum & Rosenthal, 2019).

The dosage of pancreatic enzymes depends on the severity of the malabsorption. Record the number and consistency of stools per day to monitor the effectiveness of enzyme therapy. If pancreatic enzyme treatment is effective, the stools should become less frequent and less fatty.

The primary health care provider may also prescribe drug

! NURSING SAFETY PRIORITY (USEN)
Action Alert

If the patient has diabetes, insulin or oral antidiabetic agents for glucose control are prescribed. Patients maintained on total parenteral nutrition (TPN) are particularly susceptible to elevated glucose levels and require regular insulin additives to the solution. Monitor blood glucose to control hyperglycemia. Check finger stick blood glucose (FSBG) or sugar (FSBS) levels every 2 to 4 hours. Chapter 55 describes in detail the care associated with TPN.

therapy to decrease gastric acid. Gastric acid destroys the lipase needed to break down fats. Controlling the acidity of the stomach with H2 blockers or proton pump inhibitors or neutralizing stomach acid with oral sodium bicarbonate may enhance the effectiveness of PERT.

Protein and fat malabsorption results in significant weight loss and decreased muscle mass in the patient with chronic pancreatitis. Therefore the nutritional interventions for acute pancreatitis are also used for chronic pancreatitis. The patient often limits food intake to avoid increased pain. For this reason, nutrition maintenance is often difficult to achieve. Patients receive either total parenteral nutrition (TPN) or total enteral nutrition (TEN), including vitamin and mineral replacement.

Collaborate with the registered dietitian nutritionist to teach the patient about long-term dietary management. He or she needs an increased number of calories, up to 4000 to 6000 calories per day, to maintain weight. Food high in carbohydrates and protein also assists in the healing process. Food high in fat is avoided

because it causes or increases diarrhea. Teach all patients to avoid alcohol. Alcohol-cessation programs may be recommended.

Surgical Management. Surgery is not a primary intervention for the treatment of chronic pancreatitis. However, it may be indicated for ongoing abdominal *pain,* incapacitating relapses of pain, or complications such as a pancreatic abscess or pancreatic pseudocyst.

The underlying pathologic changes determine the procedure indicated. Using laparoscopy, the surgeon incises and drains an abscess or pseudocyst. Laparoscopic cholecystectomy or choledochotomy (incision of the common bile duct) may be indicated if biliary tract disease is an underlying cause of pancreatitis. If the pancreatic duct sphincter is fibrotic, the surgeon performs a sphincterotomy (incision of the sphincter) to enlarge it. Endoscopic sphincterotomy may be used for patients who are poor surgical candidates.

In some cases laparoscopic distal pancreatectomy may be appropriate for resection of the distal pancreas or pancreas head. Endoscopic pancreatic necrosectomy and natural orifice transluminal endoscopic surgery (NOTES) are becoming more common for removing necrosed pancreatic tissue. Both procedures are performed through the GI wall without a visible skin incision. The NOTES procedure is discussed in Surgical Management in the Inflammation Concept Exemplar: Cholecystitis section.

In a few cases, pancreas transplantation may be done. However, this procedure is performed most often for patients with severe, uncontrolled diabetes. Chapter 59 discusses pancreas transplantation.

Care Coordination and Transition Management

Home Care Management. Collaborate with the hospital-based case manager (CM) or discharge planner about home care or follow-up in another setting. A community-based CM may continue to follow the patient after hospital discharge. If the patient is discharged to home, the living area should be limited to one floor until he or she regains strength and can increase activity. Teach patients and families that toilet facilities must be easily accessible because of chronic steatorrhea and frequent defecation. If they are not easily accessible, a bedside commode is obtained for the home.

Self-Management Education. Because there is no known cure for chronic pancreatitis, patient and family education is aimed at preventing acute episodes of the disease, providing long-term care, and promoting health maintenance. The Patient and Family Education: Preparing for Self-Management: Prevention of Exacerbations of Chronic Pancreatitis box outlines self-management to help prevent exacerbations of the disease.

PATIENT AND FAMILY EDUCATION: PREPARING FOR SELF-MANAGEMENT
Prevention of Exacerbations of Chronic Pancreatitis

- Avoid things that make your symptoms worse, such as drinking caffeinated beverages.
- Avoid alcohol ingestion; refer to self-help group for assistance.
- Avoid nicotine.
- Eat bland, low-fat, high-protein, and moderate-carbohydrate meals; avoid gastric stimulants such as spices.
- Eat small meals and snacks high in calories.
- Take the pancreatic enzymes that have been prescribed for you with meals.
- Rest frequently; restrict your activity to one floor until you regain your strength.

PATIENT AND FAMILY EDUCATION: PREPARING FOR SELF-MANAGEMENT

Enzyme Replacement for the Patient With Chronic Pancreatitis

- Take pancreatic enzymes with meals and snacks and follow with a glass of water.
- Administer enzymes after antacid or H₂ blockers. (Decreased pH inactivates drug.)
- Swallow the tablets or capsules without chewing, to minimize oral irritation and allow the drug to be released slowly.
- If you cannot swallow the capsule, pierce the gelatin casing and place contents in applesauce.
- Do not mix enzyme preparations in protein-containing foods.
- Wipe your lips after taking enzymes to avoid skin irritation.
- Do not crush enteric-coated preparations.
- Follow up on all scheduled laboratory testing. (Pancreatic enzyme replacements can cause an increase in uric acid levels.)

Remind the patient and family members or significant others of the importance of adhering to pancreatic enzyme replacement. The patient must take the prescribed enzymes with meals and snacks to aid in the digestion of food and promote the absorption of fats and proteins (see the Patient and Family Education: Preparing for Self-Management: Enzyme Replacement for the Patient With Chronic Pancreatitis box).

The frequency of defecation (whether continent or incontinent) poses challenging skin care problems. Instruct the patient to keep the skin dry and free of the abrasive fatty stools, which damage the skin. The skin should be cleaned thoroughly after each stool, and a moisture barrier applied to prevent breakdown and maintain skin integrity. Many products on the market actively repel stool from the skin. Remind the patient to report any skin breakdown so therapeutic interventions to promote skin integrity can be started. Abdominal fistulas are common and present a difficult challenge because pancreatic secretions irritate the skin.

If the patient develops diabetes mellitus as a result of chronic pancreatitis, management of elevated glucose levels after discharge from the hospital may require oral antidiabetic agents or insulin injections. If this is the case, collaborate with the certified diabetes educator (CDE) to provide in-depth teaching concerning diabetes, its signs and symptoms, medical management, drug therapy, nutrition therapy, blood glucose monitoring, and general care.

Chronic illnesses are devastating for families. The high costs of medical insurance, medical treatment, and drug therapy cause serious financial problems. Often the patient with chronic pancreatitis is unable to work. Collaborate with the CM about ways to assist the patient with resources for financial help.

Health Care Resources. The patient may require several home visits by nurses, depending on the severity of the chronic health problems and home maintenance and support needs. The nurse assesses the patient for pain, enzyme therapy, and psychosocial adaptation to a chronic illness. Refer him or her and the family to a counselor or a self-help group, such as Alcoholics Anonymous (www.aa.org) and Al-Anon (www.al-anon.org), if appropriate.

PANCREATIC CANCER

Pathophysiology Review

Cancer of the pancreas is a leading cause of cancer deaths each year in the United States. It is difficult to diagnose early because the pancreas is hidden and surrounded by other organs. Most often, the tumor is discovered in the late stages of development and may be a well-defined mass or diffusely spread throughout the pancreas. Treatment has limited results, and 5-year survival rates are low (American Cancer Society, 2020).

The tumor may be a primary cancer, or it may result from metastasis from cancers of the lung, breast, thyroid, kidney, or skin. Primary tumors are generally adenocarcinomas and grow in well-differentiated glandular patterns. They grow rapidly and spread to surrounding organs (stomach, duodenum, gallbladder, and intestine) by direct extension and invasion of lymphatic and vascular systems. This highly metastatic lesion may eventually invade the lung, peritoneum, liver, spleen, and lymph nodes.

Signs and symptoms depend on the site of origin or metastasis. The head of the pancreas is the most common site. The tumors are usually small lesions with poorly defined margins. Jaundice results from tumor compression and obstruction of the common bile duct and from gallbladder dilation, causing the organ to enlarge.

Cancers of the body and tail of the pancreas are usually large and invade the entire tail and body. These tumors may be palpable abdominal masses, especially in the thin patient. Through metastatic spread via the splenic vein, metastasis to the liver may cause hepatomegaly (enlargement of the liver). Regardless of where it originates, it spreads rapidly through the lymphatic and venous systems to other organs.

Venous thromboembolism is a common complication of pancreatic cancer. Necrotic products of the pancreatic tumor are believed to have thromboplastic properties resulting in the blood's hypercoagulable state. In addition, the patient is at high risk because of decreased mobility and extensive surgical manipulation.

The exact cause of pancreatic cancer is unknown. Table 54.6 highlights the major risk factors associated with the disease.

❖ Interprofessional Collaborative Care

Care for the patient with pancreatic cancer usually takes place in the hospital setting, and eventually with hospice.

TABLE 54.6 Risk Factors Associated With Pancreatic Cancer

- Diabetes mellitus
- Chronic pancreatitis
- Cirrhosis
- High intake of red meat, especially processed meat
- Long-term exposure to chemicals such as gasoline and pesticides
- Obesity
- Older age
- Male gender
- Cigarette smoking
- Family history
- Genetic mutations (e.g., *p16*, *BRCA2*)

⏭ KEY FEATURES

Pancreatic Cancer

- **Jaundice**
- **Icterus**
- Clay-colored (light) stools
- Dark urine
- Abdominal *pain,* usually vague, dull, or nonspecific, that radiates into the back
- Weight loss
- Anorexia
- Nausea or vomiting
- Glucose intolerance
- Splenomegaly (enlarged spleen)
- Flatulence
- Gastrointestinal bleeding
- New-onset diabetes mellitus
- Ascites (abdominal fluid)
- Leg or calf pain (from thrombophlebitis)
- Weakness and fatigue

◆ **Assessment: Recognize Cues.** Pancreatic cancer often presents in a slow and vague manner. The presenting symptoms depend somewhat on the location of the tumor. The first sign may be jaundice, which suggests late, advanced disease (see the Key Features: Pancreatic Cancer box).

No specific blood tests are diagnostic of pancreatic cancer. Serum *amylase* and *lipase* levels and *alkaline phosphatase* and *bilirubin* levels are increased. The degree of elevation depends on the acuteness or chronicity of the pancreatic and biliary damage. Elevated *carcinoembryonic antigen* (CEA) levels occur in most patients with pancreatic cancer. This test may provide early information about the presence of tumor cells. The tumor marker CA 19-9 has been found to be a useful serologic test for monitoring a proven diagnosis and continuing surveillance for potential spread or recurrence (Pagana & Pagana, 2018).

Abdominal *ultrasound* and *contrast-enhanced CT* are the most commonly used imaging techniques for confirming a tumor and can differentiate the tumor from a cyst. Endoscopic ultrasonography can also be performed to sample tissue for diagnosis and provide information on tumor type and size (Bujanda & Herreros-Villanueva, 2017). *Endoscopic retrograde cholangiopancreatography* (ERCP) also provides visual diagnostic data. An alternative to ERCP is a percutaneous transhepatic biliary cholangiogram with placement of a percutaneous transhepatic biliary drain (PTBD). This drain decompresses the blocked biliary system by draining bile internally, externally, or both. Aspiration of pancreatic ascitic fluid by abdominal paracentesis may reveal cancer cells and elevated amylase levels.

◆ **Interventions: Take Action.** Management of the patient with pancreatic cancer is geared toward preventing tumor spread and decreasing pain. These measures are not curative, only palliative. The cancers are often metastatic and recur despite treatment.

Nonsurgical Management. As in other types of cancer, chemotherapy or radiation is used to relieve pain by shrinking the tumor. It may be used before, after, or instead of surgery.

Chemotherapy has had limited success in increasing survival time. In most cases, combining agents has been more successful than single-agent chemotherapy. 5-Fluorouracil (5-FU), a commonly used drug, may be given alone or with gemcitabine for locally advanced, or unresectable, pancreatic cancers. Observe for adverse drug effects, such as fatigue, rash, anorexia, and diarrhea. Chapter 20 discusses nursing implications of chemotherapy in more detail.

Other targeted therapies being investigated include growth factor inhibitors, antiangiogenesis factors, and kinase inhibitors. Kinase inhibitors are a newer group of drugs that focus on cancer cells with little or no effect on healthy cells. Chapter 20 describes general nursing interventions associated with chemotherapy.

To control pain, the patient takes high doses of opioid analgesics (usually morphine) as prescribed before the pain escalates and peaks. Because of the poor prognosis, drug dependency is not a consideration. Chapter 5 describes in detail the care of the patient with chronic cancer pain.

Intensive external beam *radiation* therapy to the pancreas may offer pain relief by shrinking tumor cells, alleviating obstruction, and improving food absorption. It does not improve survival rates. The patient may experience discomfort during and after the radiation treatments. Chapter 20 describes radiation therapy in more detail.

For patients experiencing biliary obstruction who are at high surgical risk, biliary stents placed percutaneously (through the skin) can ensure patency to relieve pain. These stents are devices made of plastic materials that keep the ducts of the biliary system open. Using another approach, self-expandable stents may be inserted endoscopically to relieve obstruction.

Surgical Management. Complete surgical resection of the pancreatic tumor offers the patient with pancreatic cancer the only effective treatment, but it is done only in patients with small tumors. Partial pancreatectomy is the preferred surgery for tumors smaller than 3 cm in diameter, depending on location and length of time since diagnosis. Recent technologic advances have expanded the role of *minimally invasive surgery (MIS)* via laparoscopy in the staging, palliation, and removal of pancreatic cancers. The procedure selected depends on the purpose of the surgery and stage of the disease. For example, if the patient has a biliary obstruction, a laparoscopic procedure to relieve it is performed. This procedure diverts bile drainage into the jejunum.

For larger tumors, the surgeon may perform either a *radical pancreatectomy* or the *Whipple procedure (pancreaticoduodenectomy).* These procedures have traditionally been done using an open surgical approach. Because of new advances in laparoscopic technology using a hand-assist or robotic-assist device, this method is beginning to replace the conventional method. Some surgeons are not yet trained in how to perform this technique. Therefore the traditional open surgical approach remains a common method of performing these surgeries.

Preoperative Care. The patient with pancreatic cancer may be at poor surgical risk because of malnutrition and debilitation. Specific care depends on the type of surgical approach being used.

Often, in the late stages of pancreatic cancer or before the Whipple procedure, the primary health care provider inserts a small catheter into the jejunum (jejunostomy) so enteral feedings may be given. This feeding method is preferred to prevent reflux and facilitate absorption. Feedings are started in low concentrations and volumes and gradually increased as tolerated. Provide feedings using a pump to maintain a constant volume and assess for diarrhea frequency to determine tolerance. Chapter 55 provides additional information about enteral feeding.

For optimal *nutrition,* TPN may be necessary in addition to tube feedings or as a single measure. When central venous access is required, a peripherally inserted central catheter (PICC) or other type of IV catheter may be necessary. Meticulous IV line care is an important nursing measure to prevent catheter sepsis. Sterile dressing changes and site observation are extremely important. Additional nursing care measures for the patient receiving TPN are given in Chapter 55. Monitor nutrition indicators such as serum prealbumin and albumin.

For the laparoscopic procedure, no bowel preparation is needed. However, either approach requires that the patient have nothing by mouth (NPO) for at least 6 to 8 hours before surgery. Surgeon preference and agency policy determine the preferred protocol for preoperative preparation.

Operative Procedures. The **Whipple procedure (radical pancreaticoduodenectomy)** is an extensive surgical procedure used most often to treat cancer of the head of the pancreas. The procedure entails removal of the proximal head of the pancreas, the duodenum, a portion of the jejunum, the stomach (partial or total *gastrectomy*), and the gallbladder, with anastomosis of the pancreatic duct (*pancreaticojejunostomy*), the common bile duct (*choledochojejunostomy*), and the stomach (*gastrojejunostomy*) to the jejunum (Fig. 54.3). In addition, the surgeon may remove the spleen (**splenectomy**).

Postoperative Care. In addition to routine postoperative care measures, the patient who has undergone an *open* radical pancreaticoduodenectomy requires intensive nursing care and is typically admitted to a surgical critical care unit. Observe for multiple potential complications of the open Whipple procedure as listed in Table 54.7.

The primary benefits of *MIS* for the patient are a shorter postoperative recovery and less pain than with traditional open procedure. The patient having the laparoscopic Whipple surgery or radical pancreatectomy is also less at risk for severe complications. For patients having one of these procedures, observe for and implement preventive measures for these common surgical complications:

- Diabetes (Check blood glucose often.)
- Hemorrhage (Monitor pulse, blood pressure, skin color, and mental status [e.g., LOC].)
- Wound infection (Monitor temperature and assess wounds for redness and induration [hardness].)
- Bowel obstruction (Check bowel sounds and stools.)
- Intra-abdominal abscess (Monitor temperature and patient's report of severe pain.)

Immediately after surgery the patient is NPO and usually has a nasogastric tube (NGT) to decompress the stomach. Monitor GI drainage and tube patency. In open surgical approaches, biliary drainage tubes are placed during surgery to remove drainage and secretions from the area and prevent stress on the anastomosis sites. Assess the tubes and drainage devices for tension or kinking and maintain them in a dependent position.

Monitor the drainage for color, consistency, and amount. The drainage should be serosanguineous. The appearance of clear,

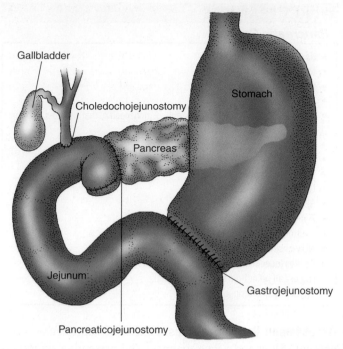

FIG. 54.3 The three anastomoses that constitute the Whipple procedure: choledochojejunostomy, pancreaticojejunostomy, and gastrojejunostomy.

TABLE 54.7	**Potential Complications of the Whipple Procedure**
Cardiovascular Complications	**GI Complications**
• Hemorrhage at anastomosis sites with hypovolemia	• Adynamic (paralytic) ileus
• Myocardial infarction	• Gastric retention
• Heart failure	• Gastric ulceration
• Thrombophlebitis	• Bowel obstruction from peritonitis
	• Acute pancreatitis
Pulmonary Complications	• Hepatic failure
• Atelectasis	• Thrombosis to mesentery
• Pneumonia	
• Pulmonary embolism	**Wound Complications**
• Acute respiratory distress syndrome	• Infection
• Pulmonary edema	• Dehiscence
	• Fistulas: pancreatic, gastric, and biliary
Metabolic Complications	
• Unstable diabetes mellitus	
• Renal failure	

colorless, bile-tinged drainage or frank blood with an increase in output may indicate disruption or leakage of an anastomosis site. Most of the disruptions of the site occur within 7 to 10 days after surgery. Hemorrhage can occur as an early or late complication.

Place the patient in the semi-Fowler position to reduce tension on the suture line and anastomosis site and to optimize lung expansion. Stress can be decreased by maintaining NGT drainage at a low or high intermittent suction level to keep the remaining stomach (if a partial gastrectomy is done) or the jejunum (if a total gastrectomy is done) free of excessive fluid buildup and pressure. The NGT also reduces stimulation of the remaining pancreatic tissue.

The development of a fistula (an abnormal passageway) is the most common and most serious postoperative complication.

Biliary, pancreatic, or gastric fistulas result from partial or total breakdown of an anastomosis site. The secretions that drain from the fistula contain bile, pancreatic enzymes, or gastric secretions, depending on which site is ruptured. *These secretions, particularly pancreatic fluid, are corrosive and irritating to the skin; and internal leakage causes chemical peritonitis.* Peritonitis (inflammation and infection of the peritoneum causing board-like abdominal rigidity) requires treatment with multiple antibiotics. *If you suspect any postoperative complications resulting from MIS or open surgical approaches, call the surgeon or Rapid Response Team immediately and provide assessment findings that support your concerns.*

Because the *open* Whipple procedure is extensive and can take many hours to complete, maintaining fluid and electrolyte balance can be difficult. Patients often have significant intraoperative blood loss and postoperative bleeding. The intestine is exposed to air for long periods, and fluid evaporates. Significant losses of fluid and electrolytes occur from the NGT and other drainage tubes. In addition, these patients may be malnourished and have low serum levels of protein and albumin, which maintain colloid osmotic pressure within the circulating system. Reduction in the serum osmotic pressure makes the patient likely to develop third spacing of body fluids, with fluid moving from the vascular to the interstitial space, resulting in shock. These problems are less likely to occur when MIS is used. Therefore, when possible, the trained surgeon prefers to perform laparoscopic Whipple procedures to shorten operating time and prevent the many complications that can occur.

> **! NURSING SAFETY PRIORITY (QSEN)**
>
> *Action Alert*
>
> To detect early signs of hypovolemia and prevent shock, closely monitor vital signs for decreased blood pressure and increased heart rate, decreased vascular pressures with a pulmonary artery catheter (Swan-Ganz catheter) (in ICU setting), and decreased urine output. Be alert for pitting edema of the extremities, dependent edema in the sacrum and back, and an intake that far exceeds output. Maintain sequential compression devices to prevent deep vein thrombosis.

Maintenance of IV isotonic fluid replacement with colloid replacements is important. Monitor hemoglobin and hematocrit values to assess for blood loss and the need for blood transfusions. Review electrolyte values for decreased serum levels of sodium, potassium, chloride, and calcium. IV fluid concentrations must be altered to correct these electrolyte imbalances. The physician prescribes replacement of electrolytes as needed.

Immediately after the Whipple procedure, the patient may have hyperglycemia or hypoglycemia as a result of stress and surgical manipulation of the pancreas. Most of the endocrine cells (responsible for insulin and glucagon secretion) are located in the body and tail of the pancreas. In some patients, up to half of the gland remains, and diabetes does not develop. However, a large number of patients have diabetes before surgery. For patients having a radical pancreatectomy, administer insulin as prescribed because the entire pancreas is removed. Monitor glucose levels frequently during the early postoperative period and administer insulin injections as prescribed.

Care Coordination and Transition Management. The patient with pancreatic cancer is usually followed by a case manager (CM), both in the hospital and in the home or other community-based setting. Collaborate with the CM to ensure that the patient receives cost-effective treatment and that his or her needs are met.

Home Care Management. The stage of progression of pancreatic cancer and available home care resources determine whether the patient can be discharged to home or whether additional care is needed in a skilled nursing facility or with a hospice provider. Home care preparations depend on the patient's physical and activity limitations and should be tailored to his or her needs. Coordinate care with the patient, family, or whoever will be providing care after discharge from the hospital (i.e., home care provider, hospice care provider, or extended-care provider).

The patient and family need compassionate emotional support to deal with issues related to this illness. The diagnosis of pancreatic cancer can frighten and overwhelm the patient and family. Help family members look realistically and objectively at the amount of physical care required. Tell family members that their own physical and emotional health is at risk during this stressful period and that supportive counseling may be needed. If the family does not have a religious affiliation or a spiritual leader (e.g., a minister or a rabbi) to provide support, suggest alternative counseling options. Refer patients and families to the certified hospital chaplain if desired. It is appropriate for the nurse to make the initial contact or appointment according to the patient's or family's wishes.

Self-Management Education. When the patient is discharged to home, many interventions are palliative and aimed at managing symptoms such as pain. In many cases the diagnosis of pancreatic cancer is made a few months before death occurs. The patient needs time to adjust to the diagnosis, which is usually made too late for cure or prolonged survival. Help the patient identify what needs to be done to prepare for death, including end-of-life care. For example, he or she may want to write a will or see family members and friends whom he or she has not seen recently. The patient needs to make known to family members or others his or her specific requests for the funeral or memorial service. These actions help prepare for death in a dignified manner. Chapter 8 discusses in detail anticipatory grieving and preparation for death, as well as symptom management during the end of life.

Health Care Resources. Regular home care nursing and assistive personnel visits may be scheduled to assist the patient and family by providing physical, psychological, and supportive care. Supply information about local palliative and hospice care (see Chapter 8) and cancer support groups.

GET READY FOR THE NEXT-GENERATION NCLEX® EXAMINATION!

Key Points
Review these Key Points for each NCLEX Examination Client Needs Category.

Safe and Effective Care Environment
- Refer patients with end-stage pancreatic cancer for palliative and hospice care. **Ethics**
- Refer patients with pancreatitis who use alcohol to community resources such as Alcoholics Anonymous. **QSEN: Patient-Centered Care**

Health Promotion and Maintenance
- Recognize that obese, middle-age women are most likely to have gallbladder disease. **QSEN: Patient-Centered Care**
- Teach patients to avoid losing weight too quickly and to keep weight under control to help prevent gallbladder disease. **QSEN: Evidence-Based Practice**
- Teach patients to avoid alcohol consumption to help prevent alcohol-induced acute pancreatitis. **QSEN: Evidence-Based Practice**
- Instruct patients about ways to prevent exacerbations of chronic pancreatitis.

Psychosocial Integrity
- Refer patients with pancreatic cancer to support services such as spiritual leaders and counselors for coping strategies and facilitation of the grieving process. **Ethics**

- Help prepare the pancreatic cancer patient and family for the death and dying process. **Ethics**

Physiological Integrity
- Be aware that autodigestion of the pancreas causes severe *pain* in patients with acute pancreatitis (see Fig. 54.2). **QSEN: Patient-Centered Care**
- Monitor serum laboratory values, especially amylase and lipase (both elevated), in patients with pancreatitis (see Table 54.4). **QSEN: Evidence-Based Practice**
- Assess for common symptoms of cholecystitis including abdominal pain and intolerance to fatty foods. **Clinical Judgment**
- Provide pain management, including opioid analgesia, for patients with acute pancreatitis. **QSEN: Patient-Centered Care**
- Recognize that acute pain relief is the first priority of care for patients with acute pancreatitis. **QSEN: Evidence-Based Practice**
- Be aware that patients with biliary and pancreatic disorders are at high risk for biliary obstruction, a serious and painful complication. **QSEN: Safety**
- Document health teaching about enzyme replacement therapy. **QSEN: Informatics**
- Assess patients with symptoms of pancreatic cancer, including jaundice and abdominal *pain*. **QSEN: Patient-Centered Care**
- Observe for and implement interventions to prevent life-threatening complications of the Whipple procedure as outlined in Table 54.5. **QSEN: Safety**

MASTERY QUESTIONS

1. Which statement by the client who is prescribed to take pancreatic enzyme replacements indicates a need for further teaching by the nurse?
   A. "I need to take the enzymes at every meal and with snacks."
   B. "After taking the enzymes, I should drink a glass of water."
   C. "I should wipe my mouth in case any of the enzyme got on my lips."
   D. "I should chew each capsule carefully so that it works in my stomach."

2. The nurse is planning care for a client who had a laparoscopic Whipple surgery. For which complications will the nurse assess? **Select all that apply**.
   A. Bleeding
   B. Wound infection
   C. Intestinal obstruction
   D. Diabetes mellitus
   E. Abdominal abscess

REFERENCES

American Cancer Society (ACS). (2020). *Cancer facts and figures—2019*. Atlanta: Author.

Bujanda, L., & Herreros-Villanueva, M. (2017). Pancreatic cancer in Lynch syndrome patients. *Journal of Cancer, 8*(18), 3667–3674.

Burchum, J. L. R., & Rosenthal, L. D. (2019). *Lehne's pharmacology for nursing care* (10th ed.). St. Louis: Elsevier.

Jarvis, C. (2020). *Physical examination & health assessment* (8th ed.). St. Louis: Elsevier Saunders.

Lew, D., Afghani, E., & Pandol, S. (2017). Chronic pancreatitis: Current status and challenges for prevention and treatment. *Digestive Diseases and Sciences, 62,* 1702–1712.

McCance, K., Huether, S., Brashers, V., & Rote, N. (2019). *Pathophysiology: The biologic basis for disease in adults and children* (8th ed.). St. Louis: Mosby.

Pagana, K. D., & Pagana, T. J. (2018). *Manual of diagnostic and laboratory tests* (6th ed.). St. Louis: Mosby.

Roberts, K. E., & Kate, V. (2016). *Transvaginal cholecystectomy*. http://emedicine.medscape.com/article/1900692-overview#a5.

55

Concepts of Care for Patients With Malnutrition: Undernutrition and Obesity

Cherie R. Rebar

http://evolve.elsevier.com/Iggy/

LEARNING OUTCOMES

1. Collaborate with the interprofessional team to coordinate high-quality care for patients with malnutrition.
2. Describe factors that place a patient at high risk for malnutrition and refer to the health care provider.
3. Implement patient-centered nursing interventions to decrease the psychosocial impact of living with malnutrition.
4. Apply knowledge of anatomy, physiology, and pathophysiology to assess patients with malnutrition.
5. Use clinical judgment to analyze assessment findings and diagnostic data in the care of patients with malnutrition.
6. Prioritize evidence-based care for patients with a malnutrition problem affecting **nutrition** and *fluid and electrolyte balance.*
7. Plan care coordination and transition management for patients with malnutrition.

KEY TERMS

anorexia The loss of appetite for food.

anorexia nervosa An eating disorder of self-induced starvation resulting from a fear of fatness, even though the patient is underweight.

bariatrics A branch of medicine that manages patients with obesity and its related diseases.

binge eating disorder An eating disorder that involves eating in binges with a feeling of loss of control over the eating behavior.

body mass index (BMI) A measure of nutrition status that does not depend on frame size; indirectly estimates total fat stores within the body by the relationship of weight to height.

body surface area (BSA) A calculated estimate of a person's total body surface area reflecting physiologic and metabolic processes including heat exchange, blood volume, and size of vital organs. Used as an indicator for appropriate dosage calculation, especially for anticancer agents.

bolus feeding A method of tube feeding that involves intermittent feeding of a specified amount of enteral product at specified times during a 24-hour period, typically every 4 hours.

bulimia nervosa An eating disorder characterized by episodes of binge eating in which the patient ingests a large amount of food in a short time, followed by purging behavior, such as self-induced vomiting or excessive use of laxatives and diuretics.

cachexia Extreme body wasting and malnutrition that develop from an imbalance between food intake and energy use.

continuous feeding A method of tube feeding in which small amounts of enteral product are continuously infused (by gravity drip or by a pump or controller device) over a specified time.

cyclic feeding A method of tube feeding similar to continuous feeding (see definition of continuous feeding) except the infusion is stopped for a specified time in each 24-hour period ("down time"); the down time typically occurs in the morning to allow bathing, treatments, and other activities.

dietary reference intakes (DRIs) Nutrition guide developed by the Institute of Medicine of the National Academies that provides a scientific basis for food guidelines in the United States and Canada.

dumping syndrome Vasomotor symptoms that typically occur within 30 minutes after eating, including vertigo, tachycardia, syncope, sweating, pallor, and palpitations.

enterostomal feeding tube A tube used for patients who need long-term enteral feeding.

food allergy A reaction to a food (or multiple foods), rooted in the immune system, that can cause a life-threatening complication like anaphylaxis.

food intolerance Inability to tolerate a food (or multiple foods), rooted in the gastrointestinal system when a food cannot be properly broken down.

gastric bypass A type of gastric restriction surgery in which gastric resection is combined with malabsorption surgery. The patient's stomach, duodenum, and part of the jejunum are bypassed so that fewer calories can be absorbed. Also known as a Roux-en-Y gastric bypass, or RNYGB.

gastrostomy A stoma created from the abdominal wall into the stomach.

jejunostomy Surgical creation of an opening between the jejunum and surface of the abdominal wall.

knee height caliper A device that uses the distance between the patient's patella and heel to estimate height.

kwashiorkor A lack of protein quantity and quality in the presence of adequate calories. Body weight is more normal, and serum proteins are low.

lactose intolerance A type of food intolerance when a patient has an inadequate amount of lactase enzyme, which converts lactose into absorbable glucose.

malnutrition Deficiencies, excesses, or imbalances in a person's intake of energy and/or nutrients.

marasmus A calorie malnutrition in which body fat and protein are wasted, and serum proteins are often preserved.

medical nutrition supplements Enteral products taken by patients who cannot or do not consume enough nutrients in their usual diet (e.g., Ensure, Boost).

nasoduodenal tube (NDT) A tube that is inserted through a nostril and into the small intestine.

nasoenteric tube (NET) Any feeding tube that is inserted nasally and then advanced into the gastrointestinal tract.

nasogastric (NG) tube A tube that is inserted through a nostril and into the stomach for liquid feeding or for withdrawing gastric contents.

nutrition screening An assessment of nutrition status that includes inspection, measured height and weight, weight history, usual eating habits, ability to chew and swallow, and any recent changes in appetite or food intake.

obesity An increase in body weight at least 20% above the upper limit of the normal range for ideal body weight, with an excess amount of body fat; in an adult, a body mass index greater than 30. Subdivided into Class I, II, or III.

overweight An increase in body weight for height compared with a reference standard (e.g., the Metropolitan Life height and weight tables) or 10% greater than ideal body weight. However, this weight may not reflect excess body fat, which in an adult is a body mass index of 25 to 30.

panniculectomy Surgical removal of the abdominal apron (panniculus).

percutaneous endoscopic gastrostomy (PEG) A stoma created from the abdominal wall into the stomach for insertion of a short feeding tube.

protein-energy undernutrition (PEU) A disorder of nutrition that may present in three forms: marasmus, kwashiorkor, and marasmic-kwashiorkor. Also called *protein-calorie malnutrition.*

refeeding syndrome Life-threatening metabolic complication that can occur when nutrition is restarted for a patient who is in a starvation state.

skinfold measurements Estimation of body fat, usually calculated through measurement of the triceps and subscapular skinfolds with a special caliper.

starvation A complete lack of nutrients.

total parenteral nutrition (TPN) Provision of intensive nutritional support for an extended time; delivered to the patient through access to central veins, usually the subclavian or internal jugular veins.

undernutrition A nutrition state of wasting, stunting, and being underweight

---

✳ PRIORITY AND INTERRELATED CONCEPTS

The priority concept for this chapter is:
- *Nutrition*

The *Nutrition* concept exemplars for this chapter are Undernutrition and Obesity.

The interrelated concept for this chapter is:
- *Fluid and Electrolyte Balance*

Eating a balanced diet yields a strong *nutrition* status, which helps the body function well through growth, the maintenance of temperature, respiration, cardiac output, muscle strength, protein synthesis, and storage and metabolism of healthy food sources. In healthy adults, most energy supplied by carbohydrates, protein, and fat undergoes digestion and is absorbed from the GI tract. The relationship between energy used and energy stored is referred to as *energy balance*. Weight is gained when food intake is more than energy used, and weight loss occurs when energy used is more than intake. The body attempts to meet its calorie requirements even if it is at the expense of protein needs; when calorie intake is insufficient, body proteins are used for energy.

Influenced by personal preference, demographic location, cultural norms, spiritual observations, financial feasibility, and availability of nutrition sources, *nutrition* status varies for each patient. Further influencing factors include age, height, weight, gender, speed of metabolism, influence of exercise or activity, medications taken, substances used (e.g., alcohol or illicit drugs), and types of fluids consumed. The estimated energy requirement (EER) is 2000 to 3000 calories per day for healthy adult men and 1600 to 2400 calories per day for healthy adult women (Office of Disease and Health Promotion, 2020). The caloric requirement may decrease if a patient needs to lose weight or increase if the patient needs to gain weight or promote healing.

NUTRITION STANDARDS FOR HEALTH PROMOTION AND MAINTENANCE

Current focuses on *nutrition* are targeted toward health promotion and the prevention of disease by healthy eating and exercise. **Dietary reference intakes (DRIs)** based on age, gender, and life stage serve as a *nutrition* guide for more than 40 nutrients that provides a scientific basis for food guidelines in the United States and Canada (National Academies of Sciences, Engineering, & Medicine, 2020). In the United States, the *Dietary*

Guidelines for Americans are revised by the U.S. Department of Agriculture (USDA) and the U.S. Department of Health and Human Services (DHHS) every 5 years. Examples of the *2015-2020 Guidelines* (8th edition) are listed in Table 55.1. At time of publication, the *2020-2025 Dietary Guidelines for Americans* are being developed based on collected evidence in the Scientific Report of the 2020 Dietary Guidelines Advisory Committee (Dietary Guidelines for Americans, 2020).

"Start Simple with MyPlate" is an initiative that reminds users about health eating styles that are built into a lifestyle (U.S. Department of Agriculture, n.d.) (Fig. 55.1). This pictorial demonstrates how to build a healthy plate of food consisting of the right proportions of fruits, vegetables, grains, proteins, and dairy products. Canada publishes Canada's Food Guide (Government of Canada, 2020), a similar visual reference.

Common Diets

Given the variance in people's preferences, place of residence, availability of foods, financial means, cultural or spiritual observations, and financial circumstances, there is not a specific "typical (or common) diet." Some people consume a highly nutrient-rich diet and remain adequately hydrated with water. Others eat excess foods heavy in fats or carbohydrates and choose to drink soda or juice on a regular basis, which can lead to obesity. Others do not have adequate access to nutrient-dense food and hydration and may experience undernutrition. Individuals with obesity or undernutrition both experience malnutrition in different ways, as the state of malnutrition occurs on a continuum.

In ideal circumstances, patients should consume a diet containing complex carbohydrates, lean proteins, and monounsaturated or polyunsaturated fats that also contains necessary vitamins and minerals. The specific foods you recommend to patients to meet their nutrition needs depends on the variances mentioned earlier.

Some adults follow vegetarian diet patterns for health, environmental, religious, cultural, or spiritual reasons (Box 55.1).

People who eat a vegan diet can develop anemia as a result of vitamin B_{12} deficiency. Teach them to include a daily source of vitamin B_{12} in their diets, such as a fortified breakfast cereal, fortified soy beverage, or meat substitute. Refer those interested in vegetarianism to www.eatright.org, which contains many credible resources regarding vegetarian health (Academy of Nutrition and Dietetics (2018).

TABLE 55.1 Examples of *2015–2020 Dietary Guidelines for Americans*

- Follow a healthy eating pattern across the lifespan.
- Focus on variety, nutrient density, and amount.
- Limit calories from added sugars and saturated fats and reduce sodium intake.
- Shift to healthier food and beverage choices.
- Support healthy eating patterns for all.

From *Dietary Guidelines for Americans 2015-2020* (8th ed.). (2015). http://health.gov/dietaryguidelines/2015/resources/2015-2020_Dietary_Guidelines.pdf.

PATIENT-CENTERED CARE: CULTURAL/ SPIRITUAL CONSIDERATIONS (QSEN)

Many adults have specific food preferences based on their ethnicity or race. Health teaching about **nutrition** should incorporate any cultural preferences voiced by the patient. However, *never assume that a patient eats only foods associated with his or her primary ethnicity.*

FOOD SENSITIVITIES

Some adults have food allergies or intolerances. A true food allergy differs from an intolerance in the sense that an allergy to a food can cause life-threatening complications like anaphylaxis. A food allergy is rooted in the immune system. The most common food allergies are milk, chocolate, eggs, soy, wheat, tree nuts, peanuts, and shellfish (McCance et al., 2019). A food intolerance involves the gastrointestinal system and occurs when the system cannot properly break down food (American Academy of Allergy, Asthma, and Immunology, 2020).

An example of a food allergy is shellfish, which can cause coughing; edema (face, lips, tongue, throat); shortness of breath;

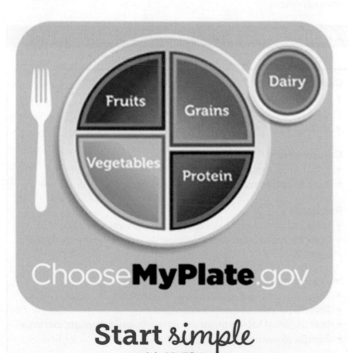

Fig. 55.1 The U.S. Department of Agriculture MyPlate. (From U.S. Department of Agriculture, 2020, www.ChooseMyPlate.gov.)

BOX 55.1 Vegetarian Types

Lacto-vegetarian—allows dairy[a]; avoids meat, poultry, seafood, eggs, and foods that contain those items

Ovo-vegetarian—allows eggs; avoids meat, poultry, seafood, and dairy[a]

Lacto-ovo vegetarian—allows eggs and dairy[a]; avoids meat, poultry, seafood

Pescatarian—allows seafood; avoids meat, poultry, dairy,[a] eggs

Vegan—consumes a plant-based diet only; avoids meat, poultry, seafood, dairy,[a] and eggs, and foods that contain those items (note = some vegans also avoid honey)

[a]Dairy = milk, cheese, yogurt, butter, etc.

or anaphylaxis in certain patients. An example of a food intolerance is lactose intolerance, in which a patient has an inadequate amount of the lactase enzyme, which converts lactose into absorbable glucose. Ingesting a milk product causes bloating, diarrhea, abdominal discomfort, and flatulence. When taking a history, ask patients specifically what kind of reaction they have to certain foods; document and plan care accordingly.

 PATIENT-CENTERED CARE: OLDER ADULT CONSIDERATIONS (QSEN)

The USDA (2015) recommends that older adults drink eight glasses of water a day and eat plenty of fiber to prevent or manage constipation. It also suggests daily calcium and vitamins D and B_{12} supplements and a reduction in sodium and cholesterol-containing foods.

NUTRITION ASSESSMENT

Nutrition status reflects the balance between nutrient requirements and intake. Evaluation of nutrition status is an important part of total patient assessment and includes:

- Review of the nutrition history
- Food and fluid intake record
- Notation of access to appropriate sources of nutrition
- Laboratory data
- Food-drug interactions
- Health history and physical assessment
- Anthropometric measurements
- Psychosocial assessment

Monitor the *nutrition* status of a patient during hospitalization as an important part of your initial assessment. Collaborate with the interprofessional health care team to identify patients at risk for nutrition problems.

Initial Nutrition Screening

The Joint Commission Patient Care Standards require that a nutrition screening occur within 24 hours of the patient's hospital admission, with a full nutrition assessment for patients identified as being at risk. The initial screening includes inspection, measured height and weight, weight history, usual eating habits, ability to chew and swallow, and any recent changes in appetite or food intake. The Full MNA® Form (Mini Nutrition Assessment) (Fig. 55.2) is a helpful and brief screening tool that can assist in identifying older adults who are malnourished or at risk for undernutrition. An even shorter version—the MNA®, which refers to the Mini Nutrition Assessment–Short Form (formerly the MNA®-SF) (Nestle Nutrition Institute, n.d.)—is also available for use in the clinical setting. See the Best Practice for Patient Safety & Quality Care: Nutrition Screening Assessment box for examples of questions to consider as part of the initial assessment.

Anthropometric Measurements

Anthropometric measurements are noninvasive methods of evaluating *nutrition* status. These measurements include obtaining height and weight and assessment of BMI. You may delegate the task of obtaining height and weight to assistive personnel (AP) under your supervision, as this is within their scope. Be sure to instruct the AP to follow up with measurements as soon as this activity is completed, as this information affects the plan of care.

Obtaining accurate measurements is important because patients tend to overestimate height and underestimate weight. Measurements taken days or weeks later may indicate an early change in nutrition status. Follow agency policy or the primary health care provider's orders for frequency of measurement.

BEST PRACTICE FOR PATIENT SAFETY & QUALITY CARE (QSEN)
Nutrition Screening Assessment

General
- Does the patient have conditions that cause nutrient loss (e.g., malabsorption syndromes, wounds, prolonged diarrhea)
- Does the patient have conditions that increase the need for nutrients (e.g., fever, burns, injury)
- Has the patient been NPO for 3 days or more?
- Is the patient receiving a modified diet or a diet restricted in one or more nutrients?
- Is the patient being enterally or parenterally fed?
- Does the patient describe food allergies, lactose intolerance, or limited food preferences?
- Has the patient experienced a recent unexplained weight loss?
- Is the patient on drug therapy, including prescription, over-the-counter, or herbal/natural products?

Gastrointestinal
- Does the patient have glossitis, stomatitis, or esophagitis?
- Does the patient have difficulty chewing or swallowing or have poor dentition?
- Does the patient have a partial or total GI obstruction?
- Does the patient report nausea, indigestion, vomiting, diarrhea, or constipation?
- Does the patient have an ostomy?

Cardiovascular
- Does the patient have ascites or edema?
- Is the patient able to perform ADLs?
- Does the patient have heart failure?

Genitourinary
- Is fluid intake about equal to fluid output?
- Is the patient hemodialyzed or peritoneally dialyzed?

Respiratory
- Is the patient receiving oxygen or on mechanical ventilatory support?
- Does the patient have chronic obstructive pulmonary disease (COPD) or asthma?

Integumentary
- Does the patient have abnormal nail or hair changes?
- Does the patient have rashes or dermatitis?
- Does the patient have dry or pale mucous membranes or decreased skin turgor?
- Does the patient have pressure injuries?

Musculoskeletal
- Does the patient have cachexia?

Modified Courtesy Ross Products Division, Abbott Laboratories, Columbus, OH.

Mini Nutritional Assessment
MNA®

Nestlé NutritionInstitute

Last name: _____   First name: _____

Sex: _____ Age: _____ Weight, kg: _____ Height, cm: _____ Date: _____

Complete the screen by filling in the boxes with the appropriate numbers.
Add the numbers for the screen. If score is 11 or less, continue with the assessment to gain a Malnutrition Indicator Score.

Screening

A Has food intake declined over the past 3 months due to loss of appetite, digestive problems, chewing or swallowing difficulties?
0 = severe decrease in food intake
1 = moderate decrease in food intake
2 = no decrease in food intake ☐

B Weight loss during the last 3 months
0 = weight loss greater than 3kg (6.6lbs)
1 = does not know
2 = weight loss between 1 and 3kg (2.2 and 6.6 lbs)
3 = no weight loss ☐

C Mobility
0 = bed or chair bound
1 = able to get out of bed / chair but does not go out
2 = goes out ☐

D Has suffered psychological stress or acute disease in the past 3 months?
0 = yes   2 = no ☐

E Neuropsychological problems
0 = severe dementia or depression
1 = mild dementia
2 = no psychological problems ☐

F Body Mass Index (BMI) = weight in kg / (height in m)^2
0 = BMI less than 19
1 = BMI 19 to less than 21
2 = BMI 21 to less than 23
3 = BMI 23 or greater ☐

Screening score (subtotal max. 14 points) ☐☐
12-14 points: Normal nutritional status
8-11 points: At risk of malnutrition
0-7 points: Malnourished

For a more in-depth assessment, continue with questions G-R

Assessment

G Lives independently (not in nursing home or hospital)
1 = yes   0 = no ☐

H Takes more than 3 prescription drugs per day
0 = yes   1 = no ☐

I Pressure sores or skin ulcers
0 = yes   1 = no ☐

J How many full meals does the patient eat daily?
0 = 1 meal
1 = 2 meals
2 = 3 meals ☐

K Selected consumption markers for protein intake
- At least one serving of dairy products (milk, cheese, yoghurt) per day   yes ☐ no ☐
- Two or more servings of legumes or eggs per week   yes ☐ no ☐
- Meat, fish or poultry every day   yes ☐ no ☐
0.0 = if 0 or 1 yes
0.5 = if 2 yes
1.0 = if 3 yes ☐.☐

L Consumes two or more servings of fruit or vegetables per day?
0 = no   1 = yes ☐

M How much fluid (water, juice, coffee, tea, milk...) is consumed per day?
0.0 = less than 3 cups
0.5 = 3 to 5 cups
1.0 = more than 5 cups ☐.☐

N Mode of feeding
0 = unable to eat without assistance
1 = self-fed with some difficulty
2 = self-fed without any problem ☐

O Self view of nutritional status
0 = views self as being malnourished
1 = is uncertain of nutritional state
2 = views self as having no nutritional problem ☐

P In comparison with other people of the same age, how does the patient consider his / her health status?
0.0 = not as good
0.5 = does not know
1.0 = as good
2.0 = better ☐.☐

Q Mid-arm circumference (MAC) in cm
0.0 = MAC less than 21
0.5 = MAC 21 to 22
1.0 = MAC greater than 22 ☐.☐

R Calf circumference (CC) in cm
0 = CC less than 31
1 = CC 31 or greater ☐

Assessment (max. 16 points) ☐☐.☐
Screening score ☐☐.☐
Total Assessment (max. 30 points) ☐☐.☐

Malnutrition Indicator Score
24 to 30 points ☐   Normal nutritional status
17 to 23.5 points ☐   At risk of malnutrition
Less than 17 points ☐   Malnourished

References
1. Vellas B, Villars H, Abellan G, *et al.* Overview of the MNA® - Its History and Challenges. *J Nutr Health Aging*. 2006; **10**:456-465.
2. Rubenstein LZ, Harker JO, Salva A, Guigoz Y, Vellas B. Screening for Undernutrition in Geriatric Practice: Developing the Short-Form Mini Nutritional Assessment (MNA-SF). *J. Geront*. 2001; **56A**: M366-377
3. Guigoz Y. The Mini-Nutritional Assessment (MNA®) Review of the Literature - What does it tell us? *J Nutr Health Aging*. 2006; **10**:466-487.

For more information: www.mna-elderly.com

Fig. 55.2 Full MNA® Form (Mini Nutrition Assessment). (Société des Produits Nestlé S.A., Vevey, Switzerland, Trademark Owners.)

Measure and weigh patients with the same scale and with the same amount of clothing (without shoes) each time. A sliding-blade **knee height caliper,** which uses the distance between the patient's patella and heel to estimate height, can be used for those who cannot stand. It is especially useful for patients who have knee or hip contractures.

The type of scale used depends on the patient's ability to stand or sit; wheelchairs scales or bed scales can be used for nonambulatory individuals. When using a bed scale, document the number of sheets, pillows, and blankets on the bed at the time of measurement. Lines, devices, and equipment should be lifted off the bed when the measurement is taking place. Normal weights for adult men and women are available from several reference standards, such as the Metropolitan Life tables. Online calculators are also available to calculate ideal body weight. *An unintentional weight loss of 5% in a month or 10% over a 6-month period significantly affects* **nutrition** *status and should be evaluated.*

> **! NURSING SAFETY PRIORITY** (QSEN)
>
> ### Action Alert
>
> Obtain weight at the same time each day, if possible, preferably before breakfast. Conditions such as heart failure and renal disease cause weight gain; dehydration and conditions such as cancer cause weight loss. *Weight is the most reliable indicator of fluid gain or loss!*

Assessment of body fat is usually calculated by the registered dietitian nutritionist (RDN) if in a hospital setting or by a fitness trainer or physical therapist in the community setting. The **body mass index (BMI)** indirectly estimates total fat stores within the body by the relationship of weight to height (Table 55.2). *Therefore an accurate height is as important as an accurate weight.* Online calculators can perform this computation, which divides a patient's weight in kilograms by the square of height in meters. The least risk for malnutrition is associated with scores between 18.5 and 24.9. BMIs above and below these values are associated with increased health risks (CDC, 2020a).

Limitations of BMI calculations include (Schnur, 2017, in Smith, 2019):

- Overestimation of amount of body fat in physically fit, athletic, or muscular patients
- Underestimation of body fat levels in older adults, active adults, and neurologically impaired individuals with decreased muscle mass
- Underestimated morbidity and obesity risk in Asian populations

> **👤 PATIENT-CENTERED CARE: OLDER ADULT CONSIDERATIONS** (QSEN)
>
> Body weight and BMI usually increase throughout adulthood until about 60 years of age. As some adults get older, they often become less hungry and eat less, even if they are healthy. Others continue usual eating patterns and are at higher risk for obesity—especially older adult females (CDC, 2020a). Do not assume that an older adult automatically eats less; personalize the nutrition assessment to accurately assess eating patterns for every patient.

TABLE 55.2	Body Mass Index (BMI) Ranges
BMI	**Weight Status**
Below 18.5	Underweight
18.5-24.9	Normal or healthy weight
25.0-29.9	Overweight
30.0 and above	Obese

From Centers for Disease Control and Prevention (CDC). (2020b). Defining adult overweight and obesity. https://www.cdc.gov/obesity/adult/defining.html.

TABLE 55.3	Calculated BSA Averages for Adults According to Age	
Age (yr)	**Average BSA (m²) for Males in United States, Rounded to Nearest Hundredth**	**Average BSA (m²) for Females in United States, Rounded to Nearest Hundredth**
20 and older (average)	2.09	1.86
20-39	2.09	1.85
40-59	2.11	1.90
60 and older	2.06	1.83

From Fryar, C.D., Kruszon-Moran, D., Gu, Q., & Ogden, C. L. (2018). Mean body weight, height, waist circumference, and body mass index among adults: United States, 1999–2000 through 2015–2016. National Health Statistics Reports; no 122. Hyattsville, MD: National Center for Health Statistics.

> **NCLEX EXAMINATION CHALLENGE 55.1**
>
> ### Health Promotion and Maintenance
>
> An older adult is admitted to the hospital. The client's height is 5 feet, 6 inches (1.68 m), and weight is 250 lb (113.3 kg). The nurse calculates the client's current body mass index (BMI) as _____. **Fill in the blank. Round your answer to the nearest whole number.**

Body surface area (BSA) (Table 55.3) is an estimate of a patient's total body surface area calculated as a biometric two-dimensional measure of a person's body size (Schnur, 2017, in Smith, 2019). It reflects physiologic and metabolic processes, included heat exchange, blood volume, and size of vital organs (Weinstein & Hagle, 2014). BSA can be used as an indicator for appropriate dosage calculation for medication and IV administration, especially for anticancer agents (Eaton and Lyman, 2019).

BSA is calculated in meters squared, combining a patient's weight and height and reflecting an estimate of their total surface (outside body layer) area (Faisal et al., 2016). If a patient has a BSA of 3 m², it means that their skin surface could be placed into a 3-meter × 3-meter box.

Calculate BSA by the Mosteller formula, which takes the square root of the height in centimeters, multiplied by the weight in kilograms, divided by 3600. The average BSA is 2.09 m² for males and 1.86 m² for females (Fryar et al., 2018). Be aware that accurate calculation of weight is imperative, as height is unlikely to change significantly, but weight is variable.

TABLE 55.4 Common Complications of Undernutrition

Cardiovascular	**Integumentary**
• Reduced cardiac output	• Dry, flaky skin
Endocrine	• Various types of dermatitis
• Cold intolerance	• Poor wound healing
Gastrointestinal	**Musculoskeletal**
• Anorexia	• Cachexia
• Diarrhea	• Decreased activity tolerance
• Impaired protein synthesis	• Decreased muscle mass
• Malabsorption	• Impaired functional ability
• Vomiting	**Neurologic**
• Weight loss	• Weakness
Immunologic	**Psychiatric**
• Susceptibility to infectious disease	• Substance misuse
	Respiratory
	• Reduced vital capacity

Skinfold measurements estimate body fat. The *triceps and subscapular* skinfolds are most commonly measured with a special caliper. Both are compared with standard measurements and recorded as percentiles. The *midarm circumference (MAC) and calf circumference (CC)* are needed if the MNA-SF tool is used. Place a flexible tape around the upper arm (or calf) at the midpoint; wrap gently to avoid compressing the tissue, and record the findings in centimeters in the electronic health record.

✴ NUTRITION CONCEPT EXEMPLAR: UNDERNUTRITION

Pathophysiology Review

Undernutrition is a multinutrient problem. If a patient does not, or cannot, consume calories and protein, he or she also misses intake of other healthy nutrients. Inadequate nutrient intake can also result when an adult is admitted to the hospital or long-term care facility. For example, decreased staffing may not allow time for patients who need to be fed, especially older adults, who may eat slowly. Many diagnostic tests, surgery, trauma, and unexpected medical complications require a period of NPO in which nutrients are not being consumed or cause **anorexia** (loss of appetite). See Table 55.4 for common complications of undernutrition and Table 55.5 for common signs and symptoms of nutrient deficiencies.

> **PATIENT-CENTERED CARE: CULTURAL/SPIRITUAL CONSIDERATIONS** (QSEN)
>
> In some cases, undernutrition results when meals provided in the health care setting differ from what the patient usually eats. Be sure to identify specific food preferences that the patient can eat and enjoy that are in keeping with his or her cultural practices.

Protein-energy undernutrition (PEU), formerly protein-calorie malnutrition (PCM), has three common forms (Morley, 2020):

• **Marasmus**: A calorie malnutrition in which body fat and protein are wasted. Serum proteins are often preserved.

• **Kwashiorkor**: A lack of protein quantity and quality in the presence of adequate calories. Body weight is more normal, and serum proteins are low.

• **Starvation**: A complete lack of nutrients. This problem can occur even when food is available but is most commonly seen in areas in which food is unavailable (e.g., during a time of famine or exposure to the elements).

Unrecognized or untreated PEU can lead to dysfunction or disability and increased morbidity and mortality.

Acute PEU may develop in patients who were adequately nourished before hospitalization but experience starvation while in a catabolic state from infection, stress, or injury. *Chronic* PEU can occur in those who have a chronic health condition such as cancer, end-stage kidney or liver disease, or chronic neurologic disease.

Eating disorders such as anorexia nervosa, bulimia nervosa, and binge eating disorder, which are seen most often in teens and young adults, can also lead to a state of undernutrition. **Anorexia nervosa** is a self-induced state of starvation resulting from a fear of fatness, even though the patient is underweight. This condition is often accompanied by a psychiatric diagnosis of *body dysmorphic disorder* (BDD). BDD is an obsessive-compulsive condition

> **PATIENT-CENTERED CARE: OLDER ADULT CONSIDERATIONS** (QSEN)
>
> Older adults are most at risk for poor **nutrition**, especially PEU. Risk factors include physiologic changes of aging, environmental factors, and health problems. See the Focused Assessment: Assessing for Undernutrition in the Older Adult box, which lists some of these major factors for which you will assess. If psychosocial concerns are present, collaborate with mental health and/or social work professionals who can assist. Chapter 4 discusses nutrition for older adults in more detail.

> **FOCUSED ASSESSMENT**
>
> ### Assessing for Undernutrition in the Older Adult
>
> **Physical Concerns**
> • Chronic conditions/illnesses
> • Constipation
> • Decreased appetite
> • Dentition—poor dental health; poor-fitting dentures; lack of teeth or dentures
> • Drugs—prescription and OTC drugs that may impair taste or appetite
> • Dry mouth
> • "Failure to thrive" (a combination of three of five symptoms, including weakness, slow walking speed, low physical activity, unintentional weight loss, exhaustion)
> • Impaired eyesight
> • Pain that is acute or persistent
> • Weight loss
>
> **Psychosocial Concerns**
> • Ability (or inability) to prepare meals due to functional decline, fatigue, memory
> • Decrease in enjoyment of meals
> • Depression
> • Income (ability to afford food)
> • Loneliness
> • Transportation access

INTERPROFESSIONAL COLLABORATION

Care of Older Adults at Risk for Undernutrition

For older adults with undernutrition, or at risk for undernutrition, assess for psychosocial concerns that can impact their desire or ability to consumer nutrient-rich foods. If any of these concerns is rooted in mental health, such as depression or loneliness, collaborate with a mental health professional, such as a counselor or psychiatric-mental health nurse practitioner who can work with the patient to enhance his or her emotional well-being. If the concerns are economic or access-related, collaborate with the case manager or social worker who can help identify ways to facilitate better access to sources of nutrition. According to the Interprofessional Education Collaborative (IPEC) Expert Panel's Competency of Roles and Responsibilities, using the unique and complimentary abilities of other team members optimizes health and patient care (IPEC, 2016; Slusser et al., 2019).

in which a patient spends an abnormal amount of time attempting to reach what he or she considers to be body perfection. In the case of a patient with anorexia nervosa, perfection is found in being thin. The condition affects the patient's ability to carry out normal ADLs and significantly impacts quality of life (Perkins, 2019). If this condition is suspected, collaborate with the primary health care provider to determine if a psychiatric consultation is needed. **Bulimia nervosa** is characterized by episodes of binge eating in which the patient ingests a large amount of food in a short time. The binge eating is followed by some form of purging behavior, such as self-induced vomiting or excessive use of laxatives and diuretics. If not treated, death can result from starvation, infection, or suicide. **Binge eating disorder** is a separate psychiatric diagnosis from bulimia nervosa. It resembles bulimia nervosa in terms of binge-eating episodes, and it involves a feeling of loss of control over the eating behavior (Kelly-Weeder et al., 2019); however, it is not accompanied by purging. Again, collaborate with the primary health care provider if this condition is suspected. Further information about eating disorders can be found in mental health nursing textbooks.

Health Promotion and Maintenance. It is estimated that 5% of hospitalized patients are diagnosed with undernutrition (Tolbert et al., 2018). This may be related to prehospitalization status, or due to lack of *nutrition* during a current illness or an injury. Malnourishment can increase length of stay and also be cause for readmission. Nurses can have a significant impact on patient length of stay when adequately advocating for the patient's nutrition status. (See the Systems Thinking and Quality Improvement box.)

 INTERPROFESSIONAL COLLABORATION

Care of Patients With Undernutrition

For patients with undernutrition, consult with a registered dietician nutritionist (RDN) who can assist with meeting nutritional needs while the patient is hospitalized, as well as help with planning for continued nutrition health after discharge. According to the Interprofessional Education Collaborative (IPEC) Expert Panel's Competency of Roles and Responsibilities, using the unique and complementary abilities of other team members optimizes health and patient care (IPEC, 2016; Slusser et al., 2019).

TABLE 55.5 Signs and Symptoms of Nutrient Deficiencies

Sign/Symptom	Potential Nutrient Deficiency
Hair	
Alopecia	Zinc
Easy to remove	Protein
Lackluster hair	Protein
"Corkscrew" hair	Vitamin C
Decreased pigmentation	Protein
Eyes	
Dryness of conjunctiva	Vitamin A
Corneal vascularization	Riboflavin
Keratomalacia	Vitamin A
Bitot spots	Vitamin A
GI Tract	
Nausea, vomiting	Pyridoxine
Diarrhea	Zinc, niacin
Stomatitis	Pyridoxine, riboflavin, iron
Cheilosis	Pyridoxine, iron
Glossitis	Pyridoxine, zinc, niacin, folic acid, vitamin B$_{12}$
Magenta tongue	Vitamin A, riboflavin
Swollen, bleeding gums	Vitamin C
Fissured tongue	Niacin
Hepatomegaly	Protein
Skin	
Dry and scaling	Vitamin A
Petechiae/ecchymoses	Vitamin C
Follicular hyperkeratosis	Vitamin A
Nasolabial seborrhea	Niacin
Bilateral dermatitis	Niacin
Musculoskeletal	
Subcutaneous fat loss	Calories
Muscle wastage	Calories, protein
Edema	Protein
Osteomalacia, bone pain, rickets	Vitamin D
Hematologic	
Anemia	Vitamin B$_{12}$, iron, folic acid, copper, vitamin E
Leukopenia, neutropenia	Copper
Low prothrombin time, prolonged clotting time	Vitamin K, manganese
Neurologic	
Disorientation	Niacin, thiamine
Confabulation	Thiamine
Neuropathy	Thiamine, pyridoxine, chromium
Paresthesia	Thiamine, pyridoxine, vitamin B$_{12}$
Cardiovascular	
Heart failure, cardiomegaly, tachycardia	Thiamine
Cardiomyopathy	Selenium
Cardiac dysrhythmias	Magnesium

Courtesy Ross Products Division, Abbott Laboratories, Columbus, OH.

SYSTEMS THINKING AND QUALITY IMPROVEMENT (QSEN)

An Interprofessional Focus on Preventing Readmissions for Patients at High Risk for Malnutrition

Beckett, C., & Walsh, S. (2019). The malnutrition readmission prevention protocol. *American Journal of Nursing, 119*(12):60–64.

Reflecting on the fact that malnutrition affects one in three hospitalized patients, the authors of this study desired to put an evidence-based protocol in place to improve patient outcomes and avoid reduced reimbursement associated with 30-day malnutrition-related readmissions. Nurses, the clinical manager of nutrition services, physicians, care coordination staff, physical therapists, quality staff, and informatics experts were tasked together as an interprofessional team to address high hospital readmission rates due to patient malnourishment.

After a comprehensive review of evidence was accomplished, the team developed the evidence-based Malnutrition Readmission Prevention Protocol, which identifies three stages of risk for malnutrition. The Protocol was used first in one facility and then implemented across a hospital system. Informatics specialists worked to create automatic alerts within the electronic health record to flag health care professionals to use the Protocol. Using this tool, patients were identified for inpatient management of nutritional supplementation, and then referral to a registered dietician nutritionist (RDN) was made. The RDN coordinated availability of 30-day supplementation to be used in the home environment following discharge. An important part of Protocol use was involving the patient (and caregiver, as appropriate) in conversations regarding inpatient and outpatient nutrition management. Follow-up calls were made by care management nurses; home visits were conducted by paramedics; and primary care providers were notified to coordinate care after discharge.

Over a 5-year period, readmissions due to malnutrition decreased from 42% to 13.3%.

Commentary: Implications for Practice and Research

Coordinating an effort where all professions involved in patient care had input into the Protocol well before implementation facilitated a collaborative effort created with best practice and favorable patient outcomes in mind. Using the Protocol together, meeting the patient's nutrition needs in the inpatient and outpatient settings greatly decreased the readmission rate related to malnutrition. Working together facilitates better outcomes when all stakeholders, including the patient and caregiver, are involved in care processes and planning.

Incidence and Prevalence. Estimates show that 6% of outpatients, 22% of hospitalized patients, and 23.1% of patients living in an extended care facility and 29.4% of patients temporarily staying in a rehabilitation setting are undernourished (Cereda et al., 2016, in Ritchie & Yukawa, 2019).

❖ Interprofessional Collaborative Care

Care for the patient with undernutrition takes place in a variety of settings, such as the home, the community, and the hospital setting if more comprehensive management is needed.

◆ Assessment: Recognize Cues

History. See the earlier Best Practice for Patient Safety & Quality Care: Nutrition Screening Assessment box to complete the initial history. For older adults, also see the Focused Assessment: Assessing for Undernutrition in the Older Adult

box. In collaboration with the registered dietitian nutritionist (RDN), also obtain information about the patient's:

- Usual daily food intake and timing of eating
- Food preferences (including cultural considerations)
- Eating behaviors/patterns
- Change in appetite
- Recent weight changes
- Economic status that may influence access to, or purchase of, food

A full *nutrition* history usually includes a 24-hour recall of food intake and the frequency with which foods are consumed. The adequacy of the diet can be evaluated by comparing the amount and types of foods consumed daily with the established standards. The registered dietitian nutritionist (RDN) then provides a more detailed analysis of nutrition intake. Be aware that patients who live in food deserts (i.e., urban areas where fresh, healthy food is in low supply or unaffordable) may have difficulty obtaining food that is densely nutritious. Also remember that an unintentional weight loss of 5% in 30 days, or 10% over a 6-month period, significantly affects *nutrition* status and should be further evaluated.

> ### ❗ NURSING SAFETY PRIORITY (QSEN)
> #### Action Alert
>
> Assess for difficulty or pain chewing or swallowing. Unrecognized dysphagia is a common problem among older adults and can cause undernutrition, dehydration, and aspiration pneumonia. See Chapter 49 for more information.

Physical Assessment/Signs and Symptoms. Assess for signs and symptoms of various nutrient deficiencies (see Table 55.5). Inspect hair, eyes, oral cavity, nails, and musculoskeletal and neurologic systems. Examine the condition of the skin, including any reddened or open areas. Anthropometric measurements may also be obtained. Monitors all food and fluid intake. A 3-day caloric intake may be collected and then calculated by the registered dietitian nutritionist (RDN). Delegate this activity to assistive personnel (AP) under your ongoing supervision, and direct AP to report the intake and output values back after obtaining them. Ask AP to report any signs of choking while the patient eats. Document the presence of mouth pain, difficulty chewing, nausea, vomiting, heartburn, or any other symptoms of discomfort with eating.

Psychosocial Assessment. The psychosocial history provides information about the patient's economic status, occupation, educational level, ethnicity/race, living and cooking arrangements, and emotional status. Determine whether financial resources are adequate for providing the necessary food. If resources are inadequate, the social worker or case manager may refer the patient and caregiver to available community services.

Laboratory Assessment. Interpret laboratory data carefully with regard to the total patient; focusing on an isolated value may yield an inaccurate conclusion. In general, laboratory values that may be decreased in the presence of undernourishment include (Pagana & Pagana, 2018):

- Cholesterol
- Hemoglobin

- Hematocrit
- Serum albumin
- Thyroxine-binding prealbumin (PAB)
- Transferrin

◆ **Analysis: Analyze Cues and Prioritize Hypothesis.** The priority collaborative problem for the patient with undernutrition is:
1. Weight loss due to inability to access, ingest or digest food, or absorb nutrients

◆ **Planning and Implementation: Generate Solutions and Take Action**

Improving Nutrition

Planning: Expected Outcomes. The patient with undernutrition is expected to have nutrients available to meet his or her metabolic needs.

Interventions. The preferred route for food intake is orally through the GI tract because it enhances the immune system, is safer, easier, less expensive, and more enjoyable.

Meal Management. Following the primary health care provider's and RDN's recommendation, provide high-calorie, nutrient-rich foods (e.g., milkshakes, cheese, supplement drinks such as Boost or Ensure). A feeding schedule of six small meals may be tolerated better than three large ones. A pureed or dental soft diet may be easier for those who have problems chewing or do not have teeth. Follow recommendations in the Best Practice for Patient Safety & Quality Care: Promoting Nutrition Intake box to provide a more enjoyable and productive eating experience for patients with undernutrition.

BEST PRACTICE FOR PATIENT SAFETY & QUALITY CARE (QSEN)

Promoting Nutrition Intake

Environment
- Remove bedpans, urinals, and emesis basins from the environment.
- Eliminate or decrease offensive odors as much as possible.
- Decrease environmental distractions as much as possible.
- Administer pain medication and/or antiemetics for nausea at least 1 hour before mealtime.

Comfort
- Allow the patient to toilet before mealtime.
- Provide mouth care before mealtime.
- Ensure that eyeglasses and hearing aids in place, if appropriate, during meals.
- Remind assistive personnel (AP) to have patient sit in a chair, if possible, at mealtime.

Function
- Ensure that meals are visually appealing, appetizing, and at appropriate temperatures.
- If needed, open cartons and packages and cut up food.
- Observe during meals for food intake, and document the percentage consumed.
- Encourage self-feeding (if able) or feed the patient slowly (delegate to AP, if desired).
- Eliminate or minimize interruptions during mealtime for nonurgent procedures or rounds.

Nutrition Supplements. If the patient cannot take in enough nutrients in food, fortified medical nutrition supplements (MNSs) (e.g., Ensure, Sustacal, Carnation Instant Breakfast [also available as a lactose-free supplement]) may be given, especially to older adults. For patients with liver and renal disease or diabetes, special products that meet these needs are available (e.g., Glucerna for patients with diabetes).

Nutrition supplements are supplied as liquid formulas, powders, soups, coffee, and puddings in a variety of flavors. Examples include Duocal for carbohydrates and fats, and Resource Beneprotein for protein. Follow the primary health care provider's prescription for nutrition supplementation.

Drug Therapy. Multivitamins, zinc, and an iron preparation are often prescribed to treat or prevent anemia in patients who are malnourished. Monitor the patient's hemoglobin and hematocrit levels for efficacy of treatment, and assess for side effects. For example, iron can cause constipation, and zinc can cause nausea and vomiting.

Total Enteral Nutrition. If a patient cannot achieve adequate *nutrition* via oral intake, total enteral nutrition (TEN) may be needed. Enteral tube feedings may be necessary to supplement oral intake or to provide total nutrition.

Patients likely to receive TEN can be divided into three groups:
- Those who can eat but cannot maintain adequate *nutrition* by oral intake of food alone
- Those with permanent neuromuscular impairment who cannot swallow
- Those who do not have permanent neuromuscular impairment but cannot eat because of their condition

Patients in the first group are often older adults or patients receiving cancer treatment. In some cases, artificial nutrition and hydration may not be desired. Check for advance directives stating whether the patient desires artificial nutrition and hydration if certain conditions exist. Legal and ethical questions often arise when patients do not have existing advance directives, are not able to make their wishes known, and do not have a designated durable power of attorney. *The decision to feed or not to feed is complex, and there is no clear right or wrong answer.* See the Ethical/Legal Considerations box for more information.

ETHICAL/LEGAL CONSIDERATIONS

Decisions about legal/ethical situations regarding feeding benefit from advice of interprofessional ethics committees in health care facilities. When clinicians are making decisions about the desirability of tube feedings in these cases, the focus should be on achieving consensus by:
- Reviewing what is known about tube feedings, especially their risks and benefits
- Reviewing the medical facts about the patient
- Investigating any available evidence that would help understand the patient's wishes
- Obtaining the input of all stakeholders in the situation
- Delaying any action until consensus is achieved

Those in the second group of patients likely to receive TEN usually have permanent swallowing problems due to a condition such as brain attack, severe head trauma, or advanced multiple sclerosis. These patients require some type of feeding tube for delivery of the enteral product on a long-term basis.

Patients in the third group receive enteral *nutrition* for as long as their illness lasts. The feeding is discontinued when the patient's condition improves and he or she can eat again.

A therapeutic combination of carbohydrates, fat, vitamins, minerals, and trace elements is available in liquid form. A prescription from the health care provider is required for enteral nutrition, but the RDN usually makes the recommendation and computes the amount and type of product needed for each patient.

NCLEX EXAMINATION CHALLENGE 55.2

Safe and Effective Care Environment

Total enteral nutrition (TEN) has been prescribed for a client with terminal cancer. When the nurse notes that no advanced directives are in place, yet a durable power of attorney exists, what is the appropriate action?

A. Withhold TEN indefinitely

B. Contact the durable power of attorney

C. Begin administration of TEN immediately

D. Turn over care to the interprofessional ethics committee

Methods of administering total enteral nutrition. TEN is administered as a "tube feeding" through a nasoenteric or enterostomal tube. It can be used in the patient's home or any health care setting.

A nasoenteric tube (NET) is a feeding tube inserted nasally and then advanced into the GI tract, such as a Dobbhoff tube. Commonly used NETs include the nasogastric (NG) tube, the smaller (small-bore) nasoduodenal tube (NDT) (Fig. 55.3), and the nasojejunal tube (NJT), which is used less often. All of these types of tubes are used for less than 4 weeks to provide short-term feeding.

Enterostomal feeding tubes are used for patients who need *long-term* enteral feeding. The surgeon directly accesses the GI tract using various surgical, endoscopic, and laparoscopic techniques. Under sedation, a gastrostomy—a stoma created from the abdominal wall into the stomach—is created. Then a percutaneous endoscopic gastrostomy (PEG) or dual-access gastrostomy-jejunostomy (PEG/J) tube (Fig. 55.4) is placed. A

jejunostomy is used for long-term feedings when it is desirable to bypass the stomach, such as with gastric disease, upper GI obstruction, and abnormal gastric or duodenal emptying. This can be accomplished via a direct percutaneous endoscopic jejunostomy (DPEJ) (see Fig. 55.4) (Simoes et al., 2018).

Tube feedings are administered by bolus feeding, continuous feeding, and cyclic feeding. Bolus feeding is an intermittent feeding of a specified amount of enteral product at set intervals during a 24-hour period, typically every 4 hours. This method can be accomplished manually or by infusion through a mechanical pump or controller device. Continuous feeding is similar to IV therapy in that small amounts are continuously infused (by gravity drip or a pump or controller device) over a specified time. Cyclic feeding is the same as continuous feeding except that the infusion is stopped for a specified time in each 24-hour period, usually 6

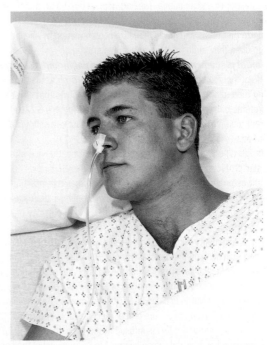

Fig. 55.3 Nasoduodenal tube. (From Lilley, L., Rainforth Collins, S., Harrington, S., & Snyder, J. [2011]. *Pharmacology and the nursing process* [6th ed.]. St. Louis: Mosby.)

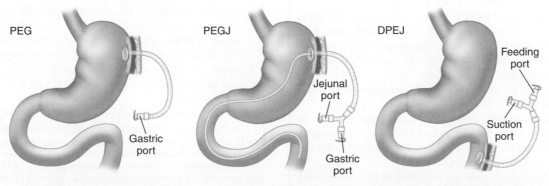

Fig. 55.4 Percutaneous endoscopic gastrostomy (PEG), dual-access gastrostomy-jejunostomy (PEG/J) tube, and direct percutaneous endoscopic jejunostomy (DPEJ). (Redrawn from Zhu, Y., Shi, L., Tang, H., & Tao, G. [2012]. Current considerations of direct percutaneous endoscopic jejunostomy. *Canadian Journal of Gastroenterology 26*[2], 92–96.)

hours or longer ("down time"). Down time typically occurs in the morning to allow bathing, treatments, and other activities. Follow the health care provider's prescription for type, rate, and method of tube feeding, as well as the amount of additional water ("free water") needed. If the patient can swallow small amounts of food, he or she may also eat orally while the tube is in place.

The nurse is responsible for the care and maintenance of the feeding tube and the enteral feeding. See the Best Practice for Patient Safety & Quality Care: Tube-Feeding Care and Maintenance box.

Complications of total enteral nutrition. The nursing priority for care of a patient receiving TEN is safety, which

includes preventing, assessing, and managing complications associated with tube feeding. Some complications of therapy result from the type of tube used to administer the feeding, and others result from the enteral product itself. The most common problem is the development of an obstructed ("clogged") tube. Use the tips in the Best Practice for Patient Safety & Quality Care: Maintaining a Patent Feeding Tube box to maintain tube patency (Drummond Hayes & Drummond Hayes, 2018).

BEST PRACTICE FOR PATIENT SAFETY & QUALITY CARE (QSEN)

Tube-Feeding Care and Maintenance

- If nasogastric or nasoduodenal feeding is prescribed, use a soft, flexible, small-bore feeding tube (smaller than 12 Fr).
- Recognize that tubes with ports minimize contamination by eliminating the need to open the feeding system to administer drugs.
- *The initial placement of the tube should be confirmed by x-ray study* even if another method of confirmation is available, such as electromagnetic feeding tube–placement device (ETPD). Evidence shows that chest x-ray is still preferable to an ETPD (Bourgault et al., 2017; Metheny & Meert, 2017).
- If correct tube placement is ever in question, a chest x-ray should again be performed.
- Secure the tube with tape or a commercial attachment device after applying a skin protectant; change the tape regularly.
- If a gastrostomy or jejunostomy tube is used, assess the insertion site for signs of infection or excoriation (e.g., excessive redness, drainage). Rotate the tube 360 degrees each day and check for in-and-out play of about ¼ inch (0.6 cm).
- Check and document residual volume every 6 hours or per agency policy by aspirating stomach contents into a syringe. If residual feeding is obtained, check with the health care provider for the appropriate intervention (usually to slow or stop the feeding for a time) or consult the American Society of Parenteral and Enteral Nutrition (ASPEN) (2020) best practice recommendations.
- Check the feeding pump to ensure proper mechanical operation.
- Ensure that the enteral product is infused at the prescribed rate (mL/hr).
- Change the feeding bag and tubing every 24 to 48 hours; label the bag with the date and time of the change with your initials. Use an irrigation set for no more than 24 hours.
- For continuous or cyclic feeding, add only 4 hours of product to the bag at a time to prevent bacterial growth. *A closed system is preferred, and each set should be used no longer than 24 hours.*
- Wear clean gloves when changing or opening the feeding system or adding product; wipe the lid of the formula can with clean gauze; wear sterile gloves when caring for patients who are critically ill or immunocompromised.
- Label open cans with date and time opened; cover and keep refrigerated. Discard any unused open cans after 24 hours.
- Do not use blue (or any color) food dye in formula because it can cause serious complications.
- To prevent aspiration, keep the head of the bed elevated at least 30 degrees during the feeding and for at least 1 hour after the feeding for bolus feeding; continuously maintain the semi-Fowler position for patients receiving cyclic or continuous feeding.
- Monitor laboratory values, especially blood urea nitrogen (BUN), serum electrolytes, hematocrit, prealbumin, and glucose.
- Monitor for complications of tube feeding, especially diarrhea.
- Monitor and document the patient's weight and intake and output per the health care provider's order or agency policy.

! NURSING SAFETY PRIORITY (QSEN)

Action Alert

If a gastrostomy or jejunostomy tube cannot be moved while you are performing your regular assessment, notify the health care provider immediately because the retention disk may be embedded in the tissue. Cover the site with a dry, sterile dressing and change the dressing at least once a day.

BEST PRACTICE FOR PATIENT SAFETY & QUALITY CARE (QSEN)

Maintaining a Patent Feeding Tube

- Recognize that a tube occlusion is more easily prevented than corrected.
- Consult with the pharmacist to be sure the prescribed medications are compatible with the enteral *nutrition* formula.
- Consult with the pharmacist to confirm that medications and formula can be cleared from the tube with appropriate flushing.
- Collaborate with the health care provider to use liquid medications instead of crushed tablets when possible, unless the liquid form of medication causes diarrhea.
- Do not mix drugs with the feeding product before giving. Crush tablets as finely as possible and dissolve in warm water. *(Check to see which tablets are safe to crush. For example, do not crush slow-acting [SA] or slow-release [SR] drugs.)*
- Flush the tube with 30 mL of water, using at least a 30-mL syringe to prevent tube rupture:
  - At least every 4 hours
  - Before and after medication administration
  - After any interruption of enteral nutrition
- If the tube becomes clogged, use 30 mL of water for flushing, applying gentle pressure with a 50-mL piston syringe.
- *Do not use* a carbonated beverage or cranberry juice; these have an acidic pH that can worsen the occlusion by causing EN formula proteins to precipitate in the tube.
- Use warm water as the best choice for unclogging.
- Attach a 30- or 60-mL piston syringe to the feeding tube; retract the plunger to facilitate dislodging the clog. Then fill the flush with warm water, reattach it to the tube, and attempt flushing. If continued resistance is experienced, move the plunger gently back and forth. Then clamp the tube to allow the warm water to penetrate the clog for approximately 20 minutes.
- If water does not unclog the tube, an experienced nurse can use an activated pancreatic enzyme solution prescribed by the health care provider, following agency policy.
- As a final attempt, commercially available enzyme declogging kits or devices can be used by an experienced nurse, again following agency policy.
- If unclogging is unsuccessful, replacement of the tube is recommended.

Data from Boullata, J., Carrera, A., Harvey, L., et al. (2017). ASPEN safe practices for enteral nutrition therapy. *Journal of Parenteral and Enteral Nutrition, 41*(1), 15–103; Drummond Hayes, K., & Drummond Hayes, D. (2018). Best practices for unclogging feeding tubes in adults. *Nursing2018, 48*(6), 66; and University of Pittsburgh Medical Center. (2017). University of Pittsburgh Medical Center Presbyterian Shadyside Procedure: Unclogging enteral feeding tubes. Pittsburgh, PA.

Patients receiving TEN are at risk for several other complications, including refeeding syndrome; tube misplacement and dislodgment; abdominal distention and nausea/vomiting; and problems with *fluid and electrolyte balance,* often associated with diarrhea. These problems can be prevented if the patient is monitored carefully and complications are detected early.

Tube misplacement and dislodgment. Misplacement or dislodgment of the tube can cause aspiration and possible death. Immediately remove any tube that you suspect is dislodged! An x-ray is the most accurate confirmation method and should always be done on initial tube insertion. After the initial placement is confirmed, check gastric residual before each intermittent feeding or drug administration, or at least every 6 hours during feeding. Do not rely on traditional methods for checking tube placement such as auscultation; pH testing of GI contents; testing of biochemical markers, such as bilirubin, trypsin, or pepsin; or assessment for carbon dioxide using capnometry (Fan et al., 2017; Hodin & Bordeianou, 2020). Once x-ray confirmation has been made, mark the tube exit point as a baseline for visual re-evaluation of placement at each assessment.

! NURSING SAFETY PRIORITY (QSEN)
Action Alert

If enteral tubes are misplaced or become dislodged, the patient is likely to aspirate. *Aspiration pneumonia is a life-threatening complication associated with TEN, especially for older adults.* Observe for fever and signs of dehydration, such as dry mucous membranes and decreased urinary output. Auscultate lungs every 4 to 8 hours to check for diminishing breath sounds, especially in lower lobes. Patients may become short of breath and report chest discomfort. If a chest x-ray confirms this diagnosis, treatment with antibiotics is started.

Abdominal distention and nausea/vomiting. Abdominal distention, nausea, and vomiting during tube feeding are often caused by overfeeding. To *prevent* overfeeding, check gastric residual volumes every 6 hours, depending on agency policy and patient assessment. If residual feeding is obtained, check with the health care provider for the appropriate intervention (usually to slow or stop the feeding for a time) or consult the American Society of Parenteral and Enteral Nutrition (ASPEN) (2020) best practice recommendations. Follow agency policy regarding holding feeding if necessary. After a period of rest, the feeding can be restarted, usually at a lower flow rate.

Fluid and electrolyte imbalances. Patients receiving enteral nutrition therapy, especially older adults and those with cardiac or renal problems, are at an increased risk for fluid imbalances. Some electrolyte imbalances can be avoided. For example, a renal patient with existing high potassium levels may be prescribed a special formula lower in potassium.

Fluid imbalances associated with enteral nutrition are usually related to the body's response to increased serum osmolarity, but fluid overload from too much tube feeding can also occur. If patients do *not* have normal renal and cardiac function, expansion of the plasma volume can lead to circulatory overload and pulmonary edema, especially in older adults. Assess for signs and symptoms, such as peripheral edema, sudden weight gain, crackles, dyspnea, increased blood pressure, and bounding pulse; report these to the health care provider.

Excessive diarrhea and/or dehydration may develop when hyperosmolar enteral preparations are delivered quickly and excessive water loss is experienced. A more iso-osmolar formula may be needed. If diarrhea continues, and especially if it has a very foul odor, evaluate for *Clostridium difficile* or other infectious organisms. Contamination can occur because of repeated and often faulty handling of the feeding solution and system.

In some cases, diarrhea may be the result of administration of multiple liquid medications, such as elixirs and suspensions that have a very high osmolarity. Examples include acetaminophen, furosemide, and phenytoin. Discuss this with the health care provider to determine whether their drug regimen can be changed to prevent diarrhea or if dilution is possible.

The two most common electrolyte imbalances associated with enteral nutrition therapy are hyperkalemia and hyponatremia. Both of these conditions may be related to hyperglycemia-induced hyperosmolarity of the plasma and the resultant osmotic diuresis. Risks for disturbances in *fluid and electrolyte balance* are discussed in detail in Chapter 13.

Refeeding syndrome. Refeeding syndrome is a potentially life-threatening complication related to fluid and electrolyte shifts during aggressive nutrition rehabilitation of the patient in a state of starvation. Prevent this complication by carefully assessing and managing nutrition needs early before a patient is severely malnourished.

! NURSING SAFETY PRIORITY (QSEN)
Critical Rescue

Recognize signs of refeeding syndrome, which include heart failure, peripheral edema, rhabdomyolysis, seizures, and hemolysis (Mehler, 2019). Laboratory values indicate hypophosphatemia and hypokalemia. Respond by contacting the health care provider immediately. More information on *fluid and electrolyte balance* can be found in Chapter 13.

Parenteral Nutrition. When a patient cannot effectively use the GI tract for *nutrition,* either partial or total parenteral nutrition therapy may be needed. This form of nutrition is introduced into the veins and differs from standard IV therapy in that any or all nutrients (carbohydrates, proteins, fats, vitamins, minerals, electrolytes, and trace elements) can be given. Parenteral nutrition can be mixed by the pharmacist using compounded bags or delivered from a multichamber bag in which commercially premixed solutions are used (King, 2019). In a multichamber bag, dextrose, amino acids, electrolytes, and lipids are preloaded in separate chambers that are mixed together right before administration. The benefit of compounding is that mixtures can be highly personalized to each patient. However, a downfall is the rate of human error that can take place in the compounding, labeling, and administration processes (King, 2019). A benefit of the multichamber bag is that shelf life is 12 months or more (compared with a 7- to 9-day shelf life for individually compounded formulations). The downfall is lack of customization to the individual patient, as multichamber bags usually contain less protein and fewer electrolytes than personalized formulations (King, 2019). At time of publication, the American Society for Parenteral and

Enteral Nutrition (ASPEN) recommends using premixed formulations or multichamber bag solutions.

Peripheral parenteral nutrition (PPN). Peripheral parenteral nutrition (PPN) is administered through a cannula or catheter in a large distal vein of the arm on a short-term basis. It is usually used for patients who can eat but are not able to take in enough nutrients to meet their needs. PPN is fat based and does not contain all of the carbohydrates a patient needs, so it is not used on a long-term basis (Baiu & Spain, 2019). The patient must have adequate peripheral vein access and be able to tolerate large volumes of fluid to have this type of nutrition therapy. PPN has an osmolarity lower than conventional parenteral nutrition and must be administered in a high volume and/or with a high fat formulation to deliver adequate nutrients (Seres, 2020). Monitor for irritation at the site of the cannula or catheter insertion, as infusion of large volumes of PPN can be irritating to tissue.

> ### ⚠ NURSING SAFETY PRIORITY (QSEN)
> #### Critical Rescue
>
> Recognize that you must monitor patients receiving fat emulsions for fever, increased triglycerides, clotting problems, and multisystem organ failure, which may indicate fat overload syndrome, especially in patients who are critically ill. Respond to any of these signs and symptoms by discontinuing the IVFE infusion and reporting the changes to the health care provider immediately.

Total parenteral nutrition. When the patient requires intensive *nutrition* support for an extended time, the health care provider prescribes centrally administered total parenteral nutrition (TPN). TPN (Fig. 55.5) is delivered through a temporary central line inserted in the neck or chest, a long-term tunneled catheter or implanted part inserted in the chest, or via a PICC line (Baiu & Spain, 2019). (See Chapter 15 for care.) This type of nutrition is hypertonic and contains a high glucose content.

TPN solutions are administered with an infusion pump. The osmolarity of the fluid and the concentrations of the specific components make controlled delivery essential. See the Best Practice for Patient Safety & Quality Care: Care and Maintenance of Total Parenteral Nutrition box for appropriate nursing interventions.

Patients receiving parenteral nutrition fluids are at risk for a wide variety of serious and potentially life-threatening complications. Complications may result from the solutions or from the peripheral or central venous catheter (see Chapter 15).

The patient with cardiac or renal dysfunction can develop problems with **fluid and electrolyte balance,** including fluid overload, heart failure, and pulmonary edema. The health care provider usually requests frequent serum electrolyte levels to detect imbalances. Potassium and sodium imbalances are common, especially when insulin is also administered as part of the therapy. Calcium imbalances, particularly hypercalcemia, are associated with TPN. The risk for metabolic and electrolyte complications is reduced when the administration rate is carefully controlled and patients are closely observed. Monitor for any of these imbalances, and report any major changes or abnormalities to the health care provider immediately.

> ## BEST PRACTICE FOR PATIENT SAFETY & QUALITY CARE (QSEN)
> ### Care and Maintenance of Total Parenteral Nutrition
>
> - Check each bag of total parenteral nutrition (TPN) solution for accuracy by comparing it with the original prescription.
> - Administer insulin as prescribed.
> - Monitor the IV pump for accuracy in delivering the prescribed hourly rate.
> - If the TPN solution is temporarily unavailable, collaborate with the health care provider so that 10% dextrose/water ($D_{10}W$) or 20% dextrose/water ($D_{20}W$) can be administered until the TPN solution can be obtained.
> - If the TPN administration is not on time ("behind"), do not attempt to "catch up" by increasing the rate.
> - Monitor and document the patient's weight daily or according to facility protocol.
> - Monitor serum electrolytes and glucose daily or per facility protocol.
> - Monitor for, report, and document complications, including problems with **fluid and electrolyte balance.**
> - Monitor and carefully record the patient's intake and output.
> - Assess the patient's IV site for signs of infection or infiltration (see Chapter 15).
> - Change the IV tubing every 24 hours or per facility protocol.
> - Change the dressing around the IV site every 48 to 72 hours or per facility protocol.
> - Before administering TPN, have a second nurse check the prescription and solution to increase patient safety.

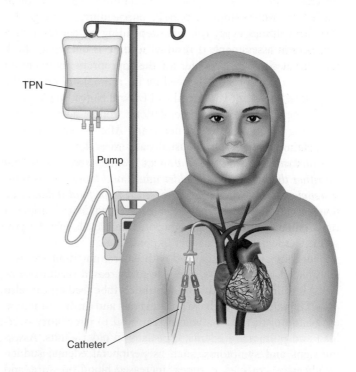

Fig. 55.5 Total parenteral nutrition.

Care Coordination and Transition Management. The patient with undernutrition, once stabilized, can be cared for in an acute care hospital, transitional care unit, nursing home, or their own home.

Home Care Management. The patient with undernutrition needs a variety of resources at home to continue consistent **nutrition** support. If he or she can consume food by the oral route, the case manager or other discharge planner can determine whether financial resources are available for nutrition supplements. If the hospital provides ambulatory nutrition counseling services, the patient may be scheduled for follow-up after discharge for assessment of weight gain.

Self-Management Education. The registered dietitian nutritionist (RDN) teaches the patient with undernutrition (and family, as indicated) about a high-calorie, high-protein diet and **nutrition** supplements. It is important for you, as the nurse, to:

- Reinforce the importance of adhering to the prescribed diet.
- Review any drugs the patient may be taking.
- Teach the importance of taking iron immediately before or during meals.
- Caution the patient that iron tends to cause constipation.
- Emphasize ways to prevent constipation, including adequate fiber intake, adequate fluids, and exercise.

Health Care Resources. The patient with undernutrition discharged to home on enteral or parenteral nutrition support needs the specialized services of a home nutrition therapy team. This team generally consists of the health care provider, nurse, registered dietitian nutritionist (RDN), pharmacist, and case manager or social worker. Several commercial companies supply these services to patients at home in addition to the feeding supplies and formulas and health teaching.

◆ **Evaluation: Evaluate Outcomes.** Evaluate the care of the patient with undernutrition based on the identified priority patient problem. The primary expected outcome is that the patient consumes available nutrients to meet the metabolic demands for maintaining weight and total protein and has adequate hydration.

✴ NUTRITION CONCEPT EXEMPLAR: OBESITY

Pathophysiology Review

The pathophysiology of obesity is complex. A number of chemicals in the body, including hormones known as *adipokines,* work together to affect appetite and fat metabolism. Dysregulation of these chemicals can result in conditions such as appetite increase, overstimulation of the autonomic nervous system, blood vessel inflammation, and ventricular hypertrophy. Complications of obesity can affect many organ systems (Table 55.6).

The terms *obesity* and *overweight* are often used interchangeably, but they refer to different health problems. For both problems, the patient often has not consumed enough healthy nutrients to achieve adequate **nutrition** and has an abnormal or excessive amount of fat accumulation (World Health Organization, 2020). Overweight is reflected by a body mass index (BMI) of 25 to 29. Obesity is reflected by a BMI of 30 or above (CDC, 2020b).

Obesity is subdivided into three categories (CDC, 2020b):

- Class I—BMI of 30 to <35
- Class II—BMI of 35 to < 40

TABLE 55.6   Common Complications of Obesity

Cardiovascular
- Coronary artery disease (CAD)
- Hyperlipidemia
- Hypertension
- Peripheral artery disease (PAD)

Endocrine
- Insulin resistance
- Metabolic syndrome
- Type II diabetes

Gastrointestinal
- Cholelithiasis

Genitourinary/Reproductive
- Erectile dysfunction in men
- Menstrual irregularities in women
- Urinary incontinence

Integumentary
- Delayed wound healing
- Susceptibility to infections

Musculoskeletal
- Chronic back and/or joint pain
- Early onset of osteoarthritis

Neurologic
- Stroke

Psychiatric
- Depression

Respiratory
- Obesity hypoventilation syndrome
- Obstructive sleep apnea

- Class III—BMI of 40 or higher (sometimes called "extreme" or "severe" obesity)

The distribution of excess body fat rather than the degree of obesity has been used to predict increased health risks. The waist circumference (WC) is a stronger predictor of coronary artery disease (CAD) than is the BMI. A WC greater than 35 inches (89 cm) in women and greater than 40 inches (102 cm) in men indicates central obesity (National Heart, Lung, and Blood Institute; National Institutes of Health; U.S. Department of Health and Human Services, n.d.). Central obesity is a major risk factor for CAD, brain attack, type 2 diabetes, some cancers (e.g., colon, breast), sleep apnea, and early death.

The waist-to-hip ratio (WHR) is also a predictor of CAD. This measure differentiates peripheral lower body obesity from central obesity. A WHR of 0.95 or greater in men (0.8 or greater in women) indicates android obesity with excess fat at the waist and abdomen.

Etiology and Genetic Risk. The causes of obesity involve complex interrelationships of many environmental, genetic, and behavioral factors. One of the most common causes of being overweight or obese is eating *high-fat and high-cholesterol diets.* Obesity is associated with diet when it contains a significant amount of *saturated* fat, which increases low-density lipoproteins (LDL, or LDL-C for low-density lipoproteins cholesterol). *Trans* fatty acids (TFAs), saturated fats, and cholesterol are linked to a higher risk for heart disease (American Heart Association, 2017). By contrast, mono-unsaturated and polyunsaturated fats are healthy fats.

Physical inactivity has been identified as another cause of overweight and obesity. The major barriers to increasing physical activity include lack of time, comfort level in a sedentary lifestyle, and decreased mobility due to health conditions.

Drug therapy also contributes to obesity when prescribed medications cause weight gain when they are taken on a long-term basis. Examples include:

- Corticosteroids
- Estrogens and certain progestins
- NSAIDs

- Antihypertensives
- Antidepressants and other psychoactive drugs
- Antiepileptic drugs
- Certain oral antidiabetic agents

PATIENT-CENTERED CARE: GENETIC/ GENOMIC CONSIDERATIONS (QSEN)

Evidence shows that genetic classifications of obesity can be (Huvenne et al., 2016):

1. Monogenic (caused by a single gene);
2. Syndromic (severe obesity associated with other phenotypes, including neurodevelopmental abnormalities like Prader-Willi syndrome);
3. Oligogenic (due to the absence of a certain phenotype); or
4. Polygenic (caused by a cumulative effect of numerous genes whose effect is increased in the environment where weight gain is prominent)

Polygenic obesity is seen most commonly. In any predisposition to obesity, environment (lifestyle) is also a strong influence. Encourage patients to focus on lifestyle modifications that are within their control, even if they believe genetics is the root cause of obesity.

Incidence and Prevalence. Worldwide, the prevalence of overweight and obesity has doubled since 1980 (Chooi et al., 2019). Approximately one third of the world's population is now classified as overweight or obese (Chooi). *This problem is a leading cause of preventable death.*

Health Promotion and Maintenance. Obesity is a major public health problem and is associated with many complications, including death. As a result of this increasing problem, the *Healthy People 2020* agenda (Office of Disease Prevention and Health Promotion, 2020) addresses the need to reduce the proportion of children, adolescents, and adults with obesity. *Healthy People 2020 Objectives for Nutrition and Weight Status* include specific population targets related to obesity and healthy **nutrition** habits (Table 55.7). *Healthy People 2030* includes initiatives that address:

- Reducing the proportion of adults with obesity
- Increasing the proportion of adults with obesity who receive counseling or education regarding weight reduction, nutrition, or physical therapy
- Increasing the consumption of whole grains
- Decreasing the consumption of calories from added sugars

In collaboration with the registered dietitian nutritionist (RDN), teach the importance of weight management and physical activity to improve health. Even a 5% weight loss can drastically decrease the risk for coronary artery disease (CAD) and diabetes mellitus. Teach patients that physical activity can be as simple as walking 20 min/day.

❖ Interprofessional Collaborative Care

Care for the patient with obesity takes place in a variety of settings, from the home, to the community, and in the hospital setting if more comprehensive management or surgery is needed. Members of the interprofessional team who collaborate most closely to care for this patient include the primary health care provider, surgeon if surgery is required, nurse,

NCLEX EXAMINATION CHALLENGE 55.3
Psychosocial Integrity

A client with obesity tells the nurse, "My genes are the only thing that have made me obese." What is the appropriate nursing response? **Select all that apply.**

A. "Genes can contribute to obesity."
B. "Tell me about your family history."
C. "Let's talk about your nutrition intake."
D. "Have you considered bariatric surgery?"
E. "How do you feel about physical activity?"
F. "What lifestyle modifications have you tried?"

TABLE 55.7 Meeting *Healthy People 2020* Select Objectives and Targets: Nutrition and Weight Status

- Increase the number of states that have state-level policies that incentivize food retail outlets to provide foods that are encouraged by the Dietary Guidelines for Americans (target 34 states)
- Increase the proportion of primary care physicians who regularly measure the body mass index of their adult patients (by 10%)
- Increase the proportion of physician office visits made by patients with a diagnosis of cardiovascular disease, diabetes, or hyperlipidemia that include counseling or education related to nutrition or weight (by 10%)
- Increase the proportion of physician office visits made by patients with a diagnosis of cardiovascular disease, diabetes, or hyperlipidemia that include counseling or education related to nutrition or weight (by 10%)
- Increase the proportion of adults who are at a healthy weight (by 10%)
- Reduce the proportion of adults who are obese (by 10%)

Data from Office of Disease Prevention and Health Promotion. (2020). *Nutrition and weight status.* https://www.healthypeople.gov/2020/topics-objectives/topic/nutrition-and-weight-status/objectives.

social worker, and registered dietitian nutritionist (RDN). For patients who experience psychological impact related to obesity, a psychologist or therapist will also have an important role in care.

◆ Assessment: Recognize Cues

History. Patients with obesity may be embarrassed or reluctant to talk about their weight or fear judgment because of the stigma that can be attached to this condition. Approach patients with obesity by using the acronym RESPECT, created by The Ohio State University (Aycock et al, 2017). Create a **r**apport with them in an **e**nvironment that is **s**afe. Ensure their safety and **p**rivacy, **e**ncourage them to set realistic goals (in the planning phase), provide **c**ompassion, and use **t**act in conversation.

See the earlier Best Practice for Patient Safety & Quality Care: Nutrition Screening Assessment box to complete the initial history. In collaboration with the registered dietitian nutritionist (RDN), also obtain the information as noted in "History" under the concept exemplar of undernutrition.

Additionally, ask about:

- Appetite
- Attitude toward food

- Presence of any chronic diseases
- Drugs taken (prescribed and over-the-counter [OTC], including herbal preparations)
- Physical activity/functional ability
- Family history of obesity
- What forms of weight loss have been tried in the past and their results

Physical Assessment/Signs and Symptoms. Obtain an accurate height and weight. Anthropometric measurements may also be obtained.

Examine the skin for reddened or open areas. Lift skinfold areas, such as pendulous breasts and abdominal aprons (*panniculus*), to observe for *Candida* (yeast) (a condition called *intertrigo*) or other infections or lesions. Infection of the panniculus is referred to as *panniculitis*.

Psychosocial Assessment. Obtain a psychosocial history to determine the patient's circumstances and emotional factors that might prevent successful weight loss or that might be worsened by intervention. Ask about the perception of current weight and weight reduction. Some patients do not view weight as a problem, which affects planning, treatment, and outcome. Ask the patient questions about his or her health beliefs related to being overweight, such as:

- What does food mean to you?
- Do you want to lose weight?
- What prevents you from losing weight?
- What do you think will motivate you to lose weight?
- How do you think you might benefit from losing weight?
- Do you have a support system in place that will encourage you during weight loss?

Some patients become very depressed regarding their weight and/or failure of weight loss efforts. If the patient reports depressed symptoms that have occurred consistently for more than 2 weeks that impact performing ADLs, referral to a mental health professional can be helpful.

◆ **Analysis: Analyze Cues and Prioritize Hypothesis.** The priority collaborative problem for the patient with obesity is:
1. Weight gain, which stresses all vital organs due to excessive intake of calories

◆ **Planning and Implementation: Generate Solutions and Take Action.** If the patient with obesity is to be hospitalized, an appropriate bariatric care room is important in the provision of high-quality, patient-centered care whether nonsurgical or surgical management is planned. Ensure that the patient has the right room so that care can be maximized to the very best benefit. Criteria for these types of rooms are located in Table 55.8.

Improving Nutrition

Planning: Expected Outcomes. The patient with obesity is expected to return to a normal BMI, while consuming dense nutrients that meet metabolic needs without overeating.

Nonsurgical Management. Weight loss may be accomplished by nutrition modification with or without the aid of drugs and in combination with a regular exercise program. Patients who may be candidates for surgical treatment include those who have:

- Repeated failure of nonsurgical interventions
- A BMI equal to or greater than 40
- Weight more than 100% above ideal body weight

TABLE 55.8	**Criteria for a Bariatric Room**
Criterion	**Specifications**
Location	Designation specifically for bariatric care
Capacity	Single-patient
Area	Minimum clear floor area of 18 m²
Clearance	Minimum distance of 1.5 m between sides and foot of bed and wall
Hand washing station	Mounted on wall, able to withstand downward static force of a predetermined maximum patient weight
Toilet room	Mounted to floor with at least 61 cm from wall to center of toilet line, and 112 cm of clear space on the opposite side of the toilet for wheelchair and caregiver access
Bathing facilities	Shower stalls—1.2 m x 1.8 m, with grab bars that support 450 kg Handheld spray nozzles mounted on a side wall Enclosure for privacy Must be separate from hand washing station and toilet room
Patient lift system	Built-in mechanical lift system
Airborne isolation room	At least one airborne isolation room per bariatric unit should be available

From Smigelski-Theiss, R., Gampong, M., & Kurasaki, J. (2017). Weight bias and psychosocial implications for acute care of patients with obesity. *AACN Advanced Critical Care, 28*(3), 254-262.

Diet programs. Diets for helping adults lose weight include fasting, very-low-calorie diets, nutritionally balanced diets, and unbalanced low-energy diets.

Short-term fasting programs and *very-low-calorie diets* (usually 200 to 800 calories/day) require an initial cardiac evaluation and supervision by the interprofessional health care team. Neither diet is ideal due to risks involved and the likelihood of regaining weight after completion of the diet. Ketosis is a risk of short-term fasting.

Nutritionally balanced diets generally provide about 1200 to 1800 calories/day with a conventional distribution of carbohydrate, protein, and fat. Vitamin and mineral supplements may be used. These diets adhere to conventional foods that are economical and easy to obtain.

Unbalanced low-energy diets, such as the low-carbohydrate diet, restrict one or more nutrients. Protein and vegetables are encouraged, but certain carbohydrates and high-fat foods are not. Although results are mixed per health research, these diets are extremely popular.

Nutrition therapy. *Nutrition* recommendations for each patient are developed through close interaction among the patient, caregiver, primary health care provider, nurse, and registered dietitian nutritionist (RDN). The diet must meet the patient's needs, habits, and lifestyle and should be realistic. At a minimum, the diet should:

- Be evidence based
- Be nutritionally balanced (see Diet Programs section)

- Have a low risk-benefit ratio
- Be practical and conducive to long-term success

Calorie estimates are easily calculated. Resting metabolic rate is determined using a gender-specific formula that incorporates the appropriate activity factor. This figure reflects the total calories needed daily for maintaining current weight. To encourage a weight loss of 1 lb (0.45 kg) a week, the registered dietitian nutritionist (RDN) subtracts 500 calories each day. To encourage a weight loss of 2 lb (0.9 kg) a week, 1000 calories each day are subtracted. The amount of weight lost varies with the patient's food intake, level of physical activity, and water losses. A reasonable expected outcome of 5% to 10% loss of body weight has been shown to improve glycemic control and reduce cholesterol and blood pressure. These benefits continue if the weight loss is sustained.

Exercise program. For most adults, adding physical activity to a healthy diet produces more weight loss than dieting alone. More of the weight lost is fat, which preserves lean body mass. An increase in exercise can reduce the waist circumference and the waist-to-hip ratio. Evidence also shows that reduction of fat in the thighs, hips, and buttocks helps to protect against cardiovascular disease and diabetes (Clifton, 2018).

A minimum-level workout should be developed so that consistency can be achieved and maintained. Encourage walking 20 minutes a day and increasing the time as endurance increases. The activity may be performed all at once or divided over the course of the day.

Drug therapy. Four medications are FDA-approved for overweight and obesity treatment. The primary health care provider will work with the patient to determine which, if any, of these drugs are appropriate. See the Common Examples of Drug Therapy: Overweight and Obesity Treatment box for information about this type of drug therapy.

Cryolipolysis. Cryolipolysis is a nonsurgical procedure also known as "fat freezing." This procedure is used to reduce fat deposits in certain body areas but is not suggested for use in patients who are overweight or have obesity (Meyer et al, 2018). Redirect patient requesting cryolipolysis to the primary health care provider for further discussion.

Behavioral management. Behavioral management of obesity helps the patient change daily eating habits to lose weight. Self-monitoring techniques include keeping a journal of foods eaten (food diary), exercise or activity patterns, and emotional and situational factors. Stimulus control involves controlling the external cues that promote overeating. Reinforcement techniques are used to self-reward the behavior change. Cognitive restructuring involves modifying negative beliefs by learning positive coping self-statements. Counseling by health care professionals must continue before, during, and after treatment. The 12-step program offered by Overeaters Anonymous (www.oa.org) has helped many adults lose weight, especially those who eat compulsively.

Complementary and integrative health. Many complementary and integrative therapies have been tested and used for obesity. These modalities aim to suppress appetite and therefore limit food intake to lose weight:

- Acupuncture
- Acupressure
- Ayurveda (a combination of holistic approaches)
- Hypnosis

Evidence about effectiveness of each of these therapies varies. Encourage the patient to speak to the primary health care provider to determine if any of these methods are recommended.

Surgical Management. Some patients seek to improve their appearance by reducing the amount of adipose tissue in selected areas of the body. A typical example of this type of surgery is

💊 COMMON EXAMPLES OF DRUG THERAPY

Overweight and Obesity Treatment

Drug	Selected Nursing Implications
Liraglutide (activates appetite regulation in the brain)	• Monitor ALT and AST; *there is an increased risk for pancreatitis when taking this drug.* • Patients taking insulin should not take this drug; *hypoglycemia can develop.* • Teach to report taking this drug to all health care providers; *alpha$_1$-adrenergic antagonists can increase or decrease the side effects of other drugs like beta blockers, calcium channel blockers, or medications used to treat erectile dysfunction.*
Naltrexone-bupropion (combines the opioid antagonist naltrexone with the antidepressant bupropion)	• Patients with uncontrolled hypertension, seizures, anorexia nervosa, or bulimia nervosa, or who are withdrawing from drugs or alcohol, should not take this drug. • Patients taking bupropion should not take this drug; *cumulative doses can increase risks for side effects.* • Monitor for suicidal ideation; *this can develop due to the antidepressant effect.*
Orlistat Inhibits lipase; thus, fats are only partially digested and absorbed	• Monitor liver enzymes; *rare cases of liver injury have been reported.* • Teach to take a multivitamin daily; *the body may not normally absorb enough vitamins found in foods due to the effect of the drug.* • Teach that loose stools, abdominal cramps, and nausea can occur unless fat intake is reduced to less than 30% of the daily intake; *the drug mechanism facilitates GI symptoms since fats are only partially digested and absorbed.*
Phentermine-topiramate (combines short-term weight loss drug phentermine with seizure medication topiramate)	• Patients with glaucoma or hyperthyroidism should not take this medication. • Determine if patient is pregnant or planning pregnancy; *this medication can cause birth defects* (**NOTE:** Patient should also not use this medication if breastfeeding).

From the National Institute of Diabetes and Digestive and Kidney Disorders. (n.d.) Prescription medications to treat overweight and obesity. https://www.niddk.nih.gov/health-information/weight-management/prescription-medications-treat-overweight-obesity.

liposuction, which can be done in a health care provider's office or ambulatory surgery center. Although the patient's appearance may improve, if weight gain continues, the fatty tissue will return. This procedure is not a solution for adults with obesity.

Bariatrics is a branch of medicine that manages patients with obesity and its related diseases. Certain adults may be considered for this type of weight loss surgery. These include patients who:

- Do not respond to traditional interventions
- Have a body mass index (BMI) of 40 or greater
- Have a BMI of 35 or greater, with other health risk factors

Surgical procedures include gastric bypass, sleeve gastrectomy, adjustable gastric band and, less commonly, the biliopancreatic diversion with duodenal switch (BPD/DS) (American Society for Metabolic and Bariatric Surgery [ASMBS], 2020). Another procedure, gastrointestinal electrical stimulation (GES), involves the implantation of a vagal-blocking device (vBloc) into the abdomen (Apovian et al., 2017) that causes early satiety, and thus, reduced intake (Shikora et al., 2019).

Depending on the procedure, the surgeon may choose to use a conventional open approach or perform minimally invasive surgery (MIS). Many patients have MIS via either the laparoscopic adjustable gastric band (LAGB) procedure or laparoscopic sleeve gastrectomy (LSG). Both procedures are classified as restrictive surgeries. The decision of whether the patient is a candidate for the MIS is based on weight, body build, history of abdominal surgery, and coexisting medical complications. With any surgical approach, patients must agree to modify their lifestyle and follow stringent protocols to lose weight and keep the weight off. After successful bariatric surgery, many patients no longer have complications of obesity, such as diabetes mellitus, hypertension, depression, or sleep apnea.

Preoperative care. Preoperative care is similar to that for any patient undergoing abdominal surgery or laparoscopy (see Chapter 9). However, patients with obesity are at increased surgical risks of pulmonary and thromboembolitic complications, as well as death. Some surgeons require a specific amount of weight loss before bariatric surgery to minimize complications. Patients also have a thorough psychological assessment and testing to detect depression, substance abuse, or other mental health/behavioral health problems that could interfere with success after surgery. Cognitive ability, coping skills, development, motivation, expectations, and support systems are also assessed. Patients who are not alert and oriented or do not have sufficient strength and mobility are not considered for bariatric surgery. *The primary role of the nurse is to reinforce health teaching in preparation for surgery.* Most bariatric surgical centers provide educational sessions for groups of patients who plan to have the procedure.

Operative procedures. *Gastric restriction* surgeries, the easiest to perform, allow for normal digestion without the risk of nutritional deficiencies. In a banding procedure, the surgeon places an adjustable band to create a small proximal stomach pouch through a laparoscope (Fig. 55.6A, Fig. 55.6B). The band may or may not be inflatable. In the vertical sleeve gastroplasty (Fig. 55.6C), about ¾ of the stomach is removed, with the sleevelike remaining stomach having a much-reduced

capacity. In the biliopancreatic diversion with duodenal switch (Fig. 55.6D), a lesser common bariatric surgery, almost 80% of the stomach is removed. The remaining pouch is connected to the bottom of the small intestine (bypassing the upper portion). Therefore, calories and nutrients are routed into the colon, where they are not absorbed (Phillips & Zieve, 2019).

The most common bariatric surgery performed in the United States is the *Roux-en-Y gastric bypass (RNYGB),* which is often done as a robotic-assistive surgical procedure. Most commonly called a gastric bypass, this procedure results in quick weight loss, but it is more invasive with a higher risk for postoperative complications. In this procedure, gastric resection is combined with malabsorption surgery. The patient's stomach, duodenum, and part of the jejunum are bypassed so that fewer calories can be absorbed (Fig. 55.6E).

Postoperative care. Postoperative care depends on the type of surgery performed. Patients having one of the MIS procedures have less pain, scarring, and blood loss. They typically have a faster recovery time and a faster return to daily activities. However, even patients having MIS are considered to have had major abdominal surgery along with all its risks, and their care is planned accordingly. These patients may require less than 24 hours in the hospital; some may need 1 to 2 days. Patients with open procedures may need several days to recover.

A major focus of postoperative care must be placed on patient and staff safety. Patients should be placed in a bariatric room (see Table 55.8). Always use additional personnel when moving the patient. Ensure that side rails are not touching the body because they can cause pressure injuries. Pressure between skinfolds and tubes and catheters can also cause skin breakdown. Monitor the skin in these areas and keep it clean and dry.

Care of the patient who has undergone any type of bariatric surgery is similar to that of any patient having abdominal or laparoscopic surgery (see Chapter 9). *The priority for postoperative care is airway management.* Patients with short and thick necks often have compromised airways and need aggressive respiratory support—possibly mechanical ventilation in the critical care unit.

In addition to the postoperative complications typically associated with abdominal and laparoscopic surgeries, patients who have undergone bariatric surgery are at risk for anastomotic leaks (a leak of digestive juices and partially digested food through an anastomosis). Implement measures to prevent complications as noted in the Best Practice for Patient Safety & Quality Care: Care of the Patient After Bariatric Surgery box.

All patients experience some degree of pain, but it is usually less severe when MIS is performed. Patients may use patient-controlled analgesia (PCA) with morphine for up to the first 24 hours. All patients receive oral opioid analgesic agents (liquid form when possible) as prescribed after the PCA is discontinued. Acute pain management is discussed in detail in Chapter 5.

Clear liquids are introduced slowly if the patient can tolerate water, and 1-ounce cups are used for each serving. A full liquid diet follows tolerance of the clear liquid diet; usually patients are discharged on full liquids. Pureed foods follow in about a week, with each meal consisting of about 5 tablespoons of food.

BEST PRACTICE FOR PATIENT SAFETY & QUALITY CARE (QSEN)

Care of the Patient After Bariatric Surgery

Cardiovascular/Respiratory Care
- Place the patient in semi-Fowler position to improve breathing and decrease risk for sleep apnea, pneumonia, or atelectasis.
- Monitor oxygen saturation; provide oxygen, bilevel, or continuous positive airway pressure (BiPAP or CPAP) ventilation as prescribed.
- Apply sequential compression stockings and administer prophylactic anticoagulant therapy as prescribed to prevent venous thromboembolisms, including pulmonary embolism (PE).

Gastrointestinal Care
- Apply an abdominal binder to prevent wound dehiscence for open surgical procedures.
- Observe for signs and symptoms of **dumping syndrome** (caused by food entering the small intestine instead of the stomach) after *gastric bypass,* such as tachycardia, nausea, diarrhea, and abdominal cramping.
- Provide six small feedings (clear and then full liquids as prescribed) and plenty of fluids to prevent dehydration in collaboration with the registered dietitian nutritionist (RDN).
- Measure and record abdominal girth daily or as prescribed.

Genitourinary Care
- Remove urinary catheter within 24 hours after surgery to prevent urinary tract infection.

Integumentary Care
- Observe skin areas and folds for redness, excoriation, or breakdown, and treat these problems early.
- Use absorbent padding between folds to prevent pressure areas and skin breakdown.
- Ensure that tubes and catheters are not causing pressure on the skin.

Musculoskeletal Care
- Collaborate with the physical therapist for transfers or ambulation assistive devices, such as walkers.
- Encourage and assist with turning every 2 hours using an appropriate weight-bearing overhead trapeze.

! NURSING SAFETY PRIORITY (QSEN)

Action Alert

Some patients who have bariatric surgery have a nasogastric (NG) tube put in place, especially after open surgical procedures. In gastroplasty procedures, the NG tube drains both the proximal pouch and the distal stomach. Closely monitor the tube for patency. *Never reposition the tube because its movement can disrupt the suture line!* The NG tube is removed on the second day if the patient is passing flatus.

After several weeks of pureed foods, soft foods are introduced. Around the eighth postoperative week, solid, nutrient-dense foods are incorporated. Remind the patient to eat and drink slowly, to consume only small meals, to stop eating before feeling full, to choose foods high in protein, and to avoid foods that are fatty or have high sugar content.

Care Coordination and Transition Management. Obesity can be a chronic, lifelong problem if weight loss is not accomplished. Diets, drug therapy, exercise, and behavior modification can

! NURSING SAFETY PRIORITY (QSEN)

Critical Rescue

Anastomotic leaks are the most common serious complication and cause of death after gastric bypass surgery. Recognize that you must monitor for symptoms of this life-threatening problem, which includes increasing back, shoulder, or abdominal pain; restlessness; and unexplained tachycardia and oliguria (scant urine). If any of these findings is present, respond by contacting the surgeon immediately!

? CLINICAL JUDGMENT CHALLENGE 55.1

Safety

A 49-year-old woman had bariatric surgery 8 weeks ago. Today, she calls the telehealth nurse and reports having nausea, abdominal cramping, and ongoing diarrhea for 2 days. In addition, she says that she feels like her heart is "racing" and she wonders if she has "the stomach flu" (gastroenteritis).

1. **Recognize Cues:** What assessment information in this client situation is the most important and immediate concern for the nurse? (Hint: Identify the **relevant** information *first* to determine what is most important.)
2. **Analyze Cues:** What client conditions are consistent with the **most relevant** information? (Hint: Think about priority collaborative problems that support and contradict the information presented in this situation.)
3. **Prioritize Hypotheses:** Which possibilities or explanations are **most likely** to be present in this client situation? Which possibilities or explanations are the most serious? (Hint: Consider all possibilities and determine their urgency and risk for this client.)
4. **Generate Solutions:** What actions would most likely achieve the desired outcomes for this client? Which actions should be **avoided** or are **potentially harmful**? (Hint: Determine the desired outcomes first to decide which interventions are appropriate and those that should be avoided.)
5. **Take Action:** Which actions are the most appropriate and how should they be implemented? In what **priority order** should they be implemented? (Hint: Consider health teaching, documentation, requested health care provider orders or prescriptions, nursing skills, collaboration with or referral to health team members, etc.)
6. **Evaluate Outcomes:** What client assessment would indicate that the nurse's actions were **effective**? (Hint: Think about signs that would indicate an improvement, decline, or unchanged client condition.)

produce short-term weight losses with reasonable safety. However, many patients who do lose weight often regain it. Treatment of obesity should focus on the long-term reduction of health risks and problems associated with obesity, improving quality of life, and promoting a health-oriented lifestyle.

Home Care Management. In collaboration with the registered dietitian nutritionist (RDN), counsel the patient on a healthful eating pattern. The physical therapist or exercise physiologist recommends an appropriate exercise program. A psychologist may recommend cognitive restructuring approaches that help alter dysfunctional eating patterns.

For patients who have surgery, additional discharge teaching is needed. The Patient and Family Education: Preparing for Self-Management: Discharge Teaching Topics for the Patient After Bariatric Surgery box lists the important areas that should be reviewed. Patients are usually followed closely by the surgeon and registered dietitian nutritionist (RDN) for several years. Encourage patients to keep all appointments and to adhere to

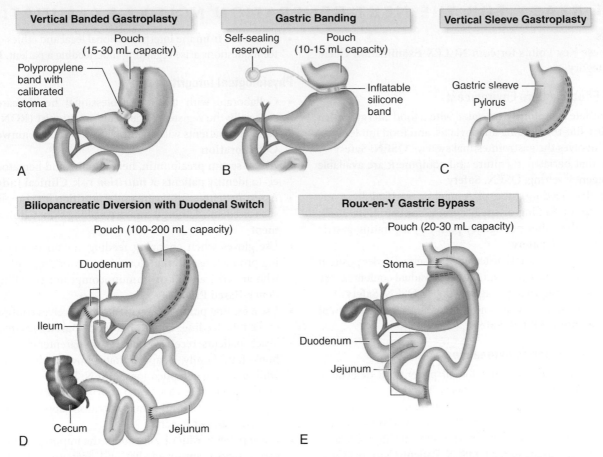

Fig. 55.6 Bariatric surgical procedures. A, Vertical banded gastroplasty. B, Gastric banding. C, Vertical sleeve gastroplasty. D, Bioliopancreatic diversion with duodenal switch. E, Roux-en-Y gastric bypass (RNYGB). (From Silvestri, L., & Silvestri, A. [2020]. *Saunders comprehensive review for the NCLEX-RN examination* [8th ed]. St. Louis: Saunders.)

the treatment plan to ensure success. Plastic surgery, such as **panniculectomy** (removal of the abdominal apron, or panniculus), may be performed if needed after weight is stabilized, usually in about 18 to 24 months.

PATIENT AND FAMILY EDUCATION: PREPARING FOR SELF-MANAGEMENT

Discharge Teaching Topics for the Patient After Bariatric Surgery

Nutrition: Diet progression, nutrient (including vitamin and mineral) supplements, hydration guidelines

Drug therapy: Analgesics and antiemetic drugs, if needed; drugs for other health problems

Wound care: Clean procedure for open or laparoscopic wounds; cover during shower or bath

Activity level: Restrictions, such as avoiding lifting; activity progression; return to driving and work

Signs and symptoms to report: Fever; excessive nausea or vomiting; epigastric, back, or shoulder pain; red, hot, and/or draining wound(s); pain, redness, or swelling in legs; chest pain; difficulty breathing

Follow-up care: Health care provider office or clinic visits, support groups and other community resources, counseling for patient (and caregiver, if needed)

Continuing education: Nutrition and exercise classes; follow-up visits with registered dietitian nutritionist (RDN)

Self-Care Management. Remind patients to coordinate with their surgeon or primary health care provider to create a manageable and appropriate physical activity plan. For patients having nonsurgical management, emphasize the need to decrease overall fat intake and to avoid reliance on appetite-reducing drugs. Keeping a food journal that documents mood and events that take place with eating can be helpful to identify eating patterns.

Teach patients who have had bariatric surgery that postsurgical bowel changes are common. Vitamin and mineral supplements are prescribed after surgery, especially vitamin D, B-complex vitamins, iron, and calcium, and adherence to this regimen is important for surgical success.

Health Care Resources. Provide the patient with a list of available community resources, such as Overeaters Anonymous (www.oa.org) and the American Obesity Association (www.obesity.org). For surgical patients, the American Society for Metabolic and Bariatric Surgery (www.asmbs.org) may be helpful.

◆ **Evaluation: Evaluate Outcomes.** Evaluate the care of the patient with obesity based on the identified priority patient problem. The primary expected outcome is that the patient consumes appropriate, nutrient-dense foods to meet metabolic demands without overeating. For surgical patients, an additional expected outcome is that the patient remains free of infection after bariatric surgery.

GET READY FOR THE NEXT-GENERATION NCLEX® EXAMINATION!

Key Points

Review these Key Points for each NCLEX Examination Client Needs Category.

Safe and Effective Care Environment

- Differentiate symptoms associated with a food allergy, which can cause life-threatening anaphylaxis, and food intolerance, which involves the gastrointestinal system. **QSEN: Safety**
- Ensure that bariatric furniture and equipment are available in the agency setting. **QSEN: Safety**
- Ensure that feeding tube placement is verified by x-ray before use for feeding or medication administration; check placement thereafter per agency policy by aspirating gastric contents. **QSEN: Safety**
- Place patients receiving tube feeding in a semi-Fowler position at all times to prevent aspiration; check residual contents every 6 hours or as designated per agency policy. QSEN: **Safety**
- Maintain feeding tube patency for patients receiving total enteral nutrition. **QSEN: Safety**

Health Promotion and Maintenance

- Perform *nutrition* screening for all patients to determine those at risk. **QSEN: Evidence-Based Practice**
- Calculate BMI as a measure of *nutrition* status and/or BSA for dosage calculation purposes. **QSEN: Evidence-Based Practice**
- Implement interventions to promote healthy nutrition intake in patients with malnourishment. **QSEN: Patient-Centered Care**

Psychosocial Integrity

- Recognize that some patients with malnutrition may not view nutrition status as a problem. **QSEN: Patient-Centered Care**
- Recognize that malnutrition can contribute to psychological distress. **QSEN: Patient-Centered Care**

- Seek input from the interprofessional legal and ethics committee if questions arise regarding tube-feeding a patient. **Ethics**

Physiological Integrity

- Collaborate with the interprofessional health care team, especially the registered dietician nutritionist (RDN), when caring for patients with malnutrition. **QSEN: Teamwork and Collaboration**
- Assess serum prealbumin, hemoglobin, and hematocrit levels to identify patients at *nutrition* risk. **Clinical Judgment**
- Assess patients with severe undernutrition for complications such as edema, lethargy, and dry, flaking skin. **Clinical Judgment**
- Use gloves when changing feeding system tubing or adding product; use sterile gloves when working with patients who are critically ill or immunocompromised. **QSEN: Evidence-Based Practice**
- Use a feeding pump for a patient who receives continuous or cyclic tube feeding. **QSEN: Evidence-Based Practice**
- Teach patients receiving enteral or parenteral nutrition at home (and family, as appropriate) how to obtain *nutrition* while avoiding complications. **QSEN: Safety**
- Teach patients who are undernourished to eat high-protein, high-calorie foods and to take nutrition supplements. **QSEN: Evidence-Based Practice**
- Teach patients with obesity about the importance of a health care provider–approved diet and exercise plan for weight reduction. **QSEN: Evidence-Based Practice**
- Assess for signs and symptoms of anastomotic leak after bariatric surgery. **Clinical Judgment**
- Teach patients who have a gastric bypass how to avoid dumping syndrome. **QSEN: Patient-Centered Care**

MASTERY QUESTIONS

1. The nurse is caring for four clients who have been recommended to consider bariatric surgery. Which assessment data require immediate nursing intervention?
   A. BMI of 23 with gastrointestinal reflux
   B. BMI of 36 with hypertension
   C. BMI of 40 with type II diabetes
   D. BMI of 43 with sleep apnea

2. What discharge teaching will the nurse provide to a client who had gastric bypass surgery? **Select all that apply.**
   A. Be certain to stay hydrated by drinking water.
   B. Solid food can be introduced back into the diet in a week.
   C. Report any back, shoulder, or abdominal pain to the surgeon.
   D. You are likely to have little urine output for the first few weeks.
   E. Each of your meals should initially contain about 5 tablespoons of food.

REFERENCES

Academy of Nutrition and Dietetics. (2018). *Vegetarianism: The basic facts*. http://www.eatright.org/resource/food/nutrition/vegetarian-and-special-diets/vegetarianism-the-basic-facts.

American Academy of Allergy, Asthma, and Immunology. (2020). *Food intolerance versus food allergy*. Retrieved from https://www.aaaai.org/conditions-and-treatments/library/allergy-library/food-intolerance.

American Heart Association. (2017). *The skinny on fats*. www.heart.org/HEARTORG/Conditions/Cholesterol/PreventionTreatmentofHighCholesterol/Know-Your-Fats_UCM_305628_Article.jsp.

American Society of. (2020). *Parenteral and enteral nutrition (ASPEN)*. Malnutrition Center. https://www.nutritioncare.org/Malnutrition/.

American Society for Metabolic and Bariatric Surgery (ASMBS). (2020). *Bariatric surgery procedures*. https://asmbs.org/patients/bariatric-surgery-procedures.

Apovian, C., et al. (2017). Two-Year outcomes of vagal nerve blocking (vBloc) for the treatment of obesity in the ReCharge Trial. *Obesity Surgery, 27*(1), 169–176.

Aycock, D., et al. (2017). Language sensitivity, the RESPECT model, and continuing education. *The Journal of Continuing Education in Nursing, 48*(11), 517–524.

Baiu, I., & Spain, D. (2019). Parenteral nutrition. *Journal of the American Medical Association, 321*(21), 2141.

Bourgault, A., Aguirre, L., & Ibrahim, J. (2017). CORTRAK-assisted feeding tube insertion: A comprehensive review of adverse events in the Maude database. *American Journal of Critical Care, 26*(2), 149–155.

Centers for Disease Control and Prevention (CDC). (2020a). *About adult BMI.* www.cdc.gov/healthyweight/assessing/bmi/adult_bmi/.

Centers for Disease Control and Prevention (CDC). (2020b). *Defining adult overweight and obesity.* Retrieved from https://www.cdc.gov/obesity/adult/defining.html.

Cereda, E., et al. (2016). Nutritional status in older persons according to healthcare setting: A systematic review and meta-analysis of prevalence data using MNA®. *Clinical Nutrition, 35*(6), 1282.

Chooi, Y., Ding, C., & Magkos, F. (2019). The epidemiology of obesity. *Metabolism Clinical and Experimental, 92*, 6–10.

Clifton, P. (2018). Relationship between changes in fat and lean depots following weight loss and changes in cardiovascular disease risk markers. *Journal of the American Heart Association, 7*(8), e008675.

Dietary Guidelines for Americans. (2020). *Work under way: Scientific Report of the 2020 Dietary Guidelines Advisory Committee.* https://www.dietaryguidelines.gov/2020-advisory-committee-report.

Drummond Hayes, K., & Drummond Hayes, D. (2018). Best practices for unclogging feeding tubes in adults. *Nursing2018, 48*(6), 66.

Eaton, K., & Lyman, G. (2019). Dosing of anticancer agents in adults. In P. Hesketh (Ed.), *UpToDate.* Waltham, MA.

Faisal, W., et al. (2016). Not all body surface area formulas are the same, but does it matter? *Journal of Global Oncology, 2*(6), 436–437.

Fan, F., Tan, S., & Ang, S. (2017). Nasogastric tube placement confirmation: Where we are and where we should be heading. *Proceedings of Singapore Healthcare, 26*(3), 189–195.

Fryar, C. D., Kruszon-Moran, D., Gu, Q., & Ogden, C. L. (2018). *Mean body weight, height, waist circumference, and body mass index among adults: United States, 1999–2000 through 2015–2016. National health statistics reports; no 122.* Hyattsville, MD: National Center for Health Statistics.

Government of Canada. (2020). *Canada's food guide.* Retrieved from https://food-guide.canada.ca/en/.

Hodin, R., & Bordeianou, L. (2020). *Inpatient placement of nasogastric and nasoenteric tubes in adults.* In A. Cochran (Ed.). *UpToDate,* Waltham, MA.

Huvenne, H., et al. (2016). Rare genetic forms of obesity: Clinical approach and current treatments in 2016. *Obesity Facts, 9*(3), 158–173.

Interprofessional Education Collaborative. (2016). Core competencies for interprofessional collaborative practice: 2016 update. Retrieved from https://nebula.wsimg.com/2f68a39520b03336b-41038c370497473?AccessKeyId=DC06780E69ED19E2B3A5&disposition=0&alloworigin=1.

Kelly-Weeder, S., et al. (2019). Binge eating and loss of control in college-age women. *Journal of the American Psychiatric Nurses Association, 25*(3), 172–180.

King, K. (2019). Trends in parenteral nutrition. *Today's Dietician, 21*(1), 36–39.

McCance, K., Huether, S., Brashers, V., & Rote, N. (2019). *Pathophysiology: The biologic basis for disease in adults and children* (9th ed.). St. Louis: Mosby.

Mehler, P. (2019). Anorexia nervosa in adults and adolescents: The refeeding syndrome. In J. Yager (Ed.), *UpToDate.* Waltham, MA.

Metheny, N., & Meert, K. (2017). Update on effectiveness of an electromagnetic feeding tube-placement device in detecting respiratory placement. *American Journal of Critical Care, 26*(2), 157–161.

Meyer, P., et al. (2018). Cryolipolysis: Patient selection and special considerations. *Clinical, Cosmetic and Investigational Dermatology, 11*, 499–503.

Morley, J. (2020). *Protein-energy undernutrition: Merck manual professional version.* https://www.merckmanuals.com/professional/nutritional-disorders/undernutrition/protein-energy-undernutrition-peu.

National Academies of Sciences, Engineering, & Medicine. (2020). *Dietary reference intakes tables and applications.* Retrieved from http://www.nationalacademies.org/hmd/Activities/Nutrition/SummaryDRIs/DRI-Tables.aspx.

National Heart, Lung, and Blood Institute; National Institutes of Health; U.S. Department of Health and Human Services (n.d.). Assessing your weight and health risk. Retrieved from https://www.nhlbi.nih.gov/health/educational/lose_wt/risk.htm

Nestle Nutrition Institute (n.d.). Mini nutritional assessment - short form (MNA-SF). Retrieved from https://www.mna-elderly.com/forms/mini/mna_mini_english.pdf

Office of Disease and Health Promotion. (2020). *Dietary guidelines 2015-2020: Appendix 2, estimated calories needs per day, by age, sex, and physical activity level.* Retrieved from https://health.gov/dietaryguidelines/2015/guidelines/appendix-2/.

Pagana, K. D., & Pagana, T. J. (2018). *Mosby's manual of diagnostic and laboratory tests* (6th ed.). St. Louis: Mosby.

Perkins, A. (2019). Body dysmorphic disorder: The drive for perfection. *Nursing2019, 49*(3), 28–33.

Phillips, M., & Zieve, D. (2019). *Biliopancreatic diversion (BPD).* Retrieved from https://medlineplus.gov/ency/imagepages/19499.htm.

Ritchie, C., & Yukawa, M. (2019). Geriatric nutrition: Nutritional issues in older adults. In K. Schmader, & D. Seres (Eds.), *UpToDate.* Waltham, MA.

Schnur, M. (2017). *Body mass index and body surface area: What's the difference? Lippincott nursing center.* Retrieved from https://www.nursingcenter.com/ncblog/august-2017/body-mass-index-and-body-surface-area-what-s-the-d.

Seres, D. (2020). *Nutrition support in critically ill patients: Parenteral nutrition.* In UpToDate, & P. Parsons (Eds.). Waltham, MA.

Shikora, S., et al. (2019). *Neurologic metabolic surgery: A review. Bulletin of the American College of surgeons.* https://bulletin.facs.org/2019/03/neurologic-metabolic-surgery-a-review/.

Simoes, P., et al. (2018). Direct percutaneous endoscopic jejunostomy: Procedural and nutrition outcomes in a large patient cohort. *Journal of Parenteral and Enteral Nutrition, 42*(5), 898–906.

Slusser, M., et al. (2019). *Foundations of interprofessional collaborative practice* (1st ed.). St. Louis: Elsevier.

Smith, L. (2019). Take a deeper look into body surface area. *Nursing2019, 49*(9), 50–54.

Tolbert, C., Mott, S., & Nepple, K. (2018). Malnutrition diagnosis during adult inpatient hospitalizations: Analysis of a multi-institutional collaborative database of academic medical centers. *Journal of the Academy of Nutrition and Dietetics, 118*(1), 125–131.

U.S. Department of Agriculture (USDA). (n.d.). Start simple with MyPlate. Retrieved from https://www.choosemyplate.gov/eathealthy/start-simple-myplate.

U.S. Department of Agriculture (USDA). (2015). *2015-2020 Dietary guidelines for Americans.* http://www.cnpp.usda.gov/2015-2020-dietary-guidelines-americans.

Weinstein, S., & Hagle, M. (2014). *Plumer's principles and practice of infusion therapy* (9th ed.). Philadelphia: Wolters Kluwer.

World Health Organization. (2020). *Obesity.* Retrieved from https://www.who.int/topics/obesity/en/.

56

Assessment of the Endocrine System

M. Linda Workman

http://evolve.elsevier.com/Iggy/

LEARNING OUTCOMES

1. Collaborate with the interprofessional team to perform a complete endocrine assessment, including issues with **nutrition, elimination,** and ***fluid and electrolyte balance***.
2. Teach adults about factors that increase the risk for endocrine problems.
3. Implement patient-centered nursing actions to help patients and families cope with the psychosocial impact caused by changes in endocrine function.
4. Apply the principles of anatomy, physiology, pathophysiology, genetics, and the aging process to perform an evidence-based assessment for the patient with a problem of the endocrine system.
5. Explain assessment findings for the patient with an endocrine problem.
6. Coordinate appropriate pretest and posttest care for patients and proper handling of specimens before, during, and after testing of the endocrine system.

KEY TERMS

gonads The male and female reproductive endocrine glands.

hormones Natural chemicals that exert their effects on specific tissues known as target tissues.

negative feedback mechanism Signals to an endocrine gland to secrete a hormone in response to a body change to cause a reaction that will result in actions to *oppose* the action of the initial condition change and restore homeostasis.

target tissues Tissues that have receptors corresponding to different hormones that when bound to the hormones respond by changing their activity.

 PRIORITY AND INTERRELATED CONCEPTS

The priority concepts for this chapter are:
- *Nutrition*
- *Elimination*

The interrelated concept for this chapter is:
- *Fluid and Electrolyte Balance*

The endocrine system works with the parts of the central nervous system and peripheral nervous system to provide control over all other body systems for optimal homeostasis. The organs and tissues of the endocrine system contain glandular cells that secrete hormones, which are natural biochemicals that exert their effects on specific target tissues. Target tissues have receptors corresponding to different hormones that when bound to the hormones respond by changing their activity. Endocrine glands are located in many body areas (Fig. 56.1) and affect all other body systems. These glands are ductless and have no direct connection between the glands and their target tissues, which may be located some distance from the endocrine gland. Instead, the hormones secreted from endocrine glands are secreted into the blood for transportation to the target tissues (McCance et al., 2019). The major endocrine glands are:

- Hypothalamus (a neuroendocrine gland)
- Pituitary gland
- Adrenal glands
- Thyroid gland
- Islet cells of the pancreas
- Parathyroid glands
- Gonads

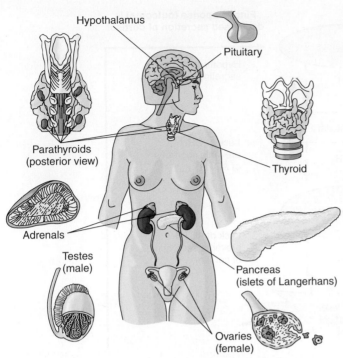

FIG. 56.1 Locations of various glands within the endocrine system.

Body functions controlled by the endocrine system for homeo stasis and regulation include metabolism, ***nutrition, elimination,*** temperature, ***fluid and electrolyte balance,*** growth, and repro- duction. Many interactions must occur between the endocrine system and all other body systems to ensure that each system maintains a constant normal balance *(homeostasis)* in response to environmental changes. For example, this regulation keeps the internal body temperature at or near 98.6°F (37°C), even when environmental temperatures vary. Other actions keep the serum sodium level between 136 and 145 mEq/L (mmol/L), regardless of whether a healthy adult eats 2 g or 12 g of sodium per day.

Table 56.1 lists hormones secreted by various endocrine glands. Although circulating hormones travel through the blood to all body areas, they exert their actions only on target tissues. Hormones recognize their target tissues and exert their actions by binding to receptors on or within the target tissue cells. In general, each receptor site type is specific for only one hormone. Hormone-receptor actions work in a "lock and key" manner in that only the correct hormone (key) can bind to and activate the receptor site (lock) (Fig. 56.2). Binding a hormone to its receptor causes the target tissue to change its activity, pro- ducing specific responses (Lazar & Birnbaum, 2016).

Endocrine system problems and disorders usually are related to:
- An excess of a specific hormone
- A deficiency of a specific hormone
- Poor hormone-receptor interactions resulting in decreased responsiveness of the target tissue

ANATOMY AND PHYSIOLOGY REVIEW

Hormones maintain homeostasis of cellular function through a series of one or more *negative feedback control mechanisms.* Secretion of any hormone depends on the body's need for the final action of that hormone. When a body condition starts to move

TABLE 56.1	**Principal Hormones of the Endocrine Glands**
Gland	**Hormones**
Hypothalamus	Corticotropin-releasing hormone (CRH)
	Thyrotropin-releasing hormone (TRH)
	Gonadotropin-releasing hormone (GnRH)
	Growth hormone–releasing hormone (GHRH)
	Growth hormone–inhibiting hormone (somatostatin GHIH)
	Prolactin-inhibiting hormone (PIH)
	Melanocyte-inhibiting hormone (MIH)
Anterior pituitary	Thyroid-stimulating hormone (TSH), also known as *thyrotropin*
	Adrenocorticotropic hormone (ACTH, corticotropin)
	Luteinizing hormone (LH), also known as *Leydig cell–stimulating hormone (LCSH)*
	Follicle-stimulating hormone (FSH)
	Prolactin (PRL)
	Growth hormone (GH)
	Melanocyte-stimulating hormone (MSH)
Posterior pituitary	Vasopressin (antidiuretic hormone [ADH])
	Oxytocin
Thyroid	Triiodothyronine (T_3)
	Thyroxine (T_4)
	Calcitonin
Parathyroid	Parathyroid hormone (PTH)
Adrenal cortex	Glucocorticoids (cortisol)
	Mineralocorticoids (aldosterone)
Ovary	Estrogen
	Progesterone
Testes	Testosterone
Pancreas	Insulin
	Glucagon
	Somatostatin

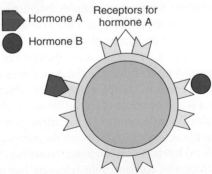

FIG. 56.2 "Lock and key" hormone-receptor binding. Hormone A fits and binds to its receptors, causing a change in cell action. Hormone B does not fit or bind to receptors; no change in cell action results.

away from the normal range and a specific response is needed to correct this change, secretion of the hormone capable of start- ing the correcting action or response is stimulated until the need (demand) is met and the body condition returns to the normal range. As the correction occurs, hormone secretion decreases (and may halt). A **negative feedback mechanism** signals an endocrine

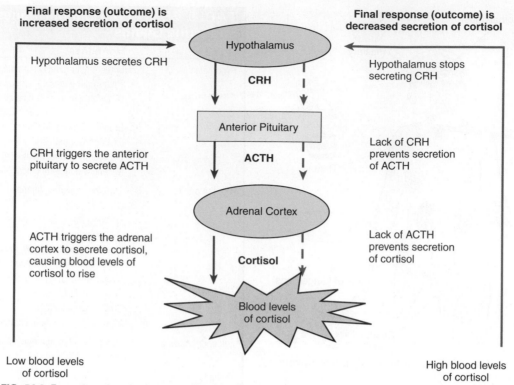

FIG. 56.3 Examples of positive and negative feedback control of hormone secretion. *ACTH,* Adrenocortico-tropic hormone; *CRH,* corticotropin-releasing hormone.

gland to secrete a hormone in response to a body change to cause a reaction that will result in actions to *oppose* the action of the initial condition change and restore homeostasis.

An example of a simple negative feedback hormone response is the control of insulin secretion. When blood glucose levels start to rise above normal, the hormone *insulin* is secreted. Insulin increases glucose uptake by the cells, causing a *decrease* in blood glucose levels. Thus the action of insulin (decreasing blood glucose levels) is the opposite of or negative to the condition that stimulated insulin secretion (elevated blood glucose levels).

Some hormones have more complex interactions for negative feedback. These interactions involve a series of reactions in which more than one endocrine gland, as well as the final target tissues, are stimulated. In this situation, the first hormone in the series may have another endocrine gland or glands as the target tissue. The final result of complex negative feedback for endocrine function is still opposite of the initiating condition.

An example of complex control is the interaction of the hypothalamus and the anterior pituitary with the adrenal cortex (Fig. 56.3). Low blood levels of cortisol from the adrenal cortex stimulate the secretion of corticotropin-releasing hormone (CRH) in the hypothalamus. CRH stimulates the anterior pituitary gland to secrete adrenocorticotropic hormone (ACTH). ACTH then triggers the release of cortisol from the adrenal cortex, the final endocrine gland in this series. The rising blood levels of cortisol inhibit CRH release from the hypothalamus. Without CRH, the anterior pituitary gland stops secretion of ACTH. In response, normal blood cortisol levels are maintained.

The normal blood level range of each hormone is well defined. Excesses or deficiencies of hormone secretion can lead to pathologic conditions affecting many body systems.

Hypothalamus and Pituitary Glands

Parts of the hypothalamus are composed of glandular tissues that have many control functions for the rest of the endocrine system. It is located beneath the thalamus in the brain, and nerve fibers connect the hypothalamus to the rest of the central nervous system. The hypothalamus shares a small, closed circulatory system with the anterior pituitary gland, known as the *hypothalamic-hypophysial portal system.* This system allows hormones produced in the hypothalamus to travel directly to the anterior pituitary gland, so only very small amounts are present in systemic circulation where they are not needed.

The function of the hypothalamus is to produce regulatory hormones (see Table 56.1). Some of these hormones are released into the blood and travel to the anterior pituitary, where they either stimulate or inhibit the release of anterior pituitary hormones.

The pituitary gland is located at the base of the brain in a protective pocket of the sphenoid bone (see Fig. 56.1). It is divided into the anterior lobe *(adenohypophysis)* and the posterior lobe *(neurohypophysis).* Nerve fibers in the hypophysial stalk directly connect the hypothalamus to the posterior pituitary (Fig. 56.4).

In response to the releasing hormones of the hypothalamus, the anterior pituitary secretes some tropic (trophic) hormones that have as their target tissues other endocrine glands. Other pituitary hormones, such as prolactin, produce their effect directly on final target tissues (Table 56.2).

The hormones of the posterior pituitary—vasopressin (antidiuretic hormone [ADH]) and oxytocin—are produced in the hypothalamus and delivered to the posterior pituitary where they are stored. These hormones are released from the posterior pituitary into the blood when needed.

TABLE 56.2 Pituitary Hormones: Target Tissues and Subsequent Actions

Hormone	Target Tissue	Actions
Anterior Pituitary		
Thyroid-stimulating hormone or thyrotropin (TSH)	Thyroid	Stimulates synthesis and release of thyroid hormone
Adrenocorticotropic hormone, corticotropin (ACTH)	Adrenal cortex	Stimulates synthesis and release of corticosteroids and adrenocortical growth
Luteinizing hormone (LH) (known as *Leydig cell–stimulating hormone* in males)	Ovary	Stimulates ovulation and progesterone secretion
	Testis	Stimulates testosterone secretion
Follicle-stimulating hormone (FSH) (known as *interstitial cell–* or *Sertoli cell–stimulating hormone* in males)	Ovary	Stimulates estrogen secretion and follicle maturation
	Testis	Stimulates spermatogenesis
Prolactin (PRL)	Mammary glands	Stimulates breast milk production
Growth hormone (GH)	Bone and soft tissue	Promotes growth through lipolysis, protein anabolism, and insulin antagonism
Melanocyte-stimulating hormone (MSH)	Melanocytes	Promotes pigmentation
Posterior Pituitary[a]		
Vasopressin (antidiuretic hormone [ADH])	Kidney	Promotes water reabsorption
Oxytocin	Uterus and mammary glands	Stimulates uterine contractions and ejection of breast milk

[a]These hormones are synthesized in the hypothalamus and are stored in the posterior pituitary gland. They are transported from the hypothalamus down the hypothalamic stalk to the posterior pituitary while bound to proteins known as *neurophysins*.

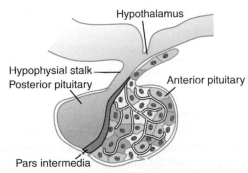

FIG. 56.1 Hypothalamus, hypophysial stalk, anterior pituitary gland, and posterior pituitary gland. (From Guyton, A., & Hall, J. [2006]. *Textbook of medical physiology* [11th ed.]. Philadelphia: Saunders.)

Other factors affect hormone release from the pituitary gland. Drugs, diet, lifestyle, and pathologic conditions can change pituitary hormone secretion (McCance et al., 2019).

Gonads

The gonads are the male and female reproductive endocrine glands. Male gonads are the testes, and female gonads are the ovaries. Function of the gonads is dormant until puberty when, under the influence of gonadotropic hormones secreted by the anterior pituitary, the glands and external genitalia mature. The testes are stimulated to produce testosterone, and the ovaries are stimulated to produce estrogen. These changes are responsible for the development of secondary sexual characteristics. The structure and function of the gonads are described in Chapter 64.

Adrenal Glands

The adrenal glands are vascular, tent-shaped organs on the top of each kidney. They have an outer cortex and an inner medulla (see Fig. 56.1). Adrenal hormones affect the entire body.

Adrenal Cortex. The adrenal cortex makes up about 90% of the adrenal gland and has cells divided into three layers. The main hormone types secreted by the cortex are the mineralocorticoids and the glucocorticoids. In addition, the cortex also secretes small amounts of sex hormones.

Mineralocorticoids are produced and secreted by the adrenal cortex to help control **fluid and electrolyte balance**. *Aldosterone* is the mineralocorticoid that maintains extracellular fluid volume and electrolyte composition. It promotes sodium and water reabsorption and potassium excretion in the kidney. Aldosterone secretion is regulated by the renin-angiotensin-aldosterone system (RAAS), serum potassium ion level, and adrenocorticotropic hormone (ACTH).

Renin is produced by specialized cells of the kidney arterioles. Its release is triggered by a decrease in extracellular fluid volume from blood loss, sodium loss, or posture changes. Hypoxemia also triggers renin release. Renin converts renin substrate (angiotensinogen), a plasma protein, to angiotensin I. Angiotensin I is then converted by an enzyme to form angiotensin II, the active form of angiotensin. In turn, angiotensin II stimulates the secretion of aldosterone. Chapter 13 (see Fig. 13.7 further explains the RAAS functions. Aldosterone causes the kidney to reabsorb sodium and water to bring the plasma volume and osmolarity back to normal.

Serum potassium level also controls aldosterone secretion. It is secreted whenever the serum potassium level increases above normal by as little as 0.1 mEq/L (mmol/L). Aldosterone then enhances kidney excretion of potassium to reduce the blood potassium level back to normal.

Glucocorticoids are produced by the adrenal cortex and are essential for life. The main glucocorticoid produced by the adrenal cortex is *cortisol*. Cortisol affects:
- The body's response to stress
- Carbohydrate, protein, and fat metabolism
- Emotional stability

TABLE 56.3   Functions of Glucocorticoid Hormones

- Prevent hypoglycemia by increasing liver glucose production (gluconeogenesis) and inhibiting peripheral glucose use
- Maintain excitability and responsiveness of cardiac muscle
- Increase lipolysis, releasing glycerol and free fatty acids
- Increase protein catabolism
- Degrade collagen and connective tissue
- Increase the number of mature neutrophils released from bone marrow
- Exert anti-inflammatory effects that decrease the migration of inflammatory cells to sites of injury
- Maintain behavior and cognitive functions

- Immune function
- Sodium and water balance

Cortisol also influences other important body processes. For example, it must be present for *catecholamine* (epinephrine, norepinephrine [NE]) action and maintaining the normal excitability of the heart muscle cells (McCance et al., 2019). Glucocorticoid functions are listed in Table 56.3.

Glucocorticoid release is regulated directly by the anterior pituitary hormone *ACTH* and indirectly by the hypothalamic corticotropin-releasing hormone *(CRH)*. The release of CRH and ACTH is affected by the serum level of free cortisol, the normal sleep-wake cycle, and stress.

As described earlier and shown in Fig. 56.3, when blood cortisol levels are low, the hypothalamus secretes CRH, which triggers the pituitary to release ACTH. Then ACTH triggers the adrenal cortex to secrete cortisol. Adequate or elevated blood levels of cortisol *inhibit* the release of CRH and ACTH. This inhibitory effect is an example of a negative feedback system.

Glucocorticoid release peaks in the morning and reaches its lowest level 12 hours after the peak. Emotional, chemical, or physical stress increases the release of glucocorticoids.

Sex hormones (androgens and estrogens) are secreted in low levels by the adrenal cortex in both genders. Adrenal secretion of these hormones is usually not significant because the gonads (ovaries and testes) secrete much larger amounts of estrogens and androgens. However, in women the adrenal gland is the major source of androgens.

Adrenal Medulla. The adrenal medulla is a sympathetic nerve ganglion that has secretory cells. Stimulation of the sympathetic nervous system causes the release of adrenal medullary hormones, the catecholamines (epinephrine and norepinephrine [NE]). These hormones travel to all areas of the body through the blood and exert their effects on target cells. The adrenal medullary hormones are not essential for life because they also are secreted by other body tissues, but they do play a role in the stress response.

The adrenal medulla secretes about 15% NE and 85% epinephrine. Hormone effects vary with the specific receptor in the cell membranes of the target tissue.

These receptors are of two types: alpha adrenergic and beta adrenergic, which are further classified as alpha$_1$ and alpha$_2$ receptors and beta$_1$, beta$_2$, and beta$_3$ receptors. NE acts mainly on alpha-adrenergic receptors, and epinephrine acts mainly on beta-adrenergic receptors.

TABLE 56.4   Catecholamine Receptors and Effects of Adrenal Medullary Hormone Stimulation on Selected Organs and Tissues

Organ or Tissue	Receptors	Effects
Heart	Beta$_1$	Increased heart rate Increased contractility
Blood vessels	Alpha	Vasoconstriction
	Beta$_2$	Vasodilation
GI tract	Alpha	Increased sphincter tone
	Beta	Decreased motility
Kidneys	Beta$_2$	Increased renin release
Bronchioles	Beta$_2$	Relaxation; dilation
Bladder	Alpha	Sphincter contractions
	Beta$_2$	Relaxation of detrusor muscle
Skin	Alpha	Increased sweating
Fat cells	Beta	Increased lipolysis
Liver	Alpha	Increased gluconeogenesis and glycogenolysis
Pancreas	Alpha	Decreased glucagon and insulin release
	Beta	Increased glucagon and insulin release
Eyes	Alpha	Dilation of pupils

Catecholamines exert their actions on many target organs (Table 56.4). Activation of the sympathetic nervous system, which then releases adrenal medullary catecholamines, is an important part of the stress response. Catecholamines are secreted in small amounts at all times to maintain homeostasis. Stress triggers increased secretion of these hormones, resulting in the "fight-or-flight" response, a state of heightened physical and emotional awareness.

Thyroid Gland

The thyroid gland is in the anterior neck, directly below the cricoid cartilage (Fig. 56.5). It has two lobes joined by a thin strip of tissue *(isthmus)* in front of the trachea.

The thyroid gland is composed of follicular and parafollicular cells. Follicular cells produce the thyroid hormones *thyroxine* (T_4) and *triiodothyronine* (T_3). Parafollicular cells produce *thyrocalcitonin (TCT or calcitonin)*, which helps regulate serum calcium levels.

Control of metabolism occurs through T_3 and T_4. Both hormones increase metabolism, which causes an increase in oxygen use and heat production in all tissues. Most circulating T_4 and T_3 are bound to plasma proteins. The free hormone moves into the cell, where it binds to its receptor in the cell nucleus. Once in the cell, T_4 is converted to T_3, the most active thyroid hormone. Conversion of T_4 to T_3 is impaired by stress, starvation, dyes, and some drugs. Cold temperatures increase the conversion. Table 56.5 lists thyroid hormone functions.

Secretion of T_3 and T_4 is controlled by the hypothalamic-pituitary-thyroid gland axis negative feedback mechanism. The

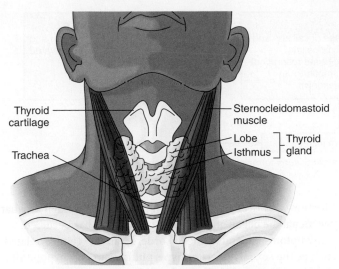

Thyroid cartilage

Trachea

Sternocleidomastoid muscle

Lobe
Isthmus } Thyroid gland

FIG. 56.5 Anatomic location of the thyroid gland.

TABLE 56.5 Functions of Thyroid Hormones in Adults

- Control metabolic rate of all cells
- Promote sufficient pituitary secretion of growth hormone and gonadotropins
- Regulate protein, carbohydrate, and fat metabolism
- Exert effects on heart rate and contractility
- Increase red blood cell production
- Affect respiratory rate and drive
- Increase bone formation and decrease bone resorption of calcium
- Act as insulin antagonists

hypothalamus secretes thyrotropin-releasing hormone (TRH). TRH triggers the anterior pituitary gland to secrete thyroid-stimulating hormone (TSH), which then stimulates the thyroid gland to make and release thyroid hormones. If thyroid hormone levels are high, release of TRH and TSH is inhibited. If thyroid hormone levels are low, TRH and TSH release is increased. Cold and stress are two factors that cause the hypothalamus to secrete TRH, which then stimulates the anterior pituitary to secrete TSH.

Dietary intake of protein and iodine is needed to produce thyroid hormones. Iodine is absorbed from the intestinal tract as iodide. The thyroid gland draws iodide from the blood and concentrates it. After iodide is in the thyroid, it combines with the amino acid *tyrosine* to form T_4 and T_3. These hormones bind to thyroglobulin and are stored in thyroid follicular cells. When stimulated, T_4 and T_3 are released into the blood. They enter all cells, where they bind to DNA receptors and turn on genes important in metabolism to regulate basal metabolic rate (BMR).

Calcium and phosphorus balance occurs partly through the actions of calcitonin (thyrocalcitonin [TCT]), which also is produced in the thyroid gland. Calcitonin lowers serum calcium and serum phosphorus levels by reducing bone resorption (release) of these minerals. Its actions are opposite of parathyroid hormone (PTH).

The serum calcium level determines calcitonin secretion. Low serum calcium levels suppress the release of calcitonin. Elevated serum calcium levels increase its secretion.

Parathyroid Glands

The parathyroid glands consist of four small glands located close to or within the back surface of the thyroid gland (see Fig. 56.1). These cells secrete parathyroid hormone (PTH).

PTH regulates calcium and phosphorus metabolism by acting on bones, the kidneys, and the GI tract (Fig. 56.6). Bone is the main storage site of calcium. PTH increases *bone resorption* (bone release of calcium into the blood from bone storage sites), thus increasing serum calcium. In the kidneys, PTH activates vitamin D, which then increases the absorption of calcium and phosphorus from the intestines. In the kidney tubules, PTH allows calcium to be reabsorbed and put back into the blood.

Serum calcium levels determine PTH secretion. Secretion decreases when serum calcium levels are high, and it increases when serum calcium levels are low. PTH and calcitonin work together to maintain normal calcium levels in the blood and extracellular fluid.

Pancreas

The pancreas has exocrine and endocrine functions. The exocrine function of the pancreas involves the secretion of digestive enzymes through ducts that empty into the duodenum. The cells in the islets of Langerhans perform the pancreatic endocrine functions (Fig. 56.7). About 1 million islet cells are found throughout the pancreas.

The islets have three distinct cell types: alpha cells, which secrete glucagon; beta cells, which secrete insulin; and delta cells, which secrete somatostatin. Glucagon and insulin affect carbohydrate, protein, and fat metabolism.

Glucagon is a hormone that increases blood glucose levels. It is triggered by decreased blood glucose levels and increased blood amino acid levels. This hormone helps prevent hypoglycemia. Chapter 59 discusses glucagon function in more detail.

Insulin promotes the movement and storage of carbohydrate, protein, and fat. It lowers blood glucose levels by enhancing glucose movement across cell membranes and into the cells of many tissues. Insulin secretion rises in response to an increase in blood glucose levels. More information on insulin is presented in Chapter 59.

Somatostatin, which is secreted not only in the pancreas but also in the intestinal tract and the brain, inhibits the release of glucagon and insulin from the pancreas. It also inhibits the release of gastrin, secretin, and other GI peptides.

NCLEX EXAMINATION CHALLENGE 56.1

Physiological Integrity

Which action **best** exemplifies the expected outcome of appropriate negative feedback control over endocrine gland hormone secretion?

A. Decreased secretion of glucagon when blood glucose approaches normal levels

B. Increased secretion of parathyroid hormone in response to a calcium-containing intravenous infusion

C. Increased secretion of thyroid-stimulating hormone in response to long-term exogenous thyroid hormone replacement therapy

D. Decreased secretion of cortisol in response to a pituitary tumor stimulating the increased secretion of adrenocorticotropic hormone

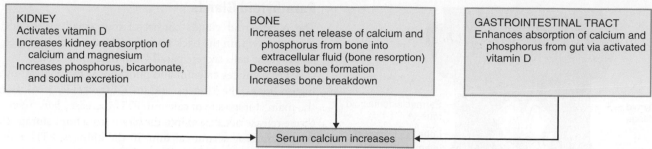

KIDNEY
Activates vitamin D
Increases kidney reabsorption of
   calcium and magnesium
Increases phosphorus, bicarbonate,
   and sodium excretion

BONE
Increases net release of calcium and
   phosphorus from bone into
   extracellular fluid (bone resorption)
Decreases bone formation
Increases bone breakdown

GASTROINTESTINAL TRACT
Enhances absorption of calcium and
   phosphorus from gut via activated
   vitamin D

Serum calcium increases

FIG. 56.6 Effects of parathyroid hormone on target tissues to maintain calcium balance.

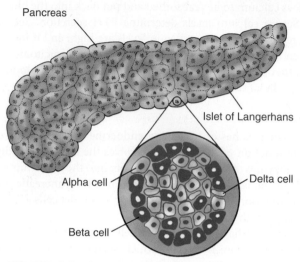

Pancreas

Islet of Langerhans

Alpha cell

Delta cell

Beta cell

FIG. 56.7 Cells of the islets of Langerhans of the pancreas.

Endocrine Changes Associated With Aging

The effects of aging on the endocrine system vary but usually result in reduced glandular function and decreased hormone secretion. The three endocrine tissues that usually have reduced function with aging are the gonads, the thyroid gland, and the endocrine pancreas (Lamberts & van den Beld, 2016; Touhy & Jett, 2020). This reduction is normally very gradual for the thyroid glands, pancreas, and male gonads. For women, reduced function of the ovaries is somewhat faster with more noticeable changes. It is difficult to distinguish normal from abnormal endocrine activity in older adults because of chronic illness, changes in diet and activity, sleep disturbances, decreased metabolism, and the use of drugs that may affect hormone function. Consider these factors when assessing the older adult with endocrine dysfunction.

Encourage the older adult to participate in regular screening examinations, including fasting and random blood glucose checks, calcium level determinations, and thyroid function testing. The Patient-Centered Care: Older Adult Considerations: Age-Related Endocrine System Changes box lists the common endocrine changes that occur in the older adult.

ASSESSMENT: RECOGNIZE CUES

Patient History

Baseline endocrine assessment data must include age and gender because certain disorders are more common in older than in younger patients, such as diabetes mellitus, loss of ovarian

function, and decreased thyroid function. Ask women at what age menarche began and whether menopause has occurred.

Symptoms of endocrine disorders can be gender related, such as the sexual effects of hyperpituitarism and hypopituitarism (see Chapter 57). Thyroid problems are more common in women (McCance et al., 2019). Assess for a history of endocrine problems, symptoms that could indicate a disorder, and hospitalizations. Ask about past and current drugs, such as cortisone, levothyroxine, oral contraceptives, and antihypertensive agents. The use of exogenous hormone drugs, when not needed for hormone replacement, can cause serious dysfunction in many endocrine glands. Use the opportunity to warn patients about the dangers of misusing hormone-based drugs such as androgens and thyroid hormones (Burchum & Rosenthal, 2019).

Nutrition History. *Nutrition* changes or GI tract disturbances may reflect many different endocrine problems. Ask about a history of nausea, vomiting, and abdominal pain. An increase or decrease in food or fluid intake may also indicate specific disorders. For example, diabetes insipidus triggers excessive thirst, and adrenal hypofunction triggers salt craving. Hunger and thirst also are associated with diabetes mellitus. Rapid changes in weight without diet changes are often associated with many endocrine disorders, including diabetes mellitus and thyroid problems.

Nutrition deficiencies from an inadequate diet, especially of protein and iodide-containing foods (saltwater fish and seafood, cheese and dairy products, iodized table salt), may be a cause of an endocrine disorder. Teach the patient about a well-balanced diet that includes at least 60 g of protein daily, less animal fat, and fewer concentrated simple sugars. Teach patients who do not eat saltwater fish on a regular basis to use iodized salt in food preparation.

Family History and Genetic Risk. Ask the patient about any family history of obesity, growth or development difficulties, diabetes mellitus, infertility, or thyroid disorders. These problems may have an autosomal dominant, recessive, or cluster pattern of inheritance.

Current Health Problems. Focus on the patient's reason for seeking health care, asking questions such as:
- When did symptoms begin?
- Did symptoms occur gradually, or start suddenly?
- Have you been treated for this problem in the past?
- How have the current problems affected your activities of daily living?

👤 PATIENT-CENTERED CARE: OLDER ADULT CONSIDERATIONS (QSEN)

Age-Related Endocrine System Changes

Change	Nursing Considerations
Decreased Antidiuretic Hormone (ADH) Production	
Urine is more dilute and may not concentrate when fluid intake is low.	The patient is at greater risk for dehydration.
	Assess the older patient more frequently for dehydration.
	If fluids are not restricted because of another health problem, teach assistive personnel (AP) to offer fluids at least every 2 hours while the patient is awake.
Decreased Ovarian Production of Estrogen	
Bone density decreases.	Teach the patient to engage in regular exercise and weight-bearing activity to maintain bone density.
Skin is thinner, drier, and at greater risk for injury.	Handle the patient carefully to avoid injury from fragile fractures.
Perineal and vaginal tissues become drier, and the risk for cystitis increases.	Avoid pulling or dragging the patient.
	Use minimal tape on the skin.
	Help patients confined to bed or chairs change positions at least every 2 hours.
	Teach patients to use skin moisturizers.
	Perform or assist the patient to perform perineal care at least twice daily.
	Unless another health problem requires fluid restriction, encourage all women to drink at least 2 liters of fluids daily.
	Teach sexually active older women to urinate immediately after sexual intercourse.
	Teach sexually active women that using vaginal lubricants with sexual activity can reduce discomfort and the risk for tissue damage.
Decreased Glucose Tolerance	
Weight becomes greater than ideal, along with:	Assess family history for obesity and type 2 diabetes.
• Elevated fasting blood glucose level	Encourage the patient to engage in regular exercise and to keep body weight within 10 lb (4.5 kg) of ideal.
• Elevated random blood glucose level	Teach patients the signs and symptoms of diabetes and instruct them to report any of these to the primary health care provider.
• Slow wound healing	Suggest diabetes testing for any patient with:
• Frequent yeast infections	• Persistent vaginal candidiasis
• Polydipsia	• Failure of a foot or leg skin wound to heal in 2 weeks or less
• Polyuria	• Increased hunger and thirst
	• Noticeable and persistent decrease in energy level
Decreased General Metabolism	
Patient has less tolerance for cold.	Teach patients to dress warmly in cool or cold weather.
Appetite is decreased.	Can be difficult to distinguish from hypothyroidism. Check for additional signs and symptoms of:
Heart rate and blood pressure (BP) are decreased.	• Lethargy
	• Constipation (as a change from usual bowel habits)
	• Decreased cognition
	• Slowed speech
	• Body temperature consistently below 97°F (36°C)
	• Heart rate below 60 beats/min

These questions can provide clues to specific endocrine disorders. Also explore changes in energy levels, *elimination* patterns, sexual and reproductive functions, and physical features.

Energy level changes occur with many endocrine problems, especially thyroid problems (see Chapter 58) and adrenal problems (see Chapter 57). Ask the patient about any change in ability to perform ADLs, and assess his or her current energy level. For instance, has he or she been sleeping longer, or are fatigue and generalized weakness present?

Elimination is affected by the endocrine system. Identify the patient's usual and past patterns of elimination to determine deviations from the normal routine. Ask about the amount and frequency of urination. Does he or she urinate frequently in large amounts? Does the patient wake during the night to urinate *(nocturia)*? Information about the frequency of bowel movements and their consistency and color may provide clues to problems in **fluid and electrolyte balance** or metabolic rate (i.e., thyroid function).

Sexual and reproductive functions are greatly affected by endocrine disturbances. Ask about any changes in the menstrual cycle, such as increased flow, duration, and frequency of menses; or a change in the regularity of menses. Ask men whether they have experienced impotence. Ask men and women about a change in *libido* (sexual desire) or fertility issues.

Physical appearance changes can reflect an endocrine problem. Discuss any changes that the patient perceives in physical features. Ask about changes in:

- Hair texture and distribution
- Facial contours and eye protrusion
- Voice quality
- Body proportions
- Secondary sexual characteristics

For example, ask a man whether he is shaving less often or a woman if she has noticed an increase in facial hair. These changes may be associated with pituitary, thyroid, parathyroid, or adrenal dysfunction.

Physical Assessment

Inspection. An endocrine problem can change physical features because of its effect on growth and development, sex hormone levels, *fluid and electrolyte balance*, and metabolism. Different clinical findings can occur with many endocrine disorders or with nonendocrine problems.

Observe the patient's general appearance, and assess height, weight, fat distribution, and muscle mass in relation to age. Heredity and age rather than health problems may be responsible for some physical features (e.g., short stature). Assess scalp and body hair growth patterns.

When examining the head, focus on abnormalities of facial structure, features, and expression, such as:

- Prominent forehead or jaw
- Round or puffy face
- Dull or flat expression
- Exophthalmos (protruding eyeballs and retracted upper lids)

Check the lower neck for a visible enlargement of the thyroid gland. Normally the thyroid tissue cannot be observed. The isthmus may be noticeable when the patient swallows. Jugular vein distention may be seen on inspection of the neck and can indicate fluid overload.

Observe skin color and look for areas of pigment loss (*hypopigmentation*) or excess (*hyperpigmentation*). Fungal skin infections, slow wound healing, bruising, and petechiae are often seen in patients with adrenal hyperfunction. Skin infections, foot ulcers, and slow wound healing often occur with diabetes mellitus. With some types of adrenal gland dysfunction, the skin over the joints, as well as any scar tissue, may show increased pigmentation due to increased levels of adrenocorticotropic hormone (ACTH) and melanocyte-stimulating hormone.

Vitiligo (patchy areas of pigment loss) is seen with primary hypofunction of the adrenal glands and is caused by autoimmune destruction of melanocytes in the skin. It is seen most often on the face, neck, arms, hands, legs, and fold areas (Jarvis, 2020). Mucous membranes may have large areas of uneven pigmentation. Document the location, color, distribution, and size of skin color changes.

Inspect the fingernails for malformation, thickness, or brittleness, all of which may suggest thyroid gland problems. Examine the extremities and the base of the spine for edema, which suggests impaired *fluid and electrolyte balance*.

Check the trunk for any abnormalities in chest size and symmetry. Truncal obesity and the presence of a "buffalo hump" between the shoulders on the back may indicate adrenocortical excess. Hormonal imbalance may also change secondary sexual characteristics. Inspect the breasts of men as well as women for size, symmetry, pigmentation, and discharge. Low testosterone levels in men induce breast enlargement (*gynecomastia*). *Striae* (reddish-purple "stretch marks") on the breasts or abdomen are often seen with adrenocortical excess.

Assess the patient's hair distribution for signs of endocrine gland dysfunction. Changes can include *hirsutism* (excessive body hair growth, especially on the face, the chest, and the center abdominal line of women), excessive scalp hair loss, or changes in hair texture (Jarvis, 2020).

Examination of the genitalia may reveal a dysfunction in hormone secretion. Observe the size of the scrotum and penis or of the labia and clitoris in relation to standards for the patient's age. The distribution and quantity of pubic hair are often affected in hypogonadism.

Palpation. The thyroid gland and the testes can be examined by palpation, most often by a primary health care provider rather than a bedside nurse. Chapters 64 and 67 discuss examination of the testes. The thyroid gland is palpated for size, symmetry, general shape, and the presence of nodules or other irregularities.

The thyroid gland is palpated by standing either behind or in front of the patient (Jarvis, 2020). Having the patient swallow sips of water during the examination helps palpate the thyroid gland, which is not easily felt when normal.

The patient sits and lowers the chin. The examiner, using the posterior approach, places both thumbs on the back of the patient's neck, with the fingers curved around to the front of the neck on either side of the trachea. When the patient swallows, the thyroid is felt as it rises. The right lobe is examined with the patient's head turned to the right, and the trachea is gently displaced by the examiner's left fingers. The right lobe is palpated with the examiner's right hand. This procedure is reversed to examine the left lobe (Jarvis, 2020).

⚠ NURSING SAFETY PRIORITY (QSEN)

Action Alert

Avoid applying pressure on or palpating the thyroid in a patient who has or is suspected to have hyperthyroidism because these actions can stimulate a sudden release of thyroid hormones and cause a thyroid storm.

Auscultation. Auscultate the chest to assess cardiac rate and rhythm to use later as a means of assessing treatment effectiveness. Some endocrine problems induce dysrhythmias. Many endocrine problems can cause dehydration and volume depletion. Document any difference in the patient's blood pressure and pulse in the lying, standing, or sitting positions (orthostatic vital signs).

When an enlarged thyroid gland is palpated, the area of enlargement is auscultated for bruits. Hypertrophy of the thyroid gland causes an increase in vascular flow, which may result in bruits.

Psychosocial Assessment

Many endocrine problems can change a patient's behaviors, personality, and psychological responses. Assess the patient's coping skills, support systems, and health-related beliefs. Ask whether the patient has noticed a change in how stress is handled, frequency of crying, or degree of patience and anger expression. Patients may not recognize these changes in themselves. Ask the family about changes in the patient's behaviors or personality.

A number of endocrine disorders affect the patient's perception of self. For example, body features can change greatly in disorders of the pituitary, adrenal, and thyroid glands. Infertility, impotence, and other changes in sexual function may result from endocrine problems. Encourage the patient to express his or her feelings and concerns about a change in appearance or in sexual function. Ask about any difficulty in coping with these changes.

Patients with endocrine problems may require lifelong drugs and follow-up care. Assess their readiness to learn and ability to carry out specific self-management skills. Patients may also face financial difficulties resulting from a prolonged medical regimen or loss of employment. A referral to social service agencies may be needed.

NCLEX EXAMINATION CHALLENGE 56.2

Safe and Effective Health Care Environment

Which assessment finding in a 40-year-old client is **most relevant** for the nurse to assess further for a possible endocrine problem?

A. He has lost 10 lb in the past month following a low-carbohydrate eating plan.

B. The client reports now needing to shave only once weekly instead of daily.

C. His new prescription for eyeglasses is for a higher strength.

D. The client's father died of a stroke at age 70 years.

❓ CLINICAL JUDGMENT CHALLENGE 56.1

Patient-Centered Care; Safety

A 27-year-old graduate student comes to student health services with reports of feeling tired all the time and having difficulty concentrating. She has gained 30 lb (13.6 kg) in the past 10 weeks without a change in eating habits and states that she is having a hard time focusing on both her class work and laboratory work. She further states that in the past 2 weeks she has fallen asleep in class several times despite sleeping 8 to 10 hours at night.

Vital signs are:
- T = 97.0°F (36.1°C)
- P = 58 beats/min
- BP = 88/40
- R = 14/min

When the nurse asks whether any other changes have been noticed, she replies that she has not had a period in 3 months and before that they had been regular. The nurse notes that the client is wearing a heavy sweater even though the day is warm.

1. **Recognize Cues:** What assessment information in this client situation is the most important and immediate concern for the nurse? (Hint: Identify the **relevant** information *first* to determine what is most important.)

2. **Analyze Cues:** What client conditions are consistent with the **most relevant** information? (Hint: Think about priority collaborative problems that support and contradict the information presented in this situation.)

Diagnostic Assessment

Laboratory Tests. Laboratory tests are an essential part of the diagnostic process for possible endocrine problems. Fluids commonly used for these tests include blood, urine, and saliva. Salivary levels of the steroid hormones (cortisol, testosterone, progesterone, and estradiol) accurately reflect blood levels of these hormones (Sluss & Hayes, 2016). Protein hormones, such as those from the pituitary gland and thyroid gland, are not assessed using saliva. Always check with the agency's laboratory for proper collection and handling of the specimen. Specialized testing for specific disorders is described in Chapters 57 to 59. The Best Practice for Patient Safety & Quality Care: Endocrine Testing box lists correct techniques for collection of specimens for general endocrine testing.

BEST PRACTICE FOR PATIENT SAFETY & QUALITY CARE (QSEN)
Endocrine Testing

For Blood Tests
- Check your laboratory's method of handling hormone test samples for tube type, timing, drugs to be administered as part of the test, etc. For example, blood samples drawn for catecholamines must be placed on ice and taken to the laboratory immediately.
- Explain the procedure and any restrictions to the patient.
- If you are drawing blood samples from an IV line, clear the line thoroughly. Do not use a double- or triple-lumen line to obtain samples; contamination or dilution from another port is possible.
- Emphasize the importance of taking a drug prescribed for the test on time. Tell the patient to set an alarm if the drug is to be taken during the night.

For Urine Tests
- Instruct the patient to begin the urine collection (whether for 2, 4, 8, 12, or 24 hours) by first emptying his or her bladder and NOT using this specimen as part of the collection. The timing for the urine collection begins *after* this specimen is discarded.
- Tell the patient to note the time of the discarded specimen and to plan to collect all urine from this time until the end of the urine collection period.
- To end the collection, instruct the patient to empty his or her bladder at the end of the timed period, even if the urge to urinate is not felt, and add that urine to the collection.
- Check with the laboratory to determine any special handling of the urine specimen (e.g., Is a preservative needed? Does the container need to be kept cold?).
- If needed, make sure that the preservative has been added to the collection container at the beginning of the collection.
- Tell the patient about any preservative and the need to avoid splashing urine from the container because some preservatives make the urine caustic.
- If the specimen must be kept cool or cold, instruct the patient to place the container in an inexpensive cooler with ice. The specimen container should not be kept with food or drinks.

Assays. An assay measures the level of a specific hormone in blood or other body fluid. The most common assays for endocrine testing are antibody-based immunologic assays and chromatographic assays, which include mass spectrometry that measures the presence of a hormone(s) based on its molecular mass and chemical composition. These assays are very sensitive and can detect even minute quantities of a given hormone. Many different hormone concentrations can be analyzed at the same time by the mass spectrometry method.

Provocative/Suppression Tests. Measurement of specific hormone blood levels does not always distinguish between the normal and the abnormal. The wide normal range for some hormones makes it necessary to trigger responses by provocative ("stimulation") or suppression tests.

For the patient who might have an underactive endocrine gland, a stimulus may be used to determine whether the gland is capable of normal hormone production. This method is called *provocative testing.* Measured amounts of selected hormones are given to stimulate the target gland to maximum production. Hormone levels are then measured and compared with expected normal values. Failure of the hormone level to rise with provocation indicates hypofunction.

Suppression tests are used when hormone levels are high or in the upper range of normal. Drugs or other substances known to normally suppress hormone production are administered. Failure of suppression of hormone production during testing indicates hyperfunction.

Urine Tests. The levels of hormones and their metabolites in the urine can be measured to determine endocrine function. Because many of the endocrine hormones are secreted in a pulsatile fashion, measurement of a specific hormone in a 24-hour urine collection, rather than as a single blood or urine sample, better reflects the function of a specific gland, such as the adrenal gland. Teach the patient how to collect a 24-hour urine sample (see also the Best Practice for Patient Safety & Quality Care: Endocrine Testing box).

Certain hormones require additives in the container at the beginning of the collection. Instruct the patient not to discard the preservative from the container and to use caution when handling it because some are caustic. Remind him or her that this collection is timed for *exactly* 24 hours. Instruct the patient to avoid taking any unnecessary drugs during endocrine testing because some drugs can interfere with the assay.

Genetic Testing. When some hormone levels are too low to be measured, genetic testing may be performed. DNA analysis or RNA assessment can determine whether a genetic mutation is responsible for the lack of hormone production or the absence of hormone receptors (Sluss & Hayes, 2016).

Tests for Glucose. Tests for functions of the islet cells of the pancreas measure the *result* of pancreatic islet cell function. Blood glucose values and the oral glucose tolerance test help diagnose diabetes mellitus. The glycosylated hemoglobin (A1C) value indicates the *average* blood glucose level over a period of 2 to 3 months. (See Chapter 59 for diabetes mellitus testing.)

Imaging Assessment. Anterior, posterior, and lateral skull x-rays may be used to view the sella turcica, the bony pocket in the skull where the pituitary gland rests. Erosion of the sella turcica indicates invasion of the wall from an abnormal growth.

MRI with contrast is the most sensitive method of imaging the pituitary gland, although CT scans can also be used to evaluate it. The thyroid, parathyroid glands, ovaries, and testes are evaluated by ultrasound. CT scans are used to evaluate the adrenal glands, ovaries, and pancreas.

Other Diagnostic Assessment. Needle biopsy is a safe and quick ambulatory surgery procedure used to indicate the composition of thyroid nodules. It is used to determine whether surgical intervention is needed.

GET READY FOR THE NEXT-GENERATION NCLEX® EXAMINATION!

Key Points
Review these Key Points for each NCLEX Examination Client Needs Category.

Safe and Effective Care Environment
- Be aware that assessment of endocrine problems requires a systematic approach because of the variety and combination of signs and symptoms. **QSEN: Evidence-Based Practice**
- Physical, psychosocial, and laboratory findings are needed for a complete and accurate endocrine assessment to avoid overlooking any problems. **QSEN: Safety**

Health Promotion and Maintenance
- Teach all patients that abusing or misusing hormones or steroids can have an adverse effect on endocrine function. **QSEN: Patient-Centered Care**
- Explain all diagnostic procedures, restrictions, and follow-up care to the patient scheduled for endocrine tests. **QSEN: Patient-Centered Care**

Psychosocial Integrity
- Encourage the patient to express concerns about a change in appearance, sexual function, or fertility as a result of a possible endocrine problem. **QSEN: Patient-Centered Care**

- Ask family members about changes in the patient's personality or behavior. **QSEN: Patient-Centered Care**

Physiological Integrity
- Be aware that the onset of endocrine problems can be slow and insidious or abrupt and life threatening.
- The presence of excess hormone production in an older adult is more likely to be caused by an actual endocrine problem than by age-related changes.
- Ask the patient about other family members with endocrine disorders, because some problems have a genetic component. **QSEN: Evidence-Based Practice**
- Ask the patient what prescribed and over-the-counter drugs are taken on a regular basis, because some drugs can alter endocrine function. **QSEN: Patient-Centered Care**
- Follow the laboratory's procedures for collecting and handling specimens for endocrine function studies. **QSEN: Evidence-Based Practice**
- Differentiate normal from abnormal laboratory test findings and signs and symptoms for patients with possible endocrine problems. **QSEN: Patient-Centered Care**

■ MASTERY QUESTIONS

1. Which statement regarding trophic (tropic) hormones is true?
   A. All are categorized as catecholamines.
   B. Responses are independent of target tissue receptors.
   C. Their target tissues are always another endocrine gland.
   D. They represent the final hormone secreted in a complex negative feedback pathway.

2. Which instruction/precaution does the nurse teach a client to **prevent harm** during a 24-hour urine specimen collection?
   A. Be sure to keep the specimen cool for the entire collection period.
   B. Avoid splashing urine in the container when a preservative is present.
   C. Add the preservative to the collection container before adding any urine.
   D. Discard the first specimen that marks the beginning of the 24-hour test period.

REFERENCES

Burchum, J., & Rosenthal, L. (2019). *Lehne's pharmacology for nursing care* (10th ed.). St. Louis: Elsevier.

Jarvis, C. (2020). *Physical examination & health assessment* (8th ed.). St. Louis: Elsevier.

Lamberts, S., & van den Beld, A. (2016). Endocrinology and aging. In S. Melmed, K. Polonsky, P. R. Larsen, & H. Kronenberg (Eds.), *Williams' textbook of endocrinology* (13th ed.). Philadelphia: Elsevier.

Lazar, M., & Birnbaum, M. (2016). Principles of hormone actions. In S. Melmed, K. Polonsky, P. R. Larsen, & H. Kronenberg (Eds.), *Williams' textbook of endocrinology* (13th ed.). Philadelphia: Elsevier.

McCance, K., Huether, S., Brashers, V., & Rote, N. (2019). *Pathophysiology: The biologic basis for disease in adults and children* (8th ed.). St. Louis: Elsevier.

Sluss, P., & Hayes, F. (2016). Laboratory techniques for recognition of endocrine disorders. In S. Melmed, K. Polonsky, P. R. Larsen, & H. Kronenberg (Eds.), *Williams' textbook of endocrinology* (13th ed.). Philadelphia: Elsevier.

Touhy, T., & Jett, K. (2020). *Ebersole and Hess' toward healthy aging: Human needs and nursing response* (10th ed.) St. Louis: Mosby.

57

Concepts of Care for Patients With Pituitary and Adrenal Gland Problems

M. Linda Workman

http://evolve.elsevier.com/Iggy/

LEARNING OUTCOMES

1. Collaborate with the interprofessional team to coordinate high-quality care and promote *fluid and electrolyte balance, cellular regulation,* and *immunity* in patients who have pituitary or adrenal disorders.
2. Apply knowledge of anatomy, physiology, and pathophysiology to assess patients with impaired pituitary or adrenal gland function affecting *fluid and electrolyte balance, cellular regulation,* or *immunity.*
3. Implement nursing actions to help the patient and family cope with the psychosocial impact caused by acute or chronic problems of the pituitary or adrenal gland.
4. Interpret clinical changes and laboratory data to determine the effectiveness of therapy for diabetes insipidus (DI) and for syndrome of inappropriate antidiuretic hormone (SIADH).
5. Use clinical judgment to prioritize evidence-based nursing care for the patient with acute adrenal insufficiency, hypercortisolism, and any other pituitary or adrenal problems.
6. Teach the patient and caregiver(s) about common drugs and other management strategies used for pituitary or adrenal gland problems.

KEY TERMS

acute adrenal insufficiency A life-threatening event in which the need for cortisol and aldosterone is greater than the body's supply. Also known as *adrenal crisis* or *addisonian crisis.*

diabetes insipidus (DI) Disorder of the posterior pituitary gland in which water loss is caused by either an antidiuretic hormone (ADH) deficiency or an inability of the kidneys to respond to ADH.

gynecomastia Male breast tissue development.

hyperaldosteronism Increased secretion of aldosterone with mineralocorticoid excess.

hypercortisolism (Cushing disease) The excess secretion of cortisol from the adrenal cortex, causing many problems.

hyperpituitarism Hormone oversecretion that occurs with anterior pituitary tumors or tissue hyperplasia (tissue overgrowth).

hypophysectomy Surgical removal of the pituitary gland.

hypopituitarism A deficiency of one and sometimes more than one pituitary hormone.

syndrome of inappropriate antidiuretic hormone (SIADH) A problem in which vasopressin (antidiuretic hormone [ADH]) is secreted even when plasma osmolarity is low or normal, resulting in water retention and fluid overload. (Also known as *Schwartz-Bartter syndrome.*)

virilization Presence of male secondary sex characteristics.

✳ PRIORITY AND INTERRELATED CONCEPTS

The priority concept for this chapter is:
- *Fluid and Electrolyte Balance*
  The *Fluid and Electrolyte Balance* concept exemplar for this chapter is Hypercortisolism (Cushing Disease).

The interrelated concepts for this chapter are:
- *Cellular Regulation*
- *Immunity*

The pituitary and adrenal glands function to secrete hormones that affect the *cellular regulation* of the entire body, including *fluid and electrolyte balance.* When these hormones are secreted in either excessive or insufficient amounts, physical and psychological changes result. The anterior pituitary hormones regulate growth, metabolism, and sexual development. The posterior pituitary hormone, *vasopressin* (antidiuretic hormone [ADH]), helps maintain *fluid and electrolyte balance.* Adrenal gland hormones are life sustaining.

A complete assessment is performed to detect specific clinical findings. The patient also often undergoes many diagnostic tests and relies on the nurse for explanations. Surgical intervention may be indicated. Priority nursing care for the patient with pituitary or adrenal gland disorders includes assessment, patient education, evaluating patient response to therapy, and providing support.

DISORDERS OF THE PITUITARY GLAND

HYPOPITUITARISM

Pathophysiology Review

The anterior pituitary gland *(adenohypophysis)* secretes the following hormones to maintain homeostasis:

- Growth hormone (GH; somatotropin)
- Thyrotropin (thyroid-stimulating hormone [TSH])
- Corticotropin (adrenocorticotropic hormone [ACTH])
- Follicle-stimulating hormone (FSH)
- Luteinizing hormone (LH)
- Melanocyte-stimulating hormone (MSH)
- Prolactin (PRL)

Hypopituitarism is a deficiency of one and sometimes more than one pituitary hormone. Most often only one pituitary hormone is deficient, a condition known as *selective hypopituitarism.* Decreased production of *all* of the anterior pituitary hormones *(panhypopituitarism)* is rare and much more serious (Mitchell-Brown & Stephens-DiLeo, 2017).

Deficiencies of *adrenocorticotropic hormone (ACTH)* or *thyroid stimulating hormone (TSH)* are the *most* life threatening because they cause a decrease in the secretion of vital hormones from the adrenal and thyroid glands. Adrenal gland hypofunction is discussed later in this chapter; hypothyroidism is discussed in Chapter 58.

Deficiency of the gonadotropins (luteinizing hormone [LH] and follicle-stimulating hormone [FSH]—hormones that stimulate the gonads to produce sex hormones) changes sexual function in both men and women. In men, gonadotropin deficiency results in testicular failure with decreased testosterone production that may cause sterility. In women, gonadotropin deficiency results in ovarian failure, *amenorrhea* (absence of menstrual periods), and infertility.

Growth hormone (GH) deficiency changes tissue growth patterns by reducing liver production of *somatomedins.* These substances, especially somatomedin C, trigger growth and maintain bone, cartilage, and other tissues throughout life.

GH deficiency results from decreased GH production, failure of the liver to produce somatomedins, or failure of tissues to respond to the somatomedins. In adults, GH deficiency alters **cellular regulation** by increasing the rate of bone destructive activity, leading to thinner bones *(osteoporosis)* and an increased risk for fractures.

The cause of hypopituitarism varies. Benign or malignant pituitary tumors can compress and destroy pituitary tissue. Pituitary function can be impaired by malnutrition or rapid loss of body fat. Shock or severe hypotension reduces blood flow to the pituitary gland, leading to hypoxia, infarction, and reduced hormone secretion. Other causes of hypopituitarism include head trauma, brain tumors or infection, radiation or surgery of the head and brain, and the last stage of human immune deficiency virus (HIV) disease, HIV-III (AIDS). *Idiopathic hypopituitarism* has an unknown cause.

Postpartum hemorrhage is the most common cause of pituitary infarction, which results in decreased hormone secretion. This clinical problem is known as *Sheehan syndrome.* The pituitary gland normally enlarges during pregnancy; if hemorrhage and hypotension occur during delivery, hemorrhage with ischemia and necrosis of the gland can occur.

❖ Interprofessional Collaborative Care

Patients with hypopituitarism require lifelong hormone replacement therapy (HRT). Such patients can be found in the community and in any care setting. It is important that HRT continues when they are admitted to an acute care setting for any reason.

◆ **Assessment: Recognize Cues.** Deficiencies of specific pituitary hormones cause changes in target organ function and even physical appearance. See the specific changes outlined in the Key Features: Pituitary Hypofunction box.

Gonadotropin (LH and FSH) deficiency changes secondary sex characteristics in men and women. Men may have facial and body hair loss. Ask about impotence and decreased *libido* (sex drive). Women may report amenorrhea, *dyspareunia* (painful intercourse), infertility, and decreased libido. Women may also have dry skin, breast atrophy, and a decrease or absence of axillary and pubic hair.

Neurologic symptoms of hypopituitarism as a result of tumor growth often first occur as changes in vision. Assess for changes in the patient's vision, especially peripheral vision. Headaches, *diplopia* (double vision), and limited eye movement are common.

Laboratory findings vary widely. Some pituitary hormone levels may be measured directly. Laboratory assessment of some pituitary hormones involves measuring the *effects* of the hormones rather than the actual hormone levels. For example, blood levels of triiodothyronine (T_3) and thyroxine (T_4) from the thyroid, testosterone and estradiol from the gonads, and prolactin levels are measured easily. If levels of any of these hormones are low, further pituitary evaluation is necessary.

Pituitary problems may cause changes in the *sella turcica* (the bony nest where the pituitary gland rests) (McCance et al., 2019). Changes include enlargement, erosion, and calcifications as a result of pituitary tumors, as well as soft-tissue lesions, seen most distinctly with CT and MRI (Pressman, 2017). An angiogram can help rule out an aneurysm or any other vascular problems in the area before surgery.

◆ **Interventions: Take Action.** Management of hypopituitarism focuses on replacement of all deficient hormones to ensure appropriate **cellular regulation** (Mitchell-Brown & Stephens-DiLeo, 2017). Men who have gonadotropin deficiency receive replacement therapy with androgens (testosterone), usually by the parenteral or transdermal route. Therapy begins with high-dose testosterone and is continued until **virilization** (presence of male secondary sex characteristics) is achieved. Positive responses include increases in penis size, libido, muscle mass, bone size, and bone strength, as well as increases in facial and body hair. After virilization is

▶▶ KEY FEATURES
Pituitary Hypofunction

Deficient Hormone	Signs and Symptoms
Anterior Pituitary Hormones	
Growth hormone (GH)	Decreased bone density
	Pathologic fractures
	Decreased muscle strength
	Increased serum cholesterol levels
Gonadotropins	*Women:*
Luteinizing hormone (LH)	Amenorrhea
Follicle-stimulating	Anovulation
hormone (FSH)	Low estrogen levels
	Breast atrophy
	Loss of bone density
	Decreased axillary and pubic hair
	Decreased libido
	Men:
	Decreased facial hair
	Decreased ejaculate volume
	Reduced muscle mass
	Loss of bone density
	Decreased body hair
	Decreased libido
	Impotence
Thyroid-stimulating	Decreased thyroid hormone levels
hormone (TSH, thyro-	Weight gain
tropin)	Intolerance to cold
	Scalp alopecia
	Hirsutism
	Menstrual abnormalities
	Decreased libido
	Slowed cognition
	Lethargy
Adrenocorticotropic	Decreased serum cortisol levels
hormone (ACTH)	Pale, sallow complexion
	Malaise and lethargy
	Anorexia
	Postural hypotension
	Headache
	Hypoglycemia
	Hyponatremia
	Decreased axillary and pubic hair (women)
Posterior Pituitary Hormones	
Antidiuretic hormone (ADH,	*Diabetes insipidus:*
vasopressin)	Greatly increased urine output
	Low urine specific gravity (<1.005)
	Hypotension
	Dehydration
	Increased plasma osmolarity
	Increased thirst
	Increased plasma electrolyte levels, especially sodium
	Urine output does not decrease when fluid intake decreases

achieved, the dose may be decreased, but continues throughout life. Therapy to increase fertility requires gonadotropin-releasing hormone (GnRH) injections, not testosterone therapy (Kaiser & Ho, 2016).

Androgen therapy is avoided in men with prostate cancer to prevent enhancing tumor cell growth. Side effects of therapy include **gynecomastia** (male breast tissue development), acne, baldness, and prostate enlargement.

Women who have gonadotropin deficiency receive HRT with a combination of estrogen and progesterone. The risk for hypertension or *thrombosis* (formation of blood clots in deep veins) is increased with estrogen therapy, especially among smokers and those who use nicotine in any form. Emphasize measures to reduce risk and the need for regular health visits. For inducing pregnancy, specific hormones may be given to trigger ovulation.

Adults with GH deficiency may be treated with subcutaneous injections of human growth hormone (hGH). Injections are given at night to mimic normal GH release (Kaiser & Ho, 2016).

HYPERPITUITARISM

Pathophysiology Review

Hyperpituitarism is hormone oversecretion that occurs with anterior pituitary tumors or tissue *hyperplasia* (tissue overgrowth). Tumors occur most often in the anterior pituitary cells that produce growth hormone (GH), prolactin (PRL), and adrenocorticotropic hormone (ACTH). Overproduction of PRL also may occur in response to tumors that overproduce GH and ACTH. Excess ACTH may occur with increased secretion of melanocyte-stimulating hormone (MSH).

👤 PATIENT-CENTERED CARE: GENETIC/ GENOMIC CONSIDERATIONS (QSEN)

One cause of hyperpituitarism is multiple endocrine neoplasia, type 1 (MEN1), in which there is inactivation of the suppressor gene *MEN1* (Online Mendelian Inheritance in Man [OMIM], 2017). MEN1 has an autosomal dominant inheritance pattern and may result in a benign tumor of the pituitary, parathyroid glands, or pancreas. In the pituitary, excessive production of growth hormone occurs and leads to acromegaly. Ask a patient with acromegaly whether either parent also has this problem or has had a tumor of the pancreas or parathyroid glands.

Most often hyperpituitarism is caused by a benign tumor *(adenoma)* within one pituitary cell type (Melmed et al., 2016). Adenomas are classified by the hormone secreted. As an adenoma gets larger and compresses brain tissue, neurologic changes, as well as endocrine problems, may occur. Symptoms may include vision changes, headache, and increased intracranial pressure (ICP). It can also be caused by a hypothalamic problem of excessive production of releasing hormones, which then overstimulate a normal pituitary gland.

Prolactin (PRL)-secreting tumors are the most common type of pituitary adenoma. Excessive PRL inhibits the secretion of gonadotropins and sex hormones in men and women, resulting in *galactorrhea* (breast milk production), amenorrhea, and infertility.

Overproduction of GH in adults results in *acromegaly* (Fig. 57.1). The onset is gradual with slow progression, and changes may remain unnoticed for years before diagnosis. Early detection and treatment are essential to prevent irreversible enlargement

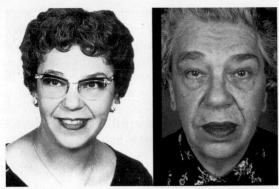

FIG. 57.1 Progression of acromegaly. (Courtesy of the Group for Research in Pathology Education [GRIPE], Oklahoma City, OK.)

of the face, hands, and feet. Other changes include increased skeletal thickness, hypertrophy of the skin, and enlargement of many organs such as the liver and heart. Some changes may be reversible after treatment, but skeletal changes are permanent.

Bone thinning and bone cell overgrowth occur slowly. Breakdown of joint cartilage and hypertrophy of ligaments, vocal cords, and eustachian tubes are common. Nerve entrapment and *hyperglycemia* (elevated blood glucose levels) are common.

Excess ACTH overstimulates the adrenal cortex. The result is excessive production of glucocorticoids, mineralocorticoids, and androgens, which leads to the development of Cushing disease or syndrome (see Fluid and Electrolyte Balance Concept Exemplar: Hypercortisolism [Cushing Disease]).

❖ Interprofessional Collaborative Care

Most care of a patient with hyperpituitarism occurs on an outpatient basis. When surgical intervention is required, hospitalization is necessary.

◆ **Assessment: Recognize Cues.** Symptoms of hyperpituitarism vary with the hormone produced in excess. Obtain the patient's age, gender, and family history. Ask about any change in hat, glove, ring, or shoe size and the presence of fatigue. The patient with high GH levels may have backache and joint pain from bone changes. Ask specifically about headaches and changes in vision.

The patient with hypersecretion of PRL often reports sexual function difficulty. Ask women about menstrual changes, decreased libido, painful intercourse, and any difficulty in becoming pregnant. Men may report decreased libido and impotence.

Usually only one hormone is produced in excess because the cell types within the pituitary gland are so individually organized and distinct. The most common hormones produced in excess with hyperpituitarism are PRL, ACTH, and GH. Changes in appearance and target organ function occur with excesses of specific anterior pituitary hormones as described in the Key Features: Anterior Pituitary Hyperfunction box.

Suppression testing can help diagnose hyperpituitarism. High blood glucose levels usually suppress the release of GH. Giving 100 g of oral glucose or 0.5 g/kg of body weight is followed by serial GH level measurements. GH levels that do not fall below 5 ng/mL (mcg/L) indicate a positive (abnormal) result associated with hyperpituitarism.

◆ **Interventions: Take Action.** The expected outcomes of management for hyperpituitarism are to return hormone levels to normal or near normal, reduce or eliminate headache and visual disturbances, prevent complications, and reverse as many of the body changes as possible.

Nonsurgical Management. Encourage the patient to express concerns about his or her altered physical appearance, such as galactorrhea, gynecomastia, and reduced sexual functioning. Reassure the patient that treatment may reverse some of these problems.

Drug therapy may be used alone or with surgery and/or radiation. Common drugs used are the dopamine agonists bromocriptine and cabergoline. These drugs stimulate dopamine receptors in the brain and inhibit the release of GH and PRL. Usually, small tumors decrease until the pituitary gland is of normal size and larger tumors decrease to some extent.

Side effects of bromocriptine include orthostatic (postural) hypotension, headaches, nausea, abdominal cramps, and constipation. Give bromocriptine with a meal or a snack to reduce GI side effects. Treatment starts with a low dose and is gradually increased until the desired level is reached. *If pregnancy occurs, the drug is stopped immediately.*

! NURSING SAFETY PRIORITY (QSEN)

Drug Alert

Teach patients taking bromocriptine to seek medical care immediately if chest pain, dizziness, or watery nasal discharge occurs because of the possibility of serious side effects, including cardiac dysrhythmias, coronary artery spasms, and cerebrospinal fluid leakage.

Other agents used for acromegaly are the somatostatin analogs, especially octreotide and lanreotide, and a growth hormone (GH) receptor blocker, pegvisomant (Burchum & Rosenthal, 2019). Octreotide inhibits GH release through negative feedback. Pegvisomant blocks GH receptor activity and blocks production of insulin-like growth factor (IGF). Combination therapy with monthly injections of a somatostatin analog and weekly injections of pegvisomant has provided good control of the disease.

Radiation therapy does not have immediate effects in reducing pituitary hormone excesses, and months to years may pass before a therapeutic effect can be seen. It is not recommended to manage acromegaly (Melmed & Kleinberg, 2016). The use of the Gamma Knife or stereotactic confocal radiotherapy method of delivering radiation to pituitary tumors has reduced the long-term side effects of this therapy.

Surgical Management. Surgical removal of the pituitary gland (**hypophysectomy**) along with any tumor is the most common treatment for hyperpituitarism. Successful surgery decreases hormone levels, relieves headaches, and may reverse changes in sexual functioning.

Preoperative Care. Explain that because nasal packing is present for 2 to 3 days after surgery, it will be necessary to breathe through the mouth, and a "mustache" dressing ("drip" pad) will be placed under the nose. Instruct the patient not to brush teeth, cough, sneeze, blow the nose, or bend forward after surgery. These activities can increase intracranial pressure (ICP) and delay healing.

Operative Procedures. Depending on tumor size and location, a transsphenoidal approach or a minimally invasive endoscopic transnasal approach with smaller instruments is used under general anesthesia instead of a more invasive procedure. Nasal packing is inserted after the transsphenoidal incision is closed, and a mustache dressing is applied. These are not needed for the minimally invasive transnasal procedure. If the tumor cannot be reached by either the endoscopic transnasal or the transsphenoidal approach, a craniotomy may be indicated (Melmed & Kleinberg, 2016) (see Chapter 41).

Postoperative Care. Monitor the patient's neurologic response and document any changes in vision or mental status, altered level of consciousness, or decreased extremity strength. Observe for complications such as transient diabetes insipidus (DI; discussed later in this chapter), cerebrospinal fluid (CSF) leakage, infection, and increased ICP.

Teach the patient to report any postnasal drip or increased swallowing, which may indicate leakage of cerebrospinal fluid (CSF). Keep the head of the bed elevated. Assess nasal drainage for quantity, quality, and the presence of glucose (present in CSF). A light yellow color at the edge of the clear drainage on the dressing is called the *halo sign* and indicates CSF. If the patient has persistent, severe headaches, CSF fluid may have leaked into the sinus area. Most CSF leaks resolve with bedrest, and surgical intervention is rarely needed.

Teach the patient to avoid coughing early after surgery because it increases pressure in the incision area and may lead to a CSF leak. Remind him or her to perform deep-breathing hourly while awake to prevent pulmonary problems. Instruct the patient to rinse the mouth frequently and to apply a lubricating jelly to dry lips to manage the dryness from mouth breathing.

Assess for indications of infection, especially meningitis, such as headache, fever, and nuchal (neck) rigidity. The surgeon may prescribe antibiotics, analgesics, and antipyretics.

If the entire pituitary gland has been removed, replacement of thyroid hormones and glucocorticoids is lifelong. See the Best Practice for Patient Safety & Quality Care: The Patient After Hypophysectomy box for specific nursing actions after hypophysectomy.

BEST PRACTICE FOR PATIENT SAFETY & QUALITY CARE (QSEN)

The Patient After Hypophysectomy

- Monitor the patient's neurologic status hourly for the first 24 hours and then every 4 hours.
- Monitor fluid balance, especially for output greater than intake.
- Encourage the patient to perform deep-breathing exercises.
- Instruct the patient not to cough, blow the nose, or sneeze.
- Instruct the patient to use dental floss and oral mouth rinses rather than toothbrushing until the surgeon gives permission.
- Instruct the patient to avoid bending at the waist to prevent increasing intracranial pressure.
- Monitor the nasal drip pad for the type and amount of drainage.
- Teach the patient methods to avoid constipation and subsequent "straining."
- Teach the patient self-administration of the prescribed hormones.

After surgery the patient needs daily self-management regimens and frequent checkups. Advise the patient to avoid activities that might interfere with healing or increase intracranial pressure (ICP). Teach him or her to avoid bending over from the waist to pick up objects or tie shoes because this position increases ICP. Teach the patient to bend the knees and then lower the body to pick up fallen objects. ICP also increases when the patient strains to have a bowel movement. Suggest techniques to prevent constipation, such as eating high-fiber foods, drinking plenty of fluids, and using stool softeners or laxatives.

Teach the patient to avoid toothbrushing for about 2 weeks after transsphenoidal surgery. Frequent mouth care with mouthwash and daily flossing provide adequate oral hygiene. A decreased sense of smell is expected after surgery and usually lasts 3 to 4 months.

Hormone replacement with vasopressin may be needed to maintain fluid balance (See discussion of Interventions in the Diabetes Insipidus section). If the anterior portion of the pituitary gland is removed, instruct the patient in cortisol, thyroid, and gonadal hormone replacement. Teach the patient to report the return of any symptoms of hyperpituitarism immediately to the primary health care provider.

DIABETES INSIPIDUS

Pathophysiology Review

Diabetes insipidus (DI) is a disorder of the posterior pituitary gland in which water loss is caused by either an antidiuretic hormone (ADH) deficiency or an inability of the kidneys to respond to ADH. The result of DI is the excretion of large volumes of dilute urine because the distal kidney tubules and collecting ducts do not reabsorb water; this leads to *polyuria* (excessive water loss through urination), dehydration, and disturbed *fluid and electrolyte balance*.

Massive water loss increases plasma osmolarity and serum sodium levels, which stimulate the sensation of thirst. Thirst promotes increased fluid intake and aids in maintaining hydration. *If the thirst mechanism is poor or if the adult cannot obtain water independently, dehydration becomes more severe and can lead to death* (Robinson & Verbalis, 2016).

> ### ! NURSING SAFETY PRIORITY (QSEN)
> **Action Alert**
>
> Ensure that no patient suspected of having DI is deprived of fluids for more than 4 hours because he or she cannot reduce urine output and severe dehydration can result.

ADH deficiency is classified as neurogenic (primary or secondary), nephrogenic, or drug related, depending on whether the problem is caused by insufficient production of ADH or an inability of the kidney to respond to the presence of ADH.

Primary neurogenic diabetes insipidus is caused by a defect in the hypothalamus or pituitary gland, resulting in a lack of ADH production or release. *Secondary neurogenic diabetes*

insipidus is not caused by an abnormal posterior pituitary gland but is a result of tumors in or near the hypothalamus or pituitary gland, head trauma, infectious processes, or brain surgery.

Nephrogenic diabetes insipidus is a problem with the kidney's response to ADH rather than a problem with ADH production. A severe kidney injury can reduce the ability of the kidney tubules to respond to ADH. Then as long as the kidney is able to continue to produce urine, DI results. In some cases, a mutation in the gene responsible for producing the ADH receptor interferes with kidney response to ADH.

Drug-related diabetes insipidus is most often caused by lithium carbonate and demeclocycline (Robinson & Verbalis, 2016). These drugs can interfere with the response of the kidneys to ADH.

> ### 👤 PATIENT-CENTERED CARE: GENETIC/GENOMIC CONSIDERATIONS (QSEN)
>
> Nephrogenic diabetes insipidus (DI) can be a genetic disorder in which the ADH receptor (vasopressin receptor) has a defect that prevents kidney tubules from interacting with ADH. The result is poor water reabsorption by the kidney, although the actual amount of hormone produced is not deficient. This problem is most commonly inherited as an X-linked recessive disorder affecting only males (OMIM, 2019). A rarer genetic problem caused by autosomal recessive inheritance of a different mutated gene results in both males and females being affected. When assessing a patient with DI, always ask whether anyone else in the family has ever had this disorder.

❖ Interprofessional Collaborative Care

◆ **Assessment: Recognize Cues.** Most symptoms of DI are related to dehydration, as shown in the Key Features: Diabetes Insipidus box. Symptoms include an increase in urination and excessive thirst. Ask about a history of recent surgery, head trauma, or drug use (e.g., lithium). Although increased fluid intake prevents serious volume depletion, the patient who is deprived of fluids or who cannot increase oral fluid intake may develop shock from fluid loss. Symptoms of dehydration (e.g., poor skin turgor, dry or cracked mucous membranes) may be present. (See Chapter 13 for discussion of dehydration.)

Water loss changes blood and urine tests. The 24-hour fluid intake and output is measured without restricting food or fluid intake. DI is considered if urine output is more than 4 L during this period and is greater than the volume ingested. The amount of urine excreted in 24 hours by patients with DI may vary from 4 to 30 L/day. Urine is dilute with a low specific gravity (less than 1.005) and low osmolarity (50 to 200 mOsm/kg) or osmolality (50 to 200 mOsm/L).

◆ **Interventions: Take Action.** Management focuses on controlling symptoms using drug therapy with desmopressin (Burchum & Rosenthal, 2019). This drug, a synthetic form of vasopressin, replaces antidiuretic hormone (ADH) and decreases urination. It is available orally, as a sublingual "melt," or intranasally in a metered spray. The frequency of dosing varies with patient responses. Teach those patients who have mild DI that they may need only one or two doses in

KEY FEATURES
Diabetes Insipidus

Cardiovascular Symptoms	**Skin Symptoms**

Cardiovascular Symptoms
- Hypotension
- Tachycardia
- Weak peripheral pulses
- Hemoconcentration

Kidney/Urinary Symptoms
- Increased urine output
- Dilute, low specific gravity

Skin Symptoms
- Poor turgor
- Dry mucous membranes

Neurologic Symptoms
- Decreased cognition[a]
- Ataxia[a]
- Increased thirst
- Irritability[a]

[a]Occurs when access to water is limited and rapid dehydration results.

24 hours. For more severe DI, one or two metered doses two or three times daily may be needed. During severe dehydration, ADH may be given IV or IM. Ulceration of the mucous membranes, allergy, a sensation of chest tightness, and lung inhalation of the spray may occur with use of the intranasal preparations. If side effects occur or if the patient has an upper respiratory infection, oral or subcutaneous vasopressin is used.

! NURSING SAFETY PRIORITY (QSEN)
Drug Alert

The parenteral form of desmopressin is 10 times stronger than the oral form, and the dosage must be reduced.

For the hospitalized patient with DI, nursing management focuses on early detection of dehydration and maintaining adequate hydration. Actions include accurately measuring fluid intake and output, checking urine specific gravity, and recording the patient's weight daily.

Urge the patient to drink fluids in an amount equal to urine output. If fluids are given IV, ensure the patency of the access catheter and accurately monitor the amount infused hourly.

The patient with permanent DI requires lifelong drug therapy. Check his or her ability to assess symptoms, and adjust dosages as prescribed for changes in conditions. Teach that polyuria and polydipsia indicate the need for another dose.

Drug therapy for DI induces water retention and can cause fluid overload (see Chapter 13). *Teach patients to weigh themselves daily to identify weight gain.* Stress the importance of using the same scale and weighing at the same time of day while wearing a similar amount and type of clothing. If weight gain of more than 2.2 lb (1 kg) along with other signs of water toxicity occurs (e.g., persistent headache, acute confusion, nausea, vomiting), instruct him or her to go immediately to the emergency department or call 911. Instruct the patient to wear a medical alert bracelet identifying the disorder and drug.

SYNDROME OF INAPPROPRIATE ANTIDIURETIC HORMONE
Pathophysiology Review

The syndrome of inappropriate antidiuretic hormone (SIADH) or *Schwartz-Bartter syndrome* is a problem in which antidiuretic hormone (ADH, vasopressin) is secreted even when plasma osmolarity is low or normal, resulting in water retention and fluid overload. A decrease in plasma osmolarity normally inhibits ADH production and secretion. SIADH occurs with many conditions (e.g., cancer therapy, pulmonary infection or impairment) and with specific drugs, including selective serotonin reuptake inhibitors (Robinson & Verbalis, 2016). Table 57.1 lists common causes of SIADH.

In SIADH, ADH continues to be released when not needed, leading to water retention and disturbances of *fluid and electrolyte balance*. Water retention results in dilutional *hyponatremia* (a decreased serum sodium level) and fluid overload. The increase in blood volume increases the kidney filtration and inhibits the release of renin and aldosterone, which increase urine sodium loss and results in greater hyponatremia.

❖ Interprofessional Collaborative Care

◆ **Assessment: Recognize Cues.** Ask the patient about his or her medical history, which may reveal conditions that can cause SIADH. Specifically obtain information about the conditions listed in Table 57.1.

Early symptoms of SIADH are related to the water-retention causing dilution of serum sodium levels (*hyponatremia*). GI disturbances, such as loss of appetite, nausea, and vomiting, may occur first, as discussed in Chapter 13. Weigh the patient and document any recent weight gain. Use this information to monitor responses to therapy. In SIADH, free water (not salt) is retained and dependent edema is not usually present, even though water is retained.

Water retention, hyponatremia, and fluid shifts affect central nervous system function, especially when the serum sodium level is below 115 mEq/L (mmol/L). The patient may have lethargy, headaches, hostility, disorientation, and a change in level of consciousness. Lethargy and headaches can progress to decreased responsiveness, seizures, and coma. Assess deep tendon reflexes, which are usually decreased.

Vital sign changes include full and bounding pulse (caused by the increased fluid volume) and hypothermia (caused by

TABLE 57.1 Conditions Causing the Syndrome of Inappropriate Antidiuretic Hormone

Malignancies
- Small cell lung cancer
- Pancreatic, duodenal, and GU carcinomas
- Thymoma
- Hodgkin lymphoma
- Non-Hodgkin lymphoma

Pulmonary Disorders
- Viral and bacterial pneumonia
- Lung abscesses
- Active tuberculosis
- Pneumothorax
- Chronic lung diseases
- Mycoses
- Positive-pressure ventilation

CNS Disorders
- Trauma
- Infection
- Tumors (primary or metastatic)
- Strokes
- Porphyria
- Systemic lupus erythematosus

Drugs
- Exogenous ADH
- Chlorpropamide
- Vincristine
- Cyclophosphamide
- Carbamazepine
- Opioids
- Tricyclic antidepressants
- General anesthetics
- Fluoroquinolone antibiotics

ADH, Antidiuretic hormone; *CNS,* central nervous system; *GU,* genitourinary.

central nervous system disturbance). Chapter 13 presents other findings that occur with hyponatremia.

Water retention causes urine volume to decrease and urine osmolarity to increase. At the same time, plasma volume increases, and plasma osmolarity decreases. Elevated urine sodium levels and specific gravity reflect increased urine concentration. Serum sodium levels decrease, sometimes to as low as 110 mEq/L (mmol/L), because of fluid retention and sodium loss.

◆ **Interventions: Take Action.** Interventions for SIADH focus on restricting fluid intake, promoting the excretion of water, replacing lost sodium, and interfering with the action of ADH. Nursing interventions include monitoring response to therapy, preventing complications, teaching the patient and family about fluid restrictions and drug therapy, and preventing injury.

Fluid restriction is essential because fluid intake further dilutes plasma sodium levels. In some cases, fluid intake may be kept as low as 500 to 1000 mL/24 hr. Use saline instead of water to dilute tube feedings, irrigate GI tubes, and give drugs by GI tube.

Measure intake, output, and daily weights to assess the degree of fluid restriction needed. A weight gain of 2.2 lb (1 kg) or more per day or a gradual increase over several days is cause for concern. A 2.2-lb (1-kg) increase is equal to a 1000-mL fluid retention (1 kg = 1 L). Prevent mouth dryness with frequent oral rinsing (warn patients not to swallow the rinses).

Drug therapy with vasopressin receptor antagonists (vaptans), such as tolvaptan or conivaptan, is used to treat SIADH when hyponatremia is present in hospitalized patients (Burchum & Rosenthal, 2019). These drugs promote water excretion without causing sodium loss. Tolvaptan is an oral drug, and

conivaptan is given IV. Tolvaptan has a black box warning that rapid increases in serum sodium levels (those greater than a 12-mEq/L [mmol/L] increase in 24 hours) have been associated with central nervous system demyelination that can lead to serious complications and death. When this drug is used at higher dosages or for longer than 30 days, there is a significant risk for liver failure and death (Robinson & Verbalis, 2016).

❗ NURSING SAFETY PRIORITY (QSEN)
Drug Alert

Administer tolvaptan or conivaptan only in the hospital setting so serum sodium levels can be monitored closely for the development of hypernatremia and other complications.

Diuretics may be used on a limited basis to manage SIADH when sodium levels are near normal and heart failure is present. With diuretics, sodium loss can be potentiated, further contributing to the problems caused by SIADH. For milder SIADH, demeclocycline, an oral antibiotic, may help reach *fluid and electrolyte balance,* although the drug is not approved for this problem.

Hypertonic saline (i.e., 3% sodium chloride [3% NaCl]) is used for SIADH when the serum sodium level is very low (Robinson & Verbalis, 2016). Give IV saline cautiously because it may add to existing fluid overload and promote heart failure. If the patient needs routine IV fluids, a saline solution is prescribed to prevent further sodium dilution.

Monitor the patient's response to therapy to prevent the fluid overload from becoming worse, leading to pulmonary edema and heart failure. Any patient with SIADH, regardless of age, is at risk for these complications. The older adult or one who also has cardiac, kidney, pulmonary, or liver problems is at greater risk.

Monitor for increased fluid overload (bounding pulse, increasing neck vein distention, lung crackles, dyspnea, increasing peripheral edema, reduced urine output) at least every 2 hours. *Pulmonary edema can occur very quickly and can lead to death.* Notify the primary health care provider of any change that indicates the fluid overload is not responding to therapy or is worse.

Providing a safe environment is needed when the serum sodium level falls below 120 mEq/L (mmol/L). The risk for neurologic changes and seizures increases as a result of osmotic fluid shifts into brain tissue. Observe for and document changes in the patient's neurologic status. Assess for subtle changes, such as muscle twitching, increasing irritability, or restlessness, before these progress to seizures or coma. Check orientation to time, place, and person every 2 hours because disorientation or confusion may be present as an early indication. Reduce environmental noise and lighting to prevent overstimulation.

The frequency of neurologic checks depends on the patient's status. For the patient being treated for SIADH who is hyponatremic but alert, awake, and oriented, checks every 2 to 4 hours may be sufficient. For the patient who has had a change in level of consciousness, perform neurologic checks at least every hour or as prescribed. Inspect the environment every shift, making sure that basic safety measures, such as side rails being securely in place, are observed.

DISORDERS OF THE ADRENAL GLAND

ADRENAL GLAND HYPOFUNCTION

Pathophysiology Review

Adrenal cortex production of steroid hormone may decrease as a result of inadequate secretion of adrenocorticotropic hormone (ACTH), dysfunction of the hypothalamic-pituitary control mechanism, or direct problems of adrenal gland tissue (Cole, 2018). Symptoms may develop gradually or occur quickly with stress. In acute adrenocortical insufficiency *(adrenal crisis)*, life-threatening symptoms may appear without warning.

Insufficiency of adrenocortical steroids causes problems through the loss of aldosterone and cortisol action. Decreased cortisol levels result in hypoglycemia. Gastric acid production and glomerular filtration decrease. Decreased glomerular filtration leads to excessive blood urea nitrogen (BUN) levels, which cause anorexia and weight loss.

Reduced aldosterone secretion causes disturbances of *fluid and electrolyte balance*. Potassium excretion is decreased, causing hyperkalemia. Sodium and water excretion are increased, causing hyponatremia and hypovolemia. Potassium retention also promotes reabsorption of hydrogen ions, which can lead to acidosis.

Low adrenal androgen levels decrease body, axillary, and pubic hair, especially in women, because the adrenals produce most of the androgens in females. The severity of symptoms is related to the degree of hormone deficiency.

Acute adrenal insufficiency *(addisonian crisis)* is a life-threatening event in which the need for cortisol and aldosterone is greater than the body's supply (Cole, 2018; McCance et al., 2019). It often occurs in response to a stressful event (e.g., surgery, trauma, severe infection), especially when the adrenal hormone output is already reduced. Problems are the same as those of chronic insufficiency but are more severe. *However, unless intervention is initiated promptly, sodium levels fall, and potassium levels rise rapidly (Pereira, 2016). Severe hypotension results from the blood volume depletion that occurs with the loss of aldosterone.* Emergency care actions for patients with acute adrenal insufficiency are listed in the Best Practice for Patient Safety & Quality Care box.

Adrenal insufficiency is classified as primary or secondary. Causes of primary and secondary adrenal insufficiency are listed in Table 57.2. A common cause of secondary adrenal insufficiency is the sudden cessation of long-term glucocorticoid therapy. This therapy suppresses production of glucocorticoids through negative feedback and causes atrophy of the adrenal cortex. Glucocorticoid drugs must be withdrawn gradually to allow for pituitary production of ACTH and activation of adrenal cells to produce cortisol.

BEST PRACTICE FOR PATIENT SAFETY & QUALITY CARE (QSEN)

Emergency Management of the Patient With Acute Adrenal Insufficiency

Hormone Replacement
- Start rapid infusion of normal saline or dextrose 5% in normal saline.
- Initial higher doses of hydrocortisone sodium or dexamethasone is administered as an IV bolus.
- Administer additional hydrocortisone sodium by continuous IV infusion over the next 8 hours.
- Give an additional dose of hydrocortisone IM concomitantly with hydration every 12 hours.
- Initiate an H_2 histamine blocker (e.g., cimetidine) IV for ulcer prevention.

Hyperkalemia Management
- Administer insulin in units equal to the same number of mg of extra dextrose in normal saline intravenously to shift potassium into cells.
- Give potassium binding and excreting resin.
- Give loop or thiazide diuretics.
- Avoid potassium-sparing diuretics, as prescribed.
- Initiate potassium restriction.
- Monitor intake and output.
- Monitor heart rate, rhythm, and ECG for signs and symptoms of hyperkalemia (slow heart rate; heart block; tall, peaked T waves; fibrillation; asystole).

Hypoglycemia Management
- Administer IV glucose as prescribed.
- Prepare to administer glucagon as needed and prescribed.
- Maintain IV access.
- Monitor blood glucose level hourly.

TABLE 57.2 Causes of Primary and Secondary Adrenal Insufficiency

Primary Causes	Secondary Causes
• Autoimmune disease[a]	• Pituitary tumors
• Tuberculosis	• Postpartum pituitary necrosis
• Metastatic cancer	• Hypophysectomy
• HIV-III (AIDS)	• High-dose pituitary or whole-brain radiation
• Hemorrhage	
• Gram-negative sepsis	• Cessation of long-term corticosteroid drug therapy[a]
• Adrenalectomy	
• Abdominal radiation therapy	
• Drugs (mitotane) and toxins	

[a]Most common cause.

❖ Interprofessional Collaborative Care

Acute adrenal insufficiency is an emergency and managed in an acute care setting. Without appropriate management, death ensues (Amrein et al., 2018).

◆ Assessment: Recognize Cues

History. Ask about symptoms and factors that cause adrenal hypofunction. Ask about any change in activity level because lethargy, fatigue, and muscle weakness are often present.

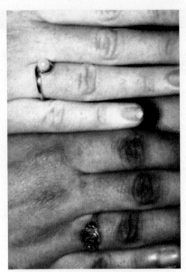

FIG. 57.2 Increased pigmentation seen in primary adrenocortical insufficiency. (From Wilson, J.D., Foster, D., Kronenberg, H., & Larsen, P.R. [1998]. *Williams' textbook of endocrinology* [9th ed.]. Philadelphia: Saunders. Courtesy Dr. H. Patrick Higgins.)

▶▶ KEY FEATURES
Adrenal Insufficiency

Neuromuscular Symptoms	Skin Symptoms
• Muscle weakness	• Vitiligo
• Fatigue	or
• Joint and/or muscle pain	• Hyperpigmentation

Gastrointestinal Symptoms	Cardiovascular Symptoms
• Anorexia	• Anemia
• Nausea, vomiting	• Hypotension
• Abdominal pain	• Hyponatremia
• Constipation or diarrhea	• Hyperkalemia
• Weight loss	• Hypercalcemia
• Salt craving	

Include questions about salt intake, because salt craving often occurs with hypofunction.

GI problems, such as anorexia, nausea, vomiting, diarrhea, and abdominal pain, often occur. Ask about weight loss during the past months. Women may have menstrual changes related to weight loss, and men may report impotence.

Ask whether the patient has had radiation to the abdomen or head. Abdominal radiation could directly damage the adrenal glands, whereas cranial radiation could interfere with hypothalamic or pituitary influences on adrenal function. Document medical problems (e.g., tuberculosis or previous intracranial surgery) and all past and current drugs, especially steroids, anticoagulants, opioids, and cancer drugs.

Physical Assessment/Signs and Symptoms. Symptoms of adrenal insufficiency vary, and the severity is related to the degree of hormone deficiency as listed in the Key Features: Adrenal Insufficiency box. In patients with primary insufficiency (problem with adrenal gland function), plasma ACTH and melanocyte-stimulating hormone (MSH) levels are elevated in response to the adrenal-hypothalamic-pituitary feedback system. (Both ACTH and MSH are made from the same prehormone molecule. Anything that stimulates increased production of ACTH often also leads to increased production of MSH.) Elevated MSH levels result in areas of *increased* pigmentation (Fig. 57.2). In primary autoimmune disease, patchy areas of *decreased* pigmentation *(vitiligo)* may occur because of destruction of skin melanocytes. Body hair may also be decreased. In secondary adrenal insufficiency (problem in the hypothalamus or pituitary gland leading to decreased ACTH and MSH levels), skin pigmentation is not changed.

Assess for hypoglycemia (e.g., sweating, headaches, tachycardia, and tremors) and fluid depletion (postural hypotension and dehydration). *Hyperkalemia* (elevated blood potassium levels) can cause dysrhythmias with an irregular heart rate and result in cardiac arrest. *Hyponatremia* (low blood sodium levels) leading to hypotension and decreased

cognition is often one of the first indicators of adrenal insufficiency (Pereira, 2016).

Psychosocial Assessment. Depending on the degree of imbalance, patients may appear lethargic, depressed, confused, and even psychotic. Assess the patient's orientation to person, place, and time. Families may report that the patient has wide mood swings and is forgetful.

Diagnostic Assessment. Laboratory findings are listed in the Laboratory Profile: Adrenal Gland Assessment box and include low serum sodium and low salivary cortisol levels, low fasting blood glucose, elevated potassium, and increased blood urea nitrogen (BUN) levels. In primary disease, the eosinophil count and ACTH level are elevated. Plasma cortisol levels do not rise during provocation tests (see Chapter 56).

Urinary 17-hydroxycorticosteroids are the glucocorticoid metabolites, and 17-ketosteroid levels reflect the adrenal androgen metabolites. Both levels are in the low or low-normal range in adrenal hypofunction.

An ACTH stimulation (provocative) test is the most definitive test for adrenal insufficiency. ACTH is given IV, and plasma cortisol levels are obtained at 30-minute and 1-hour intervals. In primary insufficiency, the cortisol response is absent or very decreased. In secondary insufficiency, it is increased. When acute adrenal insufficiency is suspected, treatment is started without stimulation testing (Stewart & Newell-Price, 2016).

Imaging Assessment. CT and MRI are most helpful in determining the cause of pituitary problems leading to adrenal insufficiency. CT and MRI can show adrenal gland atrophy, but not its cause.

◆ **Interventions: Take Action.** Nursing interventions focus on promoting fluid balance, monitoring for fluid deficit, and preventing hypoglycemia. Because hyperkalemia can cause dysrhythmias with an irregular heart rate and result in cardiac arrest, assessing cardiac function is a nursing priority. Assess vital signs every 1 to 4 hours, depending on the patient's condition and the presence of dysrhythmias or postural hypotension. Weigh the patient daily and record intake and output. Monitor laboratory values to identify hemoconcentration

⚑ LABORATORY PROFILE

Adrenal Gland Assessment

Test	Normal Range	Hypofunction	Hyperfunction
Sodium	136-145 mEq/L (mmol/L)	Low	High
Potassium	3.5-5.0 mEq/L (mmol/L)	High	Low
Glucose (fasting)	70-110 mg/dL (4-6 mmol/L)	Normal to low	Normal to high
Calcium	Total: 9-10.5 mg/dL (2.25-2.75 mmol/L) Ionized: 4.5-5.6 mg/dL (1.05-1.30 mmol/L)	High	Low
Bicarbonate	23-30 mEq/L (mmol/L)	High	Low
BUN	10-20 mg/dL (3.6-7.1 mmol/L)	High	Normal
Cortisol (serum)	6 a.m. to 8 a.m.: 5-23 mcg/dL (138-635 nmol/L) 4 p.m. to 6 p.m.: 3-13 mcg/dL (83-359 nmol/L)	Low	High
Cortisol (salivary)	7 a.m. to 9 a.m.: 100-750 ng/dL 3 p.m. to 5 p.m.: <401 ng/dL	Low	High

BUN, Blood urea nitrogen.
Data from Pagana, K., & Pagana, T. (2018). *Mosby's manual of diagnostic and laboratory tests* (6th ed.). St. Louis: Elsevier.

(e.g., increased hematocrit or BUN). Chapter 13 discusses dehydration in detail.

Cortisol and aldosterone deficiencies are corrected by hormone replacement therapy described in the Common Examples of Drug Therapy: Adrenal Hypofunction box. Hydrocortisone corrects glucocorticoid deficiency. Oral cortisol replacement regimens and dosages vary. The most common drug used for this purpose is prednisone. In general, divided doses are given, with two-thirds given on arising in the morning and one-third at 6:00 p.m. to mimic the normal release of this hormone.

⚠ NURSING SAFETY PRIORITY (QSEN)

Drug Alert

Prednisone and prednisolone are soundalike drugs, and care is needed not to confuse them. Although they are both corticosteroids, they are not interchangeable because prednisolone is more potent than prednisone.

An additional mineralocorticoid hormone, such as fludrocortisone, may be needed to maintain or restore *fluid and electrolyte balance* (especially sodium and potassium). Dosage adjustment may be needed, especially in hot weather when more sodium is lost because of excessive perspiration. *Salt restriction or diuretic therapy should not be started without considering whether it might lead to an adrenal crisis.*

NCLEX EXAMINATION CHALLENGE 57.3

Safe and Effective Care Environment

Which electrolyte laboratory values indicate to the nurse monitoring a client with adrenal insufficiency undergoing IV therapy with hydrocortisone that the client is responding positively to this drug therapy?

A. Serum sodium 147 mEq/L (mmol/L); serum potassium 7.1 mEq/L (mmol/L)
B. Serum sodium 137 mEq/L (mmol/L); serum potassium 4.9 mEq/L (mmol/L)
C. Serum sodium 127 mEq/L (mmol/L); serum potassium 2.8 mEq/L (mmol/L)
D. Serum sodium 119 mEq/L (mmol/L); serum potassium 6.2 mEq/L (mmol/L)

💊 COMMON EXAMPLES OF DRUG THERAPY

Adrenal Hypofunction

Drug	Nursing Implications
Cortisone	Instruct the patient to take the drug with meals or a snack *to avoid gastric irritation.*
Hydrocortisone	Instruct the patient to report signs or symptoms of excessive drug therapy (e.g., rapid weight gain, round face, fluid retention), *which indicate Cushing syndrome and a possible need for a dosage adjustment.*
Prednisone	Instruct the patient to report illness *because the usual daily dosage may not be adequate during periods of illness or severe stress.*
Fludrocortisone	Monitor the patient's blood pressure *to assess for the potential side effect of hypertension.* Instruct the patient to report weight gain or edema *because sodium intake may need to be restricted.*

✳ FLUID AND ELECTROLYTE BALANCE CONCEPT EXEMPLAR: HYPERCORTISOLISM (CUSHING DISEASE)

Pathophysiology Review

Hypercortisolism (Cushing disease) is the excess secretion of cortisol from the adrenal cortex, causing many problems. The disorder can be caused by a problem in the adrenal cortex itself, a problem in the anterior pituitary gland, or a problem in the hypothalamus. In addition, one of the most common causes of hypercortisolism is glucocorticoid therapy.

The presence of excess glucocorticoids, regardless of the cause, affects metabolism and all body systems. An increase in total body fat results from slow turnover of plasma fatty acids.

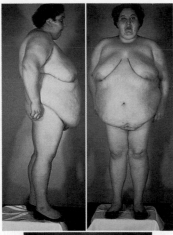
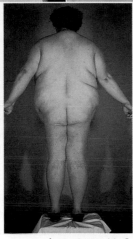

FIG. 57.3 Typical appearance of a patient with Cushing disease or syndrome. Note truncal obesity, moon face, buffalo hump, thinner arms and legs, and abdominal striae. (From Wenig, B.M., Heffess, C.S., & Adair, C.F. [1997]. *Atlas of endocrine pathology.* Philadelphia: Saunders.)

TABLE 57.3	Conditions Causing Increased Cortisol Secretion

Endogenous Secretion (Cushing Disease)

- Bilateral adrenal hyperplasia[a]
- Pituitary adenoma increasing the production of ACTH (pituitary Cushing disease)
- Malignancies: carcinomas of the lung, GI tract, pancreas
- Adrenal adenomas or carcinomas

Exogenous Administration (Cushing Syndrome)

- Therapeutic use of ACTH or glucocorticoids—most commonly for treatment of:
  - Asthma
  - Autoimmune disorders
  - Organ transplantation
  - Cancer chemotherapy
  - Allergic responses
  - Chronic fibrosis

[a]Most common cause.
ACTH, Adrenocorticotropic hormone.

This fat is redistributed, producing truncal obesity, "buffalo hump," and "moon face" (Fig. 57.3) (Jarvis, 2020). Increases in the breakdown of tissue protein result in decreased muscle mass and muscle strength, thin skin, and fragile capillaries. Effects on minerals lead to bone density loss.

High levels of corticosteroids reduce lymphocyte production and shrink organs containing lymphocytes, such as the spleen and the lymph nodes. White blood cell (WBC) cytokine production is decreased. These changes reduce immunity and increase the risk for infection.

In most cases, increased androgen production also occurs and causes acne, *hirsutism* (increased body hair growth), and occasionally clitoral hypertrophy. Increased androgens disrupt the normal ovarian hormone feedback mechanism, decreasing the ovary's production of estrogens and progesterone. *Oligomenorrhea* (scant or infrequent menses) occurs as a result.

Etiology. Cushing disease or syndrome is a group of clinical problems caused by an excess of cortisol. Table 57.3 lists causes of cortisol excess. When the anterior pituitary gland oversecretes adrenocorticotropic hormone (ACTH), this hormone causes hyperplasia of the adrenal cortex in both adrenal glands and an excess of glucocorticoid production (shown in Fig. 56.3 in Chapter 56). This problem is *pituitary Cushing disease* because the tissue causing the problem is the pituitary, not the adrenal gland. When excess glucocorticoids are caused by a problem in the actual adrenal cortex, usually a benign tumor (adrenal adenoma), the problem is called *adrenal Cushing disease (or primary Cushing disease)* and usually occurs in only one adrenal gland. When glucocorticoid excess results from drug therapy for another health problem, it is known as *Cushing syndrome* (also called secondary Cushing syndrome).

Incidence and Prevalence. The most common non–drug therapy related cause of Cushing disease is a pituitary adenoma. Women are more likely than men to develop Cushing disease. Cushing syndrome from chronic use of exogenous corticosteroids is more common because these drugs are often used to control serious chronic inflammatory conditions (Nieman, 2018).

❖ Interprofessional Collaborative Care
◆ Assessment: Recognize Cues

History. Ask about the patient's other health problems and drug therapies because glucocorticoid drug therapy is common. Regardless of cause, the patient has many changes because of the widespread effect of excessive cortisol. He or she may report weight gain and an increased appetite. Ask about changes in activity or sleep patterns, fatigue, and muscle weakness. Ask about bone pain or a history of fractures, because osteoporosis results from hypercortisolism. Ask about a history of frequent infections and easy bruising. Women often stop menstruating. GI problems include ulcer formation from increased hydrochloric acid secretion and decreased production of protective gastric mucus.

Physical Assessment/Signs and Symptoms. The patient with hypercortisolism has specific, predictable physical changes, although

KEY FEATURES

Hypercortisolism (Cushing Disease/Syndrome)

General Appearance
- Moon face
- Buffalo hump
- Truncal obesity
- Weight gain

Cardiovascular Symptoms
- Hypertension
- Frequent dependent edema
- Bruising
- Petechiae

Immune System Symptoms
- Increased risk for infection
- Reduced immunity
- Decreased inflammatory responses
- Signs and symptoms of infection and inflammation possibly masked

Musculoskeletal Symptoms
- Muscle atrophy (most apparent in extremities)
- Osteoporosis with:
  - Fragile fractures
  - Decreased height and vertebral collapse
  - Aseptic necrosis of the femur head
  - Slow or poor healing of bone fractures

Skin Symptoms
- Thinning skin
- Increased facial and body hair
- Striae and increased pigmentation

all body systems are affected as described in the Key Features: Hypercortisolism (Cushing Disease/Syndrome) box (see Fig. 57.3). Changes in fat distribution may result in fat pads on the neck, back, and shoulders (buffalo hump); an enlarged trunk with thin arms and legs; and a round face (moon face). Other changes include muscle wasting and weakness. Assess for and document changes and use these findings to prioritize patient problems.

Skin changes result from blood vessel fragility and include bruises, thin or translucent skin, and wounds that have not healed. Reddish-purple *striae* (stretch marks) occur on the abdomen, thighs, and upper arms because of the destructive effect of cortisol on collagen.

Acne and a fine coating of hair may occur over the face and body. In women, look for the presence of hirsutism, clitoral hypertrophy, and male pattern balding related to androgen excess.

Cardiac changes occur as a result of disturbed **fluid and electrolyte balance**. Both sodium and water are reabsorbed and retained, leading to hypervolemia and edema formation. Blood pressure is elevated, and pulses are full and bounding.

Musculoskeletal changes occur as a result of nitrogen depletion and mineral loss. Muscle mass decreases, especially in arms and legs (see Fig. 57.3). Muscle weakness increases the risk for falls. Bone is thinner, and osteoporosis is common, increasing the risk for fractures.

Glucose metabolism is affected by hypercortisolism. Fasting blood glucose levels are high because the liver releases glucose and the insulin receptors are less sensitive; therefore blood glucose does not move as easily into the tissues.

Immune changes caused by excess cortisol result in reduced **immunity**. Excess cortisol reduces the number of circulating lymphocytes, inhibits macrophage activity, reduces antibody synthesis, and inhibits production of cytokines and inflammatory chemicals (e.g., histamine). Infection risk is increased; and the patient may not have fever, purulent exudate, or redness in the affected area when an infection is present.

Psychosocial Assessment. Hypercortisolism can result in emotional instability, and patients often say that they do not feel like themselves. Ask about mood swings, irritability, new-onset confusion, or depression. Ask the patient whether he or she has been crying or laughing inappropriately or has had difficulty concentrating. The excess hormones stimulate the central nervous system, heightening the awareness of and responses to sensory stimulation. The patient often reports sleep difficulties and fatigue. All of these changes along with the physical changes strongly suggest hypercortisolism (Nieman, 2018).

Laboratory Assessment. Laboratory tests include blood, salivary, and urine cortisol levels. These are high in patients with any type of hypercortisolism. Plasma ACTH levels vary, depending on the cause of the problem. In pituitary Cushing disease, ACTH levels are elevated. In adrenal Cushing disease or when Cushing syndrome results from chronic steroid use, ACTH levels are low.

Salivary cortisol levels may be used to detect hypercortisolism because these levels accurately reflect blood levels, especially late-night specimens. A normal salivary cortisol level is lower than 2.0 ng/mL. Higher levels indicate hypercortisolism.

Urine is tested to measure levels of free cortisol and the metabolites of cortisol and androgens (17-hydroxycorticosteroids and 17-ketosteroids). In Cushing disease, levels of urine cortisol and androgens are all elevated in a 24-hour specimen. Cortisol-to-creatinine ratios in the first specimen of the day can replace the 24-hour test for screening. A ratio greater than 25 nmol/mmol is a positive test result (Stewart & Newell-Price, 2016)

Dexamethasone suppression testing can screen for hypercortisolism and may take place overnight or over a 3-day period. Set doses of dexamethasone are given. A 24-hour urine collection follows drug administration. When urinary 17-hydroxycorticosteroid excretion and cortisol levels are suppressed by dexamethasone, Cushing disease is *not* present.

Additional laboratory findings that accompany hypercortisolism include:
- Increased blood glucose level
- Decreased lymphocyte count
- Increased sodium level
- Decreased serum calcium level

Imaging Assessment. Imaging for hypercortisolism includes CT scans, MRI, and arteriography. These images can identify lesions of the adrenal or pituitary glands, lung, GI tract, or pancreas (Mendiratta-Lala et al., 2017).

◆ **Analysis: Analyze Cues and Prioritize Hypotheses.** The priority problems for patients with Cushing disease or Cushing syndrome are:

1. Fluid overload due to hormone-induced water and sodium retention
2. Potential for injury due to skin thinning, poor wound healing, and bone density loss
3. Potential for infection due to hormone-induced reduced **immunity**

◆ **Planning and Implementation: Generate Solutions and Take Action.** Expected outcomes of hypercortisolism management are the reduction of plasma cortisol levels, removal of tumors, and restoration of normal or acceptable body appearance. When the disorder is caused by pituitary or adrenal problems, cure is possible. When caused by drug therapy for another health problem, the focus is to prevent complications from hypercortisolism.

Restoring Fluid Volume Balance

Planning: Expected Outcomes. The patient with hypercortisolism is expected to achieve and maintain a normal or near-normal *fluid and electrolyte balance*.

Interventions. Interventions for patients with fluid volume excess focus on ensuring patient safety, restoring *fluid and electrolyte balance*, and providing supportive care. Depending on the cause, surgical management may be used to reduce cortisol production.

Nonsurgical interventions focus on patient safety, drug therapy, nutrition therapy, and monitoring; these interventions are the basis of nonsurgical action for hypercortisolism and fluid overload.

Patient safety includes preventing fluid overload from becoming worse, leading to pulmonary edema and heart failure. Any patient with fluid overload, regardless of age, is at risk for these complications. The older adult or one who has coexisting cardiac problems, kidney problems, pulmonary problems, or liver problems is at greater risk.

Monitor for indicators of fluid overload (bounding pulse, increasing neck vein distention, lung crackles, increasing peripheral edema, reduced urine output) at least every 2 hours. *Pulmonary edema can occur quickly and lead to death.* Notify the primary health care provider of any change that indicates fluid overload either is not responding to therapy or is worse.

The patient with fluid volume excess and dependent edema is at risk for skin breakdown. Use a pressure-reducing or pressure-relieving overlay on the mattress. Assess skin pressure areas, especially the coccyx, elbows, hips, and heels, daily for redness or open areas. For patients receiving oxygen by mask or nasal cannula, check the skin around the mask, nares, and ears and under the elastic band. Help the patient change positions every 2 hours or ensure that others assigned to perform the intervention are diligent in this action.

Drug therapy involves the use of drugs that interfere with adrenocorticotropic hormone (ACTH) production or adrenal hormone synthesis for temporary relief and are categorized as *steroidogenesis inhibitors*. Metyrapone, aminoglutethimide, ketoconazole, mitotane, and etomidate use different pathways to decrease cortisol production (Stewart & Newell-Price, 2016; Tritos & Biller, 2018). For patients with hypercortisolism resulting from increased ACTH production, cyproheptadine may be used because it interferes with ACTH production. For adults with increased ACTH production who have type 2 diabetes and who do not respond to other drug therapies, another drug is mifepristone, which is a synthetic steroid that blocks glucocorticoid receptors. Two additional drugs currently under investigation for use as steroid inhibitors are levoketoconazole and osilodrostat (Tritos & Biller, 2018).

> ### ! NURSING SAFETY PRIORITY (QSEN)
> **Drug Alert**
>
> Mifepristone cannot be used during pregnancy because it also blocks progesterone receptors and would cause termination of the pregnancy (Burchum & Rosenthal, 2019).

A drug to manage hypercortisolism resulting from a pituitary adenoma is pasireotide. This subcutaneous drug binds to somatostatin receptors on the adenoma and inhibits tumor production of corticotropin. Lower levels of corticotropin lead to lower levels of cortisol production in the adrenal glands. The drug is ineffective for patients whose tumors do not have somatostatin receptors.

Monitor the patient for response to drug therapy, especially weight loss and increased urine output. Observe for symptoms of problems with *fluid and electrolyte balance*, especially changes in ECG patterns. Assess laboratory findings, especially sodium and potassium values, whenever they are drawn.

Nutrition therapy for the patient with hypercortisolism may involve restrictions of both fluid and sodium intake to control fluid volume. Often sodium restriction involves only "no added salt" to ordinary table foods when fluid overload is mild. For more pronounced fluid overload, the patient may be restricted to anywhere from 2 g/day to 4 g/day of sodium. When sodium restriction is ongoing, teach the patient and family how to check food labels for sodium content and how to keep a daily record of sodium ingested. Explain to the patient and family the reason for any fluid restriction and the importance of adhering to the prescribed restriction.

Monitor intake and output and weight to assess therapy effectiveness. Ensure that assistive personnel (AP) understand that these measurements need to be accurate, not just estimated, because treatment decisions are based on the findings. Schedule fluid offerings throughout the 24 hours. Teach AP to check urine for color and character and to report these findings. Check the urine specific gravity (a specific gravity below 1.005 may indicate fluid overload). If IV therapy is used, infuse only the amount prescribed.

Fluid retention may not be visible. Rapid weight gain is the best indicator of fluid retention and overload. Each 1 lb (about 500 g) of weight gained (after the first ½ lb) equates to 500 mL of retained water. Weigh the patient at the same time daily (before breakfast), using the same scale. Have the patient wear the same type of clothing for each weigh-in.

Surgical management of adrenocortical hypersecretion depends on the cause of the problem. When adrenal hyperfunction is due to increased pituitary secretion of ACTH, removal of a pituitary adenoma using minimally invasive techniques may be attempted. Sometimes a total *hypophysectomy* (surgical removal of the pituitary gland) is needed. (See earlier discussion of Hypophysectomy in the Hyperpituitarism section.) If hypercortisolism is caused by an adrenal tumor, an *adrenalectomy* (removal of the adrenal gland) may be needed.

Preoperative care starts with correcting disturbances of *fluid and electrolyte balance* before surgery. Continue to monitor blood potassium, sodium, and chloride levels. Dysrhythmias from potassium imbalance may occur, and cardiac monitoring is needed. Hyperglycemia is controlled before surgery.

The patient with hypercortisolism is at risk for complications of infections and fractures. Prevent infection with handwashing and aseptic technique. Decrease the risk for falls by raising top side rails and encouraging the patient to ask for assistance when getting out of bed. A high-calorie, high-protein diet is prescribed before surgery.

Glucocorticoid preparations are given before surgery. The patient continues to receive glucocorticoids during surgery to prevent adrenal crisis because the removal of the tumor results in a sudden drop in cortisol levels. Before surgery, discuss the need for long-term hormone replacement therapy (HRT).

Operative procedures include a unilateral adrenalectomy when one gland is involved or a bilateral adrenalectomy when ACTH-producing tumors cannot be treated by other means or when both adrenal glands are diseased. Surgery is most often performed by laparoscopic adrenalectomy, a minimally invasive surgical approach (DiDalmazi & Reincke, 2018). If necessary, an open surgery through the abdomen or the lateral flank can be performed.

Postoperative care after adrenalectomy includes monitoring in an ICU. Immediately after surgery, assess the patient every 15 minutes for shock (e.g., hypotension; a rapid, weak pulse; and a decreasing urine output) resulting from insufficient glucocorticoid replacement. Monitor vital signs, central venous pressure, pulmonary wedge pressure, intake and output, daily weights, and serum electrolyte levels.

After a bilateral adrenalectomy, patients require lifelong glucocorticoid and mineralocorticoid HRT, starting immediately after surgery. In unilateral adrenalectomy, HRT continues until the remaining adrenal gland increases hormone production. This therapy may be needed for up to 2 years after surgery.

Preventing Injury. The patient is at risk for injury from skin breakdown, bone fractures, and GI bleeding. Prevention of these injuries is a major nursing care focus.

Planning: Expected Outcomes. The patient with hypercortisolism is expected to avoid injury.

Interventions. Priority nursing interventions for prevention of injury focus on skin assessment and protection, coordinating care to ensure gentle handling, and patient teaching regarding drug therapy for prevention of GI ulcers.

Skin injury is a continuing risk even after surgery has corrected the cortisol excess because the changes induced in the skin and blood vessels remain for weeks to months. Assess the skin for reddened areas, excoriation, breakdown, and edema. If mobility is decreased, turn the patient every 2 hours and pad bony prominences.

Instruct the patient to avoid activities that can result in skin trauma. Teach him or her to use a soft toothbrush and an electric shaver. Instruct patients to keep the skin clean and dry it thoroughly after washing. Excessive dryness can be prevented by using a moisturizing lotion.

Adhesive tape often causes skin breakdown. Use tape sparingly and remove it carefully. After venipuncture, the patient may have increased bleeding because of blood vessel fragility. Apply pressure over the site until bleeding has stopped.

Fragile fractures from bone density loss and osteoporosis are possible for months to years after cortisol levels return to normal. When helping the patient move in bed, use a lift sheet instead of grasping him or her. Remind the patient to call for help when walking. Review the use of walkers or canes, if needed. Teach AP to use a gait belt when walking with a patient who has bone density loss.

Collaborate with a registered dietitian nutritionist (RDN) to teach the patient about nutrition therapy. A high-calorie diet that includes increased amounts of calcium and vitamin D is needed. Milk, cheese, yogurt, and green leafy and root vegetables add calcium to promote bone density. Advise the patient to avoid caffeine and alcohol, which increase the risk for GI ulcers and reduce bone density.

GI bleeding is common with hypercortisolism. Cortisol (1) inhibits production of the thick, gel-like mucus that protects the stomach lining, (2) decreases blood flow to the area, and (3) triggers the release of excess hydrochloric acid. Although surgery reduces cortisol levels, the normal mucus and increased blood flow may take weeks to return. Interventions focus on drug therapy to reduce irritation, protect the GI mucosa, and decrease secretion of hydrochloric acid.

Antacids buffer stomach acids and protect the GI mucosa. Teach the patient that these drugs should be taken on a regular schedule rather than on an as-needed basis.

Some agents block the H_2 receptors in the gastric mucosa. When histamine binds to these receptors, a series of actions release hydrochloric acid. Drugs that block the H_2-receptor site include cimetidine, famotidine, and nizatidine. Omeprazole and esomeprazole inhibit the gastric proton pump and prevent the formation of hydrochloric acid.

Instruct the patient to reduce alcohol or caffeine consumption, smoking, and fasting because these actions cause gastric irritation. NSAIDs and drugs that contain aspirin or other salicylates can cause gastritis and intensify GI bleeding. These should be avoided or limited.

Preventing Infection. Glucocorticoids reduce both the inflammation and the immune responses of *immunity*, increasing the risk for infection. For the patient who is taking glucocorticoid replacement therapy, the risk is ongoing. For the patient who is recovering from surgery to prevent hypercortisolism, the infection risk continues for weeks after surgery.

Planning: Expected Outcomes. The patient with hypercortisolism is expected to remain free from infection and avoid situations that increase the risk for infection.

Interventions. Protect the patient with reduced *immunity* from infection. All personnel must use extreme care during all nursing procedures. Thorough handwashing is important. Anyone with an upper respiratory tract infection who enters the patient's room must wear a mask. Observe strict aseptic technique when performing dressing changes or any invasive procedure.

Continually assess the patient for possible infection. Symptoms may not be obvious because excess cortisol suppresses infection indicators caused by inflammation. Fever and pus formation depend on the presence of white blood cells (WBCs). The patient who has reduced *immunity* may have a severe infection without pus and with only a low-grade fever.

Monitor the patient's daily complete blood count (CBC) with differential WBC count, especially neutrophils. Inspect the mouth during every shift for lesions and mucosa breakdown. Assess the lungs every 8 hours for crackles, wheezes, or reduced breath sounds. Assess all urine for odor and cloudiness. Ask about any urgency, burning, or pain on urination.

Take vital signs at least every 4 hours to assess for fever. A temperature elevation of even 1°F (or 0.5°C) above baseline is significant for a patient who has reduced *immunity*, and indicates infection until otherwise proven.

Perform pulmonary hygiene every 2 to 4 hours. Listen to the lungs for crackles, wheezes, or reduced breath sounds. Urge the patient to deep breathe or use an incentive spirometer every hour while awake.

NCLEX EXAMINATION CHALLENGE 57.4

Safe and Effective Care Environment

A nurse caring for a client with Cushing syndrome who must remain on continued glucocorticoid therapy for another health problem will use which of the following actions to **prevent harm**?

A. Urging the client to salt his or her food
B. Testing voided urine for the present of glucose
C. Using nonadhesive methods to secure an IV access
D. Ensuring the prescribed glucocorticoid drug is given on an empty stomach

---

Care Coordination and Transition Management

Home Care Management. The patient with hypercortisolism usually has muscle weakness and fatigue for some weeks after surgery and remains at risk for falls and other injury. These problems may necessitate one-floor living for a short time; and a home health aide may be needed to assist with hygiene, meal preparation, and maintenance.

Self-Management Education. The patient taking exogenous glucocorticoids who is discharged to home remains at continuing risk for impaired *fluid and electrolyte balance*, especially fluid volume excess. Teach him or her and the family to monitor and record the patient's weight daily to show the primary health care provider at any checkups. Also instruct the patient to call the primary health care provider for weight gain of more than 3 lb in a week or more than 1 to 2 lb in a 24-hour period.

After bilateral adrenalectomy, lifelong HRT is needed to prevent adrenal insufficiency. Without the adrenal glands the patient completely depends on the exogenous drug. If the drug is stopped, even for a day or two, no other glands produce the glucocorticoids and the patient develops acute adrenal insufficiency, a life-threatening condition. Management of this problem is described in the Adrenal Gland Hypofunction section. Teach the patient and family about adherence to the drug regimen and its side effects as

---

PATIENT AND FAMILY EDUCATION: PREPARING FOR SELF-MANAGEMENT
Cortisol Replacement Therapy

- Take your medication in divided doses, as prescribed (e.g., the first dose in the morning and the second dose between 4 p.m. and 6 p.m.) for best effects.
- Take your medication with meals or snacks to prevent stomach irritation.
- Weigh yourself daily and keep a record to show your primary health care provider.
- Increase your dosage as directed by your primary health care provider for increased physical stress or severe emotional stress.
- Never skip a dose of medication. If you have persistent vomiting or severe diarrhea and cannot take your medication by mouth for 24 to 36 hours, call your primary health care provider. If you cannot reach your primary health care provider, go to the nearest emergency department. You may need an injection to take the place of your usual oral medication.
- Always wear your medical alert bracelet or necklace.
- Make regular visits for health care follow-up.
- Learn (and have a family member learn) how to give yourself an intramuscular injection of hydrocortisone in case you cannot take your oral drug.

---

described in the Patient and Family Education: Preparing for Self-Management: Cortisol Replacement Therapy box.

Protecting the patient with reduced *immunity* from infection at home is important. Urge him or her to use proper hygiene and social distancing and to avoid crowds or others with infections. Encourage the patient and all people living in the same home with him or her to have yearly influenza vaccinations. Stress that the patient should immediately notify the primary health care provider if he or she has a fever or any other sign of infection.

Health Care Resources. Immediately after returning home, the patient may need a support person to stay and provide more attention than could be given by a visiting nurse or home care aide. Contact with the interprofessional health care team is needed for follow-up and identification of potential problems. The patient taking corticosteroid therapy may have symptoms of adrenal insufficiency if the dosage is inadequate. Suggest that the patient obtain and wear a medical alert bracelet listing the condition and the drug replacement therapy.

◆ **Evaluation: Evaluate Outcomes.** Evaluate the care of the patient with hypercortisolism based on the identified priority patient problems. The expected outcomes of interventions are that the patient will:

- Maintain fluid and electrolyte balance as indicated by blood pressure at or near the normal range, stable body weight, and normal serum sodium and potassium levels
- Remain free from injury as indicated by having intact skin, minimal bruising, absence of bone fractures, and no occult blood in vomitus, stools, or GI secretions
- Remain free from infection as indicated by absence of fever, purulent drainage, cough, pain or burning on urination
- Participate in infection prevention strategies of social distancing and obtaining appropriate immunizations
- Not experience acute adrenal insufficiency

HYPERALDOSTERONISM

Pathophysiology Review

Hyperaldosteronism is an increased secretion of aldosterone with mineralocorticoid excess. Primary hyperaldosteronism (Conn syndrome) in adults results from excessive secretion of aldosterone from one or both adrenal glands, usually caused by an adrenal adenoma. In secondary hyperaldosteronism, excessive secretion of aldosterone is caused by the high levels of angiotensin II that are stimulated by high plasma renin levels. Some causes include kidney hypoxia, diabetic nephropathy, and excessive use of some diuretics.

Increased aldosterone levels cause disturbances of *fluid and electrolyte balance*, which then trigger the kidney tubules to retain sodium and excrete potassium and hydrogen ions. Hypernatremia, hypokalemia, and metabolic alkalosis result. Sodium retention increases blood volume, which raises blood pressure, increasing the risk for strokes, heart attacks, and kidney damage. (See Chapter 13 for discussion of specific electrolyte imbalances.)

Hypokalemia and elevated blood pressure are the most common problems that patients with hyperaldosteronism develop. He or she may have headache, fatigue, muscle weakness, dehydration, and loss of stamina. *Polydipsia* (excessive fluid intake) and *polyuria* (excessive urine output) occur less frequently. *Paresthesias* (sensations of numbness and tingling) may occur if potassium depletion is severe.

Hyperaldosteronism is diagnosed on the basis of laboratory studies and imaging with CT or MRI. Serum potassium levels are decreased, and sodium levels are elevated. Plasma renin levels are low, and aldosterone levels are high. Hydrogen ion loss leads to metabolic alkalemia (elevated blood pH). Urine has a low specific gravity and high aldosterone levels.

❖ Interprofessional Collaborative Care

Surgery is a common treatment for hyperaldosteronism, and one or both adrenal glands may be removed. The patient's potassium level must be corrected before surgery. Drugs used to increase potassium levels include spironolactone, a potassium-sparing diuretic and aldosterone antagonist. Potassium supplements may be used to increase potassium levels before surgery.

The patient who has undergone a unilateral adrenalectomy may need temporary glucocorticoid replacement; replacement is lifelong when both adrenal glands are removed. Glucocorticoids are given before surgery to prevent adrenal crisis.

When surgery cannot be performed, spironolactone therapy is continued to control hypokalemia and hypertension. Because spironolactone is a potassium-sparing diuretic, hyperkalemia can occur in patients who have impaired kidney function or excessive potassium intake. Advise the patient to avoid potassium supplements and foods rich in potassium, such as meat, fish, and many (but not all) vegetables and fruits. Hyponatremia can occur with spironolactone therapy, and the patient may need increased dietary sodium. Instruct patients to report symptoms of hyponatremia, such as muscle weakness, dizziness, lethargy, or drowsiness. Instruct them to report any additional side effects of spironolactone therapy, including gynecomastia, diarrhea, headache, rash, urticaria (hives), confusion, erectile dysfunction, hirsutism, and amenorrhea. Additional drug therapy to control hypertension is often needed.

❓ CLINICAL JUDGMENT CHALLENGE 57.1

Patient-Centered Care, Safety, Physiological Integrity

The client is a 64-year-old man who was brought to the emergency department by his wife, who claims he is "just not acting right." When asked to elaborate, the wife explains that over the past 4 days the client has become quieter, mumbles that his head and stomach hurt, and now does not recognize the neighbor who has been coming over daily for a short visit. The wife further explains that her husband is a nuclear physicist.

On assessment, the nurse finds the client somewhat responsive to his name, although he does not talk; he is unable to lift his arm for a blood pressure measurement. His pulse is difficult to palpate and is both irregular and slow. Blood pressure is 92/50 mm Hg. He has no obvious facial drooping but appears too confused to stick out his tongue when asked or to try to shrug his shoulders. Pulse oximetry is 94% with a respiratory rate of 14 breaths/min. When the nurse asks about his medication use, the wife reports that he is very healthy and takes only aspirin 81 mg every day. Then she remembers that until 10 days ago, he was taking dexamethasone 10 mg twice daily for about 4 weeks for his back pain. He stopped taking the drug and went back to work on Monday (today is Sunday) because he was pain free.

1. **Recognize Cues:** What assessment information in this client situation is the most important and immediate concern for the nurse? (Hint: Identify the **relevant** information *first* to determine what is most important.)
2. **Analyze Cues:** What client conditions are consistent with the **most relevant** information? (Hint: Think about priority collaborative problems that support and contradict the information presented in this situation.)
3. **Prioritize Hypotheses:** Which possibilities or explanations are **most likely** to be present in this client situation? Which possibilities or explanations are the most serious? (Hint: Consider all possibilities and determine their urgency and risk for this client.)
4. **Generate Solutions:** What actions would most likely achieve the desired outcomes for this client? Which actions should be **avoided** or are **potentially harmful**? (Hint: Determine the desired outcomes first to decide which interventions are appropriate and those that should be avoided.)
5. **Take Action:** Which actions are the most appropriate and how should they be implemented? In what **priority order** should they be implemented? (Hint: Consider health teaching, documentation, requested health care provider orders or prescriptions, nursing skills, collaboration with or referral to health team members, etc.)
6. **Evaluate Outcomes:** What client assessment would indicate that the nurse's actions were **effective**? (Hint: Think about signs that would indicate an improvement, decline, or unchanged client condition.)

GET READY FOR THE NEXT-GENERATION NCLEX® EXAMINATION!

Key Points
Review these Key Points for each NCLEX Examination Client Needs Category.

Safe and Effective Care Environment
- Handle all patients with bone density loss carefully, using lift sheets whenever possible. **QSEN: Safety**
- Ensure that hormone replacement drugs are given as close to the prescribed times as possible. **QSEN: Safety**
- Teach the patient with diabetes insipidus the indicators of dehydration.

Health Promotion and Maintenance
- Instruct the patient with adrenal insufficiency to wear a medical alert bracelet and to carry simple carbohydrates with him or her at all times. **QSEN: Patient-Centered Care**
- Teach the patient and family about the symptoms of infection and when to seek medical advice. **QSEN: Patient-Centered Care**
- Teach patients who have permanent endocrine hypofunction the proper techniques and timing of hormone replacement therapy. **QSEN: Patient-Centered Care**
- Instruct patients taking bromocriptine to seek medical care immediately if chest pain, dizziness, or watery nasal discharge occurs. **QSEN: Safety**

Psychosocial Integrity
- Explain all treatment procedures, restrictions, and follow-up care to the patient. **QSEN: Patient-Centered Care**
- Allow patients who experience a change in physical appearance to mourn this change. **QSEN: Patient-Centered Care**

Physiological Integrity
- During the immediate period after a hypophysectomy, teach the patient to avoid activities that increase intracranial pressure (e.g., bending at the waist, straining to have a bowel movement, coughing). **QSEN: Patient-Centered Care**
- Measure intake and output accurately on patients who have either diabetes insipidus or syndrome of inappropriate antidiuretic hormone (SIADH). **QSEN: Evidence-Based Practice**
- Instruct patients who are taking a corticosteroid for more than a week not to stop the drug suddenly. **QSEN: Safety**
- Ensure that no patient suspected of having DI is deprived of fluids for more than 4 hours. **QSEN: Evidence-Based Practice**
- Teach patients with diabetes insipidus the proper way to self-administer desmopressin orally or by nasal spray. **QSEN: Patient-Centered Care**

MASTERY QUESTIONS

1. Which precaution is **most important** for the nurse to teach a female client to **prevent harm** while undergoing drug therapy with estrogen and progesterone for hypopituitarism?
   A. "Use a barrier method of contraception to prevent an unplanned pregnancy."
   B. "Wear a hat with a brim and use sunscreen when outdoors."
   C. "Do not smoke or use nicotine in any form."
   D. "Avoid drinking caffeinated beverages."

2. Which assessment has the **highest priority** for the nurse to perform for a client with syndrome of inappropriate antidiuretic hormone (SIADH) receiving tolvaptan therapy for 24 hours?
   A. Evaluating serum sodium levels
   B. Evaluating serum potassium levels
   C. Examining the skin and sclera for jaundice
   D. Examining the IV site for indications of phlebitis

3. Which of the following are the **priority** precautions the nurse will teach the client who remains at continuing risk for adrenal hypofunction and is taking hormone replacement therapy to **prevent harm** related to the disorder? **Select all that apply.**
   A. "Avoid crowds and people who are ill."
   B. "Check your heart rate for irregular or skipped beats twice daily."
   C. "Do not choose low-sodium versions of prepared foods."
   D. "Get up slowly from sitting or lying positions."
   E. "Keep a source of glucose, such as candy, with you at all times."
   F. "Never skip your hormone replacement drugs."

4. A client preparing for surgery to remove a cortisol-secreting tumor from the adrenal gland asks the nurse whether the physical changes from the excessive cortisol will go away as a result of the surgery so she can look like herself again. What is the nurse's **best** response?
   A. "The surgery is to remove the tumor, not reconstructive surgery."
   B. "You will notice a great difference in your appearance starting within a week after surgery."
   C. "All the changes will resolve but may take a year or longer to completely disappear."
   D. "The fatty changes and acne will resolve with time but the stretch marks only fade."

REFERENCES

Amrein, K., Martucci, G., & Hahner, S. (2018). Understanding adrenal crisis. *Intensive Care Medicine, 44*(5), 652–655.

Burchum, J., & Rosenthal, L. (2019). *Lehne's pharmacology for nursing care* (10th ed.). St. Louis: Elsevier.

Cole, S. (2018). Evaluation and treatment of adrenal dysfunction in the primary care environment. *Nursing Clinics of North America, 53,* 385–394.

Di Dalmazi, G., & Reincke, M. (2018). Adrenal surgery for Cushing's syndrome: An update. *Endocrinology and Metabolism Clinics, 47*(2), 385–394.

Jarvis, C. (2020). *Physical examination & health assessment* (8th ed.). St. Louis: Elsevier.

Kaiser, U., & Ho, K. (2016). Pituitary physiology and diagnostic evaluation. In S. Melmed, K. Polonsky, P. R. Larsen, & H. Kronenberg (Eds.), *Williams' textbook of endocrinology* (13th ed.). Philadelphia: Saunders.

McCance, K., Huether, S., Brashers, V., & Rote, N. (2019). *Pathophysiology: The biologic basis for disease in adults and children* (8th ed.). St. Louis: Mosby.

Melmed, S., & Kleinberg, D. (2016). Pituitary masses and tumor. In S. Melmed, K. Polonsky, P. R. Larsen, & H. Kronenberg (Eds.), *Williams' textbook of endocrinology* (13th ed.). Philadelphia: Saunders.

Melmed, S., Polonsky, K., Larsen, P. R., & Kronenberg, H. (Eds.). (2016). *Williams' textbook of endocrinology* (13th ed.). Philadelphia: Saunders.

Mendiratta-Lala, M., Avram, A., Turcu, A., & Dunnick, R. (2017). Adrenal imaging. *Endocrinology and Metabolism Clinics, 46*(3), 741–759.

Mitchell-Brown, F., & Stephens-DiLeo, R. (2017). Managing panhypopituitarism in adults. *Nursing, 47*(12), 26–31.

Nieman, L. (2018). Diagnosis of Cushing's syndrome in the modern era. *Endocrinology and Metabolism Clinics, 47*(2), 259–273.

Online Mendelian Inheritance in Man (OMIM). (2017). *Multiple endocrine neoplasia type 1.* www.omim.org/entry/131100.

Online Mendelian Inheritance in Man (OMIM). (2019). *Diabetes insipidus, nephrogenic, X-linked.* www.omim.org/entry/304800.

Pagana, K., & Pagana, T. (2018). *Mosby's manual of diagnostic and laboratory tests* (6th ed.). St. Louis: Elsevier.

Pereira, K. (2016). Hyponatremia signals acute adrenal insufficiency. *American Nurse Today, 11*(7), 30.

Pressman, B. (2017). Pituitary imaging. *Endocrinology and Metabolism Clinics, 46*(3), 713–740.

Robinson, A., & Verbalis, J. (2016). Posterior pituitary. In S. Melmed, K. Polonsky, P. R. Larsen, & H. Kronenberg (Eds.), *Williams' textbook of endocrinology* (13th ed.). Philadelphia: Saunders.

Stewart, P., & Newell-Price, J. (2016). The adrenal cortex. In S. Melmed, K. Polonsky, P. R. Larsen, & H. Kronenberg (Eds.), *Williams' textbook of endocrinology* (13th ed.). Philadelphia: Saunders.

Tritos, N., & Biller, B. (2018). Medical therapy for Cushing's syndrome in the twenty-first century. *Endocrinology and Metabolism Clinics, 47*(2), 427–440.

58

Concepts of Care for Patients With Problems of the Thyroid and Parathyroid Glands

M. Linda Workman

http://evolve.elsevier.com/Iggy/

LEARNING OUTCOMES

1. Collaborate with the interprofessional team to coordinate high-quality care and promote **cellular regulation** and optimal **nutrition** in patients who have thyroid or parathyroid disorders.
2. Apply knowledge of anatomy, physiology, and pathophysiology to assess patients with impaired thyroid or parathyroid function affecting **nutrition** or **cellular regulation**.
3. Implement nursing interventions to help the patient and family cope with the psychosocial impact caused by acute or chronic problems of the thyroid gland or parathyroid glands.
4. Interpret clinical changes and laboratory data to determine the effectiveness of therapy for thyroid gland and parathyroid gland disorders.
5. Teach the patient and caregiver(s) about common drugs and other management strategies used for thyroid gland or parathyroid gland problems.
6. Use clinical judgment to prioritize evidence-based nursing care for the patient with severe hypothyroidism and the patient with thyroid storm.

KEY TERMS

euthyroid A condition of having normal or near-normal thyroid function.

exophthalmos Abnormal protrusion of the eyes.

goiter Visibly enlarged thyroid gland.

Graves disease Autoimmune disorder, often occurring after an episode of thyroid inflammation, in which the production of autoantibodies (thyroid-stimulating immunoglobulins [TSIs]) that attach to the thyroid-stimulating hormone (TSH) receptors on the thyroid gland greatly increases thyroid hormone production.

Hashimoto thyroiditis (HT) Autoimmune disorder in which infection and inflammation of the thyroid gland causes the production of autoantibodies to thyroglobulin and tissues within the thyroid gland, which results in extensive tissue destruction and reduced secretion of thyroid hormones.

hyperparathyroidism Disorder in which parathyroid secretion of parathyroid hormone is increased, resulting in hypercalcemia and hypophosphatemia.

hyperthyroidism (thyrotoxicosis) Excessive thyroid hormone secretion from the thyroid gland

hypoparathyroidism A rare disorder in which parathyroid function is decreased and serum calcium levels cannot be maintained.

hypothyroidism Reduced or absent hormone secretion from the thyroid gland that results in whole-body decreased metabolism from inadequate **cellular regulation**.

myxedema coma (hypothyroid crisis) A serious complication of untreated or poorly treated hypothyroidism with dangerously reduced cardiopulmonary and neurologic functioning, although few affected adults become comatose.

pretibial myxedema Dry, waxy swelling of the front surfaces of the lower legs that resembles benign tumors or keloids; associated with hyperthyroidism.

tetany Hyperexcitability of nerves and muscles.

thyroid storm (thyroid crisis) A life-threatening event that occurs in patients with uncontrolled hyperthyroidism, most often with Graves disease.

thyroiditis An inflammation of the thyroid gland.

PRIORITY AND INTERRELATED CONCEPTS

The priority concept for this chapter is:
- *Cellular Regulation*
  The *Cellular Regulation* concept exemplar for this chapter is Hypothyroidism.

The interrelated concepts for this chapter are:
- *Nutrition*
- *Gas Exchange*

The thyroid gland and parathyroid glands secrete hormones that affect whole-body metabolism, *cellular regulation*, *nutrition*, *gas exchange*, electrolyte balance, and excitable membrane activity. Problems of either gland can lead to symptoms in many body systems and can range from mild to life threatening.

CELLULAR REGULATION CONCEPT EXEMPLAR: HYPOTHYROIDISM

Hypothyroidism is reduced or absent hormone secretion from the thyroid gland that results in whole-body decreased metabolism from inadequate *cellular regulation*. In its early stages the disorder can be missed because the onset is gradual and undramatic (Moore, 2018). Aging also affects thyroid function, as shown in the Patient-Centered Care: Older Adult Considerations box.

Pathophysiology Review

Symptoms of hypothyroidism are widespread and reflect overall decreased metabolism from low levels of thyroid hormones (THs). Thyroid cells may fail to produce sufficient levels of THs for several reasons. Sometimes the cells themselves are damaged and no longer function normally. At other times the thyroid cells are functional, but the adult does not ingest enough of the substances needed to make thyroid hormones, especially iodide and tyrosine. When the production of thyroid hormones is too low or absent, the blood levels of THs are very low, and the patient has a decreased metabolic rate. This lowered metabolism causes the hypothalamus and anterior pituitary gland to make stimulatory hormones, especially thyroid-stimulating hormone (TSH), in an attempt to trigger hormone release from the poorly responsive thyroid gland. The TSH binds to thyroid cells and causes the thyroid gland to enlarge, forming a **goiter** (visibly enlarge thyroid gland [Fig. 58.1]), although thyroid hormone production does not increase. The presence of a goiter is common to many thyroid problems and does not definitively indicate either hypothyroidism or hyperthyroidism.

Most tissues and organs are affected by the low metabolic rate and reduced *cellular regulation* caused by hypothyroidism. Cellular energy is decreased, and metabolites that are compounds of proteins and sugars called *glycosaminoglycans (GAGs)* build up inside cells. This GAG buildup increases the mucus and water, forms cellular edema, and changes organ texture. The edema is mucinous and called *myxedema*, rather than edema caused by water alone. This edema changes the patient's

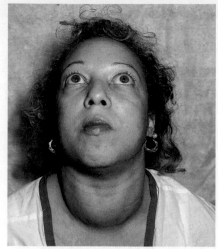

FIG. 58.1 Goiter.

appearance (Fig. 58.2). Nonpitting edema forms everywhere, especially around the eyes, in the hands and feet, and between the shoulder blades. The tongue thickens, and edema forms in the larynx, making the voice husky. General physiologic function is decreased.

Myxedema coma, sometimes called *hypothyroid crisis*, is a serious complication of untreated or poorly treated hypothyroidism with dangerously reduced cardiopulmonary and neurologic functioning, although few affected adults become comatose (McCance et al., 2019). The decreased metabolism

PATIENT-CENTERED CARE: OLDER ADULT CONSIDERATIONS (QSEN)

Age-Related Change	Nursing Adaptation
Thyroid hormone secretion decreases with age, resulting in reduced circulating hormone levels.	Do not rely solely on laboratory values to assess whether and to what degree hypothyroidism may be present (or the effects of therapy). Although secretion is reduced, clearance also is reduced, allowing circulating hormones to be present longer. Use symptom changes to evaluate hormone replacement therapy effectiveness.
Muscle mass decreases and body fat increases from age-related decreased metabolism.	Avoid using change in muscle strength as an indicator of reduced thyroid function.
Age-related changes in cardiovascular and neurologic function make the older adult more sensitive to hormone replacement therapy (HRT).	When hypothyroidism is present and thyroid HRT is started, doses should be lower and increases made more slowly to avoid inducing cardiovascular and neurologic toxicities. Always assess older adults on thyroid HRT for angina, chest pain, dysrhythmias, hypertension, or indicators of increased central nervous system activity.

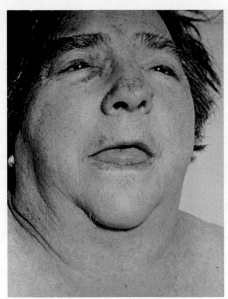

FIG. 58.2 Myxedema.

TABLE 58.1 Causes of Hypothyroidism

Primary Causes
Decreased Thyroid Tissue
- Surgical or radiation-induced thyroid destruction
- Autoimmune thyroid destruction
- Congenital poor thyroid development
- Cancer (thyroidal or metastatic)

Decreased Synthesis of Thyroid Hormone
- Endemic iodine deficiency
- Drugs:
  - Lithium
  - Propylthiouracil
  - Sodium or potassium perchlorate
  - Aminoglutethimide

Secondary Causes
Inadequate Production of Thyroid-Stimulating Hormone
- Pituitary tumors, trauma, infections, or infarcts
- Congenital pituitary defects
- Hypothalamic tumors, trauma, infections, or infarcts

causes the heart muscle to become flabby and the chamber size to increase. The result is decreased cardiac output with decreased perfusion and *gas exchange* in the brain and other vital organs, which makes the already slowed cellular metabolism worse, resulting in tissue and organ failure. *The mortality rate for myxedema coma is extremely high, and this condition is a life-threatening emergency.* Myxedema coma can be caused by a variety of events, drugs, or conditions.

Etiology. Most cases of hypothyroidism in the United States occur as a result of an autoimmune problem resulting from Hashimoto thyroiditis (HT), in which infection and inflammation of the thyroid gland causes the production of autoantibodies to thyroglobulin and tissues within the thyroid gland, which results in extensive tissue destruction and reduced secretion of thyroid hormones (McCance et al., 2019). In North America, other common causes include thyroid surgery and radioactive iodine (RAI) treatment of hyperthyroidism. Worldwide, hypothyroidism is common in areas where the soil and water have little natural iodide, causing endemic goiter. Hypothyroidism is also caused by a variety of other conditions (Table 58.1).

Incidence and Prevalence. Hypothyroidism occurs most often in women between 30 and 60 years of age. Women are affected 7 to 10 times more often than men (McCance et al., 2019).

❖ Interprofessional Collaborative Care

Depending on the severity of the symptoms at the time of diagnosis, initial therapy for hypothyroidism may start in an acute care environment or in the community. When symptoms are severe or if myxedema coma is present, an intensive care environment may be required. Drug therapy is lifelong, and patients must learn to manage their disorders in the community.

◆ Assessment: Recognize Cues

History. A decrease in thyroid hormones produces many symptoms related to decreased metabolism from inadequate *cellular regulation*. However, changes may have occurred slowly, and the patient may not have noticed them. Ask him or her to compare activity now with that of a year ago. The patient often reports an increase in time spent sleeping, sometimes up to 14 to 16 hours daily. Generalized weakness, anorexia, muscle aches, and paresthesias may also be present. Constipation and cold intolerance are common. Ask whether more blankets at night or extra clothing, even in warm weather, has been needed. Some changes may be subtle and are often missed, especially in older adults.

Both men and women may report a decreased libido. Women may have had difficulty becoming pregnant or have changes in menses (heavy, prolonged bleeding or amenorrhea). Men may have problems with impotence and infertility.

Ask about current or previous use of drugs, such as lithium, thiocyanates, aminoglutethimide, sodium or potassium perchlorate, or cobalt. All of these drugs can impair thyroid hormone production. In particular, the cardiac drug amiodarone often has damaging effects on the thyroid gland (Brent & Weetman, 2016; Burchum & Rosenthal, 2019). Also ask whether the patient has ever been treated for hyperthyroidism and what specific treatment was used.

Physical Assessment/Signs and Symptoms. Observe the patient's overall appearance. Fig. 58.2 shows the typical appearance of an adult with hypothyroidism. Common changes include coarse features, edema around the eyes and face, a blank expression, and a thick tongue. The patient's overall muscle movement is slow. He or she may not speak clearly because of tongue thickening and may take a longer time to respond to questions because of reduced cognitive functioning. The Key Features: Hypothyroidism box lists common signs and symptoms of the disorder.

▶▶ KEY FEATURES

Hypothyroidism

Pulmonary Symptoms
- Hypoventilation
- Pleural effusion
- Dyspnea

Cardiovascular Symptoms
- Bradycardia
- Dysrhythmias
- Enlarged heart
- Decreased activity tolerance
- Hypotension

Metabolic Symptoms
- Decreased basal metabolic rate
- Decreased body temperature
- Cold intolerance

Reproductive Symptoms
Women
- Changes in menses (amenorrhea or prolonged menstrual periods)
- Anovulation
- Decreased libido

Men
- Decreased libido
- Impotence

Gastrointestinal Symptoms
- Anorexia
- Weight gain
- Constipation
- Abdominal distention

Psychosocial Symptoms
- Apathy
- Depression
- Paranoia

Skin Symptoms
- Cool, pale or yellowish, dry, coarse, scaly skin
- Thick, brittle nails
- Dry, coarse, brittle hair
- Decreased hair growth, with loss of eyebrow hair
- Poor wound healing

Neuromuscular Symptoms
- Slowing of intellectual functions:
- Slowness or slurring of speech
- Impaired memory
- Inattentiveness
- Lethargy or somnolence
- Confusion
- Hearing loss
- Paresthesia (numbness and tingling) of the extremities
- Decreased tendon reflexes
- Muscle aches and pain

Other Symptoms
- Periorbital edema
- Facial puffiness
- Nonpitting edema of the hands and feet
- Hoarseness
- Goiter (enlarged thyroid gland)
- Thick tongue
- Increased sensitivity to opioids and tranquilizers
- Weakness, fatigue
- Decreased urine output
- Easy bruising
- Iron deficiency anemia

TABLE 58.2   Goiter Classification

Goiter Grade	Description
0	There is no palpable or visible goiter.
1	Mass is not visible with neck in the normal position. Goiter can be palpated and moves up when the patient swallows.
2	Mass is visible as swelling when the neck is in the normal position. Goiter is easily palpated and is usually asymmetric.

Cardiac and respiratory functions are decreased, leading to reduced *gas exchange*. Heart rate may be below 60 beats/min, and respiratory rate may be slow. Body temperature is often lower than 97°F (36.1°C).

Weight gain is very common, even when the adult is not overeating. Weigh the patient and ask whether the result is the same or different from his or her weight a year ago.

Depending on the cause of hypothyroidism, the patient may have a goiter. Remember, some types of hypothyroidism do not induce a goiter, and some types of hyperthyroidism do. The presence of a goiter *suggests* a thyroid problem but does not indicate whether the problem is excessive hormone secretion or too little hormone secretion. Goiters are classified by size (Table 58.2).

Psychosocial Assessment. Hypothyroidism causes many problems in psychosocial functioning. Depression is the most common reason for seeking medical attention. Family members often bring the patient for the initial evaluation. The patient may be too lethargic, apathetic, or drowsy to recognize changes in his or her condition. Families may report that the patient is withdrawn and has reduced cognition. Assess his or her attention span and memory, both of which can be impaired by hypothyroidism. The mental slowness can contribute to social isolation.

Laboratory Assessment. Laboratory findings for hypothyroidism show a dramatic reduction of serum triiodothyronine (T_3) and thyroxine (T_4) levels. TSH levels are high in primary hypothyroidism but can be decreased or near normal in patients with secondary hypothyroidism (see the Laboratory Profile: Thyroid Function box). Patients older than 80 years may have lower-than-normal levels of thyroid hormones without symptoms of hypothyroidism, and hormone replacement is not used until other symptoms are present (Touhy & Jett, 2020).

◆ **Analysis: Analyze Cues and Prioritize Hypotheses.** The priority problems for patients who have hypothyroidism are:
1. Decreased *gas exchange* and oxygenation due to decreased energy, obesity, muscle weakness, and fatigue
2. Hypotension and reduced perfusion due to decreased heart rate from decreased myocardial metabolism
3. Potential for the complication of myxedema coma

◆ **Planning and Implementation: Generate Solutions and Take Action.** Respiratory and cardiac problems are serious, and their management is a priority. *The most common cause of death among patients with myxedema coma is respiratory failure.*

Improving Gas Exchange

Planning: Expected Outcomes. With appropriate management, the patient with hypothyroidism is expected to have improved *gas exchange*.

Interventions. Observe and record the rate and depth of respirations and adequacy of *gas exchange*. Measure oxygen saturation by pulse oximetry, and apply oxygen if the patient has hypoxemia. Auscultate the lungs for a decrease in breath sounds or presence of crackles. If hypothyroidism is severe, the patient may require ventilatory support. Severe respiratory distress occurs with myxedema coma.

Sedating a patient with hypothyroidism can make gas exchange worse and is avoided if possible. When sedation is needed, the dosage is reduced because hypothyroidism increases sensitivity to these drugs. For the patient receiving sedation, assess for adequate gas exchange.

LABORATORY PROFILE

Thyroid Function

Test	Normal Range	Hypothyroidism	Hyperthyroidism
Serum T_3	70-205 ng/dL (1.2-3.4 nmol/L)	Decreased	Increased
Serum T_4 (total)	4-12 mcg/dL (59-142 nmol/L)	Decreased	Increased
Free T_4 index	0.8-2.8 ng/dL (10-36 pmol/L)	Decreased	Increased
TSH stimulation test (thyroid stimulation test)	>10% in RAIU or >1.5 mcg/dL	No response in primary hypothyroidism Normal response in secondary hypothyroidism	Does not apply because this test is used only to differentiate primary from secondary hypothyroidism
Thyroid-stimulating immunoglobulins (TSI)	<130% of basal activity	No change	Elevated in Graves disease Normal in other types of hyperthyroidism
Thyrotropin receptor antibodies (TRAbs)	Titer: 0%	No response	80%-95% indicates Graves disease
TSH	0.3-5 mcU/mL (0.35 mU/L)	High in primary disease Low in secondary or tertiary disease	Low in Graves disease High in secondary or tertiary hyperthyroidism

RAIU, Radioactive iodine uptake; *T₃,* Triiodothyronine; *T₄,* thyroxine; *TSH,* thyroid-stimulating hormone.
Data from Pagana, K., & Pagana, T. (2018). *Mosby's manual of diagnostic and laboratory tests* (6th ed.). St. Louis: Elsevier.

Preventing Hypotension

Planning: Expected Outcomes. The patient is expected to have adequate cardiovascular function and tissue perfusion with *gas exchange*.

Interventions. The patient may have decreased blood pressure, bradycardia, and dysrhythmias. Nursing priorities are monitoring for condition changes and preventing complications. Monitor blood pressure and heart rate and rhythm and observe for indications of shock (e.g., hypotension, decreased urine output, changes in mental status).

If hypothyroidism is chronic, the patient may have cardiovascular disease. *Instruct the patient to report episodes of chest pain or chest discomfort immediately.*

The patient requires lifelong thyroid hormone replacement. Synthetic hormone preparations are usually prescribed. The most common is levothyroxine. Therapy is started with low doses and gradually increased over a period of weeks. *The patient with more severe symptoms of hypothyroidism is started on the lowest dose of thyroid hormone replacement.* This precaution is especially important when the patient has known cardiac problems. Starting at too high a dose or increasing the dose too rapidly can cause severe hypertension, heart failure, and myocardial infarction. With myxedema coma, the drug may need to be given IV because of the severely reduced motility and absorption of the GI tract.

! NURSING SAFETY ALERT (QSEN)

Drug Alert

Teach patients and families who are beginning thyroid replacement therapy to take the drug *exactly* as prescribed and not to change the dose or schedule without consulting the primary health care provider.

Assess for chest pain and dyspnea during initiation of therapy. The final dosage is determined by blood levels of TSH and the patient's physical responses. The dosage and time required for symptom relief vary with each patient. Monitor for and teach the patient and family about the symptoms of hyperthyroidism, which can occur with replacement therapy.

Preventing Myxedema Coma. Any patient with hypo-thyroidism who has other health problem or who is newly diagnosed is at risk for myxedema coma. Factors leading to myxedema coma include acute illness, surgery, chemotherapy, discontinuation of thyroid replacement therapy, and use of sedatives or opioids. Problems that often occur with this condition include:
- Greatly reduced level of consciousness and cognition
- Respiratory failure
- Hypotension
- Hyponatremia
- Hypothermia
- Hypoglycemia

! NURSING SAFETY ALERT (QSEN)

Action Alert

Myxedema coma can lead to shock, organ damage, and death. Assess the patient with hypothyroidism at least every 8 hours for changes that indicate increasing severity, especially changes in mental status, and report these promptly to the primary health care provider.

Treatment is instituted quickly according to the patient's symptoms and without waiting for laboratory confirmation. Management interventions are listed in the Best Practice for Patient Safety & Quality Care: Emergency Care of the Patient With Myxedema Coma box.

Care Coordination and Transition Management. Hypothyroidism is usually chronic with patients living in the community and managed on an outpatient basis. Patients in acute care settings, subacute care settings, and rehabilitation centers may have long-standing hypothyroidism in addition to other

BEST PRACTICE FOR PATIENT SAFETY & QUALITY CARE (QSEN)

Emergency Care of the Patient With Myxedema Coma

- Maintain a patent airway.
- Replace fluids with IV normal or hypertonic saline as prescribed.
- Give levothyroxine sodium IV as prescribed.
- Give glucose IV as prescribed.
- Give corticosteroids as prescribed.
- Check the patient's temperature hourly.
- Monitor blood pressure hourly.
- Cover the patient with warm blankets.
- Monitor for changes in mental status.
- Turn every 2 hours.
- Institute Aspiration Precautions.

health problems. Ensure that whoever is responsible for overseeing the patient's daily care is aware of the condition and understands its management.

Home Care Management. The patient with hypothyroidism does not usually require changes in the home unless cognition has decreased to the point that he or she poses a danger to himself or herself. Activity intolerance and fatigue may necessitate one-floor living for a short time. If symptoms have not improved before discharge, discuss the need for extra heat or clothing because of cold intolerance. The patient may need help with the drug regimen. Discuss this issue with the family and patient and develop a plan for drug therapy. One person should be clearly designated as responsible for drug preparation and delivery so doses are neither missed nor duplicated.

Self-Management Education. *The most important educational need for the patient with hypothyroidism is about hormone replacement therapy and its side effects.* Emphasize the need for lifelong drugs, and review the symptoms of both hyperthyroidism and hypothyroidism. Teach the patient to wear a medical alert bracelet. Teach the patient and family when to seek medical interventions for dosage adjustment and the need for periodic blood tests of hormone levels. Instruct the patient not to take any over-the-counter drugs without consulting his or her primary health care provider because thyroid hormone preparations interact with many other drugs.

Advise the patient to maintain *nutrition* by eating a well-balanced diet with adequate fiber and fluid intake to prevent constipation. Caution him or her that use of fiber supplements may interfere with the absorption of thyroid hormone. Thyroid hormones should be taken on an empty stomach, at least 4 hours before or after a meal. Remind the patient about the importance of adequate rest.

Help the family understand that the time required for resolution of hypothyroidism varies. During this time the patient may continue to have mental slowness. Teach the family to orient the patient often and to explain everything clearly, simply, and as often as needed.

Teach the patient to monitor himself or herself for therapy effectiveness. The two easiest parameters to check are need for sleep and bowel elimination. When the patient requires more sleep and is constipated, the dose of replacement hormone may need to be increased by the primary health care provider. When the patient

FOCUSED ASSESSMENT

The Patient With Hypothyroidism

Assess cardiovascular status:
- Vital signs, including apical pulse, pulse pressure, presence or absence of orthostatic hypotension, and the quality and rhythm of peripheral pulses
- Presence or absence of peripheral edema
- Weight gain or loss

Assess cognition and mental status:
- Level of consciousness, with orientation to time, place, and person
- Ability to accurately read a seven-word sentence containing no words greater than three syllables
- Ability to count backward from 100 by 3s

Assess condition of skin and mucous membranes:
- Moistness of skin, most reliable on chest and back
- Skin temperature and color

Assess neuromuscular status:
- Reactivity of patellar and biceps reflexes
- Oral temperature
- Handgrip strength
- Steadiness of gait
- Presence or absence of fine tremors in the hand

Ask about:
- Sleep in the past 24 hours
- Patient warm enough or too warm indoors
- 24-hour diet recall and 24-hour activity recall
- Over-the-counter and prescribed drugs taken
- Last bowel movement

Assess patient's understanding of illness and adherence with therapy:
- Symptoms to report to primary health care provider
- Drug therapy plan (correct timing and dose)

has difficulty getting to sleep and has more bowel movements than normal for him or her, the dose may need to be decreased.

Health Care Resources. With severe hypothyroidism, the patient at home may need a support person to stay and provide day and night attention. Contact with the interprofessional health care team is needed for follow-up and identification of potential problems. The patient taking thyroid drugs may have symptoms of hypothyroidism if the dosage is inadequate or symptoms of hyperthyroidism if the dose is too high. A home care nurse uses the guidelines listed in the Focused Assessment: The Patient With Hypothyroidism box at every home visit for the patient with hypothyroidism.

◆ **Evaluation: Evaluate Outcomes.** Evaluate the care of the patient with hypothyroidism based on the identified priority

NCLEX EXAMINATION CHALLENGE 58.1

Safe and Effective Care Environment

An assistive personnel reports that a nursing home client who has hypothyroidism has a pulse of 48 beats/min this morning. Which assessments have the highest **priority** for the nurse to perform **immediately**? **Select all that apply.**

A. Checking body temperature
B. Testing deep tendon reflex responses
C. Measuring oxygen saturation by pulse oximetry
D. Checking blood pressure, heart rate, and rhythm
E. Determining level of consciousness and cognition
F. Identifying presence or absence of the swallowing reflex
G. Examining feet and ankles for indications of peripheral edema

patient problems. The expected outcomes are that with proper management the patient should:

- Maintain normal cardiovascular function with a pulse above 60 beats/min and a blood pressure within normal limits for age and general health
- Maintain adequate respiratory function and **gas exchange** with SpO$_2$ above 90%
- Demonstrate improvement in cognition

HYPERTHYROIDISM

Pathophysiology Review

Hyperthyroidism (thyrotoxicosis) is excessive thyroid hormone secretion from the thyroid gland. The same symptoms and terms are used even if the cause is ingestion of synthetic thyroid hormones when thyroid function is normal. Excessive thyroid hormones reduce **cellular regulation** by increasing metabolism in all body organs, which then produces many different symptoms. Hyperthyroidism can be temporary or permanent, depending on the cause.

The excessive thyroid hormones stimulate most body systems, causing hypermetabolism and increased sympathetic nervous system activity. Symptoms are listed in the Key Features: Hyperthyroidism box.

Thyroid hormones stimulate the heart, increasing rate and stroke volume. These responses increase cardiac output, blood pressure, and blood flow (McCance et al., 2019).

> ## KEY FEATURES
> ### Hyperthyroidism
>
> **Cardiopulmonary Symptoms**
> - Palpitations
> - Chest pain
> - Increased systolic blood pressure
> - Tachycardia
> - Dysrhythmias
> - Rapid, shallow respirations
>
> **Metabolic Symptoms**
> - Increased basal metabolic rate
> - Heat intolerance
> - Low-grade fever
> - Fatigue
>
> **Neurologic Symptoms**
> - Blurred or double vision
> - Eye fatigue
> - Increased tears
> - Injected (red) conjunctiva
> - Photophobia
> - Eyelid retraction, eyelid lag
> - Globe lag
> - Hyperactive deep tendon reflexes
> - Tremors
> - Insomnia
>
> **Skin Symptoms**
> - Diaphoresis (excessive sweating)
> - Fine, soft, silky body hair
> - Smooth, warm, moist skin
> - Thinning of scalp hair
>
> **Gastrointestinal Symptoms**
> - Weight loss
> - Increased appetite
> - Increased stools
>
> **Reproductive Symptoms**
> - Amenorrhea
> - Increased libido
>
> **Psychosocial Symptoms**
> - Decreased attention span
> - Restlessness and irritability
> - Emotional instability
> - Manic behavior
>
> **Other Symptoms**
> - Goiter
> - Wide-eyed or startled appearance (exophthalmos)[a]
> - Enlarged spleen
> - Muscle weakness and wasting

[a] Present in Graves disease only.

Elevated thyroid hormone levels affect protein, fat, and glucose metabolism. Protein buildup and breakdown are increased; but breakdown exceeds buildup, causing a net loss of body protein known as a *negative nitrogen balance*. Glucose tolerance is decreased, and the patient has *hyperglycemia* (elevated blood glucose levels). Fat metabolism is increased, and body fat decreases. Although the patient has an increased appetite, the increased metabolism causes weight loss and **nutrition** deficits.

Thyroid hormones are produced in response to the stimulation hormones secreted by the hypothalamus and anterior pituitary glands. Thus oversecretion of thyroid hormones changes the secretion of hormones from the hypothalamus and the anterior pituitary gland through negative feedback (see Chapter 56). Thyroid hormones also have some influence over sex hormone production. Women have menstrual problems and decreased fertility. Both men and women with hyperthyroidism have an increased *libido* (sexual interest).

Etiology and Genetic Risk. Hyperthyroidism has many causes. The most common form of the disease is Graves disease, also called *toxic diffuse goiter*. **Graves disease** is an autoimmune disorder, often occurring after an episode of thyroid inflammation, in which the production of autoantibodies (thyroid-stimulating immunoglobulins [TSIs]) that attach to the thyroid-stimulating hormone (TSH) receptors on the thyroid gland greatly increases thyroid hormone production (Davies et al., 2016; Hooley & Reagan, 2016; McCance et al., 2019). This increases the number of glandular cells, which enlarges the gland, forming a goiter, and overproduces thyroid hormones (thyrotoxicosis).

In Graves disease, all the general symptoms of hyperthyroidism are present. In addition, other changes specific to Graves disease may occur, including **exophthalmos** (abnormal protrusion of the eyes) and **pretibial myxedema** (dry, waxy swelling of the front surfaces of the lower legs that resembles benign tumors or keloids).

Hyperthyroidism caused by multiple thyroid nodules is termed *toxic multinodular goiter (TMNG)*. The nodules may be enlarged thyroid tissues or benign tumors (adenomas). These patients usually have had a goiter for years. The symptoms are milder than those seen in Graves disease, and the patient does not have exophthalmos or pretibial myxedema.

Hyperthyroidism also can be caused by excessive use of thyroid replacement hormones. This type of problem is called *exogenous hyperthyroidism*.

> ## 👤 PATIENT-CENTERED CARE: GENETIC/ GENOMIC CONSIDERATIONS (QSEN)
>
> Graves disease is associated with other autoimmune disorders, such as diabetes mellitus, vitiligo, and rheumatoid arthritis and often occurs in both members of identical twins (Online Mendelian Inheritance in Man [OMIM], 2016). Susceptibility to Graves disease is associated with several gene mutations (*GRD1, GRD2, GRDX1, GRDX2*). The pattern of inheritance is autosomal recessive with sex limitation to females. Ask the patient with Graves disease whether any other family members also have the problem.

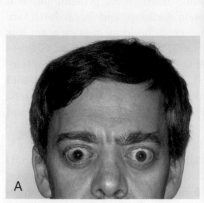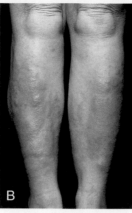

FIG. 58.3 A, Exophthalmos. B, Pretibial myxedema. (From Belchetz, P., & Hammond, P. [2003]. *Mosby's color atlas and text of diabetes and endocrinology.* Edinburgh: Mosby.)

Incidence and Prevalence. Hyperthyroidism is a common endocrine disorder. Graves disease can occur at any age but is diagnosed most often in women between 20 and 40 years of age (Davies et al., 2016). Toxic multinodular goiter usually occurs after the age of 50 years and affects women four times more often than men (McCance et al., 2019).

❖ Interprofessional Collaborative Care

◆ Assessment: Recognize Cues

History. Many changes and problems occur because the reduced *cellular regulation* of hyperthyroidism affects all body systems, although changes may occur over such a long period that patients may be unaware of them. Record age, gender, and usual weight. The increased metabolic rate affects *nutrition.* The patient may report a recent unplanned weight loss, an increased appetite, and an increase in the number of bowel movements per day.

Heat intolerance is often the first symptom the patient notices. He or she may have increased sweating even when environmental temperatures are comfortable for others, and often wears lighter clothing in cold weather. The patient may also report palpitations or chest pain as a result of the cardiovascular effects. Ask about changes in breathing patterns because dyspnea (with or without exertion) is common.

Visual changes may be the earliest problem the patient or family notices, especially exophthalmos with Graves disease (Fig. 58.3). Ask about changes in vision, such as blurring or double vision and tiring of the eyes.

Ask about changes in energy level or in the ability to perform ADLs. Fatigue and insomnia are common. Families may report that the patient has become irritable or depressed.

Ask women about changes in menses, because amenorrhea or a decreased menstrual flow is common. Initially both men and women may have an increase in libido, but this changes as the patient becomes more fatigued.

Ask about previous thyroid surgery or radiation therapy to the neck, because some adults remain hyperthyroid after surgery or are resistant to radiation therapy. Ask about past and current drugs, especially the use of thyroid hormone replacement or antithyroid drugs.

Physical Assessment/Signs and Symptoms. Exophthalmos is common in patients with Graves disease. The wide-eyed or "startled" look is due to edema in the extraocular muscles and increased fatty tissue behind the eye, which pushes the eyeball forward and may cause problems with focusing. Pressure on the optic nerve may impair vision. If the eyelids fail to close completely and the eyes are unprotected, they may become dry, and corneal ulcers may develop. Observe the eyes for excessive tearing and a bloodshot appearance. Ask about sensitivity to light (*photophobia*).

Two other eye problems are common in all types of hyperthyroidism: eyelid retraction (eyelid lag) and globe (eyeball) lag. In eyelid lag, the upper eyelid fails to descend when the patient gazes slowly downward. In globe lag, the upper eyelid pulls back faster than the eyeball when the patient gazes upward. During assessment, ask the patient to look down and then up, and document the response.

Observe the size and symmetry of the thyroid gland. The generalist medical-surgical nurse does not palpate the thyroid gland although it is superficially located. In goiter, a generalized thyroid enlargement, the thyroid gland may increase to four times its normal size (see Fig. 58.1). *Not all patients with a goiter have hyperthyroidism.* Bruits (turbulence from increased blood flow) may be heard in the neck with a stethoscope.

❗ NURSING SAFETY PRIORITY (QSEN)

Action Alert

Do not palpate a goiter or thyroid tissue in a patient with hyperthyroid symptoms. This action can stimulate the sudden release of excessive thyroid hormones and trigger a life-threatening episode of thyroid storm (crisis).

The cardiovascular problems of hyperthyroidism include increased systolic blood pressure, tachycardia, and dysrhythmias. Usually the diastolic pressure is decreased, causing a widened pulse pressure.

Inspect the hair and skin. Fine, soft, silky hair and smooth, warm, moist skin are common. Many patients notice thinning of scalp hair. Muscle weakness and hyperactive deep tendon reflexes are common. Observe motor movements of the hands for tremors. The patient may appear restless, irritable, and fatigued.

Psychosocial Assessment. Wide mood swings, irritability, decreased attention span, and manic behavior are common. Hyperactivity often leads to fatigue because of the inability to sleep well. Some patients describe their activity as having two modes (i.e., either "full speed ahead" or "completely stopped"). Ask whether he or she cries or laughs without cause or has difficulty concentrating. Family members often report a change in the patient's mental or emotional status.

Laboratory Assessment. Testing for hyperthyroidism involves measurement of blood levels for triiodothyronine (T_3), thyroxine (T_4), and thyroid-stimulating hormone (TSH). Antibodies to the TSH receptor (thyrotropin receptor [TRAbs]) are measured to diagnose Graves disease. The most common changes in laboratory tests for hyperthyroidism are listed in the Laboratory Profile: Thyroid Function box.

Other Diagnostic Assessment. Thyroid scan evaluates the position, size, and functioning of the thyroid gland. Radioactive iodine (RAI [^{123}I]) is given by mouth, and the uptake of iodine by the thyroid gland (radioactive iodine uptake [RAIU]) is measured. The half-life of ^{123}I is short, and radiation precautions are not needed. Pregnancy should be ruled out before the scan is performed. The normal thyroid gland has an uptake of 5% to 35% of the given dose at 24 hours. RAIU is increased in hyperthyroidism and can be used to identify active thyroid nodules. It is no longer the most common test for thyroid function (Davies et al., 2016).

Ultrasonography of the thyroid can determine its size and general composition of any masses or nodules. This outpatient procedure takes about 30 minutes to perform and is painless.

ECG usually shows supraventricular tachycardia. Other ECG changes include atrial fibrillation, dysrhythmias, and premature ventricular contractions.

◆ **Interventions: Take Action.** Because Graves disease is the most common form of hyperthyroidism, the interventions discussed in the following sections include those specific for the problems that occur with Graves disease. In North America, the most common interventions are drug therapy and radioablation. Surgery is reserved for severe disease that is not responsive to other forms of management. Medical management is used to decrease the effect of thyroid hormone on cardiac function and to reduce thyroid hormone secretion. The priorities for nursing care focus on monitoring for complications, reducing stimulation, promoting comfort, and teaching the patient and family about therapeutic drugs and procedures.

Nonsurgical Management. Monitoring includes measuring the patient's apical pulse, blood pressure, and temperature at least every 4 hours. Instruct the patient to report immediately any palpitations, dyspnea, vertigo, or chest pain. Increases in temperature may indicate a rapid worsening of the patient's condition and the onset of **thyroid storm (thyroid crisis)**, a life-threatening event that occurs in patients with uncontrolled hyperthyroidism, most often with Graves disease. It presents with uncontrolled hyperthyroidism and is characterized by high fever and severe hypertension (Hooley & Reagan, 2016; Schreiber, 2017). *Immediately report a temperature increase of even 1°F.* If this task is delegated to assistive personnel (AP), instruct them to report the patient's temperature to you as soon as it has been obtained. If temperature is elevated, immediately assess the patient's cardiac status. If the patient has a cardiac monitor, check for dysrhythmias.

Reducing stimulation helps prevent increasing the symptoms of hyperthyroidism and the risk for cardiac complications. Encourage the patient to rest. Keep the environment quiet by closing the door to the room, limiting visitors, and postponing nonessential care or treatments.

Promoting comfort includes reducing the room temperature to decrease discomfort caused by heat intolerance. Instruct AP to ensure that the patient always has a fresh pitcher of ice water and to change the bed linen whenever it becomes damp from diaphoresis. Suggest that the patient take a cool shower or sponge bath several times each day. For patients with exophthalmos, prevent eye dryness by encouraging the use of artificial tears.

Drug therapy with antithyroid drugs is the initial treatment for hyperthyroidism and causes some patients to go into remission for as long as 10 years (Davies et al., 2016). The Common Examples of Drug Therapy: Hyperthyroidism box lists teaching priorities for the patient receiving drug therapy for hyperthyroidism. The preferred drugs are the thionamides, especially methimazole. Propylthiouracil is used less often because of its liver toxic effects (Davies et al., 2016; Felicilda-Reynaldo & Kenneally, 2016). These drugs block thyroid hormone production by preventing iodide binding in the thyroid gland. The response to these drugs is delayed because the patient may have large amounts of stored thyroid hormones that continue to be released.

Iodine preparations may be used for short-term therapy before surgery. They decrease blood flow through the thyroid gland, reducing the production and release of thyroid hormone. Improvement usually occurs within 2 weeks, but it may be weeks before metabolism returns to normal. This treatment can result in hypothyroidism, and the patient is monitored closely for the need to adjust the drug regimen.

Beta-adrenergic blocking drugs such as propranolol may be used as supportive therapy. These drugs relieve diaphoresis, anxiety, tachycardia, and palpitations but do not inhibit thyroid hormone production. See Chapters 32 and 33 for a discussion of the actions and nursing implications of these agents.

COMMON EXAMPLES OF DRUG THERAPY

Hyperthyroidism

Drugs	Nursing Implications
Propylthiouracil Mothimazole	Teach patient to avoid crowds and people who are ill *because the drug reduces the immune response, increasing the risk for infection.*
	Teach patients to check for weight gain, slow heart rate, and cold intolerance, *which are indications of hypothyroidism and the need for a lower drug dose.*
	Teach patients taking propylthiouracil to report darkening of the urine or a yellow appearance to the skin or whites of the eyes, *which indicate possible liver toxicity or failure, a serious side effect of propylthiouracil.*
	Remind women taking methimazole to notify their primary health care providers if they become pregnant *because the drug causes birth defects and should not be used during pregnancy.*
Lugol solution Saturated solution of potassium iodide (SSKI)	Administer these drugs orally 1 hour *after* a thionamide has been given *because initially the iodine agents can cause an increase in the production of thyroid hormones. Giving a thionamide first prevents this initial increase in thyroid hormone production.*
	Check patient for a fever or rash and ask about a metallic taste, mouth sores, sore throat, or GI distress *as these are indications of iodism, a toxic effect of the drugs, and may require that the drug be discontinued.*

Although similar in action, methimazole and propylthiouracil are *not* interchangeable. The dosages for propylthiouracil are much higher than those for methimazole.

Methimazole can cause birth defects and should not be used during the first trimester of pregnancy. Instruct women to notify their primary health care provider if pregnancy occurs.

Radioactive iodine (RAI) therapy is not used in pregnant women because ¹³¹I crosses the placenta and can damage the fetal thyroid gland. The patient with hyperthyroidism may receive RAI in the form of oral ¹³¹I. The dosage depends on the thyroid gland's size and sensitivity to radiation. The thyroid gland picks up the RAI, and some of the cells that produce thyroid hormone are destroyed by the local radiation. Because the thyroid gland stores thyroid hormones to some degree, the patient may not have complete symptom relief until 6 to 8 weeks after RAI therapy. Additional drug therapy for hyperthyroidism is still needed during the first few weeks after RAI treatment.

RAI therapy is performed on an outpatient basis. One dose may be sufficient, although some patients need a second or third dose. The radiation dose is low and is usually completely eliminated within a month; however, the source is unsealed, and some radioactivity is present in the patient's body fluids and stool for a few weeks after therapy. Radiation precautions are needed to prevent exposure to family members and other people. Teach patients the precautions listed in the Patient and Family Education: Preparing for Self-Management: Safety Precautions for the Patient Receiving an Unsealed Radioactive Isotope box to use during the first few weeks after receiving ¹³¹I.

The degree of thyroid destruction varies. Some patients become hypothyroid as a result of treatment. The patient then needs lifelong thyroid hormone replacement. All patients who have undergone RAI therapy should be monitored regularly for changes in thyroid function.

Surgical Management. Surgery to remove all or part of the thyroid gland is used to manage Graves and other types of hyperthyroidism that do not respond to nonsurgical management strategies. It is also used when a large goiter causes tracheal or esophageal compression. Removal of all (*total thyroidectomy*) or part (*subtotal thyroidectomy*) of the thyroid tissue decreases the production of thyroid hormones. After a total thyroidectomy, patients must take lifelong thyroid hormone replacement.

Preoperative Care. The patient is treated with thionamide drug therapy first to have near-normal thyroid function (euthyroid) before thyroid surgery. Iodine preparations also are used to decrease thyroid size and vascularity, thereby reducing the risk for hemorrhage and the potential for thyroid storm during surgery. (Thyroid storm is discussed earlier in the Nonsurgical Management section, and later in the Thyroid Storm section of Hyperthyroidism.)

PATIENT AND FAMILY EDUCATION: PREPARING FOR SELF-MANAGEMENT
Safety Precautions for the Patient Receiving an Unsealed Radioactive Isotope

- Use a toilet that is not used by others for at least 2 weeks after receiving the radioactive iodine.
- Sit to urinate (males and females) to avoid splashing urine on the seat, walls, and floor.
- Flush the toilet (with the lid closed) three times after each use.
- If urine is spilled on the toilet seat or floor, use paper tissues or towels to clean it up, bag them in sealable plastic bags, and take them to the hospital's radiation therapy department.
- Men with urinary incontinence should use condom catheters and a drainage bag rather than absorbent gel-filled briefs or pads.
- Women with urinary incontinence should use facial tissue layers in their clothing to catch the urine rather than absorbent gel-filled briefs or pads. These tissues should then be flushed down the toilet exclusively used by the patient.
- Using a laxative on the second and third days after receiving the radioactive drug helps you excrete the contaminated stool faster (this also decreases the exposure of your abdominal organs to radiation).
- Wear only machine-washable clothing and wash these items separately from others in your household.
- After washing your clothing, run the washing machine for a full cycle on empty before it is used to wash the clothing of others.
- Avoid close contact with pregnant women, infants, and young children for the first week after therapy. Remain at least 3 feet (about 1 m) away from these people and limit your exposure to them to no more than 1 hour daily.
- Some radioactivity will be in your saliva during the first week after therapy. Precautions to avoid exposing others to this contamination (both household members and trash collectors) include:
  - Not sharing toothbrushes or toothpaste tubes
  - Using disposable tissues rather than cloth handkerchiefs and either flushing used ones down the toilet or keeping them in a plastic bag and turning them in to the radiation department of the hospital for disposal

Hypertension, dysrhythmias, and tachycardia must be controlled before surgery. The patient with hyperthyroidism may need to follow a high-protein, high-carbohydrate diet for days or weeks before surgery.

Teach the patient to perform deep-breathing exercises. Stress the importance of supporting the neck when coughing or moving by placing both hands behind the neck to reduce strain on the incision.

Explain the surgery and the care after surgery to the patient. Remind him or her that a drain and a dressing may be in place after surgery.

Operative Procedures. Many thyroidectomies are now performed as minimally invasive surgeries or mini-incision surgeries. With these surgeries, as with the traditional open approach, the parathyroid glands and recurrent laryngeal nerves are avoided to reduce the risk for complications and injury.

With a subtotal thyroidectomy, the remaining thyroid tissues are sutured to the trachea. With a total thyroidectomy, the entire thyroid gland is removed, but the parathyroid glands are left with an intact blood supply to prevent causing hypoparathyroidism.

Postoperative Care. *Monitoring the patient for complications is the most important nursing action after thyroid surgery.* Monitor vital signs every 15 minutes until the patient is stable and then every 30 minutes. Increase or decrease the monitoring of vital signs based on changes in the patient's condition.

Assess the patient's level of discomfort and give prescribed drugs for pain control as needed. Use pillows to support the head and neck. Place the patient, while he or she is awake, in a semi-Fowler position. Avoid positions that cause neck extension.

Help the patient deep-breathe every 30 minutes to 1 hour. Suction oral and tracheal secretions when necessary.

Thyroid surgery can cause hemorrhage, respiratory distress with reduced *gas exchange,* parathyroid gland injury (resulting in *hypocalcemia* [low serum calcium levels] and **tetany** [hyperexcitability of nerves and muscles]), damage to the laryngeal nerves, and thyroid storm. Remain alert to the potential for complications and identify symptoms early.

Hemorrhage is most likely to occur during the first 24 hours after surgery. Inspect the neck dressing and behind the patient's neck for blood. A drain may be present, and a moderate amount of serosanguineous drainage is normal. Hemorrhage may be seen as bleeding at the incision site or as respiratory distress caused by tracheal compression.

*Respiratory distress and reduced *gas exchange* can result from swelling, tetany, or damage to the laryngeal nerve, resulting in spasms. Laryngeal *stridor* (harsh, high-pitched respiratory sounds) is heard in acute respiratory obstruction. Keep emergency tracheostomy equipment in the patient's room. Check that oxygen and suctioning equipment are nearby and in working order.

Hypocalcemia and tetany may occur if the parathyroid glands

! NURSING SAFETY PRIORITY (QSEN)
Critical Rescue

> Monitor the patient to identify symptoms of obstruction and poor *gas exchange* (stridor, dyspnea, falling oxygen saturation, inability to swallow, drooling) after thyroid surgery. If any indications are present, respond by immediately initiating the Rapid Response Team.

are removed, damaged, or their blood supply is impaired during thyroid surgery, resulting in decreased parathyroid hormone (PTH) levels. Ask the patient hourly about tingling around the mouth or of the toes and fingers. Assess for muscle twitching as a sign of calcium deficiency. Calcium gluconate or calcium chloride for IV use should be available in an emergency situation. (For information on the later signs of hypocalcemia, see the discussion of postoperative care in the Hyperparathyroidism section and the Assessment discussion in the Hypoparathyroidism section. Hypocalcemia is also discussed in Chapter 13.)

Laryngeal nerve damage may occur during surgery. This problem results in hoarseness and a weak voice. Assess the patient's voice at 2-hour intervals and document any changes. Reassure the patient that hoarseness is usually temporary.

Thyroid storm or **thyroid crisis** is a life-threatening event that occurs in patients with uncontrolled hyperthyroidism, most often with Graves disease. Symptoms develop quickly, and the problem is fatal if left untreated (Schreiber, 2017). It is often triggered by stressors such as trauma, infection, diabetic ketoacidosis, and pregnancy. Other conditions that can lead to thyroid storm include vigorous palpation of the goiter, exposure

to iodine, and radioactive iodine (RAI) therapy. Although thyroid storm after surgery is less common because of drug therapy before thyroid surgery, it can still occur.

Symptoms of thyroid storm are caused by excessive thyroid hormone release, which dramatically increases metabolic rate. *Key symptoms include fever, tachycardia, and systolic hypertension.* The patient may have abdominal pain, nausea, vomiting, and diarrhea. Often he or she is very anxious and has tremors. As the crisis progresses, the patient may become restless, confused, or psychotic and may have seizures, leading to coma. *Even with treatment, thyroid storm may lead to death.*

! NURSING SAFETY PRIORITY (QSEN)
Critical Rescue

> When caring for a patient with hyperthyroidism, even after a thyroidectomy, assess temperature often because an increase of even 1°F (1.8°C) may indicate an impending thyroid crisis. If a temperature increase occurs, respond by reporting it immediately to the primary health care provider.

Emergency measures to prevent death vary with the intensity and type of changes. Interventions focus on maintaining airway patency, promoting adequate ventilation and *gas exchange*, reducing fever, and stabilizing the hemodynamic status. The Best Practice for Patient Safety & Quality Care box outlines interventions for emergency management of thyroid storm.

Eye and vision problems of Graves disease are not corrected by treatment for hyperthyroidism, and management is symptomatic. Teach the patient with mild problems to elevate the head of the bed at night and use artificial tears. If *photophobia* (sensitivity to light) is present, dark glasses may be helpful. For those who cannot close the eyelids completely, recommend gently taping the lids closed at bedtime to prevent irritation and injury.

If pressure behind the eye continues and forces the eye forward, blood supply to the eye can be compromised, leading to ischemia and blindness. In severe cases, short-term glucocorticoid therapy is prescribed to reduce swelling and halt the

BEST PRACTICE FOR PATIENT SAFETY & QUALITY CARE (QSEN)
Emergency Care of the Patient During Thyroid Storm

- Maintain a patent airway and adequate ventilation.
- Give oral antithyroid drugs as prescribed: methimazole or propylthiouracil.
- Administer sodium iodide solution IV daily as prescribed.
- Give propranolol IV as prescribed, slowly over 3 minutes. The patient should be connected to a cardiac monitor, and a central venous pressure catheter should be in place.
- Give glucocorticoids as prescribed: hydrocortisone, prednisone, or dexamethasone.
- Monitor continually for cardiac dysrhythmias.
- Monitor vital signs every 30 minutes.
- Provide comfort measures, including a cooling blanket.
- Give nonsalicylate antipyretics as prescribed.
- Correct dehydration with normal saline infusions.
- Apply cooling blanket or ice packs to reduce fever.

infiltrative process. Prednisone is given in high doses at first and then is tapered down according to the patient's response. Other management strategies include external radiation combined with lower-dose glucocorticoid therapy. Surgical intervention (orbital decompression) may be needed if loss of sight or damage to the eyeball is possible. Rituximab injections have been successful on a limited basis for this problem (Davies et al., 2016).

Health teaching includes reviewing with the patient and family the symptoms of hyperthyroidism and instructing the patient to report any increase or recurrence of these. Also teach about the symptoms of hypothyroidism (discussed in the next section) and the need for thyroid hormone replacement. Reinforce the need for regular follow-up because hypothyroidism can occur several years after radioactive iodine therapy.

THYROIDITIS

Thyroiditis is an inflammation of the thyroid gland. There are three types: acute, subacute, and chronic. Chronic thyroiditis (Hashimoto disease) is the most common type.

Acute thyroiditis is caused by bacterial invasion of the thyroid gland. Symptoms include pain, neck tenderness, malaise, fever, and *dysphagia* (difficulty swallowing). It usually resolves with antibiotic therapy.

Subacute or granulomatous thyroiditis results from a viral infection of the thyroid gland after a cold or other upper respiratory infection. Symptoms include fever, chills, dysphagia, and muscle and joint pain. Pain can radiate to the ears and the jaw. The thyroid gland feels hard and enlarged on palpation. Thyroid function can remain normal, although hyperthyroidism or hypothyroidism may develop.

Chronic thyroiditis (Hashimoto thyroiditis [HT]) is a common type of hypothyroidism that affects women more often than men. HT is an autoimmune disorder that is usually triggered by a bacterial or viral infection. The thyroid is invaded by antithyroid antibodies and lymphocytes, causing selective thyroid tissue destruction. When large amounts of the gland are destroyed, hypothyroidism results.

Symptoms of Hashimoto thyroiditis include dysphagia and painless enlargement of the gland. Diagnosis is based on circulating antithyroid antibodies and needle biopsy of the thyroid gland. Serum thyroid hormone levels and TSH levels vary with disease stage and type.

THYROID CANCER

Pathophysiology Review

The four distinct types of thyroid cancer are papillary, follicular, medullary, and anaplastic (American Cancer Society, 2020; Canadian Cancer Society, 2019). The initial sign of thyroid cancer is a single, painless lump or nodule in the thyroid gland. Additional signs and symptoms depend on the presence and location of *metastasis* (spread of cancer cells).

Papillary carcinoma, the most common type of thyroid cancer, occurs most often in younger women. It is a slow-growing tumor that can be present for years before spreading to nearby lymph nodes. When the tumor is confined to the thyroid gland, the chance for cure is good with a partial or total thyroidectomy.

Follicular carcinoma occurs most often in older adults. It invades blood vessels and spreads to bone and lung tissue.

When it adheres to the trachea, neck muscles, great vessels, and skin, *dyspnea* (difficulty breathing) and *dysphagia* (difficulty swallowing) result. When the tumor involves the recurrent laryngeal nerves, the patient may have a hoarse voice.

Medullary carcinoma is most common in patients older than 50 years. It often occurs with multiple endocrine neoplasia (MEN) type 2, a familial endocrine disorder (OMIM, 2014). The tumor usually secretes a variety of hormones.

Anaplastic carcinoma is a rapidly growing, aggressive tumor that invades nearby tissues. Symptoms include stridor (harsh, high-pitched respiratory sounds), hoarseness, and dysphagia.

A hallmark of thyroid cancer is an elevated serum thyroglobulin (Tg) level. The normal Tg level is 0.5 to 53.0 ng/mL (mcg/L) for men and 0.5 to 43.0 ng/mL (mcg/L) for women.

❖ Interprofessional Collaborative Care

Radiation therapy is used most often for anaplastic carcinoma because this cancer has usually metastasized at diagnosis. The patient is treated with *ablative* (enough to destroy the tissue) amounts of RAI. (See the earlier Patient and Family Education: Preparing for Self-Management box for precautions to teach the patient receiving unsealed RAI therapy.) If spread has occurred to the neck or mediastinum, external radiation is also used. If thyroid cancer does not respond to RAI, chemotherapy is initiated.

Surgery is the treatment of choice for other types of thyroid cancer. A total thyroidectomy is usually performed with dissection of lymph nodes in the neck if regional lymph nodes are involved. (See the postoperative care discussion in the Surgical Management section for Hyperthyroidism.) Suppressive doses of thyroid hormone are usually taken for 3 months after surgery. Thyroglobulin levels are monitored after surgery. A rising level indicates probable presence of cancer cells.

The patient is hypothyroid after treatment for thyroid cancer. Nursing interventions then focus on teaching him or her about the management of hypothyroidism. (See the discussion of patient-centered collaborative care in the Cellular Regulation Concept Exemplar: Hypothyroidism section.)

HYPOPARATHYROIDISM

Pathophysiology Review

The parathyroid glands maintain calcium and phosphate balance (see Fig. 56.6 in Chapter 56). Serum calcium level is normally maintained within a narrow range. Parathyroid secretion of parathyroid hormone (PTH) act directly on the kidney, causing increased kidney reabsorption of calcium and increased phosphorus excretion.

Hypoparathyroidism is a rare disorder in which parathyroid function is decreased and serum calcium levels cannot be maintained, and *hypocalcemia* (low serum calcium levels) results. Problems are directly related to a lack of parathyroid hormone (PTH) secretion or to decreased effectiveness of PTH on target tissue.

Iatrogenic hypoparathyroidism, the most common form, is caused by the removal of all parathyroid tissue during total thyroidectomy or surgical removal of the parathyroid glands.

Idiopathic hypoparathyroidism can occur spontaneously. The exact cause is unknown, but an autoimmune basis is suspected, and it may occur with other autoimmune disorders.

Hypomagnesemia (decreased serum magnesium levels) may cause hypoparathyroidism. Low magnesium levels are seen in patients with malabsorption syndromes, chronic kidney disease (CKD), and malnutrition. Low magnesium levels suppress PTH secretion and may interfere with the effects of PTH on the bones, kidneys, and calcium regulation.

❖ Interprofessional Collaborative Care

◆ **Assessment: Recognize Cues.** Ask about any head or neck surgery or radiation therapy because these treatments may injure the parathyroid glands and cause hypoparathyroidism. Also ask whether the neck has ever sustained a serious injury in a car crash or by strangulation. Assess whether the patient has any symptoms of hypoparathyroidism, which may range from mild tingling and numbness to muscle tetany. Tingling and numbness around the mouth or in the hands and feet reflect mild-to-moderate hypocalcemia. Severe muscle cramps, spasms of the hands and feet, and seizures (with no loss of consciousness or incontinence) reflect a more severe hypocalcemia. The patient or family may notice mental changes ranging from irritability to psychosis.

The physical assessment may show excessive or inappropriate muscle contractions that cause finger, hand, and elbow flexion. This can signal an impending attack of tetany. Check for Chvostek and Trousseau signs; positive responses indicate potential tetany (see Figs. 13.13 and 13.14 in Chapter 13). Bands or pits may encircle the teeth, which indicates a loss of tooth calcium and enamel.

Diagnostic tests for hypoparathyroidism include electroencephalography (EEG), blood tests, and CT scans. EEG changes revert to normal with correction of hypocalcemia. Serum calcium, phosphorus, magnesium, vitamin D, and urine cyclic adenosine monophosphate (cAMP) levels may be used in the diagnostic workup for hypoparathyroidism (see the Laboratory Profile: Parathyroid Function box). The CT scan can show brain calcifications, which indicate chronic hypocalcemia.

◆ **Interventions: Take Action.** Nonsurgical management of hypoparathyroidism focuses on correcting hypocalcemia, vitamin D deficiency, and hypomagnesemia. For patients with acute and severe hypocalcemia, IV calcium is given as a 10% solution of calcium chloride or calcium gluconate over 10 to 15 minutes. Acute vitamin D deficiency is treated with daily oral calcitriol. Acute hypomagnesemia is corrected with IV magnesium sulfate. Long-term oral therapy for hypocalcemia involves the intake of calcium, 0.5 to 2 g daily, in divided doses.

Long-term therapy for vitamin D deficiency is replacement with oral ergocalciferol daily. The dosage is adjusted to keep the patient's calcium level in the low-normal range (slightly hypocalcemic), enough to prevent symptoms of hypocalcemia. It must also be low enough to prevent increased urine calcium levels, which can lead to stone formation.

Nursing management includes teaching about the drug regimen and interventions to reduce anxiety. Teach the patient to eat foods high in calcium but low in phosphorus. Milk, yogurt, and processed cheeses are avoided because of their high phosphorus

LABORATORY PROFILE

Parathyroid Function

Test	Normal Range	Hypoparathyroidism	Hyperparathyroidism
Serum calcium	Total: 9.0-10.5 mg/dL (2.25-2.62 mmol/L) Ionized (active): 4.5-5.6 mg/dL (1.05-1.30 mmol/L)	Decreased	Increased in primary hyperparathyroidism
Serum phosphorus	3.0-4.5 mg/dL (0.97-1.45 mmol/L)	Increased	Decreased
Serum magnesium	1.3-2.1 mEq/L (0.65-1.07 mmol/L)	Decreased	Increased
Serum parathyroid hormone	C-terminal: 50-330 pg/mL (ng/L) N-terminal: 8-24 pg/mL (ng/L) Whole: 10-65 pg/mL (ng/L)	Decreased	Increased
Vitamin D (calciferol)	25-80 ng/mL (75-200 nmol/L)	Decreased	Variable

Pagana, K., & Pagana, T. (2018). *Mosby's manual of diagnostic and laboratory tests* (8th ed.). St. Louis: Elsevier.

content. *Stress that therapy for hypocalcemia is lifelong.* Advise the patient to wear a medical alert bracelet. With adherence to the prescribed drug and diet regimen, the calcium level usually remains high enough to prevent a hypocalcemic crisis.

HYPERPARATHYROIDISM

Pathophysiology Review

Hyperparathyroidism is a disorder in which parathyroid secretion of parathyroid hormone is increased, resulting in *hypercalcemia* (excessive serum calcium levels) and *hypophosphatemia* (inadequate serum phosphorus levels). In bone, excessive PTH levels increase bone *resorption* (bone loss of calcium) by decreasing *osteoblastic* (bone production) activity and increasing *osteoclastic* (bone destruction) activity. This process releases calcium and phosphorus into the blood and reduces bone density. With chronic calcium excess and hypercalcemia, calcium is deposited in soft tissues.

Although the exact trigger is unknown, primary hyperparathyroidism results when one or more parathyroid glands do not respond to the normal feedback of serum calcium levels. Common causes of secondary hyperparathyroidism include a benign tumor in one parathyroid gland and chronic kidney disease (CKD) (Gasu & Lim, 2017). Table 58.3 lists other causes.

❖ Interprofessional Collaborative Care

◆ **Assessment: Recognize Cues.** Symptoms of hyperparathyroidism may be related either to the effects of excessive PTH or to the effects of the accompanying hypercalcemia.

Ask about any bone fractures, recent weight loss, arthritis, or psychological stress. Ask whether the patient has received radiation treatment to the head or neck. The patient with chronic disease may have a waxy pallor of the skin, and bone deformities in the extremities and back.

High levels of PTH cause kidney stones and deposits of calcium in the soft tissue of the kidney. Bone lesions are caused by an increased rate of bone destruction and may result in fractures, bone cysts, and osteoporosis.

GI problems (e.g., anorexia, nausea, vomiting, epigastric pain, constipation, weight loss) are common when serum

TABLE 58.3 Causes of Parathyroid Dysfunction

Causes of Hyperparathyroidism	Causes of Hypoparathyroidism
• Parathyroid tumor or cancer • Congenital hyperplasia • Neck trauma or radiation • Vitamin D deficiency • Chronic kidney disease with hypocalcemia • Parathyroid hormone–secreting carcinomas of the lung, kidney, or GI tract	• Surgical or radiation-induced thyroid ablation • Parathyroidectomy • Congenital dysgenesis • Idiopathic (autoimmune) hypoparathyroidism • Hypomagnesemia

calcium levels are high. Elevated serum gastrin levels are caused by hypercalcemia and lead to peptic ulcer disease. Fatigue and lethargy may be present and worsen as the serum calcium levels increase. When serum calcium levels are greater than 12 mg/dL (3.0 mmol/L), the patient may have psychosis with confusion, followed by coma and death if left untreated. (See Chapter 13 for more information about hypercalcemia.)

As listed in the Laboratory Profile: Parathyroid Function box, serum PTH, calcium, and phosphorus levels and urine cyclic adenosine monophosphate (cAMP) levels are the laboratory tests used to detect hyperparathyroidism. X-rays may show kidney stones, calcium deposits, and bone lesions. Loss of bone density occurs in the patient with chronic hyperparathyroidism. Other diagnostic tests include arteriography, CT scans, venous sampling of the thyroid for blood PTH levels, and ultrasonography. Explain the procedures and care for the patient undergoing diagnostic tests.

◆ **Interventions: Take Action.** Surgical management is the treatment of choice for patients with hyperparathyroidism. For those who are not candidates for surgery, drug therapy can help control the problems. Priority nursing interventions focus on monitoring and preventing injury.

Nonsurgical Management. *Diuretic and hydration therapies* help reduce serum calcium levels in patients who have milder disease. Usually furosemide, a diuretic that increases kidney excretion of calcium, is used along with IV saline in large volumes to promote calcium excretion.

Drug therapy for patients who have more severe symptoms of hyperparathyroidism or who have hypercalcemia related to parathyroid cancer involves the use of cinacalcet, a calcimimetic. When taken orally, the drug binds to calcium-sensitive receptors on parathyroid tissue, reducing PTH production and release. The result is decreased serum calcium levels, stabilization of other minerals, and decreased progression of PTH-induced bone complications. Another drug approved for CKD-associated hyperparathyroidism in patients undergoing dialysis is etelcalcetide. It is a synthetic calcium-sensing receptor agonist given IV three times weekly at the end of a dialysis session (Hussar, 2018). Both cinacalcet and etelcalcetide require serum calcium monitoring for hypocalcemia on a regular basis for the duration of therapy.

For patients who do not respond to cinacalcet, oral phosphates are used to inhibit bone resorption and interfere with calcium absorption. IV phosphates are used only when serum calcium levels must be lowered rapidly. Calcitonin decreases the release of skeletal calcium and increases kidney excretion of calcium. It is not effective when used alone because of its short duration of action. Therapeutic effects are enhanced if calcitonin is given with glucocorticoids.

Monitor cardiac function and intake and output every 2 hours during hydration therapy. Continuous cardiac monitoring may be necessary. Compare recent ECG tracings with the patient's baseline tracings. Especially look for changes in the T waves and the QT interval, as well as changes in the rate and rhythm. Monitor serum calcium levels, and immediately report any sudden drop to the primary health care provider. Sudden drops in calcium levels may cause tingling and numbness in the muscles.

Preventing injury is important because the patient with chronic hyperparathyroidism often has significant bone density loss and is at risk for fragile fractures. Teach assistive personnel (AP) to handle the patient carefully and to use a lift sheet to reposition the patient rather than pulling him or her.

Surgical Management. Surgical management of hyperparathyroidism is a parathyroidectomy. Before surgery the patient is stabilized, and calcium levels are decreased to near normal.

The operative procedure can be performed as minimally invasive surgery or mini-incision surgery or with a traditional transverse incision in the lower neck. All four parathyroid glands are examined for enlargement. If a tumor is present on one side but the other side is normal, the surgeon removes the glands containing tumor and leaves the remaining glands on the opposite side intact. If all four glands are diseased, they are all removed.

Nursing care before and after surgical removal of the parathyroid glands is the same as that for thyroidectomy. See the Preoperative Care and Postoperative Care sections under Hyperthyroidism for specific nursing interventions.

NCLEX EXAMINATION CHALLENGE 58.3
Health Promotion and Maintenance

A client at continuing risk for hyperparathyroidism is prescribed to take furosemide 40 mg and to drink at least 3 to 4 L of fluid daily. He tells the nurse he believes taking a "water pill" and then drinking so much seems wrong. How will the nurse respond?

A. "This combination of a water pill and drinking more protects you from buildup of excess sodium in the kidney."

B. "The furosemide makes you lose water and you need to increase your intake to keep from becoming dehydrated."

C. "The drug helps you to get rid of calcium and drinking more helps dilute your blood calcium so the level doesn't get too high."

D. "You are correct. I will check with your primary health care provider to determine whether you should restrict your fluid intake."

The remaining glands, which may have atrophied as a result of PTH overproduction, require several days to several weeks to return to normal function. A hypocalcemic crisis can occur during this critical period, and the serum calcium level is assessed frequently after surgery. Check serum calcium levels whenever they are drawn until calcium levels stabilize. Monitor for indications of hypocalcemia, such as tingling and twitching in the extremities and face. Check for Trousseau and Chvostek signs, either of which indicates potential tetany (see Figs. 13.13 and 13.14 in Chapter 13).

The recurrent laryngeal nerve can be damaged during surgery. Assess the patient for changes in voice patterns and hoarseness.

When hyperparathyroidism is caused by *hyperplasia* (tissue overgrowth), three glands plus half of the fourth gland are usually removed. If all four glands are removed, a small portion of a gland may be implanted in the forearm, where it produces PTH and maintains calcium homeostasis. If all these maneuvers fail, the patient will need lifelong treatment with calcium and vitamin D because the resulting hypoparathyroidism is permanent.

GET READY FOR THE NEXT-GENERATION NCLEX® EXAMINATION!

Key Points
Review these Key Points for each NCLEX Examination Client Needs Category.

Safe and Effective Care Environment
- Keep the environment of a patient at risk for thyroid storm cool, dark, and quiet. **QSEN: Safety**
- Keep emergency suctioning and tracheotomy equipment in the room of a patient who has had thyroid or parathyroid surgery. **QSEN: Safety**
- Use a lift sheet to move or reposition a patient with hypocalcemia. **QSEN: Safety**

Health Promotion and Maintenance
- Teach all patients to take antithyroid drugs or thyroid hormone replacement therapy as prescribed. **QSEN: Patient-Centered Care**
- Teach patients to use signs and symptoms (e.g., the number of bowel movements per day, the ability to sleep) as indicators of therapy effectiveness and when the dose of thyroid hormone replacement may need to be adjusted. **QSEN: Patient-Centered Care**

Psychosocial Integrity

- Remind patients and family members that changes in cognition and behavior related to thyroid problems are usually temporary. **QSEN: Patient-Centered Care**
- Encourage the patient who has a permanent change in appearance (e.g., exophthalmia) to mourn the change. **QSEN: Patient-Centered Care**

Physiological Integrity

- Be aware that:
  - The presence of a goiter indicates a problem with the thyroid gland but can accompany either hyperthyroidism or hypothyroidism.
  - Although similar in action, methimazole and propylthiouracil are not interchangeable.
  - Methimazole can cause birth defects and should not be used during pregnancy, especially during the first trimester. Instruct women to notify their primary health care provider if pregnancy occurs.

- When stridor, dyspnea, or other symptoms of obstruction appear after thyroid surgery, notify the Rapid Response Team. **QSEN: Safety**
- When caring for a patient with hyperthyroidism, even after a thyroidectomy, immediately report a temperature increase of even 1°F because it may indicate an impending thyroid crisis. **QSEN: Evidence-Based Practice**
- Assess the cardiopulmonary status of any patient with hypothyroidism for decreased perfusion or decreased *gas exchange* at least every 8 hours. **QSEN: Patient-Centered Care**
- Use sedating drugs or opioids sparingly with patients who have hypothyroidism. **QSEN: Patient-Centered Care**
- Monitor the hydration status of patients who have hypercalcemia. **QSEN: Patient-Centered Care**
- Assess the patient with hypoparathyroidism for manifestations of hypocalcemia, especially numbness or tingling around the mouth and a positive Chvostek sign or Trousseau sign (see Figs. 13.13 and 13.14 in Chapter 13). **QSEN: Patient-Centered Care**

▌ MASTERY QUESTIONS

1. Performance of which assessment is a **priority** for the nurse before giving a client the first oral dose of hormone replacement for hypothyroidism?
   A. Measuring heart rate and rhythm
   B. Checking core body temperature
   C. Asking about previous allergic drug reactions
   D. Listening to bowel sounds in all four abdominal quadrants

2. Which assessment findings in a client with hyperthyroidism indicate to the nurse that the client is in danger of thyroid storm? **Select all that apply.**
   A. Increased salivation
   B. Client report of increased palmar sweating
   C. Decreased pulse pressure from 40 mm Hg to 36 mm Hg
   D. Diminished bowel sounds in all four abdominal quadrants

   E. An increase in temperature from 99.5°F (37.5°C) to 101.3°F (38.5°C)
   F. Serum sodium level increase from 136 mEq/L (mmol/L) to 139 mEq/L (mmol/L)
   G. Increase in premature ventricular heart contractions from 4 per minute to 28 per minute

3. The nurse reviewing the laboratory values of a client with hypoparathyroidism finds a serum calcium level of 7.9 mg/dL (1.76 mmol/L). Which parameter is most important for the nurse to assess to **prevent harm**?
   A. Temperature
   B. Heart rate and rhythm
   C. Deep tendon reflexes
   D. Level of consciousness

REFERENCES

Asterisk (*) indicates a classic or definitive work on this subject.

American Cancer Society (ACS). (2020). *Cancer facts and figures-2020*. Report No. 00-300M-No. 500820. Atlanta: Author.

Brent, G., & Weetman, A. (2016). Hypothyroidism and thyroiditis. In S. Melmed, K. Polonsky, P. R. Larsen, & H. Kronenberg (Eds.), *Williams' textbook of endocrinology* (13th ed.). Philadelphia: Saunders.

Burchum, J., & Rosenthal, L. (2019). *Lehne's pharmacology for nursing care* (10th ed.). St. Louis: Elsevier.

Canadian Cancer Society, Statistics Canada. (2019). *Canadian cancer Statistics, 2019*. Toronto, ON: Canadian Cancer Society. https://www.cancer.ca/~/media/cancer.ca/CW/cancer%20information/cancer%20101/Canadian%20cancer%20statistics/Canadian-Cancer-Statistics-2019-EN.pdf?la=en.

Davies, T., Laurberg, P., & Bahn, R. (2016). Thyrotoxicosis. In S. Melmed, K. Polonsky, P. R. Larsen, & H. Kronenberg (Eds.), *Williams' textbook of endocrinology* (13th ed.). Philadelphia: Saunders.

Felicilda-Reynaldo, R., & Kenneally, M. (2016). Antithyroid drugs for hyperthyroidism. *MEDSURG Nursing, 25*(1), 50–54.

Gasu, V., & Lim, F. (2017). Secondary hyperparathyroidism in chronic kidney disease. *American Nurse Today, 12*(7), 20–23.

Hooley, J., & Reagan, S. (2016). Hyperthyroidism: A storm brewing. *American Nurse Today, 11*(10). https://www.americannursetoday.com/hyperthyroidism-a-storm-brewing/.

Hussar, D. (2018). New drugs, part 3: Drugs for hyperparathyroidism. *Nursing, 48*(10), 32–42.

McCance, K., Huether, S., Brashers, V., & Rote, N. (2019). *Pathophysiology: The biologic basis for disease in adults and children* (8th ed.). St. Louis: Elsevier.

Moore, D. (2018). Hypothyroidism and nursing care. *American Nurse Today, 13*(2), 44–46.

*Online Mendelian Inheritance in Man (OMIM). (2014). *Multiple endocrine neoplasia, Type II A; MEN2A* www.omim.org/entry/171400.

Online Mendelian Inheritance in Man (OMIM). (2016). *Graves disease, susceptibility to, 1*. www.omim.org/entry/275000.

Pagana, K., & Pagana, T. (2018). *Mosby's manual of diagnostic and laboratory tests* (6th ed.). St. Louis: Elsevier.

Schreiber, M. (2017). Thyroid storm. *MEDSURG Nursing, 26*(2), 143–145.

Touhy, T., & Jett, K. (2020). *Ebersole and Hess' toward nursing healthy aging* (10th ed.). St. Louis: Mosby.

59

Concepts of Care for Patients With Diabetes Mellitus

Sharon A. Watts

http://evolve.elsevier.com/Iggy/

LEARNING OUTCOMES

1. Collaborate with the interprofessional team to coordinate high-quality care and promote *glucose regulation* in patients who have diabetes mellitus (DM).
2. Teach the patient and caregiver(s) about how impaired *glucose regulation* from DM and its complications affect home safety.
3. Prioritize evidence-based care for patients with common complications of DM affecting *glucose regulation*.
4. Teach the patient and caregiver(s) about common drugs and other therapies used to manage DM and its complications.
5. Teach patients with DM about self-care management when in the community.
6. Teach adults at risk for impaired *glucose regulation* how to prevent or delay development of type 2 DM.
7. Implement patient and family-centered nursing interventions to help adults cope with the psychosocial impact caused by DM and its complications.
8. Use clinical judgment to analyze relevant assessment data when planning care for patients who have impaired *glucose regulation* and DM.
9. Implement evidence-based nursing actions to improve *glucose regulation* and prevent complications of DM.

KEY TERMS

diabetes mellitus A common, complex, chronic disorder of impaired nutrient metabolism, especially glucose, that can affect the function of every body system.

diabetic ketoacidosis (DKA) A severe acute complication of diabetes; characterized by uncontrolled hyperglycemia, metabolic acidosis, and increased production of ketones.

diabetic peripheral neuropathy Progressive deterioration of nerve function with the loss of *sensory perception*.

gastroparesis A delay in gastric emptying.

glucagon A hormone important in glucose regulation that has balancing actions opposite those of insulin and prevents hypoglycemia.

gluconeogenesis Conversion of protein substances into glucose.

glucose regulation Process of maintaining optimal blood glucose levels; also known as *glycemic control*.

glycogenesis Production and storage of glycogen.

glycogenolysis Breakdown of stored glycogen into glucose.

glycosylated hemoglobin (A1C) A standardized test that measures how much glucose permanently attaches to the hemoglobin molecule; is often used to indicate the effectiveness of blood glucose control measures.

hyperglycemia Higher-than-normal blood glucose level.

hyperglycemic-hyperosmolar state (HHS) A severe acute hyperosmolar (increased blood osmolarity) state caused by hyperglycemia.

hypoglycemia Lower-than-normal blood glucose level.

hyperinsulinemia Chronically high blood insulin levels.

ketogenesis Conversion of fats to acid products.

ketone bodies ("ketones") Abnormal acidic breakdown products that collect in the blood when insulin is not available, leading to the *acid-base balance* problem of metabolic acidosis.

Kussmaul respiration A deep and rapid respiratory pattern triggered by acidosis to reduce blood hydrogen ion concentration by "blowing off" carbon dioxide.

lipolysis Breakdown of body fats.

metabolic syndrome Simultaneous presence of metabolic factors that increase risk for developing type 2 DM and cardiovascular disease.

proliferative diabetic retinopathy Growth of new fragile retinal blood vessels (neovascularization) that bleed easily and obscure vision.

proteolysis Breakdown of body proteins.

PRIORITY AND INTERRELATED CONCEPTS

The priority concept for this chapter is:
- *Glucose Regulation*

The *Glucose Regulation* concept exemplar for this chapter is Diabetes Mellitus.

The interrelated concepts for this chapter are:
- *Nutrition*
- *Tissue Integrity*
- *Sensory Perception*
- *Perfusion*
- *Immunity*
- *Fluid and Electrolyte Balance*
- *Acid-Base Balance*

GLUCOSE REGULATION CONCEPT EXEMPLAR: DIABETES MELLITUS

Diabetes mellitus (DM) is a common, chronic, complex disorder of impaired nutrient metabolism, especially glucose, that can affect the function of every body system. Although all nutrients are affected, glucose regulation is impaired first, which then changes protein and fat metabolism. *Glucose regulation* is the process of maintaining optimal blood glucose levels, also known as *glycemic control* (Fig. 59.1). With impaired glucose regulation, many acute and chronic health problems occur as life-shortening complications. In the United States and Canada the percentage of hospitalized patients who have DM is over 40%, which is much greater than the percentage of people with DM in the general population, allowing the disorder to have a large impact on health care costs and resources (Schneider et al., 2016; Watts et al., 2018). Thus a major focus of management is to identify the presence of DM to help the adult manage the disorder and maintain glycemic control for prevention of complications.

Nurses play a critical role in helping patients and families understand the disorder and actively participate in its management. As part of the team you will help plan, organize, and coordinate care with other team members to promote the patient's health and well-being. These management activities may take place in almost any setting. The desired outcome is to help patients maintain blood glucose levels in the normal range *(euglycemia)* without causing either hyperglycemia (higher than normal blood glucose level) or hypoglycemia (lower than normal blood glucose level).

Pathophysiology Review

Classification of Diabetes.
Diabetes mellitus (DM) has many subtypes, and all have the main feature of chronic hyperglycemia resulting from impaired processes in *glucose regulation* that include reduced insulin secretion or reduced insulin action or both. The disease is classified by the underlying problem causing a lack of insulin or its action and the severity of the insulin deficiency. Table 59.1 outlines the types of DM. This chapter focuses on the two most common types of DM. Regardless of the specific type of DM, the organ-damaging consequences and complications of impaired glucose regulation are the same.

The Endocrine Pancreas. The pancreas regulates digestion through its exocrine functions and ensures *glucose regulation* through its endocrine functions. The endocrine pancreas has about 1 million small glands, the islets of Langerhans, scattered through the organ. Inside the islets are two types of cells important to glucose regulation. These are the *alpha* cells, which secrete glucagon, and the *beta* cells, which produce insulin and amylin (Fig. 59.2).

Glucagon is a hormone that has balancing actions opposite those of insulin. It prevents *hypoglycemia* by triggering the release of glucose from storage sites in the liver and skeletal muscle. It is sometimes called the "hormone of starvation" because it is secreted when food intake is low to release glucose from the liver to keep blood glucose levels in the normal range.

Insulin prevents *hyperglycemia* by allowing body cells to take up, use, and store carbohydrate, fat, and protein. It is sometimes called the "hormone of plenty" because it is secreted when food intake is high and works to move glucose from the blood into cells to keep blood glucose levels in the normal range. Active insulin is a protein made up of 51 amino acids. It is first produced as inactive *proinsulin,* a prohormone that is converted in the liver to active insulin. Movement of glucose into most cells requires the presence of specific membrane receptors along with insulin. Insulin is like a "key" that opens "locked" membranes to glucose, allowing blood glucose to move into cells to generate energy. Insulin starts this action by binding to membrane insulin receptors, which changes membrane permeability to glucose (Fig. 59.3).

Insulin is secreted daily in a two-step manner, with low-level secretion during fasting (basal insulin secretion) and in a two-phase release after eating *(prandial).* An early burst of insulin secretion occurs within 10 minutes of eating, followed by an increasing release that lasts until the blood glucose level returns to normal.

Glucose Regulation and Homeostasis. Although glucose is a critical nutrient, chronically high blood glucose levels cause many serious problems, and low blood glucose levels can rapidly lead to injury or death. Thus *glucose regulation* that maintains blood glucose levels within a relatively normal range is important (see Fig. 59.1). Several organs and hormones play a role in maintaining glucose regulation. During fasting, when the stomach is empty, blood glucose is maintained between 60 and 150 mg/dL (3.3 and 8.3 mmol/L) by a balance between glucose uptake by cells and glucose production by the liver. Insulin plays a pivotal role in this process.

Glucose is the main fuel for central nervous system (CNS) cells. Because the brain cannot produce or store much glucose, it needs a continuous supply from the blood to prevent neuron dysfunction and cell death. (Other organs can use both glucose and fatty acids to generate energy.) Glucose is stored as glycogen in the liver and skeletal muscles, and free fatty acids (FFAs) are stored as triglyceride in fat cells. During a prolonged fast or after illness, proteins are broken down, and some of the amino acids are converted into glucose.

Insulin exerts many effects on metabolism and cellular processes in all tissues and organs. The main metabolic effects of

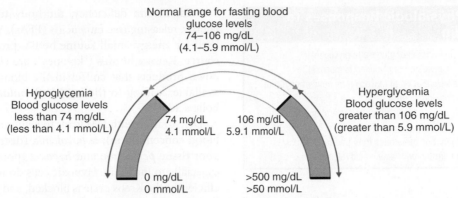

Normal range for fasting blood
glucose levels
74–106 mg/dL
(4.1–5.9 mmol/L)

Hypoglycemia
Blood glucose levels
less than 74 mg/dL
(less than 4.1 mmol/L)

74 mg/dL
4.1 mmol/L

106 mg/dL
5.9.1 mmol/L

Hyperglycemia
Blood glucose levels
greater than 106 mg/dL
(greater than 5.9 mmol/L)

0 mg/dL
0 mmol/L

>500 mg/dL
>50 mmol/L

FIG. 59.1 Fasting blood glucose levels. When *glucose regulation* is adequate, fasting levels remain in the normal range. With insufficient insulin usage, hyperglycemia results. Excess insulin or insufficient glucose results in hypoglycemia.

TABLE 59.1 Classification of Diabetes Mellitus

Type 1 Diabetes (T1DM)
- Beta cell destruction leading to absolute insulin deficiency
- Autoimmune
- Idiopathic

Type 2 Diabetes (T2DM)
Ranges from insulin resistance with relative insulin deficiency to secretory deficit with insulin resistance

Maturity-Onset Diabetes of the Young (MODY)
- Inherited mutation in one of at least six known genes that results in loss of insulin function and hyperglycemia
- Usually diagnosed in younger adults but can be found at any time in adulthood
- Resembles type 1 DM with insulin requirements and potential for diabetic ketoacidosis (DKA)
- Is **not** an autoimmune problem

Gestational Diabetes Mellitus (GDM)
- Glucose intolerance with onset in or first recognition during pregnancy (All pregnant women should be screened.)

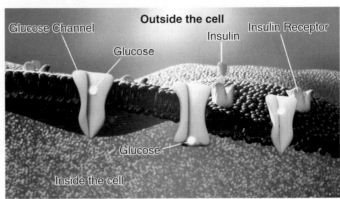

FIG. 59.3 Insulin attaches to receptors on target cells, where it promotes glucose transport into the cells through the cell membranes. (© Elsevier Animation Collection.)

insulin are to stimulate glucose uptake in skeletal muscle and heart muscle and to suppress liver production of glucose and very-low-density lipoprotein (VLDL). In the liver, insulin promotes the production and storage of glycogen (**glycogenesis**) at the same time that it inhibits glycogen breakdown into glucose (**glycogenolysis**). It increases protein and lipid (fat) synthesis and inhibits **ketogenesis** (conversion of fats to acids) and **gluconeogenesis** (conversion of proteins to glucose). In muscle, insulin promotes protein and glycogen synthesis. In fat cells, it promotes triglyceride storage. Overall, insulin keeps blood glucose levels from becoming too high and helps keep blood lipid levels in the normal range.

In the *fasting state* (not eating for 8 hours), insulin secretion is suppressed, which leads to increased gluconeogenesis in the liver and kidneys, along with increased glucose generation by the breakdown of liver glycogen. In the fed state, insulin released from pancreatic beta cells reverses this process. Instead, glycogen breakdown and gluconeogenesis are inhibited. At the same time, insulin also enhances glucose uptake and use by cells and reduces both body fat breakdown (**lipolysis**) and body protein breakdown (**proteolysis**). When more glucose is present in liver cells than can be used for energy or stored as glycogen, insulin causes the excess glucose to be converted to free fatty acids (FFAs). These extra FFAs are deposited in fat cells.

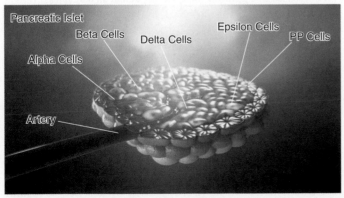

FIG. 59.2 Hormone secreting cells of the islets of Langerhans in the pancreas. Alpha cells secrete glucagon; beta cells secrete insulin. (© Elsevier Animation Collection.)

TABLE 59.2 Physiologic Responses to Insufficient Insulin

- Decreased glycogenesis (conversion of glucose to glycogen)
- Increased glycogenolysis (conversion of glycogen to glucose)
- Increased gluconeogenesis (formation of glucose from noncarbohydrate sources such as amino acids and lactate)
- Increased lipolysis (breakdown of triglycerides to glycerol and free fatty acids)
- Increased ketogenesis (formation of ketones from free fatty acids)
- Proteolysis (breakdown of protein with amino acid release in muscles)

Glucose in the blood after a meal is controlled by the emptying rate of the stomach and delivery of nutrients to the small intestine, where they are absorbed into circulation. *Incretin hormones* (e.g., *glucagon-like peptide 1 [GLP-1]*), secreted in response to food in the stomach, have several actions. They increase insulin secretion, inhibit glucagon secretion, and slow the rate of gastric emptying, thereby preventing hyperglycemia after meals.

Balancing *(counterregulatory)* hormones increase blood glucose by actions opposite those of insulin when more energy is needed. Glucagon is the main balancing hormone. Other hormones that increase blood glucose levels are epinephrine, norepinephrine, growth hormone, and cortisol. The combined actions of insulin and balancing hormones (discussed in the next section) participate in *glucose regulation* and keep blood glucose levels in the range of 60 to 100 mg/dL (3.3 to 5.6 mmol/L) to support brain function. When blood glucose levels fall, insulin secretion stops and glucagon is released. Glucagon causes glucose release from the liver. Liver glucose is made through breakdown of glycogen to glucose and conversion of amino acids into glucose. When liver glucose is unavailable, the breakdown of body fat and the breakdown of body proteins, especially muscle, provide acids as fuel for energy.

Absence of Insulin. *Glucose regulation* requires insulin to move glucose into many body tissues. The lack of insulin action in diabetes, from either a lack of production or a problem with insulin use at its cell receptors, prevents some cells from using glucose for energy. The body then breaks down fat and protein in an attempt to provide energy and increases levels of balancing hormones to make glucose from other sources. Table 59.2 outlines responses to insufficient insulin.

Without insulin, glucose builds up in the blood, causing hyperglycemia, which disturbs *fluid and electrolyte balance*, leading to the classic symptoms of diabetes: polyuria, polydipsia, and polyphagia.

Polyuria is frequent and excessive urination and results from an osmotic diuresis caused by excess glucose in the urine. With diuresis, electrolytes are excreted in the urine, and water loss is severe. Dehydration results, and *polydipsia* (excessive thirst) occurs. Because the cells receive no glucose, cell starvation triggers *polyphagia* (excessive eating). Despite eating, the adult with diabetes remains in metabolic starvation until insulin is available to move glucose into the cells.

With insulin deficiency, the body turns to stored fat for energy, releasing free fatty acids (FFAs). When this stored fat is used for energy, small ketone bodies provide a backup energy source. Ketone bodies ("ketones") are abnormal acidic breakdown products that collect in the blood when insulin is not available, leading to the *acid-base balance* problem of metabolic acidosis.

Dehydration with DM leads to *hemoconcentration* (increased blood concentration); *hypovolemia* (decreased blood volume); poor tissue *perfusion*; and *hypoxia* (poor tissue oxygenation), especially to the brain. Hypoxic cells do not metabolize glucose efficiently, the Krebs cycle is blocked, and lactic acid production increases, causing more acidosis.

The excess acids caused by absence of insulin increase hydrogen ion (H^+) and carbon dioxide (CO_2) levels in the blood, causing anion-gap metabolic acidosis. These products trigger the brain to increase the rate and depth of respiration in an attempt to "blow off" carbon dioxide and acid. This type of breathing is known as Kussmaul respiration. Acetone is exhaled, giving the breath a "rotting citrus fruit" odor. When the lungs can no longer offset acidosis, the blood pH drops. Arterial blood gas studies show a *metabolic acidosis* (decreased pH with decreased arterial bicarbonate [HCO_{3-}] levels) and *compensatory respiratory alkalosis* (decreased partial pressure of arterial carbon dioxide [$Paco_2$]).

Insulin lack first causes potassium depletion. With the increased fluid loss from hyperglycemia, excessive potassium is excreted in the urine, leading to low serum potassium levels. High serum potassium levels may occur in acidosis because of the shift of potassium from inside the cells to the blood in exchange for hydrogen ions. Serum potassium levels in DM, then, may be low *(hypokalemia),* high *(hyperkalemia),* or normal, depending on hydration, the severity of acidosis, and the patient's response to treatment. Chapter 14 discusses *acid-base balance* and acidosis in more detail.

NCLEX EXAMINATION CHALLENGE 59.1
Physiological Integrity

Which hormones help **prevent** hypoglycemia? **Select all that apply**.
A. Aldosterone
B. Cortisol
C. Epinephrine
D. Growth hormone
E. Glucagon
F. Insulin
G. Norepinephrine
H. Proinsulin

Acute Complications of Diabetes. Three glucose-related emergencies can occur in patients with DM:
- Diabetic ketoacidosis (DKA) caused by absence of insulin and generation of ketoacids
- Hyperglycemic-hyperosmolar state (HHS) caused by insulin deficiency and profound dehydration
- Hypoglycemia from too much insulin or too little glucose

All three problems require emergency treatment and can be fatal if treatment is delayed or incorrect. These problems and their management are described later in this chapter.

Chronic Complications of Diabetes. Changes in large blood vessels *(macrovascular)* and small blood vessels *(microvascular)* in tissues and organs result from DM and can lead to organ complications and early death. These blood vessel changes lead to complications from poor tissue **perfusion** and tissue ischemia. Macrovascular complications include coronary heart disease, cerebrovascular disease, and peripheral vascular disease, all of which lead to early morbidity and mortality. Microvascular complications of blood vessel structure and function lead to *nephropathy* (kidney dysfunction), *neuropathy* (nerve dysfunction), and *retinopathy* (vision problems). Such problems are responsible for increased morbidity and reduced quality of life. Causes of these diabetic vascular complications include:

- Chronic hyperglycemia thickens basement membranes, which causes organ damage.
- Glucose toxicity directly or indirectly affects functional cell integrity.
- Chronic ischemia in small blood vessels causes tissue hypoxia and microischemia.

Chronic high blood glucose levels are the main cause of microvascular complications and allow premature development of macrovascular complications. Additional risk factors contributing to poor health outcomes for adults with DM include smoking, physical inactivity, obesity, hypertension, and high blood fat and cholesterol levels.

Hyperglycemia from poor **glucose regulation** leads to long-term complications of DM. Intensive therapy to maintain glycemic control with blood glucose levels as close to normal as possible delays the onset and progression of retinopathy, nephropathy, neuropathy, and macrovascular disease for patients with DM. For every percentage point decrease in A1C (glycosylated hemoglobin), a significant reduction of kidney and eye complications occurs.

Macrovascular Complications

Cardiovascular Disease. Patients with diabetes, prediabetes, or metabolic syndrome are at increased risk for cardiovascular disease (CVD) (McCance et al., 2019; Rariden, 2019; Wisnewski, 2017). Because DM is so strongly associated with CVD, it is a target for aggressive CVD risk factor reduction.

Patients with DM, especially type 2 DM, often have the traditional CVD risk factors of obesity, high blood lipid levels, hypertension, and sedentary lifestyle. Cigarette smoking and a positive family history also increase risk for CVD. Kidney disease, indicated by *albuminuria* (presence of albumin in the urine), and retinopathy are associated with increased risk for coronary heart disease and mortality from coronary artery disease.

Cardiovascular complication rates can be reduced through aggressive management of hypertension, hyperglycemia, and hyperlipidemia. The American Diabetes Association (ADA) recommends that blood pressure be maintained below 140/90 mm Hg, with a target of 130/80 mm Hg in younger adults if that level can be achieved without excessive burden. Lipid profile screening is recommended starting at first diagnosis and every 1 to 2 years thereafter. Patients with DM who do not have overt CVD are recommended to maintain low-density lipoprotein (LDL) cholesterol below 100 mg/dL (2.60 mmol/L), and patients with indications of CVD are recommended to maintain LDL at less than 70 mg/dL (1.8 mmol/L) (ADA, 2019a). Lifestyle modifications that focus on reducing saturated fat, *trans* fat, and cholesterol intake; increasing intake of omega-3 fatty acids, fiber, and plant sterols; weight loss (if indicated); and increasing physical activity are recommended (ADA, 2019e).

Priority nursing activities focus on interventions to reduce modifiable risk factors associated with CVD. Modifiable risk factors include smoking cessation, diet, exercise, blood pressure control, and maintaining prescribed lipid-lowering drug therapy and aspirin use.

Cerebrovascular Disease. The risk for stroke is two to four times higher in adults with DM compared with those who do not have the disease (McCance et al., 2019). Diabetes also increases the likelihood of severe carotid atherosclerosis. Hypertension, hyperlipidemia, nephropathy, peripheral vascular disease, and alcohol and tobacco use further increase the risk for stroke in adults with DM.

Reduced Immunity. The combination of vascular changes and hyperglycemia reduces **immunity** by reducing white blood cell activity, inhibiting gas exchange in tissues, and promoting the growth of microorganisms. As a result, any adult who has DM is at an increased risk for developing an infection on exposure to bacteria and other organisms. In addition, infections become serious more quickly and can lead to major complications and sepsis (McCance et al., 2019).

Microvascular Complications

Eye and Vision Complications. Blindness is 25 times more common in patients with DM. Diabetic retinopathy (DR) is strongly related to the duration of diabetes. After 20 years of DM, nearly all patients with the disease have some degree of retinopathy (ADA, 2019g). Unfortunately, DR has few symptoms until vision loss occurs.

DR is related to problems that block retinal blood vessels and cause them to leak, leading to retinal hypoxia. Nonproliferative diabetic retinopathy causes structural problems in retinal vessels with areas of poor retinal circulation, edema, hard fatty deposits in the eye, and retinal hemorrhages. Fluid and blood leak from the vessels and cause retinal edema and hard exudates. Nonproliferative DR develops slowly and rarely reduces vision to the point of blindness.

Proliferative diabetic retinopathy is the growth of new retinal blood vessels, also known as *neovascularization*. When retinal blood flow is poor and hypoxia develops, retinal cells secrete growth factors that stimulate formation of new blood vessels in the eye. These new vessels are thin, fragile, and bleed easily, leading to vision loss.

Visual **sensory perception** loss from DR has several mechanisms. Central vision may be impaired by macular edema with increased blood vessel permeability and deposits of hard exudates at the center of the retina. This problem is the main cause of vision loss in the adult with DM. Vision loss also occurs from macular degeneration, corneal scarring, and changes in lens shape or clarity.

Hyperglycemia may cause blurred vision, even with eyeglasses. Because hypoglycemia can cause temporary vision changes, it is important to wait until blood glucose levels are normal before assessing for refractory changes. Cataracts occur at a younger age and progress faster among patients with DM. Open-angle glaucoma also is more common in patients with DM. The management of cataracts and glaucoma is discussed in Chapter 42.

Control of blood glucose, blood pressure, and blood lipid level is important in preventing DR. Thus patients with DM should have routine ophthalmic evaluations to detect vision problems early before vision loss occurs.

> ### 👤 PATIENT-CENTERED CARE: OLDER ADULT CONSIDERATIONS QSEN
>
> Older patients with diabetic retinopathy also have general age-related vision changes, which reduce the ability to perform self-care. They may have blurred vision, distorted central vision, fluctuating vision, and loss of color perception. Assess the ability of patients with vision changes to measure and inject insulin and to monitor blood glucose levels to determine if adaptive devices are needed to assist in self-management (Touhy & Jett, 2020).

Diabetic Peripheral Neuropathy. Diabetic peripheral neuropathy (DPN) is a progressive deterioration of nerve function that results in loss of *sensory perception*. It is a common complication of DM and often involves all body areas. Damage to sensory nerve fibers results first in pain, which is eventually followed by loss of sensation. Damage to motor nerve fibers results in muscle weakness. The onset is slow, affects both sides of the body, progresses, and is permanent. Late complications include foot ulcers and deformities. Damage to nerve fibers in the autonomic nervous system can cause dysfunction in every organ. The combination of factors leading to the nerve damage in diabetic neuropathy consists of:

- Hyperglycemia, long duration of DM, hyperlipidemia
- Damaged blood vessels leading to reduced neuronal oxygen and other nutrients
- Increased genetic susceptibility to nerve damage
- Smoking, nicotine, and alcohol use

Hyperglycemia leads to DPN through blood vessel changes and reduced tissue *perfusion* that cause nerve hypoxia, which leads to poor nerve impulse transmission. Excessive glucose is converted to sorbitol, which collects in nerves and impairs motor nerve conduction (McCance et al., 2019). Common diabetic neuropathies are listed in Table 59.3.

Diabetic Autonomic Neuropathy. Cardiovascular autonomic neuropathy (CAN) affects sympathetic and parasympathetic nerves of the heart and blood vessels. This problem is underdiagnosed in diabetes and contributes to left ventricular dysfunction, painless myocardial infarction (MI), and exercise intolerance (Wooten & Melchior, 2020). Most often, CAN leads to *orthostatic* (postural) hypotension and *syncope* (brief loss of consciousness on standing). These problems are from failure of the heart and arteries to respond to position changes by increasing heart rate and vascular tone. As a result, blood flow to the brain is interrupted briefly. Orthostatic hypotension and syncope increase the risk for falls, especially among older adults (Touhy & Jett, 2020).

TABLE 59.3   Features of Diabetic Neuropathy

	Complication	Symptom
Distal symmetric polyneuropathy	Sensory alterations	Paresthesias: burning/tingling sensations, starting in toes and moving up legs Dysesthesias: burning, stinging, or stabbing pain Anesthesia: loss of sensation
	Motor alterations in intrinsic muscles of foot	Foot deformities: high arch, claw toes, hammertoes; shift of weight bearing to metatarsal heads and tips of toes
Autonomic neuropathy	Anhidrosis	Drying, cracking of skin
	Gastrointestinal	Delayed gastric emptying, gastric retention, early satiety, bloating, nausea, vomiting, anorexia, constipation, diarrhea, diffuse sweating while eating Nocturnal diarrhea
	Neurogenic bladder	Atonic bladder, urinary retention
	Impotence	Erectile dysfunction
	Cardiovascular autonomic neuropathy (CAN)	Early fatigue, weakness with exercise, orthostatic hypotension
	Defective balancing hormones	Loss of warning signs of hypoglycemia

Autonomic neuropathy can affect the entire GI system. Common GI problems from diabetic neuropathy include gastroesophageal reflex, delayed gastric emptying and gastric retention, early satiety, heartburn, nausea, vomiting, and anorexia. Sluggish movement of the small intestine can lead to bacterial overgrowth, which causes bloating, gas, and both diarrhea and constipation. Constipation, the most common GI problem with DM, is intermittent and may alternate with bouts of diarrhea. **Gastroparesis** (delay in gastric emptying) is a cause of hypoglycemia related to the mismatch of nutrient absorption and insulin action.

Urinary problems from neuropathy cause incomplete bladder emptying and urine retention, which leads to urinary infection and kidney problems. Early symptoms include frequency and urgency. Later symptoms are inability to sense bladder fullness and incontinence.

Diabetic Nephropathy. *Nephropathy* is a pathologic change in the kidney that reduces kidney function and leads to kidney failure. Diabetes is the leading cause of end-stage kidney disease (ESKD) and kidney failure in the United States. Risk factors include a 10- to 15-year history of DM, poor blood glucose control, uncontrolled hypertension, and genetic predisposition. Kidney disease causes progressive albumin excretion and declining glomerular filtration rate (GFR). The onset of diabetic kidney disease may be delayed or prevented by maintaining optimum blood *glucose regulation* (ADA, 2019c).

Chronic high blood glucose levels cause hypertension in kidney blood vessels and excess kidney tissue *perfusion*. The blood vessels become leakier, especially in the glomerulus, allowing filtration of albumin and other proteins that deposit in the kidney tissues and blood vessels. Narrowed blood vessels decrease kidney oxygenation,

TABLE 59.4 Differentiation of Type 1 and Type 2 Diabetes

Features	Type 1	Type 2
Former names	Juvenile-onset diabetes Ketosis-prone diabetes Insulin-dependent diabetes mellitus (IDDM)	Adult-onset diabetes Ketosis-resistant diabetes Non–insulin-dependent diabetes mellitus (NIDDM)
Age at onset	Usually younger than 30 yr	May occur at any age in adults
Symptoms	Abrupt onset, thirst, hunger, increased urine output, weight loss	Frequently none; thirst, fatigue, blurred vision, vascular or neural complications
Etiology	Viral infection, autoimmunity	Not known, genetic predisposition
Pathology	Pancreatic beta cell destruction	Insulin resistance Dysfunctional pancreatic beta cell
Antigen patterns	*HLA-DR, HLA-DQ*	None
Antibodies	Often present at diagnosis	None
Endogenous insulin and C-peptide	None to very low	Low, normal, or high
Inheritance	Complex	Autosomal dominant, multifactorial
Nutritional status	Usually nonobese	60% to 80% obese
Insulin	All dependent on insulin	Required for 20% to 30%
Medical therapy	Mandatory	Mandatory

leading to kidney cell hypoxia and cell death, which can progress to chronic kidney disease (see Chapter 63 for a detailed presentation of chronic kidney disease and end-stage kidney disease). Hypertension speeds the progression of diabetic nephropathy.

Sexual Dysfunction. Sexual dysfunction can develop in both men and women with DM as a result of damage to both nerve tissue and vascular tissue. This is made worse by poorly controlled blood glucose levels. Other factors include obesity, hypertension, tobacco use, and some prescribed drugs.

In men sexual dysfunction manifests with both erectile dysfunction (ED) and retrograde ejaculation. Women may experience deceased vaginal lubrication, uncomfortable or painful sexual intercourse, and decreases in libido and sexual response.

Cognitive Dysfunction. Older adults with DM are at higher risk for developing all types of dementia compared with adults who do not have the disease (ADA, 2019i). Chronic hyperglycemia with microvascular disease contributes to neuron damage, brain atrophy, and cognitive impairment. These problems are more frequent and more severe in patients with longer-duration DM and increase the complications of neuropathy and retinopathy.

Etiology and Genetic Risk

Type 1 Diabetes. Type 1 diabetes mellitus (DM) is an autoimmune disorder in which beta cells are destroyed in a

genetically susceptible person (Table 59.4). The immune system fails to recognize normal body cells as "self," and immune system cells and antibodies take destructive actions against the insulin-secreting cells in the islets. People with certain tissue types are more likely to develop autoimmune diseases, including type 1 DM. Viral infections, such as mumps and coxsackievirus infection, may trigger autoimmune destructive actions (McCance et al., 2019).

> **PATIENT-CENTERED CARE: GENETIC/ GENOMIC CONSIDERATIONS (QSEN)**
>
> Inheritance of genes encoding for the HLA-DR and HLA-DQA and DQB tissue types increases the risk for type 1 DM (McCance et al., 2019). However, inheritance of these genes only *increases the risk,* and most people with these tissue types do *not* develop type 1 DM. Development of DM is an interactive effect of genetic predisposition and exposure to certain environmental factors. During assessment, always ask whether any family members have been diagnosed with either type 1 or type 2 diabetes or any other autoimmune disorder.

Type 2 Diabetes and Metabolic Syndrome. Type 2 DM is a progressive disorder in which the person initially has insulin resistance that progresses to decreased beta cell secretion of insulin. *Insulin resistance* (a reduced cell receptor response to insulin) develops from obesity and physical inactivity in a genetically susceptible adult (ADA, 2019h). It occurs before the onset of type 2 DM and often is accompanied by the cardiovascular risk factors of hyperlipidemia, hypertension, and increased clot formation. Many but not all patients with type 2 DM are obese. The specific causes of type 2 DM are not known, although insulin resistance and beta cell failure have many genetic and nongenetic causes. Heredity plays a major role in the development of type 2 DM, although not all gene variations that increase the risk for type 2 DM are known.

Metabolic syndrome is the simultaneous presence of metabolic factors that increase risk for developing type 2 DM and cardiovascular disease. Features of the syndrome include:

- Abdominal obesity: waist circumference of 40 inches (100 cm) or more for men and 35 inches (88 cm) or more for women
- Hyperglycemia: fasting blood glucose level of 100 mg/dL or more or on drug treatment for elevated blood glucose levels
- Hypertension: systolic blood pressure of 130 mm Hg or more or diastolic blood pressure of 85 mg Hg or more or on drug treatment for hypertension
- Hyperlipidemia: triglyceride level of 150 mg/dL or more or on drug treatment for elevated triglycerides; high-density lipoprotein (HDL) cholesterol less than 40 mg/dL for men or less than 50 mg/dL for women

Any of these health problems also increases the rate of atherosclerosis and the risk for stroke, CVD, and early death.

Incidence and Prevalence. In the United States, more than 34 million people are living with DM, and 27.8% (7.3 million) are undiagnosed. Another 86 million have prediabetes (Centers for Disease Control and Prevention [CDC], 2020). (*Prediabetes* is defined as impaired fasting glucose [IGF], an A1C between 5.7 and 6.4, or impaired glucose tolerance [IGT]. Over a 3- to 5-year period, adults with prediabetes have a 5-fold to 15-fold higher risk for developing type 2 DM than do those with normal blood glucose levels.) In Canada, about 2.2 million adults have diabetes (Statistics Canada, 2019).

PATIENT-CENTERED CARE: VETERANS HEALTH CONSIDERATIONS (QSEN)

A possible additional risk factor for type 2 DM is exposure to the main component of agent orange, dioxin, which was used during the military conflicts in Korea and Viet Nam. The risk for type 2 diabetes appears higher among U.S. military members who were assigned to those geographic areas. The risk increases with higher exposures (U.S. Department of Veterans Affairs, 2016). Development of DM among veterans who served in areas where agent orange was used occurs at earlier ages and with less obesity.

Assess veterans who were exposed to agent orange at every health care visit for indications of diabetes so the disease can be identified early and interventions implemented to prevent or delay complications. Encourage veterans to use DM prevention strategies of maintaining a healthy weight and engaging in regular physical activity.

About 90% to 95% of adults with diabetes have type 2 DM (CDC, 2020). It can be diagnosed even in preadolescents but is most common among middle-age and older adults, affecting about 12.3% of adults over the age of 20 years and 25.9% of adults age 65 years or older (Touhy & Jett, 2020). With the prevalence of obesity rising in North America, diabetes is likely to become even more common (ADA, 2019h).

PATIENT-CENTERED CARE: CULTURAL/ SPIRITUAL CONSIDERATIONS (QSEN)

Racial and ethnic minorities have a higher prevalence and greater burden of DM compared with non-Hispanic whites. The DM rate is 13% among blacks and 12% in the Hispanic population compared with non-Hispanic white Americans. At nearly 15.1%, American Indians and Alaska Indians have the highest age-adjusted prevalence of DM among U.S. racial and ethnic groups (CDC, 2020). Be alert to the risk for DM whenever you are interviewing or assessing adults who belong to these higher-risk groups. *The increase in obesity and sedentary lifestyles in the North American population intensifies this growing problem. The ADA has identified patients who should be tested for diabetes (Table 59.5).*

Health Promotion and Maintenance. Diabetes mellitus (DM) causes many devastating complications. Control of DM and its preventable complications is a major focus for health promotion activities. No interventions prevent type 1 DM, but health promotion activities that focus on controlling hyperglycemia can reduce its long-term complications.

Adopting a healthy lifestyle that includes a low-calorie diet and increasing physical activity with weight loss improves metabolic and cardiac risk factors (ADA, 2019e; Watts & Howard, 2016) and can prevent or delay the onset of type 2 DM (ADA, 2019k). These improvements include reducing hypertension, increasing heart rate variability between resting rate and exercise rate, lowering triglyceride levels, increasing high-density lipoprotein cholesterol ("healthy" or "good" cholesterol) levels, and reducing low-density lipoprotein cholesterol ("lousy" or "bad" cholesterol) levels. Smoking cessation and avoidance of excess alcohol consumption also are important in preventing complications of DM.

Teach patients with DM that keeping their blood glucose levels within prescribed target ranges can prevent or delay complications. Urge them to regularly follow up with their primary health care provider or diabetes health care provider, to have their eyes and vision tested yearly by an ophthalmologist, and

TABLE 59.5 Indications for Testing People for Type 2 Diabetes

- Testing for diabetes is considered at any age in adults with a BMI greater than 25 kg/m² (or greater than 23 kg/m² in Asian Americans) with one or more of these additional risk factors:
  - Have a first-degree relative with diabetes
  - Are physically inactive
  - Are members of a high-risk ethnic population (e.g., African American, Hispanic American, American Indian, or Pacific Islander)
  - Give birth to a baby weighing more than 9 lb (4.1 kg) or have been diagnosed with GDM
  - Are hypertensive (>140/90 mm Hg)
  - Have a high-density lipoprotein (HDL) cholesterol level less than 35 mg/dL (0.90 mmol/L) and/or a triglyceride level greater than 250 mg/dL (2.82 mmol/L)
  - Have polycystic ovary syndrome
  - Have A1C greater than 5.7%, or IFG or IGT on previous testing
  - Have a history of vascular disease
- If the tested adult has normal glucose values at this time but other conditions and risk factors remain the same, testing should be repeated at 3-year intervals.

BMI, Body mass index; *GDM,* gestational diabetes mellitus; *IFG,* impaired fasting glucose, *IGT,* impaired glucose tolerance.
Data from American Diabetes Association (ADA). (2019b). Classification and diagnosis of diabetes: Standards of medical care in diabetes—2019. *Diabetes Care, 42*(Suppl. 1), S13-S28; and American Diabetes Association (ADA). (2019k). Prevention or delay of type 2 diabetes: Standards of medical care in diabetes—2019. *Diabetes Care, 42*(Suppl. 1), S29-S33.

to have urine albumin levels assessed yearly. Early detection of changes in the eye or kidney allows adjustments in treatment plans that can slow or halt progression of retinopathy and nephropathy. Urge adults to maintain an appropriate weight range for height and body build and to engage in physical activity at least 150 minutes per week (ADA, 2019e). Encourage daily foot inspection and the prompt reporting of ulcers or open areas to the primary health care provider to reduce the risk for deep wounds or the need for amputation.

❖ Interprofessional Collaborative Care

Although adults who have DM are often hospitalized for complications of the disease, diagnosis and management generally occur in a clinic or health care provider's office. Much of the essential education about management is performed in the community, as is the overall management of the disorder. Because DM is a chronic disorder and predisposes to other health problems, you can expect to interact with and care for these patients in any health care setting.

INTERPROFESSIONAL COLLABORATIVE CARE

The Patient With Diabetes Mellitus

The complicated and chronic nature of DM requires the coordination of an interprofessional team approach for optimum outcomes. The interprofessional team members to help patients achieve desired outcomes include primary health care providers, endocrinologists, diabetes health care providers, certified diabetes educators, ophthalmologists, other medical practitioners, registered nurses, pharmacists, registered dietitian nutritionists (RDNs), podiatrists, physical therapists, and wound care specialists.

TABLE 59.6 Criteria for the Diagnosis of Diabetes

A1C >6.5%. The test should be performed in a laboratory using a method that is NGSP certified and standardized to the DCCT assay.

AND

Fasting blood glucose greater than or equal to 126 mg/dL (7.0 mmol/L). *Fasting* is defined as no caloric intake for at least 8 hours.

OR

Two-hour blood glucose equal to or greater than 200 mg/dL (11.1 mmol/L) during oral glucose tolerance testing. The test should be performed using a glucose load containing the equivalent of 75 g anhydrous glucose dissolved in water.

OR

In a patient with classic manifestations of hyperglycemia or hyperglycemic crisis, a casual or random blood glucose concentration greater than 200 mg/dL (11.1 mmol/L). *Casual* is defined as any time of the day without regard to time since last meal. The classic symptoms of diabetes include polyuria, polydipsia, and unexplained weight loss.

NOTE: In the absence of unequivocal hyperglycemia, the first three criteria should be confirmed by repeat testing.

Data from American Diabetes Association (ADA). (2019b). Classification and diagnosis of diabetes: Standards of medical care in diabetes—2019. *Diabetes Care, 42*(Suppl. 1), S132-S28.
DCCT, Diabetes Control and Complications Trial; *NGSP,* National Glycohemoglobin Standardization Program.

◆ Assessment: Recognize Cues

History. Ask about risk factors and symptoms related to DM. Ask women how large their children were at birth, because many women who develop type 2 DM had gestational diabetes mellitus (GDM) or glucose intolerance during pregnancy (ADA, 2019b). Teach women with a history of GDM and those who have prediabetes about lifestyle changes to prevent DM (ADA, 2019b).

Assessing weight and weight change is important because excess weight and obesity are risk factors for type 2 DM. The patient with type 1 DM often has weight loss with increased appetite during the weeks before diagnosis. For both types of DM, patients usually have fatigue, polyuria, and polydipsia. Ask about recent major or minor infections and assess overall ***immunity***. Ask women about frequent vaginal yeast infections. Assess whether patients have noticed that small skin injuries become infected more easily or take longer to heal. Also ask whether they have noticed any changes in vision or in the sense of touch.

Laboratory Assessment

Diagnosis of Diabetes. Diabetes can be diagnosed by assessing the blood glucose levels listed in the Laboratory Profile: Blood Glucose Values box. A test result indicating DM should be repeated to rule out laboratory error unless symptoms of hyperglycemia or hyperglycemic crisis are also present. Table 59.6 lists criteria for the diagnosis of DM.

The diagnosis of DM includes elevated glycosylated hemoglobin levels. **Glycosylated hemoglobin (A1C)** is a standardized test that measures how much glucose permanently attaches to the hemoglobin molecule and indicates the effectiveness of blood glucose control measures. Because glucose binds to proteins, including hemoglobin, through a process called

⚡ LABORATORY PROFILE

Blood Glucose Values

Test	Normal Range	Significance of Abnormal Results
Fasting blood glucose test	100 mg/dL (5.6 mmol/L) Older adults: Levels rise 1 mg/dL per decade of age	Levels >100 mg/dL (5.6 mmol/L) but <126 mg/dL (7.0 mmol/L) indicate impaired fasting glucose (IFG). Levels >126 mg/dL (7.0 mmol/L) obtained on at least two occasions are diagnostic of diabetes, even in older adults.
Glucose tolerance test (2-hr postload result)	<140 mg/dL (7.8 mmol/L)	Levels >140 mg/dL (7.8 mmol/L) and <200 mg/dL (11.1 mmol/L) indicate impaired glucose tolerance (IGT). Levels >200 mg/dL (11.1 mmol/L) indicate provisional diagnosis of diabetes.
Glycosylated hemoglobin (A1C) test	4%-6%	Levels of 5.7% to 6.4% indicate prediabetes and an increased risk for development of diabetes. Levels >6.5% indicate diabetes. Levels >8% indicate poor diabetes control and need for adherence to regimen or changes in therapy.

Data from Pagana, K., & Pagana, T. (2018). *Mosby's manual of diagnostic and laboratory tests* (6th ed.). St. Louis: Elsevier.

glycosylation, the higher the blood glucose level is over time, the more glycosylated the hemoglobin becomes.

Fasting plasma glucose (FPG) (fasting blood glucose [FBG]), along with A1C, is used to diagnose DM in nonpregnant adults. A diagnosis of DM is made with two separate test results greater than 126 mg/dL (7 mmol/L) (ADA, 2019b). *Random* or *casual plasma* glucose greater than 200 mg/dL (7.0 mmol/L) is used to diagnose DM in patients with classic hyperglycemia symptoms or hyperglycemic crisis.

The *oral glucose tolerance test (OGTT)* is a sensitive test for the diagnosis of DM. It is often used to diagnose gestational diabetes mellitus (GDM) during pregnancy and is not routinely used for general diagnosis (ADA, 2019f).

Other blood tests for diabetes can help determine whether a patient has type 1 or type 2 DM. Type 1 DM results from autoimmune destruction of the beta cells of the pancreas. Markers of this destruction include islet cell autoantibodies (ICAs), autoantibodies to insulin, zinc transporter antibodies (ZnT8), and autoantibodies to glutamic acid decarboxylase (GAD65). ICAs are present in 85% to 90% of patients with new-onset type 1 DM (McCance et al., 2019).

Screening for Diabetes. Testing to detect prediabetes and type 2 DM is recommended for patients older than 45 years and those defined as overweight (body mass index [BMI] greater than 25 kg/m²) (Touhy & Jett, 2020). Testing is considered for

TABLE 59.7 Correlation Between A1C Level and Mean Blood Glucose Levels

A1C (%)	MEAN BLOOD GLUCOSE	
	mg/dL	mmol/L
6	126	7.0
7	154	8.6
8	183	10.2
9	212	11.8
10	240	13.4
11	269	14.9
12	298	16.5

younger patients who are overweight if they have additional risk factors for DM or other health problems associated with it. Screening for DM usually is done with laboratory testing of both A1C levels and fasting plasma glucose levels (ADA, 2019b).

Ongoing Assessment. *Glycosylated hemoglobin assays* are useful as a good indicator of the average blood glucose levels. Measurement of A1C shows the average blood glucose level during the previous 120 days—the life span of red blood cells. A1C testing can help assess long-term glycemic control and predict the risk for complications. *Unlike the fasting blood glucose test, A1C test results are not altered by the eating habits on the day before the test.* This testing is performed at diagnosis and at specific intervals to evaluate the treatment plan. A1C testing is recommended at least twice yearly in patients who are meeting expected treatment outcomes and have stable blood glucose control. Quarterly assessment is recommended for patients whose therapy has changed or who are not meeting prescribed glycemic levels (ADA, 2019d). Table 59.7 shows the correlation between A1C and mean blood glucose levels.

Fructosamine assays are useful for short-term follow-up of treatment changes or in patients with hemoglobin abnormalities in which A1C does not accurately reflect glucose levels. When glucose binds to amino groups on serum proteins, especially albumin, the glycosylated protein product is called fructosamine. This product increases with elevated blood glucose levels as hemoglobin does but can indicate blood glucose control over a shorter period.

NCLEX EXAMINATION CHALLENGE 59.2
Physiological Integrity

The nurse reviewing the preadmission testing laboratory values for a 62-year-old client scheduled for a total knee replacement finds an A1C value of 6.2%. How will the nurse interpret this finding?

A. The client's A1C is completely normal.
B. The client has type 1 diabetes mellitus.
C. The client has type 2 diabetes mellitus.
D. The client has prediabetes mellitus.

◆ **Analysis: Analyze Cues and Prioritize Hypotheses.** The priority collaborative problems for patients with diabetes DM include:

1. Potential for injury due to hyperglycemia
2. Potential for poor wound healing due to endocrine and vascular effects of diabetes
3. Potential for injury due to diabetic neuropathy
4. Potential for kidney disease due to reduced kidney *perfusion*
5. Potential for the complications of hypoglycemia, diabetic ketoacidosis, and hyperglycemic-hyperosmolar state (HHS) and coma

◆ **Planning and Implementation: Generate Solutions and Take Action**

Preventing Injury From Hyperglycemia

Planning: Expected Outcomes. The patient is expected to manage DM and prevent disease progression by maintaining blood glucose levels in his or her target range.

Interventions

Nonsurgical Management. Management of DM involves **nutrition** interventions, blood glucose monitoring, a planned exercise program, and often, drugs to lower blood glucose levels. Nurses, the interprofessional team members, and the patient plan, coordinate, and deliver care.

The American Diabetes Association (ADA) has proposed these treatment outcomes for glycosylated hemoglobin (A1C) and blood glucose levels (ADA, 2019d):

- A1C levels are maintained at 7.0% or below (or as prescribed).
- The majority of premeal blood glucose levels are 70 to 130 mg/dL (3.9 to 7.2 mmol/L).
- Peak after-meal blood glucose levels are less than 180 mg/dL (<10.0 mmol/L).

Drug therapy. Drug therapy is indicated when a patient with type 2 DM does not achieve blood glucose control with diet changes, regular exercise, and stress management. Several categories of drugs may be used to lower blood glucose levels. Patients with type 1 DM require insulin therapy for blood glucose control and may use other antidiabetic drugs, as well.

Drugs are started at the lowest effective dose and increased over time until the patient reaches desired blood glucose control or the maximum dosage. Glycemic control may require the use of more than one category of drug. Insulin therapy is indicated for the patient with type 2 DM when blood glucose goals cannot be met with the use of two or three different antidiabetic agents, including GLP-1 agonists (ADA, 2019j).

Antidiabetic drugs are not a substitute for dietary modification and exercise. Teach the patient about continuing dietary changes and regular exercise while taking antidiabetic drugs.

! NURSING SAFETY PRIORITY (QSEN)
Drug Alert

To avoid drug interactions, teach the patient who is taking an antidiabetic drug to consult with his or her diabetes health care provider or pharmacist before using *any* over-the-counter drugs.

Drug selection is based on cost, the patient's ability to manage multiple drug dosages, associated risks for side effects, and response to the drugs. Shorter-acting agents (e.g., glitinides) are preferred for older patients, those with irregular eating schedules, or those with liver, kidney, or cardiac problems. Longer-acting drugs (e.g., glimepiride) with once-a-day dosing are better for adherence. Beta cell function in type 2 DM declines over time, and some drugs become less effective. Management of type 2 DM may eventually require insulin therapy either alone or with other antidiabetic drugs.

Some antidiabetic drugs are oral agents, and other types require subcutaneous injection. See the Common Examples of Drug Therapy: Diabetes Mellitus box for common antidiabetic drugs in each category.

Insulin stimulators (also known as insulin secretagogues) stimulate insulin release from pancreatic beta cells and are used for patients who are still able to produce insulin. This class include sulfonylureas and meglitinide analogs.

Sulfonylurea agents lower fasting blood glucose levels by triggering the release of insulin from beta cells. Many drugs interact with sulfonylureas. Be sure to consult a drug reference source or pharmacologist when instructing patients who are prescribed a drug from this class. Meglitinide analogs are insulin stimulators and have actions and adverse effects similar to those of sulfonylureas. They tend to increase meal-related insulin secretion.

Metformin, a biguanide, decreases liver glucose production and decreases intestinal absorption of glucose. It also improves insulin sensitivity, which increases peripheral glucose uptake and utilization.

> **! NURSING SAFETY PRIORITY (QSEN)**
> **Drug Alert**
>
> Metformin can cause lactic acidosis in patients with kidney impairment and should not be used by anyone with kidney disease (Burchum & Rosenthal, 2019). To prevent lactic acidosis and acute kidney injury, the drug is withheld before and after using contrast medium or any surgical procedure requiring anesthesia until adequate kidney function is established.

Insulin sensitizers, also known as thiazolidinediones (TZDs or "glitazones"), increase cellular use of glucose, which lowers blood glucose levels. These drugs are associated with an increased risk for heart-related deaths, bone fracture, and macular edema. The Food and Drug Administration (FDA) has issued a black box warning indicating that these drugs are not to be used by patients who have symptomatic heart failure or other specific types of cardiovascular disease. (A *black box warning* is a government designation indicating that a drug has a serious side effect and must be used with caution.)

Alpha-glucosidase inhibitors prevent after-meal hyperglycemia by delaying absorption of carbohydrate from the intestine. They inhibit enzymes in the intestinal tract, reducing the rate of starch digestion and glucose absorption. These actions prevent a sudden blood glucose surge after meals. These drugs do not cause hypoglycemia unless given with sulfonylureas or insulin.

However, side effects of GI upset and flatulence can deter adherence to the use of these drugs.

Incretin mimetics work like the natural "gut" hormones, glucagon-like peptide-1 (GLP-1) and glucose-dependent insulinotropic polypeptide (GIP), that are released by the intestine in response to food intake and act with insulin for *glucose regulation.* Drugs in this class include the GLP-1 agonists dulaglutide, exenatide, exenatide extended-release, liraglutide, lixisenatide, and semaglutide (Burchum & Rosenthal, 2019; Keresztes & Peacock-Johnson, 2019). These drugs are used in addition to diet and exercise to improve glycemic control in adults with type 2 DM.

> **! NURSING SAFETY PRIORITY (QSEN)**
> **Drug Alert**
>
> Extended-release exenatide and dulaglutide are injected subcutaneously *once weekly.* Be sure to emphasize this dosing schedule to avoid overdoses.

Dipeptidyl peptidase-4 (DPP-4) inhibitors work by preventing the inactivation of the incretins GLP and GIP. These peptides are rapidly metabolized and inactivated by the enzyme DPP-4. Drugs that inhibit the DPP-4 enzyme allow naturally produced incretin hormones to remain available for blood *glucose regulation.* The DPP-4 inhibitors used to control type 2 DM are sitagliptin, saxagliptin, linagliptin, and alogliptin.

> **! NURSING SAFETY PRIORITY (QSEN)**
> **Drug Alert**
>
> DPP-4 inhibitors and the incretin mimetics have an increased risk for pancreatitis. Warn patients taking these drugs to immediately report to the diabetes health care provider any signs of jaundice; sudden onset of intense abdominal pain that radiates to the back, left flank, or left shoulder; or gray-blue discoloration of the abdomen or periumbilical area.
>
> Saxagliptin and alogliptin have an increased risk for heart failure. Warn patients to report a sudden weight gain or new-onset shortness of breath.

Amylin analogs are drugs similar to amylin, a naturally occurring hormone produced by pancreatic beta cells that works with and is secreted with insulin in response to blood glucose elevation. Amylin levels are deficient in patients with type 1 DM. Pramlintide, an analog of amylin, is approved for patients with DM who are treated with insulin. It works by three mechanisms: delaying gastric emptying, reducing after-meal blood glucose levels, and triggering satiety (in the brain). (Satiety leads to decreased caloric intake and eventual weight loss.)

> **! NURSING SAFETY PRIORITY (QSEN)**
> **Drug Alert**
>
> Do not mix pramlintide and insulin in the same syringe because the pH of the two drugs is not compatible.

COMMON EXAMPLES OF DRUG THERAPY

Diabetes Mellitus

Drug Category	Nursing Implications
Insulin Stimulators (Secretagogues)	
Lower blood glucose levels by triggering the release of preformed insulin from beta cells.	
Second-generation sulfonylurea agents • Glipizide • Glyburide • Glimepiride Meglitinide analogs • Repaglinide • Nateglinide	Teach patient the signs and symptoms of hypoglycemia (hunger, headache, tremors, sweating, confusion) *because these drugs lower blood glucose levels even when hyperglycemia is not present.* Instruct patients to take these drugs with or just before meals *to prevent hypoglycemia.* Instruct patients taking a sulfonylurea to check with their health care provider or a pharmacist before taking any over-the-counter drug or supplement *because these drugs interact with many other drugs.*
Biguanides	
Lower blood glucose by inhibiting liver glucose production, decreasing intestinal absorption of glucose, and increasing insulin sensitivity.	
• Metformin	Instruct patients not to drink alcohol while taking this drug *to reduce the risk for lactic acidosis.* Remind patients that this drug must be stopped before certain imaging tests using contrast agents and not started again for 48 hours after testing *because of the increased risk for kidney damage and lactic acidosis.* Warn patients that GI problems are common side effects of this drug class.
Insulin Sensitizers	
Lower blood glucose by decreasing liver glucose production and improving the sensitivity of insulin receptors.	
Thiazolidinediones (TZDs) • Pioglitazone • Rosiglitazone	Teach patients with any cardiovascular disease to weigh themselves daily and report a weight gain of more than 2 lb (1 kg) in one day or 4 lb (2 kg) in a week to the prescriber *because these drugs increase the risk for heart failure.* Instruct patients to report vision changes immediately *because these drugs increase the risk for macular edema.* Warn patients that weight gain and peripheral edema are common side effects of these drugs.
Alpha-Glucosidase Inhibitors	
Prevent after-meal hyperglycemia by inhibiting enzymes in the intestinal tract from breaking down starches into glucose. This action delays the digestion of starches and the absorption of glucose from the small intestine.	
• Acarbose • Miglitol	Teach patients to take these drugs only with a meal *because the action is in the intestinal tract.* Warn patients that abdominal discomfort and bloating, flatulence, nausea, diarrhea, and indigestion are common side effects of this drug class.
Incretin Mimetics (GLP-1 Agonists)	
Act like natural "gut" hormones that work with insulin to lower blood glucose levels by reducing pancreatic glucagon secretion, reducing liver glucose production, and delaying gastric emptying.	
• Dulaglutide • Exenatide • Exenatide extended release • Liraglutide • Lixisenatide • Semaglutide	Teach patients the signs of hypoglycemia (hunger, headache, tremors, sweating) *because these drugs lower blood glucose levels even when they are normal if used in conjunction with insulin, sulfonylureas, or meglitinides.* Instruct patient how to inject themselves *because these drugs are only available as subcutaneous formulations.* Instruct patients to read exenatide and dulaglutide pens carefully *because the extended-release form is only injected **weekly** rather than daily.* Teach patients to report persistent abdominal pain and nausea to the health care provider *because these drugs increase the risk for pancreatitis.*
DPP-4 Inhibitors	
DPP-4 is an enzyme that breaks down the natural gut hormones (GLP-1 and GIP). DPP-4 inhibitors are oral agents that prevent the enzyme DPP-4 from breaking down the natural gut hormones (GLP-1 and GIP), which then allows these natural substances to work with insulin to lower glucagon secretion from the pancreas, leading to reduced liver glucose production. These oral drugs also reduce blood glucose levels by delaying gastric emptying and slowing the rate of nutrient absorption into the blood.	
• Alogliptin • Linagliptin • Saxagliptin • Sitagliptin	Teach patient the signs and symptoms of hypoglycemia (hunger, headache, tremors, sweating, confusion) *because these drugs lower blood glucose levels even when hyperglycemia is not present if used in conjunction with insulin, sulfonylureas, or meglitinides.* Instruct patients to be alert for rash or other sign of allergic reaction *because this class of drugs is associated with a moderate incidence of drug allergy.* Teach patients to report persistent abdominal pain and nausea to the health care provider *because these drugs increase the risk for pancreatitis.* Instruct patients to notify the primary health care provider if shortness of breath, dyspnea on exertion, or cough, especially when lying down, is experienced *because this class of drugs is associated with heart failure.*

💊 COMMON EXAMPLES OF DRUG THERAPY—Cont'd

Diabetes Mellitus

Drug Category	Nursing Implications
Amylin Analogs	
These drugs are similar to amylin, a naturally occurring hormone produced by beta cells in the pancreas that is co-secreted with insulin and lowers blood glucose levels by decreasing endogenous glucagon, delaying gastric emptying, and triggering satiety.	
• Pramlintide	Teach patient the signs and symptoms of hypoglycemia (hunger, headache, tremors, sweating, confusion) *because these drugs lower blood glucose levels even when hyperglycemia is not present when used in conjunction with insulin.*
	Instruct patient how to inject themselves *because these drugs are only available as subcutaneous formulations.*
	Warn patients that nausea and vomiting are common side effects of this drug class.
	Do not mix in the same syringe with insulin *because their pH is not compatible.*
Sodium-Glucose Cotransport Inhibitors	
Lower blood glucose levels by preventing kidney reabsorption of glucose and sodium that was filtered from the blood into the urine. This filtered glucose is excreted in the urine rather than moved back into the blood.	
• Canagliflozin	Teach patients the signs and symptoms of hypoglycemia (hunger, headache, tremors, sweating, confusion) *because these drugs lower blood glucose levels even when hyperglycemia is not present if used in conjunction with insulin, sulfonylureas, or meglitinides.*
• Dapagliflozin	
• Empagliflozin	
• Ertugliflozin	Teach the patient the signs and symptoms of dehydration (increased thirst, lightheadedness, dry mouth and mucous membranes, orthostatic hypotension) *because these drugs increase urine output and increase dehydration risk.*
	Teach patients the signs and symptoms of hyponatremia (muscle weakness, abdominal cramping, rapid heart rate, orthostatic hypotension) *because these drugs increase sodium loss.*
	Teach patients the signs and symptoms of urinary tract infection (frequency, pain and burning on urination, foul urine odor) *because the increased glucose in the urinary tract predisposes to infection.*
	Instruct women to be alert for genital itching and vaginal discharge *because these drugs increase the risk for genital yeast infection.*
	Teach patients to report any swelling, tenderness or redness of the genitals or perineal skin *because these drugs increase the risk for Fournier gangrene with perineal fasciitis.*

Sodium-glucose co-transport inhibitors lower blood glucose levels by preventing kidney reabsorption of glucose that was filtered from the blood into the urine. The filtered glucose is excreted in the urine rather than moved back into the blood. These oral drugs include canagliflozin, dapagliflozin, empagliflozin, and ertugliflozin (Hussar, 2019).

❗ NURSING SAFETY PRIORITY (QSEN)

Drug Alert

The FDA has issued a warning that use of empagliflozin increases the risk for acute kidney injury and impaired renal function (Aschenbrenner, 2017). In addition, canagliflozin is associated with an increased risk for lower limb amputations. Other warnings about the sodium-glucose co-transport inhibitors include the potential for genital and perineal necrotizing fasciitis.

Combination agents combine drugs with different mechanisms of action. For example, Glucovance combines glyburide with metformin. Combining drugs with different mechanisms of action may be highly effective in maintaining desired blood glucose control. Some patients may need a combination of antidiabetic agents and insulin to control blood glucose levels.

Insulin therapy. Insulin therapy is required for type 1 DM and often is used for type 2 DM. The safety of insulin therapy in older patients may be affected by reduced vision, mobility and coordination problems, and decreased memory, increasing the risk for dosage errors.

NCLEX EXAMINATION CHALLENGE 59.3

Health Promotion and Maintenance

Which precaution is a **priority** for the nurse to teach a client prescribed semaglutide to **prevent harm**?

A. Only take this drug once weekly.
B. Report any vision changes immediately.
C. Do not mix in the same syringe with insulin.
D. This drug can only be given by a health care professional.

Many types of insulin and regimens are available to achieve normal blood glucose levels. Because insulin is a small protein that is quickly inactivated in the GI tract, it is usually injected.

Types of insulin vary with the source and manufacturing techniques. Insulin analogs are synthetic human insulins in which the structure of the insulin molecule is altered to change the rate of absorption and duration of action within the body (e.g., Lispro insulin).

Rapid-, short-, intermediate-, and long-acting forms of insulin can be injected separately, and some can be mixed in the same syringe. Insulin is available in concentrations of 100 units/mL (U-100), 200 units/mL (U-200), 300 units/mL (U-300), and 500 units/mL (U-500). Insulin concentrations above 100 units/mL are reserved for when very large doses of insulin are required.

Teach the patient that the insulin types, the injection technique, and the site of injection all affect the absorption, onset, degree, and duration of insulin activity. Reinforce that changing insulins may affect blood glucose control and should be done only under supervision of the diabetes health care provider. Table 59.8 outlines the timed activity of human insulin.

Insulin regimens try to replicate the normal insulin release pattern from the pancreas. The pancreas produces a constant *(basal)* amount of insulin that balances liver glucose production with glucose use and maintains normal blood glucose levels between meals. The pancreas also produces additional meal-time *(prandial)* insulin to prevent blood glucose elevation after meals. The insulin dose required for blood glucose control varies among patients. Starting doses may be much lower for older adults or for very thin patients. For multiple-dose regimens or continuous subcutaneous insulin infusion (CSII), basal insulin makes up about 40% of the total daily dosage, with the remainder divided into premeal doses of rapid-acting insulin analogs or regular insulin. Basal insulin coverage is provided by intermediate-acting insulin (NPH) or long-acting insulin analogs such as insulin glargine, insulin detemir, or insulin degludec. Dosages are adjusted based on the results of blood glucose monitoring.

Single daily injection protocols require insulin injection only once daily. This protocol may include one injection of intermediate- or long-acting insulin or an injection of combination short- and intermediate-acting insulin. Some patients with type 2 DM combine once-daily insulin injection for basal coverage with oral agent therapy to stimulate bolus insulin secretion.

Multiple-component insulin therapy combines short- and intermediate-acting insulin injected twice daily. Two-thirds of the daily dose is given before breakfast, and one-third before the evening meal. Ratios of intermediate-acting and regular insulin are based on results of blood glucose monitoring.

Intensified regimens include a basal dose of intermediate- or long-acting insulin and a mealtime bolus dose of short- or rapid-acting insulin designed to bring the *next* blood glucose value into the target range. Blood glucose elevations above the target range are treated with "correction" doses of short- or rapid-acting insulin. The patient's blood glucose patterns determine insulin dosage. Frequency of blood glucose monitoring is based on the timed action of insulin and may occur as often as eight times daily. Blood glucose testing 2 hours after meals and within 10 minutes before the next meal helps determine the adequacy of the previous bolus dose. The patient determines the effects of basal insulin by monitoring blood glucose levels before breakfast (fasting) and before the evening meal.

Patients on intensified insulin regimens need extensive education to achieve target blood glucose values. They need to know how to adjust insulin doses and understand **nutrition** therapy for dietary flexibility and meeting target blood glucose values. Patients must also be able to correctly monitor blood glucose levels so that therapy decisions are based on accurate data.

Regardless of the specific insulin regimen, adherence to insulin injection schedules is critical in achieving the glycemic control needed to reduce long-term complications. At times, skipping an occasional insulin dose may be related to an unusual meal pattern for a day or a change in exercise.

Insulin absorption is affected by many factors including injection site; timing, type, or dose of insulin used; and physical activity.

Injection site area affects the speed of insulin absorption. Fig. 59.4 shows common insulin injection areas. Absorption is fastest in the abdomen, which is, except for a 2-inch radius around the navel, the preferred injection site. Rotating injection sites allows each injection site to heal completely before the site is used again. Rotation *within* one anatomic site is preferred to rotation from one area to another to prevent day-to-day variability in absorption.

Absorption rate is determined by insulin properties. Longer duration of action makes absorption less reliable. Larger doses prolong the absorption. Factors that increase blood flow from the injection site, such as applying heat locally, massaging the area, and exercising the injected area, increase insulin absorption. Scarred areas are less sensitive to pain, but these sites usually slow insulin absorption.

Injection depth changes insulin absorption. Usually injections are made into the subcutaneous tissue. IM injection has a faster absorption and is not used for routine insulin use. Most patients lightly grasp a fold of skin and inject at a 90-degree angle; however, a 45-degree angle is used for frail older adults and those who are very thin. Aspiration for blood is not needed. Patients who are overweight can use 4-mm or 5-mm needles to inject insulin at a 90-degree angle without pinching a skinfold before injection.

Timing of injection affects blood glucose levels. The interval between premeal injections and eating, known as "lag time," affects blood glucose levels after meals. Insulins that have rapid onsets of action are given within 10 minutes before mealtime when blood glucose is in the target range. If hyperglycemia or hypoglycemia is not present, these insulins can be given at any time from 10 minutes before mealtime to just before eating or even immediately after eating. Regular insulin is given at least 20 to 30 minutes before eating when glucose levels are within the target range. When blood glucose levels are *above* the target range, lag time is increased to permit insulin to have a greater glucose-lowering effect before food enters the stomach. When blood glucose levels are *below* the target range, teach patients to inject insulin *immediately* before eating, and to delay rapid-acting insulin injection until sometime *after* eating the meal.

Mixing insulins can change the time of peak action. Mixtures of short- and intermediate-acting insulins produce a more normal blood glucose response in some patients than does a single dose. The patient's response to mixed insulin may differ from the response to the same insulins given separately.

> **⚠ NURSING SAFETY PRIORITY** (QSEN)
> **Drug Alert**
>
> Do not mix any other insulin type with insulin glargine, insulin detemir, or any of the premixed insulin formulations such as Humalog Mix 75/25.

NCLEX EXAMINATION CHALLENGE 59.4
Safe and Effective Care Environment

How will the nurse modify insulin injection technique for a client who is 5 feet 10 inches tall and weighs 106 lb (48.1 kg)?

A. Use a 6-mm needle and inject at a 90-degree angle.
B. Use a 6-mm needle and inject at a 45-degree angle.
C. Use a 12-mm needle and inject at a 90-degree angle.
D. Use a 12-mm needle and inject at a 45-degree angle.

TABLE 59.8 Timed Activity of Pharmaceutical Insulin

Preparation	Onset (hr)	Peak (hr)	Duration (hr)
Rapid-Acting Insulin Analogs			
Insulin aspart injection	0.25	1-3	3-5
Insulin glulisine injection	0.3	0.5-1.5	3-4
Human lispro injection	0.25	0.5-1.5	5
Human lispro injection U-200	0.25	0.5-1.5	5
Insulin human inhalation powder	0.25	1-1.25	2.5
Short-Acting Insulin			
Regular human insulin injection	0.5	2-4	5-12
Humulin R (Concentrated U-500)	1.5	4-12	24
Intermediate Acting Insulin			
Isophane insulin NPH injection	1-4	4-12	10-24+
70% human insulin isophane suspension/30% human insulin injection	0.5	2-12	24
70% insulin aspart protamine suspension/30% insulin aspart injection	0.25	1-4	24
75% insulin lispro protamine suspension/25% insulin lispro injection	0.25	1-2	24
Long-Acting Insulin Analogs			
Insulin glargine injection	2-4	None	24
Insulin glargine injection U-300	2-4	12	24
Insulin detemir injection	1	6-8	5.7-24
Insulin degludec injection U-100, U-200	1	9	42

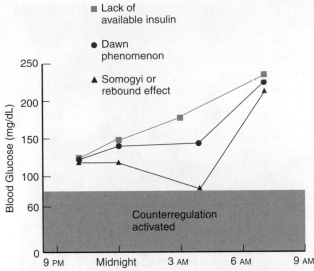

FIG. 59.5 Three blood glucose phenomena in patients with diabetes.

Hypoglycemia from insulin excess has many causes. Its effects and treatment are discussed in the Interventions for Preventing Hypoglycemia section.

Two conditions of fasting hyperglycemia (in addition to a lack of insulin) can occur (Fig. 59.5). *Dawn phenomenon* results from a nighttime release of adrenal hormones that causes blood glucose elevations at about 5 to 6 a.m. It is managed by providing more insulin for the overnight period (e.g., giving the evening dose of intermediate-acting insulin at 10 p.m. instead of with the evening meal). *Somogyi phenomenon* is morning hyperglycemia from the counterregulatory response to nighttime hypoglycemia. It is managed by ensuring adequate dietary intake at bedtime and evaluating the insulin dose and exercise programs to prevent conditions that lead to hypoglycemia. Both problems are diagnosed by blood glucose monitoring during the night. Help identify these problems and teach the patient and family about management.

Alternative methods of insulin administration are available in addition to traditional subcutaneous injections. These include continuous insulin infusion, needleless injection systems, and dry powder inhalers.

Continuous subcutaneous infusion of a basal dose of insulin (CSII) with additional insulin at mealtimes is more effective in controlling blood glucose levels than other schedules. It allows flexibility in meal timing, because if a meal is skipped, the additional mealtime dose of insulin is not given. CSII is given by an externally worn pump containing a reservoir of rapid-acting insulin and is connected to the patient by an infusion set. Teach him or her to adjust the amount of insulin based on data from blood glucose monitoring. Rapid-acting insulin analogs are used with insulin infusion pumps (Fig. 59.6).

Problems with CSII include skin infections that can occur when the infusion site is not cleaned or the infusion set is not changed every 2 to 3 days. Ketoacidosis may occur more often because of infection, obstruction of the infusion, or mechanical pump problems. Stress the need for ketone testing when blood glucose levels are greater than 300 mg/dL (16.7 mmol/L).

Patients using CSII need intensive and extensive education to operate the pump, adjust the settings, and respond appropriately to alarms. Removing the pump for any time can result

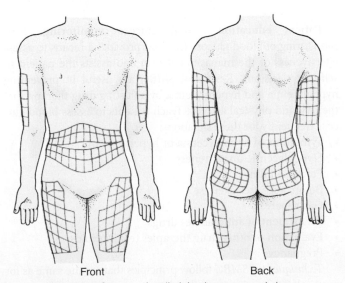

Front   Back

FIG. 59.4 Common insulin injection areas and sites.

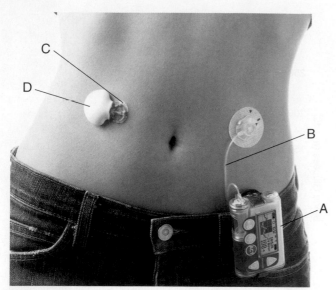

FIG. 59.6 MiniMed Paradigm REAL-Time Insulin Pump and Continuous Glucose Monitoring System. (A) Pump. (B) Injection cannula. (C) Glucose sensor. (D) Data transmitter. (Courtesy Medtronic Diabetes, Northridge, CA.)

in hyperglycemia. Provide supplemental insulin schedules for times when the pump is not operational.

Injection devices include a needleless system and an insulin pen in addition to traditional insulin syringes. With a needleless device, the needle is replaced by an ultrathin liquid stream of insulin forced through the skin under high pressure. Insulin given by jet injection is absorbed at a faster rate and has a shorter duration of action. Most types of insulin are available in pen devices, which are more convenient for multiple daily injection regimens.

A dry powder inhaler insulin delivery system with single-use cartridges is available for rapid-acting insulin. Its use is limited to adults with type 1 or type 2 DM who do not have respiratory problems and who are nonsmokers. Pulmonary testing is required before initiating this therapy. Its onset of action is about 12 minutes. Complications of this therapy include new-onset respiratory problems such as bronchospasms.

Patient education: drugs. Provide specific instructions about insulin therapy, new drug therapies, and self-monitoring of blood glucose (SMBG).

Insulin storage varies by use. Teach patients to refrigerate insulin that is not in use to maintain potency, prevent exposure to sunlight, and inhibit bacterial growth. Insulin in use may be kept at room temperature for up to 28 days to reduce injection site irritation from cold insulin.

To prevent loss of drug potency, teach the patient to avoid exposing insulin to temperatures below 36°F (2.2°C) or above 86°F° (30°C), to avoid excessive shaking, and to protect insulin from direct heat and light. Insulin should not be allowed to freeze. Teach patients to discard any unused insulin after 28 days.

Teach patients to always have a spare supply of each type of insulin used. Prefilled syringes are stable for up to 30 days when refrigerated. Store prefilled syringes in the upright position, with the needle pointing upward or flat, so insulin particles do not clog it. Teach patients to roll prefilled syringes between the hands before using to gently mix and warm the dose.

Proper dose preparation is critical for insulin effectiveness and safety. Teach patients that the person giving the insulin needs to inspect the vial before each use for changes (e.g., clumping, frosting, precipitation, or change in clarity or color) that may indicate loss in potency. Preparations containing NPH insulin are uniformly cloudy after gently rolling the vial between the hands. Other insulins should be clear. If potency is questionable, another vial or pen of the same insulin type should be used.

Syringes are usually used to inject insulin. Standard insulin syringes are marked in insulin units. They are available in 1-mL (100-U), ½-mL (50-U), and ³⁄₁₀-mL (30-U) sizes. The unit scale on the barrel of the syringe differs with the syringe size and manufacturer. Insulin syringe needles are measured in 28, 29, 30, and 31 gauges and in lengths of 6 mm, 8 mm, and 12.7 mm. To ensure accurate insulin measurement, instruct the patient to always buy the same type of syringe. The Patient and Family Education: Preparing for Self-Management: Subcutaneous Insulin Administration box reviews instructions for drawing up a single insulin injection.

Disposable needles are used only once. Teach the patient to discard the syringe and needle after one use. Information on needle disposal can be obtained at www.safeneedledisposal.org.

Pen-type injectors hold small, lightweight, prefilled insulin cartridges. These devices allow greater accuracy than traditional insulin syringes, especially when measuring small doses. Discuss proper storage for prefilled insulin pens or cartridges. Ensure that the product is appropriate for the patient's unique needs. *Pen-type injectors are not designed for independent use by visually impaired patients or by those with cognitive impairment.* Ensure that the patient understands the correct use for the selected syringe or cartridge.

! NATIONAL PATIENT SAFETY GOALS

The Institute for Safe Medication Practices (ISMP) and The Joint Commission's National Patient Safety Goals identify insulin as a *High-Alert* drug. (High-Alert drugs are those that have an increased risk for causing patient harm if given in error.) The ISMP cautions that digital displays on some insulin pens can be misread. If the pen is held upside down, as a left-handed person might do, a dose of 52 units actually appears to be a dose of 25 units, and a dose of 12 units looks like a dose of 21 units.

Patient education: blood glucose monitoring. Self-monitoring of blood glucose (SMBG) provides a means to assess effectiveness of the management plan and assists the patient in self-care decisions. Results of SMBG are useful in preventing hypoglycemia and hyperglycemia by adjusting drug therapy, diet therapy, and physical activity. Teach patients to assess blood glucose frequently for these situations:

- Symptoms of hypoglycemia or hyperglycemia
- Hypoglycemic unawareness
- Periods of illness
- Before and after exercise
- Gastroparesis
- Adjustment of antidiabetes drugs
- Evaluation of other drug therapies (e.g., steroids)
- Pregnancy

Techniques for SMBG follow principles that are the same as for most self-monitoring systems. Meter systems now require a very

PATIENT AND FAMILY EDUCATION: PREPARING FOR SELF-MANAGEMENT

Subcutaneous Insulin Administration

With Vial and Syringe

- Wash your hands.
- Inspect the bottle for the type of insulin and the expiration date.
- Gently roll the bottle of intermediate-acting insulin in the palms of your hands to mix the insulin.
- Clean the rubber stopper with an alcohol swab.
- Remove the needle cover and pull back the plunger to draw air into the syringe. The amount of air should be equal to the insulin dose. Push the needle through the rubber stopper and inject the air into the insulin bottle.
- Turn the bottle upside down and draw the insulin dose into the syringe.
- Remove air bubbles in the syringe by tapping on the syringe or injecting air back into the bottle. Redraw the correct amount.
- Make certain the tip of the plunger is on the line for your dose of insulin. Magnifiers are available to assist in measuring accurate doses of insulin.
- Remove the needle from the bottle. Recap the needle if the insulin is not to be given immediately.
- Select a site within your injection area that has not been used in the past month.
- Clean your skin with an alcohol swab. Lightly grasp an area of skin and insert the needle at a 90-degree angle.
- Push the plunger all the way down. This will push the insulin into your body. Release the pinched skin.
- Pull the needle straight out quickly. Do not rub the place where you gave the shot.
- Dispose of the syringe and needle without recapping in a puncture-proof container.

With a Pen Device

- Wash your hands.
- Check the drug label to be sure it is what was prescribed.
- Remove the cap.
- Look at the insulin to be sure it is evenly mixed if it contains NPH and that there is no clumping of particles.
- Wipe the tip of the pen where the needle will attach with an alcohol swab.
- Remove the protective pull tab from the needle and screw it onto the pen until snug.
- Remove both the plastic outer cap and inner needle cap.
- Look at the dose window and turn the dosage knob to the appropriate dose.
- Holding the pen with the needle pointing upward, press the button until at least a drop of insulin appears. This is the "cold shot," "air shot," or "safety shot." Repeat this step if needed until a drop appears.
- Dial the number of units needed.
- Hold the pen perpendicular to and against the intended injection site with your thumb on the dosing knob.
- Press the dosing knob slowly all the way to dispense the dose.
- Hold the pen in place for 6 to 10 seconds, then withdraw from the skin.
- Replace the outer needle cap; unscrew until the needle is removed, and dispose of the needle in a hard plastic or metal container.
- Replace the cap on the insulin pen.

by hematocrit values (anemia falsely elevates glucose values; polycythemia falsely depresses them) and may be unreliable in the hypoglycemic or severely hyperglycemic ranges.

Accuracy of the blood glucose monitor is ensured when the manufacturer's directions are followed. Common user errors involve failure to obtain a sufficient blood drop, poor storage of test strips, using expired strips, and not changing the code number on the meter to match the strip bottle code. Meter selection is based on cost of the meter and strips, ease of use, and availability of repair and servicing. Provide training, explain and demonstrate procedures, assess visual acuity, and check the patient's ability to perform the procedure using "teach-back" strategies. Newer meters have fewer steps, include error signals for inadequate sample size, and can store hundreds of SMBG results.

Accuracy and precision vary widely among capillary blood glucose monitoring devices. If the meter requires calibration, teach patients to properly calibrate the machine. Instruct them to recheck the calibration and retest if they obtain a test result that is unusual for them and whenever they are in doubt about test accuracy. Continued retraining of patients performing SMBG helps ensure accurate results because performance accuracy deteriorates over time. Laboratory glucose determinations are more accurate than SMBG.

Frequency of testing varies with the drug schedules, the patient's prescribed therapy, and his or her expected target outcomes. Patients taking multiple insulin injections or using insulin pump therapy may need to monitor glucose levels three or more times daily. For patients taking less-frequent injections of insulin, noninsulin therapy, or diet therapy alone, daily SMBG is useful for evaluation of therapy.

Blood glucose therapy target goals for self-management are set individually for each patient based on duration of disease, age and life expectancy, other chronic conditions, severity of cardiovascular disease, and presence of hypoglycemia unawareness (Faminu, 2018). The health care team works with him or her to reach target blood glucose levels. Recommendations for patients with type 1 DM include an A1C value less than 7%, premeal glucose levels of 70 to 130 mg/dL (3.9 to 7.2 mmol/L), and postmeal glucose levels less than 180 mg/dL (10.0 mmol/L) (ADA, 2019d). However, looser target ranges may be prescribed on the basis of age, cognitive impairment, and other health problems.

Infection control measures are needed for SMBG. The chance of becoming infected from blood glucose monitoring processes is reduced by handwashing before monitoring and by not reusing lancets. *Instruct patients to not share their blood glucose monitoring equipment* because infection can be spread by the lancet holder even when the lancet itself has been changed Regular cleaning of the meter is critical for infection control. Remind staff who perform blood glucose testing and family members who help with testing to wear gloves.

Many meters allow data to be downloaded to a computer or smart phone. Some meters allow entry of additional data such as insulin dose, amounts of carbohydrate eaten, or exercise. A radio link to an insulin pump allows automatic transfer of glucose readings to a calculator that helps the patient decide on an appropriate insulin dose. Some patients use smart phone applications to record and trend or graph serial

small blood sample, which allows for alternate testing sites (e.g., arm, thigh, hand). The selected site is pricked, a drop is drawn into a testing strip or disk impregnated with chemicals, and the glucose value is displayed or "spoken" (in mg/dL or mmol/L) on a screen.

Data obtained from SMBG are evaluated along with other A1C levels or periodic laboratory blood glucose test results. Even when SMBG is performed correctly, the results are affected blood glucose levels, insulin dosages, food intake, and other data.

Once the patient learns the technical aspects of meter use, help him or her use the results of SMBG to achieve glycemic control. Postmeal glucose monitoring provides information about the effects of the size and content of their meals. SMBG allows the patient to assess effects of exercise on glucose control and provides critical information to help patients who take insulin to exercise safely. Teach patients how to make agreed-on adjustments in the treatment plan when SMBG results are consistently out of range for a 3-day period when no change in meal plan, drugs, or activity has occurred.

Alternate site testing uses blood obtained from sites other than the fingertip and is available on many meters and meter-smart phone interfaces. Older meters have wider variation between fingertip and alternate sites, and variation is most evident during times when glucose levels change rapidly. Teach patients about the lag time for blood glucose levels between the fingertip and other sites when blood glucose levels are changing rapidly and that the fingertip reading is the only safe choice at those times.

! NURSING SAFETY PRIORITY (QSEN)

Action Alert

Teach patients with a history of hypoglycemic unawareness *not* to test at alternative sites.

Continuous blood glucose monitoring (CGM) systems monitor glucose levels in interstitial fluid to provide real-time glucose information to the user. Many systems consist of three parts: a disposable sensor that measures glucose levels, a transmitter that is attached to the sensor, and a receiver that displays and stores glucose information. After an initiation or warm-up period, the sensor gives glucose values every 1 to 5 minutes. Sensors may be used for 3 to 7 days, depending on the manufacturer. CGM provides information about the current blood glucose level, short-term feedback about results of treatment, and warnings when glucose readings become dangerously high or low. Most available sensors require at least two capillary glucose readings per day for calibration of the sensor. Sensor accuracy depends on these calibrations. There may be a lag time between the capillary glucose measurement and the glucose sensor value. If the blood glucose value is changing rapidly, the time between capillary and interstitial glucose values may be as long as 30 minutes. For this reason, capillary glucose readings need to be checked on all extreme values or if symptoms of hypoglycemia are present before any corrective treatment is given. *With older or less sophisticated systems, give insulin only after confirming the results of any continuous glucose monitoring system.*

Nutrition therapy. Effective self-management of DM requires that *nutrition*, including the meal plan, education, and counseling programs, be individualized for each patient. A registered dietitian nutritionist (RDN) is a member of the interprofessional team. The nurse, RDN, patient, and family work together on a realistic and flexible meal plan. Plans that consider the patient's cultural background, financial status, and lifestyle are more likely to be successful. The desired outcomes of nutrition and diet therapy are listed in Table 59.9.

TABLE 59.9   Desired Outcomes of Nutrition Therapy for the Patient With Diabetes

- Achieving and maintaining blood glucose levels in the normal range or as close to normal as is safely possible
- Achieving and maintaining a blood lipid profile that reduces the risk for cardiovascular disease
- Achieving blood pressure levels in the normal range or as close to normal as is safely possible
- Preventing or slowing the rate of development of the chronic complications of diabetes by modifying nutrient intake and lifestyle
- Addressing patient *nutrition* needs, taking into account personal and cultural preferences and willingness to change
- Maintaining the pleasure of eating by limiting food choices only when indicated by scientific evidence
- Meeting the *nutrition* needs of unique times of the life cycle, particularly for pregnant and lactating women and for older adults with diabetes
- Providing self-management training for patients treated with insulin or insulin stimulators for exercising safely, including the prevention and treatment of hypoglycemia and managing diabetes during acute illness

Principle of medical nutrition or Medical Nutrition Management (MNT) is recommended for use with all adults with DM. For overweight or obese adults with type 2 DM, even modest weight loss through reduced caloric intake is beneficial. Blood pressure, blood glucose levels, and lipid profiles are improved by weight loss (ADA, 2019d).

The RDN develops a meal plan based on the patient's usual food intake, weight management goals, and lipid and blood glucose patterns. Consistency in the daily timing and amount of food eaten helps control blood glucose. Patients using insulin therapy need to eat at times that are coordinated with the timed action of insulin. Teach patients using intense insulin therapy to adjust premeal insulin to allow for timing and quantity changes in their meal plan.

No specific percentage of calories from carbohydrates, protein, or fat is ideal for all adults with DM. Recommendations for the distribution of these nutrients is individualized based on food preferences, eating patterns, and metabolic goals (ADA, 2019e; Watts & Howard, 2016).

Carbohydrate intake avoids nutrient deficient sources ("empty calories") and focuses on sources from vegetables, fruits, whole grains, legumes, and dairy products. Adults with diabetes should eat at least 25 g of fiber daily. Teach patients with DM or prediabetes to avoid sugar-sweetened beverages (including high fructose corn syrup) and sucrose to prevent weight gain and adverse effects on metabolism.

Dietary fat and cholesterol intake for adults with DM focuses on the quality of fat rather than on the quantity of fat. A Mediterranean-style diet rich in monounsaturated fatty acids (MUFAs) can lower cardiac risk factors. Such diets include avocados, nuts and seeds, olives, and dark chocolate. Omega-3 fatty acids, including EPA (eicosapentaenoic acid) and DHA (docosahexaenoic acid) from fish or fish oil supplements are recommended as part of a healthy diet to prevent heart disease, as is ALA (alpha-linolenic acid) derived from plant sources. Current recommendations from the ADA to limit *trans* fats, saturated fats, and cholesterol are the same as for the general population (ADA, 2019a; ADA 2019e).

Alcohol consumption affects blood glucose levels, especially with high alcohol use or when DM is poorly controlled. Teach patients that two alcoholic beverages for men and one for women can be ingested with, and in addition to, the usual meal plan. (One alcoholic beverage equals 12 ounces of beer, 5 ounces of wine, or 1½ ounces of distilled spirits.) The risk for delayed hypoglycemia is increased when drug therapy includes insulin or an insulin stimulator.

! NURSING SAFETY PRIORITY (QSEN)

Action Alert

Because of the potential for alcohol-induced delayed hypoglycemia, instruct the patient with DM to ingest alcohol only with or shortly after meals. Even with this precaution patients must remain alert for delayed hypoglycemia following alcohol ingestion.

Patient education for nutrition is based each patient's **nutrition** recommendations that consider blood glucose monitoring results, total blood lipid levels, and A1C levels. These tests help determine whether current meal and exercise patterns need adjustment or whether present habits need reinforcement. A specific nutrition prescription is developed for each patient.

Reinforce nutrition information provided by the RDN. The patient with DM must understand how to adjust food intake during illness, planned exercise, social occasions, and when the usual time of eating is delayed. Share dietary information with the person who prepares the meals. The RDN sees each patient yearly to identify changes in lifestyle and make appropriate diet therapy changes. Some patients, such as those with weight-control problems or low incomes, may need more frequent dietary evaluation and counseling.

Carbohydrate (CHO) counting is a simple approach to **nutrition** and meal planning that uses label information of the nutritional content of packaged food items. Estimation of CHO content when dining out can be taught by the RDN. Because fat and protein have little effect on after-meal blood glucose levels, CHO counting focuses on the nutrient that has the greatest impact on these levels. It uses total grams of CHO, regardless of the food source. This method is effective in achieving blood glucose control when daily CHO intake is consistent.

Patients using intensive insulin or pump therapies can use CHO counting to determine insulin coverage. After the amount of insulin needed to cover the usual meal is determined, insulin may be added or subtracted for changes in CHO intake. An initial formula of 1 unit of rapid-acting insulin for each 15 g of CHO provides flexibility to meal plans. The patient determines the grams of CHO in a specific meal or snack by reading labels or weighing and measuring each item. The total grams of CHO are used to calculate the bolus dose of insulin based on the prescribed insulin-to-carbohydrate ratio.

Special considerations for type 1 diabetes include developing insulin regimens that conform to the patient's preferred meal routines, food preferences, and exercise patterns. Patients using rapid-acting insulin by injection or an insulin pump must learn to adjust insulin doses based on the CHO content of the meals and snacks. Insulin-to-carbohydrate ratios are developed and are used to provide mealtime insulin doses. Blood glucose monitoring before and 2 hours after meals determines whether the insulin-to-carbohydrate ratio is correct. For patients who are on fixed insulin regimens and do not adjust premeal insulin dosages, consistency in the timing of meals and the amount of CHO eaten at each meal is critical to prevent hypoglycemia.

Exercise can cause hypoglycemia if insulin is not decreased before activity. For planned exercise, hypoglycemia is prevented by a reduction in insulin dosage. For unplanned exercise, intake of additional CHO is usually needed. A 70-kg adult would need about 10 to 15 g additional CHO per hour of moderate-intensity activity. More CHO is needed for intense activity.

It is important for patients using insulin to avoid weight gain. Hyperinsulinemia (chronic high blood insulin levels) can occur with intensive management schedules and may result in weight gain. These patients may need to manage hyperglycemia by restricting calories rather than increasing insulin. Weight gain can be minimized by following the prescribed meal plan, getting regular exercise, and avoiding overtreatment of hypoglycemia.

Special considerations for type 2 DM focus on lifestyle changes. Many patients with type 2 DM are overweight and insulin resistant. **Nutrition** therapy stresses lifestyle changes that reduce calories eaten and increase calories expended through physical activity. Many patients also have abnormal blood fat levels and hypertension (metabolic syndrome), making reductions of saturated fat, cholesterol, and sodium desirable. A moderate caloric restriction (250 to 500 calories less daily) and an increase in physical activity improve *glucose regulation* and weight control. Decreases of more than 10% of body weight can significantly improve A1C.

When patients with type 2 DM need insulin, consistency in timing and CHO content of meals is important. Division of the total daily calories into three meals or into smaller meals and snacks is based on patient preference.

👤 PATIENT-CENTERED CARE: OLDER ADULT CONSIDERATIONS (QSEN)

Factors that increase the risk for poor **nutrition** in older adults with DM include dental issues, finances, changes in appetite, and changes in the ability to obtain and prepare food. Older adults may have reduced awareness of hypoglycemia and hyperglycemia and dehydration, increasing the risk for hyperglycemic-hyperosmolar state (HHS) (Touhy & Jett, 2020). They may eat out or live in situations in which they have little control over meal preparation. Visits by home health nurses can help older patients follow a diabetic meal plan.

Changing the eating habits of 60 to 70 years is difficult and requires a realistic approach. The nurse, RDN, and patient assess the patient's usual eating patterns. Teach the older patient taking antidiabetic drugs the importance of eating meals and snacks at the same time every day and eating the same amount of food from day to day.

Exercise therapy. Regular exercise is an essential part of DM management and improves carbohydrate metabolism and insulin sensitivity. Increased physical activity and weight loss reduce the risk for type 2 DM in patients with prediabetes.

Plasma glucose levels remain stable during exercise in adults without DM because of the balance between glucose use by exercising muscles and glucose production by the liver. The patient with type 1 DM cannot make the hormonal changes needed to maintain stable blood glucose levels during exercise. Without an adequate insulin supply, cells cannot use glucose. Low insulin levels trigger release of glucagon and epinephrine (balancing hormones) to increase liver glucose production, further raising blood glucose levels. Without insulin, FFAs become the source of energy. Exercise in the patient with uncontrolled DM results in hyperglycemia and ketone body formation. Prolonged elevated blood glucose levels occur after vigorous exercise.

Exercise also can cause hypoglycemia because of increased muscle glucose uptake and inhibited glucose release from the liver during exercise and for up to 24 hours after exercise. Replacement of muscle and liver glycogen stores, along with increased insulin sensitivity after exercise, causes insulin requirements to drop.

Benefits of exercise include better blood **glucose regulation** and reduced insulin requirements for patients with type 1 DM. Exercise also increases insulin sensitivity, which enhances cell uptake of glucose and promotes weight loss.

Regular exercise decreases risk for cardiovascular disease. It decreases most blood lipid levels and increases high-density lipoproteins (HDLs, the "good" cholesterol). Exercise decreases blood pressure and improves cardiac function. Regular physical activity prevents or delays type 2 DM by reducing body weight, insulin resistance, and glucose intolerance.

👤 PATIENT-CENTERED CARE: OLDER ADULT CONSIDERATIONS (QSEN)

The ability of the heart and lungs to deliver oxygen to organs declines with age. Muscle strength declines gradually. Range of motion and flexibility decrease, altering gait and increasing the risk for falls. Remaining active can limit loss of muscle mass and function.

Changes in activity levels should be gradual. Formal evaluation by a physical therapist may be needed. Emphasize that the focus for any activity program is on changing sedentary behavior to active behavior at any level. Encourage sedentary older adults to begin with low-intensity physical activity. Start low-intensity activities in short sessions (less than 10 minutes); include warm-up and cool-down components with active stretching.

Exercise adjustments are needed when some long-term DM complications are present. Vigorous aerobic or resistance exercise should be avoided in the presence of diabetic retinopathy. Teach the patient with retinopathy about activities that increase blood pressure. Heavy lifting, rapid head motion, or jarring activities can cause vitreous hemorrhage or retinal detachment. Decreased sensation in the extremities increases the risk for skin breakdown and joint damage. Teach patients with peripheral neuropathy to wear proper footwear and examine their feet daily for lesions or injury. Teach anyone with a foot injury or open sore to engage in non–weight-bearing activities such as swimming, bicycling, or arm exercises. Those with autonomic neuropathy are at increased risk for exercise-induced injury from poor temperature control, postural hypotension, and impaired thirst with risk for dehydration. Encourage high-risk patients to start with short periods of low-intensity exercise and to increase the intensity and duration slowly. Patient conditions that often require activity adjustment include:

- Uncontrolled hypertension
- Severe autonomic neuropathy
- Severe peripheral neuropathy or foot lesions
- Unstable proliferative retinopathy

In the absence of contraindications, advise adults with DM to perform at least 150 minutes per week of moderate-intensity aerobic physical activity divided into 3 days (ADA, 2019e). Teach patients to avoid going more than 2 consecutive days without aerobic physical activity. Urge patients with type 2 DM to perform resistance exercise at least twice weekly, targeting all major muscle groups.

A 5- to 10-minute warm-up period with stretching and low-intensity exercise before exercise prepares the muscles, heart, and lungs for a progressive increase in exercise intensity. After exercising, a cool-down of at least 5 to 10 minutes is performed to gradually bring the heart rate down to pre-exercise level.

Guidelines for exercise are based on blood glucose levels and urine ketone levels. Teach patients to test blood glucose before exercise, at intervals during exercise, and after exercise to determine if it is safe to exercise, and to evaluate the effects of exercise. The absence of urine ketones indicates that enough insulin is available for glucose transport. *When urine ketones are present, the patient should **NOT** exercise.* Ketones indicate that current insulin levels are not adequate and that exercise would elevate blood glucose levels. Carbohydrate foods should be ingested to raise blood glucose levels above 100 mg/dL (5.6 mmol/L) before engaging in exercise. The Patient and Family Education: Preparing for Self-Management: Exercise box lists tips to teach about exercise.

❗ NURSING SAFETY PRIORITY (QSEN)
Action Alert

Teach patients with type 1 DM to perform vigorous exercise *only* when blood glucose levels are 100 to 250 mg/dL (5.6 to 13.8 mmol/L) and no ketones are present in the urine.

Blood glucose control in hospitalized patients. Hyperglycemia in hospitalized patients occurs from loss of **glucose regulation** caused by illness, decreased physical activity, withholding of antidiabetic drugs, use of drugs such as corticosteroids, and changes in nutrition therapy. Hyperglycemia is associated with poor outcomes.

Problems with hyperglycemia in hospitalized patients lead to higher infection rates, longer hospital stays, increased need for intensive care, and greater mortality. Admission glucose levels greater than 198 mg/dL (10.9 mmol/L) are linked with greater

PATIENT AND FAMILY EDUCATION: PREPARING FOR SELF-MANAGEMENT

Exercise

- Remember that exercise helps control blood glucose levels and blood lipid levels and helps reduce complications of diabetes.
- Perform level of exercise recommended to you by your diabetes health care provider.
- Wear appropriate footwear designed for exercise.
- Examine your feet daily and after exercising.
- Stay hydrated and do not exercise in extreme heat or cold.
- Do not exercise within 1 hour of insulin injection or near time of peak insulin action.
- Prevent hypoglycemia during exercise by:
  - Do not exercise unless blood glucose level is at least 80 and less than 250 mg/dL.
  - Have a carbohydrate snack before exercising if 1 hour has passed since the last meal or if the planned exercise is of high intensity.
  - Carry a simple sugar to eat during exercise if symptoms of hypoglycemia occur.
- Carry identification information about diabetes during exercise.
- Check your blood glucose levels more often on days you exercise and remember that extra carbohydrate and less insulin may be needed during the 24-hour period following exercise.

risk for mortality and complications. Hypoglycemia, defined as blood glucose values lower than 40 mg/dL (2.2 mmol/L), also is a risk factor for mortality.

Current guidelines recommend treatment protocols that maintain blood glucose levels between 140 and 180 mg/dL (7.8 and 10.0 mmol/L) for critically ill patients. For most non–critically ill patients, premeal glucose targets are lower than 140 mg/dL (7.8 mmol/L), with random blood glucose values less than 180 mg/dL (10.0 mmol/L). To prevent hypoglycemia, insulin regimens are reviewed if blood glucose levels fall below 100 mg/dL (5.6 mmol/L) and are modified when blood glucose levels are less than 70 mg/dL (3.9 mmol/L) (ADA, 2019d).

Continuous IV insulin solutions are the most effective method for achieving glycemic targets in the intensive care setting. Scheduled subcutaneous injection with basal, meal, and correction elements is used to maintain glucose control in non–critically ill patients. Use of correction dose or "supplemental insulin" to correct premeal hyperglycemia in addition to scheduled prandial and basal insulin is determined by the patient's insulin sensitivity and current blood glucose level.

Prevention of hypoglycemia is also part of managing blood glucose levels. Causes of inpatient hypoglycemia include an inappropriate insulin type, mismatch between insulin type and/or timing of food intake, and altered eating plan without insulin dosage adjustment. Many facilities have protocols for hypoglycemia treatment that direct staff to provide carbohydrate replacement if the patient is alert and able to swallow or to administer concentrated dextrose IV or glucagon by subcutaneous injection if the patient cannot swallow, using the 15-15 Rule (see the Nutrition Therapy section under the Interventions for Preventing Hypoglycemia heading later in this chapter for specific 15-15 rule interventions). There is confusion about

whether to give or to hold insulin from a patient who is NPO. Giving rapid-acting or short-acting insulin, as well as amylin and incretin mimetics, will cause hypoglycemia if a patient is not eating. Basal insulin (often at a reduced dose) should be given when the patient is NPO because it controls baseline glucose levels. Insulin mixtures are not given because they contain some short-acting or rapid-acting insulin and will cause hypoglycemia.

Surgical Management. The most common surgical intervention for DM is pancreas transplantation. When successful, this procedure eliminates the need for insulin injections, blood glucose monitoring, and many dietary restrictions. It can eliminate the acute complications related to blood *glucose regulation* but is only partially successful in reversing long-term complications. Pancreatic transplant is successful when the patient no longer needs insulin therapy and all blood measures of glucose are normal.

Transplantation requires lifelong drug therapy to prevent graft rejection. These drug regimens have side effects that restrict their use to patients who have serious progressive complications from DM. Some antirejection drugs increase blood glucose levels. A pancreas-alone transplant is most often considered for patients with severe metabolic complications and for those with consistent failure of insulin-based therapy to prevent acute complications.

Pancreas transplantation is considered in patients with DM and end-stage kidney disease (ESKD) who have had or plan to have a kidney transplant. Pancreas graft survival is better when performed at the time of the kidney transplant. Pancreatic transplantation may be performed as a pancreas transplant alone (PTA), pancreas after kidney transplant (PAK), and simultaneous pancreas and kidney transplant (SPK).

The 1-year survival rate for patients receiving a whole pancreas in North America is above 95%, with most patients remaining free of insulin injection and diet restrictions. The degree of HLA tissue-type matching affects the results.

Operative procedures. Most pancreatic transplants involve cadaver donors using a whole pancreas still attached to the exit of the pancreatic duct. The recipient's pancreas is left in place, and the donated pancreas is placed in the pelvis. The insulin released by the pancreas graft is secreted into the bloodstream. The new pancreas also produces about 800 to 1000 mL of fluid daily, which is diverted to either the bladder or the bowel.

Excretion of pancreatic fluids can impair *fluid and electrolyte balance*, and drainage of these fluids into the urinary bladder causes irritation. When the pancreas is attached to the bladder, the loss of fluid rich in bicarbonate may cause acidosis.

Rejection management. Pancreatic transplantation requires a combination of drugs to reverse and prevent rejection. Patients undergoing antirejection therapy first receive drugs to prevent viral, bacterial, and fungal infection because of the risk for opportunistic infections from overall reduced *immunity*. When the regimen includes steroid therapy the patient will require dosage adjustments in insulin to achieve desired levels of glucose control. Long-term antirejection therapy reduces *immunity* and increases the risk for infection, cancer, and atherosclerosis.

Enhancing Surgical Recovery

Planning: Expected Outcomes. The patient with DM undergoing a surgical procedure is expected to recover completely without complications.

Interventions. The patient with DM is at higher risk for complications. Anesthesia and surgery cause a stress response with release of counterregulatory hormones that elevate blood glucose by suppressing insulin action and increasing the risk for ketoacidosis. Hyperglycemic-hyperosmolar state (HHS) is a complication of surgery and is associated with increased mortality. Diuresis from hyperglycemia can cause dehydration and increases the risk for acute kidney injury.

Complications of DM increase the risk for surgical problems. Patients with DM are at higher risk for hypertension, ischemic heart disease, cerebrovascular disease, myocardial infarction (MI), and cardiomyopathy. The patient with DM is at risk for acute kidney injury and urinary retention after surgery, especially if he or she has albumin in the urine (indicator of kidney damage). Nerve function to the intestinal wall and sphincters can be reduced, leading to delayed gastric emptying and reflux of gastric acid, which increases the risk for aspiration with anesthesia. Autonomic neuropathy may cause paralytic ileus after surgery.

Preoperative Care. Before surgery, blood glucose levels are optimized to reduce the risk for complications. Sulfonylureas are discontinued 1 day before surgery. Metformin is stopped at least 24 hours before surgery and restarted only after kidney function is documented as normal. All other oral drugs are stopped the day of surgery. Patients taking long-acting insulin may need to be switched to intermediate-acting insulin forms 1 to 2 days before surgery.

Preoperative blood glucose levels should be less than 200 mg/dL (11.1 mmol/L). Higher levels are associated with increased infection rates and impaired wound healing.

Intraoperative Care. IV infusion of insulin, glucose, and potassium is standard therapy for perioperative management of DM, and infusion rates are based on hourly capillary glucose testing. The object is to keep the glucose level between 140 and 180 mg/dL (7.8 and 10.0 mmol/L) during surgery to prevent hypoglycemia and reduce risks from hyperglycemia. Higher insulin doses may be needed because stress releases glucagon and epinephrine. Patients usually receive about 5 g of glucose per hour during surgery to prevent hypoglycemia, ketosis, and protein breakdown.

Postoperative Care. Hyperglycemia leads to increased mortality after surgical procedures. American Association of Clinical Endocrinologists (AACE) and ADA guidelines recommend insulin dosing to maintain blood glucose between 140 and 180 mg/dL (7.8 and 10.0 mmol/L) for critically ill patients (ADA, 2019d).

Continue glucose and insulin infusions as prescribed until the patient is stable and can tolerate oral feedings. Short-term insulin therapy may be needed after surgery for the patient who usually uses oral agents. For those receiving insulin therapy, dosage adjustments may be required until the stress of surgery subsides.

Opioid analgesics slow GI motility and alter blood glucose levels. The older patient who receives opioids is at risk for confusion, paralytic ileus, hypoventilation, hypotension, and urinary retention. Patient-controlled analgesia (PCA) systems reduce respiratory complications and confusion. (See Chapter 5 for pain interventions and Chapter 9 for general preoperative care.)

Monitoring. Patients with autonomic neuropathy or vascular disease need close monitoring to avoid hypotension or respiratory arrest. Those who take beta blockers for hypertension need close monitoring for hypoglycemia because these drugs mask symptoms of hypoglycemia. Patients with increased blood protein or nitrogen in the blood may have problems with fluid management. Check central venous pressure or pulmonary artery pressure as needed.

Balancing hormones are often activated and cause increased blood glucose levels before patients become febrile. *Hyperglycemia often occurs before a fever.*

> **! NURSING SAFETY PRIORITY** (QSEN)
> ### Action Alert
>
> When a patient who has had reasonably controlled blood glucose levels in the hospital develops an unexpected rise in blood glucose values, check for wound infection.

Fluid and electrolyte balance is often disrupted by surgery. *Hyperkalemia* (high blood potassium level) is common in patients with mild to moderate kidney failure and can lead to cardiac dysrhythmia. In other patients, *hypokalemia* (low blood potassium level) may occur and be made worse by insulin and glucose given during surgery. Monitor the cardiac rhythm and serum potassium values.

Cardiovascular monitoring by continuous ECG is often used for older patients with DM, those with long-standing type 1 DM, and those with heart disease. Patients with DM are at higher risk for MI after surgery. Changes in ECG or potassium level may indicate a silent MI.

Kidney monitoring, especially observing fluid balance, helps detect acute kidney injury. Management of infections may require the use of nephrotoxic antibiotics. Ensure adequate hydration when these drugs are used. Check for impending kidney failure by assessing *fluid and electrolyte balance.*

Nutrition. Patients requiring clear or full liquid diets should receive about 200 g of carbohydrate daily in equally divided amounts at meals and snack times. Initial liquids should *not* be sugar free. Most patients require 25 to 35 calories per kg of body weight every 24 hours. After surgery, food intake is initiated as quickly as possible, with progression from clear liquids to solid foods occurring as rapidly as tolerated to promote healing and metabolic balance. When oral foods are tolerated, make sure the patient eats at least 150 to 200 g of carbohydrate daily to prevent hypoglycemia.

If total parenteral nutrition (TPN) is used after surgery, severe hyperglycemia may occur. Monitor blood glucose often to determine the need for supplemental insulin.

Preventing Injury From Peripheral Neuropathy

Planning: Expected Outcomes. The patient with DM is expected to identify factors that increase the risk for injury, practice proper foot care, and maintain intact skin on the feet.

Interventions. Patients with DM need intensive education about foot care because foot injury is a common complication. Once a failure of *tissue integrity* has occurred and an ulcer has developed, there is an increased risk for wound progression that may eventually lead to amputation. Most lower extremity

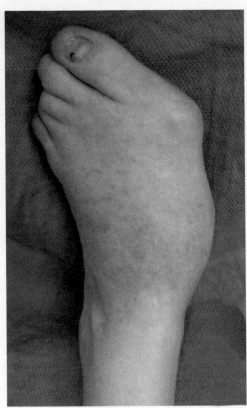

FIG. 59.7 "Charcot foot" type of diabetic foot deformity. (From Frykberg, R.G., Zgonis, T., Armstrong, D.G., Driver, V.R., Giurini, J.M., Kravitz, S.R., et al. [2006]. Diabetic foot disorders: A clinical practice guideline—2006 revision. *The Journal of Foot and Ankle Surgery, 45*[5], S1-S66.)

TABLE 59.10   Foot Risk Categories

Risk Categories	Management Categories
Risk Category 0 • Has protective sensation • No evidence of peripheral vascular disease • No evidence of foot deformity or loss of *tissue integrity*	**Management Category 0** • Comprehensive foot examination once a year • Patient education to include advice on appropriate footwear
Risk Category 1 • Does not have protective sensation • May have evidence of foot deformity	**Management Category 1** • Evaluation every 3-6 months • Consider referral to a specialist to assess need for specialized treatment and follow-up • Patient education
Risk Category 2 • Does not have protective sensation • Evidence of peripheral vascular disease	**Management Categories 2 and 3** • Evaluation every 1-3 months • Referral to a specialist • Prescription footwear • Consider vascular consultation for combined follow-up • Patient education
Risk Category 3 • History of ulcer or amputation	

amputations in adults with DM are preceded by foot ulcers, and the 5-year mortality rate after leg or foot amputation is high (CDC, 2020). Neuropathy is the main factor for development of a diabetic ulcer, and inadequate *perfusion* is the main cause of poor healing.

Motor neuropathy damages the nerves of foot muscles, resulting in foot deformities. These deformities create pressure points that gradually reduce *tissue integrity* with skin breakdown and ulceration. Thinning or shifting of the fat pad under the metatarsal heads decreases cushioning and increases areas of pressure. In claw toe deformity, toes are hyperextended and increase pressure on the metatarsal heads ("ball" of the foot). These changes predispose the patient to callus formation, ulceration, and infection. The *Charcot foot* is a type of diabetic foot deformity with many abnormalities, often including a *hallux valgus* (turning inward of the great toe) (Fig. 59.7). The foot is warm, swollen, and painful. Walking collapses the arch, shortens the foot, and gives the foot a "rocker bottom" shape.

Autonomic neuropathy causes loss of normal sweating and skin temperature regulation, resulting in dry, thinning skin. Skin cracks and fissures increase the infection risk. Sensory neuropathy may cause tingling or burning, but more often it produces numbness and reduced *sensory perception*. Without sensation, the patient does not notice injury and loss of *tissue integrity* in the foot. Peripheral arterial disease reduces blood flow to the foot, increasing the risk for ulcer formation and slowing ulcer healing (McCance et al., 2019).

Foot injuries are caused by walking barefoot, wearing ill-fitting shoes, sustaining thermal injuries from heat (e.g., hot water bottles, heating pads, baths), or chemical burns from over-the-counter corn treatments. These injuries lead to loss of *tissue integrity* and to amputation.

Ulcers result from continued pressure. Ulcers on the sole and ball of the foot are from standing or walking. Those on the top or sides of the foot usually are from shoes. The increased pressure causes calluses. Ulcers usually form over or around the great toe, under the metatarsal heads, and on the tops of claw toes.

Loss of *tissue integrity* with broken skin increases the risk for infection. Skin tends to break in areas of pressure. Infection is common in diabetic foot ulcers and, once present, is difficult to treat. Infection also impairs *glucose regulation*, leading to higher blood glucose levels and reduced *immunity*, which further increases the risk for infection.

Prevention of High-Risk Conditions. Neuropathy of the feet and legs can be delayed by keeping blood glucose levels near normal. Poor glucose control increases the risk for neuropathy and amputation. Urge smoking cessation to reduce the risk for vascular complications.

The risk for ulcers or amputation increases with duration of diabetes. Other risk factors are male gender; poor glucose control; and cardiovascular, retinal, or kidney complications. Foot-related risks include poor gait and stepping mechanics, peripheral neuropathy, increased pressure (callus, erythema, hemorrhage under a callus, limited joint mobility, foot deformities, or severe nail pathology), peripheral vascular disease, and a history of ulcers or amputation (ADA, 2019g).

Peripheral Neuropathy Management. Foot assessment techniques are listed in the Focused Assessment: The Diabetic Foot box. A thorough assessment of the feet should be performed by a health care professional at least annually. Table 59.10 lists foot risk categories.

FOCUSED ASSESSMENT
The Diabetic Foot

Assess the patient's risk for diabetic foot problems:
- History of previous ulcer
- History of previous amputation

Assess the foot for abnormal skin and nail conditions:
- Dry, cracked, fissured skin
- Ulcers
- Toenails: thickened, long nails; ingrown nails
- Tinea pedis; onychomycosis (mycotic nails)

Assess the foot for status of circulation:
- Symptoms of claudication
- Presence or absence of dorsalis pedis or posterior tibial pulse
- Prolonged capillary filling time (greater than 25 seconds)
- Presence or absence of hair growth on the top of the foot

Assess the foot for evidence of deformity:
- Calluses, corns
- Prominent metatarsal heads (metatarsal head is easily felt under the skin)
- Toe contractures: clawed toes, hammertoes
- Hallux valgus or bunions
- Charcot foot ("rocker bottom")

Assess the foot for loss of strength:
- Limited ankle joint range of motion
- Limited motion of great toe

Assess the foot for loss of protective sensation:
- Numbness, burning, tingling
- Semmes-Weinstein monofilament testing at 10 points on each foot

Data from American Diabetes Association (ADA). (2019g). Microvascular complications and foot care: Standards of medical care in diabetes—2019. *Diabetes Care, 42*(Suppl. 1), S124-S138.

PATIENT AND FAMILY EDUCATION: PREPARING FOR SELF-MANAGEMENT
Foot Care Instructions

- Inspect your feet daily, especially the area between the toes.
- Wash your feet daily with lukewarm water and soap. Dry thoroughly.
- Apply a moisturizer to your feet (but not between your toes) after bathing.
- Change into clean cotton socks every day.
- Do not wear the same pair of shoes 2 days in a row and wear only shoes made of breathable materials, such as leather or cloth.
- Check your shoes for foreign objects (nails, pebbles) before putting them on. Check inside the shoes for cracks or tears in the lining.
- Buy shoes that have plenty of room for your toes. Buy shoes later in the day, when feet are normally larger. Break in new shoes gradually.
- Wear socks to keep your feet warm.
- Trim your nails straight across with a nail clipper and smooth them with an emery board.
- See your diabetes health care provider immediately if you have blisters, sores, or infections. Protect the area with a dry, sterile dressing. Do not use tape to secure dressing to the skin.
- Do not treat blisters, sores, or infections with home remedies.
- Do not smoke or use nicotine products.
- Do not step into the bathtub without checking the temperature of the water with your wrist or thermometer.
- Do not use very hot or cold water. Never use hot-water bottles, heating pads, or portable heaters to warm your feet.
- Do not treat corns, blisters, bunions, calluses, or ingrown toenails yourself.
- Do not go barefooted.
- Do not wear sandals with open toes or straps between the toes.
- Do not cross your legs or wear garters or tight stockings that constrict blood flow.
- Do not soak your feet.

Data from American Diabetes Association (ADA). (2019g). Microvascular complications and foot care: Standards of medical care in diabetes—2019. *Diabetes Care, 42*(Suppl. 1), S124–S138.

Sensory examination of the foot with Semmes-Weinstein monofilaments is a practical measure of loss of sensation, which increases the risk for foot ulcers. The nylon monofilament is mounted on a holder standardized to exert a 10-g force. An adult who cannot feel the 10-g pressure at any point is at increased risk for ulcers. A diabetes health care provider most often performs this examination.

Footwear. Patients with any degree of peripheral neuropathy are at risk for loss of *tissue integrity* and need to wear protective shoes fitted by an experienced shoe fitter, such as a certified podiatrist. The shoe should be ½ to ⅝ inch longer than the longest toe. Heels should be less than 2 inches high. Tight shoes damage tissue. Instruct the patient to change shoes by midday and again in the evening. Socks must fit properly and be appropriate for the planned activity. Socks should feel soft and have no thick seams, creases, or holes. They should pad the foot and absorb excess moisture. White socks are recommended because the presence of blood or drainage is more easily recognized than on colored socks.

Teach patients to avoid tight stockings or those that have constricting bands. Patients with toe deformities need custom shoes with high, wide toe boxes and extra depth. Those with severely deformed feet need specially molded shoes. New shoes need a long break-in period with frequent foot inspection for irritation or blistering.

Foot care. Teach patients about preventive foot care and the need for examination of the feet and legs at each visit to a diabetes health care provider or primary health care provider. A mirror placed on the floor can help the patient visually examine the plantar surface of the foot. Identify patients with high-risk foot conditions. Explain problems caused by loss of protective sensation, the importance of monitoring the feet daily, proper care of the feet (including nail and skin care), and how to select appropriate footwear.

Assess the patient's ability to inspect all areas of the foot and to perform foot care. Teach family members how to inspect and care for the patient's feet using the guidelines in the Patient and Family Education: Preparing for Self-Management: Foot Care Instructions box if the patient is unable to do this independently.

Wound care. The standards of care for diabetic ulcers are a moist wound environment, débridement of necrotic tissue, and elimination of pressure (offloading). Eliminating pressure on an infected area is essential for wound healing. Teach patients with foot ulcers to not wear a shoe on the affected foot while the ulcer is healing. Those with poor *sensory perception* may keep walking on an ulcer because it does not hurt, causing pressure necrosis that delays healing and increases ulcer size. Pressure is reduced by specialized orthotic devices, custom-molded shoe inserts, or shoe adjustments that redistribute weight.

Offloading redistributes force away from ulcer sites and pressure points to wider areas of the foot. Available products include total-contact casting, half shoes, removable cast walkers, wheelchairs, and crutches. Total-contact casts redistribute pressure over the bottom of the foot. Casting material is molded to the foot and leg to spread pressure along the entire surface of contact, reducing vertical force. The almost complete elimination of motion of the total-contact cast reduces plantar shear forces. *Teach the patient that foot ulcers will recur unless weight is permanently redistributed.*

Reducing the Risk for Kidney Disease

Planning: Expected Outcomes. The patient with diabetes is expected to maintain a normal urine elimination pattern.

Interventions

Prevention. Diabetic kidney disease is more likely to develop in patients with poor blood glucose control. Progression to end-stage kidney disease can be delayed or prevented by normalizing blood pressure using drugs from either the angiotensin-converting enzyme inhibitor (ACEI) class or the angiotensin receptor blocker (ARB) class. Once used to "protect" the kidney, neither class of drug is recommended for patients with DM who have normal blood pressure and normal albumin excretion (ADA, 2019c). Hypertension greatly accelerates the progression of diabetic kidney disease.

Stress the need for evaluation of kidney function according to the ADA Standards of Care. An annual test to quantify urine albumin is performed for patients who have had type 1 DM for over 5 years and in all those with type 2 DM starting at diagnosis (ADA, 2019c). Persistent albuminuria in the range of 30 to 299 mg/24 hours is the earliest stage of nephropathy in type 1 DM and a marker for the development of nephropathy in type 2 DM.

Aggressive control of blood glucose, cholesterol levels, and hypertension in patients without albuminuria can avoid nephropathy. Once albuminuria develops, management focuses on controlling blood pressure and blood glucose and avoiding nephrotoxic agents.

Control of blood pressure, cholesterol, and blood glucose levels requires the patient's participation. Prescribed drugs must be taken according to schedules, and dietary restriction must be maintained. Educate patients about the roles of blood pressure and blood glucose levels in kidney disease. Teach them about maintaining normal blood glucose and cholesterol levels and keeping blood pressure levels below 140/80 mm Hg. Stress the need for yearly screening for albuminuria.

Smoking cessation is important in halting the progression of diabetic kidney disease. Teach the patient about the risks of smoking and refer him or her to appropriate resources for assistance in smoking cessation, as described in Chapter 24.

Drugs can affect kidney function either through toxic effects on the kidney or by an acute but reversible reduction in function. The most common prescribed nephrotoxic drugs are antifungal agents and aminoglycoside antibiotics. Other common nephrotoxic drugs are NSAIDs such as ibuprofen or naproxen. Teach the patient to check with his or her diabetes health care provider or a pharmacist before taking over-the-counter drugs or herbal remedies.

Radiocontrast media can also affect kidney function, especially in patients with preexisting kidney problems. Monitor IV hydration before and after a contrast agent is used, to prevent contrast-induced nephropathy in patients with DM.

Drug Therapy. Use of angiotensin-converting enzyme inhibitors (ACEIs) or angiotensin receptor blockers (ARBs) is recommended for all patients with persistent albuminuria or advanced stages of nephropathy (ADA, 2019c). ACE inhibitors reduce the level of albuminuria and the rate of progression of kidney disease, although they do not appear to prevent albuminuria. Monitor serum potassium levels for development of hyperkalemia (ADA, 2019c).

Dialysis for patients with DM and kidney failure is the same as for patients without diabetes (see Chapter 63). The dosage of insulin needs to be adjusted when dialysis starts.

NCLEX EXAMINATION CHALLENGE 59.5
Health Promotion and Maintenance

A client with diabetes who now has chronic albuminuria asks the nurse how this change will affect his health. How will the nurse answer this question?

A. "You will need to limit your intake of dietary albumin and other proteins to reduce the albuminuria."

B. "This change indicates beginning kidney problems and requires good blood glucose control to prevent more damage."

C. "Your risk for developing urinary tract infections is greatly increased, requiring the need to take daily antibiotics for prevention."

D. "From now on you will need to limit your fluid intake to just 1 L daily and completely avoid caffeine to protect your kidneys."

Preventing Complications from Hypoglycemia, Diabetic Ketoacidosis, and Hyperglycemic-Hyperosmolar Stage (HHS)

Planning: Expected Outcomes. The patient is expected to have blood glucose levels within the normal range, avoiding levels below 70 mg/dL (3.9 mmol/L) and never higher than 200 mg/dL (11.1 mmol/L).

Interventions for Preventing Hypoglycemia. Hypoglycemia is a low blood glucose level that induces specific symptoms and resolves when blood glucose concentration is raised. Once plasma glucose levels fall below 70 mg/dl (3.9 mmol/L), a sequence of events begins with release of counterregulatory hormones, stimulation of the autonomic nervous system, and production of *neurogenic* and *neuroglycopenic* symptoms. Peripheral autonomic symptoms, including sweating, irritability, tremors, anxiety, tachycardia, and hunger, serve as an early warning system and occur before the symptoms of confusion, paralysis, seizure, and coma occur from brain glucose deprivation. *Neuroglycopenic symptoms* occur when brain glucose *gradually declines* to a low level. *Neurologic symptoms* result from autonomic nervous activity triggered by a *rapid decline* in blood glucose (Table 59.11).

Central nervous system (CNS) function depends on a continuous supply of glucose in the blood. The brain cannot make glucose and stores only a few minutes' supply as glycogen. This needed supply is not maintained when the blood glucose level falls below critical levels.

TABLE 59.11 Symptoms of Hypoglycemia

Neuroglycopenic Symptoms	Neurogenic Symptoms
• Weakness	• Adrenergic:
• Fatigue	• Shaky or tremulous
• Difficulty thinking	• Heart pounding
• Confusion	• Nervous or anxious
• Behavior changes	• Cholinergic:
• Emotional instability	• Sweaty
• Seizures	• Hungry
• Loss of consciousness	• Tingling
• Brain damage	
• Death	

The first defense against falling blood glucose levels in the adult without DM is decreased insulin secretion, decreased glucose use, and increased glucose production. Normally, insulin secretion decreases when blood glucose levels drop to about 83 mg/dL (4.5 mmol/L). Balancing (counterregulatory) hormones are activated at about 67 mg/dL (3.7 mmol/L), a level above the threshold for symptoms of hypoglycemia. The main balancing hormone is glucagon. Both glucagon and epinephrine raise blood glucose levels by stimulating liver glycogen breakdown and conversion of protein to glucose. Epinephrine also limits insulin secretion.

Type 1 DM disrupts the body's response to hypoglycemia, usually within 1 to 5 years of diagnosis, because insulin comes from an injection rather than from the pancreas. As blood glucose levels fall after the injection, insulin levels do not decrease. Over time, the pancreas loses its ability to secrete glucagon in response to hypoglycemia. Eventually the response of epinephrine to falling blood glucose levels does not occur until the blood glucose level is very low, which greatly increases the risk for severe hypoglycemia.

A second problem with long-standing type 1 DM is *hypoglycemic unawareness,* in which patients no longer have the warning symptoms of early hypoglycemia that could prompt them to take preventive action. This problem occurs most often in patients who have had type 1 DM for 30 years or longer. Hypoglycemic unawareness also can occur in patients who have had type 2 DM for many years with a long-standing history of hypoglycemia.

The blood glucose level at which symptoms of hypoglycemia occur varies among patients. Thus clinical criteria used to categorize hypoglycemia are based on symptom severity rather than blood glucose levels. In mild hypoglycemia, the patient remains alert and able to self-manage symptoms. In severe hypoglycemia, neurologic function is so impaired that he or she needs another person's help to increase blood glucose levels.

Blood Glucose Management. Monitor blood glucose levels before giving antidiabetic drugs, before meals, before bedtime, and when the patient is symptomatic. All patients who take insulin, those taking long-acting insulin stimulators (glyburide), and those taking metformin in combination with glyburide are at risk for hypoglycemia. This risk is increased if they are older, have liver or kidney impairment, or are taking drugs that enhance the effects of antidiabetic drugs. In the hospital setting,

mealtime insulin *must* be coordinated with timely monitoring and food delivery to avoid episodes of hypoglycemia (Watts & Nemes, 2018). Blood glucose should be checked no more than 1 hour before a meal, and rapid-acting insulin given just before the meal to avoid hypoglycemia.

The most common causes of hypoglycemia are:
- Too much insulin compared with food intake and physical activity
- Insulin injected at the wrong time relative to food intake and physical activity
- The wrong type of insulin injected at the wrong time
- Decreased food intake resulting from missed or delayed meals
- Delayed gastric emptying from gastroparesis
- Decreased liver glucose production after alcohol ingestion
- Decreased insulin clearance due to progressive kidney failure

Nutrition Therapy. In hospitalized patients, most protocols for management of hypoglycemia follow the 15-15 rule for hypoglycemia management (Watts et al., 2020). With this rule, 15 g of CHO are given if the blood glucose level is less than 70 mg/dL (3.9 mmol/L) (or 30 g if less than 50 mg/dL [2.8 mmol/L]) or if the patient is experiencing symptoms of hypoglycemia. If the patient can swallow, give a liquid form of CHO, although any fast-acting CHO source can be used (avoid high-potassium options such as orange juice). If the blood glucose recheck within 15 minutes is still low, the same treatment is given again. If at any time the patient is unable to swallow, an IV dose of concentrated dextrose or subcutaneous glucagon is indicated. Specific recommendations are listed in the Patient and Family Education: Preparing for Self-Management box for management of hypoglycemia at home.

The blood glucose level determines the form and amount of glucose used. The response should be apparent in 10 to 20 minutes; however, test plasma glucose again in about 60 minutes because additional management may be needed. Fluid is absorbed much more quickly from the GI tract than are solids. Concentrated sweet fluids, such as chocolate, may slow absorption because of the fat content.

Management of hypoglycemia is most effective with ingestion of glucose or glucose-containing foods rather than foods containing complex carbohydrates. *Adding protein to CHO does not improve blood glucose response and does not prevent subsequent hypoglycemia.* Commercially available products provide predictable glucose absorption.

Drug Therapy. Subcutaneous or IM glucagon and concentrated IV dextrose are given to patients who cannot swallow. Glucagon is the main balancing hormone to insulin and is used as first-line therapy for severe hypoglycemia. Take care to prevent aspiration in patients receiving glucagon, because it often causes vomiting. Give concentrated dextrose carefully to avoid extravasation because it is hyperosmolar and can damage tissue. The effects of glucagon and dextrose are temporary. Evaluate response by monitoring blood glucose levels for several hours because symptoms may persist. A target blood glucose level is 70 to 110 mg/dL (3.9 to 6.2 mmol/L).

PATIENT AND FAMILY EDUCATION: PREPARING FOR SELF-MANAGEMENT

Management of Hypoglycemia at Home

For mild hypoglycemia (hungry, irritable, shaky, weak, headache, fully conscious; blood glucose usually less than 70 mg/dL [3.9 mmol/L]):

- Treat the symptoms of hypoglycemia with 15 g of carbohydrate. You may use one of these:
  - Glucose tablets or glucose gel (dosage is printed on the package)
  - A half cup (120 mL) of fruit juice or of regular (nondiet) soft drink
  - 8 ounces (240 mL) of skim milk
  - 6 to 10 hard candies
  - 4 cubes of sugar or 4 teaspoons of sugar
  - 6 saltines
  - 3 graham crackers
  - 1 tablespoon (15 mL) of honey or syrup
- Retest blood glucose in 15 minutes.
- Repeat this treatment if glucose remains less than 70 mg/dL (3.9 mmol/L). Symptoms may persist after blood glucose has normalized.
- Eat a small snack of carbohydrate and protein if your next meal is more than an hour away.

For moderate hypoglycemia (cold, clammy skin; pale; rapid pulse; rapid, shallow respirations; marked change in mood; drowsiness; blood glucose usually less than 40 mg/dL [2.2 mmol/L]):

- Treat the symptoms of hypoglycemia with 30 g of rapidly absorbed carbohydrate.
- Retest glucose in 15 minutes.
- Repeat treatment if glucose is less than 60 mg/dL (3.4 mmol/L).
- Eat additional food, such as low-fat milk, after 10 to 15 minutes.

For severe hypoglycemia (unable to swallow; unconsciousness or convulsions; blood glucose usually less than 20 mg/dL [1.0 mmol/L]):

- Treatment administered by family members:
  - Give prescribed dose of glucagon as intramuscular or subcutaneous injection.
  - Give a second dose in 10 minutes if the person remains unconscious.
  - Notify the diabetes health care provider immediately and follow instructions.
  - If still unconscious, transport the person to the emergency department.
  - Give a small meal when the person wakes up and is no longer nauseated.

❗ NURSING SAFETY PRIORITY (QSEN)

Critical Rescue

Assess patients to recognize the presence and severity of hypoglycemia. For the patient with *severe* hypoglycemia (unable to swallow, unconscious or convulsing, blood glucose usually less than 20 mg/dL [1.0 mmol/L]), respond by:
1. Giving prescribed dose of glucagon subcutaneously or IM.
2. Repeating the dose in 10 minutes if the patient remains unconscious
3. Notifying the diabetes health care provider immediately, and following instructions

---

Prevention Strategies. Teach the patient how to prevent hypoglycemia by avoiding its four common causes: (1) excess insulin, (2) deficient intake or absorption of food, (3) exercise when insulin action is peaking, and (4) alcohol intake.

Insulin excess from variable absorption of insulin can cause hypoglycemia even when insulin is injected correctly. Differences in insulin formulation can result in hypoglycemia.

Deficient food intake from inadequate or incorrectly timed meals can result in hypoglycemia. Educate about the importance of regular timing and quantity of food eaten, especially carbohydrates.

Exercise often causes blood glucose levels to fall. Prolonged exercise increases muscle glucose uptake for several hours after exercise. Teach the patient about blood glucose monitoring and carbohydrate consumption before and during exercise (if necessary). Also teach him or her to exercise at times when insulin activity is not peaking.

Alcohol inhibits liver glucose production and leads to hypoglycemia. It interferes with the hormone response to hypoglycemia and impairs glycogen breakdown. Instruct the patient to ingest alcohol only with or shortly *after* eating a meal with enough carbohydrate to prevent hypoglycemia.

Patient and Family Education. Help each patient develop a personal treatment plan for hypoglycemia. The exact glucose rise from a set amount of carbohydrate (CHO) varies; however, using the estimate that each 5 g of CHO raises blood glucose about 20 mg/dL is a good starting plan. For example, the patient may be directed to take:

- 20 to 30 g of CHO if the blood glucose level is 50 mg/dL (2.8 mmol/L) or less
- 10 to 15 g of CHO if the blood glucose level is 51 to 70 mg/dL (2.9 to 3.9 mmol/L)

Encourage the patient to wear a medical alert bracelet or have a wallet card describing how to manage diabetes emergencies. This information is helpful if the patient becomes hypoglycemic and is unable to perform self-care.

Teach the patient and family about the symptoms of hypoglycemia (see Table 59.11). Stress that delaying a meal for more than 30 minutes raises the risk for hypoglycemia when using some insulin regimens. Instruct him or her to keep a CHO source nearby at all times. Teach the patient and family how to inject glucagon. The changes in cognition associated with hypoglycemia may cause confusion among family members with those seen in severe hyperglycemia; review the differences in the common signs and symptoms of these two emergencies (Table 59.12).

👤 PATIENT-CENTERED CARE: OLDER ADULT CONSIDERATIONS (QSEN)

Older patients are at increased risk for hypoglycemia. Age-related declines in kidney function reduce the elimination of sulfonylureas and insulin, thus potentiating their hypoglycemic effects. Older adults have reduced epinephrine and glucagon release in response to low blood glucose levels and often have hypoglycemic unawareness. The presence of impaired motor skills when glucose is low reduces the ability to take steps to return glucose levels to normal.

Instruct the older patient's family to check blood glucose values when symptoms such as unsteadiness, light-headedness, poor concentration, trembling, or sweating occur (Touhy & Jett, 2020). Remind them to make sure that sufficient foods are eaten at appropriate times. Encourage a patient with a poor appetite to eat a small snack at bedtime to prevent hypoglycemia during the night.

TABLE 59.12 Differentiation of Hypoglycemia and Hyperglycemia

Feature	Hypoglycemia	Hyperglycemia
Skin	Cool, clammy, "sweaty"	Warm, dry, vasodilated
Dehydration	Absent	Present
Respirations	No particular or consistent change	Rapid, deep[a]; Kussmaul type; acetone odor (rotten "fruity" odor) to breath
Mental status	Anxious, nervous,[a] irritable, mental confusion,[a] seizures, coma	Varies from alert to stuporous, obtunded, or frank coma
Symptoms	Weakness,[a] double vision, blurred vision, hunger, tachycardia, palpitations	None specific for DKA Acidosis; hypercapnia; abdominal cramps, nausea and vomiting Dehydration: decreased neck vein filling, orthostatic hypotension, tachycardia, poor skin turgor
Glucose	<70 mg/dL (3.9 mmol/L)	>250 mg/dL (13.8 mmol/L)
Urine or blood ketones	Negative	Positive

DKA, Diabetic ketoacidosis.
[a]Classic symptoms.

Interventions for Preventing Diabetic Ketoacidosis.

Diabetic ketoacidosis (DKA) is a complication of diabetes characterized by uncontrolled hyperglycemia, metabolic acidosis, and increased production of ketones. This condition results from the combination of insulin deficiency and an increase in hormone release that leads to increased liver and kidney glucose production (Fig. 59.8). Laboratory diagnosis of DKA is shown in Table 59.13. All of these changes increase ketoacid production with resultant ketonemia and metabolic acidosis. The most common precipitating factor for DKA is infection. *Death occurs in up to 10% of these cases even with appropriate treatment.*

Hyperglycemia leads to osmotic diuresis with dehydration and electrolyte loss. Classic symptoms of DKA include polyuria, polydipsia, polyphagia, a rotting citrus fruit odor to the breath, vomiting, abdominal pain, dehydration, weakness, confusion, shock, and coma. Mental status can vary from total alertness to profound coma. As ketones rise, blood pH decreases, and acidosis occurs. Kussmaul respirations cause respiratory alkalosis in an attempt to correct metabolic acidosis by exhaling carbon dioxide. Initial serum sodium levels may be low or normal.

Blood Glucose Management. Monitor for symptoms of DKA (see Table 59.13 and Fig. 59.8). Document and use these findings to determine therapy effectiveness. *First assess the airway, level of consciousness, hydration status, electrolytes, and blood glucose level.* Check the patient's blood pressure, pulse, and respirations every 15 minutes until stable. Record urine output, temperature, and mental status every hour. When a central venous catheter is present, assess central venous pressure every 30 minutes or as prescribed. After treatment starts and these values are stable, monitor and record vital signs every 4 hours. Use blood glucose values to assess therapy and determine when to switch from saline to dextrose-containing solutions.

Fluid and Electrolyte Management. *Closely assess the patient's fluid and electrolyte balance.* Assess for acute weight loss, thirst, decreased skin turgor, dry mucous membranes, and oliguria with a high specific gravity. Assess for weak and rapid pulse, flat neck veins, increased temperature, decreased central venous pressure, muscle weakness, postural hypotension, and cool, clammy, and pale skin to determine if the patient is at risk for dehydration.

The first outcome of fluid therapy is to restore blood volume and maintain **perfusion** to vital organs. Typically initial infusion rates are 15 to 20 mL/kg/hr during the first hour.

The second outcome of replacing total body fluid losses is achieved more slowly. Usually hypotonic fluids are infused at 4 to 14 mL/kg/hr after the initial fluid bolus. When blood glucose levels reach 250 mg/dL (13.8 mmol/L), give 5% dextrose in 0.45% saline. This solution helps prevent hypoglycemia and cerebral edema, which can occur when serum osmolarity declines too rapidly.

During the first 24 hours of treatment, the patient needs enough fluids to replace the actual volume lost, as well as any ongoing losses, and the total may be as much as 6 to 10 L. Assess cardiac, kidney, and mental status to avoid fluid overload. Watch for symptoms of heart failure and pulmonary edema. Assess the status of fluid replacement by monitoring blood pressure, intake and output, and changes in daily weight.

Drug Therapy. Insulin therapy is used to lower serum glucose by about 50 to 75 mg/dL/hr (2.8 to 4.2 mmol/L/hr). Unless the episode of DKA is mild, regular insulin by continuous IV infusion is the usual management. An initial IV bolus dose is given, followed by an IV continuous infusion. Continuous insulin infusion is used because insulin half-life is short and subcutaneous insulin has a delayed onset of action (Fayfman et al., 2017). Subcutaneous insulin is started when the patient can take oral fluids and ketosis has stopped. DKA is considered resolved when blood glucose is less than 200 mg/mL (11.2 mmol/L) along with a serum bicarbonate level higher than 18 mEq/L (mmol/L), venous pH is higher than 7.30, and a calculated anion gap is less than 12 mEq/L (mmol/L). Assess therapy effectiveness by monitoring blood glucose levels and serial electrolyte levels.

Mild-to-moderate hyperkalemia is common in patients with hyperglycemia. Insulin therapy, correction of acidosis, and volume expansion decrease serum potassium concentration. To prevent hypokalemia, potassium replacement is initiated after serum levels fall below normal (5.0 mEq/L [mmol/L]). *Assess for signs of hypokalemia, including fatigue, malaise, confusion, muscle weakness, shallow respirations, abdominal distention or paralytic ileus, hypotension, and weak pulse.* An ECG shows conduction changes related to alterations in potassium. Hypokalemia is a common cause of death in the treatment of DKA.

! NURSING SAFETY PRIORITY (QSEN)
Action Alert

Before giving IV potassium-containing solutions, ensure that urine output is at least 30 mL/hr.

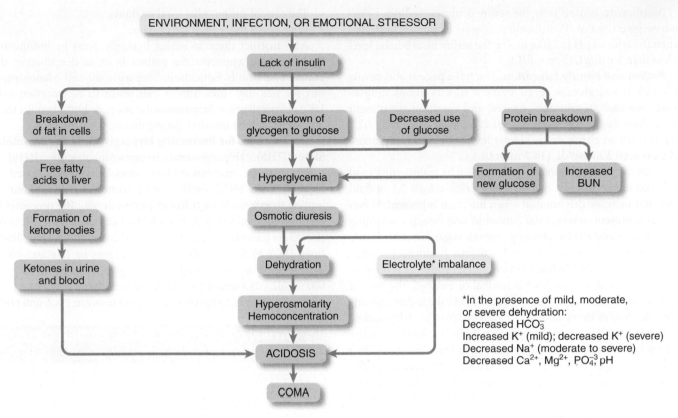

FIG. 59.8 Pathophysiologic mechanism of diabetic ketoacidosis (DKA). *BUN*, Blood urea nitrogen; *Ca²⁺*, calcium; HCO₃⁻, bicarbonate; *K⁺*, potassium; *Mg²⁺*, magnesium; *Na⁺*, sodium; PO₄⁻³, phosphate.

TABLE 59.13	Differences Between Diabetic Ketoacidosis and Hyperglycemic-Hyperosmolar State	
	Diabetic Ketoacidosis (DKA)	**Hyperglycemic-Hyperosmolar State (HHS)**
Onset	Sudden	Gradual
Precipitating factors	Infection Other stressors Inadequate insulin dose	Infection Other stressors Poor fluid intake
Symptoms	Ketosis: Kussmaul respiration, "rotting fruit" breath, nausea, abdominal pain Dehydration or electrolyte loss: polyuria, polydipsia, weight loss, dry skin, sunken eyes, soft eyeballs, lethargy, coma	Altered central nervous system function with neurologic symptoms Dehydration or electrolyte loss: same as for DKA
Laboratory Findings		
Serum glucose	>300 mg/dL (16.7 mmol/L)	>600 mg/dL (33.3 mmol/L)
Osmolarity/osmolality	Variable	>320 mOsm/L (mOsm/kg)
Serum ketones	Positive at 1:2 dilutions	Negative
Serum pH	<7.35	>7.4
Serum HCO₃⁻	<15 mEq/L (mmol/L)	>20 mEq/L (mmol/L)
Serum Na⁺	Low, normal, or high	Normal or low
BUN	>30 mg/dL (10 mmol/L); elevated because of dehydration	Elevated
Creatinine	>1.5 mg/dL (60 mcmol/L); elevated because of dehydration	Elevated
Urine ketones	Positive	Negative

BUN, Blood urea nitrogen; HCO₃⁻, bicarbonate; *Na⁺*, sodium.

Bicarbonate is used only for severe acidosis. Sodium bicarbonate, given by slow IV infusion over several hours, is indicated when the arterial pH is 7.0 or less or the serum bicarbonate level is less than 5 mEq/L (5 mmol/L).

Patient and Family Education. Teach the patient and family to check blood glucose levels every 4 to 6 hours as long as symptoms such as anorexia, nausea, and vomiting are present and as long as glucose levels exceed 250 mg/dL (13.8 mmol/L). Teach them to check urine ketone levels when blood glucose levels exceed 300 mg/dL (16.7 mmol/L).

Teach the patient to prevent dehydration by maintaining food and fluid intake. Suggest that he or she drink at least 2 L of fluid daily and increase this amount when infection is present. When nausea is present, instruct the patient to take liquids containing both glucose and electrolytes (e.g., regular sugar-sweetened soda pop, diluted fruit juice, and sports drinks [Gatorade]). Small amounts of fluid may be tolerated even when vomiting is present. When the blood glucose level is normal or elevated, the patient should take 8 to 12 ounces (240 to 360 mL) of calorie-free and caffeine-free liquids every hour while awake to prevent dehydration.

Liquids containing carbohydrate (CHO) can be taken if the patient cannot eat solid food. Ingesting at least 150 g of CHO daily reduces the risk for starvation ketosis. After consulting the diabetes health care provider, urge the patient to take additional rapid-acting (lispro) or short-acting (regular) insulin based on blood glucose levels.

Instruct the patient and family to consult the diabetes health care provider or primary health care provider when these problems occur:

- Blood glucose exceeds 250 mg/dL (13.8 mmol/L) and does not respond to therapy.
- Ketonuria lasts for more than 24 hours.

PATIENT AND FAMILY EDUCATION: PREPARING FOR SELF-MANAGEMENT

Sick-Day Rules

- Notify your primary health care provider or diabetes health care provider that you are ill.
- Monitor your blood glucose at least every 4 hours.
- Test your urine for ketones when your blood glucose level is greater than 240 mg/dL (13.8 mmol/L).
- Continue to take insulin or other antidiabetic agents, unless instructed otherwise by your primary health care provider.
- To prevent dehydration, drink 8 to 12 ounces (240 to 360 mL) of sugar-free liquids every hour that you are awake. If your blood glucose level is below your target range, drink fluids that contain sugar.
- Continue to eat meals at regular times.
- If unable to tolerate solid food because of nausea, consume more easily tolerated foods or liquids equal to the carbohydrate content of your usual meal.
- Call your diabetes health care provider for any of these problems:
  - Persistent nausea and vomiting
  - Moderate or high ketones
  - Blood glucose elevation after two supplemental doses of insulin
  - High (101.5°F [38.6°C]) temperature or increasing fever; fever for more than 24 hours
- Treat diarrhea, nausea, vomiting, fever as directed by your diabetes health care provider.
- Get plenty of rest.

- The patient cannot take food or fluids.
- Illness lasts more than 1 to 2 days.

Also instruct them to detect hyperglycemia by monitoring blood glucose whenever the patient is ill, as described in the Patient and Family Education: Preparing for Self-Management box for sick-day rules. Illness can result in dehydration with DKA, hyperglycemic-hyperosmolar state, or both. Insulin therapy should not be omitted during illness.

Interventions for Preventing Hyperglycemic-Hyperosmolar State (HHS). Hyperglycemic-hyperosmolar state (HHS) is a hyperosmolar (increased blood osmolarity) state caused by hyperglycemia. HHS results from a sustained osmotic diuresis leading to extremely high blood glucose levels. The processes of HHS are outlined in Fig. 59.9. Both HHS and diabetic ketoacidosis (DKA) are caused by hyperglycemia and dehydration. HHS differs from DKA in that ketone levels are absent or low and blood glucose levels are much higher. Blood glucose levels may exceed 600 mg/dL (33.3 mmol/L), and blood osmolarity may exceed 320 mOsm/L. Table 59.13 lists the differences between DKA and HHS.

👤 PATIENT-CENTERED CARE: OLDER ADULT CONSIDERATIONS (QSEN)

HHS occurs most often in older patients with type 2 DM, many of whom are unaware they have the disease (Touhy & Jett, 2020). Mortality rates in older patients with HHS have been reported to be as high as 16% (Fayfman et al., 2017). The onset of HHS is slow and may not be recognized. The older patient often seeks medical attention later and is sicker than the younger patient. HHS does not occur in well-hydrated patients. Older patients are at greater risk for dehydration and HHS because of age-related changes in thirst perception, poor urine-concentrating abilities, and use of diuretics. Assess all older adults for dehydration, regardless of whether they are known to have DM.

Myocardial infarction, sepsis, pancreatitis, stroke, and some drugs (glucocorticoids, diuretics, phenytoin, beta blockers, and calcium channel blockers) also may cause or contribute to HHS. Central nervous system (CNS) changes range from confusion to complete coma. Unlike DKA, patients with HHS may have seizures and reversible paralysis. The degree of neurologic impairment is related to serum osmolarity, with coma occurring once serum osmolarity is greater than 350 mOsm/L (350 mmol/L). Normal serum osmolarity is between 270 mOsm (270 mmol/L) and 300 mOsm/L (300 mmol/L).

The development of HHS rather than DKA is related to residual insulin secretion. In HHS, the patient secretes just enough insulin to prevent ketosis but not enough to prevent hyperglycemia. The hyperglycemia of HHS is more severe than that of DKA, greatly increasing blood osmolarity, leading to extreme diuresis with severe dehydration and electrolyte loss.

Fluid Therapy. The expected outcomes of therapy are to rehydrate the patient and restore normal blood glucose levels within 36 to 72 hours. The choice of fluid replacement and the rate of infusion are critical in managing HHS. The severity of the CNS problems is related to the level of blood hyperosmolarity and cellular dehydration. Re-establishing fluid balance in brain cells is a difficult and slow process, and many patients do not recover baseline CNS function until hours after blood glucose levels have returned to normal.

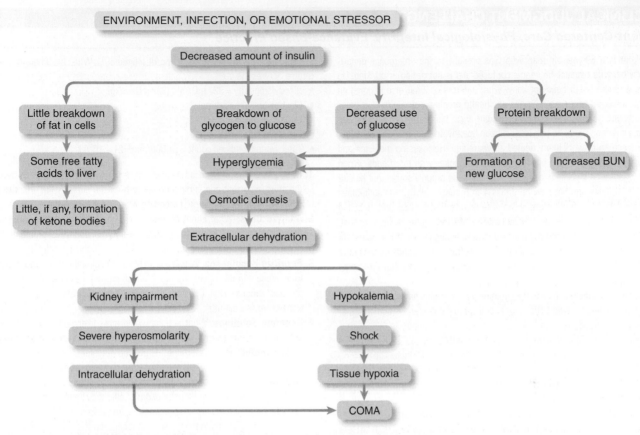

FIG. 59.9 Pathophysiologic mechanism of hyperglycemic-hyperosmolar state (HHS). *BUN,* Blood urea nitrogen.

The *first* priority for fluid replacement in HHS is to increase blood volume. In shock or severe hypotension, normal saline is used. Otherwise half-normal saline is used. Infuse fluids at 1 L/hr until central venous pressure or pulmonary capillary wedge pressure begins to rise or until blood pressure and urine output are adequate. The rate is then reduced to 100 to 200 mL/hr. Half of the estimated fluid deficit is replaced in the first 12 hours, and the rest is given over the next 36 hours. Body weight, urine output, kidney function, and the presence or absence of pulmonary congestion and jugular venous distention determine the rate of fluid infusion. *Assess the patient hourly for signs of cerebral edema (i.e., abrupt changes in mental status, abnormal neurologic signs, and coma).* Lack of improvement in level of consciousness may indicate inadequate rates of fluid replacement or reduction in plasma osmolarity. Regression after initial improvement may indicate a too-rapid reduction in plasma osmolarity. A slow but steady improvement in CNS function is the best evidence that fluid management is satisfactory.

! NURSING SAFETY PRIORITY (QSEN)

Critical Rescue

Continually monitor the patient being managed for hyperglycemic-hyperosmolar state to recognize status changes. When you notice changes in the level of consciousness; changes in pupil size, shape, or reaction; or seizures, respond by immediately notifying the diabetes health care provider.

Continuing Therapy. IV insulin is administered after adequate fluids have been replaced. Usually an initial bolus dose is given followed by continuous IV infusion until blood glucose levels fall to 250 mg/dL (13.9 mmol/L). A reduction of blood glucose of 50 to 70 mg/dL (2.8 to 4.0 mmol/L) per hour is the expected outcome. Monitor the patient closely for hypokalemia because potassium levels drop quickly with insulin therapy. Check serum electrolytes every 1 to 2 hours until stable, and monitor cardiac rhythm continuously for signs of hypokalemia or hyperkalemia. Patient education and interventions to minimize dehydration are similar to those for ketoacidosis.

Care Coordination and Transition Management

Self-Management Education. DM is a chronic disease requiring those affected to be actively involved in managing self-care. Education about blood glucose control for those with or at risk for DM occurs in a variety of health care settings. The interprofessional team of certified diabetes educators, primary health care providers, nurses, registered dietitian nutritionists (RDNs), pharmacists, social workers, and psychologists all participate in the education at every health care encounter. The patient must be an active participant at all levels for self-management to be successful (Faminu, 2019; Harris, 2019).

Assessing Learning Needs and Readiness to Learn. First assess the patient's learning needs and readiness to learn to establish what the patient already knows and what he or she needs to know. Assess the needs of both patient and family before teaching as described in Table 59.14.

? CLINICAL JUDGMENT CHALLENGE 59.1

Patient-Centered Care, Physiological Integrity, Evidence-Based Practice

The client is a 69-year-old man who was brought to the emergency department by his wife because he seems confused and is not eating or drinking. He knows who she is but does not know what day it is or what else is going on in their home. When asked if he has any health problems, the wife says no—that although he has gained a lot of weight since his retirement 4 years ago from construction work, he has always been healthy. In fact, he has not seen a doctor since an at-work injury healed 28 years ago. He takes no medicine and his current hobbies include bowling and playing poker with his friends. When asked whether he smokes or drinks alcohol, the wife proudly states that he quit smoking 10 years ago but now he drinks 4 to 5 beers nightly, and sometimes more when he is with his friends. The wife reports that he has been hobbling around a little the past few days because of an infected big toe on his right foot. Yesterday he was nauseated and did not feel well enough to eat anything except a little chicken broth and only drank one cup of coffee as his liquids for the entire day. Their daughter, who lives about 3 hours away, suggested that they come to the hospital.

On assessment the nurse finds the client responsive to his name, and he keeps stating that he feels "awful." His pulse is difficult to palpate and is both irregular and very fast. Blood pressure is 90/50 mm Hg. Pulse oximetry is 96% with a respiratory rate of 24 breaths/min. Temperature is 102.2°F (39°C). His affected toe is edematous and red with a red streak extending about 3 inches up his foot. Other findings include dry skin with poor turgor (tenting of skin on the forehead is present 2 minutes after pinching it up), sunken appearance to the eyeballs, and sticky coating over tongue and teeth.

His wife says he is 5 feet 9 inches (1.75 m) tall. His weight in the emergency department is 232 lb (105.2 kg), which his wife says is about 15 lb (6.8 kg) less than his weight at home earlier this week. When asked, the wife reports that he hasn't "peed" today.

A stat blood glucose level is 720 mg/dL (40 mmol/L). When his laboratory work returns, the results are:

- Blood osmolarity = 322 mOsm/L (322 mOsm/kg)
- Electrolytes = low normal
- pH = 7.39
- Ketone bodies = negative
- Total white blood cell count = 21,000/mm³ (21 × 10⁹/L)

1. **Recognize Cues:** What assessment information in this client situation is the most important and immediate concern for the nurse? (Hint: Identify the **relevant** information *first* to determine what is most important.)
2. **Analyze Cues:** What client conditions are consistent with the **most relevant** information? (Hint: Think about priority collaborative problems that support and contradict the information presented in this situation.)
3. **Prioritize Hypotheses:** Which possibilities or explanations are **most likely** to be present in this client situation? Which possibilities or explanations are the most serious? (Hint: Consider all possibilities and determine their urgency and risk for this client.)
4. **Generate Solutions:** What actions would most likely achieve the desired outcomes for this client? Which actions should be **avoided** or are **potentially harmful**? (Hint: Determine the desired outcomes first to decide which interventions are appropriate and those that should be avoided.)
5. **Take Action:** Which actions are the most appropriate and how should they be implemented? In what **priority order** should they be implemented? (Hint: Consider health teaching, documentation, requested health care provider orders or prescriptions, nursing skills, collaboration with or referral to health team members, etc.)
6. **Evaluate Outcomes:** What client assessment would indicate that the nurse's actions were **effective**? (Hint: Think about signs that would indicate an improvement, decline, or unchanged client condition.)

TABLE 59.14 Assessment of Learning Needs for the Patient With Diabetes

- Health and medical history
- Nutrition history and practices
- Physical activity and exercise behaviors
- Prescription and over-the-counter drugs and complementary and integrative therapies and practices
- Factors that influence learning such as education and literacy levels, perceived learning needs, motivation to learn, and health beliefs
- Diabetes self-management behaviors, including experience with self-adjusting the treatment plan
- Previous diabetes self-management training, actual knowledge, and skills
- Physical factors, including age, mobility, visual acuity, hearing, manual dexterity, alertness, attention span, and ability to concentrate or special needs or limitations requiring adaptive support and use of alternative skills
- Psychosocial concerns, factors, or issues, including family and social support
- Current mental health status
- History of substance use, including alcohol, tobacco (especially smoking), and recreational drugs
- Occupation, vocation, education level, financial status, and social, cultural, and religious practices
- Access to and use of health care resources

Provide information that applies directly to the patient. Ask about his or her concerns and what specifically he or she wants to learn. Start with what the patient already knows, and build on that base. Make sure that the patient's knowledge is current and applies to his or her type of DM.

When the patient is not ready to learn needed self-management behaviors, ask his or her permission to teach a family member about DM management. Provide written materials on DM management, as well as telephone numbers for the patient to call when he or she is ready to learn.

Assessing Physical, Cognitive, and Emotional Limitations. Assessing the patient's literacy is essential in developing a plan of care and providing self-management education (Watts et al., 2017). It is important to measure the patient's ability to read and understand written materials and perform math calculations. Match the literacy level of materials to the literacy level of the patient.

Assess the patient's ability to read printed information, insulin labels, and markings on syringes and equipment. Many older adult patients have age-related vision problems that are made worse by blurred vision caused by changing blood glucose levels.

Assess manual dexterity for any physical limitations that may alter the teaching plan. A hand injury, tremors, or severe arthritis often leads to dosing errors with a standard syringe and may require a change in insulin preparation.

Learning styles vary. Successful self-management education provides written handouts, discusses steps involved in a procedure such as insulin administration or self-monitoring of blood glucose (SMBG), and encourages the learner to touch and manipulate equipment. Confirm that the patient understands your instructions by using "teach-back" techniques.

Tailor educational sessions to the time available and to the condition of the patient. Hospitalized adults require only basic education when they are acutely ill. In these situations, it is appropriate to teach basic survival skills or focused problem-solving skills while reserving more detailed education for follow-up sessions.

Survival Skills Information. The initial phase of education involves teaching just the information necessary for the survival of any adult diagnosed with DM. Survival information includes:

- Simple information on pathophysiology of DM
- Learning how to prepare and inject insulin or how to take other antidiabetic drugs
- Recognition, treatment, and prevention of hypoglycemia and hyperglycemia
- Basic diet information
- Monitoring of blood glucose and urine ketones
- Sick-day management rules
- Where to buy DM supplies and how to store them
- When and how to notify the diabetes health care provider or primary health care provider

In-Depth Education. In-depth education and counseling involve teaching more detailed information about survival skills and actions for avoiding long-term complications. Educational sessions with the patient and family are needed to individualize the DM regimen for their needs and abilities.

The adult with DM must be able to discuss the action of insulin and the effects of insulin deficiency, as well as be able to explain the effects of diet, drugs, and activity on blood glucose. The patient is expected to relate maintaining normal blood glucose levels to preventing complications. This includes relating changes in glucose level to the possible need for a change in insulin dosage.

Provide education about the symptoms of hypoglycemia along with the prescribed treatment options if the patient takes any drugs that will lower blood glucose levels. Educate patients and families about common causes of hypoglycemia described earlier. Review indications of hypoglycemia at each visit. Advise patients to check their blood glucose levels before driving and to make sure they have easy-to-reach snacks and/or fast-acting sugars with them at all times. Remind them to contact their diabetes health care provider if they experience low blood glucose levels more than twice a week.

Ask patients taking an antidiabetic drug to identify the drug(s) and describe the prescribed schedule. Determine if the patient is able to inject insulin or other injectable antidiabetic drugs accurately by having him or her demonstrate injection techniques. Ask the patient to discuss the onset, peak, and duration of the insulin used. The patient must be able to state when insulin is to be injected, where it is injected, and how it is stored. Review formulas for self-adjustment in insulin (when supported by the diabetes health care provider), and explain blood glucose monitoring requirements needed to evaluate

the effects of additional insulin. Stress the dangers of skipping doses. Review drug interactions, especially with older patients taking oral antidiabetic drugs.

Teach patients receiving diet therapy alone, glucose-lowering drugs, or fixed insulin doses to eat the consistent amounts of carbohydrate (CHO) at meals and snacks. Patients who adjust mealtime doses of insulin or those on insulin pump therapy can be taught to match their insulin dose to the CHO content of their diet. The patient needs to understand what to eat, how much to eat, and when to eat. Stress the importance of eating on time, the dangers of skipping meals, and how to maintain food intake during illness. Ask the patient to describe the meal plan and explain the adjustments needed to meet diabetic diet requirements. Include the family member usually responsible for buying groceries and preparing meals in this teaching.

Teach the patient the skills needed to perform self-monitoring of blood glucose (SMBG), how to interpret results, and when to adjust behaviors and therapy based on the information. In addition, show patients who use insulin how to use SMBG to adjust dosages in order to achieve glucose control while avoiding episodes of hypoglycemia.

Teach patients sick-day procedures when initially diagnosed with DM. Hyperglycemia often develops before infection symptoms and can serve as a warning sign that infection is developing. Provide guidelines for the frequency of glucose testing, ketone testing, and insulin adjustment for those patients able to self-adjust insulin doses.

Psychosocial Preparation. The diagnosis of DM may represent a loss of control and flexibility. Life becomes ordered, and routines must be followed. Some events surrounding DM are predictable. Injecting insulin and not eating for several hours causes hypoglycemia. Poorly controlled DM leads to complications and premature death. Tight control of blood glucose prevents complications.

Patients are more likely to adhere to disease management activities when the strategies make sense and seem effective. The patient's belief that the activity is important, having confidence in himself or herself, and having support promote adherence to management strategies. Mastery of blood glucose monitoring helps the patient feel control over the disease. Knowing the effects of extra activities, extra food, or extra insulin is helpful in learning to adjust the regimen. Feeling a sense of control over the condition promotes a positive attitude about DM. Success in injecting insulin provides concrete evidence that he or she can master the disease. Teach by breaking a task into small, achievable units to ensure mastery. For example, a patient may begin learning how to inject insulin by first obtaining an accurate dose.

Devote as much teaching time as possible to insulin injection and blood glucose monitoring. Patients with newly diagnosed DM may fear giving themselves injections. After this technique is mastered, he or she may be less anxious and more able to attend to other tasks.

Home Care Management. Patients with DM self-manage their disease. Each day they decide what to eat, whether to exercise, and whether to take prescribed drugs. Maintaining blood glucose control depends on the accuracy of self-management skills. The role of the nurse is to provide support and education and to empower the patient to make informed

FOCUSED ASSESSMENT

The Insulin-Dependent Patient With Diabetes During a Home or Clinic Visit

- Assess overall mental status, wakefulness, ability to participate in a conversation.
- Take vital signs and weight:
  - Fever could indicate infection.
  - Are blood pressure and weight within target range? If not, why?
- Ask the patient about any change in vision; check current visual acuity.
- Inspect oral mucous membranes, gums, and teeth.
- Ask about injection areas used; inspect areas being used; assess whether the patient is using areas and rotating sites appropriately.
- Inspect skin for intactness, wounds that have not healed, new sores, ulcers, bruises, or burns; assess any previously known wounds for infection, progression of healing.
- Ask the patient how often and how he or she performs foot care.
- Assess lower extremities and feet for peripheral pulses, lack of or decreased sensation, abnormal sensations, breaks in skin integrity, condition of toes and nails.
- Ask about the color and consistency of stools and frequency of bowel movements; assess abdomen for bowel sounds.
- Review patient's home health diary:
  - Is blood glucose within targeted range? If not, why?
  - Is glucose monitoring being recorded often enough?
  - Is the patient's food intake adequate and appropriate? If not, why?
  - Is exercise occurring regularly? If not, why?
- Assess the patient's ability to perform self-monitoring of blood glucose.
- Assess the patient's procedures for obtaining and storing insulin and syringes, cleaning equipment, disposing of syringes and needles.
- Assess the patient's insulin preparation and injection technique.
- Assess the patient's knowledge of drug therapy and which side effects to look for.

TABLE 59.15 Outcome Criteria for Diabetes Teaching

Before self-management begins at home, the patient with diabetes or the significant other should be able to:

- Tell why insulin or a noninsulin antidiabetic drug is being prescribed
- Name which insulin or noninsulin antidiabetic drug is being prescribed, and name the dosage and frequency of administration
- Discuss the relationship between mealtime and the action of insulin or the other antidiabetic agent
- Discuss plans to follow diabetic diet instructions
- Prepare and inject insulin accurately
- Test blood for glucose or state plans for having blood glucose levels monitored
- Test urine for ketones and state when this test should be done
- Describe how to store insulin
- List symptoms that indicate a hypoglycemic reaction
- Tell which carbohydrate sources are used to treat hypoglycemic reactions
- Tell which symptoms indicate hyperglycemia
- Tell which dietary changes are needed during illness
- State when to call the diabetes health care provider or the nurse (frequent episodes of hypoglycemia, symptoms of hyperglycemia)
- Describe the procedures for proper foot care

Patient With Diabetes During a Home or Clinic Visit box during any home or clinic visit.

◆ **Evaluation: Evaluate Outcomes.** Evaluate the care of the patient with DM based on the identified priority patient problems. Outcome success for diabetes education is the ability of the patient to maintain blood glucose levels within their established target range. General outcome criteria are listed below and in Table 59.15. The expected outcomes include that with successful education the patient will be able to:

- Achieve blood glucose control by following the recommended diet, following the prescribed drug regimen, and reaching and maintaining optimum body weight
- Avoid acute and chronic complications of diabetes
- Avoid injury
- Recover from surgery without infection and with good wound healing
- Experience relief of pain
- Remain free of foot lesions, infections, and deformities
- Maintain optimal vision
- Maintain a urine output in the expected range
- Have an optimal level of mental status functioning
- Have decreased episodes of hypoglycemia
- Have decreased episodes of hyperglycemia

decisions. Self-management education allows patients to identify their problems and provides techniques to help them make decisions, take appropriate actions, and adjust these actions as needed.

Provide information about resources. The patient must know whom to contact in case of emergency. Older adults who live alone need to have daily telephone contact with a friend or neighbor. The patient may also need help shopping and preparing meals. He or she may have limited access to transportation and may not have sufficient supplies of food, particularly in bad weather. Because of the likelihood of vision problems in older patients, they may need help in preparing insulin syringes for injection or in monitoring blood glucose. Make referrals to home care or public health agencies as needed. Assess the areas listed in the Focused Assessment: The Insulin-Dependent

---

GET READY FOR THE NEXT-GENERATION NCLEX® EXAMINATION!

Key Points

Review these Key Points for each NCLEX Examination Client Needs Category.

Safe and Effective Care Environment

- Ensure that meals are available with or immediately after the patient receives an antidiabetic drug or insulin. **QSEN: Safety**

- Collaborate with the diabetes health care provider, diabetes nurse educator, registered dietitian nutritionist, pharmacist, social worker, and case manager to individualize patient care for the adult with diabetes in any care setting. **QSEN: Patient-Centered Care**
- Never dilute or mix insulin glargine with any other insulin or solution. **QSEN: Safety**

- Instruct the patient and family about complications and when to seek assistance. **QSEN: Safety**
- Assess patients' visual acuity and peripheral tactile sensation to determine needed adjustments in teaching self-medication and self-monitoring of blood glucose levels. **QSEN: Safety**
- Teach patients with peripheral neuropathy to use a bath thermometer to test water for bathing, to avoid walking barefoot, and to inspect their feet daily. **QSEN: Safety**
- Teach the patient and family about the symptoms of infection and when to seek medical advice. **QSEN: Safety**
- Instruct patients to wear a medical alert bracelet or carry a wallet ID. **QSEN: Safety**
- Instruct patients to always carry a glucose source. **QSEN: Safety**

Health Promotion and Maintenance

- Encourage all patients to maintain weight within an appropriate range. **QSEN: Patient-Centered Care**
- Encourage patients with diabetes to participate regularly in exercise or physical activity appropriate to their health status. **QSEN: Evidence-Based Practice**
- Instruct all patients with diabetes to avoid becoming dehydrated and to drink at least 2 L of water each day unless another medical condition requires fluid restriction. **QSEN: Patient-Centered Care**
- Teach patients to self-manage hypoglycemia with 15 to 30 g of carbohydrate (especially glucose), depending on the severity of the low blood glucose level, and to avoid overtreatment. Tell them to recheck blood glucose level in 15 minutes and re-treat as needed. **QSEN: Patient-Centered Care**
- Use return demonstration with "teach-back" strategies when teaching the patient about drug regimen, insulin injection, blood glucose monitoring, and foot assessment. **QSEN: Patient-Centered Care**
- Refer patients newly diagnosed with diabetes to local resources and support groups. **QSEN: Patient-Centered Care**

Psychosocial Integrity

- Allow the patient the opportunity to express concerns about the diagnosis of diabetes or the treatment regimen. **QSEN: Patient-Centered Care**
- Pace your education sessions to match the learning needs and style of the patient. **QSEN: Patient-Centered Care**
- Urge patients newly diagnosed with DM to attend diabetes education classes to become a fully engaged partner in management of the disease. **QSEN: Patient-Centered Care**

Physiological Integrity

- Assess the patient's A1C for indications of adherence to prescribed regimens and their effectiveness. **QSEN: Evidence-Based Practice**
- Explain all procedures, restrictions, drugs, and follow-up care to the patient and family. **QSEN: Patient-Centered Care**
- Teach patients to inject an accurate dose of insulin using a pre-filled or disposable insulin pen. **QSEN: Patient-Centered Care**
- Instruct patients who are taking sulfonylurea drugs or insulin stimulators about an increased risk for hypoglycemic reactions. **QSEN: Patient-Centered Care**
- Start carbohydrate replacement per the diabetes health care provider's prescription or standing protocols immediately on identifying a patient with hypoglycemia. **QSEN: Evidence-Based Practice**
- Give glucagon subcutaneously or IM or concentrated dextrose IV to patients identified with hypoglycemia who cannot swallow. **QSEN: Evidence-Based Practice**
- Use blood glucose values to assess therapy effectiveness and determine when to switch from saline to dextrose-containing solutions in a patient with diabetic ketoacidosis. **QSEN: Evidence-Based Practice**
- Immediately report indications of cerebral edema (abrupt changes in mental status; changes in level of consciousness; changes in pupil size, shape, or reaction; seizures) in a patient with HHS to the diabetes health care provider. **QSEN: Patient-Centered Care**

▮ MASTERY QUESTIONS

1. Which physiological processes directly prevent severe hypoglycemia in a healthy adult without diabetes who is NPO for 12 hours? **Select all that apply.**
   A. Gluconeogenesis
   B. Glycogenesis
   C. Glycogenolysis
   D. Ketogenesis
   E. Lipogenesis
   F. Lipolysis

2. Which precaution is a **priority** for the nurse to teach a client prescribed pramlintide to **prevent harm**?
   A. Only take this drug once weekly.
   B. Do not drink alcohol when taking this drug.
   C. Do not mix in the same syringe with insulin.
   D. Report any genital itching to your primary health care provider.

3. Which health promotion activity(ies) will the nurse recommend to **prevent harm** in a client with type 2 diabetes? **Select all that apply.**
   A. "Avoid all dietary carbohydrate and fat."
   B. "Have your eyes and vision assessed by an ophthalmologist every year."
   C. "Reduce your intake of animal fat and increase your intake of plant sterols."
   D. "Be sure to take your antidiabetes drug right before you engage in any type of exercise."
   E. "Keep your feet warm in cold weather by using either a hot water bottle or a heating pad."
   F. "Avoid foot damage from shoe-rubbing by going barefoot or wearing flip-flops when you are at home."

4. When preparing to administer a prescribed subcutaneous dose of NPH insulin from an open vial taken from a medication drawer to a client with diabetes, the nurse notes the solution is cloudy. What action will the nurse perform to ensure client **safety**?

A. Warm the vial in a bowl of warm water until it reaches normal body temperature.

B. Return the vial to the pharmacy and open a fresh vial of NPH insulin.

C. Roll the vial between the hands until the insulin is clear.

D. Check the expiration date and draw up the insulin dose.

5. While making rounds the nurse finds a client with type 1 diabetes mellitus pale, sweaty, and slightly confused; the client can swallow. The client's blood glucose level check is 48 mg/dL (2.7 mmol/L). What is the nurse's best **first** action to **prevent harm**?

A. Call the pharmacy and order a STAT does of glucagon.

B. Immediately give the client 30 g of glucose orally.

C. Start an IV and administer a small amount of a concentrated dextrose solution.

D. Recheck the blood glucose level and call the Rapid Response Team.

REFERENCES

American Diabetes Association (ADA). (2019a). Cardiac disease and risk management: Standards of medical care in diabetes-2019. *Diabetes Care, 42*(Suppl. 1), S103–S123.

American Diabetes Association (ADA). (2019b). Classification and diagnosis of diabetes: Standards of medical care in diabetes-2019. *Diabetes Care, 42*(Suppl. 1) S132-S28.

American Diabetes Association (ADA). (2019c). Comprehensive medical evaluation and assessment of comorbidities: Standards of medical care in diabetes-2019. *Diabetes Care, 42*(Suppl. 1), S34–S45.

American Diabetes Association (ADA). (2019d). Glycemic targets: Standards of medical care in diabetes-2019. *Diabetes Care, 42*(Suppl. 1), S61–S70.

American Diabetes Association (ADA). (2019e). Lifestyle management: Standards of medical care in diabetes-2019. *Diabetes Care, 42*(Suppl. 1), S46–S60.

American Diabetes Association (ADA). (2019f). Management of diabetes in pregnancy: Standards of medical care in diabetes-2019. *Diabetes Care, 42*(Suppl. 1), S165–S172.

American Diabetes Association (ADA). (2019g). Microvascular complications and foot care: Standards of medical care in diabetes-2019. *Diabetes Care, 42*(Suppl. 1), S124–S138.

American Diabetes Association (ADA). (2019h). Obesity management for the treatment of type 2 diabetes: Standards of medical care in diabetes-2019. *Diabetes Care, 42*(Suppl. 1), S81–S89.

American Diabetes Association (ADA). (2019i). Older adults: Standards of medical care in diabetes-2019. *Diabetes Care, 42*(Suppl. 1), S139–S147.

American Diabetes Association (ADA). (2019j). Pharmacologic approaches to glycemic treatment: Standards of medical care in diabetes-2019. *Diabetes Care, 42*(Suppl. 1), S90–S102.

American Diabetes Association (ADA). (2019k). Prevention or delay of type 2 diabetes: Standards of medical care in diabetes-2019. *Diabetes Care, 42*(Suppl. 1), S29–S33.

Aschenbrenner, D. (2017). Diabetes drug receives new indication. *American Journal of Nursing, 117*(4), 24–25.

Burchum, J., & Rosenthal, L. (2019). *Lehne's pharmacology for nursing care* (10th ed.). St. Louis: Elsevier.

Centers for Disease Control and Prevention (CDC). (2020). *National diabetes statistics report-2020.* https://www.cdc.gov/diabetes/pdf/data/statistics/national-diabetes-statistics-report.pdf.

Faminu, F. (2019). Diabetes: Setting and achieving glycemic goals. *Nursing2019, 49*(3), 49–54.

Fayfman, M., Pasquel, F., & Umpierrez, G. (2017). Management of hyperglycemic crisis. *Medical Clinics of North America, 101*, 587–606.

Harris, A. (2019). Diabetes self-management education provision by an interprofessional collaborative practice team: A quality improvement project. *Nursing Clinics of North America, 54*(1), 149–158.

Hussar, D. (2019). New drugs, 2019: Part 1. *Nursing2019, 49*(2), 28–36.

Keresztes, P., & Peacock-Johnson, A. (2019). Type 2 diabetes: A pharmacologic update. *American Journal of Nursing, 119*(3), 32–40.

McCance, K., Huether, S., Brashers, V., & Rote, N. (2019). *Pathophysiology: The biologic basis for disease in adults and children* (8th ed.). St. Louis: Mosby.

Pagana, K., & Pagana, T. (2018). *Mosby's manual of diagnostic and laboratory tests* (6th ed.). St. Louis: Elsevier.

Rariden, C. (2019). Prediabetes: A wake-up call. *Nursing2019, 49*(4), 38–44.

Schneider, A., Kalyani, R., Golden, S., Stearns, S., Wruck, L., Yeh, H., et al. (2016). Diabetes and prediabetes risk of hospitalization: The atherosclerosis risk in communities (ARIC) study. *Diabetes Care, 39*(5), 772–779.

Statistics Canada. (2019). *Health: All subtopics for health-Diabetes by age-group and sex.* http://www.statcan.gc.ca/tables-tableaux/sum-som/l01/cst01/health53a-eng.htm.

Touhy, T., & Jett, K. (2020). *Ebersole & Hess' toward healthy aging* (10th ed.). St. Louis: Mosby.

U.S. Department of Veterans Affairs. (2016). *Diabetes type 2 and agent orange.* http://www.publichealth.va.gov/exposures/agentorange/conditions/diabetes.asp.

Watts, S., & Howard, J. (2016). Prediabetes: What nurses need to know. *American Journal of Nursing, 116*(7), 54–58.

Watts, S., & Nemes, D. (2018). Best practice nursing management of nosocomial hypoglycemia: Lessons learned. *Medsurg Nursing, 27*(2), 98–102.

Watts, S., Nemes, D., Davian, T., & Pensiero, A. (2020). 10 years of inpatient diabetes certification-Lessons learned. *American Nurse Journal, 15*(1), 20–23.

Watts, S., Stevenson, C., & Adams, M. (2017). Improving health literacy in patients with diabetes. *Nursing2017, 47*(1), 25–31.

Watts, S., Stevenson, C., & Russell, L. (2018). Diabetes basics for the inpatient nurse. *Medsurg Nursing, 27*(3), 161–165 185.

Wisnewski, C. (2017). Diabetes and cardiovascular disease: A deadly duo. *American Journal of Nursing, 117*(9), 12–17.

Wooton, A., & Melchior, L. (2020). Diabetes-associated cardiac autonomic neuropathy. *The Nurse Practitioner, 45*(2), 24–31.

60

Assessment of the Renal/ Urinary System

Carolyn Gersch

http://evolve.elsevier.com/Iggy/

LEARNING OUTCOMES

1. Collaborate with the interprofessional team to perform a complete urinary and renal system assessment, including *elimination, fluid and electrolyte balance,* and *acid-base balance.*
2. Provide a safe environment for patients and staff when performing a physical assessment of the renal and urinary systems.
3. Explain how physiologic changes of the urinary/renal system affect *elimination* and the associated care of older adults.
4. Implement patient-centered nursing interventions to help patients and families cope with the psychosocial impact caused by a urinary *elimination* health problem.
5. Apply knowledge of anatomy and physiology to perform an evidence-based assessment for the patient with a urinary *elimination* health problem.
6. Use clinical judgement to analyze assessment findings for the patient with a urinary or renal system health problem.
7. Teach the patient and caregivers about diagnostic procedures associated with assessment of kidney and urinary health problems.

KEY TERMS

bruit An audible swishing sound produced when the volume of blood or the diameter of the blood vessel changes.

calculi Stone formation.

continence The ability to voluntarily control emptying of the bladder or colon.

cystitis A bladder inflammation, most often with infection.

elimination The excretion of waste from the body by the GI tract (as feces) and kidneys (as urine).

external urethral sphincter Skeletal muscle that surrounds the urethra and helps to control the exit of urine.

incontinence The involuntary loss of urine or stool.

internal urethral sphincter is smooth detrusor muscle of the bladder neck and elastic tissue that helps to control the exit of urine.

microalbuminuria The presence of very small amounts of albumin in the urine that are not measurable by usual urinalysis procedures.

nocturnal polyuria Increased urination at night.

renal threshold The point at which the kidney is overwhelmed with glucose and can no longer reabsorb; also called *transport maximum.*

proteinuria The presence of protein in the urine.

uremia The buildup of nitrogenous waste products in the blood (azotemia).

urethral meatus The opening at the endpoint of the urethra.

urgency A sense of a nearly uncontrollable need to urinate.

✳ PRIORITY AND INTERRELATED CONCEPTS

The priority concept for this chapter is:
- *Elimination*

The interrelated concepts for this chapter are:
- *Fluid and Electrolyte Balance*
- *Acid-Base Balance*

The concept of *elimination* is the excretion of waste from the body by the GI tract as feces and by the kidneys as urine. See Chapter 3 for an overview of the concept of elimination and how it relates to the concepts of *fluid and electrolyte balance* and *acid-base balance.* In this chapter, the focus is on elimination of waste via the renal system. The kidneys and urinary tract make up the renal system, which is responsible for urine elimination.

The kidneys are responsible for filtering water and wastes from the bloodstream. The filtered-out particles and excess fluid are excreted out of the body into the urinary tract via the ureters, bladder, and ureters ridding the body of these wastes. Structural or functional problems within the renal system may alter **fluid and electrolyte balance** and **acid-base balance.**

The kidneys help maintain health in many ways. *Most important, they maintain body fluid volume and composition and create urine for waste* **elimination.** In addition, the kidneys help regulate blood pressure, **acid-base balance;** produce erythropoietin for red blood cell (RBC) synthesis; and convert vitamin D to an active form.

ANATOMY AND PHYSIOLOGY REVIEW

Kidneys

Structure. The two kidneys are located behind the peritoneum, outside of the abdominal cavity, one on either side of the spine (Fig. 60.1). The adult kidney is 4 to 5 inches (10 to 13 cm) long, 2 to 3 inches (5 to 7 cm) wide, and about 1 inch (2.5 to 3 cm) thick. The left kidney is slightly longer and narrower than the right kidney. Larger-than-usual kidneys may indicate obstruction or polycystic disease. Smaller-than-usual kidneys may indicate chronic kidney disease (CKD).

Variation in kidney shape and number is relatively common and does not always indicate a problem in kidney function. Some adults have more than two kidneys or may have only one large, horseshoe-shaped kidney. As long as tests of kidney function are normal, these variations are of no significance (Brenner, 2016).

Several layers of tissue surround the kidney, providing protection and support. The outer surface of the kidney is a layer of fibrous tissue called the *capsule* (Fig. 60.2). It covers most of the kidney except the *hilum,* which is the indented area where the

kidney blood vessels and nerves enter and exit. It is also where the ureter exits. The capsule is surrounded by layers of fat and connective tissue.

Underneath the capsule fibrous layer are two layers of functional kidney tissue: the cortex and the medulla. The *renal cortex* is the outer tissue layer. The *medulla* is the medullary tissue lying below the cortex in the shape of many fans. Each "fan" is called a pyramid. Pyramids are separated by the *renal columns,* cortical tissue that dips down into the interior of the kidney.

The tip of each pyramid is called a *papilla.* The papillae drain urine into the collecting system. A cuplike structure called a *calyx* collects the urine at the end of each papilla. The calices join together to form the *renal pelvis,* which narrows to become the ureter.

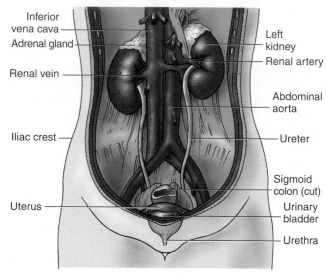

FIG. 60.1 Anatomic location of the kidneys and structures of the urinary system.

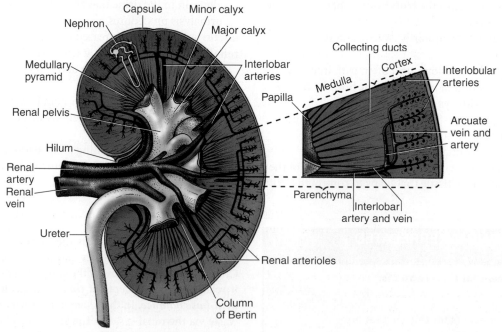

FIG. 60.2 Bisection of the kidney showing its major structures.

The kidneys have a rich blood supply and receive a blood flow from 600 to 1300 mL/min. The blood supply to each kidney comes from the renal artery, which branches off from the abdominal aorta. The renal artery divides into progressively smaller arteries, supplying blood to areas of the kidney tissue and the nephrons. The smallest arteries *(afferent arterioles)* feed the nephrons directly to form urine.

Venous blood from the kidneys starts with the capillaries surrounding each nephron. These capillaries drain into progressively larger veins, with blood eventually returned to the inferior vena cava through the renal vein.

Microscopic Anatomy. The **nephron** is the functional unit of the kidney and forms urine by filtering waste products and water from the blood. There are about 1 million nephrons per kidney, and each nephron separately performs filtration and makes urine from blood.

There are two types of nephrons: *cortical nephrons* and *juxtamedullary nephrons.* The cortical nephrons are short and lie totally within the renal cortex. The juxtamedullary nephrons (about 20% of all nephrons) are longer, and their tubes and blood vessels dip deeply into the medulla. The purpose of these nephrons is to concentrate urine during times of low fluid intake to allow continued excretion of body waste with less fluid loss (McCance & Huether, 2019).

Blood supply to the nephron is delivered through the *afferent arteriole* (i.e., the smallest, most distal portion of the renal arterial system). From the afferent arteriole, blood flows into the *glomerulus,* which is a series of specialized capillary loops. It is through these capillaries that water and small particles are filtered from the blood to make urine. The remaining blood leaves the glomerulus through the *efferent arteriole,* which is the first vessel in the kidney's venous system. From the efferent arteriole, blood exits into either the *peritubular capillaries* around the tube of the cortical nephrons or the *vasa recta* around the tube of juxtamedullary nephrons.

Each nephron is a tubelike structure with distinct parts (Fig. 60.3). The tube begins with the Bowman capsule, a saclike structure that surrounds the glomerulus. The tubular tissue of the Bowman capsule narrows into the *proximal convoluted tubule (PCT).* The PCT twists and turns, finally straightening into the descending limb of the *loop of Henle.* The descending loop of Henle dips in the direction of the medulla but forms a hairpin loop and comes back up into the cortex as the ascending loop of Henle.

The two segments of the ascending limb of the loop of Henle are the thin segment and the thick segment. The *distal convoluted tubule (DCT)* forms from the thick segment of the ascending limb of the loop of Henle. The DCT ends in one of many collecting ducts located in the kidney tissue. The urine in the collecting ducts passes through the papillae and empties into the renal pelvis.

Special cells in the afferent arteriole, efferent arteriole, and DCT are known as the *juxtaglomerular complex* (Fig. 60.4). These cells produce *renin,* which is a hormone that helps regulate blood flow, glomerular filtration rate (GFR), and blood pressure. Renin is secreted when sensing cells in the DCT (called the *macula densa*) sense changes in blood volume and

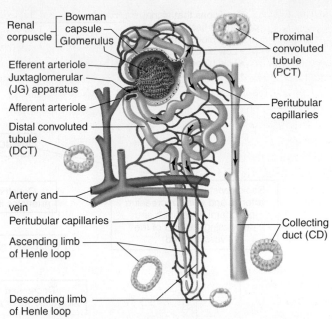

FIG. 60.3 Anatomy of the nephron—the functional unit of the kidney. The differences in appearance in tubular cells seen in a cross section reflect the differing functions of each nephron segment. Note that the particular nephron labeled here is a juxtamedullary nephron. (From Patton, K. T., & Thibodeau, G. A. [2018]. *The human body in health & disease* [7th ed.]. St. Louis: Mosby.)

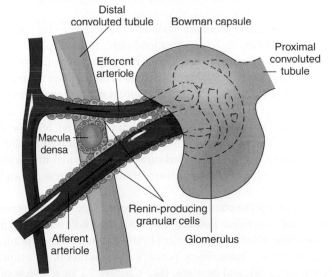

FIG. 60.4 Juxtaglomerular complex showing juxtaglomerular cells and the macula densa.

pressure. The macula densa touches the renin-producing cells. Renin is produced when the macula densa cells sense that blood volume, blood pressure, or blood sodium level is low. Renin then converts renin substrate (angiotensinogen) into angiotensin I. This leads to a series of reactions that cause secretion of the hormone aldosterone (Fig. 60.5). Aldosterone increases kidney reabsorption of sodium and water, restoring blood pressure, blood volume, and blood sodium levels (McCance & Huether, 2019). It also promotes excretion of potassium (see Chapter 13).

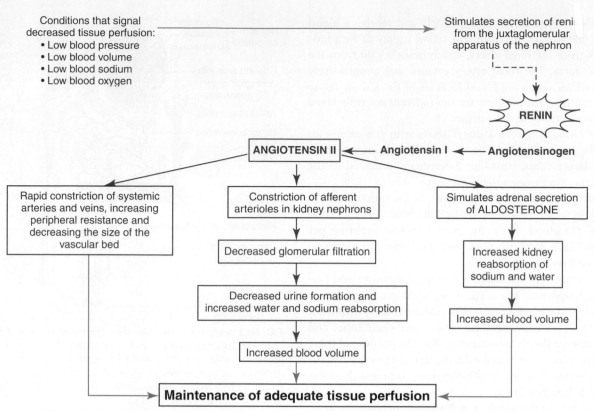

FIG. 60.5 Role of aldosterone, renin substrate (angiotensinogen), angiotensin I, and angiotensin II in the renal regulation of water and sodium.

The glomerular capillary wall has three layers (Fig. 60.6): the endothelium, the basement membrane, and the epithelium. The endothelial and epithelial cells lining these capillaries are separated by pores that filter water and small particles from the blood into the Bowman capsule. This fluid is called the *filtrate.*

Function. The kidneys have both regulatory and hormonal functions. The regulatory functions control ***fluid and electrolyte balance*** and ***acid-base balance.*** The hormonal functions control red blood cell (RBC) formation, blood pressure, and vitamin D activation.

Regulatory Functions. The kidney processes that maintain ***fluid and electrolyte balance*** and ***acid-base balance*** through urine ***elimination*** are glomerular filtration, tubular reabsorption, and tubular secretion. These processes use filtration, diffusion, active transport, and osmosis. (See Chapter 13 for a review of these actions.) Table 60.1 lists the functions of nephron tubules and blood vessels.

Glomerular filtration is the first process in urine formation. As blood passes from the afferent arteriole into the glomerulus, water, electrolytes, and other small particles (e.g., creatinine, urea nitrogen, glucose) are filtered across the glomerular membrane into the Bowman capsule to form *glomerular* filtrate. As the filtrate enters the proximal convoluted tubule (PCT), it is called *tubular filtrate* or *early urine.*

Large particles, such as blood cells, albumin, and other proteins, are too large to filter through the glomerular capillary walls. *Therefore these substances are not normally present in the excreted final urine.*

BOWMAN CAPSULE

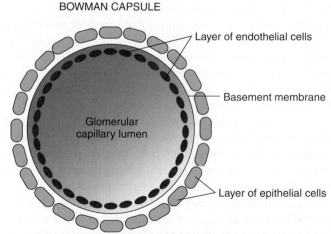

FIG. 60.6 Glomerular capillary wall.

Filtration rate is expressed in milliliters per minute. Normal glomerular filtration rate (GFR) averages 125 mL/min, totaling about 180 L daily. If the entire amount of filtrate were excreted as urine, death would occur from dehydration. Actually, only about 1 to 3 L are excreted each day as urine. The rest is reabsorbed back into the blood (McCance & Huether, 2019).

GFR is controlled by blood pressure and blood flow. The kidneys self-regulate their own blood pressure and blood flow, which keeps GFR constant. GFR is controlled by selectively constricting and dilating the afferent and efferent arterioles. When the afferent arteriole is constricted or the efferent arteriole is dilated, pressure in the glomerular capillaries falls and

TABLE 60.1　Vascular and Tubular Components of the Nephron

Structure	Anatomic Features	Physiologic Aspects
Vascular Components		
Afferent arteriole	Delivers arterial blood from the branches of the renal artery into the glomerulus	Autoregulation of renal blood flow via vasoconstriction or vasodilation Renin-producing granular cells
Glomerulus	Capillary loops with thin, semipermeable membrane	Site of glomerular filtration Glomerular filtration occurs when hydrostatic pressure (blood pressure) is greater than opposing forces (tubular filtrate and oncotic pressure)
Efferent arteriole	Delivers arterial blood from the glomerulus into the peritubular capillaries or the vasa recta	Autoregulation of renal blood flow via vasoconstriction or vasodilation Renin-producing granular cells
Peritubular capillaries (PTCs) and vasa recta (VR)	PTCs: surround tubular components of cortical nephrons VR: surround tubular components of juxtamedullary nephrons	Tubular reabsorption and tubular secretion allow movement of water and solutes to or from the tubules, interstitium, and blood
Tubular Components		
Bowman capsule (BC)	Thin membranous sac surrounding ⅞ of the glomerulus	Collects glomerular filtrate (GF) and funnels it into the tubule
Proximal convoluted tubule (PCT)	Evolves from and is continuous with Bowman capsule Specialized cellular lining facilitates tubular reabsorption	Site for reabsorption of sodium, chloride, water, glucose, amino acids, potassium, calcium, bicarbonate, phosphate, and urea
Loop of Henle	Continues from PTC Juxtamedullary nephrons dip deep into the medulla Permeable to water, urea, and sodium chloride	Regulation of water balance
Descending limb (DL)	Continues from the loop of Henle Permeable to water, urea, and sodium chloride	Regulation of water balance
Ascending limb (AL)	Emerges from DL as it turns and is redirected up toward the renal cortex	Potassium and magnesium reabsorption in the thick segment Thin segment is impermeable to water
Distal convoluted tubule (DCT)	Evolves from AL and twists, so the macula densa cells lie adjacent to the juxtaglomerular cells of afferent arteriole	Site of additional water and electrolyte reabsorption, including bicarbonate Potassium and hydrogen secretion
Collecting ducts	Collect formed urine from several tubules and deliver it into the renal pelvis	Receptor sites for antidiuretic hormone regulation of water balance

filtration decreases. When the afferent arteriole is dilated or the efferent arteriole is constricted, pressure in the glomerular capillaries rises and filtration increases. This way the kidney maintains a constant GFR, even when systemic blood pressure changes. When systolic pressure drops below 65 to 70 mm Hg, these self-regulation processes do not maintain GFR.

Tubular reabsorption is the second process in urine formation. Tubular reabsorption of most of the filtrate (early urine) keeps normal urine output at 1 to 3 L/day and prevents dehydration. As the filtrate passes through the tubular parts of the nephron, water and electrolytes are reabsorbed from the tubular lumen of the nephron and into the peritubular capillaries. This process returns much of the water, electrolytes, and other particles to the blood.

The tubules return about 99% of filtered water back into the body (Fig. 60.7). Most water reabsorption occurs in the proximal convoluted tubule (PCT). Water reabsorption continues as the filtrate flows down the descending loop of Henle. The thin and thick segments of the ascending loop of Henle are *not* permeable to water, and no water reabsorption occurs here.

The distal convoluted tubule (DCT) can be permeable to water, and some water reabsorption occurs as the filtrate continues to flow through the tubule. The membrane of the DCT may be made more permeable to water when *vasopressin* (antidiuretic hormone [ADH]) and aldosterone are present. Vasopressin increases tubular permeability to water, allowing water to leave the tube and be reabsorbed into the capillaries. Vasopressin also increases arteriole constriction. Arteriole constriction alters blood pressure, which then affects the amounts of fluid and particles that exit glomerular capillaries. Aldosterone promotes the reabsorption of sodium in the DCT. Water reabsorption occurs as a result of the movement of sodium (where sodium goes, water follows).

The ability of the kidneys to vary the volume or concentration of urine helps regulate water balance regardless of fluid intake. In this way, the healthy kidney can prevent dehydration when fluid intake is low and can prevent circulatory overload when fluid intake is high.

In addition to water, electrolytes are reabsorbed as needed to maintain **fluid and electrolyte balance** in the blood. Most sodium, chloride, and water reabsorption occurs in the proximal convoluted tubule (PCT). The collecting ducts are the other site of sodium, chloride, and water reabsorption. Here reabsorption is caused by aldosterone. Potassium is mostly reabsorbed in the PCT and thick segment of the loop of Henle.

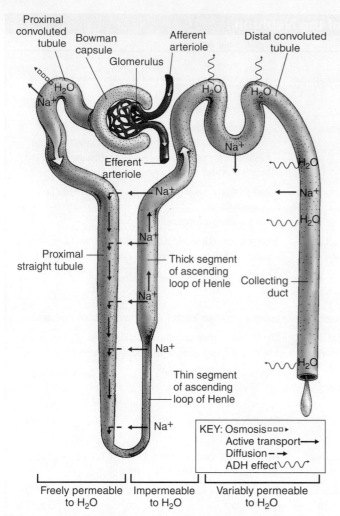

FIG. 60.7 Sodium and water reabsorption by the tubules of a cortical nephron. *ADH,* Antidiuretic hormone; *Na+,* sodium.

Bicarbonate, calcium, and phosphate are mostly reabsorbed in the PCT. Bicarbonate reabsorption helps **acid-base balance** and maintains a normal blood pH. Blood levels of calcitonin and parathyroid hormone (PTH) (see Chapters 13 and 58) control calcium balance.

Some types of particles in the tubular filtrate are also returned to the blood by *tubular reabsorption.* About 50% of all urea in the filtrate is reabsorbed; creatinine is not reabsorbed.

The kidney reabsorbs some of the glucose filtered from the blood. However, there is a limit to how much glucose the kidney can reabsorb. The point where the kidney is overwhelmed with glucose and can no longer reabsorb is called the **renal threshold** or *transport maximum* for glucose reabsorption. The renal threshold for glucose is >180 mg/dL (10 mmol/L). This means that at a blood glucose level of 180 mg/dL (10 mmol/L) or less, all glucose is reabsorbed and returned to the blood, with no glucose present in final urine. When blood glucose levels are greater than 180 mg/

> **! NURSING SAFETY PRIORITY** (QSEN)
>
> ***Action Alert***
>
> Report the presence of glucose or proteins in the urine of a patient undergoing a screening examination to the primary health care provider because this is an abnormal finding and requires further assessment.

dL (10 mmol/L), some glucose stays in the filtrate and is present in the urine (McCulloch, 2018). Normally, almost all glucose and most proteins are reabsorbed and thus are not present in the urine.

Tubular secretion is the third process of urine formation. It allows substances to move from the blood into the urine. During tubular secretion, substances move from the peritubular capillaries in reverse, across capillary membranes, and into the cells that line the tubules. From the cells, these substances are moved into the urine and excreted from the body. Potassium (K^+) and hydrogen (H^+) ions are some of the substances moved in this way to maintain **fluid and electrolyte balance** and **acid-base balance** (pH).

Hormonal Functions. The kidneys produce renin, prostaglandins, erythropoietin, and activated vitamin D (Table 60.2). Other kidney products, such as the kinins, change kidney blood flow, regulate blood pressure, and influence capillary permeability. The kidneys also help break down and excrete insulin and many other drugs.

Renin, as discussed in the Microscopic Anatomy section, assists in blood pressure control. It is formed and released when there is a decrease in blood flow, blood volume, or blood pressure through the renal arterioles or when too little sodium is present in kidney blood. These conditions are detected through the receptors of the juxtaglomerular complex.

Renin release causes the production of *angiotensin II* through a series of steps (see Fig. 60.5). Angiotensin II increases systemic blood pressure with powerful blood vessel constricting effects and triggers the release of aldosterone from the adrenal glands. Aldosterone increases the reabsorption of sodium in the distal tubule of the nephron. Therefore more water is reabsorbed, which increases blood volume and blood pressure. When blood flow to the kidney is reduced, this system also prevents fluid loss and maintains circulating blood volume (see Chapter 13).

Prostaglandins are produced in the kidney and many other tissues. Those produced specifically in the kidney help regulate glomerular filtration, kidney vascular resistance, and renin production. They also increase sodium and water excretion.

Erythropoietin is produced and released in response to decreased oxygen in the kidney's blood supply. It triggers red blood cell (RBC) production in the bone marrow. When kidney function is poor, erythropoietin production decreases and anemia results.

Vitamin D activation occurs through a series of steps. Some of these steps take place in the skin when it is exposed to sunlight, and then more processing occurs in the liver. From there, vitamin D is converted to its active form in the kidney. Activated vitamin D is needed to absorb calcium in the intestinal tract and regulate calcium balance (McCance & Huether, 2019).

Ureters

Each kidney usually has a single ureter, which is a hollow tube that connects the renal pelvis with the urinary bladder. The ureter is about ½ inch (1.25 cm) in diameter and about 12 to 18 inches (30 to 45 cm) in length. The diameter of the ureter narrows in three areas:

- In the upper third of the ureter, at the point at which the renal pelvis becomes the ureter, is a narrowing known as the ureteropelvic junction (UPJ).
- The ureter also narrows as it bends toward the abdominal wall (aortoiliac bend).

TABLE 60.2 Kidney Hormones and Hormones Influencing Kidney Function

	Site	Action
Kidney Hormones		
Renin	Renin-producing granular cells	Raises blood pressure as result of angiotensin (local vasoconstriction) and aldosterone (volume expansion) secretion
Prostaglandins	Kidney tissues	Regulate intrarenal blood flow by vasodilation or vasoconstriction
Bradykinins	Juxtaglomerular cells of the arterioles	Increase blood flow (vasodilation) and vascular permeability
Erythropoietin	Kidney parenchyma	Stimulates bone marrow to make red blood cells
Activated vitamin D (1,25-dihydrocholecalciferol)	Kidney parenchyma	Promotes absorption of calcium in the GI tract
Hormones Influencing Kidney Function		
Vasopressin (antidiuretic hormone [ADH])	Released from posterior pituitary	Makes DCT and CD permeable to water to maximize reabsorption and produce a concentrated urine
Aldosterone	Released from adrenal cortex	Promotes sodium reabsorption and potassium secretion in DCT and CD; water and chloride follow sodium movement
Natriuretic hormones	Cardiac atria, cardiac ventricles, brain	Cause tubular secretion of sodium

CD, Collecting duct; *DCT,* distal convoluted tubule.

- Each ureter narrows at the point at which it enters the bladder; this point is called the ureterovesical junction (UVJ).

The ureter tunnels through bladder tissue for a short distance and then opens into the bladder at the trigone (Fig. 60.8).

The ureter has three layers: an inner lining of mucous membrane *(urothelium),* a middle layer of smooth muscle fibers, and an outer layer of fibrous tissue. The middle layer of muscle fibers is controlled by several nerve pathways from the lower spinal cord.

Contractions of the smooth muscle in the ureter move urine from the kidney pelvis to the bladder. Stretch receptors in the kidney pelvis regulate this movement. For example, a large volume of urine in the kidney pelvis triggers the stretch receptors, which respond by increasing ureteral contractions and ureter peristalsis.

Urinary Bladder

Structure. The urinary bladder is a muscular sac (see Fig. 60.8) that lies directly behind the pubic bone. In men, the bladder is in front of the rectum. In women, it is in front of the vagina.

The bladder is composed of the *body* (the rounded sac portion) and the *bladder neck* (posterior urethra), which connects to the bladder body. The bladder has three linings: an inner lining of epithelial cells *(urothelium),* middle layers of smooth muscle *(detrusor muscle),* and an outer lining. The *trigone* is an area on the posterior wall between the points of ureteral entry (ureterovesical junctions [UVJs]) and the urethra.

The **internal urethral sphincter** is the smooth detrusor muscle of the bladder neck and elastic tissue. The **external urethral sphincter** is skeletal muscle that surrounds the urethra. In men, the external sphincter surrounds the urethra at the base of the prostate gland. In women, the external sphincter is at the base of the bladder. The pudendal nerve from the spinal cord controls the external sphincter.

Function. The bladder stores urine, provides continence, and enables voiding. The secretions of the urothelium lining the bladder resist bacteria.

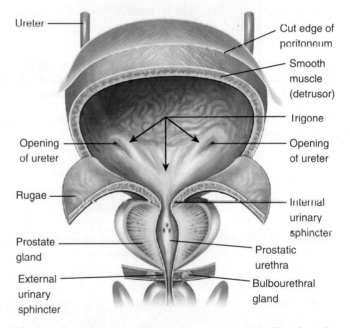

FIG. 60.8 Gross anatomy of the urinary bladder. (Modified from Patton, K.T., & Thibodeau, G.A. [2013]. *Anatomy & physiology* [8th ed.]. St. Louis: Mosby.)

Continence is the ability to voluntarily control bladder emptying. It occurs during bladder filling through the combination of detrusor muscle relaxation, internal sphincter muscle tone, and external sphincter contraction. As the bladder fills with urine, stretch sensations are transmitted to spinal sacral nerves.

Maintaining continence occurs by the interaction of the nerves that control the muscles of the bladder, bladder neck, urethra, and pelvic floor, as well as by factors that close the urethra. In the continent person, the smooth muscle of the detrusor remains relaxed during a period of urine filling and storage. Sympathetic nervous system fibers prevent detrusor muscle contraction. The control centers for voiding are located in the cerebral cortex, the brainstem, and the lower spinal cord. For urethral closure to be adequate for continence, the mucosal surfaces must be in contact and must be adhesive. Contact depends on the presence and proper function of the involved nerves and muscles. Adhesion depends on the secretion of mucus-like substances.

Micturition (voiding, urination) is a reflex of autonomic control that triggers contraction of the detrusor muscle (closing the ureter at the UVJ to prevent backflow) at the same time as relaxation of the external sphincter and the muscles of the pelvic floor. Voluntary urine *elimination* (voiding) occurs as a learned response and is controlled by the cerebral cortex and the brainstem. Contraction of the external sphincter inhibits the micturition reflex and prevents voiding.

Urethra

The urethra is a narrow tube lined with mucous membranes. Its purpose is to allow urine *elimination* from the bladder. The ure-thral meatus, or opening, is the endpoint of the urethra. In men, the urethra is about 6 to 8 inches (15 to 20 cm) long, with the meatus located at the tip of the penis. The male urethra has three sections:

- The prostatic urethra, which extends from the bladder through the prostate gland
- The membranous urethra, which extends from the prostate to the wall of the pelvic floor
- The cavernous urethra, which is external and extends through the length of the penis

In women, the urethra is 1 to 1.5 inches (2.5 to 3.75 cm) long and exits through the pelvic floor. The meatus lies slightly below the clitoris and directly in front of the vagina and rectum.

Kidney and Urinary Changes Associated With Aging

Kidney Changes. Changes occur in the kidney as a result of the aging process that can affect urine *elimination* and health (see the Patient-Centered Care: Older Adult Considerations: Changes in the Renal System Related to Aging box). The kidney loses cortical tissue and nephrons and gets smaller with age as a result of reduced blood flow to the kidney (Denic et al., 2016; Touhy & Jett, 2016). The medulla is not affected by aging, and the juxtamedullary nephron functions are preserved. The glomerular and tubular linings thicken. Both the number of glomeruli and their surface areas decrease with aging. Tubule length decreases. The changes reduce the older adult's ability to filter blood and excrete waste products.

👤 PATIENT-CENTERED CARE: OLDER ADULT CONSIDERATIONS (QSEN)

Changes in the Renal System Related to Aging

Physiologic Change	Nursing Interventions	Rationales
Decreased glomerular filtration rate (GFR)	Monitor hydration status.	The ability of the kidneys to regulate water balance decreases with age.
	Ensure adequate fluid intake.	The kidneys are less able to conserve water when necessary.
	Use caution when administering potentially nephrotoxic agents or drugs	Dehydration reduces kidney blood flow and increases the nephrotoxic potential of many agents. Acute or chronic kidney failure may result.
Nocturia	Ensure adequate nighttime lighting and a hazard-free environment.	Falls and injuries are common among older patients seeking bathroom facilities.
	Ensure the availability of a bedside toilet, bedpan, or urinal.	Using these items instead of getting up to go the bathroom can help prevent falls.
	Discourage excessive fluid intake for 2-4 hr before the patient goes to bed.	Excessive fluid intake at night may increase nocturia.
	Evaluate drugs and timing.	Some drugs increase urine output and increase the risk for falling when toileting.
Decreased bladder capacity	Encourage the patient to use the toilet, bedpan, or urinal at least every 2 hr.	Emptying the bladder on a regular basis may avoid overflow urinary incontinence.
	Respond as soon as possible to the patient's indication of the need to void.	A quick response may alleviate episodes of urinary stress incontinence.
Weakened urinary sphincters and shortened urethra in women	Provide thorough perineal care after each voiding.	The shortened urethra increases the potential for bladder infections.
		Good perineal hygiene may prevent skin irritations and urinary tract infection (UTI).
Tendency to retain urine	Observe the patient for urinary retention (e.g., bladder distention) or urinary tract infection (e.g., dysuria, foul odor, confusion).	Urinary stasis may result in a UTI, which may lead to bloodstream infections, urosepsis, or septic shock.
	Provide privacy, assistance, and voiding stimulants such as warm water over the perineum as needed.	Nursing interventions can help initiate voiding.
	Evaluate drugs for possible contribution to retention.	Anticholinergic drugs promote urinary retention.

Blood flow to the kidney declines by about 10% per decade as blood vessels thicken. This means that blood flow to the kidney is not as adaptive in older adults, leaving nephrons more vulnerable to damage during episodes of either hypotension or hypertension.

Glomerular filtration rate (GFR) decreases with age. By age 65 years, the GFR is about 65 mL/min (half the rate of a young adult) and increases the risk for fluid overload. This decline is more rapid in patients with diabetes, hypertension, or heart failure. The combination of reduced kidney mass, reduced blood flow, and decreased GFR contributes to reduced drug clearance and a greater risk for drug reactions and kidney damage from drugs and contrast media in older adults.

Tubular changes with aging decrease the ability to concentrate urine, resulting in urgency (a sense of a nearly uncontrollable need to urinate) and nocturnal polyuria (increased urination at night). The regulation of sodium, acids, and bicarbonate is less efficient. Along with an age-related impairment in the thirst mechanism, these changes increase the risk for disturbances of *fluid and electrolyte balance,* such as dehydration and hypernatremia (increased blood sodium levels) in the older adult. Hormonal changes include a decrease in renin secretion, aldosterone levels, and activation of vitamin D.

Urinary Changes. Changes in detrusor muscle elasticity lead to decreased bladder capacity and reduced ability to retain urine (Touhy & Jett, 2016). The urge to void may cause immediate bladder emptying because the urinary sphincters lose tone and often become weaker with age. In women, weakened muscles in the pelvic floor shorten the urethra and promote incontinence. In men, an enlarged prostate gland makes starting the urine stream difficult and may cause urinary retention.

> ### 👤 PATIENT-CENTERED CARE: CULTURAL/ SPIRITUAL CONSIDERATIONS (QSEN)
>
> African Americans have more rapid age-related decreases in GFR than do white adults. Kidney excretion of sodium is less effective in hypertensive African Americans who have high sodium intake, and the kidneys have about 20% less blood flow as a result of anatomic changes in small blood vessels and intrarenal responses to renin. Thus African-American patients are at greater risk for kidney failure than are white patients (Jarvis, 2020). Yearly health examinations should include urinalysis, checking for the presence of microalbuminuria, and evaluating serum creatinine.

ASSESSMENT: RECOGNIZE CUES

Patient History

Demographic information, such as age, gender, race, and ethnicity, is important to consider as nonmodifiable risk factors in the patient with any kidney or urinary *elimination* problem. A sudden onset of hypertension in patients older than 50 years suggests possible kidney disease. Clinical changes in polycystic kidney disease typically occur in patients in their 40s or 50s. In men older than 50 years, altered urine patterns accompany prostate disease.

Anatomic gender differences make some disorders worse or more common. For example, men rarely have ascending urinary tract infections. Women have a shorter urethra and more commonly develop cystitis (bladder inflammation, most often with infection) because bacteria pass more readily into the bladder.

Modifiable risk factors, as well as socioeconomic status, level of education, language, and health beliefs, should be considered when assessing renal function. *Socioeconomic status* may influence health care practices. Prevention, early detection, and treatment of kidney or urinary problems may be limited by inability to access to health care, lack of transportation, insufficient or no insurance, and/or reduced income. These barriers may also result in difficulty following medical advice, having prescriptions filled, adhering to dietary instructions, and keeping follow-up appointments.

Educational level may affect health-seeking practices and the patient's understanding of a disease or its symptoms. Recurring urinary tract infections can result from not completing a course of antibiotic therapy or from not following up to ensure that the infection is cleared.

The language used by patients may be different from that used by the health care professional. When obtaining a history, listen to and explore the terms used by the patient. By using the patient's own terms, you may help him or her provide a more complete description of the problem and may decrease the patient's discomfort when discussing bodily functions.

The patient's health beliefs affect the approach to health and illness. Cultural background or religious affiliation may influence the belief system, as well as comfort when discussing issues about *elimination* (Jackson et al., 2013).

Ask the patient about previous kidney or urologic problems, including tumors, infections, stones, or urologic surgery. A history of any chronic health problems, especially diabetes mellitus or hypertension, increases the risk for development of kidney disease because these disorders damage kidney blood vessels.

Ask the patient about environmental, food, or medication allergies. Exposure to certain contrast media during imaging can harm the kidneys. Iodinated contrast medium used for CT scans is associated with both acute and chronic kidney injury (Lambert et al., 2017). High-osmolarity contrast agents can also contribute to kidney function impairment. Exposure to gadolinium-enhanced MRI can result in nephrogenic systemic fibrosis.

Ask the patient about chemical exposures at the workplace or with hobbies. Exposure to hydrocarbons (e.g., gasoline, oil), heavy metals (especially mercury and lead), and some gases (e.g., chlorine, toluene) can impair kidney function. Use this opportunity to teach patients who come into contact with chemicals at work or during leisure-time activities to avoid direct skin or mucous membrane contact with these chemicals. Use of heroin, cocaine, methamphetamine, ecstasy, and volatile solvents (inhalants) has also been associated with kidney damage.

Specifically ask the patient whether he or she has ever been told about the presence of protein or albumin in the urine. The question, "Have you ever been told that your blood pressure is high?" may prompt a response different from the one to the question, "Do you have high blood pressure?" Ask women about health problems during pregnancy (e.g., proteinuria, high blood pressure, gestational diabetes, urinary tract infections). Obtain information about:

- Chemical or environmental toxin exposure in occupational, diagnostic, or other settings
- Recent travel to geographic regions that pose infectious disease risks
- Recent trauma or injury, particularly to the abdomen or pelvic or genital areas
- A history of altered patterns of urinary *elimination*

Nutrition History. Ask the patient with known or suspected kidney or urologic disorders about diet and any recent dietary changes. Note any excessive intake or omission of certain food categories. Ask about food and fluid intake. Assess how much and which types of fluids the patient drinks daily, especially fluids with a high-calorie or caffeine content. Use this opportunity to teach the patient the importance of drinking sufficient fluid to cause urine to be dilute (clear or very light yellow). If another medical problem does not require fluid restriction, ingestion of about 2 L of fluid daily is recommended. If the patient has followed a diet for weight reduction, the details of the diet plan are important and collaboration with a dietitian may be needed. A high-protein intake can result in temporary kidney problems. For example, a patient at risk for calculi (stone) formation who ingests large amounts of protein or has a poor fluid intake may form new stones.

Ask about any change in appetite or taste. These symptoms can occur with the buildup of nitrogenous waste products from kidney failure. Changes in thirst or fluid intake may also cause changes in the volume of urine *elimination*. Endocrine disorders may also cause changes in thirst, fluid intake, and urine output. (See Chapter 56 for a discussion of endocrine influences on fluid balance.)

Medication History. Identify all of the patient's prescription drugs because many can impair kidney function (Burchum & Rosenthal, 2019). Ask about the duration of drug use and whether there have been any recent changes in prescribed drugs. Drugs for diabetes mellitus, hypertension, cardiac disorders, hormonal disorders, cancer, arthritis, and psychiatric disorders are potential causes of kidney problems. Antibiotics, such as gentamicin, may also cause acute kidney injury. Drug-drug interactions and drug–contrast media interactions also may lead to kidney dysfunction (Lambert et al., 2017).

Explore the past and current use of over-the-counter (OTC) drugs or agents, including dietary supplements, vitamins and minerals, herbal agents, laxatives, analgesics, acetaminophen, and NSAIDs. Many of these agents affect kidney function and urine *elimination*. For example, dietary supplementation with synthetic creatine, used to increase muscle mass, has been associated with compromised kidney function. High-dose or long-term use of NSAIDs or acetaminophen can seriously reduce kidney function. Some agents are associated with hypertension, hematuria, or proteinuria, which may occur before kidney dysfunction.

Family History and Genetic Risk. The family history of the patient with a suspected kidney or urologic problem is important because some disorders have a familial pattern. Ask whether siblings, parents, or grandparents have had kidney problems. Past terms used for kidney disease include *Bright disease*, *nephritis*, and *nephrosis*. Although nephritis is a current term for an inflammatory process in the kidney and nephrosis is a current term for a degenerative process in the kidney, these terms have been used by lay adults for years to describe any type of kidney problem. Polycystic kidney disease, which is a genetic disorder, can occur in either gender.

Current Health Problem. The effects of kidney failure are seen in all body systems. Document all of the patient's current health problems. Ask the patient to describe all health concerns, because some kidney disorders cause problems in other body systems. Recent upper respiratory problems, achy muscles or joints, heart disease, or GI conditions may be related to problems of kidney function.

Assess the kidney and urologic system by asking about any changes in the appearance (color, odor, clarity) of the urine, pattern of urine *elimination,* ability to initiate or control voiding, and other unusual symptoms. For example, urine that is reddish, rust-colored, brown or black, greenish, or different from the usual yellowish color may prompt the patient to seek health care assistance. Urine typically has a mild but distinct odor of ammonia. An increase in the intensity of color, a change in odor quality, or a decrease in urine clarity may suggest infection.

Ask about changes in urination patterns, such as incontinence (involuntary bladder emptying), nocturia (urination at night), urgency (nearly uncontrollable urge to urinate), frequency, or an increase or decrease in the amount of urine. The normal urine output for adults is about 1500 to 2000 mL/day or within 500 mL of the volume of fluid ingested daily. Ask about how closely the urine output is to the volume of fluid ingested. A bladder diary may be useful. Ask whether:

- Initiating urine flow is difficult
- A burning sensation or other discomfort occurs with urination
- The force of the urine stream is decreased
- Persistent dribbling or leaking of urine is present

The onset of pain in the flank, in the lower abdomen or pelvic region, or in the perineal area triggers concern and usually prompts the patient to seek assistance. Ask about the onset, intensity, and duration of the pain; its location; precipitating and relieving factors; and its association with any activity or event.

Pain associated with kidney or ureteral irritation is often severe and spasmodic. Pain that radiates into the perineal area, groin, scrotum, or labia is described as *renal colic*. This pain occurs with distention or spasm of the ureter, such as in an obstruction or the passing of a stone. Renal colic pain may be intermittent or continuous and may occur with pallor, diaphoresis, and hypotension. These general symptoms occur because of the location of the nerve tracts near or in the kidneys and ureters (Brenner, 2016).

Because the kidneys are close to the GI organs and the nerve pathways are similar, GI symptoms may occur with kidney problems. These renointestinal reflexes often complicate the description of the kidney problem.

Uremia is the buildup of nitrogenous waste products in the blood from inadequate *elimination* as a result of kidney failure. Symptoms include anorexia, nausea and vomiting, muscle cramps, *pruritus* (itching), fatigue, and lethargy.

Physical Assessment

The physical assessment of the patient with a known or suspected kidney or urologic disorder includes general appearance, a review of body systems, and specific structure and functions of the kidney and urinary system.

Assess the patient's general appearance and check the skin for the presence of any rashes, bruising, or yellowish discoloration. The skin and tissues may show edema associated with kidney disease, especially in the *pedal* (foot), *pretibial* (shin), and sacral tissues and around the eyes. Use a stethoscope to listen to the lungs to determine whether fluid is present. Weigh the patient and measure blood pressure as a baseline for later comparisons.

Assess the levels of consciousness and alertness. Record any deficits in memory, concentration, or thought processes. Family members may report subtle changes. Cognitive changes may be the result of the buildup of waste products when kidney disease is present.

Assessment of the Kidneys, Ureters, and Bladder. Assess the kidneys, ureters, and bladder during an abdominal assessment (Jarvis, 2020). Auscultate before percussion and palpation because these activities can alter bowel sounds and obscure abdominal vascular sounds.

Inspect the abdomen and the flank regions with the patient in both the supine and sitting positions. Observe the patient for asymmetry (e.g., swelling) or discoloration (e.g., bruising or redness) in the flank region, especially in the area of the costovertebral angle (CVA). The CVA is located between the lower portion of the twelfth rib and the vertebral column.

Listen for a bruit by placing a stethoscope over each renal artery on the midclavicular line. A **bruit** is an audible swishing sound produced when the volume of blood or the diameter of the blood vessel changes. It often occurs with blood flow through a narrowed vessel, as in renal artery stenosis.

Kidney palpation is usually performed by a health care provider. It can help locate masses and areas of tenderness in or around the kidney. The health care provider will lightly palpate the abdomen in all quadrants, ask about areas of tenderness or pain, and examine nontender areas first (Fig. 60.9). The outline of the bladder may be noted as high as the umbilicus in patients with severe bladder distention.

> **! NURSING SAFETY PRIORITY** (QSEN)
>
> **Action Alert**
>
> Performing palpation on a patient with a suspected abdominal tumor or aneurysm may harm the patient.

Because the kidneys are located deep and posterior, palpation is easier in thin patients who have little abdominal musculature. For palpation of the right kidney, the patient is placed in a supine position while the examiner places one hand under

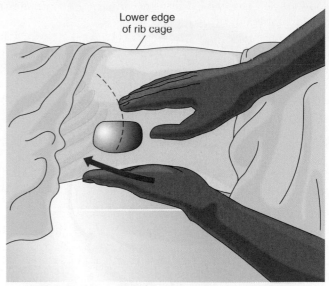

FIG. 60.9 Advanced technique for palpation of the kidney.

the right flank and the other hand over the abdomen below the lower right part of the rib cage. The lower hand is used to raise the flank, and the upper hand depresses the abdomen as the patient takes a deep breath (Fig. 60.9). The left kidney is deeper and often cannot be palpated. A transplanted kidney is readily palpated in either the lower right or left abdominal quadrant. The normal kidney is smooth, firm, and nontender.

A distended bladder sounds dull when percussed. After gently palpating to determine the outline of the distended bladder, begin percussion on the lower abdomen and continue in the direction of the umbilicus until dull sounds are no longer produced. If you suspect bladder distention, use a portable bladder scanner (Fig. 60.10) to determine the amount of retained urine.

If the patient reports flank pain or tenderness, the nontender flank should be percussed first. For percussion, the patient is placed in a sitting, side-lying, or supine position. Percussion, generally performed by the health care provider, is done by forming one hand into a clenched fist and the other hand lies flat over the CVA of the patient. Using the hand in a fist, a quick, firm thump is administered to the hand over the CVA area (Jarvis, 2020). Costovertebral tenderness often occurs with kidney infection or inflammation. Patients with inflammation or infection in the kidney or nearby structures may describe their pain as severe or as a constant, dull ache.

Assessment of the Urethra. Using a good light source and wearing gloves, inspect the urethra by examining the meatus and the tissues around it. Record any unusual discharge such as blood, mucus, or pus. Inspect the skin and mucous membranes of surrounding tissues. Record the presence of lesions, rashes, or other abnormalities of the penis or scrotum or of the labia or vaginal opening. Urethral irritation is suspected when the patient reports discomfort with urination. Use this opportunity to remind women to clean the perineum by wiping from front to back, never from back to front. Teach them that the front-to-back technique keeps organisms in stool from coming close to the urethra and decreases the risk for infection.

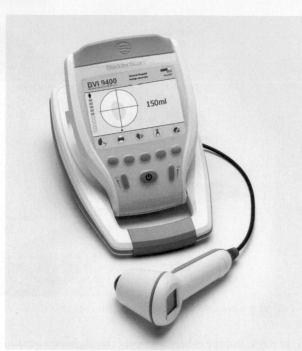

FIG. 60.10 "BladderScan" BVI 9400, a handheld portable bladder scanner. (Courtesy Verathon Corporation, Bothell, WA.)

👤 PATIENT-CENTERED CARE: CULTURAL/ SPIRITUAL CONSIDERATIONS (QSEN)

Women from some cultures or religions may have undergone female circumcision. This procedure alters the appearance of the vulvar-perineal area and increases the risk for urinary tract infections. It also makes urethral inspection or catheterization difficult. Document any noted anatomic changes and ask the patient to describe hygiene practices for this area.

Psychosocial Assessment

Concerns about the urologic system may evoke fear, anger, embarrassment, anxiety, guilt, or sadness in the patient. Childhood learning often includes the idea that toileting should take place in private and not be discussed with other people. Urologic disorders may bring up forgotten memories of difficult toilet training and bedwetting or of childhood experiences of exploring one's body. The patient may ignore symptoms or delay seeking health care because of emotional responses or cultural taboos about the urogenital area.

NCLEX EXAMINATION CHALLENGE 60.1

Physiological Integrity

When obtaining a health history and physical assessment from a 68-year-old male client who has a history of an enlarged prostate, which finding does the nurse consider significant? **Select all that apply.**

A. Distended bladder
B. Absence of a bruit
C. Frequency of urination
D. Dribbling urine after voiding
E. Chemical exposure in the workplace

Diagnostic Assessment
Laboratory Assessment
Blood Tests. Serum creatinine is produced when muscle and other proteins are broken down. Because protein breakdown is usually constant, the serum creatinine level is a good indicator of kidney function. Serum creatinine levels are slightly higher in men than in women because men tend to have a larger muscle mass than do women. Similarly, adults with greater muscle mass or muscle mass turnover (e.g., athletes) may have a slightly higher-than-average serum creatinine level. Muscle mass and the amount of creatinine produced decrease with age. However, because of decreased rates of creatinine clearance, the serum creatinine level remains relatively constant in older adults unless kidney disease is present.

No common pathologic condition other than kidney disease increases the serum creatinine level. When the serum creatinine level is doubled, it indicates a 50% reduction in glomerular filtration rate (Pagana & Pagana, 2018); therefore *any* elevation of serum creatinine values is important and should be assessed further. Creatinine is excreted solely by the kidneys.

❗ NURSING SAFETY PRIORITY (QSEN)
Action Alert

A serum creatinine of 1.5 mg/dL (110 mcmol/L) or greater places a patient at risk for acute kidney injury (AKI) from iodinated contrast media and some drugs (Lambert et al., 2017). Monitor both baseline and trend values to recognize risk for and actual kidney damage, especially among patients exposed to agents that can cause kidney dysfunction. If indicated, respond by promptly informing the primary health care provider of increases in serum creatinine greater than 1.5 times the baseline and urine output values of less than 0.5 mL/kg/hr for 6 or more hours. Using the baseline and trending creatinine levels is important, especially in older adults and young children as they have lower creatinine levels due to reduced muscle mass than the normal adult.

Blood urea nitrogen (BUN) measures the effectiveness of kidney excretion of urea nitrogen, a by-product of protein breakdown in the liver. Urea nitrogen is produced mostly from liver metabolism of food sources of protein. The kidneys filter urea nitrogen from the blood and excrete the waste as part of urine *elimination.*

Other factors influence the BUN level, and an elevation does not always mean that kidney disease is present (see the Laboratory Profile: Kidney Function Blood Studies box). For example, rapid cell destruction from infection, cancer treatment, or steroid therapy may elevate BUN level. In addition, blood is a protein. Blood in the tissues rather than in the blood vessels is reabsorbed as if it were a general protein. Thus reabsorbed blood protein is processed by the liver and increases BUN levels. This means that injured tissues can result in increased BUN levels even when kidney function is normal. In addition, BUN is increased by protein turnover in exercising muscle and is elevated as a result of concentration during dehydration.

The liver must function properly to produce urea nitrogen. When liver and kidney dysfunction are present, urea nitrogen levels are actually *decreased* because the liver failure limits urea production. The BUN level is not always elevated with kidney disease and is not the best indicator of kidney function. However, an elevated BUN level suggests kidney dysfunction.

Blood urea nitrogen to serum creatinine ratio can help determine whether non–kidney-related factors, such as low cardiac output or red blood cell destruction, are causing the elevated BUN level. When blood volume is deficient (e.g., dehydration) or cardiac output is low, the BUN level rises more rapidly than the serum creatinine level. As a result, the ratio of BUN to creatinine is *increased*.

When both the BUN and serum creatinine levels increase at the same rate, the BUN/creatinine ratio remains normal. However, elevations of *both* serum creatinine and BUN levels suggest kidney dysfunction that is not related to dehydration or poor perfusion.

Cystatin-C measures glomerular filtration rate. Cystatin-C is a protein produced by nucleated cells in the body. Since cystatin-C is produced at a constant rate, it can be used as an indicator of glomerular filtration rate. When the glomerular filtration rate is reduced, cystatin-C increases. Increased levels can be considered a predictor of chronic renal disease. Cystatin-C is not influenced by factors that influence BUN and creatinine levels, making it potentially a better indicator of glomerular filtration rate. Research is still in progress as to the efficacy of cystatin-C in the role of identifying renal disease and other health alterations such as cardiovascular disease and metabolic syndrome (Pagana & Pagana, 2018).

Blood osmolarity is a measure of the overall concentration of particles in the blood and is a good indicator of hydration status. The kidneys excrete or reabsorb water to keep blood osmolarity in the range of 280 to 300 mOsm/kg (mmol/kg). Osmolarity is slightly higher in older adults. When blood osmolarity is decreased, vasopressin (antidiuretic hormone [ADH]) release is inhibited. Without vasopressin, the distal tubule and collecting ducts are *not* permeable to water. As a result, water is *excreted*, not reabsorbed, and blood osmolarity increases. When blood osmolarity increases, vasopressin is released. Vasopressin increases the permeability of the distal tubule to water. Then water is reabsorbed, and blood osmolarity decreases.

Urine Tests

Urinalysis. Urinalysis is a part of any complete physical examination and is especially useful for patients with suspected kidney or urologic disorders (see the Laboratory Profile: Urinalysis box). Ideally, the urine specimen is collected at the morning's first voiding. Specimens obtained at other times may be too dilute. The specimen may be collected by several techniques (Box 60.1).

Urine color comes from urochrome pigment. Color variations may result from increased levels of urochrome or other pigments, changes in the concentration or dilution of the urine, and the presence of drug metabolites in the urine. Urine smells faintly like ammonia and is normally clear without *turbidity* (cloudiness) or haziness.

Specific gravity is the concentration of particles (i.e., electrolytes, wastes) in urine. A high specific gravity indicates concentrated urine from dehydration, decreased kidney blood flow, or excess vasopressin associated with stress, surgery, anesthetic agents, and certain drugs (e.g., morphine, some oral antidiabetic drugs) or syndrome of inappropriate antidiuretic hormone (SIADH) (see Chapter 57). Low specific gravity indicates dilute urine that may occur from high fluid intake, diuretic drugs, or diabetes insipidus (DI) (see Chapter 57).

Specific gravity of urine is compared with distilled water, which has a specific gravity of 1.000. The normal specific gravity of urine ranges from 1.005 to about 1.030. Kidney disease diminishes the concentrating ability of the kidney, and chronic kidney disease may be associated with a low (dilute) specific gravity.

pH is a measure of urine acidity or alkalinity. A pH value less than 7 is acidic, and a value greater than 7 is alkaline. Urine pH is affected by diet, drugs, systemic disturbances of **acid-base balance**, and kidney tubular function. For example, a high-protein diet produces acidic urine, whereas a high intake of citrus fruit produces alkaline urine. The normal pH of urine ranges from 4.6 to 8.0 with an average of 6.0 (Pagana & Pagana, 2018).

Urine specimens become more alkaline when left standing unrefrigerated for more than 1 hour, when bacteria are present,

---

⑤ LABORATORY PROFILE

Kidney Function Blood Studies

Test	Normal Range for Adults	Canadian Normal Range	Significance of Abnormal Findings
Serum creatinine	*Males:* 0.6-1.2 mg/dL *Females:* 0.5-1.1 mg/dL *Older adults:* may be decreased	*Males:* 53-106 mcmol/L *Females:* 44-97 mcmol/L	An *increased level* indicates kidney impairment. A *decreased level* may be caused by decreased muscle mass.
Blood urea nitrogen (BUN)	10-20 mg/dL *Older adults:* slightly higher	3.6-7.1 mmol/L	An *increased level* may indicate liver or kidney disease, dehydration or decreased kidney perfusion, a high-protein diet, infection, stress, steroid use, GI bleeding, or other situations in which blood is in body tissues. A *decreased level* may indicate malnutrition, fluid volume excess, or severe hepatic damage.
BUN/creatinine ratio (BUN divided by creatinine)	6-25 15.5 optimum level for adults	6-25	An *increased ratio* may indicate fluid volume deficit, obstructive uropathy, catabolic state, or a high-protein diet. A *decreased ratio* may indicate fluid volume excess.

Data from Pagana, K., & Pagana, T. (2018). *Mosby's manual of diagnostic & laboratory test* (6th ed.). St. Louis: Mosby; and Pagana, K., Pagana, T., & Pike-McDonald, S. (2018). *Mosby's Canadian manual of diagnostic and laboratory tests.* St. Louis: Elsevier.

◢ LABORATORY PROFILE

Urinalysis

Test	Normal Range for Adults	Significance of Abnormal Findings
Color	Yellow	*Dark amber* indicates concentrated urine. *Very pale yellow* indicates dilute urine. *Dark red* or *brown* indicates blood in the urine. Brown may indicate increased bilirubin level. Red also may indicate the presence of myoglobin. *Other color* changes may result from diet or drugs.
Odor	Specific aroma, similar to ammonia	*Foul smell* indicates possible infection, dehydration, or ingestion of certain foods or drugs.
Turbidity	Clear	*Cloudy urine* indicates infection, sediment, or high levels of urine protein.
Specific gravity	1.005-1.030; usually 1.010-1.025 *Older adult:* decrease with age	*Increased* in decreased kidney perfusion, inappropriate ADH secretion, or heart failure. *Decreased* in chronic kidney disease, diabetes insipidus, malignant hypertension, diuretic administration, and lithium toxicity.
pH	Average: 6; range: 4.6-8	*Changes* are caused by diet, drugs, infection, age of specimen, acid-base imbalance, and kidney disease.
Glucose	Fresh specimen, negative 50-300 mg/day in a 24-hr specimen	*Presence* reflects hyperglycemia or a decrease in the kidney threshold for glucose.
Ketones	None	*Presence* occurs with diabetic ketoacidosis, prolonged fasting, and anorexia nervosa.
Protein	0-8 mg/dL (50-80 mg in 24-hr specimen at rest <250 mg in 24-hr specimen with exercise	*Increased* amounts may indicate stress, infection, recent strenuous exercise, or glomerular disorders.
Bilirubin (urobilinogen)	None	*Presence* suggests liver or biliary disease or obstruction.
Red blood cells (RBCs)	0-2 per high-power field	*Increased* is normal with catheterization or menses but may reflect tumor, stones, trauma, glomerular disorders, cystitis, or bleeding disorders.
White blood cells (WBCs)	0-4 per low-power field	*Increased* may indicate an infection or inflammation in the kidney and urinary tract, kidney transplant rejection, or exercise.
Casts	None	*Increased* indicates bacteria, protein, or urinary calculi.
Crystals	None	*Presence* may indicate that the specimen has been allowed to stand.
Bacteria	<1000 colonies/mL	*Increased* indicates the need for urine culture to determine the presence of urinary tract infection.
Parasites	None	*Presence* of *Trichomonas vaginalis* indicates infection, usually of the urethra, prostate, or vagina.
Leukocyte esterase	None	*Presence* suggests urinary tract infection.
Nitrites	None	*Presence* suggests urinary *Escherichia coli*.

Data from Pagana, K., & Pagana, T. (2018). *Mosby's manual of diagnostic & laboratory test* (6th ed.). St. Louis: Mosby; and Pagana, K., Pagana, T., & Pike-McDonald, S. (2018). *Mosby's Canadian manual of diagnostic and laboratory tests*. St. Louis: Elsevier.

or when a specimen is left uncovered. Alkaline urine increases cell breakdown; thus the presence of red blood cells may be missed on analysis. Ensure that urine specimens are covered and delivered to the laboratory promptly. Urine specimens delayed 2 or more hours require refrigerated or other specific storage and transport precautions to ensure the integrity of the urine specimen (Pagana & Pagana, 2018). During systemic acidosis or alkalosis, the kidneys, along with blood buffers and the lungs, normally respond to keep serum pH normal. Chapter 14 discusses *acid-base balance* and imbalance.

Protein is not normally present in the urine. Microalbumin levels greater than 80 mcg/24 hr (0.08 g/24 hr) are abnormal. Protein molecules are too large to pass through intact glomerular membranes. When glomerular membranes are not intact, protein molecules pass through and are excreted with urine *elimination.*

Increased membrane permeability is caused by infection, inflammation, or immunologic problems. Some systemic problems cause production of abnormal proteins, such as globulin. Detection of abnormal protein types requires electrophoresis.

A random finding of **proteinuria** (usually albumin in the urine) followed by a series of negative (normal) findings does not imply kidney disease. If infection is the cause of the proteinuria, urinalyses after resolution of the infection should be negative for protein. Persistent proteinuria needs further investigation.

Microalbuminuria is the presence of albumin in the urine that is not measurable by a urine dipstick or usual urinalysis procedures. Specialized assays are used to quickly analyze a freshly voided urine specimen for microscopic levels of albumin. The normal microalbumin levels in a freshly voided specimen should be less than 2.0 mg/dL. Higher levels indicate microalbuminuria

BOX 60.1   Collection of Urine Specimens

Nursing Interventions	Rationales
Voided Urine	
Collect the first specimen voided in the morning.	Urine is more concentrated in the early morning.
Send the specimen to the laboratory as soon as possible.	After urine is collected, cellular breakdown results in more alkaline urine.
Refrigerate the specimen if a delay is unavoidable.	Refrigeration delays the alkalinization of urine. Bacteria are more likely to multiply in an alkaline environment.
Clean-Catch Specimen	
Explain the purpose of the procedure to the patient.	Correct technique is needed to obtain a valid specimen.
Instruct the patient to self-clean before voiding:	Surface cleaning is necessary to remove secretions or bacteria from the urethral meatus.
Instruct the female patient to separate the labia and use the sponges and solution provided to wipe with three strokes over the urethra. The first two wiping strokes are over each side of the urethra; the third wiping stroke is centered over the urethra (from front to back).	
Instruct the male patient to retract the foreskin of the penis and to similarly clean the urethra, using three wiping strokes with the sponge and solution provided (from the head of the penis downward).	
Instruct the patient to initiate voiding after cleaning. The patient then stops and resumes voiding into the container.	A midstream collection further removes secretions and bacteria because urine flushes the distal portion of the internal urethra.
At no time should any part of the patient's anatomy touch the lip or inner aspect of the container.	
Only 1 oz (30 mL) is needed; the remainder of the urine may be discarded into the commode.	
Ensure that the patient understands the procedure.	An improperly collected specimen may result in inappropriate or incomplete treatment.
Help the patient as needed.	The patient's understanding and the nurse's assistance ensure proper collection.
Catheterized Specimen	
For nonindwelling (straight) catheters:	The one-time passage of a urinary catheter may be necessary to obtain an uncontaminated specimen for analysis or to measure the volume of residual urine.
Use sterile technique and follow facility procedures for urinary catheterization.	These procedures minimize bacterial entry.
For indwelling catheters:	Urine is collected from an indwelling catheter or tubing when patients have catheters for continence or long-term urinary drainage.
• Apply a clamp to the drainage tubing, distal to the injection port for 15-30 minutes	Clamping allows urine to collect in the tubing at the location where the specimen is obtained.
• Clean the injection port cap of the catheter drainage tubing with an appropriate antiseptic and allow to dry. Povidone-iodine solution or alcohol is acceptable.	Surface contamination is prevented by following the cleaning procedures.
• Attach a sterile 5-mL syringe into the port and aspirate the quantity of urine required.	A minimum of 5 mL is needed for culture and sensitivity (C&S) testing.
• Inject the urine sample into a sterile specimen container.	A sterile container is used for C&S specimens.
• Remove the clamp to resume drainage.	
• Properly dispose of the syringe.	
24-Hour Urine Collection	
Instruct the patient thoroughly.	A 24-hr collection of urine is necessary to quantify or calculate the rate of clearance of a particular substance.
Provide written materials to assist in instruction.	Instructional materials for patients, signs, etc. remind patients and staff to ensure that the total collection is completed.
Place signs appropriately.	
Inform all personnel or family caregivers of test in progress.	
Check laboratory or procedure manual on proper technique for maintaining the collection (e.g., on ice, in a refrigerator, or with a preservative).	Proper technique prevents breakdown of elements to be measured.
On initiation of the collection, ask the patient to void, discard the urine, and note the time. If a Foley catheter is in use, empty the tubing and drainage bag at the start time and discard the urine.	Proper techniques ensure that *all* urine formed within the 24-hr period is collected.
Collect all urine of the next 24 hr.	
Twenty-four hours after initiation, ask the patient to empty the bladder and add that urine to the container.	
Do not remove urine from the collection container for other specimens.	Urine in the container is not considered a "fresh" specimen and may be mixed with preservative.

and could mean mild or early kidney disease, especially in patients with diabetes mellitus. In 24-hour urine specimens, levels greater than 80 mcg/24 hr (0.08 g/24 hr) indicate microalbuminuria.

Glucose in the urine may indicate a high level of glucose in the blood, typically greater than 220 mg/dL (12 mmol/L). Changes in the renal threshold for glucose may occur temporarily in patients who have infection or severe stress.

Ketone bodies are formed from the incomplete metabolism of fatty acids. Three types of ketone bodies are acetone, acetoacetic acid, and beta-hydroxybutyric acid. *Normally there are no ketones in urine.* Ketone bodies are produced when fat is used instead of glucose for cellular energy. Ketones present in the blood are partially excreted in the urine.

Leukoesterase is an enzyme found in some white blood cells, especially neutrophils. When the number of these cells increases in the urine or they are damaged (lysed), the urine then contains leukoesterase. A normal reading is no leukoesterase in the urine. A positive test (+ sign) is an indication of a urinary tract infection.

Nitrites are not usually present in urine. Many types of bacteria, when present in the urine, convert nitrates (normally found in urine) into nitrites. A positive nitrites test enhances the sensitivity of the leukoesterase test to detect urinary tract infection (Pagana & Pagana, 2018).

Sediment is precipitated particles in the urine. These particles include cells, casts, crystals, and bacteria. Normally, urine contains few, if any, cells. Types of cells abnormally present in the urine include tubular cells (from the tubule of the nephron), epithelial cells (from the lining of the urinary tract), red blood cells (RBCs), and white blood cells (WBCs). WBCs may indicate a urinary tract or kidney infection. RBCs may indicate *glomerulonephritis, acute tubular necrosis, pyelonephritis,* kidney trauma, or kidney cancer.

Casts are clumps of materials or cells. When cells, bacteria, or proteins are present in the urine, minerals and sticky materials clump around them and form a cast of the distal renal tubule and collecting duct. Casts are described by the type of particle they have surrounded (e.g., hyaline [protein-based] or cellular [from RBCs, WBCs, or epithelial cells]) or the stage of cast breakdown (whole cell or granular from cell breakdown). Although an isolated urinalysis with sediment from casts may be the result of strenuous exercise, repeated findings with sediment are more likely to be associated with disease.

Urine crystals come from mineral salts as a result of diet, drugs, or disease. Common salt crystals are formed from calcium, oxalate, urea, phosphate, magnesium, or other substances. Some drugs, such as the sulfates, can also form crystals. Crystals can form into calculi.

Bacteria multiply quickly, so the urine specimen must be analyzed promptly to avoid falsely elevated counts of bacterial colonization. Normally urine is sterile, but it can be easily contaminated by perineal bacteria during collection.

Recent advances in technology and molecular biology have led to new diagnostic tests using urine, including identification of biomarkers of disease and profiling for specific proteins. Markers such as cystatin-C are being investigated to identify early-onset kidney dysfunction, target therapy, and predict responsiveness to intervention. Other markers for angiogenesis and kidney cell adhesion, regulation, and apoptosis (i.e., connective tissue growth factor [CTGF], neutrophil gelatinase-associated lipocalin [NGAL]) will likely contribute to clinical diagnostics in the future.

Urine for Culture and Sensitivity. Urine is analyzed for the number and types of organisms present. Symptoms of infection and unexplained bacteria in a urine specimen are indications for urine culture and sensitivity testing. Bacteria from urine are placed in a medium with different antibiotics. In this way, we can know which antibiotics are effective in killing or stopping the growth of the organisms (organisms are "sensitive") and which are not effective (organisms are "resistant"). A clean-catch or catheter-derived specimen is best for culture and sensitivity testing as these procedures reduce the chance of perineal surface organisms contaminating the specimen.

Composite Urine Collections. Some urine collections are made for a specified number of hours (e.g., 24 hours) for precise analysis of urine levels of substances, such as creatinine or urea nitrogen, sodium, chloride, calcium, catecholamines, or other components (see the Laboratory Profile: 24-Hour Urine Collection box). For a composite urine specimen, *all* urine within the designated time frame must be collected. If other urine must be obtained while the collection is in progress, measure and record the amount collected but not added to the timed collection.

The urine collection may need to be refrigerated or stored on ice to prevent changes in the urine during the collection time. Follow the procedure from the laboratory for urine storage, including whether a preservative is to be added. The urine collection must be free from fecal contamination. Menstrual blood and toilet tissue also contaminate the specimen and can invalidate the results.

The collection of all urine for a 24-hour period is often challenging. With hospitalized patients, the cooperation of staff personnel, the patient, family members, and visitors is essential. Placing signs in the bathroom, instructing the patient and family, and emphasizing the need to save the urine are helpful.

Creatinine Clearance. Creatinine clearance is a measure of glomerular filtration rate (GFR) and kidney function. The patient's age, gender, height, weight, diet, and activity level influence the expected amount of excreted creatinine. Thus these factors are considered when interpreting creatinine clearance test results. Decreases in the creatinine clearance rate may require reducing drug doses and often signifies the need to further explore the cause of kidney deterioration.

Commonly, creatinine clearance is calculated from serum creatinine, age, weight, urine creatinine, gender, and race. Creatinine clearance can be based on the excretion of injected inulin or other substances that are not reabsorbed into the blood. Creatinine clearance to estimate GFR can also be based on a 24-hour urine collection, although urine can be collected for shorter periods (e.g., 8 or 12 hours). The analysis compares the urine creatinine level with the blood creatinine level; therefore a blood specimen for creatinine must also be collected. The range for normal creatinine clearance is 107 to 139 mL/min for men (1.78 to 2.32 mL/sec) and 87 to 107 mL/min (1.45 to 1.78 mL/sec) for women tested with a 24-hour urine collection (Pagana & Pagana, 2018). Values decrease

LABORATORY PROFILE
24-Hour Urine Collection

Component	Normal Range for Adults	Canadian Range for Adults	Significance of Abnormal Findings
Creatinine	*Males:* 1-2 g/24 hr *Females:* 0.6-1.8 g/24 hr *Older adults:* slightly lower	*Males:* 124-230 mcmol/kg/24 hr *Females:* 97-177 mcmol/kg/24 hr	*Decreased amounts* indicate deterioration in function caused by kidney disease. *Increased amounts* occur with infections, exercise, diabetes mellitus, and meat meals.
Urea nitrogen	12-20 g/24 hr	0.43-0.71 mmol/24 hr	*Decreased amounts* occur when kidney damage or liver disease is present. *Increased amounts* commonly result from a high-protein diet, dehydration, trauma, or sepsis.
Sodium	40-220 mEq/24 hr	40-220 mmol/day	*Decreased* in hemorrhage, shock, hyperaldosteronism, and prerenal acute kidney injury. *Increased* with diuretic therapy, excessive salt intake, hypokalemia, and acute tubular necrosis.
Chloride	110-250 mEq/24 hr	110-250 mmol/24 hr	*Decreased* in certain kidney diseases, malnutrition, pyloric obstruction, prolonged nasogastric tube drainage, diarrhea, diaphoresis, heart failure, and emphysema. *Increased* with hypokalemia, adrenal insufficiency, and massive diuresis.
Calcium	100-300 mg/24 hr	2.50-7.50 mmol/kg/24 hr	*Decreased* with hypocalcemia, hypoparathyroidism, nephrosis, and nephritis *Increased* with calcium kidney stones, hyperparathyroidism, sarcoidosis, certain cancers, immobilization, and hypercalcemia.
*Total catecholamines	<100 mcg/24 hr	<591 mmol/24 hr	*Increased* with pheochromocytoma, neuroblastomas, stress, or heavy exercise.
Protein	<80 mg/24 hr	10-150 mg/24 hr	*Increased* in glomerular disease, nephrotic syndrome, diabetic nephropathy, urinary tract malignancies, and irritations.

Data from Pagana, K., & Pagana, T. (2018). *Mosby's manual of diagnostic & laboratory test* (6th ed.). St. Louis: Mosby; Pagana, K., Pagana, T., & Pike-McDonald, J. (2018). *Mosby's Canadian manual of diagnostic and laboratory tests.* St. Louis: Elsevier; and United States Library of Medicine.

progressively per decade of life for adults older than 40 years because of age-related decline in GFR. However, these expensive and time-consuming methods are usually reserved for when a decision for starting renal replacement therapy (dialysis) is needed.

Current guidelines suggest that clinical laboratories report an estimate of GFR (eGFR) based on the Modification of Diet in Renal Disease (MDRD) study equation. The MDRD equation does not require urine to estimate GFR; the calculation requires the serum creatinine level, age, and numbers specific to gender and ethnicity. The calculation is an accurate way to measure urine creatinine clearance. The estimated GFR (eGFR) for the MDRD equation is >60 mL/min/1.73 m^2 (Pagana & Pagana, 2018).

Urine Electrolytes. Urine samples can be analyzed for electrolyte levels (e.g., sodium, chloride). Normally the amount of sodium excreted in the urine is nearly equal to that consumed. Urine sodium levels can vary depending on the amount of water and salt consumed. Normal values for a 24-hour urine sample ranges from 40 to 220 mEq/day (or 40 to 220 mmol/day). A value of greater than 20 mEq/L for a routine urine specimen is considered normal (Pagana & Pagana, 2018).

Urine Osmolarity. Osmolarity measures the concentration of particles in solution. The particles in urine contributing to osmolarity include electrolytes, glucose, urea, and creatinine.

NCLEX EXAMINATION CHALLENGE 60.2
Physiological Integrity

A client is on a 24-hour urine collection. At midpoint during the collection, the client tells the nurse that some of the urine was discarded. What action will the nurse take? **Select all that apply.**

A. No action is required.
B. Reinforce client education.
C. Notify the laboratory staff.
D. Restart the urine collection.
E. Document the discarded urine.
F. Notify the health care provider.

Urine osmolarity can vary from 50 to 1200 mOsm/kg or L (mmol/kg or L), depending on the patient's hydration status and kidney function. With average fluid intake, the range for urine osmolarity is 300 to 900 mOsm/kg or L (mmol/kg or L). Electrolytes, acids, and other normal metabolic wastes are continually produced. These particles are the solute load that must be excreted in the urine on a regular basis. This is referred to as *obligatory solute excretion*. If the patient loses excessive fluids, the kidney response is to save water while excreting wastes by excreting small amounts of highly concentrated urine. Diet, drugs, and activity can change urine osmolarity. Urine with an increased osmolarity is concentrated urine with less water and more solutes. Urine with a decreased osmolarity is dilute urine with more water and fewer solutes.

Bedside Sonography/Bladder Scanners. The use of portable ultrasound scanners in the hospital and rehabilitation setting by nurses is a noninvasive method of estimating bladder volume (see Fig. 60.10). Bladder scanners are used to screen for postvoid residual volumes and determine the need for intermittent catheterization based on the amount of urine in the bladder rather than the time between catheterizations. There is no discomfort with the scan, and no patient preparation beyond an explanation of what to expect is required.

Explain the reason the procedure is being done and what sensations the patient might experience during the procedure. For example, "This test will measure the amount of urine in your bladder. I will place a gel pad just above your pubic area and then place the probe, which is a little bigger and heavier than a stethoscope, on the gel."

Before scanning, select the male or female icon on the bladder scanner. Using the female icon allows the scanner software to subtract the volume of the uterus from any measurement. Use the male icon on all men and on women who have undergone a hysterectomy.

Place an ultrasound gel pad right above the pubic bone or moisten the round dome of the scan head area with 5 mL of conducting gel to improve ultrasound conduction. Use gel on the scanner head for obese patients and those with heavy body hair in the area to be scanned. Place the probe midline over the abdomen about 1.5 inches (4 cm) above the pubic bone. Aim the scan head so the ultrasound is projected toward the expected location of the bladder, typically toward the patient's coccyx. Press and release the scan button. The scan is complete with the sound of a beep, and a volume is displayed. Two readings are recommended for best accuracy. An aiming icon on the portable bladder scanner indicates whether the bladder image is centered on the crosshairs of the scan head. If the crosshairs on the aiming icon are not centered on the bladder, the measured volume may not be accurate.

Imaging Assessment. Many imaging procedures are used to diagnose abnormalities within the renal-urinary system (Box 60.2). Explain the procedures, prepare, and provide follow-up care to the patient. Patient education materials for many urologic tests have been developed by organizations, such as the Society for Urologic Nurses and Associates, and are freely available. Encourage the patient to use reliable and credible sources for online information.

Kidney, Ureter, and Bladder X-rays. An x-ray of the kidneys, ureters, and bladder (KUB) is a plain film of the abdomen obtained without any specific patient preparation. The KUB study shows gross anatomic features and obvious stones, strictures, calcifications, or obstructions in the urinary tract. This test identifies the shape, size, and position of the organs in relation to other parts of the urinary tract. Other tests are needed to diagnose functional or structural problems.

There is no discomfort or risk from this procedure. Tell the patient that the x-ray will be taken while in a supine position. No specific follow-up care is needed.

BOX 60.2 Radiologic and Special Diagnostic Tests for Patients With Disorders of the Kidney and Urinary System

Test	Purpose
Radiography of kidneys, ureters, and bladder (KUB) (plain film of abdomen)	To screen for the presence of two kidneys To measure kidney size To detect gross obstruction in kidneys or urinary tract
Computed tomography (CT) with contrast, CT arteriography or angiography	To measure kidney size To evaluate contour to assess for injury, masses, or obstruction in kidneys or the urinary tract To assess renal blood flow
Magnetic resonance imaging (MRI)	Similar to CT Useful for staging of cancers
Ultrasonography (US) Can be used with contrast media	To identify the urine volume in the bladder, size of the kidneys or obstruction (e.g., tumors, stones) in the kidneys or lower urinary tract Assess blood flow to and from the kidney
(Nuclear) renal scan	To evaluate renal perfusion To estimate glomerular filtration rate To provide functional information without exposing the patient to iodinated contrast medium
Cystoscopy	To identify abnormalities of the bladder wall and urethral and ureteral occlusions To treat small obstructions or lesions via fulguration, lithotripsy, or removal with a stone basket
Cystography and cystourethrography With or without retrograde studies With or without contrast medium	To outline bladder's contour when full and examine structure during voiding To examine the structure of the urethra To detect backward urine flow
Metabolic imaging with positron emission tomography (PET)	To evaluate cysts, tumors, and other lesions, eliminating the need for biopsy in some patients

---

Computed Tomography. Inform the patient that a CT scan provides three-dimensional information about the kidneys, ureters, bladder, and surrounding tissues. The CT scan is performed in a special room, usually in the radiology department. It can provide information about tumors, cysts, abscesses, other masses, and obstruction. CT can also be used to image the kidney's vascular system (i.e., CT angiography). Some hospitals require patients having CT scans to be NPO for some period before the scan, although there is no specific evidence guiding this practice.

Determine whether the scan requires contrast medium (often called *dye*). The most common contrast agents used for imaging of the kidney are radiopaque, contain iodine, are nonionic, and have varying osmolarity. These include iohexol, iopromide, and iodixanol. Oral or injected contrast medium is usually given before starting the imaging procedure. Dye use may be omitted in patients at risk for contrast-induced acute kidney injury, but the images produced are less distinct.

When contrast is used, ensure that there is sufficient oral or IV intake to dilute and excrete the contrast media. Typically, the radiologist will specify a total fluid intake of 1 L or a variable rate to maintain urine output at 1 to 2 mL/kg/hr for up to 6 hours. When no contrast is used, there is no special postprocedural care.

Contrast medium is potentially kidney damaging (nephrotoxic). *Contrast-induced nephropathy* is the onset of *acute kidney failure* within 48 hours after the administration of iodinated contrast medium (Lambert et al., 2017). The risk for *contrast-induced nephropathy* is greatest in patients who are older or dehydrated, have pre-existing chronic kidney disease (CKD), or have comorbidities of diabetes, heart failure, or current hypotension (Pagana & Pagana, 2018). Patients who take nephrotoxic drugs are also at risk. The best practice for patient safety and quality care lists assessment questions to ask before a patient undergoes testing with contrast material.

In addition, patients taking metformin are at risk for lactic acidosis when they receive iodinated contrast media. Metformin should be discontinued at least 24 hours before the time of a procedure and for at least 48 hours after the procedure. Kidney function should be re-evaluated before the patient resumes metformin therapy.

> ## ! NURSING SAFETY PRIORITY (QSEN)
> ### Drug Alert
>
> Ensure that the patient who is prescribed metformin does not receive the drug after a procedure requiring IV contrast material until adequate kidney function has been determined.

> ## BEST PRACTICE FOR PATIENT SAFETY & QUALITY CARE (QSEN)
>
> ### Assessing the Patient About to Undergo a Kidney Test or Procedure Using Contrast Medium
>
> Before the procedure:
> - Ask the patient:
>   - Have you had contrast medium before? If so, did you have a reaction? If so, describe the reaction (e.g., hives, facial edema, difficulty breathing, bronchospasm). If the patient has had a reaction before, he or she is at higher risk for having another reaction.
>   - Do you have a history of asthma? Patients with asthma have been shown to be at greater risk for contrast reactions than the general public. When reactions do occur, they are more likely to be severe.
>   - Do you have hay fever or food or drug allergies? Contrast reactions have been reported to be as high as 15% in patients with hay fever or food or drug allergies, especially to seafood, eggs, milk, or chocolate.
>   - Are you taking metformin. Metformin must be discontinued at least 24 hours before any study using contrast media because the life-threatening complication of lactic acidosis, although rare, could occur.
>   - When have you last eaten or drank anything?
> - Assess for a history of renal impairment and for conditions that have been implicated in increasing the chance of developing kidney injury or impairment after contrast media (e.g., diabetic nephropathy, class IV heart failure, dehydration, concomitant use of potentially nephrotoxic drugs such as the aminoglycosides or NSAIDs, and cirrhosis).
> - Assess hydration status by checking blood pressure, heart and respiratory rates, mucous membranes, skin turgor, and urine concentration.

All patients at risk for contrast-induced nephrotoxicity need regular assessment and collaboration with the primary health care provider to maintain hydration and decrease the risk for kidney injury following a CT scan with IV contrast administration. IV fluids of normal saline are the most effective before the procedure to prevent contrast-induced nephrotoxic effects during radiologic procedures (Sethi et al., 2018). Diuretics may be given immediately after the contrast is injected to enhance excretion in patients who are well hydrated.

> ## ! NURSING SAFETY PRIORITY (QSEN)
> ### Drug Alert
>
> When a CT scan with contrast is prescribed, report the patient's history of immediate hypersensitivity reactions associated with the administration of contrast media to the radiologist and health care provider.

Magnetic Resonance Imaging. MRI provides improved imaging between normal and abnormal tissue in the renal system compared with a CT scan. As with all MRIs, the patient with metal implants (pins, pacemaker, joint replacement, aneurysmal clips, or other cosmetic or medical devices) is not eligible for this test because the magnet can move the metal implant, resulting in harm to the patient. A variation of MRI is magnetic resonance angiography (MRA). This noninvasive procedure is used to detect blockages in large arteries and can determine renal artery stenosis.

Gadolinium-based contrast agents are used with MRI similar to CT scans. The contrast agent is injected intravenously and excreted via the kidneys. These agents have been linked with nephrogenic systemic fibrosis (Pagana & Pagana, 2018) and should not be used in patients with renal impairment, usually defined as a serum creatinine above 1.5 mg/dL (110 mcmol/L) or an estimated GFR less than 45 mL/min. Adults older than 60 years should be carefully evaluated for renal impairment.

Kidney Ultrasonography. Inform the patient that ultrasonography does not cause discomfort and is without risk. This test usually requires a full bladder. Ask the patient to drink 500 to 1000 mL of water, if needed, about 2 to 3 hours before the test to help fill the bladder. The patient should not void after drinking the water until the test is complete. This test applies sound waves to structures of different densities to produce images of the kidneys, ureters, and bladder and surrounding tissues. Ultrasonography allows assessment of kidney size, cortical thickness, and status of the calices. The test can identify obstruction in the urinary tract, tumors, cysts, and other masses without the use of contrast. In addition, it can determine blood flow into and out of the kidney using Doppler color flow imaging.

The patient undergoing kidney ultrasound is usually placed in the prone position. Sonographic gel is applied to the skin over the back and flank areas to enhance sound wave conduction. A transducer in contact with and moving across the skin delivers sound waves and measures the echoes. Images of the internal structures are produced. Assisting the patient to a position of comfort and skin care to remove the gel is all that is needed after ultrasonography.

Renal Scan. This imaging test is used to examine the perfusion, function, and structure of the kidneys by the IV administration of a radioisotope. It does not use an iodinated contrast agent and thus may be used in preference to a CT scan when the patient is allergic to iodine or has impaired kidney function that places him or her at risk for kidney injury from IV contrast.

No fasting or sedation is used. A peripheral IV catheter is inserted to give the radioisotope contrast agent. While the patient lies in a prone or sitting position, a camera is passed over the kidney area and records the isotope uptake on film, minutes after the radioisotope is given. After initial images, the patient may be given furosemide or captopril to better visualize kidney function and blood flow. The isotope is eliminated 6 to 24 hours after the procedure. Encourage the patient to drink fluids to aid in excretion of the isotope. Because only tracer doses of radioisotopes are used, no precautions are needed related to radioactive exposure.

! **NURSING SAFETY PRIORITY** (QSEN)

Drug Alert

A renal scan is contraindicated in women who are pregnant unless the benefits outweigh the risks.

Renal Arteriography (Angiography). Renal arteriography allows visualization of the renal arteries using a radiopaque contrast medium that enters the renal blood vessels and generates images to determine blood vessel size and abnormalities. The contrast medium is injected through the femoral or brachial artery as x-ray pictures are taken. This test has largely been replaced by other imaging techniques (e.g., nuclear renal scans, ultrasonography, computed tomography) and is seldom used as a stand-alone diagnostic procedure. The most common use of renal arteriography is at the time of a renal angioplasty or other intervention.

Cystoscopy and Cystourethroscopy

Patient Preparation. Cystoscopy and cystourethroscopy are endoscopic procedures used to evaluate the bladder, urethra, and lower portions of the ureters. An endoscopy scope is inserted through the urethra into the bladder providing direct visualization. These procedures require completion of a preoperative checklist and a signed informed consent statement. The urologist provides a complete description of and reasons for the procedure, and the nurse reinforces this information. Cystoscopy may be performed for diagnosis or treatment. This test is used to examine for bladder trauma (cystoscopy) or urethral trauma (cystourethroscopy) and to identify causes of urinary tract obstruction. Cystoscopy also may be used to remove bladder tumors or plant radium seeds into a tumor, dilate the urethra and ureters with or without stent placement, stop areas of bleeding, or resect an enlarged prostate gland.

Cystoscopy may be performed under general anesthesia or under local anesthesia with sedation. The patient's age and general health and the expected duration of the procedure are considered in the decision about anesthesia. A light evening meal may be eaten. Usually the patient is NPO after midnight on the night before the cystoscopy. A bowel preparation with laxatives or enemas is performed the evening before the procedure so that bowel contents do not interfere with the procedure.

Procedure. The cystoscopy is performed in a designated cystoscopic examination room. If the procedure is performed in a surgical suite under general anesthesia, the usual surgical support personnel are present (see Chapter 9). This procedure is often performed in clinics, ambulatory surgery or short-procedure units, or a urologist's office.

Assist the patient onto a table and, after sedation, place the patient in the lithotomy position. After the anesthesia is given and the area cleansed and draped, the urologist inserts a cystoscope through the urethra into the urinary bladder. This examination commonly includes the use of both the cystoscope and urethroscope.

Follow-up Care. After this procedure with general anesthesia, the patient is returned to a postanesthesia care unit (PACU) or area. If local anesthesia and sedation were used, the patient may be returned directly to the hospital room. Patients undergoing cystoscopic examinations as outpatients are transferred to an area for monitoring before discharge to home. Monitor for airway patency and breathing, changes in vital signs (including temperature), and changes in urine output. Also observe for the complications of bladder puncture, excessive bleeding, and infection. Bladder puncture is accompanied by severe pain, including abdominal pain, nausea, and vomiting.

A catheter may or may not be present after cystoscopy. The patient without a catheter has urinary frequency as a result of irritation from the procedure. The urine may be pink tinged, but gross bleeding is not expected. Bleeding or the presence of clots may obstruct the catheter and decrease urine output. Monitor urine output and notify the urologist of obvious blood clots or a decreased or absent urine output. Irrigate the Foley catheter with sterile saline, if prescribed. Notify the urologist if the patient has a fever (with or without chills) or an elevated white blood cell (WBC) count, which suggests infection. Urge the patient to take oral fluids to increase urine output (which helps prevent clotting) and reduce the burning sensation on urination.

Cystography and Cystourethrography. These tests are a series of x-rays or a continuous radiographic visualization by fluoroscopy. During the imaging, radiopaque contrast medium fills the bladder and the bladder is emptied. Images show structure and function of the bladder and urethra. Tumors, rupture or perforation of the bladder and urethra, abnormal backflow of urine, and distortion from trauma or other pelvic masses can be seen.

Patient Preparation and Procedure. Explain the procedure to the patient. A urinary catheter is temporarily needed to instill contrast medium directly into the bladder for both procedures. The contrast medium enhances x-ray visibility of the lower urinary tract and is not absorbed into the bloodstream, reducing the risk for contrast-induced kidney injury.

After bladder filling, x-rays are taken from the front, back, and side positions. For the voiding cystourethrogram (VCUG), the patient is requested to void and x-rays are taken during the voiding. A VCUG can determine whether urine refluxes (flow backward) into the ureter. The cystogram is used in cases of trauma when urethral or bladder injury is suspected or for patients with recurrent *pyelonephritis* (kidney infection).

Follow-up Care. Monitor for infection as a result of catheter placement. In this test, the contrast medium is not nephrotoxic because it does not enter the bloodstream and does not reach the kidney. Encourage fluid intake to dilute the urine and reduce the burning sensation from catheter irritation after removal. Monitor for changes in urine output because pelvic or urethral trauma may be present.

Retrograde Procedures. *Retrograde* means going against the normal flow of urine. A retrograde examination of the ureters and pelvis *(pyelogram)*, the bladder *(cystogram)*, and the urethra *(urethrogram)* involves instilling radiopaque contrast medium into the lower urinary tract. Because the contrast agent is instilled directly to obtain an outline of the structures desired, the agent does not enter the bloodstream. Therefore the patient is not at risk for contrast-induced kidney injury.

The patient is prepared for retrograde procedures (retrograde pyelography, retrograde cystography, and retrograde urethrography) in the same way as for cystoscopy. Retrograde x-rays are obtained during the cystoscopy. After placement of the cystoscope by the urologist, catheters are placed into each ureter and contrast is instilled into each ureter and renal pelvis. The catheters are removed by the urologist, and x-rays are taken to outline these structures as the agent is excreted. The procedure identifies obstruction or structural abnormalities.

For patients undergoing retrograde cystoscopy or urethrography, radiopaque contrast medium is instilled similarly into the bladder or urethra. Cystography and urethrography identify structural problems, such as fistulas, diverticula, and tumors.

After retrograde procedures, monitor the patient for infection caused by placing instruments in the urinary tract. Because these procedures are performed during cystoscopic examination, follow-up care is the same as that for cystoscopy, including monitoring for bladder puncture or perforation.

Other Diagnostic Assessments

Urodynamic Studies. Urodynamic studies examine the processes of voiding and include:

- Tests of bladder capacity, pressure, and tone
- Studies of urethral pressure and urine flow
- Tests of perineal voluntary muscle function

These tests are often used along with voiding urographic or cystoscopic procedures to evaluate problems with urine flow and disorders of the lower urinary tract.

Cystometrography (CMG) can determine how well the bladder wall (detrusor) muscle functions and how sensitive it is to stretching as the bladder fills. This test provides information about bladder capacity, bladder pressure, and voiding reflexes.

Explain the procedure and inform the patient that a urinary catheter will be needed temporarily during the procedure. Ask the patient to void normally. Record the amount and time of voiding. Insert a urinary catheter to measure the residual urine volume. The cystometer is attached to the catheter, and fluid is instilled via the catheter into the bladder. The point at which the patient first notes a feeling of the urge to void and the point at which he or she notes a strong urge to void are recorded. Bladder capacity and bladder pressure readings are recorded graphically. The patient is asked to void when the bladder instillation is complete (about 500 mL). The residual urine after voiding is recorded, and the catheter is removed. Electromyography of the perineal muscles may be performed during this examination.

For any procedure that involves inserting instruments into the urinary tract, monitor for infection. Record the patient's temperature, the character of the urine, and urine output volume.

Urethral pressure profile (also called a *urethral pressure profilometry* [UPP]) can provide information about the nature of urinary incontinence or urinary retention.

Explain the procedure and inform the patient that a urinary catheter will be needed temporarily during the procedure. A special catheter with pressure-sensing capabilities is inserted into the bladder. Variations in the pressure of the smooth muscle of the urethra are recorded as the catheter is slowly withdrawn.

As with any study involving inserting instruments into the urinary tract, monitor the patient for symptoms of infection.

Urine stream testing is used to evaluate pelvic muscle strength and the effectiveness of pelvic muscles in stopping the flow of urine. It is useful in assessing urinary incontinence.

Explain the procedure and reassure the patient that efforts will be made to ensure privacy. The patient is asked to begin urinating. Three to five seconds after urination begins, the examiner gives the patient a signal to stop urine flow. The length of time required to stop the flow of urine is recorded.

Cleaning the perineal area, as after any voiding, is all that is necessary after the urine stream test.

Electromyography (EMG) of the perineal muscles tests the strength of the muscles used in voiding. This information may help identify methods of improving continence. Inform the patient that some mild, temporary discomfort may accompany placement of the electrodes.

In EMG of the perineal muscles, electrodes are placed in either the rectum or the urethra to measure muscle contraction and relaxation. After the completion of EMG, administer analgesics as prescribed to promote the patient's comfort.

NCLEX EXAMINATION CHALLENGE 60.3
Safe and Effective Care Environment

The nurse is admitting a client undergoing a CT scan with contrast. Which finding does the nurse report as a possible **immediate** hypersensitivity reaction? **Select all that apply.**

A. Nausea
B. Pruritis
C. Urticaria
D. Laryngeal stridor
E. Flushing of the skin

Kidney Biopsy

Patient Preparation. Explain that a kidney biopsy can help determine a cause of unexplained kidney problems and help direct or change therapy. Most kidney biopsies are performed percutaneously (through skin and other tissues) using ultrasound or CT guidance. The patient signs an informed consent. Patients are NPO for 4 to 6 hours before the procedure.

Because of the risk for bleeding after the biopsy, coagulation studies such as platelet count, activated partial thromboplastin time (aPTT), prothrombin time (PT), and bleeding time are performed before surgery. Hypertension is aggressively managed before and after the procedure because high blood pressure can make stopping the bleeding after the biopsy more difficult. Uremia also increases the risk for bleeding, and dialysis may be prescribed before a biopsy. A blood transfusion may be needed to correct anemia before biopsy.

Procedure. In a percutaneous biopsy, the nephrologist or radiologist obtains tissue samples without an incision. Patients receive sedation and are monitored throughout the procedure. The patient is placed in the prone position on the procedure table. The entry site is selected after taking preliminary images. The area is prepped and sterilely draped. A local anesthetic is injected, and the physician then inserts the biopsy device into the tissues toward the kidney. Needle depth and placement are confirmed by ultrasound or CT. While the patient holds his or her breath, the needle is advanced into the renal cortex. Samples are then taken with a spring-loaded coring biopsy needle and sent for pathologic study (Pagana & Pagana, 2018).

Follow-up Care. After a percutaneous biopsy, the major risk is bleeding into the kidney or the tissues external from the kidney at the biopsy site. For 24 hours after the biopsy, monitor the dressing site, vital signs (especially fluctuations in blood pressure), urine output, hemoglobin level, and hematocrit. Even if the dressing is dry and there is no hematoma, the patient could be bleeding from the site. An internal bleed is not readily visible but is suspected with flank pain, decreasing blood pressure, decreasing urine output, or other signs of hypovolemia or shock. With severe bleeding, some patients develop bruising along the flank and back accompanied by pain.

The patient follows a plan of strict bedrest, lying in a supine position with a back roll for additional support for 2 to 6 hours after the biopsy. The head of the bed may be elevated, and the patient may resume oral intake of food and fluids. After bedrest, the patient may have limited bathroom privileges if there is no evidence of bleeding.

Monitor for hematuria, the most common complication of kidney biopsy. Hematuria occurs microscopically in most patients, but 5% to 9% have gross hematuria. This problem usually resolves without treatment 48 to 72 hours after the biopsy but can persist for 2 to 3 weeks. In rare cases, transfusions and surgery are required. There should be no obvious blood clots in the urine.

The patient may have some local pain after the biopsy. If aching originates at the biopsy site and begins to radiate to the flank, back, and around the front of the abdomen, bleeding may have started, or a hematoma is forming around the kidney. This pattern of pain with bleeding occurs because blood in the tissues around the kidney increases pressure on local nerve tracts.

If bleeding occurs, IV fluid, packed red blood cells, or both may be needed to prevent shock. In general, a small amount of bleeding creates enough pressure to compress bleeding sites. This is called a *tamponade effect*. If tamponade does not occur and bleeding is extensive, surgery for hemostasis or even nephrectomy may be needed. A hematoma in, on, or around the kidney may become infected, requiring treatment with antibiotics and surgical drainage.

If no bleeding occurs, the patient can resume general activities after 24 hours. Instruct the patient to avoid lifting heavy objects, exercising, or performing other strenuous activities for 1 to 2 weeks after the biopsy procedure. Driving may also be restricted. Refer to Chapter 9 for general postoperative care for the patient who has undergone an open kidney biopsy.

NCLEX EXAMINATION CHALLENGE 60.4

Safe and Effective Care Environment

Which assessment finding would require the nurse to take **immediate** action in a client who is 1 hour post kidney biopsy? **Select all that apply**.

A. Pink-tinged urine
B. Nausea and vomiting
C. Increased bowel sounds
D. Reports of flank pain
E. The patient is ambulating to the bathroom

❓ CLINICAL JUDGMENT CHALLENGE 60.1

Safety; Patient-Centered Care

The nurse is assessing a 42-year-old female client who is scheduled for surgical repair of a hip fracture from a car crash 4 hours ago. The client was traveling approximately 40 miles per hour when she struck a guard rail after a deer ran into the roadway. The client was wearing a seat belt at the time of the accident. The client reports pain in the left hip area with noted swelling. There is a 2-cm abrasion over the right eye and a contusion on the left upper forearm. When the client voids, the nurse assesses that the urine is rust colored and the client states "It burns when I urinate." The client has a history of anxiety.

1. **Recognize Cues:** What assessment information in this client situation is the most important and immediate concern for the nurse? (Hint: Identify the **relevant** information *first* to determine what is most important.)
2. **Analyze Cues:** What client conditions are consistent with the **most relevant** information? (Hint: Think about priority collaborative problems that support and contradict the information presented in this situation.)

GET READY FOR THE NEXT-GENERATION NCLEX® EXAMINATION!

Key Points

Review these Key Points for each NCLEX Examination Client Needs Category.

Safe and Effective Care Environment

- Wear gloves when handling urine or drainage from the genitourinary tract. **QSEN: Safety**
- Evaluate the patient for potential adverse or allergic reactions to radiopaque contrast agents, iodine, or gadolinium. **QSEN: Safety**
- Assess the patient for use of drugs that increase risk for kidney dysfunction. **QSEN: Safety**
- Assess the patient for bleeding, increased pain, and symptoms of perforation or infection after any invasive test of kidney/urinary function. **QSEN: Safety**
- Inform primary health care providers about any symptoms of complications following invasive or noninvasive tests of urinary and kidney structure or function. **QSEN: Safety**

Health Promotion and Maintenance

- Teach patients to clean the perineal area after voiding, after having a bowel movement, and after sexual intercourse. **QSEN: Evidence-Based Practice**
- Urge all patients to maintain an adequate fluid intake (sufficient to dilute urine to a light yellow color) unless another health problem requires fluid restriction. **QSEN: Evidence-Based Practice**

Psychosocial Integrity

- Allow the patient to express fear or anxiety about renal system diagnostic tests and renal system alterations. **QSEN: Patient-Centered Care**
- Provide privacy for patients undergoing examination or testing of the renal system. **QSEN: Patient-Centered Care**
- Use language and terminology that the patient can understand during discussions of kidney/urinary assessment. **QSEN: Patient-Centered Care**

Physiological Integrity

- Ask the patient about kidney problems in any other family members because some problems have a genetic component. **QSEN: Patient-Centered Care**
- Explain all diagnostic procedures, restrictions, and follow-up care to the patient scheduled for tests. **QSEN: Patient-Centered Care**
- Interpret laboratory data to distinguish between dehydration and kidney impairment. **QSEN: Evidence-Based Practice**
- Describe how to obtain different types of urine specimens. **QSEN: Evidence-Based Practice**
- Document renal and urinary system assessment in the patient's electronic health record. **QSEN: Patient-Centered Care**
- Assess urine and serum tests of kidney function closely after renal system diagnostic tests. **QSEN: Evidence-Based Practice**

MASTERY QUESTIONS

1. Which client being managed for dehydration does the nurse consider at greatest risk for possible reduced kidney function?
   A. An 80-year-old man who has benign prostatic hyperplasia
   B. A 62-year-old woman with a known allergy to contrast media
   C. A 48-year-old woman with established urinary incontinence
   D. A 45-year-old man receiving oral and intravenous fluid therapy

2. Which client assessment data is essential for the nurse to report to the health care provider before a renal scan is performed?
   A. Pink-tinged urine
   B. Reports pregnancy
   C. Reports claustrophobia
   D. History of an aneurysm clip

3. Which lab finding is indicative of renal function alterations and not dehydration? Select all that apply.
   A. BUN 20 mL/dL
   B. Creatinine 2.3 mL/dL
   C. Hemoglobin 14 g/dL
   D. Cystatin-c 105 mg/mL
   E. BUN/creatinine ratio 10
   F. Creatinine clearance 175 mL/min

4. Which symptom(s) in a client during the first 12 hours after a kidney biopsy indicates to the nurse a possible complication from the procedure?
   A. The client experiences nausea and vomiting after drinking juice.
   B. The biopsy site is tender to light palpation.
   C. The abdomen is distended, and the client reports abdominal discomfort.
   D. The heart rate is 118, blood pressure is 108/50, and peripheral pulses are thready.

REFERENCES

Brenner, B. M. (Ed.). (2016). *Brenner & Rector's the kidney* (10th ed.) Philadelphia: Saunders.

Burchum, J., & Rosenthal, L. (2019). *Lehne's pharmacology for nursing care* (10th ed.). St. Louis: Elsevier.

Denic, A., Glassock, R., & Rule, A. (2016). *Structural and functional changes with the aging kidney*, *23*(1). https://doi.org/10.1053/j.ackd.2015.08.004.

Jackson, C., Botelho, E., Josepf, J., & Tennstedt, S. (2013). Accessing and evaluating urologic health information: Differences by race/ethnicity and gender. *Urologic Nursing*, *33*(6), 282–287.

Jarvis, C. (2020). *Physical examination & health assessment* (8th ed.). St. Louis: Elsevier.

Lambert, P., Chasson, K., Horton, S., Petrin, C., Marshall, E., Bowdon, S., et al. (2017). Reducing acute kidney injury due to contrast material: How nurses can improve patient safety. *Critical Care Nurse*, *37*(1), 13–26.

McCance, K., & Huether, S. (2019). *Pathophysiology: The biologic basis for disease in adults and children* (8th ed.). St. Louis: Mosby.

McCulloch, D. (2018). Estimation of blood glucose control in diabetes mellitus. In D. Nathan, & J. Wolfsdorf (Eds.), *UpToDate*. Waltham, MA.

National Institute of Diabetes and Digestive and Kidney Diseases (NIDDK). (2018). *Kidney disease*. Retrieved from https://www.niddk.nih.gov/health-information/kidney-disease.

National Kidney Foundation. (2017). *How your kidneys work*. Retrieved from https://www.kidney.org/kidneydisease/howkidneyswrk.

Pagana, K., & Pagana, T. (2018). *Mosby's manual of diagnostic and laboratory test reference* (6th ed.). St. Louis: Mosby.

Pagana, K., Pagana, T., & Pike-McDonald, S. (2018). *Mosby's Canadian manual of diagnostic and laboratory tests*. St. Louis: Elsevier.

Sethi, A., Kohli, J., Patel, A., & Rudnick, M. (2018). Chapter 13 Contract-induced nephropathy. In E. Lerma, M. Sparks, & J. Topf (Eds.), *Nephrology secrets: First south asia edition (e-book)*.

Touhy, T., & Jett, K. (2016). *Ebersole & Hess' toward healthy aging: Human needs & nursing response*. St. Louis: Elsevier.

U.S. Renal data systems. (2018). *2018 USRDS Annual data report. Epidemiology of kidney disease in the United States*. Bethesda, MD: National Institutes of Health, National Institute of Diabetes and Digestive and Kidney Diseases. http://www.usrds.org/adr.aspx.

61

Concepts of Care for Patients With Urinary Problems

Carolyn Gersch

http://evolve.elsevier.com/Iggy/

LEARNING OUTCOMES

1. Collaborate with the interprofessional team to coordinate high-quality care and promote urinary *elimination* in patients who have problems in the urinary tract.
2. Teach the patient and caregiver(s) how home safety is affected by impaired *elimination* resulting from problems in the urinary tract.
3. Identify community resources for patients requiring assistance with incontinence or any chronic urinary tract problem.
4. Teach adults how to decrease the risk for urinary tract infections.
5. Implement nursing interventions to help patients and families cope with the psychosocial impact caused by urinary incontinence or any other chronic problem of the urinary tract.
6. Apply knowledge of anatomy and physiology to assess patients with urinary problems affecting *elimination.*
7. Use clinical judgement to analyze information from laboratory data and assessment findings in the care of patients with urinary problems.
8. Plan evidence-based nursing care to promote *elimination* and prevent complications in patients with urinary problems.

KEY TERMS

anuria Absence of urine output.

bacteremia Also called *urosepsis;* spread of the infection from the urinary tract to the bloodstream.

bacteriuria Presence of bacteria in the urine.

continence Control over the time and place of urine *elimination.*

cystitis Inflammation of the bladder.

cystocele Herniation of the bladder into the vagina.

dysuria Pain or burning with urination.

frequency Urge to urinate frequently in small amounts.

hematuria Presence of red blood cells (RBCs) in the urine; blood in the urine.

hydronephrosis Enlargement of the kidney caused by blockage of urine lower in the tract and filling of the kidney with urine.

hydroureter Enlargement of the ureter.

incontinence Involuntary loss of urine.

intracorporeal Inside the body.

intravesical Inside the bladder.

interstitial cystitis A painful inflammatory bladder condition.

lithotripsy Extracorporeal *shock wave lithotripsy* (SWL) is the use of sound, laser, or dry shock waves to break the stone into small fragments.

nephrolithiasis Formation of stones in the kidney.

oliguria Scant urine output.

pyuria Presence of white blood cells (WBCs) in the urine.

radical cystectomy Removal of the bladder and surrounding tissue.

renal colic Term used to describe the severe flank pain resulting from stones.

stent Small tube that is placed in the ureter by ureteroscopy to dilate the ureter and enlarge the passageway for the stone or stone fragments.

trabeculation Abnormal thickening of the bladder wall caused by urinary retention and obstruction.

ureterolithiasis Formation of stones in the ureter.

urethritis Inflammation of the urethra that can result from infectious and noninfectious conditions.

urgency Feeling that urination will occur immediately.

urolithiasis Presence of *calculi* (stones) in the urinary tract.

urosepsis Also called *bacteremia;* spread of the infection from the urinary tract to the bloodstream.

PRIORITY AND INTERRELATED CONCEPTS

The priority concept for this chapter is:
- *Elimination*

The *Elimination* concept exemplar for this chapter is Urinary Incontinence.

The interrelated concepts for this chapter are:
- *Pain*
- *Immunity*
- *Tissue Integrity*

The urinary tract includes the ureters, bladder, and urethra. Although these structures play no role in the making of urine, their functions are essential for the urine made by the kidneys to be eliminated from the body. Both infectious and noninfectious problems in the urinary tract can disrupt urinary *elimination* and affect control of fluids, electrolytes, nitrogenous wastes, and blood pressure.

Any urinary problem can affect the storage or *elimination* of urine. Both acute and chronic urinary problems are common and costly. For urinary tract infections (UTIs) there were more than 7 million office visits, 1 million emergency department visits, and more than 100,000 hospitalizations costing over $1.6 billion in the United States between 2008 and 2011 (Simmering et al., 2017). In addition, many other people sought treatment for kidney and ureter stones, urinary incontinence, urologic trauma, and cancer involving the urinary system. Although life-threatening complications are rare with urinary problems, patients may have functional, physical, and psychosocial changes that reduce quality of life. Nursing interventions are directed toward prevention, early detection, and early management of urologic disorders.

 ELIMINATION CONCEPT EXEMPLAR: URINARY INCONTINENCE

Pathophysiology Review

Continence is the control over the time and place of *elimination*. Urinary continence is specific to control over urinary elimination and is a learned behavior. Efficient bladder emptying (i.e., coordination between bladder contraction and urethral relaxation) is needed for continence. Continence occurs when pressure in the urethra is greater than pressure in the bladder. For normal voiding to occur, the urethra must relax and the bladder must contract with enough pressure and duration to empty completely. Voiding normally occurs in a smooth and coordinated manner under conscious control.

Urinary incontinence (UI) is an involuntary loss of urine severe enough to cause social or hygienic problems. It is *not* a normal consequence of aging or childbirth and often is a stigmatizing and an underreported health problem. Many adults suffer in silence, are socially isolated, and may be unaware that treatment is available. In addition, the cost of incontinence can be enormous (Zhang, 2018).

Urinary incontinence has several possible causes (Table 61.1). Except for infection, temporary causes of incontinence usually do not involve a disorder of the urinary tract. The most common types of adult urinary incontinence are stress incontinence, urge incontinence, overflow incontinence, functional incontinence, and a mixed form of incontinence.

Stress incontinence is the most common type urinary incontinence in younger women (Lukacz et al., 2017). Its main feature is the inability to retain urine when laughing, coughing, sneezing, jogging, or lifting. In the continent adult, the urethra can be relaxed and tightened under conscious control because skeletal muscles of the pelvic floor surround it. When an adult feels the urge to urinate, the conscious contraction of the urethra can override a bladder contraction if the urethral contraction is strong enough. Patients with *stress incontinence* cannot tighten the urethra enough to overcome the increased bladder pressure caused by contraction of the detrusor muscle.

Urge incontinence is the loss of urine for no apparent reason after suddenly feeling the need or urge to urinate. Normally when the bladder is full, contraction of the smooth muscle fibers of the bladder detrusor muscle signals the brain that it is time to urinate. Continent adults override that signal and relax the detrusor muscle for the time it takes to locate a toilet. Those who suffer from urge incontinence cannot suppress the signal and have a sudden strong urge to void and can leak large amounts of urine at this time. Urge incontinence is also known as an *overactive bladder (OAB)* and is more common in older women.

Overflow incontinence occurs when the detrusor muscle fails to contract and the bladder becomes overdistended. This type of incontinence (*reflex incontinence* or *underactive bladder*) occurs when the bladder has reached its maximum capacity and some urine must leak out to prevent bladder rupture. It is important to note that more than one type of incontinence can exist at the same time. This is called *mixed incontinence* and is a combination of stress and urge incontinence.

Functional incontinence occurs as a result of factors other than the abnormal function of the bladder and urethra. A common factor is the loss of cognitive function in patients affected by dementia.

Etiology. Urinary incontinence may have temporary or permanent causes (see Table 61.1) Evaluation of the patient with urinary incontinence means considering all possible causes, beginning with those that are temporary and correctable. Surgical and traumatic causes of urinary incontinence are related to procedures or surgery in the lower pelvic structures, which are areas that contain complex nerve pathways. Radical urologic, prostatic, and gynecologic procedures for treatment of pelvic cancers may result in urinary incontinence. Injury to segments S2 to S4 of the spinal cord may cause incontinence from impairment of normal nerve pathways.

Inappropriate bladder contraction may result from disorders of the brain and nervous system or from bladder irritation due to chronic infection, stones, chemotherapy, or radiation therapy. Other causes of bladder contraction failure include neuropathies associated with diabetes mellitus, syphilis, and previous treatment with neurotoxic anticancer drugs. Constipation can lead to temporary urinary incontinence. Some drugs or drug-drug interactions from polypharmacy, such as anticholinergics, calcium channel blockers, diuretics, and sedatives, can cause or worsen urinary incontinence.

TABLE 61.1 Types of Urinary Incontinence

Type and Description	Causes	Symptoms	Management
Stress Incontinence Involuntary loss of urine during activities that increase abdominal and detrusor pressure Inability to tighten the urethra sufficiently to overcome the increased detrusor pressure Leakage of urine	Weakening of bladder neck supports, associated with childbirth Intrinsic sphincter deficiency, such as epispadias (abnormal location of the urethra on the dorsum of the penis) or myelomeningocele Acquired anatomic damage to the urethral sphincter from repeated incontinence surgeries, prostatectomy, radiation therapy, and trauma Vaginal prolapse from vaginal birth or aging	Urine loss with physical exertion, cough, sneeze, or exercise Usually only small amounts of urine are lost with each exertion Normal voiding habits (≤8 times per day, ≤2 times per night) Postvoid residual usually ≤50 mL Pelvic examination shows hypermobility of the urethra or bladder neck with Valsalva maneuvers	Weight reduction for patients who are obese Smoking cessation Pelvic muscle therapy Vaginal cone therapy Bladder training Estrogen therapy for postmenopausal women Electrical stimulation Magnetic resonance therapy Pessary devices Surgery includes slings, bladder suspension, injection of bulking agents, prostatectomy Electrical stimulation device
Urge Incontinence Overactive bladder (OAB) Involuntary loss of urine associated with a strong desire to urinate Inability to suppress the signal from the bladder muscle to the brain that it is time to urinate	Idiopathic Neurologic disorders, such as stroke Benign prostatic hypertrophy Bladder inflammation or infection Bladder irritants, such as artificial sweeteners, caffeine, alcohol, citric intake, drugs, nicotine Bladder cancer Medications that cause increased bladder contractility	An abrupt and strong urge to void (urinary urgency) Urinary frequency Nocturia May have loss of large amounts of urine with each occurrence	Bladder training Pelvis muscle therapy Weight reduction for patients who are obese Avoid bladder irritants, such as caffeine and alcohol Smoking cessation Drug therapy if bladder training is not successful: anticholinergics, tricyclic antidepressants with anticholinergic and alpha-adrenergic agonist activity, beta-adrenergic agonist, and onabotulinumtoxinA Electrical stimulation device Surgery includes transurethral resection of the prostate or prostatectomy
Mixed Incontinence Combination of stress and urge incontinence	Causes associated with stress and urge incontinence	Symptoms associated with stress and urge incontinence	See management for stress and urge incontinence
Overflow Incontinence (reflex incontinence) Involuntary loss of urine associated with overdistention of the bladder when the bladder capacity has reached its maximum Detrusor underactivity Bladder outlet obstruction	Urethral obstruction such as benign prostatic hypertrophy or uterine prolapse Diabetic neuropathy Some neurologic disorders, such as multiple sclerosis or spinal cord damage Medication side effects	Bladder distention, Constant dribbling of urine Sense of incomplete emptying of the bladder Pelvic discomfort Palpable bladder	Bladder training Bladder compression (Credé method) Intermittent self-catheterization Drug therapy if bladder training unsuccessful: bethanechol chloride Nonsurgical treatment unless surgery is required to remove the obstruction: i.e., prostatectomy or repair of uterine prolapse

Functional Incontinence Leakage of urine caused by factors other than disease of the lower urinary tract	Decreased cognition such as with dementia
	Impaired mobility, such as paralysis or inability to walk to the toilet; some neurologic disorders
		Quantity and timing of urine leakage vary
		Patterns difficult to discern
			Habit training
			Prompted voiding is used to establish a predictable pattern of bladder emptying to prevent incontinence
			Applied devices:
			  Intravaginal pessaries
			  Penile clamps
			  Condom catheter
			  Intermittent or long-term catheterization

Incidence and Prevalence. Urinary incontinence is a major health problem. The incidence of UI increases with age (Milson & Gyhagen, 2018). Up to 45% of women older than 65 years report some degree of urinary incontinence (Engberg & Li, 2017).

Risk for urinary incontinence increases with chronic conditions such as diabetes mellitus, stroke, cognitive impairment, and impaired mobility. Urinary incontinence occurs not only with older age but with a history of vaginal delivery, particularly if the first child was delivered after age 30. Conditions of pelvic prolapse in women, prostate problems in men, diabetes, heart failure, spinal cord or nerve injury, and obesity also increase the risk for urinary incontinence (Lukacz et al., 2017).). Both central nervous system diseases (i.e., dementia, multiple sclerosis, Parkinson disease) and musculoskeletal disorders (i.e., osteoporosis, osteoarthritis, paresthesia, pain or paralysis) contribute to cognitive and mobility impairment, resulting in the onset and severity of urinary incontinence (Engberg & Li, 2017; McCance & Huether, 2019). Because urinary incontinence is common among older adults, routine screening for incontinence is recommended for all adults 65 years and older (Touhy & Jett, 2016). Older adults who are institutionalized with UI have a higher risk for mortality (Damien et al., 2017). Patients with mild cognitive impairment are 30% more likely to have urinary incontinence (Aoki et al., 2017).

❖ Interprofessional Collaborative Care

Urinary incontinence can occur in any setting and is very common in the community. Usually the adult with incontinence is treated using self-management strategies. Even when surgical intervention is used, hospitalization for incontinence is rare. Because urinary incontinence carries a burden of impaired comfort, activity disruption, shame or embarrassment, and loss of *tissue integrity,* it has a great impact on quality of life for most adults.

◆ Assessment: Recognize Cues

History. Incontinence may be underreported because health care professionals do not ask patients about urine loss. Ask patients about incontinence as many patients are hesitant to initiate the subject. (Lukacz et al., 2017). Effective screening includes asking patients to respond "always," "sometimes," or "never" to these questions:

- Do you ever leak urine or water when you don't want to?
- Do you ever leak urine or water when you cough, sneeze, laugh, or exercise?
- Do you ever leak urine or water on the way to the toilet?
- Do you ever use pads, tissue, or cloth in your underwear to catch urine?

If any answer is "always" or "sometimes," perform a focused assessment (see the Focused Assessment: The Patient with Urinary Incontinence box).

Physical Assessment/Signs and Symptoms. Assess the abdomen to estimate bladder fullness, rule out palpable hard stool, and evaluate bowel sounds. Urinary incontinence is confirmed by evaluating the force and character of the urine stream during voiding. Ask the patient to cough while wearing a perineal pad to assess for stress incontinence; a wet pad on forceful coughing indicates stress incontinence.

For women, inspect the external genitalia to determine whether there is apparent urethral or uterine prolapse, cystocele (herniation of the bladder into the vagina), or rectocele. These conditions occur with pelvic floor muscle weakness. A primary health care provider puts on an examination glove and inserts two fingers into the vagina to assess the strength of these muscles. Strength is described as *weak, adequate,* or *strong* based on the amount of pressure felt by the primary health care provider

FOCUSED ASSESSMENT

The Patient With Urinary Incontinence

Note the presence of risk factors for urinary incontinence:
- Age
- If female, menopausal status
- Central or peripheral neurologic disease with associated impairment in cognition or mobility
- Diabetes mellitus
- History of vaginal delivery; vaginal prolapse
- Urologic procedures
- Prescribed and over-the-counter drugs that affect cognition or mobility
- Bowel patterns; fecal impaction
- Stress/anxiety level

Detail the symptoms of urinary incontinence:
- Leakage
- Frequency
- Urgency
- Nocturia
- Sensation of full bladder before leakage

Obtain a 24-hour intake-and-output record or a voiding diary:
- Time and amount of oral intake and continent voiding
- Time and estimated amount of incontinent leakages
- Activity around the time of leakage

Assess the patient's:
- Mobility
- Self-care ability
- Cognitive ability
- Communication patterns

Assess the environment for barriers to toileting:
- Privacy
- Restrictive clothing
- Access to toilet

as the patient tightens vaginal muscles. Describe and document the color, consistency, and odor of any secretions from the genitourinary orifices. The urine stream interruption test (i.e., asking a patient to voluntarily start and stop urine flow during a void at least twice) is another method of determining pelvic muscle strength. For men, inspect the urethral meatus for any discharge.

A digital rectal examination (DRE) is performed by the primary health care provider on both male and female patients. It provides information about the nerve integrity to the bladder. The examiner determines whether there is tactile sensation in the anal area by observing whether the rectal sphincter is relaxed or contracted on digital insertion. Because nerve supply to the bladder is similar to nerve supply to the rectum, the presence of tactile sensation and a rectal sphincter that contracts suggest that the nerve supply to the bladder is intact. Impaction of stool is a cause of transient urinary incontinence and can be detected during a rectal examination. The primary health care provider assesses for prostate enlargement in men as a possible cause of incontinence.

Laboratory Assessment. A urinalysis is useful to rule out urinary tract infection. This test is the first step in the assessment of incontinent patients of any age. The presence of red blood cells (RBCs), white blood cells (WBCs), leukocyte esterase, or nitrites is an indication for culturing the urine. Any infection is treated before further assessment of incontinence.

Imaging Assessment. Determine the amount of postvoid residual urine (urine remaining in the bladder right after voiding) by portable ultrasound (bladder scanner). If prescribed, catheterizing the patient immediately after voiding can also be used to assess residual volume. Additional imaging is needed when surgery is being considered. CT is most useful for locating abnormalities in kidneys and ureters. A voiding cystourethrogram (VCUG) or urodynamic testing may be performed to assess the size, shape, support, and function of the urinary tract system. Urodynamic testing (see Chapter 60) may take several hours and more than one visit. Electromyography (EMG) of the pelvic muscles may be a part of the urodynamic studies.

◆ **Analysis: Analyze Cues and Prioritize Hypotheses.** The priority collaborative problems for patients with urinary incontinence include:
1. Altered urinary *elimination* due to incontinence
2. Potential for altered *tissue integrity*

◆ **Planning and Implementation: Generate Solutions and Take Action**

Planning: Expected Outcomes. The expected outcomes for altered urinary incontinence are to maintain optimal urinary *elimination, tissue integrity,* and comfort. Nursing interventions for the management of the different types of urinary incontinence focus on restoring continence, psychosocial comfort, tissue integrity, and patient education.

Promoting Urinary Elimination. With appropriate therapy, the patient with altered urinary elimination due to incontinence is expected to develop continence of urine *elimination.* Indicators include that the patient consistently or often demonstrates these actions:

- Stress urinary incontinence: No urine leakage between voidings and no urine leakage with increased abdominal pressure (e.g., sneezing, laughing, lifting)
- Urge urinary incontinence: Responds to urge in a timely manner, gets to toilet between urge and passage of urine, and avoids substances that stimulate the bladder (e.g., caffeine, alcohol)
- Overflow urinary incontinence: Recognizes the urge to void, maintains a predictable pattern of voiding, empties bladder completely, and keeps urine volume in the bladder under 300 mL
- Functional urinary incontinence: Uses urine containment or collection measures to ensure dryness and manages clothing independently

Nonsurgical Management. Maintaining a diary can be beneficial for patients with stress incontinence to determine patterns of the incontinent events. Patients may use collection devices, absorbent pads, and undergarments during the often lengthy process of assessment and treatment of urinary incontinence and by patients who elect not to pursue further interventions.

Nutrition Therapy. Nutrition therapy plays a role in specific types of urinary incontinence. Nutrition therapy with weight reduction is helpful for patients who are obese because stress incontinence is made worse by increased abdominal pressure from obesity (Lukacz et al., 2017). Teach the patient to avoid bladder irritants in the diet, such as caffeine and alcohol, that can contribute to urgency and frequency. Stress the importance of maintaining an adequate fluid intake, especially water. Refer the patient to a registered dietitian as needed.

Drug Therapy. Drug therapy with topical estrogen to the perineal and vaginal orifice is used to treat postmenopausal women with stress incontinence. Estrogen may increase the blood flow and tone of the muscles around the vagina and urethra, thus improving the patient's ability to contract those muscles during times of increased intra-abdominal stress.

Because the hypertonic bladder contracts involuntarily in patients with urge incontinence, drugs that relax the smooth muscle and increase the bladder's capacity are prescribed (see the Common Examples of Drug Therapy: Urinary Incontinence box). The most commonly prescribed drugs are anticholinergics (also known as *antimuscarinics* because they target specific receptors in the cholinergic family of receptors), which include darifenacin, fesoterodine, oxybutynin, propiverine (only available in Canada), solifenacin, tolterodine, and trospium. Some of these drugs are available over the counter. This class of drugs has serious side effects, particularly for older adults, and is used along with behavioral interventions. These drugs inhibit the nerve fibers that stimulate bladder contraction. In addition, tricyclic antidepressants with anticholinergic and alpha-adrenergic agonist activity, such as imipramine, have been used successfully in younger patients for enuresis.

A beta-adrenergic agonist, mirabegron, has demonstrated effectiveness in reducing urge incontinence. The evidence comparing different drug categories for effectiveness in managing incontinence is limited, and no single drug or class is recommended over another.

Another drug therapy for urge incontinence is onabotulinumtoxinA (Botox). This drug is injected during cystoscopy into multiple areas of the detrusor muscle of the bladder. Usually 10 to 30 different sites are injected during one treatment session. This treatment relaxes the detrusor muscle and relieves the urge to urinate (Hubb et al., 2018). Some patients have relief of incontinence for as long as 6 to 9 months after injection. Side effects may include urinary retention, painful urination, and an increased incidence of urinary tract infections. For most patients who experience urinary retention, the condition is temporary but does require intermittent self-catheterization.

Drugs are prescribed for short-term management of urinary retention seen in overflow incontinence, often after surgery. They are not used in long-term management of overflow incontinence caused by a hypotonic bladder. The most commonly used drug is bethanechol chloride, an agent that increases bladder pressure.

! NURSING SAFETY PRIORITY (QSEN)

Drug Alert

Teach patients taking the extended-release forms of anticholinergic drugs to swallow the tablet or capsule whole without chewing or crushing. Chewing or crushing the tablet/capsule destroys the extended-release feature, allowing the entire dose to be absorbed quickly, which increases adverse drug side effects.

Devices. Devices can be used to assist with continence. A pessary (plastic device, often ring shaped, that helps hold internal organs in place) inserted into the vagina may help with a prolapsed uterus or bladder when this condition is contributing to urinary incontinence. A prolapse occurs when the supportive tissue in the vagina weakens and stretches, allowing pelvic organs to protrude into the vaginal lumen. The pessary presses against the wall of the vagina to reposition pelvic organs. Generally, a pessary is removed and cleaned with soap and water on a monthly basis by the patient, but the nurse can do it for adults with cognitive or musculoskeletal impairment.

Urethral occlusion devices (urethral plugs) can be helpful for activity-induced incontinence. One device, the Reliance insert, is like a small tampon that the patient inserts into the urethra. After insertion, the patient inflates a tiny balloon, which rests at the bladder neck and prevents the flow of urine. To void, the patient pulls a string to deflate the balloon and removes the device. The applicator is reusable, although the tampon part is disposed of after each void.

Applied devices for functional urinary incontinence include intravaginal pessaries for women and penile clamps for men. The intravaginal pessary supports the uterus and vagina and helps maintain the correct position of the bladder. (See Chapter 66 for further discussion of pessaries.) The penile clamp is applied around the outside of the penis to compress the urethra and prevent urine leakage. Adverse outcomes from pessaries and penile clamps include reduced *tissue integrity* with tissue damage from pressure and infection from colonization of damaged tissues. Both devices require that the patient have either manual dexterity or a caregiver to apply and remove the device. Instruct the patient or caregivers in the use of these devices.

Male patients may use an external collecting device, such as a condom catheter. In acute care settings, the Pickwick, a female external collecting device, has demonstrated promise in effectively collecting urine and preventing tissue damage due to urinary leakage (Beeson & Davis, 2018). The Pickwick female external catheter is a tube that lies between the labia next to the urethral opening and extends between the buttocks. The tube is secured to the suprapubic area and is attached to low, continuous suction to wick away urine as it leaks from the urethral opening. This external urinary collection device is effective for patients who are lying down or in the sitting position.

Electrical Stimulation. Electrical stimulation with either an intravaginal or intrarectal electrical stimulation device is available to treat urge, stress, and mixed incontinence. Treatment consists of stimulating sensory nerves to decrease the sensation of urgency. It is done as an office-based procedure one to three times weekly for 6 to 8 weeks.

Magnetic Resonance Therapy. Magnetic resonance therapy involves targeted urinary tract nerves and muscles for depolarization. The patient sits on a chair containing a magnetic device that induces depolarization and helps reduce stress-induced incontinence similar to drug-induced relaxation of muscle and nerves.

Pelvic Muscle Therapy. Pelvic muscle (Kegel) exercise therapy for women with stress incontinence strengthens the muscles of the pelvic floor (circumvaginal muscles). These muscles become strengthened, as any other skeletal muscle

COMMON EXAMPLES OF DRUG THERAPY

Urinary Incontinence

Drug Category	Nursing Implications
Hormones	
Thought to enhance nerve conduction to the urinary tract, improve blood flow, and reduce tissue deterioration of the urinary tract	
Estrogen vaginal cream daily or an estrogen-containing ring inserted monthly	Teach patients to use only a thin application of the cream *to minimize excessive absorption and distribution and avoid systemic side effects.*
	Teach patients that it takes 4-6 weeks to achieve continence benefits and that benefits disappear about 4 weeks after discontinuing regular use *because knowing the drug responses increases the likelihood of its correct use.*
Anticholinergics	
Suppress involuntary bladder contraction and increase bladder capacity	
Darifenacin	Ask whether the patient has glaucoma before starting any drugs from this class *because anticholinergics can increase intraocular pressure and make glaucoma worse.*
Fesoterodine	
Oxybutynin	Suggest that patients increase fluid intake and use hard candy to moisten the mouth *to reduce the dry mouth side effect.*
Solifenacin	Teach patients to increase fluid intake and the amount of dietary fiber *to prevent constipation associated with this drug category.*
Tolterodine	Teach patients to monitor urine output and to report an output significantly lower than intake to the primary health care
Trospium	provider *because all of these drugs can cause urinary retention, especially for men with an enlarged prostate.*
	Instruct patients taking the extended-release forms of these drugs not to chew or crush the tablet/capsule *to avoid both ruining the time-release feature and increasing the risk for a bolus dose with more side effects.*
Alpha-Adrenergic Agonists	
Increase contractile force of the urethral sphincter, increasing resistance to urine outflow	
Midodrine[a]	Teach the patient to monitor his or her blood pressure periodically when starting the *drug because this drug can cause severe supine hypertension and should not be used in patients with severe cardiac disease.*
Beta₃ Agonists	
Relax the detrusor smooth muscle to increase bladder capacity and urine storage	
Mirabegron	Teach the patient to periodically obtain a blood pressure and to inform the health care provider if the systolic or diastolic values increase more than 10 mm Hg or above 180/110 *because this drug has the potential to increase blood pressure.*
	If the patient is taking warfarin, avoid this drug or schedule additional blood testing for potential increased risk for bleeding *because this drug uses the same metabolic pathway as warfarin and can potentiate warfarin's effects, leading to a prolonged international normalized ratio (INR) and increase the risk for bleeding.*
Antidepressants: Tricyclics and Serotonin-Norepinephrine Reuptake Inhibitors (SNRIs)	
Increase norepinephrine and serotonin levels, which are thought to strengthen the urinary sphincters; also have anticholinergic actions	
Tricyclics:	Warn patients not to combine these drugs with other antidepressant drugs *to avoid a drug-drug interaction that can lead to a hypertensive crisis.* Instruct patients to inform their primary health care provider if they take drugs to manage hypertension.
Imipramine	
Amitriptyline	
SNRI:	Teach patients to change positions slowly, especially in the morning *to avoid dizziness from orthostatic hypotension, which increases the risk for falls.*
Duloxetine[a]	Teach patients the same interventions as for anticholinergic agents *because these drugs have anticholinergic activity and can produce the same side effects.*

[a]These drugs are used off label and do not have U.S. Food and Drug Administration (FDA) approval for use to treat incontinence. However, they are commonly used to manage incontinence syndromes.

does, by frequent, systematic, and repeated contractions. Pelvic floor muscle training improves not only continence but also quality of life in women with stress urinary incontinence (Aoki et al., 2017). The most important step in teaching pelvic muscle exercises is to help the patient learn which muscles to exercise. During the pelvic examination in women and the rectal examination in men or women, instruct the patient to tighten the pelvic muscles around your fingers. Then provide feedback about the strength of the contraction. Starting and stopping the urine stream or stopping the passage of flatus indicates that the patient has correctly identified the pelvic muscles. Biofeedback devices, such as electromyography or perineometers, measure the strength of contraction. A perineometer is a tampon-shaped instrument inserted into the vagina to measure the strength of pelvic muscle contractions. The graph shows the amplitude of

muscle contraction to the patient for biofeedback. Alternatively, retention of a vaginal weight also shows that the patient has identified the proper muscle (see discussion on vaginal cone therapy).

Instructions for pelvic muscle exercises are provided in the Patient and Family Education: Preparing for Self-Management: Pelvic Muscle Exercises box. Although improvement may take several months, most patients notice a positive change after 6 weeks. Teach patients to continue the exercises 10 times daily to improve and maintain pelvic muscle strength.

Pelvic muscle exercises are also effective for urge incontinence and are taught in the same way as for stress incontinence. Improved urethral resistance helps the patient overcome abnormal detrusor contractions long enough to get to the toilet.

PATIENT AND FAMILY EDUCATION: PREPARING FOR SELF-MANAGEMENT

Pelvic Muscle Exercises

- The pelvic muscles are composed of a sling of muscles that support your bladder, urethra, and vagina. Like any other muscles in your body, you can make your pelvic muscles stronger by alternately contracting (tightening) and relaxing them in regular exercise periods. By strengthening these muscles, you will be able to stop your urine flow more effectively.
- To identify your pelvic muscles, sit on the toilet with your feet flat on the floor about 12 inches apart. Begin to urinate, and then try to stop the urine flow. Do not strain down, lift your bottom off the seat, or squeeze your legs together. When you start and stop your urine stream, you are using your pelvic muscles.
- To perform pelvic muscle exercises, tighten your pelvic muscles for a slow count of 10 and then relax for a slow count of 10. Do this exercise 15 times while you are lying down, sitting up, and standing (a total of 45 exercises). Repeat—and this time rapidly contract and relax the pelvic muscles 10 times. This should take no more than 10 to 12 minutes for all three positions, or 3 to 4 minutes for each set of 15 exercises.
- Begin with 45 exercises a day in three sets of 15 exercises each. You will notice faster improvement if you can do this twice a day, or a total of 20 minutes each day. Remember to exercise in all three positions so your muscles learn to squeeze effectively despite your position. At first, it is helpful to have a designated time and place to do these exercises because you will have to concentrate to do them correctly. After you have been doing them for several weeks, you will notice improvement in your control of urine. However, many people report that improvement may take as long as 3 months.

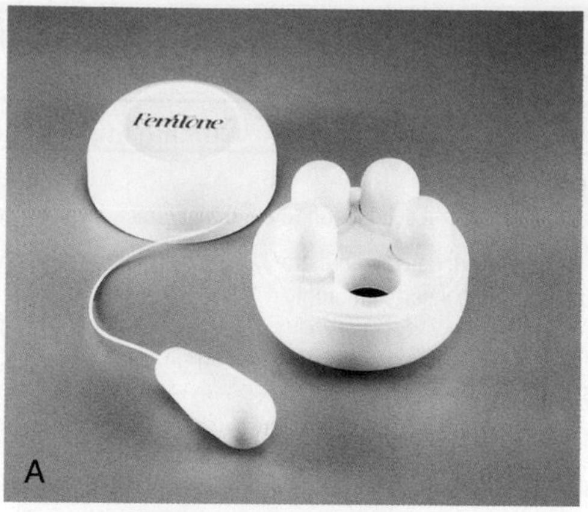

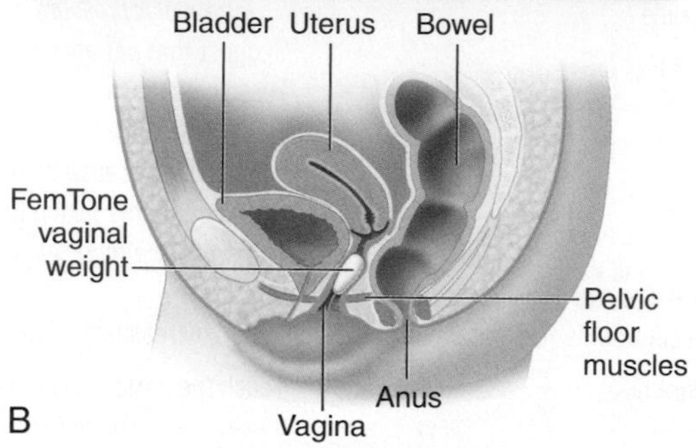

FIG. 61.1 A, FemTone vaginal weights, or cones. The number on the top of each cone represents increasing weight up to the heaviest cone, a 5. B, Diagram showing the correct positioning of a vaginal weight, or cone, in place. (A Courtesy ConvaTec, A Bristol-Meyers Squibb Company, a Division of E.R. Squibb & Sons, Inc., Princeton, NJ.)

Vaginal Cone Therapy. *Vaginal cone weight therapy* involves using a set of five small, cone-shaped weights (Touhy & Jett, 2016). They are of equal size but of varying weights and are used together with pelvic muscle exercise. The woman inserts the lightest cone, labeled 1, into her vagina (Fig. 61.1A), with the string to the outside, for a 1-minute test period. If she can hold the first cone in place without its slipping out while she walks around, she proceeds to the second cone, labeled 2, and repeats the procedure. The patient begins her treatment with the heaviest cone she can comfortably hold in her vagina for the 1-minute test period. Treatment periods are 15 minutes twice a day. When the patient can comfortably hold the cone in her vagina for 15 minutes, she progresses to the next heaviest weight. Treatment is completed with the cone labeled 5.

Weighted vaginal cones can help strengthen the pelvic muscles and decrease stress incontinence but may not help pelvic prolapse. Vaginal cones do not require a prescription.

Behavioral Interventions. Other interventions for urinary incontinence may include behavior modification or training (i.e., bladder training [see the Best Practice for Patient Safety & Quality Care: Bladder Training and Habit Training to Reduce Urinary Incontinence box]). Bladder training involves a great deal of patient participation and often begins with a thorough explanation of the problem of urge incontinence. Instead of the bladder being in control of the patient, the patient learns to control the bladder. For the program to succeed, the patient must be alert, aware, and able to resist the urge to urinate (Aoki et al., 2017).

Start a schedule for voiding, beginning with the longest interval that is comfortable for the patient, even if the interval is only 30 minutes. Instruct the patient to void every 30 minutes and to ignore any urge to urinate between the set intervals. Once the patient is comfortable with the starting schedule, increase the interval by 15 to 30 minutes. Instruct the patient to follow the new schedule until achieving success again. As the interval increases, the bladder gradually tolerates more volume. Teach relaxation and distraction techniques to maximize success in the retraining. Provide positive reinforcement for maintaining the prescribed schedule.

Habit training (scheduled toileting) is a type of bladder training that is successful in reducing incontinence in cognitively impaired patients. To use habit training, caregivers help the patient void at specific times (e.g., every 2 hours on the even hours). The goal is to get the patient to the toilet before incontinence occurs. The focus is on reducing incontinence and resulting loss of tissue integrity. When a reduction in incontinence has been achieved, the focus may change to increasing bladder capacity by gradually lengthening the voiding intervals, but this is only secondary.

Prompted voiding, a supplement to habit training, attempts to increase the patient's awareness of the need to void and to prompt him or her to ask for toileting assistance. Habit training otherwise relies completely on a time schedule.

BEST PRACTICE FOR PATIENT SAFETY & QUALITY CARE (QSEN)

Bladder Training and Habit Training to Reduce Urinary Incontinence

Bladder Training

- Assess the patient's awareness of bladder fullness and ability to cooperate with training regimen.
- Assess the patient's 24-hour urine *elimination* pattern for 2 to 3 consecutive days (bladder diary).
- Base the initial interval of toileting on the voiding pattern (e.g., 45 minutes).
- Teach the patient to void every 45 minutes on the first day and to ignore or suppress the urge to urinate between the 45-minute intervals.
- Take the patient to the toilet or remind him or her to urinate at the 45-minute intervals.
- Provide privacy for toileting and run water in the sink to promote the urge to urinate at this time.
- If the patient is not consistently able to resist the urge to urinate between the intervals, reduce the intervals by 15 minutes.
- Continue this regimen for at least 24 hours or for as many days as it takes for the patient to be comfortable with this schedule and not urinate between the intervals.
- When the patient remains continent between the intervals, increase the intervals by 15 minutes daily until a 3- to 4-hour interval is comfortable for the patient.
- Praise successes. If incontinence occurs, work with the patient to re-establish an acceptable toileting interval.

Habit Training

- Assess the patient's 24-hour voiding pattern for 2 to 3 days.
- Base the initial interval of toileting on the voiding pattern (e.g., 2 hours).
- Help the patient to the toilet or provide a bedpan/urinal every 2 hours (or whatever has been determined to be an appropriate toileting interval for the individual patient).
- During the toileting, remind the patient to void and provide cues such as running water.
- If the patient is incontinent between scheduled toileting, reduce the time interval by 30 minutes until the patient is continent between voidings.
- Help the patient to toilet and prompt to void at prescribed intervals.
- Do not leave the patient on the toilet or bedpan for longer than 5 minutes.
- Ensure that all nursing staff members comply with the established toileting schedule and do not apply briefs or encourage the patient to "just wet the bed."
- Reduce toileting interval by 30 minutes if there are more than two incontinence episodes in 24 hours.
- If the patient remains continent at the toileting interval, attempt to increase the interval by 30 minutes until a 3- to 4-hour continence interval is reached.
- Praise the patient for successes and spend extra time socializing with the patient.
- Discuss daily record of continence with staff to provide reinforcement and encourage compliance with toileting schedule.
- Include assistive personnel in all aspects of the habit training.

! NURSING SAFETY PRIORITY (QSEN)

Action Alert

Habit training is undermined when absorbent briefs are used in place of timed toileting. Do not tell patients to "just wet the bed." A common cause of falls in health care facilities is related to patient efforts to get out of bed unassisted to use the toilet. Collaborate with all staff members, including assistive personnel (AP), to consistently implement the toileting schedule for habit training.

For overflow incontinence, the most effective common behavioral interventions are bladder compression and intermittent self-catheterization. Bladder compression uses techniques that promote bladder emptying and include the Credé method, the Valsalva maneuver, double-voiding, and splinting.

For the Credé method, teach the patient how to press over the bladder area, increasing the pressure, or to trigger nerve stimulation by tugging at pubic hair or massaging the genital area. These techniques manually help the bladder empty. In the Valsalva maneuver, breathing techniques increase chest and abdominal pressure. This increased pressure is then directed toward the bladder during exhalation. (The Valsalva maneuver is contraindicated in patients who have some cardiac problems because it can trigger a vagal response and cause bradycardia.) With the technique of double-voiding, the patient empties the bladder and then, within a few minutes, attempts a second bladder emptying.

For women who have a large cystocele (prolapse of the bladder into the vagina), a technique called splinting both compresses the bladder and moves it into a better position. The woman inserts her fingers into her vagina, gently lifts the cystocele, and begins to urinate. A pessary, described earlier, can also provide relief from cystocele-related incontinence.

Intermittent self-catheterization is often used to help patients with long-term problems of incomplete bladder emptying. It is effective, can be learned fairly easily, and remains the preferred method of bladder emptying in patients who have incontinence as a result of a neurogenic bladder (Beauchemin et al., 2018). These points are important in teaching the technique:

- Proper handwashing and cleaning of the catheter reduce the risk for infection.
- A small lumen and good lubrication of the catheter prevent urethral trauma.
- A regular schedule for bladder emptying prevents distention and mucosal trauma.

Patients must be able to understand instructions and have the manual dexterity to manipulate the catheter. Caregivers or family members in the home can also be taught to perform intermittent catheterization using clean (rather than sterile) technique with good outcomes (Beauchemin et al., 2018).

Surgical Interventions. Stress incontinence may be treated by a surgical sling or bladder suspension procedure (Table 61.2). A sling procedure creates a sling around the bladder neck and urethra using strips of body tissue or synthetic mesh. Midurethral sling procedures are particularly effective for stress urinary incontinence (Clemens, 2018). Bladder suspension procedures are more extensive than sling procedures, and the surgeon sutures tissue near the bladder neck to a pubic bone ligament to provide support and prevent sagging. A third surgical procedure is the injection of bulking agents into the urethral wall to provide resistance to urine outflow. Bulking agents include collagen, carbon-coated zirconium beads, and silicone implants. Interventions for the patient with overflow (reflex) incontinence caused by obstruction of the bladder outlet may include surgery to relieve the obstruction. The most

TABLE 61.2 Surgical Procedures for Stress Incontinence

Procedure	Purpose	Nursing Considerations
Anterior vaginal repair (colporrhaphy)	Elevates the urethral position and repairs any cystocele	Because the operation is performed by vaginal incision, it is often done in conjunction with a vaginal hysterectomy. Recovery is usually rapid, and a urethral catheter is in place for 24-48 hr.
Retropubic suspension (Marshall-Marchetti-Krantz or Burch colposuspension)	Elevates the urethral position and provides longer-lasting results	The operation requires a low abdominal incision and a urethral or suprapubic catheter for several days after. Recovery takes longer, and urinary retention and detrusor instability are the most frequent complications.
Needle bladder neck suspension (Pereyra or Stamey procedure)	Elevates the urethral position and provides longer-lasting results without a long operative time	The combined vaginal approach with a needle and a small suprapubic skin incision does not allow direct vision of the operative site; however, the high complication rates may be due to the selection of patients who, because of their medical condition, are not good candidates for longer retropubic procedures.
Pubovaginal sling procedures	A sling made of synthetic or fascial material is placed under the ureterovesical junction to elevate the bladder neck.	The operation uses an abdominal, vaginal, or combined approach to treat intrinsic sphincter deficiencies. Temporary or permanent urinary retention is common after surgery.
Midurethral sling procedures	A tensionless vaginal sling is made from polypropylene mesh (or other materials) and placed near the ureterovesical junction to increase the angle, which inhibits movement of urine into the urethra with lower intravesical pressures.	This ambulatory surgery procedure uses a vaginal approach to improve symptoms of stress incontinence. Temporary or permanent urinary retention is common after surgery.
Artificial sphincters	A mechanical device to open and close the urethra is placed around the anatomic urethra.	The operation is done more frequently in men. The most common complications include mechanical failure of the device, erosion of tissue, and infection.
Periurethral injection of collagen or Siloxane	Implantation of small amounts of an inert substance through several small injections provides support around the bladder neck.	The procedure can be done in an ambulatory care setting and can be repeated as often as needed. Certain compounds may migrate after injection; an allergy test to bovine collagen must be performed before implantation.

common procedures are prostate removal (see Chapter 67) and repair of uterine prolapse (see Chapter 66).

Preoperative Care. Teach the patient about the procedure, and clarify the surgeon's explanation of events surrounding the surgery. In contrast to stress urinary incontinence, urge urinary incontinence requires extensive preoperative testing for diagnosis and selection of surgery. The patient may need emotional support during this extensive diagnostic work-up. Surgical procedures and preoperative and postoperative management are described in Table 61.2.

Postoperative Care. After surgery, assess for and intervene to prevent or detect complications. For prevention of movement or traction on the bladder neck, secure the urethral catheter with tape or a tube holder. If a suprapubic catheter is used instead of a urethral catheter, monitor the dressing for urine leakage and other drainage. Catheters are usually in place until the patient can urinate easily and has residual urine volume of less than 50 mL after voiding. (See Chapter 9 for general care before and after surgery.)

Maintaining Tissue Integrity. A major concern with the use of wearable protective pads is the risk for skin breakdown (loss of *tissue integrity*). Some patients develop incontinence-associated dermatitis (IAD) even when the skin is kept free of contact with urine (Gray et al., 2016). The wearable pads generate heat and sweat in the area that can cause dermatitis. Materials and costs of protective pads vary. Some are reusable; others are disposable. Avoid use of the word "diaper" when discussing these adult pants because of the association of diapers with a baby. More acceptable terms are "briefs" and "pads." Identifying

patients at risk for IAD is important to prevent IAD episodes and maintain tissue integrity. Risk factors may include patients with functional, physical, cognitive, and mobility alterations (Bliss et al., 2017). See Chapter 23 for more information about IAD.

When external devices (condom catheter or female urinary collection device) or containment materials are needed, discuss the possible options and help the patient make a selection that is best for his or her lifestyle and resources. Containment is achieved with absorbent pads and briefs designed to collect urine and keep the patient's skin and clothing dry. Many types and sizes of pads are available:

- Shields or liners inserted inside a panty
- Undergarments that are full-size pads with waist straps
- Plastic-lined protective underpants
- Combination pad and pant systems
- Absorbent bed pads

Correct use of external devices and containment materials is essential to ensure *tissue integrity* is maintained (Beeson & Davis, 2018).

Catheterization for control of functional incontinence may be intermittent or involve a long-term catheter. Intermittent catheterization is preferred to a long-term catheter because of the reduced risk for infection (Beauchemin et al., 2018). A long-term urinary catheter is appropriate for patients with altered *tissue integrity* who need a dry environment for healing, for those who are terminally ill and need comfort, and for those who are critically ill and require precise measurement of urine output.

CLINICAL JUDGMENT CHALLENGE 61.1

Patient-Centered Care; Evidence-Based Practice

The client is a 45-year-old woman who reports leakage of urine when she sneezes, coughs, and laughs. She states that the problem started several years ago and it occurred only a once or twice a month but now it occurs almost daily. She is able to drive and does not have any motor or sensory dysfunctions; however, she is embarrassed and now is afraid to go anywhere in case she "wets her pants." She states that the problem is because she is getting older and asks how other woman her age handle the leakage. She currently works at home and seldom goes to church or out with her spouse because of the urine leakage. Currently, the client reports using toilet paper in her undergarments so that no one will find out she has a problem with urine leakage. Client history includes seasonal allergies, vaginal deliveries of three full-term infants, and type II diabetes mellitus.

1. **Recognize Cues:** What assessment information in this client situation is the most important and immediate concern for the nurse? (Hint: Identify the **relevant** information *first* to determine what is most important.)
2. **Analyze Cues:** What client conditions are consistent with the **most relevant** information? (Hint: Think about priority collaborative problems that support and contradict the information presented in this situation.)
3. **Prioritize Hypotheses:** Which possibilities or explanations are **most likely** to be present in this client situation? Which possibilities or explanations are the most serious? (Hint: Consider all possibilities and determine their urgency and risk for this client.)
4. **Generate Solutions:** What actions would most likely achieve the desired outcomes for this client? Which actions should be **avoided** or are **potentially harmful**? (Hint: Determine the desired outcomes first to decide which interventions are appropriate and those that should be avoided.)
5. **Take Action:** Which actions are the most appropriate and how should they be implemented? In what **priority order** should they be implemented? (Hint: Consider health teaching, documentation, requested health care provider orders or prescriptions, nursing skills, collaboration with or referral to health team members, etc.)
6. **Evaluate Outcomes:** What client assessment would indicate that the nurse's actions were **effective**? (Hint: Think about signs that would indicate an improvement, decline, or unchanged client condition.)

PATIENT AND FAMILY EDUCATION: PREPARING FOR SELF-MANAGEMENT

Urinary Incontinence

- Maintain a normal body weight to reduce the pressure on your bladder.
- Do not try to control your incontinence by limiting your fluid intake. Adequate fluid intake is necessary for kidney function and health maintenance.
- If you have a catheter in your bladder, follow the instructions given to you about maintaining the sterile drainage system.
- If you are discharged with a suprapubic catheter in your bladder, inspect the entry site for the tube daily, clean the skin around the opening gently with warm soap and water, and place a sterile gauze dressing on the skin around the tube. Report any redness, swelling, drainage, or fever to your primary health care provider.
- Do not put anything into your vagina, such as tampons, drugs, hygiene products, or exercise with weights, until you check with your primary health care provider at your 6-week checkup after surgery.
- Do not have sexual intercourse until after your 6-week postoperative checkup.
- Do not lift or carry anything heavier than 5 lb or participate in any strenuous exercise until your primary health care provider gives you postoperative clearance. In some cases, this could be as long as 3 months.
- Avoid exercises, such as running, jogging, step or dance aerobic classes, rowing, cross-country ski or stair-climber machines, and mountain biking. Brisk walking without any additional hand, leg, or body weights is allowed. Swimming is allowed after all drains and catheters have been removed and your incision is completely healed.
- If Kegel exercises are recommended, ask your nurse for specific instructions.

Care Coordination and Transition Management. Community-based care for the patient with urinary incontinence considers personal, physical, emotional, and social resources. Important personal resources for self-care include mobility and manual dexterity. When planning care, consider who will be the primary caregiver and which factors may influence the effectiveness of the plan. Nonpharmacologic and nonsurgical treatments provide significant clinical benefits with low risk for adverse effects but that these interventions are also associated with poor adherence (Clemens, 2018). Ongoing relationships with primary health care providers may improve adherence.

Home Care Management. Assess the home environment for barriers that limit access to the bathroom. Eliminate hazards that might slow walking or lead to a fall. Such hazards include throw rugs, furniture with legs that extend into the walking area, slippery waxed or polished floors, and poor lighting.

If the patient must climb stairs to reach a bathroom, handrails should be installed and stairs kept free of obstacles. Toilet seat extenders may help provide the right level and height of seating so that maximal abdominal pressure may be applied for voiding.

Portable commodes may be obtained when ambulatory access to toilets is impractical. Physical and occupational therapists are valuable resources for assisting with home care management.

Self-Management Education. Teach the patient and family about the cause of the specific type of incontinence and discuss available treatment options for its management. The teaching plan should address the prescribed drugs (purpose, dosage, method and route of administration, and expected and potential side effects). Instruct the patient and family about the importance of weight reduction and dietary modification to help control incontinence of urine *elimination.* Remind the patient who smokes that nicotine can contribute to bladder irritation and that coughing can cause urine leakage.

For urge urinary incontinence, teach the patient to avoid foods that irritate the bladder such as caffeine and alcohol. Spacing fluids at regular intervals throughout the day (e.g., 120 mL every hour or 240 mL every 2 hours) and limiting fluids after the dinner hour (e.g., only 120 mL at bedtime) help avoid fluid overload on the bladder and allow urine to collect at a steady pace. Remind patients that maintaining an ideal body weight helps avoid the pressure that abdominal fat places on pelvic organs, thus reducing incontinence.

For patients who require external devices or containment materials, discuss the options available and work with the patient to determine the best selection. For patients who will use intermittent catheterization or those with artificial urinary sphincters, demonstrate the correct technique to the patient or caregiver. Having the patient return demonstrate correct technique is essential to prevent complications (Beauchemin et al., 2018).

Psychosocial Preparation. The embarrassment of incontinence can be devastating to self-esteem, body image, and relationships. Sexual intimacy is often adversely affected, and the unpredictable nature of incontinence creates anxiety. Patients may be embarrassed to seek help and, even when resources are identified, they may need help to feel comfortable in using them. Buying supplies at a local store may threaten privacy.

Acknowledge the personal concerns of the patient and caregiver. Never make their concerns seem trivial. As he or she learns the specifics of the plan that will allow control of urinary incontinence, the confidence to resume social interactions should return. Many continence supplies can be purchased online and delivered to the home to maintain privacy.

Health Care Resources. Referral to home care agencies for help with personal care and to continence clinics that specialize in evaluation and treatment may be helpful. In many continence clinics, nurses collaborate with physicians and other health care professionals to evaluate and manage patients. The treatment plan is specific for each patient; supplies and products are custom selected.

Patients may benefit from education and from the support of others who experience similar concerns. The National Association for Continence (NAFC) (www.nafc.org), and the Wound, Ostomy, and Continence Nurses (www.wocn.org) publish newsletters and educational materials written with easy-to-understand explanations. The American Urological Association (www.auanet.org) provides information on many areas of urologic dysfunction. Local hospitals often have local NAFC-approved support groups.

NCLEX EXAMINATION CHALLENGE 61.1

Physiological Integrity

For which client would the nurse expect to teach intermittent catheterization?

A. 35-year-old woman who has multiple sclerosis and incontinence

B. 48-year-old man who is admitted for pneumonia and is on complete bed-rest

C. 61-year-old woman who is admitted following a fall at home and has new-onset dysrhythmia

D. 74-year-old man who has lung cancer with brain metastasis and has advanced dementia

---

◆ **Evaluation: Evaluate Outcomes.** Evaluate the care of the patient with urinary incontinence based on the identified priority patient problems. The expected outcomes are that the patient will:

• Maintain optimal urinary elimination through a reduction in the number of urinary incontinence episodes

• Maintain tissue integrity of the skin and mucous membranes in the perineal area

• Demonstrate knowledge of proper use of drugs and correct procedures for self-catheterization, use of the artificial sphincter, or care of an indwelling urinary catheter

• Demonstrate effective use of the selected exercise or bladder-training program

• Select and use incontinence interventions, devices, and products

CYSTITIS

Pathophysiology Review

Cystitis is an inflammatory condition of the bladder. Commonly, it refers to inflammation from an infection of the bladder. However, cystitis can be caused by inflammation without infection. For example, drugs, chemicals, or local radiation therapy cause bladder inflammation without an infecting organism. Irritants, such as feminine hygiene spray, spermicidal jellies, or long-term use of a catheter can cause cystitis without infection. Cystitis may sometimes occur as a complication of other disorders, such as gynecologic cancers, pelvic inflammatory disorders, endometriosis, Crohn's disease, diverticulitis, lupus, or tuberculosis.

An infection can occur in any area of the urinary tract and the kidney. Such infections are known as *urinary tract infections* or *UTIs*. An acute UTI is the invasion of the urinary tract by an infectious organism. A recurrent UTI is defined as having two or more infections in 6 months or three or more infections in 1 year. These distinctions in UTIs are important because they have different approaches to management (Feng et al., 2018). Contributing factors associated with cystitis and other UTIs are listed in Table 61.3.

👤 PATIENT-CENTERED CARE: GENDER HEALTH CONSIDERATIONS (QSEN)

Bladder infections are more common in women than men. Up to 60% of women have experienced a UTI in their lifetime with most infections being a bladder infection. Women are 30 times more likely to have a UTI than men (Tan & Chlebicki, 2016).

A UTI is further categorized as *uncomplicated* or *complicated* (Table 61.4). With an uncomplicated UTI, there is no anatomic or functional abnormality of the urinary tract or condition that increases the risk for infection or possibility of treatment failing to resolve the infection (such as the presence of a multi–drug-resistant organism or urologic dysfunction). Some factors and conditions that contribute to a diagnosis of complicated UTI are pregnancy, male gender, obstruction, diabetes, neurogenic bladder, chronic kidney disease, and reduced **immunity** (Nicolle, 2016). In men, a UTI is generally considered complicated even with normal structure and function because most UTIs occur in older men or in association with anal intercourse or intercourse with a female who has infectious vaginitis, resulting in exposure to potentially virulent pathogens. Complicated cystitis or other UTI requires greater vigilance to avoid or detect adverse events from the infection and a longer course of antimicrobial treatment. A diagnosis of complicated UTI may require additional testing to identify and manage other related health problems (comorbidities).

The presence of bacteria in the urine is bacteriuria and may occur with cystitis or any UTI. When the patient has bacteriuria but no symptoms of infection, it is called *colonization* or *asymptomatic bacteriuria (ABU)* and is more common in older adults. This problem may progress to acute infection or renal insufficiency when the patient has other conditions, and only then does it require treatment (Avelluto & Bryman, 2018).

TABLE 61.3 Factors Contributing to Urinary Tract Infections

Factor	Mechanism
Obstruction	Incomplete bladder emptying creates a continuous pool of urine in which bacteria can grow, prevents flushing out of bacteria, and allows bacteria to ascend more easily to higher structures.
	Bacteria have a greater chance of multiplying the longer they remain in residual urine.
	Overdistention of the bladder damages the mucosa and allows bacteria to invade the bladder wall.
Stones (calculi)	Large stones can obstruct urine flow.
	The rough surface of a stone irritates mucosal surfaces and creates a spot where bacteria can establish and grow.
	Bacteria can live within stones and cause reinfection.
Vesicoureteral reflux	The urethra is colonized with bacteria. These bacteria are noninfectious until they move to upstream anatomy (bladder, ureters, kidneys) and colonize or form an infection with reflux (backward-flowing urine).
	Reflux of sterile urine can cause kidney scarring, which may promote kidney dysfunction.
Diabetes mellitus	Excess glucose in urine provides a rich medium for bacterial growth.
	Peripheral neuropathy affects bladder innervation and leads to a flaccid bladder and incomplete bladder emptying.
Characteristics of urine	Urine pH can promote different species of bacterial growth.
	Concentrated urine allows bacterial growth and adhesion to urinary tract anatomy.
Gender	**Women**
	Susceptibility to urethral colonization with coliform or pathogenic bacteria is increased, especially as estrogen levels fall during menopause.
	Use of douches, perfumed pads or toilet tissue, diaphragms, or spermicide (including spermicide-coated condoms) in women can inflame periurethral tissue and contribute to colonization.
	Bladder displacement during pregnancy predisposes women to cystitis and the development of pyelonephritis.
	A diaphragm or pessary that is too large can obstruct urine flow or traumatize the urethra.
	Men
	With increased age, the prostate enlarges and may obstruct the normal flow of urine, producing stasis.
	With increased age, prostatic secretions lose their antibacterial characteristics and predispose to bacterial proliferation in the urine.
	Sexually transmitted infections may cause urethral strictures that obstruct the flow of urine and predispose to urinary stasis.
Age	Urinary stasis may be caused by incomplete bladder emptying as a result of an enlarged prostate in men and cystocele and vaginal prolapse in women.
	Neuromuscular conditions that cause incomplete bladder emptying, such as Parkinson disease and stroke, affect older adults more frequently.
	The use of drugs with intentional or unintentional anticholinergic properties in older adults contributes to delayed bladder emptying.
	Fecal incontinence contributes to urethral contamination.
	Low estrogen in menopausal women adversely affects the cells of the vagina and urethra, making them more susceptible to infections.
	Overall *immunity* declines with age, increasing the risk for uncomplicated infections to become complicated.
Sexual activity	Sexual intercourse is the strongest risk factor for uncomplicated cystitis, particularly in young women.
	Irritation of the perineum and urethra during intercourse can promote migration of bacteria from the perineal area to the urinary tract in some women.
	Inadequate vaginal lubrication may exacerbate potential urethral irritation.
	Bacteria may be introduced into the male urethra during anal intercourse or during vaginal intercourse with a woman who has infectious vaginitis.
Recent use of antibiotics	Antibiotics change *immunity* and normal protective flora, providing opportunity for pathogenic bacterial overgrowth and colonization.
Virulence factors	The more virulent the organism, the more severe the infection.

The urinary and genitourinary tracts are normally sterile, apart from the distal urethra. Several host defenses help protect against infection in the urinary tract. Mucin produced by cells lining the bladder helps maintain mucosal integrity and prevents cellular damage. Mucin also prevents bacteria from adhering to urothelial cells. Urine pH also contributes to sustaining sterile urine. White blood cells in the urinary tract are the *immunity* cells that engulf and destroy pathogens. Urine proteins, such as secreted antibodies, also are protective. In men, the prostate gland secretes additional protective proteins. Frequent voiding is another defense against bacterial growth and adherence by preventing urine stasis and flushing out organisms.

Etiology and Genetic Risk. UTIs, like other infections, result from interactions between a pathogen and the host. Usually a high bacterial *virulence* (ability to invade and infect) is needed to overcome normal host defenses and *immunity.* However, an adult with reduced immunity is more likely to become infected even with bacteria that have low virulence. With UTI, bacteria (and, infrequently, fungi) move up the urinary tract from the external

TABLE 61.4 Urinary Tract Infection Types

Type	Description
Acute uncomplicated cystitis	Acute UTI — bladder involvement only No signs/symptoms of upper UTI No anatomic or functional abnormality of the urinary tract or condition that increases the risk for infection or possibility of treatment failing to resolve the infection
Acute complicated cystitis	Involves more than the bladder Symptoms of upper UTI: fever, flank pain, chills/rigors, malaise, costovertebral angle tenderness, and pelvic and/or perineal pain in men

urethra to the bladder to cause infectious cystitis. Less commonly, spread of infection through the blood and lymph fluid can occur, although this cause of UTI is not common. Invading bacteria with special adhesions are more likely to cause ascending UTIs that start in the urethra or bladder and move up into the ureter and kidney.

Infectious cystitis is typically caused by pathogens from the bowel or, in some cases, the vagina. Greater than 80% of UTIs are caused by *Escherichia coli.* Less common organisms include *Staphylococcus saprophyticus, Klebsiella pneumoniae,* and organisms from the *Proteus* and *Enterobacter* species (McLellan & Hunstad, 2016; Nicolle, 2016). Other infecting microbes causing infectious cystitis are viruses, mycobacteria, parasites, and yeast (fungus), especially *Candida* species. Reflux from the colonized distal urethra can also contribute to UTI in vulnerable patients. Irritation, trauma, or instrumentation of the urinary tract decreases host defenses and contributes to UTIs through the ascending migration of uropathogens.

Catheters are the most common factor associated with new-onset UTIs in the hospital and long-term care settings (Conway et al., 2017; Panchisin, 2016). Within 48 hours of catheter insertion, bacterial colonization along the urethra and the catheter itself begins. Risks for infection associated with a catheter increases 3% to 10% per day the catheter is in place (Ferguson, 2018).

The way that a catheter-associated urinary tract infection (CAUTI) occurs varies between genders. Bacteria from a woman's perineal area are more likely to ascend to the bladder by moving along the urethra. The shorter urethra in women aids in the ascending organisms' migration. In men, bacteria tend to gain access to the bladder from the catheter itself (Conway et al., 2017). Any break in the closed urinary drainage system allows bacteria to move through the lumen of the catheter. The external catheter surface also provides route for migration. Best practices to reduce the risk for catheter contamination and catheter-associated UTIs are listed in the Best Practice for Patient Safety & Quality Care: Minimizing Catheter-Associated Urinary Tract Infection (CAUTI) box and in Box 61.1.

BEST PRACTICE FOR PATIENT SAFETY & QUALITY CARE (QSEN)
Minimizing Catheter-Associated Urinary Tract Infection (CAUTI)

- Maintain good hand hygiene during insertion and manipulation of the catheter system to avoid contamination.
- Insert urinary catheters for appropriate use only, including:
  - Acute urinary retention or bladder obstruction.
  - Accurate measurement of urine volume in critically ill patients if needed.
  - Perioperative situations only as needed, such as urogenital, gynecological, laparoscopic, and orthopedic surgeries. Avoid routine use of indwelling catheters for surgical patients.
  - To assist in healing of open sacral or perineal wounds in incontinent patients. Avoid use of indwelling catheters to manage patients who are incontinent.
  - Consider intermittent catheterization or other alternatives to indwelling catheters for patients with spinal cord injuries or conditions.
  - To provide comfort at end of life.
- Ensure that only properly trained personnel insert and maintain catheters.
- Use routine hygiene to clean periurethral area; antiseptic cleaning solutions are NOT recommended.
- Leave catheters in place only as long as needed. The strongest predictor of a CAUTI is the length of time the catheter dwells in a patient.
- Assess the need for urinary catheter daily and document patient needs or indications.
- For example, remove catheters in postanesthesia care or as soon as possible after surgery when intraoperative indications have resolved.
- Use aseptic technique and sterile equipment in the acute care setting when inserting a urinary (intermittent or indwelling) catheter.
- Maintain a closed system by ensuring that catheter tubing connections are sealed securely; disconnections can introduce pathogens into the urinary tract.
- Obtain urine samples aseptically.

- If breaks in the system occur, replace the catheter and entire collecting system.
- Maintain unobstructed urine flow:
  - Keep the catheter and collecting tube free from kinking.
  - Keep the urine collection bag below the level of the bladder and do not rest the bag on the floor.
  - Empty the bag regularly, using a separate, clean container for each patient.
  - Ensure that the drainage spigot does not come into contact with nonsterile surfaces.
- Secure the catheter to the patient's thigh (women) or lower abdomen (men); catheter movement can cause urethral friction and irritation.
- Consider the use of antiseptic or antimicrobial catheters for patients requiring urinary catheters for more than 3 to 5 days. These catheters reduce bacterial colonization (i.e., biofilm) along the catheter.
- Consider appropriate alternatives to an indwelling catheter:
  - External (condom) devices in cooperative men without obstruction or urinary retention
  - Intermittent catheterization in patients requiring drainage for neurogenic bladder or postoperative urinary retention
- Use portable ultrasound devices to assess urine volume to reduce unnecessary catheterization.
- Implement best practices in quality improvement to ensure that core recommendations for use, insertion, and maintenance are implemented. Examples of projects that improve patient care and reduce CAUTI include:
  - Nurse-initiated protocols for urinary catheter removal
  - Compliance with hand hygiene
  - Impact of educational programs on CAUTI occurrence
  - Compliance with documentation for catheter placement or maintenance
  - Number of CAUTI per 1000 catheter days or patient days on unit
  - Track number of catheters inserted

Adapted from https://www.cdc.gov/nhsn/acute-care-hospital/cauti/.

BOX 61.1 Catheter-Associated Urinary Tract Infection (CAUTI) Prevention

A catheter-associated urinary tract infection (CAUTI) is the fourth leading cause of health care–associated infections occurring in acute care settings in the United States. Up to 25% of patients admitted to an acute care setting have a catheter, which places the individual at risk for infection. The estimated cost of a CAUTI is $758 for each individual with an overall annual cost of $340 million for the United States alone. Costs associated with a CAUTI are not reimbursed. CAUTI causes harm to the patients and reduces positive outcomes. Implementing a CAUTI prevention program increases the nurses' knowledge about prevention methods, reduces the incidence of CAUTI, and improves patient outcomes (Ferguson, 2018). Implementing a CAUTI prevention program is also one way to meet the National Patient Safety Goal specific to prevention CAUTI (The Joint Commission, 2019).

👤 PATIENT-CENTERED CARE: OLDER ADULT CONSIDERATIONS (QSEN)

In women, there is a 20% incidence of UTIs for those between ages 18 and 24 annually and 50% of women will have a UTI by 35 years of age (Simmering et al., 2017). In men, the incidence of UTI is significantly lower than in women; however, the incidence greatly increases as men become older (Lee & Le, 2018). Skin and mucous membrane changes from a lack of estrogen appear to account for much of the increased risk in older women, together with overall decreased *immunity*. Prostate disease increases risk for UTIs in men. Often the older adult does not have the typical symptoms of UTI (i.e., flank pain, dysuria, fever). More common symptoms are grossly bloody, foul-smelling urine with increasing frequency of urination (Touhy & Jett, 2016). When UTI leads to urosepsis, mental status changes occur. Ask about these additional symptoms of UTI whenever you are assessing an older adult.

Organisms other than bacteria cause cystitis. Fungal infections, such as those caused by *Candida*, can occur during long-term antibiotic therapy because antibiotics change normal protective flora that reduce the adherence and volume of pathogenic bacteria. Patients with reduced *immunity* (those who are severely immunosuppressed, are receiving corticosteroids or other immunosuppressive agents, or have diabetes mellitus or acquired immune deficiency syndrome) are at higher risk for fungal UTIs.

Viral and parasitic infections are rare and usually transfer to the urinary tract from an infection at another body site. For example, *Trichomonas*, a parasite found in the vagina, can also be found in the urine. Treatment of the vaginal infection also resolves the UTI.

Noninfectious cystitis may result from chemical exposure, such as to drugs (e.g., cyclophosphamide); from radiation therapy; and from *immunity* problems, as with systemic lupus erythematosus (SLE).

Interstitial cystitis is a rare, chronic inflammation of the entire lower urinary tract (bladder, urethra, and adjacent pelvic muscles) that is related to genetic and *immunity* dysfunction rather than infection. The condition affects women more often than men, and the diagnosis is difficult to make. Symptoms are pain associated with bladder filling or voiding, usually accompanied by frequency, urgency, and nocturia (Kim, 2016). Pain occurs in suprapubic or pelvic areas, sometimes radiating to the groin, vulva, or rectum.

Although cystitis is not life threatening, infection of the urinary tract can lead to life-threatening complications, including pyelonephritis and sepsis. Severe kidney damage from an ascending UTI is a rare complication. Patients with predisposing factors, such as anatomic abnormalities, pregnancy, obstruction, reflux, calculi, or diabetes, are at greater risk for complications.

The urinary tract is often the infection source in severe sepsis or septic shock. The spread of the infection from the urinary tract to the bloodstream is termed *bacteremia* or urosepsis. Catheter-associated urinary tract infections are the leading cause of urosepsis, which has a mortality rate of 10% (Ferguson, 2018). Sepsis, regardless of the source, is a systemic reaction to infection that prolongs hospitalization and can lead to shock, multiple organ failure, and other profound complications (see Chapter 34).

Incidence and Prevalence. The incidence of UTI is second only to upper respiratory infections in primary care and affects 150 million people worldwide annually (McLellan & Hunstad, 2016). Total costs for UTIs are estimated at $2.8 billion annually. In addition to a high prevalence in primary care, UTIs are one of the most common health care–associated infections (Feng et al., 2018).

The hallmark symptoms of UTI are frequency (an urge to urinate frequently in small amounts), dysuria (pain or burning with urination), and urgency (feeling that urination will occur immediately).

Health Promotion and Maintenance. Although infectious cystitis is common, in many cases it is preventable. When catheters must be used in institutional settings, strict attention to sterile technique during insertion is essential to reduce the risk for UTIs (see the Best Practice for Patient Safety & Quality Care: Minimizing Catheter-Associated Urinary Tract Infection box). Long-term placement of urinary catheters requires aseptic technique for insertion. When *intermittent catheterization* was used in home care settings, the use of clean technique resulted in a similar rate of UTI compared with sterile technique. Clean technique, using single-use catheters, for catheter insertion is recommended in home settings where multiple resistant organisms are less likely to be present. Multiuse catheters for home use are no longer recommended. Sterile technique must be used in health care facilities to reduce the risk for infection (Beauchemin et al., 2018).

❗ NURSING SAFETY PRIORITY (QSEN)
Action Alert

Ensuring that urinary catheters are used appropriately and discontinued as early as possible is required (The Joint Commission, 2019). Do not allow catheters to remain in place for staff convenience.

Certain changes in fluid intake patterns, urinary *elimination* patterns, and hygiene patterns can help prevent or reduce cystitis in the general population. For example, a liberal water intake of 2.2 L for women and 3 L for men can promote general health. Another strategy to promote health is to have sufficient fluid intake to cause 1.5 L of clear or light yellow urine daily. Strategies to prevent cystitis and other UTIs are listed in the Patient and Family Education: Preparing for Self-Management: Preventing a Urinary Tract Infection box. Although some of these strategies do not have consistent evidence to support a reduced risk for UTI when followed, they are low risk and reasonable.

! NATIONAL PATIENT SAFETY GOALS
Prevention of CAUTI

The Joint Commission (2019) has implemented a national patient safety goal (NPSG) designed to decrease the incidence of indwelling catheter–associated urinary tract infections. Elements of performance include ongoing education for staff to decrease the risk and incidence of CAUTI. Each hospital should have written criteria regarding the use and care of indwelling urinary catheters. These criteria include the evidence-based guidance to minimize use when possible and limit indwelling duration. Be sure to review the facility specific protocol to minimize CAUTI.

❖ Interprofessional Collaborative Care

Cystitis and UTIs can occur in any setting and are very common in the community. Usually the adult with cystitis is treated at home using self-management strategies.

◆ Assessment: Recognize Cues

Physical Assessment/Signs and Symptoms. Frequency, urgency, and dysuria are the common symptoms of a urinary tract infection (UTI), but other symptoms may be present (see the Key Features:

PATIENT AND FAMILY EDUCATION: PREPARING FOR SELF-MANAGEMENT
Preventing a Urinary Tract Infection

- Drink fluid liberally, as much as 2 to 3 L daily if not contraindicated by health conditions.
- Be sure to get enough sleep, rest, and nutrition daily to maintain immunologic health.
- If spermicides are used, consider changing to another method of contraception.
- *[For women]* Clean your perineum (the area between your legs) from front to back.
- *[For women]* Avoid using or wearing irritating substances such as douches, scented lubricants for intercourse, bubble bath, tight-fitting underwear, and scented toilet tissue. Wear loose-fitting cotton underwear.
- *[For women]* Empty your bladder before and after intercourse.
- *[For both women and men]* Gently wash the perineal area before intercourse.
- Do not routinely delay urination because the flow of urine can help remove bacteria that may be colonizing the urethra or bladder.
- If you experience burning when you urinate, if you have to urinate frequently, or if you find it difficult to begin urinating, notify your primary health care provider right away, especially if you have a chronic medical condition (e.g., diabetes) or are pregnant.

▶▶ KEY FEATURES
Urinary Tract Infection

Common Symptoms	Complicated Cystitis Symptoms
• Frequency	• Fever
• Urgency	• Chills and rigors
• Dysuria	• Nausea or vomiting
• Suprapubic pain or tenderness, low back pain	• Malaise
• Nocturia	• Flank pain and costovertebral angle tenderness
• Incontinence	
• Hematuria	**Symptoms That May Occur in the Older Adult**
• Pyuria	• Sudden or worsening: dysuria, urinary incontinence, nocturia, urgency, and frequency. A general sense of lack of well-being.
• Bacteriuria	
• Retention	
• Suprapubic tenderness or fullness	• Note: Changes in mental status and falls are not reliable predictors of UTIs. These changes need to be fully assessed to determine the underlying cause.
• Feeling of incomplete bladder emptying	

Urinary Tract Infection box). Urine may be cloudy, foul smelling, or blood tinged. Ask the patient about risk factors for UTI during the assessment (see Table 61.3). For noninfectious cystitis, the Pelvic Pain and Urgency/Frequency Patient Symptom Scale (PUF, 2011) can identify patients with interstitial cystitis.

For patients with a urinary catheter, in addition to common signs of UTI (e.g., fever with or without chills; leukocytosis; suprapubic or flank pain; urine with sediment, blood, or foul odor), new onset of hypotension or changes in mental status can indicate a UTI. Diagnostic testing for UTIs in older adults should not be based on mental status changes alone but should be performed when UTI symptoms are present (Hooten & Gupta, 2018). If a catheter has been in place for more than 2 weeks, it may be necessary to first replace the catheter before obtaining a urine specimen for culture (McGoldrick, 2016).

Before performing the physical assessment, ask the patient to void so that the urine can be examined and the bladder emptied before palpation. Assess vital signs to help identify the presence of infection (e.g., fever, tachycardia, tachypnea). Inspect the lower abdomen and palpate the bladder. Distention after voiding indicates incomplete bladder emptying.

Using Standard Precautions, record any lesions around the urethral meatus and vaginal opening. To help differentiate between a vaginal and a urinary tract infection, note whether there is any vaginal discharge or irritation. Vaginal discharge and irritation are more indicative of vaginal infection. Women often report burning with urination when urine touches labial tissues that are inflamed or have lost *tissue integrity* with ulcerations by vaginal infections or sexually transmitted infections (STIs). Maintain privacy with drapes during the examination.

The prostate is palpated by digital rectal examination (DRE) by the primary health care provider for size, change in shape or consistency, and tenderness. A large prostate gland can obstruct urine outflow and contribute to urostasis and bacterial colonization of the urinary tract, contributing to the risk for a complicated UTI.

Laboratory Assessment. Laboratory assessment for a UTI begins with a clean-catch urine specimen that is divided into two containers. If the patient cannot produce a clean-catch specimen, you may need to obtain the specimen with a small-diameter (6 Fr) catheter. For a routine urinalysis, 10 mL of urine is needed; smaller quantities are sufficient for culture.

One container is used for a urinalysis. The combination of a positive leukocyte esterase and nitrate from a urinalysis is 68% to 88% sensitive in the diagnosis of a UTI. The presence of white blood cells (WBCs) (**pyuria**), red blood cells (RBCs) (**hematuria**), or casts (clumps of material or cells) also may indicate UTI (Pagana & Pagana, 2018). The presence of more than 20 epithelial cells/high-power field (HPF) suggests contamination, and a new specimen may be collected for culture and sensitivity.

If the urinalysis suggests a UTI and there are no risk factors or conditions for complicated UTI in a woman, treatment can be started. If the UTI is complicated, the second specimen is analyzed as a urine culture. A culture may also be performed when a patient with a UTI does not respond to usual therapy, when the diagnosis is uncertain, to assess for sensitivity, or to determine resolution of UTI (Hooten & Gupta, 2018). Urinalysis is less specific in diagnosing a UTI in an older adult, especially one who has a urinary catheter.

A urine culture confirms the type of organism and the number of colonies. Urine culture is expensive, and initial results take at least 24 hours. A UTI is confirmed when more than 10^5 colony-forming units/mL are in the urine from any patient. In noncatheterized patients who have symptoms of UTI (e.g., fever, dysuria, new-onset frequency or urgency, suprapubic or flank pain, or hematuria), as few as 10^3 colony-forming units/mL in a voided specimen can confirm the infection. For patients with a catheter who are symptomatic, 10^2 colony-forming units/mL are diagnostic of a complicated UTI. The presence of many different types of organisms in low colony counts usually indicates that the specimen is contaminated. Sensitivity testing follows culture results when complicating factors are present (e.g., stones or recurrent infection), when the patient is older, or to ensure that appropriate antibiotics are prescribed.

Occasionally the serum WBC count may be elevated, with the differential WBC count showing a "left shift" (see Chapter 16). This shift indicates that the number of immature WBCs is increasing and the number of mature WBCs is decreasing in response to continued infection. Thus the number of "bands," or immature WBCs, is elevated, which indicates reduced ***immunity***. Left shift most often occurs with urosepsis and rarely occurs with uncomplicated cystitis, because cystitis is a local rather than a systemic infection.

Other Diagnostic Assessment. The diagnosis of UTI and cystitis is based on history, physical examination, and laboratory data. If urinary retention and obstruction of urine outflow are suspected, pelvic ultrasound or CT may be needed to locate the site of obstruction or the presence of calculi. Voiding cystourethrography (see Chapter 60) is needed when urine reflux is suspected.

Cystoscopy (see Chapter 60) may be performed when the patient has recurrent UTIs (more than three annually). A urine culture is performed first to ensure that no infection is present. If infection is present, the urine is sterilized with antibiotic therapy before the procedure to reduce the risk for sepsis. Cystoscopy identifies abnormalities that increase the risk for cystitis. Such abnormalities include bladder calculi, bladder diverticula, urethral strictures, foreign bodies (e.g., sutures from previous surgery), and trabeculation (an abnormal thickening of the bladder wall caused by urinary retention and obstruction). Retrograde pyelography, along with the cystoscopic examination, shows outlines and images of the drainage tract.

Cystoscopy is needed to accurately diagnose interstitial (noninfectious) cystitis. A urinalysis usually shows WBCs and RBCs but no bacteria. Common findings in interstitial cystitis are a small-capacity bladder, the presence of Hunner ulcers (a type of bladder lesion), and small hemorrhages after bladder distention.

◆ Interventions: Take Action

Nonsurgical Management. The expected outcome is to maintain an optimal urine ***elimination*** pattern. Nursing interventions for the management of cystitis focus on ***pain*** relief and teaching about drug therapy, fluid intake, and prevention measures. In a hospital setting, timely administration of antibiotics can prevent or reduce complications from urosepsis.

Drug Therapy. Drugs used to treat bacteriuria and relieve ***pain*** include urinary antiseptics or antibiotics, analgesics, and antispasmodics. Cure of a UTI depends on the antimicrobial levels achieved in the urine. Fluconazole is the drug of choice for treatment of *Candida* (fungal) infections. Antispasmodic drugs decrease bladder spasms and promote complete bladder emptying.

Antibiotic therapy is used for bacterial UTIs (see the Common Examples of Drug Therapy: Urinary Tract Infections box). Guidelines for uncomplicated cystitis recommend nitrofurantoin, trimethoprim/sulfamethoxazole, or fosfomycin as first-line therapy for those patients at low risk of resistance to antimicrobials (Hooten & Gupta, 2018). Longer antibiotic treatment (7 to 21 days) and sometimes different agents are required for hospitalized patients and those with complicated UTIs (e.g., men, pregnant women, and patients with anatomic, functional or metabolic derangements that affect the urinary tract).

! NURSING SAFETY PRIORITY (QSEN)

Drug Alert

Sulfamethoxazole/trimethoprim should be stopped at the first appearance of a skin rash. A rash may indicate the onset of Stevens-Johnson syndrome (aching joints and muscles; bilateral blistering skin) or toxic epidermal necrolysis (redness, blistering, and peeling skin and mucous membranes).

Antibiotics are one of the drug categories most frequently involved in the error of administration to patients who have documented allergies to these drugs.

COMMON EXAMPLES OF DRUG THERAPY

Urinary Tract Infections

Drug	Nursing Implications
Trimethoprim[a]/sulfamethoxazole	Ask patients about drug allergies, especially to sulfa drugs, before beginning drug therapy *because allergies to sulfa drugs are common and require changing drug therapy.* Teach patients to drink a full glass of water with each dose and to have an overall fluid intake of 3 L daily *because these drugs can form crystals that precipitate in the kidney tubules. Fluids can prevent this complication.* Teach patients to keep out of the sun or to wear protective clothing outdoors and use a sunscreen *because these drugs increase sun sensitivity and can lead to severe sunburn.* Caution patients to complete the drug regimen even if the symptoms improve or disappear sooner *to prevent bacterial resistance and infection recurrence.*
Ciprofloxacin, levofloxacin ofloxacin	Teach patients taking the extended-release drugs to swallow them whole and not to crush or chew the tablets *because this action ruins the extended effect.* Warn patients not to take the drug within 2 hours of taking an antacid *to prevent interference with drug absorption.* Teach patients how to take their pulse, to monitor it twice daily while on this drug, and to notify the primary health care provider if new-onset irregular heartbeats occur *to identify serious drug-induced dysrhythmias.* Teach patients to keep out of the sun or to wear protective clothing outdoors and use a sunscreen *to avoid serious sunburns from increased sun sensitivity.* Caution patients to complete the drug regimen even if the symptoms improve or disappear sooner *to reduce bacterial resistance and infection recurrence.*
Amoxicillin Amoxicillin/clavulanate	Ask patients about drug allergies to penicillin before beginning drug therapy *because allergies to this drug category are common.* Teach patients to take the drug with food *to reduce the risk for GI upset.* Instruct patients to call the primary health care provider if severe or watery diarrhea develops *to recognize the complication of pseudomembranous colitis, which may require discontinuing the drug.* Suggest that women who take oral contraceptives use an additional method of birth control while taking this drug *because these drugs may reduce the effectiveness of estrogen-containing contraceptives.* Caution patients to complete the drug regimen even if the symptoms improve or disappear sooner *to prevent bacterial resistance and infection recurrence.*
Cefdinir, cefaclor, or cefpodoxime	Ask about drug allergies to penicillin or cephalosporins before beginning drug therapy *because these drugs are structurally similar to penicillin and anyone with allergies to penicillin is likely to be allergic to the cephalosporins.* Instruct patients to call the prescriber if severe or watery diarrhea develops *to recognize the complication of pseudomembranous colitis, which may require discontinuing the drug.* Caution patients to complete the drug regimen even if the symptoms improve or disappear sooner *to prevent bacterial resistance and infection recurrence.* Instruct patients to follow the directions on the label if the medication needs to be reconstituted. Add water as directed and shake well *to ensure that all particles are mixed thoroughly and the correct dose is taken.* Avoid taking this drug when also taking metoclopramide or any other drug that increases GI motility *to prevent interference with drug absorption.* Teach patients to shake the bottle well before measuring the drug *to thoroughly mix the suspension.* Suggest that patients obtain a calibrated spoon for liquid drugs and not to use household spoons *to ensure accurate dosing.* Teach patients to drink a full glass of water with each dose and to have an overall fluid intake of at least 3 L daily *to avoid having the drug precipitate in the kidneys and cause kidney damage.* Caution patients to complete the drug regimen even if the symptoms improve or disappear sooner *to prevent bacterial resistance and infection recurrence.*
Phenazopyridine	Remind patients that this drug will not treat an infection, only the symptoms *because these drugs have no antibacterial activity.* Teach patients to take the drug with or immediately after a meal *to reduce the risk for GI upset.* Warn patients that urine will turn red or orange *to reduce anxiety about this change.*
Hyoscyamine	Teach patients to notify the primary health care provider if blurred vision or other eye problems, confusion, dizziness or fainting spells, fast heartbeat, fever, or difficulty passing urine occurs *because these symptoms indicate drug toxicity.* Teach patients to wear dark glasses in sunlight or other bright-light areas *because these drugs dilate the pupil and increase eye sensitivity to light.*

[a]Trimethoprim can be given alone to patients with a sulfa allergy.

Low-dose antibiotic therapy over 6 to 12 months is sometimes used for chronic, recurring infection caused by structural abnormalities or stones or for long-term management of the older patient with frequent UTIs. For women who have recurrent UTIs after intercourse, antibiotics may be prescribed to be taken after intercourse. The three most common drug treatment regimens are (1) one low-dose tablet of trimethoprim, (2) sulfamethoxazole/trimethoprim, or (3) nitrofurantoin.

Recent evidence demonstrates that severe UTIs leave inflammatory-related damage to the bladder wall and change the genetic material of the cells. This makes the bladder more susceptible to infection. These inflammatory changes may be controlled by COX_2 inhibitors. More research is needed to determine short and long-term efficacy (O'Brien et al., 2016).

PATIENT-CENTERED CARE: GENDER HEALTH CONSIDERATIONS (QSEN)

Pregnant women with a bacterial UTI require prompt and aggressive treatment because a UTI can lead to acute pyelonephritis during pregnancy. Pyelonephritis in pregnancy can cause preterm labor and adversely affect the fetus. Remind patients who are pregnant to contact their health care provider whenever symptoms of UTI are present.

Fluid Intake. Urge patients to drink enough fluid to maintain dilute urine throughout the day and night unless fluid restriction is needed for another health problem. Some urologists recommend sufficient fluid intake to result in at least 1.5 L of urine output or 7 to 12 voidings daily. Food can provide 20% or more of fluid intake, particularly the intake of fruits and vegetables.

Cranberry-containing products appear to decrease the ability of bacteria to adhere to the epithelial cells lining the urinary tract. In some patients, this may result in preventing UTI or decreasing the incidence of recurrent symptomatic UTIs; however, evidence is conflicting (Feng et al., 2018). Cranberry juice can be an irritant to the bladder with interstitial cystitis and should be avoided by patients with this condition. Avoiding spices, soy products, and tomato products may decrease bladder irritation and *pain* during cystitis (Feng et al., 2018).

Comfort Measures. A warm sitz bath two or three times a day for 20 minutes may provide *pain* relief and some relief of local symptoms. If burning with urination is severe or urinary retention occurs, teach the patient to sit in the sitz bath and urinate into the warm water. Urinary tract analgesics or antispasmodics may also provide comfort (see the Common Examples of Drug Therapy: Urinary Tract Infections box).

Surgical Management. Surgery for cystitis treats the conditions that increase the risk for recurrent UTIs (e.g., removal of obstructions and repair of vesicoureteral reflux). Procedures may include cystoscopy (see Chapter 60) to identify and remove calculi or obstructions.

Care Coordination and Transition Management. Assess the patient's level of understanding of the problem. The patient's knowledge about factors that promote the development of cystitis determines the teaching interventions planned.

Teach the patient how to take prescribed drugs. Stress the need for correct spacing of doses throughout the day and the need to complete all of the prescribed antibiotics. If the drug will change the color of the urine, as it does with phenazopyridine, inform the patient to expect this change.

Patients may associate discomfort with sexual activities and have feelings of guilt and embarrassment. Open and sensitive discussions with a woman who has recurrences of UTI after sexual intercourse can help her find techniques to handle the problem (see the earlier Patient and Family Education: Preparing for Self-Management: Preventing a Urinary Tract Infection box). Explore with her the factors that contribute to her infections, such as sexual penetration when the bladder is full, diaphragm use, and her general *immunity* responses against infection. Some positions during intercourse may reduce urethral irritation and subsequent cystitis. Remind the patient that vigorous cleaning of the perineum with harsh soaps and vaginal douching may irritate the perineal tissues and *increase* the risk for UTI. At the patient's request, discuss the problem with her and her partner to help them find ways of maintaining their intimate relationship.

NCLEX EXAMINATION CHALLENGE 61.2

Health Promotion and Maintenance

The nurse is caring for an 80-year-old female client with recurrent cystitis. Which teaching will the nurse include in the plan of care? **Select all that apply.**

A. Drink citrus juices daily.
B. Douche regularly; a minimum of two times weekly.
C. Encourage fluid intake of 2-3 L of fluid throughout the day.
D. Instruct her to always wipe the perineum from front to back after each toilet use.
E. Reinforce that she should complete the entire course of antibiotics as prescribed.
F. Instruct her to empty her bladder immediately before and after having intercourse.

URETHRITIS

Pathophysiology Review

Urethritis is an inflammation of the urethra and can result from infectious and noninfectious conditions. The incidence is highest among adults ages 20 to 24 years. The most common cause of infectious urethritis is sexually transmitted infections (STIs). These include gonorrhea or nonspecific urethritis caused by *Ureaplasma* (a gram-negative bacterium), *Chlamydia* (a sexually transmitted gram-negative bacterium), or *Trichomonas vaginalis* (a protozoan found in both the male and female genital tract). Urethritis is also known as *pyuria-dysuria syndrome, frequency-dysuria syndrome, trigonitis syndrome,* and *urethral syndrome.*

Many women with urethritis have symptoms similar to cystitis, vaginitis, or cervicitis. Men with urethritis may report symptoms of cystitis, as well as heaviness in the genitals (*orchalgia*).

Noninfectious urethritis in postmenopausal women may be related to uretero-genital tissue changes resulting from low estrogen levels.

Symptoms of urethritis include discharge of mucopurulent or purulent material, dysuria, and itching or discomfort of the area (urethral pruritus). The discharge can be any color, depending on the infecting organism or source of irritation. Additional symptoms may include fever (with or without chills) and urgent or frequent urination.

❖ Interprofessional Collaborative Care

Ask the patient about a history of STI, painful or difficult urination, discharge from the penis or vagina, and discomfort in the lower abdomen. Urinalysis may show pyuria (white blood cells [WBCs] in the urine) without a large number of bacteria. Similarly, a urethral smear may show WBCs. All patients with urethritis should be tested for *N. gonorrhoeae* and *C. trachoma* with an endourethral (in men) or endocervical (women) smear. Testing for *Chlamydia* may be done with the same sample. STI testing for VDRL serology and HIV is suggested by the Centers for Disease Control and Prevention (Barrow et al., 2020; CDC, 2016). A pregnancy test is performed for women who have had unprotected intercourse. In women, a pelvic examination may reveal tissue changes from low estrogen levels in the vagina. Urethroscopy may show low estrogen changes with inflammation of urethral tissues.

Noninfectious urethritis symptoms usually resolve spontaneously over time, regardless of treatment. Postmenopausal women often have improvement in urethral symptoms with the use of estrogen vaginal cream. Estrogen cream applied locally to the vagina increases the amount of estrogen in the urethra as well, reducing irritating symptoms. Urethritis from STIs is treated with antibiotic therapy. More information on STIs can be found in Chapter 69.

UROLITHIASIS

Pathophysiology Review

Urolithiasis is the presence of *calculi* (stones) in the urinary tract. Stones often do not cause symptoms until they pass into the lower urinary tract, where they can cause excruciating pain. Nephrolithiasis is the formation of stones in the kidney; formation of stones in the ureter is ureterolithiasis. Stones are particles in the urine that occur in amounts too high to stay dissolved (become supersaturated) in urine. As a result of supersaturation, the particles precipitate and collect to form calculi.

The most common condition associated with stone formation is dehydration. Everyone excretes crystals in the urine at some time, but less than 10% of adults form stones. Most stones contain calcium as one part of the stone complex. Struvite (15%), uric acid (8%), and cystine (3%) are more rare compositions of stones. Formation of stones involves two conditions:

1. Supersaturation of the urine with the particular element (e.g., calcium, uric acid) that first becomes crystallized and later becomes the stone
2. Formation of a *nidus* (deposit of crystals that can be the point of infection) along the lining of the kidney and urinary tract

In addition, some patients may have decreased amounts of inhibitor substances in the urine that would otherwise prevent supersaturation with crystal aggregation. This type of metabolic risk factor can be inherited.

In addition to low urine volume, high urine acidity (as with uric acid and cystine stones) or alkalinity (as with calcium phosphate and struvite stones), as well as drugs (e.g., topiramate, corticosteroids, indinavir, acetazolamide), contribute to stone formation.

One example of a metabolic problem causing stone formation begins when excessive amounts of calcium are absorbed through the intestinal tract, leading to hypercalciuria. As blood circulates through the kidneys, the excess calcium is filtered into the urine, causing supersaturation of calcium in the urine. If fluid intake is poor, such as when a patient is dehydrated, supersaturation is more likely to occur.

Any stone may result in obstruction within the urinary tract, which can threaten both glomerular filtration rate (GFR) and kidney perfusion. When the stone occludes the ureter and blocks the flow of urine, the ureter dilates. Enlargement of the ureter is called hydroureter.

The pain associated with ureteral spasm is excruciating and may cause the patient to go into shock from stimulation of nearby nerves. Hematuria (bloody urine) may result from damage to the urothelial lining. If the obstruction is not removed, urinary stasis can lead to infection and impair kidney function on the side of the blockage. As the blockage persists, hydronephrosis (enlargement of the kidney caused by blockage of urine lower in the tract and filling of the kidney with urine) and permanent kidney damage may develop.

Etiology and Genetic Risk. The vast majority of adults who form stones have a metabolic risk factor. The cause of stone formation in a susceptible adult (e.g., one who has a metabolic risk factor) is dehydration. Table 61.5 lists some metabolic problems that cause stone formation. Patients who have a family history of stones, are obese, or have diabetes or gout (hyperuricemia) have increased risk for initial stone formation (Sofia, 2016). Because a metabolic problem is so strongly associated with stone formation and is a nonmodifiable risk factor, an adult of any age who develops a stone is always at high risk for future stone development.

Diet may be considered a risk for stone formation. Increased sodium intake has been associated with stone formation (Sofia, 2016) (Table 61.6).

🔲 PATIENT-CENTERED CARE: GENETIC/GENOMIC CONSIDERATIONS (QSEN)

Family history has a strong association with stone formation and recurrence because of inherited metabolic variations. More than 30 genetic variations are associated with the formation of kidney stones, although single gene disorders are rare. More commonly, nephrolithiasis is a complex disease, with genetic variation in intestinal calcium absorption, kidney calcium transport, or kidney phosphate transport all associated with stone formation (Online Mendelian Inheritance in Man [OMIM], 2016). Always ask a patient with a renal stone whether other family members also have this problem.

TABLE 61.5 Metabolic Defects That Commonly Cause Kidney Stones

Metabolic Deficit	Etiology
Hypercalcemia	
Primary	Absorptive: Increased intestinal calcium absorption
	Renal: Decreased kidney tubular excretion of calcium
Secondary	Resorptive: Hyperparathyroidism, vitamin D intoxication, kidney tubular acidosis, prolonged immobilization
Hyperoxaluria	
Primary	Genetic: Autosomal-recessive trait resulting in high oxalate production
Secondary	Dietary: Excess oxalate from foods such as spinach, rhubarb, Swiss chard, cocoa, beets, wheat germ, pecans, peanuts, okra, chocolate, and lime peel
Hyperuricemia	
Primary	Gout is an inherited disorder of purine metabolism (20% of patients with gout have uric acid calculi)
Secondary	Increased production or decreased clearance of purine from myeloproliferative disorders, thiazide diuretics, carcinoma
Struvite	Made of magnesium ammonium phosphate and carbonate apatite; formed by urea splitting by bacteria, most commonly, *Proteus mirabilis;* needs an alkaline urine to form
Cystinuria	Autosomal-recessive defect of amino acid metabolism that precipitates insoluble cystine crystals in the urine

Incidence and Prevalence. The incidence of stone disease is high and varies with geographic location, race, and family history. About 12% of adults will have at least one episode of renal stone disease (Sofia, 2016). The incidence of most stone types is higher in men, although struvite stones are twice as common in women. This difference in struvite stone formation incidence is thought to be related to the fact that women have more UTIs and struvite stones are associated with UTI. Recurrence rates vary depending on the type of treatment, although any adult who has had a stone is much more likely to have recurrence. Recurrence of stones occurs in patients with a family history of stone disease and in those who had their first occurrence by age 25 years.

👤 PATIENT-CENTERED CARE: CULTURAL/ SPIRITUAL CONSIDERATIONS (QSEN)

The incidence of stone disease is most common in the southeastern United States, Japan, and western Europe. Calcium stone disease is more common in men than in women and tends to occur in young adults or during early middle adulthood. Initial onset of stone disease occurs more often in younger adults than older adults (Sofia, 2016). For patients in these higher-risk groups, nursing care includes teaching family members, as well as patients, to avoid dehydration. Collaborate with the interprofessional health care team about referring patients with recurrent stone formation to evaluate metabolic risk factors.

❖ Interprofessional Collaborative Care

◆ **Assessment: Recognize Cues.** Ask the patient about a personal or family history of urologic stones. Obtain a diet history, focusing on fluid intake patterns and supplemental vitamin or mineral intake. If he or she has a history of stone formation, ask about past treatment, whether chemical analysis of the stone was performed, and which preventive measures are followed.

TABLE 61.6 Dietary Treatment for Kidney and Urinary Stones

Stone Type	Dietary Interventions	Rationales
Calcium oxalate	Avoid oxalate sources, such as spinach, black tea, and rhubarb.	Reduction of urinary oxalate content may help prevent these stones from forming. Urinary pH is not a factor.
	Decrease sodium intake.	High sodium intake reduces kidney tubular calcium reabsorption.
Calcium phosphate	Limit intake of foods high in animal protein to 5-7 servings per week and never more than 2 per day.	Reduction of protein intake reduces acidic urine and prevents calcium precipitation.
	Some patients may benefit from a reduced calcium intake (milk, other dairy products).	Reduction of urine calcium concentration may prevent calcium precipitation and crystallization.
	Decrease sodium intake.	High sodium intake reduces kidney tubular calcium reabsorption.
Struvite (magnesium ammonium phosphate)	Limit high-phosphate foods, such as dairy products, organ meats, and whole grains.	Reduction of urinary phosphate content may help prevent these stones from forming.
Uric acid (urate)	Decrease intake of purine sources, such as organ meats, poultry, fish, gravies, red wines, and sardines.	Reduction of urinary purine content may help prevent these stones from forming.
Cystine	Limit sodium and animal protein intake (as above).	It reduces urinary cystine levels.
	Encourage oral fluid intake (500 mL every 4 hours while awake and 750 mL at night).	Increased fluid helps dilute the urine and prevents the cystine crystals from forming.

The major symptom of stones is severe pain, commonly called **renal colic.** Flank pain suggests that the stone is in the kidney or upper ureter. Flank pain that extends toward the abdomen or to the scrotum and testes or the vulva suggests that stones are in the ureters or bladder. Pain is most intense when the stone is moving or the ureter is obstructed.

Renal colic begins suddenly and is often described as "unbearable." Nausea, vomiting, pallor, and diaphoresis often accompany the pain. However, a large stationary stone in the kidney (staghorn calculus) rarely causes much pain because it is not moving. Frequency and dysuria occur when a stone reaches the bladder. **Oliguria** (scant urine output) or **anuria** (absence of urine output) suggests obstruction, possibly at the bladder neck or urethra.

> **! NURSING SAFETY PRIORITY** (QSEN)
>
> **Action Alert**
>
> Urinary tract obstruction is an emergency and must be treated immediately to preserve kidney function.

Assess the patient for bladder distention. He or she may appear pale, ashen, and diaphoretic and may have excruciating pain. Vital signs may be elevated with pain; body temperature and pulse are elevated with infection. Blood pressure may decrease if the severe pain causes shock.

Urinalysis is performed in patients with suspected stones. Measurement of urine specific gravity and osmolarity can provide a clue about the adequacy of fluid intake. Urine pH can help in the determination of stone type. High urine acidity (low urine pH) is associated with uric acid and cystine stones; high urine alkalinity (high urine pH) is associated with calcium phosphate and struvite stones. A 24-hour urine analysis can determine whether supersaturation of common stone particles is present. Hematuria during renal colic is common, and blood may make the urine appear smoky or rusty. RBCs are usually caused by stone-induced trauma to the lining of the ureter, bladder, or urethra. WBCs and bacteria may be present as a result of urinary stasis. Increased *turbidity* (cloudiness) and odor indicate that infection may also be present. Microscopic examination of the urine may identify possible stone-forming crystals.

The serum WBC count is elevated with infection. Increases in the serum levels of calcium, phosphate, or uric acid levels indicate that excess minerals that may contribute to stone formation are present.

The current standard for confirming urinary stones is an unenhanced helical CT scan of the abdomen and pelvis. Most stones are radiopaque; and the size, location, and surrounding anatomic structures are easily seen. In settings where a CT is not available, a routine abdominal x-ray (KUB) is useful (Fig. 61.2). Ultrasound may be used in pregnant women suspected to have stones, but it is not sensitive for ureteral stones and is not used for general screening.

◆ **Interventions: Take Action.** Nursing interventions focus on *pain* relief and preventing infection and urinary obstruction. Most patients expel the stone without invasive procedures. Size

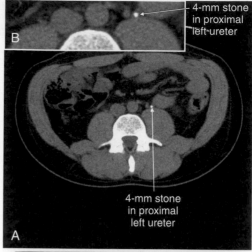
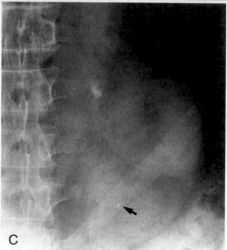

FIG. 61.2 **A** and **B,** Urinary stones on CT scan. **C,** Urinary stones on x-ray of the kidneys, ureters, and bladder (KUB). (**A** and **B** from Broder, J. K. [2011]. *Diagnostic imaging for the emergency physician.* Philadelphia: Saunders. **C** from Pollack, H. M. [2000]. *Clinical urography* [2nd ed.]. Philadelphia: Saunders.)

(i.e., less than 5 mm) is the most important factor for whether a stone will pass on its own; its composition and location are also factors. The larger the stone and the higher up in the urinary tract it is, the less likely it is to pass. When the stone is passed, it should be captured and sent to the laboratory for analysis. Other interventions are needed when the stone does not pass spontaneously (Fig. 61.3).

Managing Pain. Nonsurgical and surgical approaches are used to help the patient with a kidney stone achieve an acceptable degree of *pain* relief.

Nonsurgical Management. Nonsurgical measures to relieve pain include strategies to enhance stone passing, as well as direct pain management.

Drug therapy is needed in the first 24 to 36 hours when pain is most severe. Opioid analgesics are used to control the severe pain caused by stones in the urinary tract and may be given IV for rapid pain relief. NSAIDs such as ketorolac or ketoprofen in the acute phase may be effective. When NSAIDs are used, there is an increased risk for kidney impairment from reduced perfusion. NSAIDs interfere with renal autoregulation, and the risk

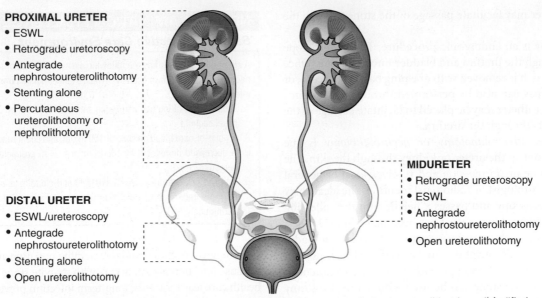

PROXIMAL URETER
- ESWL
- Retrograde ureteroscopy
- Antegrade nephrostoureterolithotomy
- Stenting alone
- Percutaneous ureterolithotomy or nephrolithotomy

MIDURETER
- Retrograde ureteroscopy
- ESWL
- Antegrade nephrostoureterolithotomy
- Open ureterolithotomy

DISTAL URETER
- ESWL/ureteroscopy
- Antegrade nephrostoureterolithotomy
- Stenting alone
- Open ureterolithotomy

FIG. 61.3 Treatment options for ureteral stones. *ESWL,* Extracorporeal shock wave lithotripsy. (Modified from Singal, R. K., & Denstedt, J. D. [1997]. Contemporary management of ureteral stones. *The Urologic Clinics of North America, 24*[1], 59–70.)

for impairment is greater among patients with pre-existing kidney dysfunction. Risk for bleeding is also increased from platelet inhibition when NSAIDs are used. Bleeding risk is particularly concerning when surgical intervention for stones is needed.

Control of *pain* is more effective when drugs are given at regularly scheduled intervals or by a constant delivery system (e.g., skin patch) instead of PRN. Spasmolytic drugs, such as oxybutynin chloride and propantheline bromide, are important for control of pain. Administer the drugs as prescribed and assess the response by asking the patient to rate the discomfort on a pain-rating scale.

Other management techniques include avoiding overhydration and underhydration in the acute phase to help make the passage of a stone less painful. Strain the urine and teach the patient to strain it to monitor for stone passage. Send any stone passed to the laboratory for analysis because preventive therapy is based on stone composition.

Antibiotics may be used to manage struvite stones because these are associated with urinary infections from urease-producing organisms such as *Proteus mirabilis, Klebsiella, Enterobacter,* or *Pseudomonas.* (*E. coli* does not produce urease.) When urease-producing bacteria remain in the urine and within the stone, urine becomes alkaline, causing phosphate to precipitate and allowing staghorn-shaped struvite stones to form rapidly.

Two drugs may be used to aid in stone expulsion: a thiazide diuretic and allopurinol. These drugs, combined with a high fluid intake, increase urine volume or decrease urine pH and help increase the excretion of stones or stone fragments. Alpha-adrenergic blockers and calcium channel blockers can shorten the time to stone passage by relaxing the smooth muscle within the ureters. Citrate may be used to alkalinize urine pH and dissolve uric acid stones. Implementing oral citrate treatment cannot be done until stone composition is known. It is typically reserved for prevention and treatment of recurrent stone formation.

A stone that has not passed within 1 to 2 months is unlikely to pass spontaneously. Other options for stone intervention are considered when infection occurs, when pain cannot be well managed, or when there is an actual or increased risk for reduced kidney function. An observation period of 1 to 2 weeks may be reasonable if the patient is comfortable or has few symptoms and stones are smaller than 5 mm.

Lithotripsy or extracorporeal *shock wave lithotripsy (SWL)* is the use of sound, laser, or dry shock waves to break the stone into small fragments. The patient receives moderate sedation and lies on a flat table with the lithotriptor aimed at the stone, which is located by fluoroscopy. A local anesthetic cream is applied to the skin site over the stone 45 minutes before the procedure. During the procedure, cardiac rhythm is monitored by ECG and the shock waves are delivered in synchrony with the R wave. Shock waves at the rate of 60 to 120/min are applied over 30 to 45 minutes (Li et al., 2013). Continuous ECG monitoring for dysrhythmia and fluoroscopic observation for stone destruction are maintained.

After lithotripsy, strain the urine to monitor the passage of stone fragments. Bruising may occur on the flank of the affected side. Occasionally a stent is placed in the ureter before SWL to ease passage of the stone fragments.

Surgical Management. Minimally invasive surgical and open surgical procedures are used if urinary obstruction occurs or if the stone is too large to be passed.

Minimally Invasive Surgical Procedures. Minimally invasive surgical (MIS) procedures include stenting, ureteroscopy, percutaneous ureterolithotomy, and percutaneous nephrolithotomy.

Stenting is performed with a **stent,** a small tube that is placed in the ureter by ureteroscopy. The stent dilates the ureter and enlarges the passageway for the stone or stone fragments. This totally internal procedure prevents the passing stone from coming in contact with the ureteral mucosa, thereby reducing pain, bleeding, and infection risk, all of which could block the ureter.

A Foley catheter may facilitate passage of the stone through the urethra.

Ureteroscopy is an endoscopic procedure. The ureteroscope is passed through the urethra and bladder into the ureter. Once the stone is seen, it is removed with grasping baskets, forceps, or loops. Lithotripsy can also be performed through the ureteroscope. A Foley catheter may be placed to facilitate passage of the stone fragments through the urethra.

Percutaneous ureterolithotomy or nephrolithotomy is the removal of a stone in the ureter or kidney through the skin. The patient lies prone or on the side and receives local or general anesthesia. The urologist or radiologist identifies the ideal entry point with fluoroscopy and passes a needle into the collecting system of the kidney. Once a tract has been made in the kidney, other equipment, such as an **intracorporeal** (inside the body) ultrasonic or laser lithotriptor, can be used to break up and remove the stone. An endoscope with a special attachment to grasp and extract the stone can be used. Often a nephrostomy tube is left in place at first to prevent the stone fragments from passing through the urinary tract.

Monitor the patient for complications after the procedure. Complications include bleeding at the site or through the tube, pneumothorax, and infection. Monitor nephrostomy tube drainage for volume and the presence of blood in the urine, which is normal for the first 24 to 48 hours after tube placement. Provide routine nephrostomy tube care, with sterile dressing changes and tube flushing (if prescribed).

Open Surgical Procedures. When other stone removal attempts have failed or when risk for a lasting injury to the ureter or kidney is possible, an *open ureterolithotomy* (into the ureter), *pyelolithotomy* (into the kidney pelvis), or *nephrolithotomy* (into the kidney) procedure may be performed. These procedures are used for a large or impacted stone.

Preoperative care. Explain to the patient how, when, and where the procedure will be performed. Describe what he or she can expect to see, hear, and feel before and after the procedure. The patient is given nothing by mouth and also receives a bowel preparation before the procedure. (See Chapter 9 for routine care before surgery.)

Operative procedures. The retroperitoneal area is entered through a large flank incision, as for nephrectomy (see Chapter 62), pyelolithotomy, or nephrolithotomy and through a lower abdominal incision for ureterolithotomy. The urinary tract is entered surgically, and the stone is removed. Before closure, tubes and drains may be placed (e.g., nephrostomy tube, ureteral stent, Penrose or other wound drainage device, Foley catheter).

Postoperative care. Follow routine procedures for assessment of the patient who has received anesthesia. See Chapter 9 for routine care after surgery. Monitor the amount of bleeding from incisions and in the urine. Maintain adequate fluid intake. Strain the urine to monitor passage of stone fragments. Teach the patient how to prevent future stones with dietary changes, including consistent daily fluid intake to avoid dehydration and supersaturation.

Preventing Infection. Infection control before invasive procedures is critical for preventing urosepsis. Interventions include giving antibiotics, either to eliminate an existing infection or to

prevent new infections, and maintaining nutrition and fluid intake. Because infection always occurs with struvite stone formation, the health care team plans for long-term infection prevention.

Drug therapy involves the use of quinolones, ampicillin, or other broad-spectrum antibiotics. When urine culture and sensitivity (C&S) results are known, more specific antibiotics may be prescribed. C&S studies are often repeated 48 hours after completion of antibiotic therapy to evaluate whether urine sterility has returned.

Urine levels of antibiotics may be measured to ensure that adequate levels have been reached. If the antibiotic is not sufficiently concentrated in urine, organisms may not be completely eliminated. Evidence of a new infection (e.g., chills, fever, altered mental status) warrants the collection of urine sample for new C&S tests.

For the patient with struvite stones, periodic and long-term monitoring of the urine for infection is needed. Urine cultures are checked monthly for as long as 1 year. Long-term use of antibiotics, while recommended, makes the development of resistant organisms more likely and antibiotic therapy less effective. Drugs that prevent bacteria from splitting urea, such as acetohydroxamic acid and hydroxyurea, are often prescribed long term for patients with struvite stones. Serum creatinine levels are monitored in patients receiving acetohydroxamic acid, and the drug is stopped if creatinine levels are above 2 mg/dL. Review interventions aimed at preventing urinary tract infection (UTI). See the earlier Patient and Family Education: Preparing for Self-Management: Preventing a Urinary Tract Infection box.

Nutrition therapy ideally includes adequate calorie intake with a balance of all food groups. Encourage a fluid intake sufficient to dilute urine to a light color throughout the 24-hour day (typically 2 to 3 L/day) unless another health problem requires fluid restriction.

Preventing Obstruction. Measures to prevent urinary obstruction by stones include a high intake of fluids (3 L/day or more) and accurate measures of intake and output. Fluid intake sufficient to provide diluted urine helps prevent dehydration, promotes urine flow, and decreases the chance of crystals forming a stone. Interventions also depend on the type of stone the patient has formed. Drugs, diet modification, and fluid intake are the major strategies used to prevent future stones.

Drug therapy to prevent obstruction depends on what is causing stone formation and the type of stone formed. Teach the patient the reason for the drug and assess for side effects or adverse drug reactions. Some drugs may need to be avoided because they may contribute to stone formation.

Drugs to treat *hypercalciuria* (high levels of calcium in the urine) include thiazide diuretics (e.g., chlorothiazide or hydrochlorothiazide). These drugs promote calcium reabsorption from the renal tubules back into the body, thereby reducing urine calcium loads. For patients with *hyperoxaluria* (high levels of oxalic acid in the urine), vitamin B_6 and thiazide diuretics may be prescribed.

Patients with hyperuricemia or chronic gout have high uric acid levels causing acidic urine and resulting in a higher risk for uric acid stone formation. Acidic urine is more likely to cause uric acid to precipitate, resulting in uric acid stones. Normal urine pH can range from 4.6 to 8.0 with the average at 6.0. Urine pH under 5.0 is considered acidic and over 8.0 alkaline. The desired urine pH range for patients with high uric acid levels and a history of uric acid stone formation is 6.5 to 7.0.

Three measures are commonly used to treat and/or prevent uric stone formation: increasing urine pH, increasing fluid intake, and decreasing uric acid production. To alkalinize the urine, drugs such as potassium citrate, 50% sodium citrate, and sodium bicarbonate are used. Drinking 2 to 3 L of water is effective in flushing out excess uric acid and reduces uric acid stone formation. Modifying the diet to restrict purines can be effective in decreasing uric acid production. Foods that contain high levels of purines include organ meats, sardines, and red meats. The use of xanthine oxidase inhibitors such as allopurinol and febuxostat can also be used to decrease the body's production of uric acid.

Cystinuria (high levels of cystine in the urine) can lead to stone formation. Cystinuria is genetic and affects children more than adults. Conservative measures are used to prevent stone formation. Drinking 2 to 3 L of water throughout the day and night is encouraged to reduce high cystine levels in the urine. Moderating sodium and protein consumption has been effective in reducing urine cystine levels. To alkalinize urine, drugs such as potassium citrate are used. However, since moderating sodium has been shown to be effective in reducing urine cystine levels, sodium bicarbonate and sodium citrate are avoided because of the sodium content in these medications. If conservative measures fail, medications such as tiopronin, D-penicillamine, and captopril are used to lower urine cystine levels (Goldfarb, 2019). *Nutrition therapy* depends on the type of stone formed (see Table 61.5). Collaborate with the registered dietitian nutritionist (RDN) to plan for and teach the appropriate diet to the patient.

Other measures can help the stone pass more quickly. Urge the patient to walk as often as possible. Walking promotes passage of stones and reduces bone calcium resorption. Check the urine pH daily and strain all urine with filter paper or a special urine sieve/strainer to collect passed stones and fragments.

Self-management education includes follow-up care to evaluate effects of intervention includes a 24-hour urine collection and serum chemical analysis. The patient often has great

---

PATIENT AND FAMILY EDUCATION: PREPARING FOR SELF-MANAGEMENT

Urinary Calculi

- Finish your entire prescription of antibiotics to ensure that you will not get a urinary tract infection.
- You may resume your usual daily activities.
- Remember to balance regular exercise with sleep and rest.
- You may return to work 2 days to 6 weeks after surgery, depending on the type of intervention, your personal tolerance, and your primary health care provider's directives.
- Depending on the type of stone you had, you may be advised to take medications or adjust your diet may to reduce the risk for further stone formation.
- Remember to drink at least 3 L of fluid a day to dilute potential stone-forming crystals, prevent dehydration, and promote urine flow.
- Monitor urine pH as directed (possibly up to three times per day).
- Expect bruising after lithotripsy. The bruising may be quite extensive and may take several weeks to resolve.
- Your urine may be bloody for several days after surgery.
- Pain in the region of the kidneys or bladder may signal the beginning of an infection or the formation of another stone. Report any pain, fever, chills, or difficulty with urination immediately to your primary health care provider or nurse.
- Keep follow up appointments to check on infection and have repeat cultures done.

---

anxiety and fear that a stone and its pain may recur. In addition to anxiety about the pain, the risk for repeated surgical interventions or permanent and serious kidney damage may be present. Psychosocial preparation is enhanced when patients know what to expect and which actions to take if problems develop. Reassure the patient that preventive and health promotion activities help prevent recurrence. See the Patient and Family Education: Preparing for Self-Management; Urinary Calculi box.

UROTHELIAL CANCER

Pathophysiology Review

Urothelial cancers are malignant tumors of the *urothelium*, which is the lining of transitional cells in the kidney, renal pelvis, ureters, urinary bladder, and urethra. Most urothelial cancers occur in the bladder, and the term *bladder cancer* describes this condition. Urothelial cancer is also known as *transitional cell carcinoma* (TCC).

In North America, most urinary tract cancers are transitional cell carcinomas of the bladder (American Cancer Society [ACS], 2019; Canadian Cancer Society, 2016). The second most common site of urinary tract cancer is the kidney and renal pelvis. Urothelial cancers are usually low grade, have multiple points of origin (*multifocal*), and are recurrent. Once the cancer spreads beyond the transitional cell layer, it is highly invasive and can spread beyond the bladder. Because of the nature of this cancer, patients may have recurrence up to 10 years after being cancer free (ACS, 2019). Less common bladder cancers include squamous cell carcinoma, adenocarcinoma, small cell carcinoma, and sarcoma (ACS, 2019).

Tumors confined to the bladder mucosa are treated by simple excision, whereas those that are deeper but not into the muscle layer are treated with excision plus intravesical (inside the bladder) chemotherapy. Cancer that has spread deeper into the bladder muscle layer is treated with more extensive surgery, often a radical cystectomy (removal of the bladder and surrounding tissue) with urinary diversion. Chemotherapy and radiation therapy are used in addition to surgery. If untreated, the tumor invades surrounding tissues; spreads to distant sites (liver, lung, and bone); and ultimately leads to death.

Exposure to toxins such as gasoline and diesel fuel, as well as to chemicals used in hair dyes and in the rubber, paint, electric cable, and textile industries, increases the risk for bladder cancer. The greatest risk factor for bladder cancer is tobacco use. Other risks include *Schistosoma haematobium* (a parasite) infection, excessive use of drugs containing phenacetin, and long-term use of cyclophosphamide.

In the United States and Canada, about 87,730 new cases of bladder cancer are diagnosed each year, and about 19,190 deaths occur each year from the disease (ACS, 2017; Canadian Cancer Society, 2016). This cancer is rare in adults younger than 40 years and is most common after 55 years of age (ACS, 2019).

As with many urologic conditions, sexual health is commonly affected by this diagnosis and treatment (ACS, 2019). To manage sexual health concerns, encourage patients to discuss sexual health and ensure that the proper interprofessional care team member provides education to patients and their partners about:

- Potential implications of treatment on sexuality
- Treatment options
- Referrals to providers who specialize in sexual dysfunction

Health Promotion and Maintenance. Many adults believe that tobacco use is associated with cancers only of organs that come into direct contact with it, such as the lungs. However, many compounds in tobacco enter the bloodstream and affect other organs, such as the bladder. Therefore encourage people who smoke to quit (see the Health Promotion and Maintenance section of Chapter 24). Just as important, encourage anyone who comes in contact with dry, liquid, or gaseous chemicals to take precautions. Some adults work with chemicals, and others may come into contact with them while engaging in hobbies. Many chemicals and fumes can enter the body through contact with skin and with mucous membranes in the respiratory tract. Use of personal protective equipment, such as gloves and masks, can reduce this contact. Also encourage anyone who works with chemicals to shower or bathe and change clothing as soon as contact is completed.

NCLEX EXAMINATION CHALLENGE 61.4

Physiological Integrity

A 68-year-old male client is seeing the primary care provider for an annual examination. Which assessment finding alerts the nurse to an increased risk for bladder cancer?

A. A 5 pack-year history of smoking 45 years ago
B. Difficulty starting and stopping the urine stream
C. A 30-year occupation as a long-distance truck driver
D. A recent colon cancer diagnosis in his 72-year-old brother

---

❖ Interprofessional Collaborative Care

◆ Assessment: Recognize Cues

Physical Assessment/Signs and Symptoms. Ask about the patient's perception of his or her general health. Document the gender and age of the patient. Ask about active and passive exposure to cigarette smoke. To detect exposure to harmful environmental agents, ask the patient to describe his or her occupation and hobbies in detail. Also ask the patient to describe any change in the color, frequency, or volume of urine *elimination* and any abdominal discomfort.

Observe the patient's overall appearance, especially skin color and nutrition status. Inspect, percuss, and palpate the abdomen for asymmetry, tenderness, and bladder distention.

Examine the urine for color and clarity. Blood in the urine is often the first indication of bladder cancer. It may be gross or microscopic and is usually painless and intermittent. Dysuria, frequency, and urgency occur when infection or obstruction is also present.

Psychosocial Assessment. Assess the patient's emotions, including the response to a tentative diagnosis of bladder cancer, and note anxiety, fear, sadness, anger, or guilt. Early symptoms are painless, and many patients ignore the blood in the urine because it is intermittent. They also may be reluctant to seek treatment if they suspect a sexually transmitted infection (STI). As a result, they may have guilt or anger about their own delays in seeking medical attention.

Assess the patient's coping methods and available support from family members. Social support may provide motivation and improve coping during recovery from treatment.

Diagnostic Assessment. The only significant finding on a routine urinalysis is gross or microscopic hematuria. Cytologic testing on voided urine specimens is usually not helpful. Bladder-wash specimens and bladder biopsies are the most specific tests for cancer.

Cystoscopy is usually performed to evaluate painless hematuria. A biopsy of a visible bladder tumor can be performed during cystoscopy. This is essential for staging and is usually performed in an ambulatory care surgery center. Cystoureterography may be used to identify obstructions, especially where the ureter joins the bladder. CT scans show tumor invasion of surrounding tissues. Ultrasonography shows masses but is less valuable for tumor staging. MRI may help assess deep, invasive tumors. See Chapter 60 for general care of the patient undergoing diagnostic testing.

◆ Interventions: Take Action.
Therapy for the patient with bladder cancer usually begins with surgical removal of the tumor for diagnosis and staging of disease. For tumors extending beyond the mucosa, surgery is followed by intravesical chemotherapy or immunotherapy. High-grade or recurrent tumors are treated with more radical surgery plus intravesical chemotherapy, radiotherapy, or both. Systemic chemotherapy is reserved for patients with distant metastases. (See Chapter 20 for general care of the patient receiving chemotherapy or radiation therapy.)

Nonsurgical Management. Prophylactic immunotherapy with intravesical instillation of bacille Calmette-Guérin (BCG), a live virus compound, is used to prevent tumor recurrence of superficial cancers. This procedure is more effective than single-agent chemotherapy. Usually the agent is instilled in an outpatient cancer clinic and allowed to dwell in the bladder for a specified length of time, usually 2 hours. When the patient urinates, live virus is excreted with the urine.

Teach patients receiving this treatment to prevent contact of the live virus with other members of the household by not sharing a toilet with others for at least 24 hours after instillation. Instruct men to urinate while sitting down to avoid splashing the urine. After 24 hours, the toilet should be completely cleaned using a solution of 10% liquid bleach. If only one toilet is available in the household, teach the patient to flush the toilet after use and follow this by adding one cup of undiluted bleach to the bowl water. The bowl is then flushed after 15 minutes, and the seat and flat surfaces of the toilet are wiped with a cloth containing a solution of 10% liquid bleach. Instruct the patient to wear gloves during the cleaning and to dispose of the cloth after sealing it in a plastic bag.

Underwear or other clothing that has come in contact with the urine during the immediate 24 hours after instillation should be washed separately from other clothing in a solution of 10% liquid bleach. Sexual intercourse is avoided for 24 hours after the instillation.

Multiagent chemotherapy is successful in prolonging life after distant metastasis has occurred but rarely results in a cure. Radiation therapy is also useful in prolonging life.

Surgical Management. The type of surgery for bladder cancer depends on the type and stage of the cancer and the patient's general health. Complete bladder removal *(cystectomy)* with additional removal of surrounding muscle and tissue offers the best chance of a cure for large, invasive bladder cancers. Four alternatives for urine *elimination* are used after cystectomy: ileal conduit; continent pouch; bladder reconstruction, also known as *neobladder;* and ureterosigmoidostomy.

Preoperative Care. Specific patient education depends on the type and extent of the planned surgical procedure. Coordinate education before surgery with the patient, surgeon, and enterostomal therapist (ET) or wound, ostomy, and continence nurse. Discuss the type of planned urinary diversion and the selection of a site for the stoma. Including the patient in this planning improves the chances for the patient to have a positive attitude about body image and a positive self-image. Use educational counseling to ensure understanding about self-care practices, methods of pouching, control of urine drainage, and management of odor.

The site selected for the stoma should be visible to the patient and avoid folds of skin, bones, and scar tissue. When possible, the waistline or belt area is avoided to reduce the risk for reducing *tissue integrity.* Prepare the patient for the number and type of drains that will be present after surgery. General care before surgery is discussed in Chapter 9.

Operative Procedures. Transurethral resection of the bladder tumor (TURBT) or partial cystectomy is performed for small, early, superficial tumors. In a partial (segmental) cystectomy, a portion of the bladder is removed when there is only a single isolated bladder tumor.

When the entire bladder must be removed (complete cystectomy), the ureters are diverted into a collecting reservoir. Techniques for urinary diversion are shown in Fig. 61.4. With an ileal conduit, the ureters are surgically placed in the ileum and urine is collected in a pouch on the skin around the stoma. More often, a continent reservoir known as a "neobladder" is created from an intestinal graft to store urine and replace the surgically removed bladder. With cutaneous ureterostomy or ureteroureterostomy, the ureter opening is brought out onto the skin. The cutaneous ureterostomies may be located on either side of the abdomen or side by side.

Postoperative Care. After cutaneous ureterostomy, an external pouch covers the ostomy to collect urine and maintain *tissue integrity.* Collaborate with the ET to focus care on the wound, the skin, and urinary drainage. (See Chapter 51 for ostomy care.)

The patient with a Kock's pouch, a continent reservoir, may have a Penrose drain and a plastic Medena catheter in the stoma. The drain removes lymphatic fluid or other secretions; the catheter ensures urine drainage so incisions can heal. The patient with a neobladder usually requires 2 to 4 days in the ICU and will have a drain at first in the event the neobladder requires irrigation. Later, irrigation can be performed with intermittent catheterization. Irrigation is performed to ensure patency. There is no sensation of bladder fullness with a neobladder because sensory nerves are not attached. As a result, the patient will need to learn new cues to void, such as prescribed times or noticing a feeling of neobladder pressure. General care after surgery is discussed in Chapter 9.

Different types of drains and nephrostomy catheters are used, sometimes on a temporary basis, to drain urine from the kidney. Some are totally internal, with no drainage to the outside. Others may drain exclusively to the outside, and urine is collected in a pouch or bag. For this type of drainage system, urine output remains constant. Decreased or no drainage is cause for concern and must be reported to the surgeon or nephrologist, as is leakage around the catheter. Some nephrostomy tubes are connected both to the new bladder (internal drainage) and to an external drainage system. With this type of system, urine output from the external portion of the catheter varies. With any drainage system, intervention is needed if the external catheter is partially or completely pulled out accidentally. Immediately notify the surgeon or nephrologist. If the catheter remains partially in place, secure it from further movement. This action may result in a reinsertion process rather than a total replacement.

Care Coordination and Transition Management

Self-Management Education. Teach the patient and family about drugs, diet and fluid therapy, the use of external pouching systems, and the technique for catheterizing a continent reservoir.

With some procedures, the patient may need electrolyte replacement to prevent long-term deficits. Teach the patient to avoid foods that are known to produce gas if the urinary diversion uses the intestinal tract. When intestinal production of gas is excessive, flatus can induce incontinence.

Patients who have a neobladder created often have extreme weight loss during the first few weeks after surgery. Collaborate with a dietitian to develop a diet plan specific to the patient to meet his or her caloric needs.

Ureterostomies divert urine directly to the skin surface through a ureteral skin opening (stoma). After ureterostomy, the patient must wear a pouch.

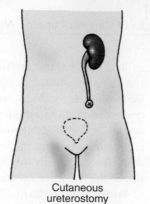
Cutaneous ureterostomy

Cutaneous ureteroureterostomy

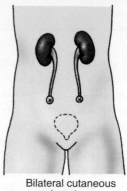
Bilateral cutaneous ureterostomy

Conduits collect urine in a portion of the intestine, which is then opened onto the skin surface as a stoma. After the creation of a conduit, the patient must wear a pouch.

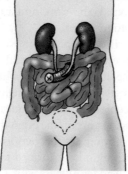
Ileal (Bricker's) conduit

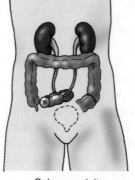
Colon conduit

Ileal reservoirs divert urine into a surgically created pouch, or pocket, that functions as a bladder. The stoma is continent, and the patient removes urine by regular self-catheterization.

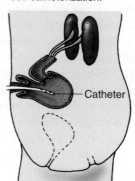
—Catheter

Continent internal ileal reservoir (Kock's pouch)

Sigmoidostomies divert urine to the large intestine, so no stoma is required. The patient excretes urine with bowel movements, and bowel incontinence may result.

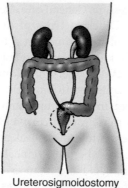
Ureterosigmoidostomy

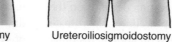
Ureteroiliosigmoidostomy

FIG. 61.4 Urinary diversion procedures used in the treatment of bladder cancer.

! NURSING SAFETY PRIORITY (QSEN)

Action Alert

Infection is common in patients who have a neobladder. Teach patients and family members the symptoms of infection and the importance of reporting them immediately to the surgeon.

Instruct the patient and family about any changes in self-care activities related to the urinary diversion. In collaboration with the enterostomal therapist, demonstrate external pouch application, local skin care, pouch care, methods of adhesion, and drainage mechanisms. If a Kock pouch has been created, teach the patient how to use a catheter to drain the pouch. For all instruction, observe at least one return demonstration or "teach-back" session by the patient or the caregiver. Ideally the patient assumes responsibility for self-care before discharge.

Help the patient prepare for the impact of urinary diversion on self-image, body image, sexual functioning, and self-esteem. Counseling provides information and support to reduce feelings of powerlessness.

Through discussions with the patient about common social situations, help the patient gain control over new toileting practices. Men with a urinary diversion into the sigmoid colon need to learn the habit of sitting to urinate. For patients of either gender, promote confidence in social situations by encouraging frequent emptying of urinary collection devices before traveling or attending social functions. Resumption of sexual activity is a major concern for many, regardless of age. Address this topic openly and with sensitivity. Cystectomy causes impotence in men, but treatment is available (see Chapter 67).

Health Care Resources. The United Ostomy Association (https://www.ostomy.org) and the ACS have educational materials that may be useful to patients. Refer patients and family members to local chapters or units of these organizations. In some areas, local support groups have meetings to help others and to send visitors to provide peer counseling and support. Home care personnel may help with follow-up, easing the transition from hospital to home. The Wound, Ostomy, and Continence Nurses Society has educational programs and a journal for the care of patients with ostomies.

GET READY FOR THE NEXT-GENERATION NCLEX® EXAMINATION!

Key Points
Review these Key Points for each NCLEX Examination Client Needs Category.

Safe and Effective Care Environment
- Use sterile technique when inserting a catheter in the acute care environment. **QSEN: Safety**
- Use Contact Precautions with any drainage from the genitourinary tract. **QSEN: Safety**
- Teach patients with urge or stress incontinence to keep pathways to the bathroom well lighted and clear of obstacles to help prevent falls. **QSEN: Safety**

Health Promotion and Maintenance
- Teach patients to clean the perineal area daily and after voiding, having a bowel movement, and after sexual intercourse. **QSEN: Patient-Centered Care**
- Encourage all patients to maintain an adequate fluid intake. **QSEN: Evidence-Based Practice**
- Teach women who have stress incontinence the proper way to perform pelvic floor–strengthening exercises. **QSEN: Patient-Centered Care**

Psychosocial Integrity
- Allow the patient the opportunity to express feelings or concerns regarding a urinary tract disorder or a cancer diagnosis. **QSEN: Patient-Centered Care**
- Use a nonjudgmental approach in caring for patients with urinary incontinence. **QSEN: Patient-Centered Care**
- Avoid referring to protective pads, briefs, or pants as "diapers." **QSEN: Patient-Centered Care**
- Recognize the need for the patient undergoing cystectomy and urinary diversion to grieve about the body image change. **QSEN: Patient-Centered Care**

Physiological Integrity
- Identify hospitalized patients at risk for bacteriuria and urosepsis. **QSEN: Evidence-Based Practice**
- Teach patients with UTI to complete all prescribed antibiotic therapy even when symptoms of infection are absent. **QSEN: Patient-Centered Care**
- Evaluate daily the need for maintaining urinary catheters and discontinue as soon as possible. **QSEN: Evidence-Based Practice**
- Teach patients the expected side effects and any adverse reactions to prescribed drugs. **QSEN: Patient-Centered Care**

MASTERY QUESTIONS

1. Which adverse drug effects will the nurse assess for in a hospitalized client who is prescribed an anticholinergic drug to manage incontinence? (*Select all that apply.*)
   A. Insomnia
   B. Blurred vision
   C. Constipation
   D. Dry mouth
   E. Loss of sphincter control
   F. Increased sweating
   G. Worsening mental function

2. A 28-year-old female client states, "I don't know why I get cystitis every year. I don't drink much at work so that I can avoid using the public toilet." Which teaching by the nurse is most likely to reduce her risk for cystitis? *Select all that apply.*
   A. Reinforce her choice to avoid using a public toilet.
   B. Teach her to shower immediately after having sexual intercourse.
   C. Suggest that she drink at least 2 to 3 L of fluid throughout the day.
   D. Urge her to change her method of birth control from oral contraceptives to a barrier method.
   E. Instruct her to always wipe her perineum from front to back after each toilet use.
   F. Reinforce that she should complete the entire course of antibiotics as prescribed.
   G. Instruct her to empty her bladder immediately before intercourse.

3. A client is diagnosed with renal colic. What would the nurse do first?
   A. Prepare the client for lithotripsy.
   B. Encourage oral intake of fluids.
   C. Strain the urine and send for urinalysis.
   D. Administer opioids as prescribed.

4. For which hospitalized client does the nurse recommend the ongoing use of a urinary catheter?
   A. A 35-year-old woman who was admitted with a splenic laceration and femur fracture (closed repair completed) following a car crash
   B. A 48-year-old man who has established paraplegia and is admitted for pneumonia
   C. A 61-year-old woman who is admitted following a fall at home and has new-onset dysrhythmia
   D. A 74-year-old man who has lung cancer with brain metastasis and is being transitioned to hospice

REFERENCES

American Cancer Society (ACS). (2019). *About bladder cancer.* Retrieved from https://www.cancer.org/cancer/bladder/about/what-is-bladder-cancer.

American Cancer Society (ACS). (2017). *Cancer facts and figures 2017. Report No. 01-300M—No. 500817.* Atlanta: Author.

Aoki, Y., Brown, H., Brubaker, L., Comu, J., Daly, J., & Cartwright, R. (2017). Urinary incontinence in women. *National Reviews Disease Primers, 3.* https://doi.org/10.1038/nrdp.2017.42.

Avelluto, G., & Bryman, P. (2018). Asymptomatic bacteriuria vs. symptomatic urinary tract infection: Identification and treatment challenges in geriatric care. *Urologic Nursing, 38*(3). https://doi.org/10.7257/1053816X.2018.38.3.129.

Barrow, R. Y., Ahmed, F., Bolan, G. A., & Workowski, K. A. (2020). Recommendations for providing quality sexually transmitted diseases clinical services. *Morbidity and Mortality Weekly Report Recommendations and Reports, 68*(No. RR-5), 1–20. https://doi.org/10.15585/mmwr.rr6805a1.

Beauchemin, L., Newman, D., Danseur, M., Jackson, A., & Ritmiller, M. (2018). Best practices for clean intermittent catheterization. *Nursing 2018, 48*(9). https://doi.org/10.1097/01.NURSE.0000544216.23783.bc.

Beeson, T., & Davis, C. (2018). Urinary management with an external female collection device. *The Journal of Wound, Ostomy and Continence Nursing, 45*(2). https://doi.org/10.1097/WON.0000000000000417.

Bliss, D., Mathiason, M., et al. (2017). Incidence and predictors of incontinence associated skin damage in nursing home residents with new onset incontinence. *The Journal of Wound, Ostomy and Continence Nursing, 44*(2). https://doi.org/10.1097/WON.0000000000000313.

Canadian Cancer Society. (2016). *Statistics Canada. Canadian cancer Statistics, 2016.* Toronto: Canadian Cancer Society.

Centers for Disease Control and Prevention (CDC). (2016). *2015 Sexually transmitted disease treatment guidelines.* www.cdc.gov/std/tg2015.

Clemens, J. (2018). Urinary incontinence in men. In S. Calderwood (Ed.), *UpToDate,* Waltham, MA.

Conway, L., Liu, J., Harris, A., & Larson, E. (2017). Risk factors for bacteremia in patients with urinary catheter-associated bacteriuria. *American Journal of Critical Care, 26*(1), 43–52.

Damien, J., Pastor-Barriuso, R., Lopez, G., & de Pedro-Cuesta, J. (2017). Urinary incontinence and mortality among older adults residing in care homes. *Journal of Advanced Nursing, 73*(2). https://doi.org/10.1111/jan.13170.

Engberg, S., & Li, H. (2017). Urinary incontinence in frail older adults. *Urologic Nursing, 37*(3).

Feng, F., Hawks, J., Kernen, J., & Kyle, E. (2018). Recurrent urinary tract infection care: Integrating complementary and alternative medicine. *Urologic Nursing, 38*(5). https://doi.org/10.7257/1053-816X.2018.38.5.231.

Ferguson, A. (2018). Implementing a CAUTI prevention program in an acute care setting. *Urologic Nursing, 38*(6). https://doi.org/10.7257/1053816X.2018.38.6.273.

Goldfarb, D (2019). Cystine stones. In S. Goldfarb (Ed.), *UpToDate,* Waltham, MA.

Gray, M., McNichol, L., & Nix, D. (2016). Incontinence-associated dermatitis: Progress, promises, and ongoing challenges. *The Journal of Wound, Ostomy and Continence Nursing, 43*(2), 188–192.

Hooten, T., & Gupta, K. (2018). Acute simple cystitis in women. In S. Calderwood (Ed.), *UpToDate,* Waltham, MA.

Hubb, A., Stachowicz, A., & Wood, S. (2018). Onabutulinumtoxin A injections for urge incontinence. *American Family Physician, 97*(3). Online.

Kim, H. (2016). Update on the pathology and diagnosis. *International Neurology Journal, 20*(1). https://doi.org/0.5213/inj.1632522.261.

Lee, H., & Le, J. (2018). *Urinary tract infections. Infectious diseases.* Retrieved from https://www.accp.com/docs/bookstore/psap/p2018b1_sample.pdf.

Li, K., Lin, T., Zhang, C., Fan, X., Xu, K., Bi, L., et al. (2013). Optimal frequency of shock wave lithotripsy in urolithiasis treatment: A systematic review and meta-analysis of randomized controlled trials. *The Journal of Urology, 190*(4), 1260–1267.

Lukacz, E., Santiago, Y., & Albo, M. (2017). Urinary incontinence in women: A review. *Journal of American Medical Association, 318*(16). https://doi.org/10.1001/jama.2017.12137.

McCance, K., & Huether, S. (2019). *Pathophysiology: The biologic basis for disease in adults and children* (8th ed.). St. Louis: Mosby.

McGoldrick, M. (2016). Frequency for changing long-term indwelling urinary catheters. *Home Healthcare, Now, 34*(2), 105–106.

McLellan, L., & Hunstad, D. (2016). Urinary tract infection: Pathogenesis and outlook. *Trends in Molecular Medicine, 22*(11). https://doi.org/10.1016/j.molmed.2016.09.003.

Milson, I., & Gyhagen, M. (2018). The prevalence of urinary incontinence. *Climacteric.* https://doi.org/10.1080/13697137.2018.1543263.

Nicolle, L. (2016). Urinary tract infections in adults. In K. Skorecki, G. Chertow, P. Marsden, M. Taal, & A. Yu (Eds.), *Brenner and rector" the kidney* (10th ed.). Philadelphia: Elsevier.

O'Brien, V., Hannan, T., Yu, L., Robertson, E., Schwartz, D., Souza, S., et al. (2016). A mucosal imprint left by prior Escherichia coli bladder infection sensitizes to recurrent disease. *National Microbiology.* https://doi.org/10.1036/nmicrobiol.2016.196.

Panchisin, T. (2016). Improving outcomes with the ANA CAUTI prevention tool. *Nursing, 46*(3), 55–59.

Simmering, J., Tang, F., Cavannaugh, J., Polgreen, L., & Polgreen, P. (2017). The increase in hospitalizations for urinary tract infections and the associated costs in the United States, 1998-2011. *Open Forum Infectious Diseases, 4*(1). https://doi.org/10.1093/ofid/ofw281.

Tan, C., & Chlebicki, M. (2016). Urinary tract infections in adults. *Singapore Medical Journal, 57*(9). In T. Touhy & K. Jett (Vol. Ed.), *Ebersole & Hess' toward healthy aging: Human needs & nursing response.* St. Louis: Elsevier. https://doi.org/10.11622/smedj.2016153.

Zhang, N. (2018). An evolutionary concept analysis of urinary incontinence. *Urologic Nursing, 38*(6). https://doi.org/10.7257/1053-816X.2018.38.6.289.

62

Concepts of Care for Patients With Kidney Disorders

Robyn Mitchell

http://evolve.elsevier.com/Iggy/

LEARNING OUTCOMES

1. Collaborate with the interprofessional team to coordinate high-quality care and promote urinary *elimination* in patients who have kidney disorders.
2. Teach the patient and caregiver(s) about home safety issues affected by impaired *elimination* and impairment of *fluid and electrolyte balance* or *acid-base balance* resulting from kidney problems.
3. Prioritize evidence-based care for patients with kidney disorders that impair urinary *elimination.*
4. Identify community resources for patients requiring assistance with any acute or chronic kidney problem.
5. Teach adults how to decrease the risk for kidney damage or kidney disease.
6. Implement nursing interventions to help the patient and family cope with the psychosocial impact caused by acute or chronic kidney disorders.
7. Apply knowledge of pathophysiology to assess patients with kidney disorders affecting *elimination, fluid and electrolyte balance,* or *acid-base balance.*
8. Use clinical judgment to analyze information from laboratory data and assessment findings in the care of patients with kidney disorders.
9. Teach the patient and caregiver(s) about common drugs and other management strategies used for kidney disorders, including *pain* control.
10. Implement evidence-based nursing interventions to prevent complications of kidney disorders and their therapies.

KEY TERMS

abscess A localized collection of pus caused by an inflammatory response to bacteria in tissues and organs.

acute glomerulonephritis Inflammation of the glomerulus that develops suddenly from an excess immunity response within the kidney tissues.

dysuria Painful urination.

hydronephrosis Abnormal enlargement of the kidney.

hydroureter Abnormal distention of the ureter.

nephrectomy Surgical removal of the kidney.

nephrosclerosis Degenerative kidney disorder resulting from changes in kidney blood vessels

nephrostomy The surgical creation of an opening directly into the kidney; performed to divert urine externally and prevent further damage to the kidney when a stricture

is causing hydronephrosis and cannot be corrected with urologic procedures.

nephrotic syndrome (NS) Immunologic kidney disorder in which glomerular permeability increases so larger molecules pass through the membrane into the urine and are then excreted; causes massive loss of protein into the urine and decreased plasma albumin levels.

polycystic kidney disease (PKD) Genetic disorder in which fluid-filled cysts develop in the kidneys.

pyelolithotomy Surgical removal of a stone from the kidney.

pyelonephritis A bacterial infection in the kidney and renal pelvis.

stricture Narrowing of the urinary tract.

ureteroplasty Surgical repair of the ureter.

✳ PRIORITY AND INTERRELATED CONCEPTS

The priority concept for this chapter is:

- *Elimination*

  The *Elimination* concept exemplar for this chapter is Pyelonephritis.

The interrelated concepts for this chapter are:

- *Fluid and Electrolyte Balance*
- *Acid-Base Balance*
- *Immunity*
- *Pain*

Healthy kidneys are the major controllers of urinary *elimination.* They perform this function by filtering wastes from the blood and selectively determining which substances remain in the body and which are eliminated. Thus the kidneys maintain homeostasis by contributing to *fluid and electrolyte balance* and *acid-base balance.* Any problem that disrupts kidney function has the potential to impair general homeostasis and all aspects of urinary elimination (Fig. 62.1). Interaction with other organs and systems is necessary for the kidneys to function effectively. In addition, when the kidneys are impaired, the buildup of toxic

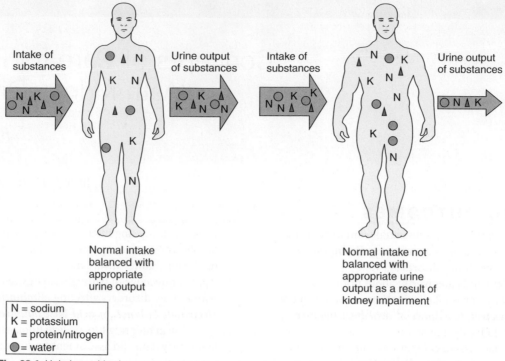

N = sodium
K = potassium
▲ = protein/nitrogen
⬤ = water

Fig. 62.1 Unbalanced body water, electrolytes, and waste products as a result of kidney problems that prevent adjustments in urinary elimination.

wastes affects all other body systems and can lead to life-threatening outcomes. This chapter describes a variety of infectious and noninfectious kidney disorders, kidney tumors, and kidney trauma. Acute kidney injury (AKI) and chronic kidney disease (CKD) are discussed in Chapter 63.

✳ ELIMINATION CONCEPT EXEMPLAR: PYELONEPHRITIS

In the healthy adult, urine is normally sterile. Urinary tract infection (UTI) is an infection in any part of this normally sterile system. Pyelonephritis is a bacterial infection that starts in the bladder and moves upward to infect the kidneys (National Institute of Diabetes and Digestive and Kidney Diseases, 2018). It can be acute or chronic. Pyelonephritis interferes with urinary *elimination,* which is the excretion of waste from the body by the urinary system (as urine). Chapter 3 provides a summary of the concept of elimination in more detail.

Pathophysiology Review

Acute pyelonephritis is an active bacterial infection, whereas *chronic pyelonephritis* results from repeated or continued upper urinary tract infections that occur almost exclusively in patients who have anatomic abnormalities of the urinary tract. Bacterial infection causes local (e.g., kidney) and systemic (e.g., fever, aches, and malaise) inflammatory symptoms.

In pyelonephritis, organisms move up from the urinary tract into the kidney tissue. This is more likely to occur when urine refluxes from the bladder into the ureters and then to the kidney. Reflux is the reverse or upward flow of urine toward the renal pelvis and kidney. Infection also can be transmitted by

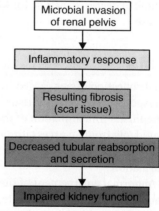

Fig. 62.2 Pathophysiology of pyelonephritis.

organisms in the blood, but this cause of pyelonephritis is rare unless the patient has impaired *immunity.*

Acute pyelonephritis involves acute tissue inflammation, local edema, tubular cell necrosis, and possible abscess formation. Abscesses, which are pockets of infection, can occur anywhere in the kidney. The infection is scattered within the kidney; healthy tissues can lie next to infected areas. Fibrosis and scar tissue develop from chronic inflammation in the kidney glomerular and tubular structures. As a result, filtration, reabsorption, and secretion are impaired, and kidney function is reduced (Fig. 62.2).

Etiology and Genetic Risk. Single episodes of *acute pyelonephritis* result from bacterial infection, with or without obstruction or reflux. *Chronic pyelonephritis* usually occurs with structural deformities, urinary stasis, obstruction, or reflux. Conditions that lead to urinary stasis include prolonged bedrest and paralysis. Obstruction can be caused by stones, kidney cancer, scarring from pelvic radiation or surgery, recurrent infection, or injury. Reflux may occur from scarring or result from anatomic anomalies. Reflux also results from bladder tumors, prostate enlargement, or urinary stones. Reduced bladder tone from diabetic neuropathy, spinal cord injury, and neurodegenerative diseases (e.g., spina bifida, multiple sclerosis) contributes to stasis and reflux.

Pyelonephritis from an ascending infection may follow manipulation of the urinary tract (e.g., placement of a urinary catheter), particularly in patients who have reduced *immunity* or diabetes. In patients with chronic kidney stone disease, stones may retain organisms, resulting in ongoing infection and kidney scarring. Drugs, such as high-dose or prolonged use of NSAIDs, can lead to papillary necrosis and reflux.

The most common pyelonephritis-causing infecting organism among community-dwelling adults is *Escherichia coli*. *Enterococcus faecalis* is common in hospitalized patients. Both organisms are in the intestinal tract. Other organisms that cause pyelonephritis in hospitalized patients include *Proteus mirabilis*, *Klebsiella* species, and *Pseudomonas aeruginosa*. When the infection is bloodborne, common organisms include *Staphylococcus aureus* and *Candida* and *Salmonella* species.

Other causes of kidney scarring contributing to increased risk for pyelonephritis are inflammatory responses resulting from *immunity* excesses with antibody reactions, cell-mediated immunity against the bacterial antigens, or autoimmune reactions.

Incidence and Prevalence. Acute pyelonephritis is most common in women who are young and sexually active (Nicolle, 2018). Hormonal changes as well as obstruction caused by the fetus during pregnancy make acute pyelonephritis more common during the second trimester and beginning of the third trimester. Care must be taken because any febrile illness in later pregnancy can precipitate premature labor and delivery (Nicolle, 2018).

Chronic pyelonephritis is rarely characterized by infection alone, so the incidence and prevalence are linked to the underlying condition or conditions that lead to relapsing inflammatory damage of the kidney. These conditions include congenital structural abnormality, neurogenic bladder dysfunction, and primary vesicoureteral reflux (Nicolle, 2018).

❖ Interprofessional Collaborative Care

Depending on the severity of the disease, pyelonephritis may be managed in any care setting and in the community. Hospitalization becomes necessary in cases of bacteremia or hemodynamic instability and when oral medication cannot be tolerated. Bacteremia occurs in approximately 10% of cases. Bacteremia is more common in older-adult women and women with diabetes (Nicolle, 2018). The focus of care for patients with chronic pyelonephritis requires continuing attention to managing the structural or functional abnormality that contributes to recurrent infection and inflammatory fibrosis.

◆ Assessment: Recognize Cues

History. Ask about recurrent urinary tract infections (UTIs), diabetes mellitus (DM), stone disease, and known defects of the genitourinary tract. Ask about disease or treatment that results in reduced *immunity*, which also increases risk for pyelonephritis. Ask about kidney function; knowledgeable patients may be able to describe their stage of chronic kidney disease (CKD) if chronic pyelonephritis has led to permanent kidney damage. Ensure that a woman is not pregnant before radiographic imaging.

Physical Assessment/Signs and Symptoms. Ask about specific symptoms of acute pyelonephritis (see the Key Features: Acute Pyelonephritis box). Chronic pyelonephritis has a less dramatic presentation but similar symptoms. Ask the patient to describe any urinary symptoms or abdominal discomfort. Inquire about any history of repeated low-grade fevers. Changes in urine color or odor may accompany bacteriuria. See the Key Features: Chronic Pyelonephritis box for kidney-related effects of chronic pyelonephritis.

The objective assessment includes inspecting the flanks and gently palpating the costovertebral angle (CVA). Inspect both CVAs for enlargement, asymmetry, edema, or redness, all of which can indicate inflammation (Jarvis, 2019). If there is no tenderness to light palpation in either CVA, the primary health care provider may firmly percuss each area. Tenderness or discomfort may indicate infection or inflammation.

Psychosocial Assessment. Any infection in an older adult can lead to acute confusion. Assess the older adult who has new-onset confusion for signs and symptoms of urinary or renal infection.

The patient with any problem in the genitourinary area may have feelings of anxiety, embarrassment, or guilt. Listen for signs of anxiety or specific fears and prevent embarrassment

---

▶▶ KEY FEATURES

Acute Pyelonephritis

- Fever
- Chills
- Tachycardia and tachypnea
- Flank, back, or loin pain
- Tenderness at the costovertebral angle (CVA)
- Abdominal, often colicky, discomfort
- Nausea and vomiting
- General malaise or fatigue
- Burning, urgency, or frequency of urination
- Nocturia
- Recent cystitis or treatment for urinary tract infection (UTI)

▶▶ KEY FEATURES

Chronic Pyelonephritis

- Hypertension
- Inability to conserve sodium
- Decreased urine-concentrating ability, resulting in nocturia
- Tendency to develop hyperkalemia and acidosis

during assessment. Feelings of guilt, often associated with sexual habits or practices, may be masked through delay in seeking treatment or through vague, nonspecific responses to specific or direct questions. Encourage patients to tell their own story in familiar, comfortable language.

Laboratory Assessment. Urinalysis shows a positive leukocyte esterase and nitrite dipstick test and the presence of white blood cells (WBCs) and bacteria. Occasional red blood cells (RBCs) and protein may be present. The urine is cultured to determine the specific organisms causing the infection and the susceptibility or resistance of the specific organisms to various antibiotics. The urine sample for culture and sensitivity testing is usually obtained by the clean-catch method. In patients with recurrent pyelonephritis, more specific testing of bacterial antigens and antibodies may help determine whether the same organism is responsible for the recurrent infections.

Blood cultures may be obtained to determine the source and spread of infectious organisms. Other blood tests include the WBC count and differential of the complete blood count, as well as C-reactive protein and erythrocyte sedimentation rate (ESR) to determine *immunity* responses and presence of inflammation. Serum tests of kidney function, such as blood urea nitrogen (BUN) and creatinine, are used as baseline and to trend recovery or deterioration. Estimate of glomerular filtration rate (GFR) also is used to trend kidney function.

Imaging Assessment. An x-ray of the kidneys, ureters, and bladder (KUB) or CT is performed to visualize anatomy, inflammation, fluid accumulation, abscess formation, and defects in kidneys and the urinary tract. These tests also identify stones, kidney tumors or cysts, or prostate enlargement. Urine reflux caused by incompetent bladder-ureter valve closure can be seen with a cystourethrogram. (See Chapter 60 for more information on imaging assessment.)

Other Diagnostic Assessment. Other diagnostic tests include examining antibody-coated bacteria in urine, testing for certain enzymes (e.g., lactate dehydrogenase isoenzyme 5), and performing radionuclide renal scans. Examining urine for antibody-coated bacteria helps identify patients who may need long-term antibiotic therapy. High-molecular-weight enzymes in urine, such as lactate dehydrogenase isoenzyme 5, are present with any kidney tissue deterioration problem and give trend data. The renal scan can identify active pyelonephritis or abscesses in or around the kidney. A kidney biopsy may be performed to rule out less obvious causes of inflammation.

NCLEX EXAMINATION CHALLENGE 62.1
Physiological Integrity

Which assessment data would the nurse anticipate in a client with acute pyelonephritis? **Select all that apply.**
A. Urinary frequency
B. Dysuria
C. Oliguria
D. Heart rate 120 beats/min
E. Uremia
F. Costovertebral angle tenderness

◆ **Analysis: Analyze Cues and Prioritize Hypotheses.** The priority collaborative problems for the patient with pyelonephritis are:
1. *Pain* (flank and abdominal) due to inflammation and infection
2. Potential for chronic kidney disease (CKD) disease due to kidney tissue destruction

◆ **Planning and Implementation: Generate Solutions and Take Action**

Managing Pain
Planning: Expected Outcomes. With proper intervention, the patient with pyelonephritis is expected to achieve an acceptable state of comfort.

Interventions. Interventions may be nonsurgical or surgical. Interventional radiologic techniques may be used to relieve obstruction or repair a stricture of the urinary tract.

Nonsurgical Management. Interventions include the use of drug therapy, nutrition and fluid therapy, and teaching to ensure the patient's understanding of the treatment.

Drug therapy can reduce pain. Acetaminophen is preferred over NSAIDs because it does not interfere with kidney autoregulation of blood flow. Reduction of fever will also reduce *pain.* Some patients may require the use of opioids in the short term for pain control.

Drug therapy with antibiotics is prescribed to treat the infection. At first the antibiotics are broad spectrum. After urine and blood culture and sensitivity results are known, more specific antibiotics may be prescribed. Antibiotics are given (usually IV in hospitalized patients; orally in community-dwelling patients) to achieve adequate blood levels or sterile blood culture results. A prophylactic antibiotic is not recommended for patients with impaired voiding or chronic catheter use because it does not limit recurrence or severity of UTI (Nicolle, 2018)

Catheter replacement is supportive for a patient requiring a urinary catheter for 2 or more weeks (e.g., for neurogenic bladder or wound healing). This involves removal and replacement of the catheter and closed drainage system before starting antibiotic therapy. This intervention reduces bioburden by removing a device with a biofilm of concentrated organisms.

Nutrition therapy involves ensuring that the patient's nutrition intake has adequate calories from all food groups for healing to occur. A registered dietitian nutritionist should be part of the interprofessional team. Fluid intake is recommended at 2 L/day, sufficient to result in dilute (pale yellow) urine, unless another health problem requires fluid restriction.

Surgical Management. Surgical interventions can correct structural problems causing urine reflux or obstruction of urine outflow or can remove the source of infection. Teach the patient the nature and purpose of the proposed surgery, the expected outcome, and how he or she can participate.

The surgical procedures may be one of these: **pyelolithotomy** (stone removal from the kidney), **nephrectomy** (removal of the kidney), ureteral diversion, or reimplantation of ureter(s) to restore proper bladder drainage.

A pyelolithotomy is needed for removal of a large stone in the kidney pelvis that blocks urine flow and causes infection. Nephrectomy is a last resort when all other measures to clear the infection have failed. For patients with poor ureter valve closure or dilated ureters, ureteroplasty (ureter repair or revision) or ureteral reimplantation (through another site in the bladder wall) preserves kidney function and eliminates infections.

Preventing Chronic Kidney Disease

Planning: Expected Outcomes. The patient is expected to conserve existing kidney function. Underlying genitourinary abnormalities must be identified, and appropriate interventions taken to manage a current infection and the risk for subsequent infections. The approach by the urologist or nephrologist depends on signs and symptoms as well as on patient history.

Interventions. Specific antibiotics are prescribed to treat the infection. Stress the importance of completing the drug therapy as directed. Discuss with the patient and family the importance of regular follow-up examinations and completing the recommended diagnostic tests.

Blood pressure control slows the progression of kidney dysfunction. Ensure that the patient is able to detect adverse changes in blood pressure using community resources such as free blood pressure readings at community settings or retail pharmacies. When pyelonephritis causes or worsens CKD, ensure a referral to a nephrologist for additional assessment and management (see CKD in Chapter 63). Encourage the patient to drink sufficient fluid during waking hours to prevent dehydration because dehydration could further reduce kidney function. When dietary protein is restricted, a registered dietitian nutritionist (RDN) can help the family select appropriate food and proportions. Collaborate with the RDN and reinforce the prescribed interventions.

Care Coordination and Transition Management. Pyelonephritis may cause fear and anxiety in the patient and family. The severity of the acute process and its potential to develop into a chronic process are frightening. The patient and the family need reassurance that treatment and preventive measures can be successful.

Home Care Management. If no surgery is performed, the patient may need help with self-care, nutrition, and drug management at home. If surgery is performed, he or she may need help with incision care, self-care, and transportation for follow-up appointments.

Self-Management Education. After assessing the patient's and family's understanding of pyelonephritis and its therapy, explain:

- Drug regimen (purpose, timing, frequency, duration, and possible side effects)
- The role of nutrition and adequate fluid intake
- Best practices for chronic urinary catheter care, if needed
- The need for a balance between rest and activity, including any limitations after surgery
- The signs and symptoms of disease recurrence
- The use of previously successful coping mechanisms and community resources

Advise the patient to complete all prescribed antibiotic regimens and to report any side effects or unusual symptoms to

TABLE 62.1 Infectious Agents Associated With Glomerulonephritis
• Group A beta-hemolytic *Streptococcus*
• Staphylococcal or gram-negative bacteremia or sepsis
• Pneumococcal, *Mycoplasma*, or *Klebsiella* pneumonia
• Syphilis
• Dengue
• Hantavirus
• Varicella
• Parvovirus
• Hepatitis B and C
• Cytomegalovirus
• Parvovirus
• Epstein-Barr virus
• Human immunodeficiency virus

Adapted from Patel, N.P. (2018, November 28). Infection-induced kidney diseases. Retrieved from U.S. National Library of Medicine, National Institutes of Health. https://www.ncbi.nlm.nih.gov/pmc/articles/PMC6282040/.

the primary health care provider rather than stopping the drugs. Ensure that interprofessional care includes nutrition counseling, because many patients have special nutrition requirements, such as those for diabetes or pregnancy.

Health Care Resources. The patient may also briefly need a home health care nurse to help with drug or nutrition therapy at home. Housekeeping services may be helpful while he or she is regaining strength.

◆ **Evaluation: Evaluate Outcomes.** Evaluate the care of the patient with pyelonephritis based on the identified priority patient problems. Expected outcomes may include that the patient will:

- Report that **pain** is controlled
- Be knowledgeable about the disease, its treatment, and interventions to prevent or reduce CKD progression

ACUTE GLOMERULONEPHRITIS

Pathophysiology Review

Glomerulonephritis (GN) is categorized into conditions that primarily involve the kidney (primary glomerular nephritis) and those in which kidney involvement is only part of a systemic disorder (secondary GN). It is a group of diseases that injure and inflame the glomerulus, the part of the kidney that filters blood. Inflamed glomeruli allow passage of protein and blood in the urine. GN is associated with high blood pressure, progressive kidney damage (leading to CKD), and edema. Anemia from reduced production of erythropoietin and high cholesterol often co-occur. GN can cause altered urinary *elimination*.

Acute glomerulonephritis (GN) develops suddenly from an excess *immunity* response within the kidney tissues. Usually an infection is noticed before kidney symptoms of acute GN are present. The onset of symptoms is about 10 days from the time of infection. Usually patients recover quickly and completely from acute GN.

Many causes of primary GN are infectious (Table 62.1). Secondary GN can be caused by multisystem diseases (Table 62.2)

TABLE 62.2 Secondary Glomerular Diseases and Syndromes

- Systemic lupus erythematosus (SLE)
- Sustained liver disease (hepatitis B or C, autoimmune hepatitis, and cirrhosis)
- Amyloidosis
- Mesangiocapillary glomerulonephritis (MCGN)
- Alport syndrome
- Vasculitis
- Goodpasture syndrome
- IgA nephropathy
- Wegener granulomatosis
- HIV-associated nephropathy
- Diabetic glomerulopathy

HIV, Human immune deficiency virus.
Data from Muthu, V.R. (2018, Jan-Feb). *Clinicopathological spectrum of glomerular diseases in adolescents: a single-center experience over 4 years.* Retrieved from U.S. National Library of Medicine, National Institutes of Health. https://www.ncbi.nlm.nih.gov/pmc/articles/PMC5830804/; and Radhakrishnan, J. (2020). Glomerular disease: evaluation and differential diagnosis in adults. *UpToDate.* Retrieved from: https://www.uptodate.com/contents/glomerular-disease-evaluation-and-differential-diagnosis-in-adults.

and can manifest as acute or chronic disease. However, the division of primary and secondary GN is complex because diagnostic findings, histologic changes, and other changes are the same in both kidney and systemic disease, with both demonstrating altered *immunity.* Drugs and inherited disorders are also implicated in GN with an acute or chronic presentation.

❖ Interprofessional Collaborative Care

◆ Assessment: Recognize Cues

History. Ask about recent infections, particularly of the skin or upper respiratory tract, and about recent travel or other possible exposures to viruses, bacteria, fungi, or parasites. Recent illnesses, surgery, or other invasive procedures may suggest infection. Ask about any systemic diseases that alter *immunity,* such as systemic lupus erythematosus (SLE), which could cause acute GN.

Physical Assessment/Signs and Symptoms. Inspect the patient's skin for lesions or recent incisions, including body piercings, because these may be the source of organisms causing GN. Assess the face, eyelids, hands, and other areas for edema because edema is present in most patients with acute GN. Assess for fluid overload and pulmonary edema that may result from fluid and sodium retention occurring with acute GN. Ask about any difficulty breathing or shortness of breath. Assess for crackles in the lung fields, an S_3 heart sound (gallop rhythm), and neck vein distention.

Ask about changes in urine *elimination* patterns and any change in urine color, volume, clarity, or odor. The patient may describe blood in the urine as smoky, reddish brown, rusty, or cola colored. Ask about dysuria or oliguria. Weigh him or her to assess for fluid retention.

Take the patient's blood pressure and compare it with the baseline blood pressure. Mild-to-moderate hypertension occurs with acute GN as a result of impaired *fluid and electrolyte*

balance with fluid and sodium retention. The patient may have fatigue, a lack of energy, anorexia, nausea, and/or vomiting if uremia from severe kidney impairment is present.

👤 PATIENT-CENTERED CARE: OLDER ADULT CONSIDERATIONS (QSEN)

Glomerulonephritis can lead to chronic kidney disease, making it essential to prevent and treat in the older adult who is at greater risk for CKD. In the older adult, symptoms of glomerulonephritis can easily be confused with an exacerbation of heart failure. Older adults with glomerulonephritis have a higher risk of mortality than younger patients with the same diagnosis, adding to the importance of early recognition and prompt intervention (Raman, 2018).

Laboratory Assessment. Urinalysis shows red blood cells *(hematuria)* and protein *(proteinuria).* An early morning specimen of urine is preferred for urinalysis because the urine is concentrated, most acidic, and filled with more intact formed elements at that time. Microscopic examination often shows red blood cell casts, as well as casts from other substances.

A 24-hour urine collection for total protein assay is obtained. The protein excretion rate for patients with acute GN may be increased from 500 mg/24 hr to 3 g/24 hr. Serum albumin levels are decreased because this protein is lost in the urine and fluid retention causes dilution.

Serum creatinine and BUN provide information about kidney function and may be elevated, indicating impairment of *elimination.* The glomerular filtration rate (GFR), either estimated from a single serum and urine creatinine value or measured by the 24-hour urine test for creatinine clearance, may be decreased to 50 mL/min. Recall that the older adult has a decline in GFR, which may make GFR results challenging to interpret.

Other Diagnostic Assessment. A kidney biopsy provides a precise diagnosis of the condition, assists in determining the prognosis, and helps in outlining treatment (see Chapter 60). The specific tissue features are determined by light microscopy, immunofluorescent stains, and electron microscopy to identify cell type, the presence of immunoglobulins, or the type of tissue deposits.

◆ Interventions: Take Action.

Interventions focus on managing infection, preventing complications, and providing appropriate patient education.

Managing infection as a cause of acute GN begins with appropriate antibiotic therapy. Penicillin, erythromycin, or azithromycin is prescribed for GN caused by streptococcal infection. Check the patient's known allergies before giving any drug. Stress personal hygiene and basic infection control principles (e.g., handwashing) to prevent spread of the organism. Teach patients the importance of completing the entire course of the prescribed antibiotic.

Modifying *immunity* with drugs can also benefit patients with acute glomerulonephritis (GN) that is not due to acute infection but is related to excessive inflammation. Corticosteroids and cytotoxic drugs (e.g., cyclosporine, cyclophosphamide) to suppress *immunity* responses may be used. Patients receiving immunosuppressants need to take precautions to avoid exposure to new infections.

Preventing complications is an important nursing intervention, especially when *fluid and electrolyte balance* is disrupted. For patients with fluid overload, hypertension, and edema, diuretics and sodium and water restrictions are prescribed. The usual fluid allowance is equal to the 24-hour urine output plus 500 to 600 mL. Patients with oliguria usually have increased serum levels of potassium and blood urea nitrogen (BUN). Potassium and protein intake may be restricted to prevent hyperkalemia and uremia as a result of the elevated BUN. Antihypertensive drugs may be needed to control hypertension (see Chapter 33).

Nausea, vomiting, or anorexia indicates that uremia is present. Dialysis is necessary if uremic symptoms or fluid volume excess cannot be controlled with nutrition therapy and fluid management (see Chapter 63). *Plasmapheresis* (removal and filtering of the plasma to eliminate antibodies) also may be used (see Chapter 37).

Coordinate care to conserve patient energy and balance activity with rest to maintain function. Relaxation techniques and diversional activities can reduce emotional stress.

Preparing for self-management includes teaching the patient and family members about the purpose of prescribed drugs, the dosage and schedule, and potential adverse effects. Ensure that they understand diet and fluid restrictions. Advise the patient to measure weight and blood pressure daily at the same time each day. Instruct him or her to notify the primary health care provider of any sudden increase in weight or blood pressure.

If short-term dialysis is required to control *fluid and electrolyte balance* or uremic symptoms, explain vascular access care and dialysis schedules and routines (see Chapter 63).

Rapidly progressive glomerulonephritis (RPGN) is a primary GN also called *crescentic glomerulonephritis* because of the presence of crescent-shaped cells in the Bowman capsule. RPGN develops acutely over several weeks or months. Patients become quite ill quickly and have symptoms of kidney impairment (fluid volume excess, hypertension, oliguria, electrolyte imbalances, and uremic symptoms). Regardless of treatment, RPGN often progresses to end-stage kidney disease (ESKD).

CHRONIC GLOMERULONEPHRITIS

Pathophysiology Review

Chronic GN, or *chronic nephritic syndrome*, develops over years to decades. Mild proteinuria and hematuria, hypertension, fatigue, and occasional edema are often the only symptoms.

Although the exact cause is not known, changes in kidney tissue result from infection, hypertension, inflammation from *immunity* excess, or poor kidney blood flow. Kidney tissue atrophies, and functional nephrons are greatly reduced. Biopsy in the late stages of atrophy may show glomerular changes, cell loss, protein and collagen deposits, and fibrosis of the kidney tissue. Microscopic examination shows deposits of immune complexes and inflammation.

The loss of nephrons reduces glomerular filtration. Hypertension and renal arteriole sclerosis are often present. The glomerular damage allows proteins to enter the urine. Chronic

GN always leads to end-stage kidney disease (ESKD) (see Chapter 63).

❖ Interprofessional Collaborative Care

◆ Assessment: Recognize Cues

History. Ask about other health problems, including systemic diseases, kidney or urologic disorders, infectious diseases (i.e., streptococcal infections), and recent exposures to infections. Ask about overall health status and whether increasing fatigue and lethargy have occurred.

Identify the patient's urine *elimination* pattern. Ask whether the frequency of voiding has increased or the quantity of urine has decreased. Ask about changes in urine color, odor, or clarity and whether dysuria or incontinence has occurred. Nocturia is a common symptom.

Assess the patient's general comfort and ask whether new-onset dyspnea has occurred, because fluid overload can occur with decreased urine output. Ask about and observe for changes in cognition (i.e., irritability, an inability to read, or incapacity during job-related functions) or disturbed concentration. Changes in memory and the ability to concentrate occur as waste products collect in the blood.

Physical Assessment/Signs and Symptoms. Assess for systemic circulatory overload. Auscultate lung fields for crackles, observe the respiratory rate and depth, and measure blood pressure and weight. Assess the heart rate, rhythm, and presence of an S_3 heart sound. Inspect the neck veins for venous engorgement and check for edema of the feet and ankles, on the shins, and over the sacrum.

Assess for uremic symptoms, such as slurred speech, ataxia, tremors, or asterixis (flapping tremor of the fingers or the inability to maintain a fixed posture with the arms extended and wrists hyperextended). Inspect skin for a yellowish color, texture changes, bruises, rashes, or eruptions. Ask about itching and document areas of dryness or any excoriation from scratching.

Psychosocial Assessment. A diagnosis of chronic GN is associated with psychosocial responses of uncertainty, loss, and fear of the need for lifestyle changes as the disease progresses. While obtaining the history, listen carefully for spoken and unspoken feelings of anger, resentment, futility, sadness, or anxiety, all of which may need further exploration.

Diagnostic Assessment. Urine output decreases and urinalysis shows protein, usually less than 2 g in a 24-hour collection. The specific gravity is fixed at a constant level of dilution (around 1.010) despite variable fluid intake. Red blood cells and casts may be in the urine.

The glomerular filtration rate (GFR) is low. The serum creatinine level is elevated; usually it is greater than 6 mg/dL (500 mcmol/L) but may be as high as 30 mg/dL (2500 mcmol/L) or more because of poor waste *elimination.* The BUN is increased, often as high as 100 to 200 mg/dL (35 to 70 mmol/L).

Decreased kidney function disturbs *fluid and electrolyte balance.* Sodium retention is common, but dilution of the plasma from excess fluid can result in a falsely normal serum sodium level (135 to 145 mEq/L [mmol/L]) or a low sodium level (less than 135 mEq/L [mmol/L]). When oliguria develops, potassium is not excreted, and hyperkalemia occurs when levels exceed 5.4 mEq/L (mmol/L).

Hyperphosphatemia develops with serum levels greater than 4.7 mg/dL (1.73 mmol/L). Serum calcium levels are usually low normal or are slightly below normal.

Disturbances of **acid-base balance** with acidosis develop from hydrogen ion retention and loss of bicarbonate. However, there may be a decrease in serum carbon dioxide (CO_2) levels as patients breathe more rapidly to compensate for the acidosis. If respiratory compensation is present, the pH of arterial blood is between 7.35 and 7.45. A pH of less than 7.35 means that the patient's respiratory system is not completely compensating for the acidosis (see Chapter 14).

The kidneys are abnormally small on x-ray or CT in chronic GN.

◆ **Interventions: Take Action.** Interventions focus on slowing the progression of the disease and preventing complications. Management is systemic and consists of diet changes, fluid intake sufficient to prevent reduced blood flow to the kidneys, and drug therapy to control the problems from uremia. Eventually **elimination** is so impaired that the patient requires dialysis or transplantation to prevent death. (Care for the patient requiring dialysis or transplantation is discussed in Chapter 63.)

NEPHROTIC SYNDROME

Pathophysiology Review

Nephrotic syndrome (NS) is an immunologic kidney disorder in which glomerular permeability increases so larger molecules pass through the membrane into the urine and are then excreted. This process causes massive loss of protein into the urine, edema formation, and decreased plasma albumin levels. Minimal change disease is the most common cause of NS and accounts for 90% of NS in children and 20% in adults. The name *minimal change* comes from the need to see changes in the glomerulus using an electron microscope since changes with a light microscope cannot be seen (Trachtman, 2018).

The most common cause of glomerular membrane changes is altered **immunity** with inflammation. Defects in glomerular filtration can also occur as a result of genetic defects of the glomerular filtering system, such as Fabry disease. Altered liver function may occur with NS, resulting in increased lipid production and hyperlipidemia.

❖ Interprofessional Collaborative Care

The main feature of NS is increased protein **elimination** with severe proteinuria (with more than 3.5 g of protein in a 24-hour urine sample). Patients also have low serum albumin levels of less than 3 g/dL (30 g/L), high serum lipid levels, fats in the urine, edema, and hypertension (see the Key Features: Nephrotic Syndrome box). Renal vein thrombosis often occurs at the same time as NS, either as a cause of the problem or as an effect. NS may progress to end-stage kidney disease (ESKD), but treatment can prevent progression.

Management varies, depending on which process is causing the disorder (identified by kidney biopsy). Excess **immunity**

⯈ **KEY FEATURES**
Nephrotic Syndrome

Key features include sudden onset of these symptoms:
- Massive proteinuria
- Hypoalbuminemia
- Edema (especially facial and periorbital)
- Lipiduria
- Hyperlipidemia
- Delayed clotting or increased bleeding with higher-than-normal values for serum activated partial thromboplastin time (aPTT), coagulation, or international normalized ratio for prothrombin time (INR, PT)
- Reduced kidney function with elevated blood urea nitrogen (BUN) and serum creatinine and decreased glomerular filtration rate (GFR)

---

may improve with suppressive therapy using steroids and cytotoxic or immunosuppressive agents. Angiotensin-converting enzyme inhibitors (ACEIs) can decrease protein loss in the urine, and cholesterol-lowering drugs can improve blood lipid levels. Heparin may reduce vascular defects and improve kidney function. Diet changes are often prescribed. If the glomerular filtration rate (GFR) is normal, dietary intake of proteins is needed. If the GFR is decreased, protein intake must be decreased. Mild diuretics and sodium restriction may be needed to control edema and hypertension. Assess the patient's hydration status because vascular dehydration is common. If plasma volume is depleted, kidney problems worsen. Acute kidney injury (AKI) may be avoided if adequate blood flow to the kidney is maintained.

NEPHROSCLEROSIS

Pathophysiology Review

Nephrosclerosis is a degenerative disorder resulting from changes in kidney blood vessels. Nephron blood vessels thicken, resulting in narrowed lumens and decreased kidney blood flow. The tissue is chronically hypoxic, with ischemia and fibrosis developing over time.

Nephrosclerosis occurs with all types of hypertension, atherosclerosis, and diabetes mellitus (DM). The more severe the hypertension, the greater the risk for severe kidney damage. Nephrosclerosis is rarely seen when blood pressure is consistently below 160/110 mm Hg. The changes caused by hypertension may be reversible or may progress to end-stage kidney disease (ESKD) within months or years. Hypertension is the second leading cause of ESKD, with many patients requiring kidney replacement therapy (e.g., dialysis or transplantation).

More recent advances in genetic testing have revealed a complex pathogenesis in nephrosclerosis. Patients were often diagnosed with nephrosclerosis thought to be caused by hypertension. However, advanced genetic evidence indicated many as having genetic focal segmental glomerulosclerosis. The apolipoprotein L1 (APOL1) allele is a risk factor for glomerulosclerosis that presents with symptoms such as nephrosclerosis. People with the APOL1 allele are usually of African ancestry. Not all patients with the ALOL1 allele will develop kidney disease, suggesting that there may be environmental factors as well. The treatment of patients with genetically caused focal segmental glomerulosclerosis is evolving (Crawford, 2018).

PATIENT-CENTERED CARE: CULTURAL/ SPIRITUAL CONSIDERATIONS (QSEN)

Patient-Centered Care

Approximately 14% of the general population is affected by chronic kidney disease. African Americans, Native Americans, and Mexican Americans are more likely to have chronic kidney disease than Caucasians. The prevalence of end-stage renal disease (ESRD) is 3.7 times higher in African Americans and 1.4 times higher in Native Americans than in Caucasians. Hispanics are 1.5 times more likely to develop ESRD than non-Hispanics (National Institute of Diabetes and Digestive and Kidney Diseases, 2016).

❖ Interprofessional Collaborative Care

Management focuses on controlling high blood pressure and reducing albuminuria to preserve kidney function. Although many antihypertensive drugs may lower blood pressure, the patient's response is important in ensuring long-term adherence to the prescribed therapy. Factors that promote adherence include once-a-day dosing, low cost, and minimal side effects.

Lack of knowledge or misinformation about hypertension poses many challenges to health care professionals working with patients who have hypertension. When kidney disease occurs, adherence to therapy is even more important for preserving health.

Many drugs can control high blood pressure (see Chapter 33), and more than one agent may be needed for best control. Angiotensin-converting enzyme inhibitors (ACEIs) are very useful in reducing hypertension and preserving kidney function. Diuretics can maintain *fluid and electrolyte balance* in the

presence of kidney function insufficiency. Hyperkalemia needs to be prevented when potassium-sparing diuretics, alone or in combination with other diuretics, are used to treat hypertensive patients with known kidney disease.

POLYCYSTIC KIDNEY DISEASE

Pathophysiology Review

Polycystic kidney disease (PKD) is a genetic disorder in which fluid-filled cysts develop in the nephrons (Fig. 62.3). Relentless development and growth of cysts from loss of cellular regulation and abnormal cell division result in progressive kidney enlargement. Patients with PKD often experience hypertension, abdominal fullness and pain, episodes of cyst bleeding, hematuria, kidney stone formation, infections, and systemic disease (Rizk, 2018).

The cysts look like clusters of grapes (see Fig. 62.3). Over time, growing cysts damage the glomerular and tubular membranes. Each cystic kidney enlarges, becoming the size of a football, and may weigh 10 lb or more each. As cysts fill with fluid and become larger, kidney function becomes less effective, and urine formation and waste *elimination* are impaired.

Most patients with PKD have high blood pressure. The cause of hypertension is related to kidney ischemia from the enlarging cysts. As the vessels are compressed and blood flow to the kidneys decreases, the renin-angiotensin system is activated, raising blood pressure. Control of hypertension is a top priority because proper treatment can disrupt the process that leads to further kidney damage, as well as avoid complications such as stroke from hypertension.

Cysts may also occur in the liver and blood vessels. The incidence of cerebral *aneurysms* (outpouching and thinning of an artery wall) is higher in patients with PKD. Aneurysms

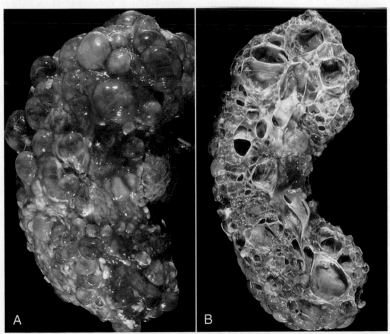

A   B

Fig. 62.3 External surface (A) and internal surface (B) of a polycystic kidney. (From Kumar, V., Abbas, A., Fausto, N., & Aster, J. [2010]. *Robbins and Cotran pathologic basis of disease* [8th ed.]. Philadelphia: Saunders.)

may rupture, causing bleeding and sudden death. For unknown reasons, kidney stones occur in many patients with PKD. Heart valve problems (e.g., mitral valve prolapse), left ventricular hypertrophy, and colonic diverticula also are common in patients with PKD.

Etiology and Genetic Risk. Kidney cysts are genetically and clinically related to many symptoms and problems. PKD can be inherited as either an autosomal dominant trait or, less often, an autosomal recessive trait. Autosomal dominant PKD is the most common inherited kidney disease, occurring in 1 in 400 to 1000 live births. People who inherit the recessive form of PKD usually die in early childhood. Rarely, a new gene mutation can cause PKD in a patient with no family history of the trait. However, the cases of gene mutation tend to be a milder form of PKD. Recent advances have made the genetic forms of cystic disorders of the kidney easier to understand. Many of the genes that cause cystic diseases of the kidney have been identified (Rizk, 2018). However, the number of genes influencing PKD is challenging and requires geneticists and genetic counselors to be a part of the interprofessional team caring for patients with or at risk for the disease.

> ### 👤 PATIENT-CENTERED CARE: GENETIC/ GENOMIC CONSIDERATIONS (QSEN)
>
> Autosomal dominant PKD (ADPKD) is the most common form of the disease in adults, who have a 50% risk of passing the mutated gene to their children. Fig. 62.4 shows a pedigree for a family with ADPKD. Recent advances in molecularly targeted therapies offer new hope for improved outcomes and eventually a cure for PKD (Rizk, 2018).

Three genes have been implicated in the cause of ADPKD. Among the genes causing ADPKD, 85% of ADPKD cases are caused by mutations in the *PKD1* gene, 15% have mutations in the *PKD2* gene, and 1% have mutations in the *GANAB* gene. The *PKD1* gene mutations cause a more severe form of PKD with more kidney cysts, earlier onset of hypertension, and more instances of ESKD (Rizk, 2018).

There is no way to prevent PKD, although early detection and management of hypertension may slow the progression of kidney damage and impaired *elimination.* Genetic counseling may be useful for adults who have one parent with PKD. Family history analysis is used to help identify people at risk (see Fig. 62.4).

Incidence and Prevalence. PKD affects about 600,000 people of all ethnic groups in the United States and causes about 5% of kidney failure (National Kidney Foundation, 2019). Men and women have an equal chance of inheriting the disease because the gene responsible for PKD is on an autosome (see Chapter 6).

❖ Interprofessional Collaborative Care

◆ Assessment: Recognize Cues.
Because PKD is a chronic disease with periods of acute problems, most management occurs in the community rather than in an acute care hospital. With acute problems or when surgery is needed, initial care is in a hospital setting, and continuing care can occur in any setting.

History. Explore the family history of a patient with suspected or actual PKD and ask whether either parent was known to have PKD or whether there is any family history of kidney disease. Important information to obtain is the age at which the problem was diagnosed in the parent and any related complications. Ask about *pain,* abdominal discomfort, constipation, changes in urine color or frequency, hypertension, headaches, and a family history of stroke or sudden death.

Physical Assessment/Signs and Symptoms. **Pain** is often the first symptom. Inspect the abdomen. A distended abdomen is common as the cystic kidneys swell and push the abdominal contents forward. Polycystic kidneys are easily palpated because of their increased size. Use *gentle* abdominal palpation because the cystic kidneys and nearby tissues may be tender and palpation is uncomfortable. The patient also may have flank pain as a dull ache or as a sharp and intermittent discomfort. Dull, aching pain is caused by increased kidney size with distention, abnormal stimulation of sensory neurons in the kidney, or infection within the cyst. Sharp, intermittent pain occurs when a cyst ruptures or a stone is present. When a cyst ruptures, the patient may have bright red or cola-colored urine. Infection is suspected if the urine is cloudy or foul smelling or if there is dysuria (pain on urination). See the Key Features: Polycystic Kidney Disease box.

Nocturia (the need to urinate excessively at night) is an early symptom and occurs because of decreased urine concentrating ability. Patients with early PKD often have hyperfiltration leading to wasting of sodium and water, which disrupts *fluid and electrolyte balance.* Later, as kidney function declines (i.e., reduced glomerular filtration rate [GFR]), the patient retains

> ### ⏩ KEY FEATURES
> #### *Polycystic Kidney Disease*
>
> - Abdominal or flank pain
> - Hypertension
> - Nocturia
> - Frequent urinary tract infections
> - Increased abdominal girth
> - Constipation
> - Hematuria (bloody urine)
> - Sodium wasting and inability to concentrate urine in early stage
> - Progression to kidney failure with anuria (Holt, 2018)

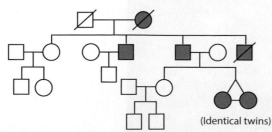

(Identical twins)

Fig. 62.4 Four-generation pedigree for autosomal dominant polycystic kidney disease (ADPKD). *Colored-in symbols* indicate family members with ADPKD. *Slashes* indicate that the person has died.

water and sodium, which causes hypertension, edema, and uremic symptoms such as anorexia, nausea, vomiting, pruritus, and fatigue (see Chapter 63). Because intracranial berry aneurysms often occur in patients with PKD, a severe headache with or without neurologic or vision changes requires attention.

Psychosocial Assessment. A PKD diagnosis is associated with psychosocial responses of uncertainty, loss, and fear due to the life-threatening complications that can occur (Rizk, 2018). The patient may have had a parent who died or relatives who required dialysis or transplantation. Listen for spoken and unspoken feelings of anger, resentment, futility, sadness, or anxiety. Such feelings may need further exploration. Feelings of guilt and concern for the patient's children may also complicate the issue.

Diagnostic Assessment. Ultrasound is the primary method for diagnosing PKD. The size of the kidney is measured by ultrasound as well as cysts within the kidney. MRI or CT may be used in order to confirm ultrasound findings or when a family member is being evaluated for potential kidney donation (Rizk, 2018).

Urinalysis may show proteinuria (protein in the urine), which indicates a decline in kidney function and impaired *elimination.* Hematuria may be gross or microscopic. Bacteria in the urine indicate infection, usually in the cysts. Obtain a urine sample for culture and sensitivity testing when there is evidence of infection. As kidney function declines, serum creatinine and blood urea nitrogen (BUN) levels rise. With further decline, creatinine clearance decreases, and the GFR is low. Changes in kidney handling of sodium may cause either sodium losses or sodium retention.

Genetic testing is not routinely performed for diagnostic assessment of PKD. It may be considered for patients who have atypical imaging findings or for those with symptoms who have no family history of PKD.

◆ **Interventions: Take Action.** Currently no treatments are effective in extending kidney function in PKD. Drug therapies to interrupt the pathways that promote malignant cyst formation such as molecular signaling for cell division or endothelial growth are being evaluated. Supportive interventions for PKD include management of hypertension and pain, reducing complications from infection and constipation, and slowing disease progression. Be attentive to the psychosocial issues of uncertainty and fear related to an inherited disorder, as well as reproductive issues. Genetic counseling is part of comprehensive care of the patient and family experiencing PKD.

When the disease progresses and the kidneys no longer function for waste *elimination,* care becomes similar to that needed for the patient with end-stage kidney disease (see Chapter 63).

Managing Blood Pressure. Blood pressure control and lifestyle and dietary modifications are necessary to reduce cardiovascular complications and slow the progression of kidney dysfunction. Nursing interventions include education for self-management. Dietary salt of less than 2 g/day is now advised. Calorie restriction with weight reduction has been shown to decrease blood pressure (Rizk, 2018).

Drug therapy with angiotensin-converting enzyme inhibitors (ACEIs) to reach a blood pressure below 130/80 mm Hg in all patients with PKD or 110/75 mm Hg in young adults with preserved kidney function is recommended (Rizk, 2018). These drugs also help control the cell growth aspects of PKD and reduce microalbuminuria. Additional antihypertensive drugs, such as calcium channel blockers, beta blockers, and vasodilators, may be used (see Chapter 33).

Teach the patient and family how to measure and record blood pressure. Help the patient establish a schedule for self-administering drugs, monitoring daily weights, and keeping blood pressure records (see the Patient and Family Education: Preparing for Self-Management: Polycystic Kidney Disease box). Explain the potential side effects of the drugs. Make available written materials, such as drug teaching cards and booklets. Work with the patient and a registered dietitian nutritionist to develop strategies to manage sodium and other dietary issues that contribute to hypertension.

Managing Pain. Because PKD-related pain is chronic, a multidisciplinary *pain* management approach is helpful. Drugs may include opioids along with acetaminophen. NSAIDs are used cautiously because they can reduce kidney blood flow. Aspirin-containing drugs are avoided to reduce bleeding risk.

Complementary therapy includes positioning and the application of dry heat to the abdomen or flank. Teach the patient methods of relaxation and comfort using deep breathing, guided imagery, or other strategies (see Chapter 5 for pain management). When pain is severe, cysts can be reduced by needle aspiration and drainage; however, they usually refill. When the quality or severity of pain abruptly increases, assess for infection.

Reducing Complications From Infection. Fever, abdominal *pain,* and either leukocytosis or serum markers of inflammation (e.g., elevated erythrocyte sedimentation rate [ESR] or C-reactive protein [CRP]) may be associated with cystic or systemic infection. Blood and urine cultures may or may not be positive with cyst infection. Early infection management

---

PATIENT AND FAMILY EDUCATION: PREPARING FOR SELF-MANAGEMENT

Polycystic Kidney Disease

- Measure and record your blood pressure daily and notify your primary health care provider about consistent changes in blood pressure.
- Take your temperature if you suspect you have a fever. If a fever is present, notify your physician or nurse.
- Weigh yourself every day at the same time of day and with the same amount of clothing; notify your primary health care provider or nurse if you have a sudden weight gain.
- Limit your intake of salt to help control your blood pressure once hyperfiltration is no longer a symptom of your disease (once chronic kidney disease [CKD] is present).
- Notify your primary health care provider or nurse if your urine smells foul or has a new occurrence of blood in it.
- Notify your primary health care provider or nurse if you have a headache that does not go away or if you have visual disturbances because these are symptoms of a stroke or bleeding in the brain.
- Monitor bowel movements to prevent constipation.

can prevent or reduce complications and acute kidney injury. Monitor serum creatinine levels because some antibiotics are nephrotoxic.

Percutaneous or surgical drainage of the cyst may be indicated. Prepare patients similarly as for kidney biopsy, described in Chapter 60.

Preventing Constipation. Teach the patient who has adequate urine output to prevent constipation by maintaining adequate fluid intake (generally 2 to 3 L daily in food and beverages), maintaining dietary fiber intake, and exercising regularly. Explain that pressure on the large intestine may occur as the polycystic kidneys increase in size. These recommendations for bowel management might change, particularly when ESKD develops. Advise the patient about the use of stool softeners and bulk agents, including careful use of laxatives, to prevent chronic constipation.

Slowing Progression of Chronic Kidney Disease. Early in the disease when patients have hyperfiltration with decreased urine concentration, nocturia, and low specific gravity, urge them to maintain adequate fluid intake to prevent dehydration, which can further reduce kidney function. Hyperfiltration may persist for several years. Maintaining adequate fluid intake can reduce the vasopressin release that reduces kidney blood flow. In patients with preserved kidney function, 3 L of fluid daily is recommended in order to slow cyst growth. Care must be taken to monitor for hyponatremia with excess water intake (Rizk, 2018).

As the disease progresses, protein intake may be limited to slow the development of ESKD. Help the patient and family understand the diet plan and why it was prescribed. Work closely with the dietitian to foster the patient's understanding.

Strategies for kidney protection include the use of a vasopressin-suppressing agent such as tolvaptan to improve blood flow, slow kidney volume growth, and sustain kidney function. Although pravastatin has shown beneficial effects on urinary albumin excretion, statins are not currently approved for treatment of PKD (Rizk, 2018).

Care Coordination and Transition Management

Health Care Resources. The PKD Foundation (www.pkdcure.org) and the National Kidney and Urologic Diseases Information Clearinghouse (NKUDIC) of the National Institute of Diabetes and Digestive and Kidney Diseases (www.niddk.nih.gov) conduct research and provide education about PKD. Many pamphlets are available; there is a fee for some materials. Chapters of the National Kidney Foundation (NKF) and the American Association of Kidney Patients (AAKP) also have resources for information and support.

HYDRONEPHROSIS AND HYDROURETER

Pathophysiology Review

Hydronephrosis and hydroureter are problems of urinary *elimination* with outflow obstruction. Urethral strictures obstruct urine outflow and may contribute to bladder distention, hydroureter, and hydronephrosis. Prompt recognition and treatment are crucial to preventing permanent kidney damage.

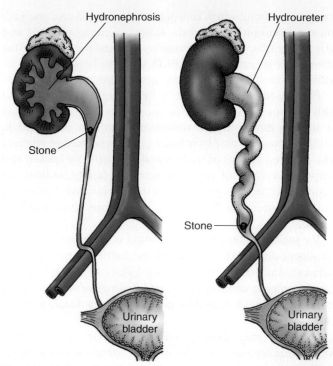

Fig. 62.5 Hydronephrosis is caused by obstruction in the upper part of the ureter. Hydroureter is caused by obstruction in the lower part of the ureter.

In **hydronephrosis**, the kidney enlarges as urine collects in the renal pelvis and kidney tissue. Because the capacity of the renal pelvis is normally 5 to 8 mL, obstruction in the renal pelvis or at the point where the ureter joins the renal pelvis quickly distends the renal pelvis. Kidney pressure increases as the volume of urine increases. Over time, sometimes in only a matter of hours, the blood vessels and kidney tubules can be damaged extensively (Fig. 62.5).

In patients with **hydroureter** (enlargement of the ureter), the effects are similar, but the obstruction is in the ureter rather than in the kidney. The ureter is most easily obstructed where the iliac vessels cross or where the ureters enter the bladder. Ureter dilation occurs above the obstruction and enlarges as urine collects (see Fig. 62.5).

Urinary obstruction causes damage when pressure builds up directly on kidney tissue. Tubular filtrate pressure also increases in the nephron as drainage through the collecting system is impaired and glomerular filtration decreases or ceases. Kidney necrosis can occur. Nitrogen waste products (urea, creatinine, and uric acid) and electrolytes (sodium, potassium, chloride, and phosphorus) are retained, and *acid-base balance* is impaired.

The cause of hydronephrosis or hydroureter is an obstruction, which can occur at any location between the collecting duct and the urethral meatus. Common causes of urinary obstruction include kidney stones, tumors, fibrosis, structural abnormalities, trauma, abscess, and cysts (Sutherland, 2018). With cancer, obstructed ureters may result from tumors pressing on the ureters, pelvic radiation, or surgical treatment. Early treatment of the causes can prevent ureteral problems and permanent kidney damage. The time needed to prevent permanent damage depends on the patient's kidney health. Permanent damage can occur in less than 48 hours in some patients and after several weeks in other patients.

❖ Interprofessional Collaborative Care

◆ **Assessment: Recognize Cues.** Obtain a history from the patient, focusing on known kidney or urologic disorders. A history of childhood urinary tract problems may indicate previously undiagnosed structural defects. Ask about his or her usual pattern of urinary *elimination,* especially amount, frequency, color, clarity, and odor. Ask about recent flank or abdominal pain. Chills, fever, and malaise may be present with a urinary tract infection (UTI).

Inspect each flank to identify asymmetry, which may occur with a kidney mass, and *gently* palpate the abdomen to locate areas of tenderness. Palpate the bladder to detect distention, or use a bedside bladder scanner (see Chapter 60). Gentle pressure on the abdomen may cause urine leakage, which reflects a full bladder and possible obstruction.

Urinalysis may show bacteria or white blood cells if infection is present. When urinary tract obstruction is prolonged, microscopic examination may show tubular epithelial cells. Blood chemistries are normal unless glomerular filtration has decreased and waste *elimination* is impaired. Blood creatinine and BUN levels increase with a reduced GFR. Serum electrolyte levels may be altered with elevated blood levels of potassium, phosphorus, and calcium along with a metabolic acidosis (bicarbonate deficit). Urinary outflow obstruction can be seen with ultrasound (US) or CT.

◆ **Interventions: Take Action.** Urinary retention and potential for infection are the primary problems. Failure to treat the cause of obstruction leads to infection and acute kidney injury (AKI).

Urologic Interventions. If obstruction is caused by a kidney stone (calculus), it can be located and removed using cystoscopic or retrograde urogram procedures. See Chapter 61 for more information about kidney stone management. After stone removal, a plastic stent is usually left in the ureter for a few weeks to improve urine flow in the area irritated by the stone. The stent is later removed by another cystoscopic procedure.

Radiologic Interventions. When an abnormal narrowing of the urinary tract (**stricture**) causes hydronephrosis and cannot be corrected with urologic procedures, a **nephrostomy** is performed. Most nephrostomy drains provide only external drainage (diversion). Other styles of nephrostomy drains enter the kidney and extend to the bladder, draining urine out to a bag or past a ureteral obstruction and into the bladder. With these, there are both internal and external parts to the nephrostomy tubing. Externally, a fully external or an internal/external diversion drain appears the same. The urine output will fluctuate more if all urine goes to the bladder before external drainage.

Patient Preparation. If possible, the patient is kept NPO for 4 to 6 hours before the procedure. Clotting studies (e.g., international normalized ratio [INR], prothrombin time [PT], and partial thromboplastic time [PTT]) should be normal or corrected. Drugs are used to reduce hypertension. The patient receives moderate sedation for the procedure.

Procedure. The patient is placed in the prone position. The kidney is located under ultrasound or fluoroscopic guidance, and a local anesthetic is given. A needle is placed into the kidney, a soft-tipped guidewire is placed through the needle, and then a catheter is placed over the wire. The catheter tip remains in the renal pelvis, and the external end is connected to a drainage bag. The procedure immediately relieves the pressure and prevents further damage. The nephrostomy tube remains in place until the obstruction is resolved.

Follow-up Care. Assess the amount of drainage in the collection bag. The amount of drainage depends on whether a ureteral catheter is also being used (with a separate drainage bag). Patients with ureteral tubes may have all urine pass through to the bladder or may have it drain into the collection bags. The type of urine drainage system placed must be clearly communicated in the chart. If urine is expected to drain into the collection bag, assess the amount of drainage hourly for the first 24 hours. If the amount of drainage decreases and the patient has back pain, the tube may be clogged or dislodged.

Monitor the nephrostomy site for leaking urine or blood. Urine drainage may be bloody for the first 12 to 24 hours after the procedure and should gradually clear. If prescribed, the nephrostomy tube can be irrigated with 5 mL sterile saline to check patency and dislodge clots. It is common for diuresis to occur when a nephrostomy is placed for obstruction. Monitor intake and output hourly for the first several hours, and inform the surgeon if the patient begins to have symptoms of dehydration (i.e., hypotension, poor skin turgor, dry mucous membranes, increased thirst). Assess for indications of infection (i.e., fever, change in urine character).

! NURSING SAFETY PRIORITY (QSEN)

Critical Rescue

After nephrostomy, monitor the patient for indications of complications (i.e., decreased or absent drainage, cloudy or foul-smelling drainage, leakage of blood or urine from the nephrostomy site, back pain) (Martin & Baker, 2019). If any indications are present, respond by notifying the surgeon immediately.

NCLEX EXAMINATION CHALLENGE 62.2

Physiological Integrity

The nurse is reviewing the client's laboratory data prior to a nephrostomy tube insertion. Which data requires the nurse to take action?

A. White blood cells in the urine
B. INR of 2.1
C. Hematocrit 44%
D. Creatinine 0.8 mg/dL

RENOVASCULAR DISEASE

Pathophysiology Review

Processes affecting the renal arteries may severely narrow the lumen and greatly reduce blood flow to the kidney tissues. Uncorrected renovascular disease, such as renal vein thrombosis

? CLINICAL JUDGMENT CHALLENGE 62.1

Patient-Centered Care; Safety

A 48-year-old client presents to the emergency department with fever, severe flank pain, and painful and restricted urinary output. The health care provider orders labs that reveal the following: creatinine 4.2 mg/dL; BUN 120 mg/dL; potassium 4.8 mEq/L; sodium 148 mEq/L. The client has a history of recurrent kidney infections and kidney stones. The client also has diabetes, anxiety, joint pain, and venous thrombosis. Current medications include metformin, escitalopram, daily vitamin supplement, and use of NSAIDs for muscular pain and associated joint pain and inflammation.

1. **Recognize Cues:** What assessment information in this client situation is the most important and immediate concern for the nurse? (Hint: Identify the **relevant** information *first* to determine what is most important.)

2. **Analyze Cues:** What client conditions are consistent with the **most relevant** information? (Hint: Think about priority collaborative problems that support and contradict the information presented in this situation.)

3. **Prioritize Hypotheses:** Which possibilities or explanations are **most likely** to be present in this client situation? Which possibilities or explanations are the most serious? (Hint: Consider all possibilities and determine their urgency and risk for this client.)

4. **Generate Solutions:** What actions would most likely achieve the desired outcomes for this client? Which actions should be **avoided** or are **potentially harmful**? (Hint: Determine the desired outcomes first to decide which interventions are appropriate and those that should be avoided.)

5. **Take Action:** Which actions are the most appropriate and how should they be implemented? In what **priority order** should they be implemented? (Hint: Consider health teaching, documentation, requested health care provider orders or prescriptions, nursing skills, collaboration with or referral to health team members, etc.)

6. **Evaluate Outcomes:** What client assessment would indicate that the nurse's actions were **effective?** (Hint: Think about signs that would indicate an improvement, decline, or unchanged client condition.)

or renal artery stenosis (RAS), atherosclerosis, or thrombosis, causes ischemia and atrophy of kidney tissue, leading to severe impairment of urinary *elimination, fluid and electrolyte balance,* and *acid-base balance.*

Patients with renovascular disease, particularly those older than 50 years, often have a sudden onset of hypertension. Patients with high blood pressure but no family history of hypertension also may potentially have RAS. RAS from atherosclerosis or blood vessel hyperplasia is the main cause of renovascular disease. Other causes include thrombosis and renal vessel aneurysms.

Atherosclerotic changes in the renal artery often occur along with sclerosis in the aorta and other major vessels. Renal artery changes are often located where the renal artery and aorta meet. Fibrotic changes of the blood vessel wall occur throughout the length of the renal artery.

◆ Interprofessional Collaborative Care

◆ **Assessment: Recognize Cues.** Hypertension usually first occurs after age 40 to 50, and often the patient does not have a family history of hypertension (see the Key Features: Renovascular Disease box). Diagnosis is made by magnetic resonance angiography (MRA), renal ultrasound, radionuclide imaging, or renal arteriography. MRA provides an excellent image of the renal vasculature and kidney anatomy. Radionuclide imaging is

▶▶ KEY FEATURES

Renovascular Disease

- Significant, difficult-to-control high blood pressure
- Poorly controlled diabetes or sustained hyperglycemia
- Elevated serum creatinine
- Decreased glomerular filtration rate (GFR)

a noninvasive way of evaluating kidney blood flow and excretory function. Combining radionuclide imaging with ingestion of an angiotensin-converting enzyme inhibitor (ACEi) such as lisinopril improves the accuracy of the test. A renal arteriogram makes the features of the renal blood vessels visible.

◆**Interventions: Take Action.** Identifying the type of defect, extent of narrowing, and condition of the surrounding blood vessels is critical for treatment choice, as is the patient's overall health. Many patients with renovascular disease also have cardiovascular disease, and both conditions require treatment.

RAS may be managed by drugs to control high blood pressure and by procedures to restore the blood supply to the kidney. Drugs may control high blood pressure but may not lead to long-term preservation of kidney function. In younger adults, a lifetime of treatment with many drugs for high blood pressure makes treatment difficult and outcomes uncertain.

Endovascular techniques are nonsurgical approaches to repair RAS. Stent placement with or without balloon angioplasty is an example of an endovascular intervention (see Chapter 33). These techniques are less risky and require less time for recovery than does renal artery bypass surgery. After the procedure, the patient usually remains under close observation for 24 hours to monitor for sudden blood pressure fluctuations as the kidneys adjust to increased blood flow.

Renal artery bypass surgery is a major procedure and requires 2 or more months for recovery. A bypass may be performed for either one or both renal arteries. A synthetic blood vessel graft is inserted to redirect blood flow from the abdominal aorta into the renal artery, beyond the area of narrowing. A splenorenal bypass can also restore blood flow to the kidney. The process is similar to other arterial bypass procedures (see Chapter 35).

DIABETIC NEPHROPATHY

Diabetic nephropathy is a vascular complication of diabetes mellitus (DM) and the leading cause of chronic kidney disease in the world. Approximately 40% of patients who are diabetic will develop diabetic kidney disease (Alicic, 2017). It occurs with either type 1 or type 2 DM. Severity of diabetic kidney disease is related to the degree of hyperglycemia the patient generally experiences. With poor control of hyperglycemia, the complicating problems of atherosclerosis, hypertension, and neuropathy (which promotes loss of bladder tone, urinary stasis, and urinary tract infection) are more severe and more likely to cause kidney damage. Chapter 59 discusses diabetic nephropathy. Management of diabetic nephropathy is the same as for chronic kidney disease (see Chapter 63).

TABLE 62.3 **Staging Kidney Tumors**
Stage I
Tumors <7 cm in largest dimension in the kidney. The renal vein, perinephric fat, and adjacent lymph nodes have no tumor.
Stage II
Tumors are >7 cm in largest dimension in the kidney. However, the tumor remains in the kidney with no lymph node involvement.
Stage III
Tumor has penetrated the major veins or perinephric tissues, yet not beyond Gerota fascia. Tumors extend into the lymph nodes but do have distant metastasis.
Stage IV
Tumors include invasion of adjacent organs beyond Gerota fascia or metastasis to distant tissues.

Adapted from Gallardo, E.A. (2017, November 13). *SEOM clinical guideline for treatment of kidney cancer.* Retrieved from U.S. National Library of Medicine, National Institutes of Health. https://www.ncbi.nlm.nih.gov/pmc/articles/PMC5785618/.

RENAL CELL CARCINOMA

Pathophysiology Review

Renal cell carcinoma (RCC) or adenocarcinoma of the kidney is the most common type of kidney cancer and occurs as a result of impaired cellular regulation. Healthy kidney tissue is damaged and replaced by cancer cells, which impairs urine *elimination* for that kidney.

Systemic effects occurring with this cancer type are called *paraneoplastic syndromes* and include anemia, erythrocytosis, hypercalcemia, liver dysfunction with elevated liver enzymes, hormonal effects, increased sedimentation rate, and hypertension.

Anemia and erythrocytosis may seem confusing; however, most patients with this cancer have *either* anemia *or* erythrocytosis, not both at the same time. There is some blood loss from hematuria, but the small amount lost does not cause anemia. The cause of the anemia and the erythrocytosis is related to kidney cell production of erythropoietin. At times, the tumor cells produce large amounts of erythropoietin, causing erythrocytosis. At other times, the tumor cells destroy the erythropoietin-producing kidney cells and anemia results.

Parathyroid hormone produced by tumor cells can cause hypercalcemia. Other hormone changes include increased renin levels (causing hypertension) and increased human chorionic gonadotropin (hCG) levels, which decrease libido and change secondary sex features.

RCC has five distinct carcinoma cell types: clear cell, papillary cell, chromophobe cell, collecting duct carcinoma, and unclassified type (McCance et al., 2019).

Kidney tumors are classified into four stages (Table 62.3). Complications include metastasis and urinary tract obstruction. The cancer usually spreads to the adrenal gland, liver, lungs, long bones, or the other kidney. When the cancer surrounds a ureter, hydroureter and obstruction may result.

The causes of nonhereditary RCC are unknown, but the risk is slightly higher for adults who use tobacco or are exposed to cadmium and other heavy metals, asbestos, benzene, and trichloroethylene. Men are slightly more likely to acquire RCC, as are persons with obesity, those with hypertension, and African Americans.

There are 73,750 new cases of kidney cancer in the United States each year (American Cancer Society [ACS], 2020a). Approximately 14,830 people die annually from kidney cancer in the United States. Kidney cancer is among the top 10 most common cancers in men and women, with the average age at diagnosis of 64 years. Kidney cancer is not common in people younger than 45 (ACS, 2020a).

❖ Interprofessional Collaborative Care

The most common treatment for RCC is a nephrectomy. When the cancer is local (i.e., only in the kidney), a nephrectomy can provide a cure. For patients with metastasis, nephrectomy is followed by targeted chemotherapy combined with cytokine treatment. Patients with RCC are at risk for CKD and cardiovascular complications. Patients need ongoing, interprofessional care with surveillance for best outcomes. Follow-up therapy is managed on an outpatient basis.

◆ Assessment: Recognize Cues

History. Ask the patient about his or her age, known risk factors (e.g., smoking or chemical exposures), weight loss, changes in urine color, abdominal or flank discomfort, and fever. Also ask whether any other family member has ever been diagnosed with cancer of the kidney, bladder, ureter, prostate gland, uterus, or ovary.

Physical Assessment/Signs and Symptoms. Some patients with RCC have flank pain, obvious blood in the urine, and a kidney mass that can be palpated. Ask about the nature of the flank or abdominal discomfort. Patients often describe the pain as dull and aching. Pain may be more intense if bleeding into the tumor or kidney occurs. Inspect the flank area, checking for asymmetry or an obvious bulge. An abdominal mass may be felt with *gentle* palpation. A renal bruit may be heard on auscultation.

Bloody urine is a *late* common sign. Blood may be visible as bright red flecks or clots, or the urine may appear smoky or cola colored. Without gross hematuria, microscopic examination may or may not reveal red blood cells (RBCs).

Inspect the skin for pallor, darkening of the nipples, and, in men, breast enlargement *(gynecomastia)* caused by changing hormone levels. Other findings may include muscle wasting, weakness, and weight loss. All tend to occur late in the disease.

Diagnostic Assessment. Urinalysis may show RBCs. Hematologic studies show decreased hemoglobin and hematocrit values, hypercalcemia, increased erythrocyte sedimentation rate, and increased levels of adrenocorticotropic hormone, human chorionic gonadotropin (hCG), cortisol, renin, and parathyroid hormone. Elevated serum creatinine and blood urea nitrogen (BUN) levels indicate impaired kidney function.

Kidney masses may be detected by CT scan or MRI. Ultrasound is also used to detect masses or for initial screening. Kidney biopsy may be considered to help target therapy.

◆ Interventions: Take Action. Treatment for kidney cancer focuses on preventing the spread of the cancer and managing

complications. Chemotherapy is not as effective when treating advanced kidney cancers. Targeted therapies that block the growth of new blood vessels that nourish cancer and immunotherapies can be effective (ACS, 2020b).

Nonsurgical Management. Microwave ablation (MWA) or cryoablation can slow tumor growth. It is a minimally invasive procedure carried out after MRI has precisely located the tumor. MWA is used most commonly for patients who have only one kidney or who are not surgical candidates.

Traditional chemotherapy has limited effectiveness against this cancer type. Use of biologic response modifiers (BRMs) such as interleukin-2 (IL-2), interferon (IFN), and tumor necrosis factor (TNF) has increased survival time (see Chapter 20) (ACS, 2020b).

Surgical Management. Renal cell carcinoma (RCC) is usually treated surgically by *nephrectomy* (kidney removal). Renal cell tumors are highly vascular, and blood loss during surgery is a major concern. Before surgery, the arteries supplying the kidney may be occluded (embolized) by the interventional radiologist to reduce bleeding during nephrectomy.

Preoperative Care. Instruct the patient about surgical routines (see Chapter 9). Explain the probable site of incision and the presence of dressings, drains, or other equipment after surgery. Reassure the patient about pain relief. Care before surgery may include giving blood and fluids IV to prevent shock.

Operative Procedures. The patient is placed on his or her side with the kidney to be removed uppermost. The trunk area is flexed to increase exposure of the kidney area. The eleventh or twelfth rib may need to be removed to provide better access to the kidney. The surgeon removes either part or all of the kidney and all visible tumor. The renal artery, renal vein, and fascia also may be removed. A drain may be placed in the wound before closure. The adrenal gland may be removed when the tumor is near this organ.

When a *radical* nephrectomy is performed, local and regional lymph nodes are also removed. The surgical approach may be transthoracic (as discussed in the previous paragraph), lumbar, or through the abdomen, depending on the size and location of the tumor. Radiation therapy may follow a radical nephrectomy.

Postoperative Care. Refer to Chapter 9 for care of the patient after surgery. Nursing priorities are focused on assessing kidney function to determine effectiveness of the remaining kidney, pain management, and preventing complications.

Monitoring includes assessing for hemorrhage and adrenal insufficiency. Inspect the patient's abdomen for distention from bleeding. Check the bed linens under the patient because blood may pool there. Hemorrhage or adrenal insufficiency causes hypotension, decreased urine output, and an altered level of consciousness.

A decrease in blood pressure is an early sign of both hemorrhage and adrenal insufficiency. With hypotension, urine output also decreases immediately. Large water and sodium losses in the urine occur in patients with adrenal insufficiency, leading to impaired **fluid and electrolyte balance.** As a result, a large urine output is followed by hypotension and oliguria (less than 400 mL/24 hr or less than 25 mL/hr). IV replacement of fluids and packed RBCs may be needed.

The second kidney is expected to provide adequate function, but this may take days or weeks. Assess urine output hourly for the first 24 hours after surgery (urine output of 0.5 mL/kg/hr or about 30 to 50 mL/hr is acceptable). A low urine output of less than 25 to 30 mL/hr suggests decreased blood flow to the remaining kidney and potential for acute kidney injury (AKI). The hemoglobin level, hematocrit values, and white blood cell count may be measured every 6 to 12 hours for the first day or two after surgery.

Monitor the patient's temperature, pulse rate, and respiratory rate at least every 4 hours. Accurately measure and record fluid intake and output. Weigh the patient daily.

The patient may be in a special care unit for 24 to 48 hours after surgery for monitoring of bleeding and adrenal insufficiency. A drain placed near the site of incision removes residual fluid. Because of the discomfort of deep breathing, the patient is at risk for atelectasis. Fever, chills, thick sputum, or decreased breath sounds suggest pneumonia.

Managing pain after surgery usually requires opioid analgesics given IV. The incision was made through major muscle groups used with breathing and movement. Liberal use of analgesics is needed for 3 to 5 days after surgery to manage pain. Oral agents may be tried when the patient can eat and drink.

Preventing complications focuses on infection and management of adrenal insufficiency. Antibiotics may be prescribed during and after surgery to prevent infection. The need for additional antibiotics is based on evidence of infection. Assess the patient at least every 8 hours for indications of systemic infection or local wound infection.

Adrenal insufficiency is possible as a complication of kidney and adrenal gland removal. Although only one adrenal gland may be affected, the remaining gland may not be able to secrete sufficient glucocorticoids immediately after surgery. Steroid replacements may be needed in some patients. Chapter 57 discusses the signs and symptoms of acute adrenal insufficiency in detail along with specific nursing interventions.

NCLEX EXAMINATION CHALLENGE 62.3

Physiological Integrity

The nurse is caring for a male client 8 hours after a nephrectomy. Which assessment data point requires **immediate** nursing intervention?

A. Abdominal distention
B. Urine output 38 mL in the last hour
C. Blood pressure 108/64 mm Hg
D. Hemoglobin 14 g/dL

KIDNEY TRAUMA

Pathophysiology Review

Trauma to one or both kidneys may occur with penetrating wounds or blunt injuries to the back, flank, or abdomen. Another cause of kidney trauma is urologic procedures. Blunt trauma accounts for most kidney injuries. Traumatic kidney injury is classified into five grades based on the severity of the injury. Grade 1 consists of low-grade injury in the form of kidney bruising, and grade 5 represents the most severe variety associated with shattering of the kidney and tearing of its blood

PATIENT AND FAMILY EDUCATION: PREPARING FOR SELF-MANAGEMENT

Preventing Kidney and Genitourinary Trauma

- Wear a seat belt.
- Practice safe walking habits.
- Use caution when riding bicycles and motorcycles.
- Wear appropriate protective clothing when participating in contact sports.
- Avoid all contact sports and high-risk activities if you have only one kidney.

supply. Adults of any age can sustain kidney trauma. Strategies to prevent trauma are reviewed in the Patient and Family Education: Preparing for Self-Management: Preventing Kidney and Genitourinary Trauma box.

◆ Interprofessional Collaborative Care

❖ **Assessment: Recognize Cues.** Obtain a history of the patient's usual health and the events involved in the trauma from the patient, a witness, or emergency personnel. Document the mechanism of injury to help determine the severity of the injury. For example, blunt trauma of the kidney from car crashes usually results in an injury of low severity. Critical information to acquire is a history of kidney or urologic disease, surgical intervention, or health problems such as diabetes or hypertension.

Ureteral or renal pelvic injury often causes diffuse abdominal pain. Urine outside of the urinary tract may be visible. Ask the patient about pain in the flank or abdomen.

Assess patients with kidney injuries carefully and thoroughly. Take the patient's blood pressure, apical and peripheral pulses, respiratory rate, and temperature. Inspect both flanks for bruising, asymmetry, or penetrating injuries. Also inspect the abdomen, chest, and lower back for bruising or wounds. Percuss the abdomen for distention. Inspect the urethra for blood.

Urinalysis shows hemoglobin or RBCs from tissue damage or kidney blood vessel rupture. Microscopic examination may also show red blood cell casts, which suggest tubular damage. Hemoglobin and hematocrit values decrease with blood loss.

Diagnostic procedures include ultrasound and CT. CT scan shows greater detail about blood vessel and tissue integrity. Hematomas within or through the kidney capsule can be seen, along with the integrity and patency of the urinary tract. If the patient is being taken to the operating room emergently, a high dose of ionic or nonionic IV contrast material can be given, followed by an abdominal x-ray (KUB) to visualize the traumatic injury and any organ damage.

❖ **Interventions: Take Action**

Nonsurgical Management. A combination of both drug and fluid therapy may be used to replace blood components and coagulation factors. Drug therapy is used for bleeding prevention or control. Fluid therapy is used to restore circulating blood volume and ensure adequate kidney blood flow. During fluid restoration, give fluids at the prescribed rate and monitor the patient for signs of shock. Take vital signs as often as every 5 to 15 minutes. Measure and record urine output hourly. Output should be greater than 0.5 mL/kg/hr.

The interventional radiologist may use percutaneous or other instrumentation to drain collections of fluid or to embolize (clot) an artery or artery segment or place a stent to repair the urethra or ureters.

! NURSING SAFETY PRIORITY (QSEN)

Action Alert

If the urethral opening is bleeding, consult with the urologist or primary health care provider before attempting urinary catheterization, to avoid making the injury worse.

Surgical Management. Most kidney injuries are managed without surgery. Many serious injuries can be treated with minimally invasive techniques such as angiographic embolization, which accesses the arteries of the kidneys through large blood vessels in the groin, similar to a cardiac catheterization. Surgery to explore the injured kidney occurs when the patient is in shock and may be losing a lot of blood from the kidney. Patients who have other significant abdominal injuries, such as injuries to the bowel, spleen, or liver, and require a laparotomy may also undergo inspection and repair of the injured kidney at the same time. The aim of surgical management is to repair the injured kidney and restore its **elimination** function. If the kidney is severely injured (grade 5 injury), a nephrectomy is performed.

Care Coordination and Transition Management. Teach the patient and family how to assess for infection and other complications following kidney trauma. The most common complications are urine leakage and delayed bleeding. Instruct the patient to check the pattern and frequency of urination and note whether the color, clarity, and amount appear normal. The development of an abscess surrounding the kidney also can occur. Instruct the patient to seek medical attention for worsening hematuria, any worrisome change, or pain with voiding. Chills, fever, lethargy, and cloudy, foul-smelling urine indicate a urinary tract infection or abscess formation. Traumatic kidney injury can also cause hypertension from changes in perfusion and activation of the renin-angiotensin-aldosterone system (see Chapter 60). Advise the patient to seek medical care promptly for all new and concerning signs or symptoms.

GET READY FOR THE NEXT-GENERATION NCLEX® EXAMINATION!

Key Points

Review these Key Points for each NCLEX Examination Client Needs Category.

Safe and Effective Care Environment

- Report any condition that obstructs urine flow. **QSEN: Safety**
- Check the blood pressure and urine output frequently in patients who have any type of kidney problem. **QSEN: Safety**
- Report immediately to the primary health care provider sudden decreases of urine output in a patient with kidney disease or trauma. Expected adult urine output is 0.5 to 1 mL/kg/hr. **QSEN: Safety**
- Teach patients with any kidney disorder about strategies to prevent kidney damage from dehydration or trauma. **QSEN: Safety**
- Instruct patients with any type of kidney problem to weigh daily and to notify the primary health care provider if there is a sudden weight gain. **QSEN: Patient-Centered Care**

Health Promotion and Maintenance

- Refer patients with polycystic kidney disease to a geneticist or a genetic counselor. **QSEN: Patient-Centered Care**
- Refer patients to community resources, support groups, and information organizations such as the National Kidney Foundation, the PKD Foundation, and the American Association of Kidney Patients. **QSEN: Patient-Centered Care**
- Encourage patients with diabetes to achieve tight glycemic control. **QSEN: Patient-Centered Care**
- Encourage patients with hypertension to follow their treatment regimens to maintain proper blood pressure **QSEN: Evidence-Based Practice**
- Teach patients to match daily urine output with fluid intake, usually at least 2 liters for kidney health unless another health problem requires fluid restriction. **QSEN: Evidence-Based Practice**

Psychosocial Integrity

- Allow the patient to express fear or anxiety regarding the potential for chronic kidney disease and end-stage kidney disease. **QSEN: Patient-Centered Care**
- Assess the patient's level of comfort in discussing issues related to *elimination* and the genitourinary area. **QSEN: Patient-Centered Care**
- Use language with which the patient is comfortable during assessment of the kidney and urinary system. **QSEN: Patient-Centered Care**
- Explain treatment procedures to patients and families. **QSEN: Patient-Centered Care**

Physiological Integrity

- Teach patients the expected side effects and any adverse reactions to prescribed drugs, especially as they relate to kidney function. **QSEN: Patient-Centered Care**
- Teach patients the indications of disease recurrence and when to seek medical help. **QSEN: Patient-Centered Care**
- Teach patients on antibiotic therapy for a UTI (pyelonephritis) to complete the drug regimen. **QSEN: Evidence-Based Practice**
- Explain the genetics of autosomal dominant polycystic kidney disease.
- Use laboratory data and signs and symptoms to determine the effectiveness of therapy for pyelonephritis, polycystic kidney disease, glomerulonephritis (GN), and renal cell carcinoma (RCC).
- Be aware of the signs and symptoms of hydronephrosis.
- Be aware of the relation between kidney disease and hypertension and the associated risk for cardiovascular events.

MASTERY QUESTIONS

1. Which question will the nurse ask the client who has a urinary tract infection to assess the risk for pyelonephritis?
   A. "What drugs do you take for asthma?"
   B. "How long have you had diabetes?"
   C. "How much fluid do you drink daily?"
   D. "Do you take your antihypertensive drugs at night or in the morning?"

2. When assessing a client with acute glomerulonephritis, which question will the nurse ask to determine if the client is following best practices to slow progression of kidney damage?
   A. "Do you avoid contact sports while you are taking cyclosporine?"
   B. "How are you evaluating the amount of daily fluid you drink?"
   C. "Have you contacted anyone from our dialysis support services?"
   D. "Have you increased your protein intake to promote healing of the damaged nephrons?"

3. When providing care to a client who has undergone a nephrostomy for hydronephrosis, which observation alerts the nurse to a possible complication? **Select all that apply.**
   A. Urine output of 15 mL for the first hour and then diminishing
   B. Tenderness at the surgical site
   C. Pink-tinged urine draining from the nephrostomy
   D. A hematocrit value 3% lower than the preoperative value
   E. Sudden onset of abdominal pain that worsens after abdominal palpation
   F. Blood pressure of 180/90 mm Hg that persists despite administration of pain medication

REFERENCES

Alicic, R. Z. (2017). Diabetic kidney disease. *Clinical Journal of the American Society of Nephrology*, 2032–2045.

American Cancer Society. (2020a). *Key Statistics about kidney cancer.* Retrieved from American Cancer Society: https://www.cancer.org/cancer/kidney-cancer/about/key-statistics.html.

American Cancer Society. (2020b). *Targeted therapies for kidney cancer.* Retrieved from American Cancer Society: https://www.cancer.org/cancer/kidney-cancer/treating/targeted-therapy.html.

Crawford, B. S. (2018). Genetics and kidney disease (APOL1). In S. W. Gilbert (Ed.), *Primer on kidney diseases* (pp. 356–360). Philadelphia: Elsevier.

Gallardo, E. A. (2017). *SEOM clinical guideline for treatment of kidney cancer.* Retrieved from US National Library of Medicine National Institute of Health. https://www.ncbi.nlm.nih.gov/pmc/articles/PMC5785618/.

Holt, N. (2018). Renal disease. In R. Hines (Eds.), *stoelting's anesthesia and co-existing disease* (7th ed.) (pp. 425–448). Philadelphia: Elsevier.

Jarvis, C. (2019). *Physical examination and health assessment.* Philadelphia: Elsevier.

Martin, R., & Baker, H. (2019). Nursing care and management of patients with a nephrostomy. *Nursing Times [Online]*, *115*(11), 40–43. Retrieved from: https://www.nursingtimes.net/clinical-archive/patient-safety/nursing-care-and-management-of-patients-with-a-nephrostomy-14-10-2019/.

McCance, K., Huether, S., Brashers, V., & Rote, N. (2019). *Pathophysiology: The biologic basis for disease in adults and children* (8th ed.). St. Louis: Mosby.

Muthu, V. R. (2018). *Clinicopathological spectrum of glomerular diseases in adolescents: A single-center experience over 4 Years.* Retrieved from US National Library of Medicine National Institute of Health. https://www.ncbi.nlm.nih.gov/pmc/articles/PMC5930804/

National Institute of Diabetes and Digestive and Kidney Diseases. (2016). *Kidney disease Statistics for the United States.* Retrieved from https://www.niddk.nih.gov/health-information/health-statistics/kidney-disease.

National Institute of Diabetes and Digestive and Kidney Diseases. (2018). *U.S. Department of health and human services.* Retrieved from Kidney Infection (Pyelonephritis): https://www.niddk.nih.gov/health-information/urologic-diseases/kidney-infection-pyelonephritis.

National Kidney Foundation. (2019). *Polycystic kidney disease.* Retrieved from National Kidney Foundation: https://www.kidney.org/atoz/content/polycystic.

Nicolle, L. E. (2018). Urinary tract infection and pyelonephritis. In S. J. Gilbert (Ed.), *National kidney Foundation's primer on kidney diseases* (pp. 427–434). Philadelphia: Elsevier.

Patel, N. P. (2018). *Infection-induced kidney diseases.* Retrieved from US National Library of Medicine National Institute of Health. https://www.ncbi.nlm.nih.gov/pmc/articles/PMC6282040/.

Raman, M. G. (2018). Comparing the impact of older age on outcome in chronic kidney disease of different etiologies: A prospective cohort study. *Journal of Nephrology*, 931–939.

Rizk, D. R. (2018). Polycystic and other cystic kidney diseases. In S. W. Gilbert (Ed.), *National kidney Foundation's primer on kidney diseases* (pp. 375–384). Philadelphia: Elsevier.

Sutherland, R. W. (2018). Obstructive uropathy. In S. W. Gilbert (Ed.), *National kidney Foundation's primer on kidney diseases* (pp. 412–419). Philadelphia: Elsevier.

Trachtman, H. H. (2018). Minimal change nephrotic syndrome. In S. W. Gilbert (Ed.), *National kidney Foundation's primer on kidney diseases* (pp. 175–180). Philadelphia: Elsevier.

University of Pennsylvania. (2019). *Glomerular diseases.* Retrieved from Penn Medicine: https://www.pennmedicine.org/for-patients-and-visitors/find-a-program-or-service/kidney/glomerular-diseases-clinic

63

Concepts of Care for Patients With Acute Kidney Injury and Chronic Kidney Disease

Robyn Mitchell

http://evolve.elsevier.com/Iggy/

LEARNING OUTCOMES

1. Collaborate with the interprofessional team to coordinate high-quality care and promote urinary *elimination* in patients who have acute kidney injury or chronic kidney disease.
2. Teach the patient and caregiver(s) about home safety issues affected by impaired *elimination* and impairment of *fluid and electrolyte balance* or *acid-base balance* resulting from acute kidney injury or chronic kidney disease.
3. Prioritize evidence-based care for patients with impaired urinary *elimination* from either acute kidney injury or chronic renal failure.
4. Identify community resources for patients requiring assistance with management of altered *elimination* as a result of acute kidney injury or chronic kidney disease.
5. Teach adults how to decrease the risk for acute kidney injury or chronic kidney disease.
6. Implement evidence-based nursing interventions to help patients and families cope with the psychosocial impact caused by acute kidney injury or chronic kidney disease.
7. Apply knowledge of anatomy and pathophysiology to assess patients with impaired kidney function from acute kidney injury or chronic kidney disease.
8. Teach the patient and caregiver(s) about common drugs and other strategies used for acute kidney injury and chronic kidney disease.
9. Implement evidence-based nursing interventions to prevent complications in patients undergoing kidney replacement therapy.
10. Use clinical judgment to analyze information from laboratory data and assessment findings in the care of patients with acute kidney injury and chronic kidney disease.

KEY TERMS

acute kidney injury (AKI) A rapid reduction in kidney function resulting in a failure to maintain waste *elimination, fluid and electrolyte balance,* and *acid-base balance.*

azotemia An excess of nitrogenous wastes (urea) in the blood.

cardiorenal syndrome Disorders of the kidney or heart that cause dysfunction in the other organ.

dialysate Solution used in dialysis that contains a balanced mix of electrolytes and water and that closely resembles human plasma.

diffusion Movement of molecules from an area of higher concentration to an area of lower concentration.

hyperpnea Abnormal increase in the depth of respiratory movements.

Kussmaul respiration Breathing pattern with respirations that are fast and deep; often associated with metabolic acidosis.

melena Blood in the stool with the appearance of black, tarry stool.

oliguria Urine output less than 400 mL/day.

pruritus Itching.

renal osteodystrophy Bone metabolism and structural damage caused by chronic kidney disease–induced low calcium levels and high phosphorus levels.

uremia The accumulation of nitrogenous wastes in the blood (azotemia); a result of renal failure, with clinical symptoms that include nausea and vomiting.

uremic frost Layer of urea crystals from evaporated sweat; may appear on the face, eyebrows, axillae, and groin in patients with advanced uremic syndrome.

uremic syndrome The systemic clinical and laboratory manifestations of end-stage kidney disease.

The kidney function of urinary *elimination* includes excretion of waste, *fluid and electrolyte balance,* regulation of *acid-base balance,* and hormone secretion. These processes are greatly impaired with kidney function loss, and every organ system is affected. Acute kidney injury (AKI) is most common in the acute care setting, whereas chronic kidney disease (CKD) is more likely to be seen in community settings or as a coexisting condition in acute care settings. The features of AKI and CKD are described in Table 63.1.

Both types of kidney problems can require kidney replacement therapy (KRT; e.g., dialysis). When kidney function is permanently or persistently impaired, as with end-stage kidney disease (ESKD), dialysis or kidney transplant is a lifesaving approach for urinary *elimination* to maintain homeostasis, *fluid and electrolyte balance,* and *acid-base balance.* ESKD reduces independence, shortens life, and decreases quality of life. Many diseases and conditions are associated with the onset and severity of kidney function loss.

When kidney function declines gradually, it is diagnosed as CKD, formerly termed *chronic renal failure (CRF).* The patient may have many years of abnormal blood urea nitrogen (BUN) and creatinine values, sometimes called *renal insufficiency,* before ESKD develops. When kidney function decline is sudden, acute kidney injury (AKI) is diagnosed. AKI can be a temporary condition that resolves, or it can progress to CKD.

Even when AKI does not progress to CKD, AKI is associated with higher morbidity and mortality, even in young patients without other chronic diseases that increase risks (Fuhrman, 2018). AKI also can occur in a patient with established CKD. When these two conditions co-occur, the loss of kidney function and waste *elimination* is usually more severe and accelerated.

Acute kidney injury affects *many* body systems. Chronic kidney disease affects *every* body system. The problems that occur with kidney function loss are related to disturbances of *fluid and electrolyte balance,* disturbances of *acid-base balance,* buildup of nitrogen-based wastes (uremia), and loss of kidney hormone function.

ACUTE KIDNEY INJURY

Pathophysiology Review

Acute kidney injury (AKI) is a rapid reduction in kidney function resulting in a failure to maintain waste *elimination, fluid and electrolyte balance,* and *acid-base balance.* AKI occurs over a few hours or days. The most current definition of AKI is an increase in serum creatinine by 0.3 mg/dL (26.2 mcmol/L) or more within 48 hours; or an increase in serum creatinine to 1.5 times or more from baseline, which is known or presumed to have occurred in the previous 7 days; or a urine volume of less than 0.5 mL/kg/hr for 6 hours (Gilbert & Weiner, 2018). Criteria for staging the severity of AKI are in Table 63.2. The Kidney Disease: Improving Global Outcomes (KDIGO) classification is a universal definition and staging system for AKI.

The creatinine level is most commonly used in the recognition of AKI. However, this value is not ideal because the creatinine level takes time to increase, which can create delays in treatment. A baseline creatinine value is also necessary to evaluate for AKI, as this provides a means for comparison.

Biomarkers that are specific to kidney injury have been approved by the Food and Drug Administration (FDA) (Gilbert & Weiner, 2018). These biomarkers indicate damage earlier than the creatinine level and do not require a baseline value for comparison. These biomarkers specific to kidney injury can be used similarly to biomarkers such as troponin in cardiac injury. These biomarkers can identify patients at high risk for developing AKI during the next 12 to 24 hours and include tissue injury metalloproteinase 2 (TIMP-2) and insulin-like growth factor binding protein 7 (IGFBP-7) (Moore, 2018). Earlier identification of risk allows for earlier intervention. Although these biomarkers show significant promise, they are not yet widely used.

Glomerular filtration rate (GFR) is accepted as the best overall indicator of kidney function, but it is not accurate during acute and critical illness (Gilbert & Weiner, 2018). Estimations of GFR from serum creatinine are affected by metabolic problems and treatments during critical illnesses. Urine output is altered when diuretics or IV fluids are used. AKI also causes systemic effects and complications described in Table 63.3. These complications increase discomfort and risk for death. Duration of oliguria or anuria closely correlates with lack of recovery of kidney function; the longer the duration of oliguria or anuria, the less likely it is that the patient will return to full or baseline kidney function.

Etiology. The causes of AKI are reduced *perfusion* to the kidneys, damage to kidney tissue, and obstruction of urine outflow. Urine outflow obstruction along with tissue damage of the kidneys and reduction of perfusion are causes of AKI. Table 63.4 lists causes of AKI along with the diseases and associated conditions. However, the diseases listed in Table 63.3 are described in greater detail in another section of this text. Risk factors for AKI include shock, cardiac surgery, hypotension, prolonged mechanical ventilation, and sepsis. Older adults or adults with diabetes, hypertension, peripheral vascular disease, liver disease, or CKD are at higher risk of AKI if hospitalized.

AKI is categorized as prerenal, intrinsic renal (also called intrarenal), and postrenal in order to better understand and treat the disorder. Prerenal AKI is caused by a source outside of the kidney creating conditions that impair renal *perfusion.* Common causes include shock, dehydration, burns, and sepsis. Intrinsic renal injury occurs inside the kidney by disorders that directly affect the renal cortex or medulla. Examples of disorders causing intrinsic renal AKI include allergic disorders, embolism or thrombosis of

TABLE 63.1 Features of Acute Kidney Injury and Chronic Kidney Disease

Characteristic	Acute Kidney Injury	Chronic Kidney Disease
Onset	Sudden (hours to days)	Gradual (months to years)
Percentage of nephron involvement	50%-95%	Varies by stage; generally symptomatic with 75% loss and dialysis with 90%-95% loss
Duration	May not progress; full recovery (return to baseline) possible ESKD occurs in 10%-20% with lifetime reliance on dialysis or kidney transplant	Progressive and permanent Treatment and lifestyle can slow progression and delay onset of ESKD
Prognosis	Good when kidney function is maintained or returns High mortality associated with renal replacement therapy requirements or prolonged illness	Progression of CKD depends on stage of GFR, stage of albuminuria, and specific conditions associated with the onset of the disorder ESKD fatal without a renal replacement therapy (dialysis or transplantation) Reduced life span and potential for complex medical regimen even with optimal treatment

CKD, Chronic kidney disease; *ESKD*, end-stage kidney disease; *GFR*, glomerular filtration rate.

TABLE 63.2 The KDIGO Classification System for Severity of Acute Kidney Injury

Stage	Serum Creatinine	Urine Output
Stage 1	1.5-1.9 times baseline OR ≥0.3 mg/dL (≥26.5 mmol/L) increase over 48 hr	<0.5 mL/kg/hr for 6-12 hr
Stage 2	2.0-2.9 times baseline	<0.5 mL/kg/hr for ≥12 hr
Stage 3	1.0 times baseline OR Increase in serum creatinine to ≥4.0 mg/dL (≥353.6 mmol/L) OR Initiation of renal replacement therapy OR In patients <18 years, decrease in eGFR to <35 mL/min/1.73 m²	Anuria lasting for ≥12 hr OR <0.3 mL/kg/hr for >24 hr

eGFR, Estimated glomerular filtration rate; *KDIGO*, Kidney Disease: Improving Global Outcomes (2012).

TABLE 63.3 Systemic Complications From Acute Kidney Injury

Metabolic
- Metabolic acidosis
- Hyperlipidemia
- Hyperkalemia
- Hyponatremia
- Hypocalcemia
- Hypophosphatemia

Cardiopulmonary
- Peripheral and pulmonary edema
- Heart failure
- Pulmonary embolism
- Pericarditis
- Pericardial effusion
- Hypertension
- Myocardial infarction

Neurologic
- Neuromuscular irritability or weakness
- Asterixis
- Seizures
- Mental status changes

Immune/Infectious
- Pneumonia
- Sepsis

Gastrointestinal
- Nausea
- Vomiting
- Decreased peristalsis
- Enteral nutrition intolerance
- Malnutrition
- Ulcer formation
- Bleeding

Hematologic
- Bleeding
- Thrombosis
- Anemia

Renal
- Chronic kidney disease (CKD)
- End-stage kidney disease (ESKD)

Other
- Hiccups
- Elevated parathyroid hormone
- Low thyroid hormone level

the renal vessels, and nephrotoxic agents. Postrenal AKI is caused by a urine flow obstruction. The obstruction can be caused by tumors, kidney stones, or strictures (McCance et al., 2019).

With prerenal or postrenal pathology, the kidney compensates with the three responses of constricting kidney blood vessels, activating the renin-angiotensin-aldosterone pathway, and releasing antidiuretic hormone (ADH). These responses increase blood volume and improve kidney *perfusion.* However, these same responses reduce urine *elimination,* resulting in oliguria (urine output less than 400 mL/day) and azotemia (the retention and buildup of nitrogenous wastes in the blood). Toxins can also cause blood vessel constriction in the kidney, leading to reduced kidney blood flow, oliguria, and azotemia.

Activated *immunity* and damage from kidney toxins (nephrotoxins) (Table 63.5) cause intracellular changes of the tubular system in kidney tissue. Inflammatory proteins and immune-mediated complexes can damage cells and tissues in the kidney. With extensive damage, tubular cells slough and nephrons lose the ability to repair themselves. The presence of tubular debris and sediment in urine from kidney tissue damage (intrarenal failure or *acute tubular necrosis*) is related to systemic ischemia, reduced kidney *perfusion,* or nephrotoxin exposure.

Even with severe AKI (i.e., stage 2 or 3 in Table 63.2), some adults return to baseline kidney function during recovery from illness. It is the responsibility of all health care professionals to be alert to the possibility of AKI and implement prevention strategies when risk factors are present. *Timely interventions to remove*

TABLE 63.4 Diseases and Conditions That Contribute to Acute Kidney Injury

Perfusion Reduction (Prerenal Causes)

- Blood or fluid loss
- Blood pressure medications
- Heart attack
- Heart disease
- Infection (e.g., sepsis, septic shock)
- Liver failure
- Use of aspirin, ibuprofen, naproxen, or other related drugs
- Severe allergic reaction (anaphylaxis)
- Severe burns
- Severe dehydration
- Renal artery stenosis
- Bleeding or clotting in the kidney blood vessels (coagulopathy)
- Atherosclerosis or cholesterol deposits that block blood flow in the kidneys

Kidney Damage (Intrinsic or Intrarenal Causes)

- Blood clots in nearby veins and arteries
- Cholesterol deposits that block blood flow in the kidneys
- Glomerulonephritis
- Hemolytic uremic syndrome
- Local infection (pyelonephritis)
- Lupus, an immune system disorder causing glomerulonephritis
- Pharmaceuticals, such as certain chemotherapy agents, antibiotics, iodinated or hyperosmolar contrast media used during imaging tests
- Scleroderma, a group of rare diseases affecting the skin and connective tissues
- Thrombotic thrombocytopenic purpura (TTP), a rare platelet disorder that increases clotting

Urine Flow Obstruction (Postrenal Causes)

- Bladder cancer
- Cervical cancer
- Colon cancer
- Prostate cancer
- Enlarged prostate
- Kidney stones
- Nerve damage involving the nerves that control the bladder
- Blood clots in the urinary tract

TABLE 63.5 Examples of Potentially Nephrotoxic Substances

Drugs

Antibiotics/Antimicrobials

- Amphotericin B
- Colistimethate
- Polymyxin B
- Rifampin
- Sulfonamides
- Tetracycline hydrochloride
- Vancomycin

Aminoglycoside Antibiotics

- Gentamicin
- Neomycin
- Tobramycin

Chemotherapy Agents

- Cisplatin
- Cyclophosphamide
- Methotrexate

NSAIDs

- Celecoxib
- Flurbiprofen
- Ibuprofen
- Indomethacin
- Ketorolac
- Meloxicam
- Nabumetone
- Naproxen
- Oxaprozin
- Tolmetin

Other Drugs

- Acetaminophen
- Captopril
- Cyclosporine
- Fluorinate anesthetics
- Metformin
- Quinine

Other Substances

Organic Solvents

- Carbon tetrachloride
- Ethylene glycol

Nondrug Chemical Agents

- Radiographic contrast media (e.g., iodinated media, hyperosmolar media, and gadolinium)
- Pesticides
- Fungicides
- Myoglobin (from breakdown of skeletal muscle)

Heavy Metals and Ions

- Arsenic
- Bismuth
- Copper sulfate
- Gold salts
- Lead
- Mercuric chloride

Nurses have an essential role in the prevention of AKI in hospitalized patients. Always be on the lookout for signs of impending kidney dysfunction through assessment and close monitoring of laboratory values. Early recognition and correction of problems causing reduced urinary *elimination* may avoid kidney tissue damage. Evaluate the patient's fluid status. Accurately measure intake and output and check body weight to identify changes in fluid balance. Note the characteristics of the urine and report new sediment, hematuria (smoky or red color), foul odor, or other worrisome changes. Report a urine output of less than 30 mL/hr for 2 hours or dark amber urine to the primary health care provider (Jarvis & Eckhardt, 2020). Waiting for 6 hours of oliguria to meet AKI criteria may allow progression of kidney damage—act early!

! NURSING SAFETY PRIORITY (QSEN)

Critical Rescue

In any acute care setting, preventing volume depletion and providing intervention early when volume depletion occurs are nursing priorities. Reduced *perfusion* from volume depletion is a common cause of AKI. Assess continually to recognize the signs and symptoms of volume depletion (low urine output, decreased systolic blood pressure, decreased pulse pressure, orthostatic hypotension, thirst, rising blood osmolarity). Respond by intervening early with oral fluids or, in the patient who is unable to take or tolerate oral fluid, requesting an increase in IV fluid rate from the primary health care provider to prevent permanent kidney damage.

---

the cause of AKI may prevent progression to ESKD and the need for lifelong renal replacement therapy (RRT) or a renal transplant.

Incidence and Prevalence. Twenty percent of all hospitalized patients and 60% of intensive care unit patients develop AKI. AKI is increasingly recognized as an in-hospital complication that is associated with shock, heart conditions, and surgery (Pavkov et al., 2018). Patients who are older or who have chronic kidney disease or diabetes are at greater risk for AKI.

Health Promotion and Maintenance. *Keep in mind that dehydration (severe blood volume depletion) reduces* **perfusion** *and can lead to AKI even in adults who have no known kidney problems.* Urge all healthy adults to avoid dehydration by drinking 2 to 3 L of water daily. This is especially important for athletes or anyone who performs strenuous exercise or work and sweats heavily.

Monitor laboratory values for any changes that reflect poor kidney function. A significant increase in creatinine, especially when the increase occurs over hours or a few days, is a concern and must be reported urgently to the primary health care provider. Other laboratory values that help monitor kidney function include serum blood urea nitrogen (BUN); serum potassium, sodium, and osmolarity; and urine specific gravity, albumin-creatinine ratio, and electrolytes. Know the baseline (steady-state) GFR because a reduced GFR makes the patient more vulnerable to AKI.

Be aware of nephrotoxic substances that the patient may ingest or be exposed to (see Table 63.5). Question any prescription for potentially nephrotoxic drugs, and validate the dose before the patient receives the drug. Many antibiotics have nephrotoxic effects. NSAIDs can cause or increase the risk for AKI. Combining two or more nephrotoxic drugs dramatically increases the risk for AKI. If a patient must receive a known nephrotoxic drug, closely monitor laboratory values, including BUN, creatinine, and drug peak and trough levels, for indications of reduced kidney function. When a nephrotoxic agent such as contrast medium will be used, additional nephrotoxic medications such as metformin should be withheld at least 24 hours before and after the procedure, if possible. Intravenous fluids should be administered before and after exposure to the contrast medium (Moore, 2018).

❖ Interprofessional Collaborative Care

AKI is managed initially in the hospital setting, most commonly in an ICU. During the acute phase of the problem, members of the interprofessional team include the nephrologist, nephrology nurse, registered dietitian nutritionist (RDN), pharmacist, and dialysis technician. The responsibilities of each of these professionals are described within the interventions sections of this chapter. When the patient is discharged before urinary *elimination* returns to normal, continuing management is needed as part of the transition to community care.

◆ Assessment: Recognize Cues

History. The accurate diagnosis of AKI, including its cause, depends on a detailed history. Know the risk factors for and criteria of AKI and chronic kidney disease (CKD). Ask about any change in urine appearance, frequency, or volume.

Ask about recent surgery or trauma, transfusions, allergic (hypersensitivity) reactions, or other factors that might lead to reduced kidney *perfusion.* Obtain a drug history, especially use of antibiotics and NSAIDs. Ask about recent imaging procedures requiring injection of a contrast medium. Coexisting conditions of advanced age, chronic kidney disease, diabetes, long-term hypertension, major or systemic infection (sepsis), peripheral vascular disease, chronic liver disease, acquired immune deficiency syndrome (AIDS [HIV-III]) and prior kidney surgery increase the risk for AKI (Gilbert & Weiner, 2018).

To identify *immunity*-mediated AKI (i.e., acute glomerulonephritis), ask about acute illnesses such as influenza, colds, gastroenteritis, and sore throats. Allergic reactions from a drug or food allergy may result in AKI as late as 10 days after exposure.

Ask about rashes, hives, or fever and evaluate the white blood cell (WBC) differential for an increased eosinophil count.

Anticipate AKI following any episode of hypotension or shock. Any problem in which the blood volume is depleted can contribute to AKI by reducing *perfusion.* Such problems include cardiac bypass surgery, extensive bowel preparations, being NPO before surgery, or dehydration from exercise. Recent use of IV vasopressors (e.g., epinephrine or norepinephrine) may contribute to AKI when blood volume is reduced (hypovolemia).

Consider whether there is a history of urinary obstructive problems. Ask the patient about any difficulty in starting the urine stream, changes in the amount or appearance of the urine, narrowing of the urine stream, nocturia, urgency, or symptoms of kidney stones. Also ask about any cancer history that may cause urinary obstruction.

👤 PATIENT-CENTERED CARE: OLDER ADULT CONSIDERATIONS (QSEN)

AKI is more common as people age. People aged 80 to 89 years of age are 55% more likely to develop AKI than people under age 50. As the kidneys age, structural and functional changes occur including fewer nephrons and sclerosis of glomeruli and the renal arteries. These changes lead to an increased risk for AKI. Older adults also have more comorbid conditions such as diabetes, hypertension, and chronic kidney disease (Johnson et al., 2019).

Further increasing the risk of AKI in the older adult is an increased exposure to nephrotoxic drugs. The use of multiple drugs is associated with drug-induced AKI, particularly in acute and critical care settings. Assess risk and take actions to reduce exposure to nephrotoxic agents, avoid hypotension and hypovolemia, evaluate drug-drug interactions for potential adverse kidney effects, and stop unnecessary drugs to maintain kidney function in older adults.

Physical Assessment/Signs and Symptoms. If a patient has a urinary catheter, assess urine output every hour after surgery until stable, during fluid resuscitation for shock or hypotension, and when the patient has a high risk for AKI following hospital admission. Even a brief period of oliguria, defined as less than 0.5 mL/kg/hr of urine output for 2 or more hours, can signal AKI.

Other symptoms of AKI are related to the buildup of nitrogenous wastes (azotemia) and decreased urine output (oliguria). As AKI progresses in severity, the patient may have symptoms of fluid overload because fluid is not eliminated. Indications of fluid overload include pulmonary crackles, dependent and generalized edema *(anasarca),* decreased oxygenation (low peripheral oxygenation or SpO_2), confusion, increased respiratory rate, and dyspnea. See Chapter 13 for assessment of fluid overload.

Evaluate vital signs to recognize early hypoperfusion and hypoxemia. Symptoms of reduced blood volume such as mean arterial pressure (MAP) below 65 mm Hg, tachycardia, thready peripheral pulses, or decreasing cognition may indicate risk for AKI from poor *perfusion*; an SpO_2 below 88% may indicate potential hypoxemic or ischemic damage to kidney tissue.

Laboratory Assessment. The many changes in laboratory values in the patient with AKI are similar to those occurring in chronic kidney disease (CKD). (See the Laboratory Profile:

Kidney Disease box.) Expect to see rising creatinine and BUN levels and abnormal blood electrolyte values. However, patients with AKI usually do *not* have the anemia associated with CKD unless there is blood loss from another condition (e.g., surgery, trauma) or when BUN levels are high enough to break (lyse) red blood cells (RBCs).

In early AKI, urine tests provide important information. Urine sodium levels may reflect an inability to concentrate urine. Urine may be dilute with a specific gravity near 1.000 or concentrated with a specific gravity greater than 1.030. The presence of urine sediment (e.g., RBCs, casts, and tubular cells), myoglobin, or hemoglobin may lead to nephron damage.

Imaging Assessment. Ultrasonography is useful in the diagnosis of kidney and urinary tract obstruction. Dilation of the renal calyces and collecting ducts, as well as stones, can be detected. Ultrasonography can show kidney size and patency of the ureters. Small kidney size may indicate an underlying CKD with loss of kidney tissue.

CT scans without contrast medium can determine adequacy of kidney *perfusion* and identify obstruction or tumors. Contrast medium is usually avoided to prevent further kidney damage (Lambert et al., 2017). An MRI may be used in place of a CT scan.

X-rays of the pelvis or kidneys, ureters, and bladder (KUB) may provide an initial view of kidneys and the urinary tract to determine the cause of AKI. Enlarged kidneys with obstruction may show hydronephrosis. X-rays can show stones obstructing the renal pelvis, ureters, or bladder. More commonly, ultrasound is used to screen for hydronephrosis.

A nuclear medicine study called *MAG3* may be used to determine the nature of the kidney failure and measure GFR. A renal scan can determine whether *perfusion* of the kidneys is sufficient. Cystoscopy or retrograde pyelography may be needed to identify obstructions of the lower urinary tract (see Chapter 60).

LABORATORY PROFILE

Kidney Disease

Test	Normal Range for Adults	Values in Kidney Disease
Serum creatinine	*Male:* 0.6-1.2 mg/dL (53-106 mmol/L) *Female:* 0.5-1.1 mg/dL (44-97 mmol/L) *Older adults:* May be slightly increased	**In chronic kidney disease:** May increase by 0.5-1.0 mg/dL (50-100 mcmol/L) every 1-2 yr **In acute kidney injury:** Increase of 1-2 mg/dL (100-200 mmol/L) every 24-48 hr May increase 1-6 mg/dL (100-600 mmol/L) in 1 wk or less
Serum sodium	136-145 mEq/L (136-145 mmol/L)	Normal, increased, or decreased
Serum potassium	3.5-5.0 mEq/L (3.5-5.0 mmol/L)	Increased
Serum phosphorus (phosphate)	3.0-4.5 mg/dL (0.97-1.45 mmol/L) *Older adults:* May be slightly decreased	Increased
Serum calcium	Total calcium: 9.0-10.5 mg/dL (2.25-2.62 mmol/L) Ionized calcium: 4.5-5.6 mg/dL (1.05-1.3 mmol/L) *Older adults:* Slightly decreased	Decreased
Serum magnesium	1.3-2.1 mEq/L (0.65-1.05 mmol/L)	Increased or decreased
Serum carbon dioxide combining power (bicarbonate) (venous)	23-30 mEq/L (23-30 mmol/L)	Decreased
Arterial blood pH	7.35-7.45	Decreased (in metabolic acidosis) or normal
Arterial blood bicarbonate (HCO_3^-)	21-28 mEq/L (21-28 mmol/L)	Decreased
Arterial blood $Paco_2$	35-45 mm Hg	Decreased
Hemoglobin	*Female:* 12-16 g/dL (7.4-9.9 mmol/L) *Male:* 14-18 g/dL (8.7-11.2 mmol/L) *Older adults:* Slightly decreased	Decreased
Hematocrit	*Female:* 37%-47% (0.37-0.47 volume fraction) *Male:* 42%-52% (0.42-0.52 volume fraction) *Older adults:* May be slightly decreased	Decreased
Blood osmolality	285-295 mOsm/kg (285-295 mmol/kg)	Elevated in volume-depleted states, increasing the risk for acute kidney injury

Data from Pagana, K., Pagana, T. & Pagana, T. (2017). *Mosby's diagnostic and laboratory test reference* (13th ed.). St. Louis: Elsevier.

Other Diagnostic Assessments. Kidney biopsy is performed if the cause of AKI is uncertain and symptoms persist or an immunologic disease is suspected. Prepare the patient before the test, particularly managing both hypotension and hypertension. Hypertension increases the risk for intrarenal hemorrhage following needle biopsy. Provide follow-up care. Be aware of all test results and understand how they might affect the treatment regimen. (See Chapter 60 for a detailed discussion of diagnostic tests related to the kidney.)

NCLEX EXAMINATION CHALLENGE 63.1
Safe and Effective Care Environment

A 62-year-old client was admitted 2 days ago with traumatic injuries and hypovolemic shock. Which lab result is **most important** for the nurse to report to the health care provider immediately?

A. Serum sodium 132 mEq/L (mmol/L)
B. Serum potassium 6.9 mEq/L (mmol/L)
C. Blood urea nitrogen 24 mg/dL (mmol/L)
D. Hematocrit 32% (0.32 volume fraction); hemoglobin 9.2 g/dL (92 g/L)

◆ **Interventions: Take Action.** Avoid hypotension and maintain normal fluid balance *(euvolemia)* to prevent and manage AKI. A reduction in kidney *perfusion* may initially not be recognized when there is no associated drop in systemic blood pressure. Autoregulation and the renin-angiotensin-aldosterone system (RAAS) effectively maintain normal kidney perfusion and glomerular filtration rate. Maintaining a mean arterial pressure (MAP) of 80 to 85 mm Hg has been shown to lower rates of AKI in patients with pre-existing hypertension. However, there is an increased risk of atrial fibrillation in patients with a mean arterial pressure (MAP) of 80 to 85 mm Hg as opposed to 65 to 70 mm Hg. Accordingly, blood pressure goals are determined based on pre-existing conditions and risk versus benefit to the patient (Moore, 2018).

Reduce exposure to nephrotoxic agents and drugs that alter kidney perfusion. When such substances cannot be avoided, monitor drug levels and communicate with the pharmacist to adjust doses to minimize harm. Contrast media can have serious toxic effects on tubular cells (Lambert et al., 2017). Ensure that kidney function is assessed before an imaging test that includes contrast media. A large volume of contrast, agents with high osmolarity (>2000 mOsm/L [mmol/L]), and frequent administration (given twice in 3 months or more often) of agents are more likely to cause contrast-induced nephropathy. Ensure that kidney function is assessed before an imaging test and that both the radiologist and the requesting primary health care provider are aware of reduced kidney function before contrast medium is given.

Communicate with the radiologist so that the lowest dose of the contrast agent is used in high-risk adults. Adequate hydration is essential to prevent contrast-induced nephropathy (Honicker & Holt, 2016; Lambert et al., 2017). The patient may receive IV fluids at a rate of 1 mL/kg/hr for 12 hours before the imaging test or at 3 mL/kg/hr for 1 hour just before the procedure to ensure hydration and dilution of the contrast medium and to speed urinary *elimination* of the agent. A common

desired outcome for patients undergoing a procedure with contrast medium is a urine output of 150 mL/hr for the first 6 hours after administration of the contrast agent.

Observations about new-onset or increased peripheral edema, increased daily weight, and reduced urine output can identify patients with a positive fluid balance from AKI who may require treatment with fluid restriction or diuretic therapy. Impairment of *acid-base balance* and electrolyte imbalance can occur and may require treatment, especially in older adults.

Blood sampling of patients at risk for AKI allows early recognition of elevated serum creatinine levels and trend data. Communicate observations about worsening kidney function early and often to the primary health care provider so interventions can promote kidney health and interrupt the progression of AKI when it occurs.

Not all patients with AKI experience oliguria. *Immunity* and inflammatory causes of AKI may allow proteins to enter the glomerulus, and these proteins can hold fluid in the filtrate, causing a *polyuria* (excess urine output) that disrupts *fluid and electrolyte balance.* During AKI with high-volume urine output, hypovolemia and electrolyte *loss* are the main problems. The patient in the diuretic phase of AKI needs a plan of care that focuses on fluid and electrolyte *replacement* and monitoring. Onset of polyuria can signal the start of recovery from AKI.

Surviving kidney tubule cells possess a remarkable ability to regenerate and proliferate, and early identification can stop progression of AKI, as well as aid in recovery of kidney function. Base the desired outcomes of care on collaboration and communication with interprofessional team members. Update the plan of care for either restriction (when fluid overload from new AKI is present) or liberal administration of fluid (to prevent AKI or promote elimination of contrast medium) based on timely and accurate team communication.

Frequent laboratory value monitoring, close surveillance of intake and output, drug therapy, nutrition, careful administration of fluids and minerals, and renal replacement therapy are commonly used to manage AKI.

NCLEX EXAMINATION CHALLENGE 63.2
Safe and Effective Care Environment

The nurse is caring for a 74-year-old client scheduled for a cardiac catheterization with contrast dye. What nursing action is appropriate? **Select all that apply.**

A. Assess creatinine clearance using a 24-hour urine collection test.
B. Assess for coexisting conditions of diabetes, heart failure, and kidney disease.
C. Collaborate with the provider about whether IV fluids should be infused before the test.
D. Notify the provider regarding changes in serum creatinine from 0.2 to 0.4 mg/dL in 24 hours.
E. Alert the provider to a glomerular filtration rate (GFR) below 60 mL/min/1.73 m^2.

Drug Therapy. The interprofessional team consults the inpatient pharmacist for drug adjustment based on kidney function. As kidney function changes, drug dosages are changed. It is important to be knowledgeable about the site of drug metabolism and especially careful when giving drugs. Continuously monitor the patient with AKI for adverse drug events and interactions of the drugs that he or she is receiving. Diuretics may be used to increase urine output in AKI. Diuretic-induced urine output does not preserve kidney function or stop AKI, but diuretics do rid the body of retained fluid and electrolytes in the patient with AKI that has not progressed to end-stage kidney disease (ESKD).

Fluid challenges are often used to promote kidney ***perfusion.*** In patients without fluid overload, 500 to 1000 mL of normal saline may be infused over 1 hour. It is important to assess the patient's response to fluid to prevent fluid overload. Fluid overload in critical illness has been shown to increase mortality (Moore, 2018). The term *fluid responsive* is used when identifying patients who have a positive response to fluid. There are many methods to evaluate fluid responsiveness, such as systolic pressure variation, pulse pressure variation, and stroke volume variation, which are obtained from the arterial or pulse oximetry waveforms. In patients with a method of monitoring stroke volume and cardiac output, a passive leg raise can determine if the patient is fluid responsive without the risk of giving fluids. The patient's leg is raised to 45 degrees for 30 to 90 seconds in order to temporarily move fluid by increasing venous return, and if the stroke volume or cardiac output improves, the patient will respond positively to more fluid volume (Brown & Semler, 2019).

Nutrition Therapy. Patients who have AKI often have a high rate of *catabolism* (protein breakdown). Increases in metabolism and protein breakdown may be related to the stress of illness and the increase in blood levels of catecholamines, cortisol, and glucagon. The rate of protein breakdown correlates with the severity of uremia and azotemia. Catabolism causes the breakdown of muscle protein and increases azotemia.

The interprofessional team's registered dietitian nutritionist (RDN) in the ICU setting calculates the patient's protein and caloric needs. A consultation may need to be requested for inpatients outside of the ICU or for those in community settings. Work with the RDN to establish a diet with specified amounts of protein, sodium, and fluids. For the patient who does not require dialysis, 0.6 g/kg of body weight or 40 g/day of protein is usually prescribed. For patients who require dialysis, the protein level needed ranges from 1 to 1.5 g/kg. The dietary sodium ranges from 60 to 90 mEq/kg (mmol/kg). If high blood potassium levels are present, dietary potassium is restricted to 60 to 70 mEq/kg (mmol/kg). The daily amount of fluid permitted is calculated to be equal to the urine volume plus 500 mL. Assess food intake every shift to ensure that caloric intake is adequate.

Many patients with AKI are too ill or their appetite is too poor to meet caloric goals. For these patients, nutrition support with oral supplements, enteral nutrition, or parenteral nutrition (PN or hyperalimentation) is needed. Nutrition support in AKI aims to provide sufficient nutrients to maintain or improve nutrition status, preserve lean body mass, restore or maintain fluid balance, and preserve kidney function.

There are several kidney-specific formulations of oral supplements and enteral solutions (e.g., Nepro, Suplena, and Novasource Renal). Most specialty formulas for patients with kidney problems are lower in sodium, potassium, and phosphorus and higher in calories than are standard feedings. Enteral nutrition, delivered with a nasogastric or nasojejunal tube (these tubes can also be placed orally), can be used for nutrition support. If PN is used, the IV solutions are mixed to meet the patient's specific needs. Because kidney function is unstable in AKI, continuously monitor intake and output and serum electrolyte levels to determine how the supplementation affects ***fluid and electrolyte balance.*** IV fat emulsion (Intralipid) infusions can provide a nonprotein source of calories. In uremic patients, fat emulsions are used in place of glucose to avoid the problems of excessive sugars.

Kidney Replacement Therapy. Kidney replacement therapy (KRT), also called renal replacement therapy (RRT), is used for patients with loss of kidney function and inadequate waste ***elimination.*** Indications for KRT include symptomatic uremia (e.g., pericarditis, neuropathy, decline in cognition), persistent or rapidly rising high potassium levels (i.e., greater than 6.5 mEq/L [mmol/L]), severe metabolic acidosis (pH less than 7.1), or fluid overload that inhibits tissue ***perfusion.*** When AKI occurs with drug or alcohol intoxication, KRT also can remove toxins.

Advancements in KRT over the past 10 years have led to multiple options for patients requiring treatment. Options for KRT include various types of intermittent and continuous hemodialysis (HD) as well as peritoneal dialysis (PD). Despite recent advances, the life expectancy for patients starting KRT ranges from 3 to 5 years. Mortality is highest in the first several months following dialysis (Gilbert & Weiner, 2018).

Immediate vascular access for KRT in patients with AKI is made by placement of a catheter specific for dialysis (Fig. 63.1). The temporary catheter is placed in a central vein, most often the internal jugular (Schell-Chaple, 2017), using best practices to avoid catheter-associated bloodstream infections (see Chapter 15). Placement of the catheter requires informed consent and a "time-out" similar to other surgical procedures (see Chapter 9, Care of Perioperative Patients). This catheter is not used to acquire blood samples, give drugs or fluid, or monitor central venous pressure. Provide site care in accordance with agency policy and best practices to avoid catheter-related bloodstream infection (CRBSI).

A long-term dialysis catheter may be placed in the radiology department using a tunneling technique under moderate sedation. Under ultrasound or fluoroscopic guidance, the physician makes a small incision where the internal jugular vein passes behind the clavicle. A 6- to 8-cm tunnel is created away from the site of the incision. A long-term hemodialysis (HD) catheter is inserted through the tunnel and into the jugular vein. Keeping a segment of the catheter within the subcutaneous tissues before entering the jugular vein reduces the risk for infection. This central catheter is used only for dialysis and requires aseptic dressing changes.

Dialysis catheters have two lumens—one for outflow and one for inflow. This allows the patient's blood to flow out and, once dialyzed, to be returned through the inflow lumen. Some catheters have a third lumen to sample venous blood or give drugs and fluid during dialysis.

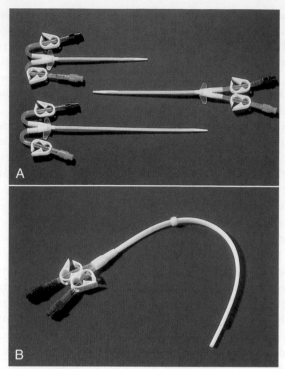

FIG. 63.1 Subclavian dialysis catheters. These catheters are radiopaque tubes that can be used for hemodialysis access. The Y-shaped tubing allows arterial outflow and venous return through a single catheter. (A) Mahurkar catheters, made of polyurethane and used for short-term access. (B) PermCath catheter, made of silicone and used for long-term access. (Courtesy Kendall Company, Bothell, WA.)

Intermittent Versus Continuous Kidney Replacement Therapy. Kidney replacement therapy (KRT) is a supportive strategy to purify blood, substituting for the normal function of the kidney. Particles are separated from blood based on the different ability of particles to pass through (diffuse) a membrane or across the peritoneal lining. KRT can be delivered intermittently, continuously, or as a hybrid of these approaches. Mortality is significant, regardless of modality, among patients who require KRT.

Intermittent KRT, sometimes called *hemodialysis,* is delivered over 3 to 6 hours. Generally a technician or dialysis nurse brings the dialysis machine to the bedside of a critically ill patient. Patients who do not need intensive care may be transported to an inpatient dialysis unit for the duration of the KRT treatment.

Intermittent KRT uses a dialysis machine to mix and monitor the *dialysate* (the fluid that helps remove the unwanted particles and waste products from blood). Dialysate is prescribed by the nephrology health care provider as an admixture to restore electrolytes and minerals to normal levels in the blood. The machine also monitors the flow of blood while it is outside of the body. Alarms are set and monitored by the dialysis technician or nurse to ensure safe and effective flow. This type of KRT is delivered three or four times weekly and requires anticoagulation in the dialysis circuit. Dialysis creates shifts of fluid and electrolytes that may not be tolerated in critically ill patients. Another form of intermittent KRT is peritoneal dialysis (PD), which is more commonly used for end-stage kidney disease.

This therapy is discussed in detail in the Peritoneal Dialysis section of this chapter.

Continuous kidney replacement therapies (CKRTs), also known as continuous renal replacement therapy (CRRT), are alternative methods for removing wastes and restoring both *acid-base balance* and *fluid and electrolyte balance.* They are used in hospitalized adults who are too unstable to tolerate the changes in blood pressure that occur with intermittent conventional hemodialysis. As with hemodialysis, blood is passed through a filter to remove waste and undesired particles. Although intermittent hemodialysis occurs for 4 hours 3 days a week, CKRTs are typically prescribed for over 24 hours (Ronco et al., 2019). Some CKRT therapies use a different approach to remove particles from the blood. Hemofiltration uses ultrafiltration, whereas diffusion is used in intermittent dialysis to remove toxins and other particles. *Ultrafiltration* is the separation of particles from a suspension by passage through a filter with very fine pores. In ultrafiltration, the separation is performed by convective transport. During intermittent hemodialysis, separation depends on differential diffusion. Some approaches to CKRT combine ultrafiltration with diffusion (combined hemofiltration and hemodialysis).

CKRT occurs only in the ICU, because of the need for frequent monitoring and the specialized skill set of the nurse to maintain safety during extracorporeal circulation (blood flow outside the body). Life-threatening complications can occur if there is an error in the preparation of electrolyte solution or if the conductivity monitors fail (Ronco et al., 2019). The American Nephrology Nurses Association provides resources for intermittent and continuous KRT policies and procedures.

Several strategies can be used to provide CKRT to critically ill patients. The most commonly used CKRTs are continuous venovenous hemofiltration (CVVH) and continuous venovenous hemodialysis (CVVHD). The different CKRT modalities use the same machines, which are set up differently based on the needs of the patient. CVVH uses ultrafiltration, whereas CVVHD uses diffusion to filter the blood. CKRT is powered by a pump that drives blood from the patient catheter into the dialyzer (filter). The ultrafiltrate fluid is then collected into a bag for disposal. There may be a second pump that acts on the ultrafiltrate tubing to create negative pressure and increase fluid removal. Replacement fluid is infused via the inflow circuit in some systems. The pump increases the risk for an air embolus, and KRT systems have alarms that detect air (Ronco et al., 2019).

Another KRT modality is a hybrid of continuous and intermittent approaches. Slow continuous ultrafiltration (SCUF) provides slow removal of fluid over 12 to 24 hours and may be useful when azotemia or uremia is not a concern. Sustained low-efficiency dialysis (SLED) uses the dialysis machine to deliver prolonged dialysis for 12 to 24 hours. Lower blood flow and dialysate flow rates remove both particles and water and may be better tolerated by the unstable or critically ill patient, with fewer episodes of hypotension. A newer type of CKRT is continuous venovenous hemodiafiltration (CVVHDF), which combines the principles of hemodialysis with hemofiltration. Another new type of CKRT is continuous venovenous high-flux hemodialysis (CVVHFD), which uses high-flux membranes in the filter (Ronco et al., 2019).

Continuous KRT is expensive and resource intensive. It requires consultation and collaboration with the nephrologist and close collaboration with a dialysis nurse. Conservative management of *fluid and electrolyte balance, acid-base balance,* and drug therapy is an acceptable and reasonable approach to manage AKI.

Posthospital Care. Patients with AKI may have many outcomes. Some patients recover and return to baseline kidney function and general health. Others have partial recovery with mild or moderate chronic kidney disease (CKD). Still others may require permanent KRT. Some die from the acute illness.

The care for a patient with AKI after discharge from the hospital varies, depending on the status of the kidney function when the patient is discharged. Resolution of kidney injury may occur over several months, and follow-up care may be provided by a nephrologist or by the primary health care provider in consultation with the nephrologist. Frequent medical visits are necessary, as are scheduled laboratory blood and urine tests to monitor kidney function. A registered dietitian nutritionist can plan modifications to the patient's diet according to the degree of kidney function and ongoing nutrition needs. Fluid restrictions and daily weights may be advised to avoid fluid overload while kidneys are recovering.

Recovery of renal function is adversely affected by KRT, putting patients at risk for developing end-stage kidney disease (ESKD). Insult to the kidney by KRT is thought to be related to the loss of autoregulation and inflammation that occurs (Ronco et al., 2019). For patients who require dialysis at discharge following AKI, follow-up care is similar to that needed for patients with ESKD from CKD (see Care Coordination and Transition Management in the Chronic Kidney Disease section). Depending on their level of independence and family support, patients may need home care nursing or social work assistance.

NCLEX EXAMINATION CHALLENGE 63.3

Health Promotion and Maintenance

The nurse is preparing a client with stage 3 CKD for discharge. Which client statement indicates the need for further teaching?

A. "I will be sure to attend my follow-up appointment with my nephrologist."

B. "I will increase my protein intake so my body can heal."

C. "I will weigh myself daily and call the doctor if my weight increases by 2 lb or more."

D. "I will take my blood pressure each day and keep a daily log."

✳ ELIMINATION CONCEPT EXEMPLAR: CHRONIC KIDNEY DISEASE

Pathophysiology Review

Unlike acute kidney injury (AKI), chronic kidney disease (CKD) is a progressive, irreversible disorder lasting longer than 3 months (Ferri, 2020). When kidney function and waste *elimination* are too poor to sustain life, CKD becomes end-stage

---

▶ KEY FEATURES

Uremia

• Metallic taste in the mouth	• Uremic frost on skin
• Anorexia	• Fatigue and lethargy
• Nausea	• Hiccups
• Vomiting	• Edema
• Muscle cramps	• Dyspnea
	• Paresthesias

---

kidney disease (ESKD). Terms used with CKD include **azotemia** (buildup of nitrogen-based wastes in the blood), **uremia** (azotemia with symptoms [see the Key Features: Uremia box]), and **uremic syndrome**. See Table 63.1 for a comparison of AKI and CKD.

Stages of Chronic Kidney Disease. CKD is classified into five stages based on glomerular filtration rate (GFR) category. Direct measurement of urine creatinine (described in Chapter 60, with a 3-hour or 24-hour urine collection) is needed for the most accurate GFR estimation. The five stages of CKD are described in Table 63.6. CKD starts with a normal GFR but increased risk for kidney damage. In the first stage, the patient may have a normal GFR (>90 mL/min/1.73 m^2) but abnormal urine findings, structural abnormalities, or genetic traits that point to kidney disease. The patient is at increased risk for kidney damage from infection, *immunity* responses with inflammation, pregnancy, dehydration, and hypotension. Careful management of conditions such as diabetes, hypertension, and heart failure (HF) can slow the onset and progression of CKD.

In stage 2 CKD, GFR is reduced, ranging between 60 and 89 mL/min/1.73 m^2, and albuminuria may be present. Kidney nephron damage has occurred, and there may be slight elevations of metabolic wastes in the blood because of nephron loss. Levels of blood urea nitrogen (BUN), serum creatinine, uric acid, and phosphorus are not sensitive enough to define this stage. Increased output of dilute urine may occur at this stage of CKD and lead to severe dehydration.

⚠ NURSING SAFETY PRIORITY (QSEN)

Action Alert

Teach patients with mild chronic kidney disease (CKD) that carefully managing fluid volume, blood pressure, electrolytes, and other kidney-damaging diseases by following prescribed drug and nutrition therapies can slow progression to end-stage kidney disease (ESKD).

In stage 3 CKD, GFR reduction continues and ranges between 30 and 59 mL/min/1.73 m^2, and albuminuria is usually present. Nephron damage is greater, and azotemia reflecting poor waste *elimination* is present. Ongoing management of the underlying conditions that cause nephron damage is essential, especially diabetes mellitus and blood pressure control. Restriction of fluids, proteins, and electrolytes is needed. Stage 3 is further divided into 3a and 3b to more accurately assess the risk for complications from CKD as GFR decreases below 45 mL/min/1.73 m^2.

TABLE 63.6 Stages of Chronic Kidney Disease

Stage	Estimated Glomerular Filtration Rate	Intervention
Stage 1		
At risk; normal kidney function, but urine findings indicate kidney disease	>90 mL/min/ 1.73 m²	Screen for risk factors and manage care to reduce risk: • Uncontrolled hypertension • Diabetes with poor glycemic control • Congenital or acquired anatomic or urinary tract abnormalities • Family history of genetic kidney diseases • Exposure to nephrotoxic substances
Stage 2		
Slightly reduced kidney function	60-89 mL/min/ 1.73 m²	Focus on reduction of risk factors
Stage 3		
Moderately reduced kidney function	30-59 mL/min/ 1.73 m²	Implement strategies to slow disease progression
Stage 4		
Severely reduced kidney function; a noticeable jaundice can occur, particularly around the eyes	15-29 mL/min/ 1.73 m²	Manage complications Discuss patient preferences and values Educate about options and prepare for renal replacement therapy
Stage 5		
End-stage kidney disease (ESKD)	<15 mL/min/ 1.73 m²	Implement renal replacement therapy or kidney transplantation

Over time, patients progress to stage 4 CKD and *end-stage kidney disease* (ESKD) (stage 5). Waste **elimination** is poor, with excessive amounts of urea and creatinine building up in the blood, and the kidneys cannot maintain homeostasis. Severe impairments of **fluid and electrolyte balance** and **acid-base balance** occur. Without kidney replacement therapy, death results from ESKD.

Three albuminuria stages also are considered in evaluating CKD. These stages are defined by the albumin-to-creatinine ratio in urine. The first stage (A1) is none to mildly increased albumin up to 29 mg/g creatinine (<3 mg/mmol) and is sometimes called *microalbuminuria*. The second (A2) stage has values of 30 to 300 mg/g creatinine (3 to 30 mg/mmol). The stage of greatest kidney damage (A3) has values >300 mg/g creatinine (>30 mg/mmol). The risk for progression of CKD, ESKD, and mortality is increased when urine albumin increases. Albumin in the urine is a marker of kidney damage, whereas GFR reflects kidney function. The combined values help identify adults at risk for progression of CKD and complications and guide interventions.

Kidney Changes. CKD with greatly reduced GFR causes many problems, including abnormal urine production, severe disruption of *fluid and electrolyte balance,* and metabolic abnormalities. Because healthy nephrons become larger and work harder, urine production and water *elimination* are sufficient to maintain essential homeostasis until about three-fourths of kidney function is lost. As the disease progresses, the ability to produce diluted urine is reduced, resulting in urine with a fixed osmolarity *(isosthenuria)*. As kidney function continues to decline, the BUN increases, and urine output decreases. Extracellular volume overload can occur in CKD because the body loses the capability to excrete sodium (Johnson et al., 2019). At this point, the patient is at risk for fluid overload with edema, pulmonary crackles, shortness of breath, and pleural or pericardial effusion (with symptoms of a friction rub on auscultation and/or decreased breath sounds or heart sounds).

Metabolic Changes. *Urea and creatinine* excretion are disrupted by CKD. Creatinine comes from proteins in skeletal muscle. The rate of creatinine excretion depends on muscle mass, physical activity, and diet. Without major changes in diet or physical activity, the serum creatinine level is constant. Creatinine is partially excreted by the kidney tubules, and a decrease in kidney function leads to a buildup of serum creatinine. Urea is made from protein metabolism and is excreted by the kidneys. The BUN level normally varies directly with protein intake.

Sodium excretion changes are common. Early in CKD, the patient is at risk for *hyponatremia* (sodium depletion) because there are fewer healthy nephrons to reabsorb sodium. Thus sodium is lost in the urine. Polyuria of mild-to-moderate CKD also causes sodium loss.

In the later stages of CKD, kidney excretion of sodium is reduced as urine production decreases. Then sodium retention and high serum sodium levels *(hypernatremia)* occur with only modest increases in dietary sodium intake. This problem leads to severe disruption of **fluid and electrolyte balance** (see Chapter 13). Sodium retention causes hypertension and edema.

Even with sodium retention, the serum sodium level may appear normal because plasma water is retained at the same time. If fluid retention occurs at a greater rate than sodium retention, the serum sodium level is falsely low because of dilution (see the Laboratory Profile: Kidney Disease box).

Potassium excretion occurs mainly through the kidney. Any increase in potassium load during the later stages of CKD can lead to hyperkalemia (high serum potassium levels). Normal serum potassium levels of 3.5 to 5 mEq/L (mmol/L) are maintained until the 24-hour urine output falls below 500 mL. High potassium levels then develop quickly, reaching 7 to 8 mEq/L (mmol/L) or greater. Life-threatening changes in cardiac rate and rhythm result from this elevation because of abnormal depolarization and repolarization. Other factors contribute to high potassium levels in CKD, including the ingestion of potassium in drugs, failure to restrict dietary potassium, tissue breakdown, blood transfusions, and bleeding or hemorrhage. (See Chapter 13 for discussion of potassium imbalance.)

Acid-base balance is affected by CKD. In the early stages, blood pH changes little because the remaining healthy nephrons increase their rate of acid excretion. As more nephrons are lost, acid excretion is reduced and metabolic acidosis results (see Chapter 14).

Many factors lead to acidosis in CKD. First, the kidneys cannot excrete excessive hydrogen ions (acids). Normally, tubular cells move hydrogen ions into the urine for excretion, but ammonium and bicarbonate are needed for this movement to occur (Johnson et al., 2019). In patients with CKD, ammonium production is decreased and reabsorption of bicarbonate does not occur. This process leads to a buildup of hydrogen ions and reduced levels of bicarbonate *(base deficit)*. High potassium levels further reduce kidney ammonium production and excretion.

As CKD worsens and acid retention increases, increased respiratory action is needed to keep blood pH normal. The respiratory system adjusts or compensates for the increased blood hydrogen ion levels (acidosis or decreased pH) by increasing the rate and depth of breathing to excrete carbon dioxide through the lungs. This breathing pattern, called **Kussmaul respiration**, increases with worsening kidney disease. Serum bicarbonate measures the extent of metabolic acidosis (bicarbonate deficit). Patients usually need alkali replacement to counteract acidosis.

Calcium and phosphorus balance is disrupted by CKD. A complex, balanced normal reciprocal relationship exists between calcium and phosphorus (used interchangeably with phosphate) and is influenced by vitamin D (see Chapter 13). The kidney produces a hormone needed to activate vitamin D, which then enhances intestinal absorption of calcium.

Normally, excess phosphorus is excreted in the urine. In CKD, renal phosphate excretion decreases, which causes elevated phosphate levels. Bone and skeletal changes can occur when the GFR decreases to 25% or less (McCance et al., 2019).

Parathyroid hormone (PTH) controls the amount of phosphorus in the blood by causing tubular excretion of phosphorus when there is an excess. An early effect of CKD is reduced phosphorus excretion (Fig. 63.2). As plasma phosphorus levels increase *(hyperphosphatemia)*, calcium levels decrease *(hypocalcemia)*. Chronic low blood calcium levels stimulate the parathyroid glands to release more PTH. With additional PTH, calcium is released from storage areas in bones *(bone resorption)*, which results in bone density loss. The extra calcium from the bone is needed to balance the excess plasma phosphorus level. The problem of low blood calcium levels is made worse with severe CKD because kidney cell damage also reduces production of active vitamin D. Deficiencies in vitamin D lead to even further decreased calcium levels because vitamin D aids in calcium absorption (McCance et al., 2019).

The problems in bone metabolism and structure caused by CKD-induced low calcium levels and high phosphorus levels are called **renal osteodystrophy**. Bone mineral loss causes bone pain, spinal sclerosis, fractures, bone density loss, osteomalacia, and tooth calcium loss.

Crystals formed from excessive calcium or phosphorus are called *metastatic calcifications* and may precipitate in many body areas. When the plasma level of the calcium-phosphorus product (serum calcium level multiplied by the serum phosphorus level) exceeds 70 mg/dL (6 mmol/L), the crystals may lodge in the kidneys, heart, lungs, blood vessels, joints, eyes (causing conjunctivitis), and brain. Itching increases with calcium-phosphorus imbalances.

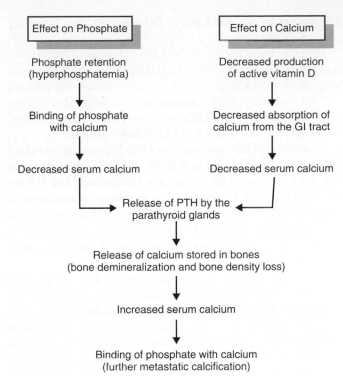

FIG. 63.2 Effects of kidney dysfunction on phosphorus and calcium balance. *PTH,* Parathyroid hormone.

Calcium is also deposited in atherosclerotic plaques in the lining of blood vessels. Vascular calcium deposits are a marker of significant risk for cardiovascular disease.

Cardiac Changes. Cardiorenal syndrome refers to disorders of the kidney or heart that cause dysfunction in the other organ. The kidney and the heart have a reciprocal relationship that can make an alteration in one cause an alteration in the other (Ferri, 2020).

Hypertension is common in most patients with CKD. It may be either the cause or the result of CKD. In patients who have other causes of hypertension such as atherosclerosis, the increased blood pressure damages the glomerular capillaries, and eventually ESKD results.

CKD itself elevates blood pressure by causing fluid and sodium overload and dysfunction of the renin-angiotensin-aldosterone system (RAAS). Hypertension alone can damage kidney arterioles, reducing **perfusion.** A decrease in kidney blood flow results in the production and release of a number of signaling chemicals, including renin, to improve blood flow to the kidney. The release of renin triggers the production of angiotensin and aldosterone. Angiotensin causes blood vessel constriction and increases blood pressure. Aldosterone stimulates kidney tubules to reabsorb sodium and water. These actions increase plasma volume and raise blood pressure. However, in the presence of CKD, an increase in blood pressure may not result in increased blood flow, and the production of renin continues, which creates a cycle of vasoconstriction in kidney arterioles and peripheral arterioles. The result is severe hypertension that is difficult to manage and worsens kidney function. Many patients with CKD have heart damage and enlargement from the long-term hypertension that results in coronary artery damage and poor coronary artery perfusion.

Hyperlipidemia occurs in CKD from changes in fat metabolism that increase triglyceride, total cholesterol, and low-density lipoprotein (LDL) levels. These changes increase the patient's risk for coronary artery disease and acute cardiac events. Problems with lipids and atherosclerosis are greatly increased for the patient with both CKD and diabetes mellitus.

Heart failure (HF) may occur in CKD because the workload on the heart is increased as a result of anemia, hypertension, and fluid overload. Left ventricular enlargement and HF are common in ESKD. Uremia may cause *uremic cardiomyopathy,* the uremic toxin effect on the myocardium. HF also may occur in these patients because of hypertension and coronary artery disease. Cardiac disease is a leading cause of death in patients with ESKD.

Pericarditis also occurs in patients with CKD. The pericardial sac becomes inflamed by uremic toxins or infection. If it is not treated, this problem leads to pericardial effusion, cardiac tamponade, and death. Symptoms include shortness of breath from low cardiac output, severe chest pain, tachycardia, narrow *pulse pressure* (close values for systolic and diastolic blood pressure), low-grade fever, and a pericardial friction rub that can be heard with a stethoscope placed over the left sternal border. Dysrhythmias may occur with uremia and uremic pericarditis. Treatment of tamponade, which is a medical emergency, requires immediate removal of pericardial fluid by placement of a needle, catheter, or drainage tube into the pericardium.

Hematologic and Immunity Changes.

Anemia is common in patients in the later stages of CKD and worsens CKD symptoms. The causes of anemia include a decreased erythropoietin level with reduced red blood cell (RBC) production, decreased RBC survival time from uremia, and iron and folic acid deficiencies (Norton et al., 2017b). The patient may have increased bleeding or bruising as a result of impaired platelet function.

CKD causes reduced *immunity,* which increases the risk for infection. Uremia disrupts white blood cell (WBC) production and function, decreasing host defenses. Protein, fluid, and electrolyte abnormalities contribute to inflammation and further immunity impairment.

Gastrointestinal Changes.

Uremia affects the entire GI system. The flora of the mouth change with uremia. The mouth contains the enzyme *urease,* which breaks down urea into ammonia. The ammonia generated remains and then causes halitosis (uremic fetor) and *stomatitis* (mouth inflammation). Anorexia, nausea, vomiting, and hiccups are common in patients with uremia. The specific cause of these problems is unknown but may be related to high BUN and creatinine levels and acidosis.

Peptic ulcer disease is common in patients with uremia, but the exact cause is unclear. Uremic colitis with watery diarrhea or constipation may also be present with uremia. Ulcers may occur in the stomach or intestine, causing erosion of blood vessels. The blood loss caused by these erosions may lead to hemorrhagic shock from severe GI bleeding.

TABLE 63.7   Selected Causes of Chronic Kidney Disease

Glomerular Disease
- Glomerulonephritis
- Basement membrane disease
- Goodpasture syndrome
- Intercapillary glomerulosclerosis

Tubular Disease
- Chronic hypercalcemia
- Chronic potassium depletion
- Fanconi syndrome
- Heavy metal (lead) poisoning

Vascular Disease of the Kidney
- Ischemic disease of the kidney
- Bilateral renal artery stenosis
- Nephrosclerosis
- Hyperparathyroidism

Inherited or Genetic Conditions
- Hypoplastic kidneys
- Medullary cystic disease
- Polycystic kidney disease

Infection
- Pyelonephritis
- Tuberculosis

Systemic Vascular Disease
- Intrarenal renovascular hypertension
- Extrarenal renovascular hypertension

Metabolic Kidney Disease
- Diabetes
- Amyloidosis
- Gout (hyperuricemic nephropathy)
- Milk-alkali syndrome
- Sarcoidosis

Connective Tissue Disease
- Progressive systemic sclerosis
- Systemic lupus erythematosus
- Polyarteritis

Urinary Tract Disease
- Obstructive uropathy

NOTE: List is not all-inclusive.

Cognitive and Functional Changes.

Although CKD may be asymptomatic in the early stages, as it progresses complications include cognitive and physical impairment. There is also increased risk for systemic drug toxicity and adverse effects from interventions used to prevent or treat CKD.

Etiology and Genetic Risk.

The causes of CKD are complex (Table 63.7). More than 100 different disease processes can result in progressive loss of kidney function (see also Chapter 62). Two main causes of CKD leading to dialysis or kidney transplantation are hypertension and diabetes mellitus. African-American patients are much more likely to develop ESKD and have hypertensive ESKD.

Incidence and Prevalence.

The number of patients being treated for CKD is increasing, particularly among older adults. About 15% of adults in the United States (37 million people) are estimated to have CKD (Centers for Disease Control and Prevention [CDC], 2019). Most adults who have CKD (9 out of 10) do not know that they have the disease (CDC, 2019). Almost 48,000 Canadians are currently being treated for kidney failure, with 1 in 10 Canadians having CKD, and millions more at risk (Kidney Foundation of Canada, 2018). Refer to the Patient and Family Education: Preparing for Self-Management box for prevention of kidney and urinary problems.

Health Promotion and Maintenance.

Health promotion activities to prevent or delay the onset of CKD focus on controlling the diseases that lead to its development, such as diabetes and hypertension. Educating and encouraging the patient to accept

PATIENT AND FAMILY EDUCATION: PREPARING FOR SELF-MANAGEMENT

Prevention of Kidney and Urinary Problems

- Be alert to the general appearance of your urine. Note any changes in its color, clarity, or odor.
- Changes in the frequency or volume of urine passage occur with changes in fluid intake. More frequent or infrequent voiding not associated with changes in fluid intake may signal health problems.
- Any discomfort or distress with the passage of urine is not normal. Pain, burning, urgency, aching, or difficulty with initiating urine flow or complete bladder emptying is of some concern. Report such symptoms to your primary health care provider.
- The kidneys need 1 to 2 L of fluid a day to flush out your body wastes. Water is the ideal flushing agent.
- Avoid sugary, high-calorie drinks; they provide low-quality calories that contribute to weight gain and sugar-induced urination.
- Changes in kidney function are often silent for many years. Periodically ask your primary health care provider to measure your kidney function with a blood test (serum creatinine) and a urinalysis.
- If you have a history of kidney disease, diabetes mellitus, or hypertension (high blood pressure) or a family history of kidney disease, you should know your serum creatinine level and your glomerular filtration rate (either estimated from serum creatinine or measured with a 24-hour creatinine urine collection). At least one checkup per year that includes laboratory blood and urine testing of kidney function is recommended.
- If you are identified as having decreased kidney function, ask about whether any prescribed drug, diagnostic test, or therapeutic procedure will present a risk to your current kidney function. Evaluate the contribution of diet to risk for kidney disease with your primary health care provider or a registered dietitian nutritionist. Check out all nonprescription drugs with your primary health care provider or pharmacist before using them.

lifestyle modifications and how to implement them are incorporated into the ongoing plan of care. Diet adjustments (e.g., sodium, protein, and cholesterol restriction), weight maintenance (i.e., achieve body mass index of 22 to 25 kg/m^2), smoking cessation, participation in 30 to 60 minutes of moderate-intensity exercise daily, and limitation of alcohol to one or two drinks daily are examples of lifestyle recommendations for the patient with CKD. Identifying patients who have diabetes or hypertension at an early stage is critical to CKD prevention (Norton et al., 2017a). Teach patients to adhere to drug and diet regimens and to engage in regular physical activity to prevent the blood vessel changes and kidney cell damage that lead to CKD. Instruct patients with diabetes to keep their blood glucose levels within the prescribed range. Teach patients with hypertension that drug therapy reduces vessel damage. Urge patients with diabetes or hypertension to have yearly testing for urine albumin-to-creatinine ratio (UACR) along with serum creatinine and BUN.

Teach adults treated for an infection anywhere in the kidney/urinary system to take all antibiotics as prescribed. Urge adults to drink at least 2 L of water daily unless a health problem requires fluid restriction. Caution adults who use NSAIDs to use the lowest dose for the briefest time period because these drugs interfere with blood flow to the kidney. High-dose and long-term NSAID use reduces kidney function.

NCLEX EXAMINATION CHALLENGE 63.4

Health Promotion and Maintenance

The nurse is caring for a 38-year-old male with hypertension and stage 1 CKD. The client reports lifestyle changes and feeling "better" and has stopped taking a prescribed diuretic. What is the appropriate nursing response?

A. "The diuretic will reduce your blood pressure, which may slow or prevent progression of your chronic kidney disease."

B. "Your primary health care provider prescribed the diuretic because it will reverse the damage caused by kidney disease."

C. "Taking medications is a personal decision, and you have the right to decline this prescription."

D. "Since you have implemented lifestyle changes, the diuretic is likely not needed."

❖ Interprofessional Collaborative Care

Although the patient with CKD may require hospitalization during exacerbation of imbalances or when other health problems require it, the vast majority of care occurs in the community. For best outcomes, the patient with CKD must be engaged in self-management. Because patients with CKD are at risk for so many adverse outcomes (not just ESKD), the interprofessional care team includes many specialists and health care professionals (e.g., nephrologists, nephrology nurses, pharmacists, registered dietitian nutritionists, mental health therapists, physical therapists, case managers, social workers, clergy or pastoral care workers). The responsibilities of these interprofessional team members are described within the interventions sections for CKD. With so many professionals involved, care coordination is essential to positive outcomes in this population (Hain, 2015). The nurse coordinates the interprofessional team to support and counsel the patient and family, often over many years of treatment. The nurse has the most contact with the patient when he or she is hospitalized or undergoing in-center dialysis treatments.

SYSTEMS THINKING AND QUALITY IMPROVEMENT (QSEN)

CKD Clinics Improving Patient Outcomes

CKD is a complex disease that affects physical, mental, and social aspects of health. This requires an understanding of available resources in order to improve patient outcomes. CKD clinics use an interprofessional approach, treating all aspects of the patient's health. Hospitals that develop and maintain clinics for patients with chronic diseases such as heart failure and CKD have fewer hospital readmissions and better patient outcomes. CKD clinics are successful because they foster care coordination and promote convenience for the patient.

The following services are recommended at a CKD clinic (Himmelfarb & Ikizler, 2018):

- Scheduling of tests (such as ultrasound and CT scans)
- Scheduling of specialist appointments as necessary
- Providing reminders for appointments and tests
- Following up with test results
- Providing a patient liaison for pharmacy and laboratory tests
- Consulting with interprofessional team members such as registered dietitian nutritionists (RDNs)
- Educating regarding disease processes, transplants, and therapies
- Referring as necessary for dialysis catheter insertion

◆ **Assessment: Recognize Cues**

History. When taking a history from a patient with risk for or actual CKD, document the patient's age and gender. Accurately measure weight and height and ask about usual weight and recent weight gain or loss. Weight gain may indicate fluid retention from poor kidney function with disrupted *fluid and electrolyte balance.* Weight loss may be the result of anorexia from uremia.

Ask about a history of kidney and urologic disorders, chronic health problems, and drug use. Chronic hypertension, diabetes, inflammatory diseases of systemic lupus erythematosus or arthritis, cancer, and tuberculosis can cause decreased kidney function. Ask the patient about family members' kidney disease, which might indicate a genetic problem.

Document the use of current and past prescribed and over-the-counter drugs because many drugs are nephrotoxic and drug interactions can cause kidney damage (Burchum & Rosenthal, 2019) (see Table 63.5). Ask whether the patient has had x-rays or CT scans with contrast medium.

Examine the patient's dietary habits and discuss any GI problems. A change in the taste of foods often occurs with CKD. Patients may report that sweet foods are not as appealing or that meats have a metallic taste. Ask about the presence of nausea, vomiting, anorexia, hiccups, diarrhea, or constipation. These symptoms may be the result of excess wastes that the body cannot eliminate because of kidney disease.

Ask about the patient's energy level and any recent injuries or bleeding. Explore changes in his or her daily routine as a possible *result* of fatigue. Fatigue is a common and often profound problem among patients with CKD, particularly among patients receiving dialysis. Weakness, drowsiness, and shortness of breath suggest impending pulmonary edema or neurologic degeneration. Ask about bruising or bleeding caused by hematologic changes from uremia.

Discuss urine *elimination* in detail, including frequency of urination, appearance of the urine, and any difficulty starting or controlling urination. These data can help identify urologic problems that may influence kidney function.

Physical Assessment/Signs and Symptoms. CKD causes changes in all body systems (see the Key Features: Severe, Chronic, and End-Stage Kidney Disease box). Most symptoms are related to changes in *fluid and electrolyte balance, acid-base balance,* and buildup of nitrogenous wastes.

Neurologic symptoms of CKD and uremic syndrome vary (see both Key Features boxes in this chapter). Observe for problems ranging from lethargy to seizures or coma, which may indicate uremic encephalopathy. Fluid overload can cause changes in cognition. Assess for sensory changes that appear in a glove-and-stocking pattern over the hands and feet *(peripheral neuropathy).* Check for weakness in upper and lower extremities *(uremic neuropathy).* Fatigue can result in decreased activity.

If untreated, encephalopathy can lead to seizures and coma. Dialysis is used emergently when neurologic problems result from CKD. The symptoms of encephalopathy may resolve with dialysis. However, improvement in neuropathy can be limited by severe or recurrent episodes of brain dysfunction. Depression may compound cognitive and neurologic problems.

KEY FEATURES
Severe, Chronic, and End-Stage Kidney Disease

Neurologic Symptoms
- Lethargy and daytime drowsiness
- Inability to concentrate or decreased attention span
- Seizures
- Coma
- Slurred speech
- Asterixis (jerky movements or "flapping" of the hands)
- Tremors, twitching, or jerky movements
- Myoclonus
- Ataxia (alteration in gait)
- Paresthesias from peripheral neuropathy

Cardiovascular Symptoms
- Cardiomyopathy
- Hypertension
- Peripheral edema
- Heart failure
- Uremic pericarditis
- Pericardial effusion
- Pericardial friction rub
- Cardiac tamponade
- Cardiorenal syndrome

Respiratory Symptoms
- Uremic halitosis
- Tachypnea
- Deep sighing, yawning
- Kussmaul respirations
- Uremic pneumonitis
- Shortness of breath
- Pulmonary edema
- Pleural effusion
- Depressed cough reflex
- Crackles

Hematologic Symptoms
- Anemia
- Abnormal bleeding and bruising
- Reduced white blood cell count
- Increased risk for infection

Gastrointestinal Symptoms
- Anorexia
- Nausea
- Vomiting
- Metallic taste in the mouth
- Changes in taste acuity and sensation
- Uremic colitis (diarrhea)
- Constipation
- Uremic gastritis (possible GI bleeding)
- Uremic fetor (breath odor)
- Stomatitis

Urinary Symptoms
- Polyuria, nocturia (early)
- Oliguria, anuria (later)
- Proteinuria
- Hematuria
- Diluted, straw-colored urine appearance (early)
- Concentrated and cloudy urine appearance (later)

Integumentary Symptoms
- Decreased skin turgor
- Yellow-gray pallor
- Dry skin
- Pruritus
- Ecchymosis
- Purpura
- Soft-tissue calcifications
- Uremic frost (late, premorbid)

Musculoskeletal Symptoms
- Muscle weakness and cramping
- Bone pain
- Fractures
- Renal osteodystrophy

Reproductive Symptoms
- Decreased fertility
- Infrequent or absent menses
- Decreased libido
- Impotence
- Sexual dysfunction

Metabolic Symptoms
- Hyperparathyroidism
- Hyperlipidemia
- Alterations in vitamin D, calcium, and phosphorus adsorption and metabolism
- Metabolic acidosis
- Hyperkalemia

Psychosocial Symptoms
- Depression
- Fatigue
- Sleep disturbances
- Sexual dysfunction
- Cognitive impairment
- Unemployment

Cardiovascular symptoms of CKD result from fluid overload, hypertension, heart failure (HF), pericarditis, potassium-induced dysrhythmias, and cholesterol/calcium (plaque, atherosclerosis) deposits in blood vessels. Assess for indications of reduced sodium and water excretion. Blood volume overload, if untreated, leads to hypertension, pulmonary edema, peripheral edema, and HF.

Assess heart rate and rhythm, listening for extra sounds (particularly an S_3), irregular patterns, or a pericardial friction rub. Unless a dialysis vascular access has been created, measure blood pressure in each arm. Assess the jugular veins for distention, and assess for edema of the feet, shins, and sacrum and around the eyes. Crackles during lung auscultation and shortness of breath with exertion and at night suggest fluid overload.

Respiratory symptoms of CKD also vary (e.g., breath that smells like urine [*uremic fetor* or uremic halitosis], deep sighing, yawning, shortness of breath). Observe the rhythm, rate, and depth of breathing. Tachypnea and hyperpnea (increased depth of breathing) occur with metabolic acidosis.

With severe metabolic acidosis, extreme increases in rate and depth of ventilation (Kussmaul respirations) occur. A few patients have pneumonitis, or *uremic lung.* In these patients, assess for thick sputum, reduced coughing, tachypnea, and fever. A pleural friction rub may be heard with a stethoscope. Patients often have pleuritic pain with breathing. Auscultate the lungs for crackles, which indicate fluid overload.

Hematologic symptoms of CKD include anemia and abnormal bleeding. Check for indicators of anemia (e.g., fatigue, pallor, lethargy, weakness, shortness of breath, dizziness). Check for abnormal bleeding by observing for bruising, petechiae, purpura, mucous membrane bleeding in the nose or gums, or intestinal bleeding (black, tarry stools [melena]).

GI symptoms of CKD include foul breath (halitosis) and mouth inflammation or ulceration. Document any abdominal pain, cramping, or vomiting. Test all stools for occult blood.

Skeletal symptoms of CKD are related to osteodystrophy from poor absorption of calcium and continuous bone calcium loss. Adults with osteodystrophy have thin, fragile bones that are at risk for fractures with even slight trauma. Vertebrae become more compact and may bend forward, leading to an overall loss of height. Ask about changes in height and bone pain. Observe for spinal curvatures and any unusual bumps or protrusions in bone areas that may indicate fractures. Handle the patient carefully during examination and care.

Urine symptoms in CKD reflect the kidneys' decreasing function. Urine amount, frequency, and appearance change. Protein, sediment, or blood may be in the urine.

The amount and composition of the urine change as kidney function decreases and waste *elimination* is disrupted. With the onset of mild-to-moderate CKD, the urine may be more dilute and clearer because tubular reabsorption of water is reduced. The actual urine output in a patient with CKD varies with the amount of remaining kidney function. The patient with severe CKD or ESKD usually has oliguria, but some patients continue to produce 1 L or more daily. Daily urine volume usually changes again after dialysis is started. A long duration of oliguria is an indication that recovery of kidney function is not to be expected.

Skin symptoms of CKD occur as a result of uremia. Pigment is deposited in the skin, causing a yellowish coloration, or darkening when skin is brown or bronze. The anemia of CKD causes sallowness, appearing as a faded suntan on lighter-skinned patients.

Skin oils and turgor are decreased in patients with uremia. A distressing problem of uremia is severe pruritus (itching). Uremic frost, a layer of urea crystals from evaporated sweat, may appear on the face, eyebrows, axillae, and groin in patients with advanced uremic syndrome. Assess for bruises *(ecchymosis),* purple patches *(purpura),* and rashes.

Psychosocial Assessment. CKD and its treatment disrupt many aspects of a patient's life. Psychosocial assessment and support are part of the nurse's role from the time that CKD is first diagnosed. With ongoing issues, a mental health professional is an important member of the care team. Ask about the patient's understanding of the diagnosis and what the treatment regimen means to him or her (e.g., diet, drugs, dialysis). Assess for anxiety and fear and for coping styles used by the patient and family. CKD affects family relations, social activity, work patterns, body image, and sexual activity. The chronic nature of severe CKD and ESKD, the many treatment options, and the uncertainties about the disease and its treatment require ongoing psychosocial assessment, psychosocial interventions, and ongoing support. Support the recommendations of the mental health professional.

Laboratory Assessment. CKD causes extreme changes in many laboratory values (see the Laboratory Profile: Kidney Disease box). Monitor these blood values: creatinine, blood urea nitrogen (BUN), sodium, potassium, calcium, phosphorus, bicarbonate, hemoglobin, and hematocrit. Also monitor GFR for trends.

A urinalysis is performed. In the early stages of CKD, urinalysis may show protein, glucose, red blood cells (RBCs) and white blood cells (WBCs), and decreased or fixed specific gravity. Urine osmolarity is usually decreased. As CKD progresses, urine output decreases dramatically, and osmolarity increases. A urine albumin-to-creatinine ratio (UACR) provides important information about kidney function and damage.

Glomerular filtration rate (GFR) can be estimated from serum creatinine levels, age, gender, race, and body size. But this type of estimation is generally used for screening rather than for staging of CKD. Estimation of GFR based on a formula that includes serum creatinine is also useful to calculate drug dose or drug frequency when reduced kidney function is a concern. However, to determine stage of CKD, a urine collection of 3 hours to 24 hours is usually done to assess creatinine clearance. A spot urine albumin-to-creatinine ratio (UACR) also is completed.

In severe CKD, serum creatinine and BUN levels may be used to determine the presence and degree of uremia. Serum creatinine levels may increase gradually over a period of years, reaching levels of 15 to 30 mg/dL (500 to 1000 mcmol/L) or more, depending on the patient's muscle mass. BUN levels are directly related to dietary protein intake. Without protein restriction, BUN levels may rise to 10 to 20 times the value of the serum creatinine level. With dietary protein restriction, BUN levels are elevated but less than those of non–protein-restricted patients. Fluid balance also affects BUN.

Imaging Assessment. Few x-ray findings are abnormal with CKD. Bone x-rays of the hand can show renal osteodystrophy. With long-term ESKD, the kidneys shrink (except for ESKD caused by polycystic kidney disease) and may be 8 to 9 cm or smaller. This small size results from atrophy and fibrosis. If CKD progresses suddenly, a kidney ultrasound or CT scan without contrast medium may be used to rule out an obstruction. (See Chapter 60 for a complete description of diagnostic tests for kidney function.)

◆ **Analysis: Analyze Cues and Prioritize Hypotheses.** The patient with CKD usually has progressive reduction of kidney function. Management generally occurs in the community setting. In the acute or long-term care setting, the focus of care is to manage problems and prevent complications of CKD. The priority collaborative problems for patients with CKD include:

1. Fluid overload due to the inability of diseased kidneys to maintain body fluid balance
2. Decreased cardiac function due to reduced stroke volume, dysrhythmias, fluid overload, and increased peripheral vascular resistance
3. Weight loss due to inability to ingest, digest, or absorb food and nutrients as a result of physiologic factors
4. Potential for injury due to effects of kidney disease on bone density, blood clotting, and drug elimination
5. Potential for psychosocial compromise due to chronic kidney disease

◆ **Planning and Implementation: Generate Solutions and Take Action**

Managing Fluid Volume

Planning: Expected Outcomes. The patient with CKD is expected to achieve and maintain an acceptable *fluid and electrolyte balance* and remain free of pulmonary edema.

Interventions. Management of the patient with CKD includes drug therapy, nutrition therapy, fluid restriction, and dialysis (when the patient reaches stage 5). Hemodialysis is performed intermittently for 3 to 4 hours, typically 3 days per week. Alternatively, some patients with ESKD receive peritoneal dialysis (PD). PD uses the peritoneum as the dialyzing membrane. The dialysate is infused through a catheter tunneled into the peritoneum. Dialysis for ESKD is described later in the Kidney Replacement Therapies section.

The purpose of fluid management is to attain fluid balance and prevent complications of fluid overload (see the Best Practice for Patient Safety & Quality Care: Managing Fluid Volume box). Monitor the patient's intake and output and hydration status. Assess for indications of fluid overload (e.g., lung crackles, edema, distended neck veins).

Drug therapy with diuretics is prescribed for patients with mild-to-severe CKD to increase urinary *elimination* of fluid. The increased urine output with this therapy helps reduce fluid overload and hypertension in patients who still have some urine output. Diuretics are seldom used in ESKD after dialysis is started, because as kidney function is reduced these drugs can accumulate and harm the remaining kidney cells and the patient's hearing. See the Common Examples of Drug Therapy: Chronic Kidney Disease box.

BEST PRACTICE FOR PATIENT SAFETY & QUALITY CARE QSEN
Managing Fluid Volume

- Weigh the patient daily at the same time each day, using the same scale, with the patient wearing the same amount and type of clothing, and graph the results.
- Observe the weight graph for trends (1 L of water weighs 1 kg).
- Accurately measure all fluid intake and output.
- Teach the patient and family about the need to keep fluid intake within prescribed restricted amounts and to ensure that the prescribed daily amount is evenly distributed throughout the 24 hours.
- Monitor for these symptoms of fluid overload at least every 4 hours during critical illness:
  - Decreased urine output
  - Rapid, bounding pulse
  - Rapid, shallow respirations
  - Presence of dependent edema
  - Auscultation of crackles or wheezes
  - Presence of distended neck veins in a sitting position
  - Decreased oxygen saturation
  - Elevated blood pressure
  - Narrowed pulse pressure
- Assess level of consciousness and degree of cognition.
- Ask about the presence of headache or blurred vision.

Assess fluid status by obtaining daily weights and reviewing intake and output. Daily weight gain in these patients indicates fluid retention rather than true body weight gain. Estimate the amount of fluid retained: 1 kg of weight equals about 1 L of fluid retained. Weigh the patient daily at the same time each day, on the same scale, wearing the same amount of clothing, and after voiding (if the patient is not anuric). Monitor weight for changes before and after dialysis.

Fluid restriction is often needed. Consider all forms of fluid intake, including oral, IV, and enteral sources, when calculating fluid intake. Help the patient spread oral fluid intake over a 24-hour period. Monitor his or her response to fluid restriction, and notify the primary health care provider if symptoms of fluid overload persist or worsen.

Pulmonary edema can result from left-sided heart failure (HF) related to fluid overload or from blood vessel injury. In left-sided HF, the heart is unable to eject blood adequately from the left ventricle, leading to an increased pressure in the left atrium and in the pulmonary blood vessels. The increased pressure causes fluid to cross the capillaries into the pulmonary tissue, forming edema (McCance et al., 2019). Pulmonary edema can also occur from injury to the lung blood vessels as a result of uremia. This condition causes inflammation and capillary leak. Fluid then leaks from pulmonary circulation into the lung tissue and alveoli. It may also leak into the pleural space, causing a *pleural effusion.*

Assess the patient for early indicators of pulmonary edema, such as restlessness, anxiety, rapid heart rate, shortness of breath, and crackles that begin at the base of the lungs. As pulmonary edema worsens, the level of fluid in the lungs rises. Auscultation reveals increased crackles and decreased breath sounds. The patient may have frothy, blood-tinged sputum. As cardiac and

COMMON EXAMPLES OF DRUG THERAPY

Chronic Kidney Disease

Drug	Nursing Implications
Loop Diuretics	
Increase urine output to manage volume overload when urinary elimination is still present.	
• Furosemide • Bumetanide • Dose varies with severity of kidney damage; not effective in ESKD	Monitor intake and output *to assess therapy effectiveness.* Generally the expected outcome is for output to be greater than intake by 500-1000/mL/24 hr. Monitor electrolytes *because these drugs result in loss of potassium;* this can be a desired effect in patients with hyperkalemia.
Vitamins and Minerals	
Used to replace those lost through dialysis or poorly absorbed as a result of dietary restrictions and to lower vitamin or mineral excesses that could lead to more problems.	
Phosphate binders form an insoluble calcium-phosphate complex to inhibit GI absorption to prevent hyperphosphatemia and renal osteodystrophy from hypocalcemia: • Calcium acetate • Calcium carbonate Noncalcium phosphate binders reduce blood phosphate levels without disturbing calcium levels: • Lanthanum carbonate • Sevelamer	Teach patients to take drugs with meals *to increase the effectiveness in slowing or preventing the absorption of dietary phosphorus.* Teach patients not to take these drugs within 2 hours of other scheduled drugs *to prevent the inhibited absorption of other drugs, especially cardiac drugs and antibiotics.* Monitor both serum phosphorus and calcium levels because *these drugs lower phosphorus and can cause hypercalcemia.* Monitor for constipation *because these can cause significant constipation, leading to fecal impaction or ileus.* Teach patients to report muscle weakness, slow or irregular pulse, or confusion to the prescriber *because these are symptoms of hypophosphatemia and indicate that dosage adjustment is required.*
Multivitamins and vitamin B supplements • Folic acid/folate • Cyanocobalamin (B_{12})	Teach patients to take the drugs after dialysis *to prevent the supplement from being removed from the blood during dialysis.* Teach patients to take iron supplements (ferrous sulfate) with meals *to reduce nausea and abdominal discomfort.*
Oral iron salts • Ferrous sulfate • Ferrous fumarate • Ferrous gluconate	Teach patients to take stool softeners daily while taking iron supplements, *which can cause constipation.* Remind patients that iron supplements change the color of the stool *because knowing the expected side effects decreases anxiety when they appear.*
Parenteral iron salts: • Iron dextran (IV) • Iron sucrose (IV)	A test dose of iron dextran is recommended *before IV administration because the incidence of allergic reactions is high.* Do not mix with drug with other parenteral drugs *because there are many incompatibilities.*
Vitamin D. • Calcitriol • Paricalcitol • Doxercalciferol	Monitor serum levels of calcium *because this active form of vitamin D suppresses parathyroid production and can lead to hypocalcemia.* Monitor serum levels of vitamin D *because this is a lipid-soluble vitamin that can be overingested and lead to toxicity. Serum calcium levels should stay below 10 mg/dL (Burchum & Rosenthal, 2019).*
Erythropoietin-Stimulating Agents (ESAs)	
Used to prevent or correct anemia caused by kidney disease through the stimulation of the bone marrow to increase red blood cell production and maturation.	
• Epoetin alfa • Darbepoetin alfa	Monitor hemoglobin values *because these drugs can overproduce blood cells, which increases blood viscosity and causes hypertension. This problem increases the risk for a myocardial infarction. Dosage is individualized to produce hemoglobin levels no higher than 10-11 g/dL (Burchum & Rosenthal, 2019).* Teach patients to report any of these side effects to the prescriber as soon as possible: chest pain, difficulty breathing, high blood pressure, rapid weight gain, seizures, skin rash or hives, or swelling of feet or ankles *because these symptoms indicate possible serious cardiac complications.*
Parathyroid Hormone Modulator	
Used to reduce parathyroid gland production of parathyroid hormone by decreasing the gland's sensitivity to calcium. This action helps maintain blood calcium and phosphorus levels closer to normal and can reduce renal osteodystrophy in patients with chronic kidney disease.	
• Cinacalcet	Monitor blood levels of calcium and phosphorus *to assess drug therapy effectiveness and recognize imbalances of these important electrolytes.* Teach the patient to monitor for and report diarrhea and muscle pain (myalgia), *which are indications of calcium and/or phosphorus imbalance.*

ESKD, End-stage kidney disease.

TABLE 63.8 Dietary Restrictions Needed for Severe Kidney Disease			
Dietary Component	With Chronic Uremia	With Hemodialysis	With Peritoneal Dialysis
Protein	0.55-0.60 g/kg/day	1.0-1.5 g/kg/day	1.2-1.5 g/kg/day
Fluid	Depends on urine output but may be as high as 1500-3000 mL/day	500-700 mL/day plus amount of urine output	Restriction based on fluid weight gain and blood pressure
Potassium	60-70 mEq or mmol daily	70 mEq or mmol daily	Usually no restriction
Sodium	1-3 g/day	2-4 g/day	Restriction based on fluid weight gain and blood pressure
Phosphorus	700 mg/day	700 mg/day	800 mg/day

pulmonary function decrease further, the patient becomes diaphoretic and cyanotic.

The patient with pulmonary edema usually is admitted to the hospital for aggressive treatment and continuous cardiac monitoring. Place the patient in a high-Fowler position and give oxygen to improve gas exchange. Drug therapy with kidney failure and pulmonary edema is difficult because of potential adverse drug effects on the kidneys (Burchum & Rosenthal, 2019). Loop diuretics such as IV furosemide are used to manage pulmonary edema. Kidney impairment increases the risk for *ototoxicity* (ear damage with hearing loss) with furosemide; thus IV doses are given cautiously and slowly. Diuresis usually begins within 5 minutes of giving IV furosemide. Measure urine output hourly until the patient is stabilized. Monitor vital signs and assess breath sounds at least every 2 hours to evaluate the patient's response to this treatment.

IV morphine can be prescribed to reduce myocardial oxygen demand by triggering blood vessel dilation and to provide sedation. Dosage adjustments are needed to achieve the desired response and avoid respiratory depression. Monitor the patient's respiratory rate, oxygen saturation, and blood pressure hourly during this therapy. Other drugs that dilate blood vessels, such as nitroglycerin, may be given as a continuous infusion to reduce pulmonary pressure from left-sided HF. Monitor vital signs at least hourly because this drug combination may cause severe hypotension.

Monitor serum electrolyte levels daily and report abnormalities to the primary health care provider so imbalances can be corrected quickly. If using ECG monitoring, identify dysrhythmias as they occur and report changes in rhythm that affect consciousness or blood pressure immediately to the provider. Monitor oxygen saturation levels by pulse oximetry and consult with the respiratory therapist for the optimal method to deliver oxygen (e.g., facemask, nasal cannula, or noninvasive mechanical support [see Chapter 25]). Monitor the patient for worsening of the condition with indications of increasing hypoxemia (decreasing SpO_2 values, restlessness, decreased cognition, or new-onset confusion). Temporary intubation and mechanical ventilation may be needed if respiratory failure occurs.

Patients with CKD who have existing cardiac problems, high blood pressure, or chronic fluid retention are at increased risk for developing pulmonary edema. They are less likely to respond quickly to treatment and are more likely to develop problems related to drug therapy. Kidney replacement therapy with ultrafiltration or dialysis may be used to reduce fluid volume.

Improving Cardiac Function

Planning: Expected Outcomes. The patient with CKD is expected to attain and maintain adequate cardiac function.

Interventions. Many patients with long-standing hypertension are at risk for CKD and accelerated progression of kidney failure once CKD occurs. *Therefore blood pressure control is essential in preserving kidney function* (Norton et al., 2017a). To control blood pressure, diuretics (especially thiazides), calcium channel blockers, angiotensin-converting enzyme inhibitors (ACEIs), alpha-adrenergic and beta-adrenergic blockers, and vasodilators may be prescribed. ACEIs are the most effective drugs to decrease cardiovascular events when patients have CKD and hypertension. Calcium channel blockers can improve the GFR and blood flow within the kidney.

More information on the specific drugs for blood pressure control can be found in Chapter 33. Indications vary, depending on the patient, and these drugs are used carefully to avoid complications. Different dosages and combinations may be tried until blood pressure control is adequate and side effects are minimized. Although there are many blood pressure guidelines available regarding goals of treatment, in CKD (diabetic and nondiabetic) with albumin excretion greater than 30 mg/24 hr, a target blood pressure of 130/80 mm Hg or lower is recommended (Ferri, 2020).

Teach the patient and family to measure blood pressure daily. Evaluate their ability to measure and record blood pressure accurately using their own equipment. Recheck measurement accuracy on a regular basis. Teach the patient and family about the relationship of blood pressure control to diet and drug therapy. Instruct the patient to weigh daily and to bring records of blood pressure measurements and drug administration times and weights for discussion with the physician, nurse, or registered dietitian nutritionist.

Assess the patient on an ongoing basis for signs and symptoms of reduced cardiac output, heart failure (HF), and dysrhythmias. These topics are discussed in Chapters 30, 31, and 32.

Enhancing Nutrition

Planning: Expected Outcomes. The patient with CKD is expected to maintain adequate nutrition, demonstrating a protein-caloric intake appropriate for his or her weight-to-height ratio, muscle tone, and laboratory values (serum albumin, hematocrit, hemoglobin).

Interventions. The nutrition needs and diet restrictions for the patient with CKD vary according to the degree of kidney function and the type of kidney replacement therapy used (Table 63.8). The purpose of nutrition therapy is to provide the food and fluids needed to prevent malnutrition and avoid complications from CKD.

Referral to a registered dietitian nutritionist (RDN) is recommended in patients with a GFR below 50 mL/min/1.73 m² and is a Medicare-covered service (Ferri, 2020). Collaborate with the RDN to teach the patient about diet changes that are needed as a result of CKD. Common changes include control of protein intake; fluid intake limitation; restriction of potassium, sodium, and phosphorus intake; taking vitamin and mineral supplements; and eating enough calories to meet metabolic need.

Protein restriction early in the course of the disease prevents some of the problems of CKD and may preserve kidney function. Protein is restricted on the basis of the degree of kidney and waste **elimination** impairment (reduced glomerular filtration rate [GFR]) and the severity of the symptoms. Buildup of waste products from protein breakdown is the main cause of uremia.

The GFR and treatment of CKD are used to guide safe levels of protein intake. In patients with a GFR below 30 mL/min/1.73 m², KDIGO has recommended that protein intake should be lowered to 0.8 g/kg/day. Protein intake greater than 1.3 g/kg/day should be avoided in adults with CKD at risk of progression (Ferri, 2020). If protein is lost in the urine, it is added to the diet in amounts equal to that lost. Protein requirements are calculated by the registered dietitian nutritionist based on actual body weight (corrected for edema), not ideal body weight.

The patient with ESKD receiving dialysis needs *more* protein because some protein is lost through dialysis. Protein requirements are tailored according to the patient's postdialysis, or "dry," weight. In general, patients receiving hemodialysis are allowed about 1 to 1.3 g of protein per kilogram per day (Ferri, 2020). Suggested protein-containing foods are meat and eggs. If protein intake is not adequate, muscle wasting can occur. BUN and serum prealbumin levels are used to monitor the adequacy of protein intake. Decreased serum prealbumin levels indicate poor protein intake.

Sodium restriction is needed in patients with little or no urine output to maintain **fluid and electrolyte balance.** Both fluid and sodium retention cause edema, hypertension, and heart failure (HF). Most patients with CKD retain sodium; a few cannot conserve sodium.

Estimate fluid and sodium retention status by monitoring the patient's body weight and blood pressure. In uremic patients not receiving dialysis, sodium is limited to 1 to 3 g daily, and fluid intake depends on urine output. In patients receiving dialysis, the sodium restriction is 2 to 4 g daily, and fluid intake is limited to 500 to 700 mL plus the amount of any urine output. Instruct the patient not to add salt at the table or during cooking. Many foods are significant sources of sodium (e.g., processed food, fast food, potato chips, pretzels, pickles, ham, bacon, sausage) and difficult to moderate or remove from one's diet. Inattention to sodium intake can increase the duration or number of dialysis treatments and contribute to *disequilibrium syndrome* (feeling unsteady or off balance) following dialysis.

Potassium restriction may be needed because high blood potassium levels can cause dangerous cardiac dysrhythmias.

Monitor the ECG for tall, peaked T waves caused by hyperkalemia. Instruct the patient with ESKD to limit potassium intake to 60 to 70 mEq (mmol) daily. Teach him or her to read labels of seasoning agents carefully for sodium and potassium content. Foods that are low in potassium and are permitted and foods that are high in potassium should be avoided (see Chapter 13). Instruct patients to avoid salt substitutes composed of potassium chloride. Those receiving peritoneal dialysis (PD) or who are producing urine may not need potassium restriction.

Phosphorus restriction for control of phosphorus levels is started early in CKD to avoid renal osteodystrophy. Monitor serum phosphorus levels. Dietary phosphorus restrictions and drugs to assist with phosphorus control may be prescribed. Phosphate binders must be taken at mealtime. Most patients with CKD already restrict their protein intake; and, because high-protein foods are also high in phosphorus, this reduces phosphorus intake. Chapter 13 lists foods high in potassium, sodium, and phosphorus. Cinacalcet, a drug to control parathyroid hormone excess, is also used to manage hyperphosphatemia and hypocalcemia.

Vitamin and mineral supplementation is needed daily for most patients with CKD. Low-protein diets are also low in vitamins, and water-soluble vitamins are removed from the blood during dialysis. Anemia also is a problem in patients with CKD because of the limited iron content of low-protein diets and decreased kidney production of erythropoietin. Thus supplemental iron is needed. Calcium and vitamin D supplements may be needed, depending on the patient's serum calcium levels and bone status.

Nutrition needs for patients undergoing peritoneal dialysis (PD) are slightly different from those for patients undergoing dialysis. Because protein is lost with the dialysate in PD, protein replacement is needed. Often 1.2 to 1.5 g of protein per kilogram of body weight per day is recommended. Patients may have anorexia and have difficulty eating enough protein. High-calorie oral supplements may also be needed (e.g., Magnacal Renal, Ensure Plus). Sodium restriction varies with fluid weight gain and blood pressure. Usually dietary potassium does not need to be restricted because the dialysate is potassium free, causing excess potassium to be removed from the blood. Any potassium restriction is determined by serum potassium levels.

Collaborate with the RDN to assess each patient's nutrition needs. Teach the patient the dietary regimen and evaluate his or her understanding of and adherence to it. Give the patient and family written examples of the diet to promote adherence. Help patients adapt diet restrictions to their budget, ethnic background, and food preferences.

Preventing Injury

Planning: Expected Outcomes. The patient with CKD is expected to remain free of injury including pathologic fractures, toxic side effects from drug therapy, infection, and bleeding.

Interventions. *Injury prevention strategies* are needed because the patient with long-standing CKD may have brittle, fragile bones that fracture easily and cause little pain. When lifting or moving a patient with fragile bones, use a lift sheet rather than pulling the patient. Teach assistive personnel (AP) the correct use of lift sheets. Observe for normal range of joint motion and for any unusual surface bumps or depressions over bony areas.

Managing drug therapy in patients with CKD is a complex clinical problem. Many over-the-counter drugs contain agents that alter kidney function. Therefore it is important to obtain a detailed drug history. Know the use of each drug, its side effects, and its site of metabolism.

Certain drugs must be avoided, and the dosages of others must be adjusted according to the degree of remaining kidney function. As the patient's kidney function decreases, consult with the nephrologist and pharmacist to determine if further dosage adjustments are necessary. Assess for side effects and indications of drug toxicity and notify the prescriber as appropriate.

! NURSING SAFETY PRIORITY (QSEN)

Drug Alert

Monitor the patient with severe CKD or ESKD closely for drug-related complications and ensure that dosages are adjusted as needed. Patients with CKD have complex needs due to multiple medications and comorbidities. Consult with the pharmacist to determine safe effective doses.

Drugs to control an excessively high phosphorus level include phosphate-binding agents. These drugs help prevent renal osteodystrophy and related injuries. Stress the importance of taking these agents and all prescribed drugs.

Hypophosphatemia (low serum phosphorus levels) is a complication of phosphate binding, especially in patients who do not eat adequately but continue to take phosphate-binding drugs. *Hypercalcemia* (high serum calcium levels) can occur in patients taking calcium-containing compounds to control phosphorus excess. In patients taking aluminum-based phosphate binders for prolonged periods, aluminum deposits may cause bone disease or neurologic problems. Monitor the patient for muscle weakness, anorexia, malaise, tremors, and bone pain.

Teach patients with kidney disease to avoid antacids containing magnesium. These patients cannot excrete magnesium and thus should avoid additional intake.

Some drugs, in addition to those used to treat kidney failure, require special attention because they either are normally excreted by the kidney or can further damage the kidney. These drugs include antibiotics, opioids, antihypertensives, diuretics, insulin, and heparin.

Monitor carefully for indicators of infection. These indicators include fever, lymph node enlargements, and elevated WBC counts, as well as positive cultures. For patients undergoing dialysis, inspect the vascular access site or PD catheter insertion site every shift for redness, swelling, pain, or drainage. If antibiotics are required, use caution in the patient with CKD. Many antibiotics are safe for patients with CKD, but those excreted by the kidney and those that are nephrotoxic require dose adjustment (Himmelfarb & Ikizler, 2018). To prevent complications of bloodstream infection from mouth bacteria, prophylactic antibiotics are given to patients with CKD before dental procedures.

Give opioid analgesics cautiously in patients with stage 3 or 4 CKD or ESKD because the effects often last longer. Patients with uremia are sensitive to the respiratory depressant effects of these drugs. Because opioids are broken down by the liver and not the kidneys, the dosages are often the same, regardless of the level of kidney function. Monitor the patient's reactions closely after opioids are given to determine whether adjustments are needed.

As CKD progresses, the patient with diabetes often requires reduced doses of insulin or antidiabetic drugs because the failing kidneys do not excrete or metabolize these drugs well. Thus the drugs are effective longer, increasing the risk for hypoglycemia. Monitor blood glucose levels at least four times daily to assess whether a dosage change is needed.

Poor platelet function and capillary fragility in CKD make anticoagulant therapy risky. Monitor patients receiving heparin, warfarin, or any anticoagulant every shift for bleeding. See Chapter 37 for more information on caring for patients at increased risk for bleeding.

Minimizing Psychosocial Compromise. Due to the chronic nature and impact of CKD, the patient with CKD may experience fatigue and psychosocial impact. These impacts can include anxiety, social isolation, and depression. The patient with CKD often experiences depression (Lotfaliany, 2018). Loss, such as loss of work or family roles, may contribute to depression. Depressive symptoms have been associated with nonadherence to CKD treatments. Sleep disturbances, also interrelated with depression, are common among adults receiving dialysis for ESKD.

Planning: Expected Outcomes. The goal for patients with CKD is to conserve energy by balancing activity and rest, have reduced anxiety and depression, and minimize the overall psychosocial impact of the disease.

Interventions. Perform an ongoing assessment of the patient's level of fatigue as well as reports of anxiety. Ask about sleep patterns and quality. Assess the coping mechanisms and successful methods of dealing with problems. Observe behavior for cues indicating increasing anxiety (e.g., anxious facial expressions, clenching of hands, tapping of feet, withdrawn posture, absence of eye contact) and provide interventions to decrease the anxiety level. Evaluate the support systems and the involvement of family and friends with the patient's care. Provide ongoing supportive interventions throughout therapy. Assess for indicators of depression including despair and loneliness.

Some causes of *fatigue* in the patient with CKD include vitamin deficiency, anemia, and buildup of urea. All patients are given vitamin and mineral supplements because of diet restrictions and vitamin losses from dialysis. Avoid giving these supplements right before hemodialysis (HD) treatment because they will be dialyzed out of the body and the patient will receive no benefit.

The anemic patient with CKD is treated with agents to stimulate red blood cell (RBC) production. The desired outcome of this therapy is to maintain a hemoglobin level around 10 g/dL (100 g/L). This therapy triggers bone marrow production of RBCs if the patient has adequate iron stores. Iron supplements may be needed in patients who are iron deficient. Many who receive these drugs report improved appetite and sexual function along with decreased fatigue. The increased production of all blood cells from this therapy may increase blood pressure. The improved appetite challenges patients in their attempts to maintain protein, potassium, and fluid restrictions and requires additional education.

Unfamiliar settings and lack of knowledge about treatments and tests can increase the patient's anxiety level. Explain all procedures, tests, and treatments. Identify the patient's knowledge needs about kidney disease. Provide instruction at a level that he or she can understand, using a variety of written and visual materials. Provide continuity of care, whenever possible, by using a consistent and trusting nurse-patient relationship to decrease anxiety and encourage the patient to discuss his or her thoughts and feelings about any current problems or concerns.

Encourage the patient to ask questions and discuss fears about the diagnosis, treatment strategies, and common outcomes. An open atmosphere that allows for discussion can decrease anxiety. Facilitate discussions with family members about the prognosis and the impact on lifestyle.

Identify community resources to maintain independence, including delivered meals, transportation, and financial or health care options.

In the general population, drugs are commonly used to manage depression. However, pharmacologic effects of drugs in adults with CKD or those receiving dialysis are altered, and additional monitoring may be needed with alternative approaches for effective care. Care coordination for patients with CKD is essential because multiple health care professions may be involved in delivering care. Care coordination helps to avoid adverse drug effects (and drug-drug interactions), avoid hospitalizations, and decrease problems related to depression.

Kidney Replacement Therapies. Kidney replacement therapy (KRT) is needed when the pathologic changes of stage 4 and stage 5 CKD are life threatening or pose continuing discomfort. When the patient can no longer be managed with conservative therapies, such as diet, drugs, and fluid restriction, dialysis is indicated. Transplantation may be discussed at any time.

Hemodialysis. Intermittent hemodialysis (HD) is the most common KRT used with ESKD (Table 63.9). Dialysis removes excess fluids and waste products and restores *fluid and electrolyte balance* and *acid-base balance*. HD involves passing the patient's blood through an artificial semipermeable membrane to perform the kidney's filtering and excretion functions. Safe HD therapy requires technicians to provide meticulous care to the machines delivering HD and nurses to implement and supervise direct care. Technical or human error can lead to avoidable complications (e.g., hemolysis, air embolism, dialysate error, contamination, exsanguination).

Patient Selection. Any patient may be considered for intermittent HD therapy. Starting HD depends on symptoms from disruptions of *fluid and electrolyte balance* and waste and toxin accumulation, not the GFR alone. Normally the decision to start dialysis is made by a nephrologist who has been monitoring a patients decreasing GFR and increasing symptoms.

TABLE 63.9 **Comparison of Hemodialysis and Peritoneal Dialysis**	
Hemodialysis	**Peritoneal Dialysis**
Advantages	
More efficient clearance of wastes	Flexible schedule for exchanges
Short time needed for treatment	Few hemodynamic changes during and following exchanges
	Fewer dietary and fluid restrictions
Complications	
Disequilibrium syndrome	Protein loss
Muscle cramps and back pain	Peritonitis
Headache	Respiratory distress
Itching	Inflammatory bowel disease
Hemodynamic and cardiac adverse events (hypotension, cell lysis contributing to anemia, cardiac dysrhythmias)	Bowel perforation
	Infection
Infection	Weight gain; discomfort from "carrying" 1-2 L in abdomen during dwell time; potential for back pain or development of hernia
Increased risk for subdural and intracranial hemorrhage from anticoagulation and changes in blood pressure during dialysis	
Anemia	
Access site complications	
Contraindications	
Hemodynamic instability or severe cardiac disease	Extensive peritoneal adhesions, fibrosis, or active inflammatory GI disease (e.g., diverticulitis, inflammatory bowel conditions)
Severe vascular disease that prevents vascular access	
Serious bleeding disorders	Ascites or massive central obesity
	Recent abdominal surgery
Access	
Arteriovenous (AV) fistula	Intra-abdominal catheter
AV graft	
Central venous catheter	
Procedure	
Complex; requires a second person trained in the technique whether completed at home or at a dialysis unit/center	Simple, easier to complete at home compared with at-home hemodialysis
Special training for center personnel and in-home use	Less complex training; typically managed by patient; can be managed by one person

Some indications for emergent dialysis include:

- Pulmonary edema
- Severe uncontrollable hypertension
- Symptomatic hyperkalemia with ECG changes
- Other severe electrolyte or acid-base disturbances
- Some overdoses
- Pericarditis

Most commonly, hemodialysis for CKD is started when uremic symptoms (e.g., intractable nausea and vomiting, confusion, seizures, or severe bleeding from platelet dysfunction) occur.

Many patients survive for years with HD therapy, and others may live only a few months. Length of survival with HD therapy depends on patient age, the cause of CKD, and the presence of other diseases, such as cardiovascular conditions or diabetes. Selection criteria include:

- Irreversible kidney failure when other therapies are unacceptable or ineffective
- No disorders that would seriously complicate HD
- Patient values and preferences
- Expected ability to continue or resume roles at home, work, or school

Dialysis Settings. Patients with CKD may receive HD treatments in many settings, depending on specific needs. Regardless of the setting for therapy, they need ongoing nursing support to maintain this complex and lifesaving treatment.

Patients may be dialyzed in a hospital-based center if they have recently started treatment or have complicated conditions that require close supervision. Stable patients not requiring intense supervision may be dialyzed in a community or freestanding dialysis center. Selected patients may participate in self-care in an ambulatory care center or with in-home HD.

In-home HD is the least disruptive treatment and allows the patient to adapt the regimen to his or her lifestyle. Newer technologies and HD equipment are making home dialysis an easier process to learn. It is growing in popularity and use. A water treatment system must be installed in the home to provide a safe, clean water supply for the dialysis process.

Procedure. Dialysis works by using the passive transfer of toxins by diffusion. **Diffusion** is the movement of molecules from an area of higher concentration to an area of lower concentration. The rate of diffusion during dialysis is most dependent on the difference in the solute concentrations between the patient's blood and the dialysate. Large molecules, such as RBCs and most plasma proteins, cannot pass through the membrane.

When HD is started, blood and **dialysate** (dialyzing solution) flow in opposite directions across an enclosed semipermeable membrane. The dialysate contains a balanced mix of electrolytes and water that closely resembles human plasma. On the other side of the membrane is the patient's blood, which contains nitrogen waste products, excess water, and excess electrolytes. During HD, the waste products move from the blood into the dialysate because of the difference in their concentrations (diffusion). Some water is also removed from the blood into the dialysate by *osmosis*. Electrolytes can move in either direction, as needed, and take some fluid with them. Potassium and sodium typically move out of the plasma into the dialysate. Bicarbonate and calcium generally move from the dialysate into the plasma. This circulating process continues for a preset length of time, removing nitrogenous wastes, reestablishing *fluid and electrolyte balance,* and restoring *acid-base balance.* Water volume may be removed from the plasma by applying positive or negative pressure to the system.

The HD system includes a dialyzer, dialysate, vascular access routes, and an HD machine. The artificial kidney, or dialyzer (Fig. 63.3), has four parts: a blood compartment, a dialysate compartment, a semipermeable membrane, and an enclosed support structure.

Dialysate is made from water and chemicals and is free of any waste products or drugs. It is usually dispensed from the

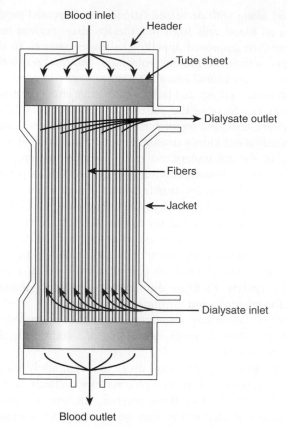

FIG. 63.3 Hollow fiber dialyzer (artificial kidney) used in hemodialysis. (From Feehally, J., Floege, J., & Johnson, R. [2007]. *Comprehensive clinical nephrology* [3rd ed.]. Philadelphia: Mosby.)

pharmacy in an acute care setting. The solution may be mixed in large or small batches by technicians in dialysis centers. Because bacteria and other organisms are too large to pass through the membrane, dialysate is not sterile. Water used in dialysate must meet specific standards and requires special treatment before mixing the dialysate. Dialysate composition may be altered for the patient's needs for management of electrolyte imbalances. During HD, the dialysate is warmed to 100°F (37.8°C) to increase the diffusion rate and prevent hypothermia.

The HD machine has built-in safety features such as the ability to record patient vital signs, blood and dialysate flows, arterial and venous pressures, delivered dialysis dose, plasma volume changes, and temperature changes. If any of these problems are detected, an alarm sounds to protect the patient from life-threatening complications.

All dialyzers function in a similar manner. Fig. 63.4 shows a comparison of fluid and particle movement across the dialyzer membranes, comparing intermittent HD with continuous kidney replacement circuits. For intermittent HD, the number and length of treatments depend on the amount of wastes and fluid to be removed, the clearance capacity of the dialyzer, and the blood flow rate to and from the machine. Fig. 63.5 shows a typical intermittent dialysis machine. Most patients receive three 4-hour treatments over the course of a week. For those with some ongoing urine production, two 5- to 6-hour treatments a week may be adequate. If the patient gains large amounts of

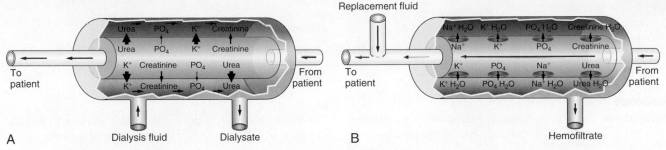

FIG. 63.4 Comparison of hemodialysis and hemofiltration fluid and solute movements across the membrane. Demonstrates this movement in hemodialysis (A) and hemofiltration (B). The *arrows* that cross the membrane indicate the predominant direction of movement of each solute through the membrane; the relative size of the *arrows* indicates the net amounts of the solute transferred. Other *arrows* indicate the direction of flow. (From Feehally, J., Floege, J., & Johnson, R. [2007]. *Comprehensive clinical nephrology* [3rd ed.]. Philadelphia: Mosby.)

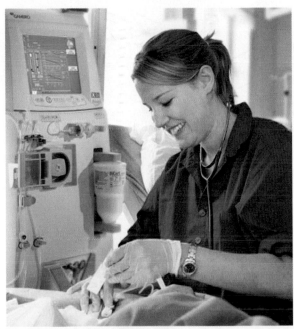

FIG. 63.5 Renal replacement therapy with an intermittent hemodialysis machine. (Courtesy Gambro Lundia AB, Lund, Sweden.)

fluid, a longer HD treatment time may be needed to remove the fluid without hypotension or other severe side effects.

Anticoagulation. Blood clotting can occur during dialysis. Anticoagulation, usually with heparin, is delivered into the blood circuit via a pump. In patients with high risk for bleeding, a reduced dose, regional anticoagulation (using citrate rather than heparin for anticoagulation or reversing heparin actions by administering protamine before returning blood to the patient), or no anticoagulation may be used. Patient response to heparin varies, and the dose is adjusted on the basis of each patient's need.

Heparin remains active in the body for 4 to 6 hours after dialysis, increasing the patient's risk for hemorrhage during and immediately after HD treatments. Invasive procedures must be avoided during that time. Monitor him or her closely for any signs of bleeding or hemorrhage. Protamine sulfate is an antidote to heparin and always should be available in the dialysis setting.

Vascular Access. Vascular access is required for hemodialysis (Table 63.10 and Fig. 63.6). The procedure requires the availability of a high blood flow: at least 250 to 300 mL/min, usually for a period of 3 to 4 hours (Norton et al., 2017b). Normal venous cannulation does not provide this high rate of blood flow.

Long-term vascular access is internal for most patients having long-term HD (see Table 63.10). The two common choices are an internal arteriovenous (AV) fistula or an AV graft (see Fig. 63.6). *AV fistulas* are formed by surgically connecting an artery to a vein. The vessels used most often are the radial or brachial artery and the cephalic vein of the nondominant arm. Fistulas increase venous blood flow to the 250 to 400 mL/min needed for effective dialysis.

Time is needed after the surgeon creates the AV fistula for it to develop into a usable access site for HD. As the AV fistula "matures," the increased pressure of the arterial blood flow into the vein causes the vessel walls to thicken. This thickening increases their strength and durability for repeated cannulation. The amount of time needed for the fistula to mature varies. Some fistulas may not be ready for use for as long as 4 months after the surgery, and a temporary vascular access (AV shunt or HD catheter) is used during this time. Fig. 63.7 shows a mature fistula.

To access a fistula, cannulate it by inserting two needles: one toward the venous blood flow and one toward the arterial blood flow. This procedure allows the HD machine to draw the blood out through the arterial needle and return it through the venous needle.

Arteriovenous grafts are used when the AV fistula does not develop or when complications limit its use. The polytetrafluoroethylene (PTFE) graft is a synthetic material (GORE-TEX). This type of graft is commonly used for older patients using HD. Figs. 63.6A and 63.7 show a patient's fistula.

Precautions. Precautions are needed to ensure the functioning of an internal AV fistula or AV graft. First assess for adequate circulation in the fistula or graft and in the lower portion of the arm. Check distal pulses and capillary refill in the arm with the fistula or graft. Then check for a bruit or a thrill by auscultation or palpation over the access site. See the Best Practice for Patient Safety & Quality Care: Caring for the Patient With an Arteriovenous Fistula or Arteriovenous Graft box.

TABLE 63.10 Types of Vascular Access for Hemodialysis

Access Type	Description	Location	Time to Initial Use
Permanent			
AV fistula	An internal anastomosis of an artery to a vein	Forearm Upper arm	2-3 mo or longer
AV graft	Looped plastic tubing tunneled beneath the skin, connecting an artery and a vein	Forearm Upper arm Inner thigh	1-3 wk after surgery
Temporary			
Dialysis catheter	A specially designed catheter with separate lumens for blood outflow and inflow	Subclavian vein, internal jugular, or femoral vein	Immediately after insertion and x-ray confirmation of placement
Subcutaneous catheter	An internal device with two access ports and a cuff or dual-lumen catheter inserted into a large central vein	Subclavian vein, internal jugular, or femoral vein	Dedicated use; do not access for blood sampling or drug administration

AV, Arteriovenous.

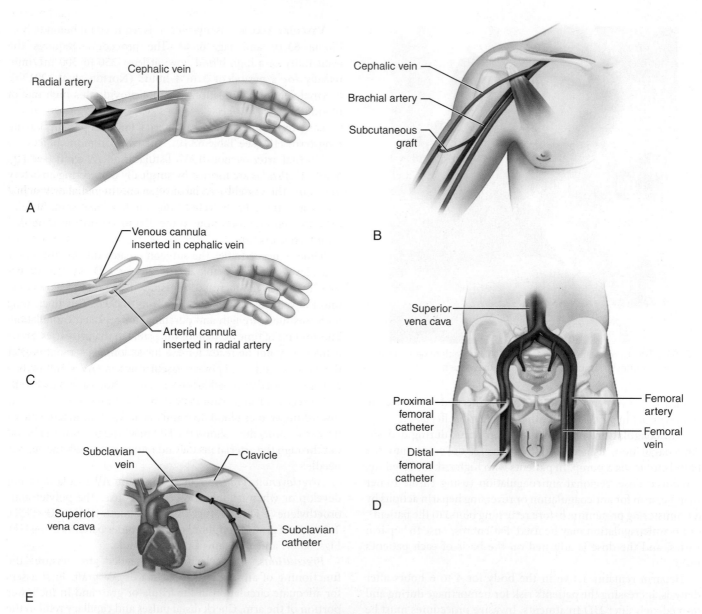

FIG. 63.6 Frequently used means for gaining vascular access for hemodialysis include arteriovenous fistula (A), arteriovenous graft (B), external arteriovenous shunt (C), femoral vein catheterization (D), and subclavian vein catheterization (E). (A) and (B) are options for long-term vascular access for hemodialysis. (C), (D), and (E) are used for short-term access for intermittent hemodialysis or for continuous renal replacement therapy in acute care.

BEST PRACTICE FOR PATIENT SAFETY & QUALITY CARE (QSEN)

Caring for the Patient With an Arteriovenous Fistula or Arteriovenous Graft

- Do not take blood pressure readings using the extremity in which the vascular access is placed.
- Do not perform venipunctures or start an IV line in the extremity in which the vascular access is placed.
- Palpate for thrills and auscultate for bruits over the vascular access site every 4 hours while the patient is awake.
- Assess the patient's distal pulses and circulation in the arm with the access.
- Elevate the affected extremity after surgery.
- Encourage routine range-of-motion exercises.
- Check for bleeding at needle insertion sites.
- Assess for indications of infection at needle sites.
- Instruct the patient not to carry heavy objects or anything that compresses the extremity in which the vascular access is placed.
- Instruct the patient not to sleep with his or her body weight on top of the extremity in which the vascular access is placed.

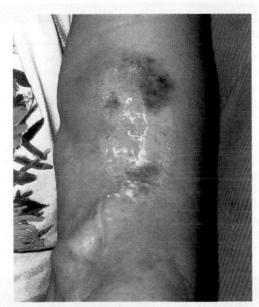

FIG. 63.7 A mature fistula for hemodialysis access. The increased pressure from the anastomosed artery forced blood into the vein. This process caused the vein to dilate enough for fistula needles to be placed for hemodialysis. When the vein is sufficiently dilated, a process that takes 8 to 12 weeks, the fistula is said to be *developed* or *mature*.

! NURSING SAFETY PRIORITY (QSEN)

Action Alert

Because repeated compression can result in the loss of the vascular access, avoid taking the blood pressure or performing venipunctures in the arm with the vascular access. Do not use an AV fistula or graft for general delivery of IV fluids or drugs.

Access Complications. Complications can occur with any type of access. Common problems include thrombosis or stenosis, infection, aneurysm formation, ischemia, and HF (Norton et al., 2017b). Table 63.11 lists strategies to prevent access complications.

Thrombosis, or clotting of the AV access, is the most frequent complication. Most grafts fail because of high-pressure arterial flow entering the venous system. The muscle layers of the veins react to this increased pressure by thickening. The venous thickening reduces or occludes blood flow. An interventional radiologist can reopen failing grafts with the injection of a thrombolytic drug to dissolve the clot. The clot usually dissolves within minutes, and often a stricture is revealed at the point where the graft and the vein connect. The stricture can be corrected by balloon angioplasty.

Most infections of the vascular access are caused by *Staphylococcus aureus* introduced during cannulation. Prepare the skin with an antibacterial agent according to agency policy before cannulation to prevent infection. When using dialysis catheters, be sure to use only the cleansing agent recommended by the catheter manufacturer. Some disinfectants can damage the catheter (Woo, 2019).

Aneurysms can form in the fistula and are caused by repeated needle punctures at the same site. Large aneurysms may cause loss of the fistula's function and require surgical repair.

Ischemia occurs in a few patients with vascular access when the fistula decreases arterial blood flow to areas below the fistula *(steal syndrome)*. Symptoms vary from cold or numb fingers to gangrene. If the collateral circulation is poor, the fistula may need to be surgically tied off, and a new one created in another area to preserve extremity circulation.

Shunting of blood directly from the arterial system to the venous system through the fistula can cause HF in patients with limited cardiac function. This complication is rare; but, if it does occur, the fistula may need to be revised to reduce arterial blood flow.

TABLE 63.11 Interventions for Preventing Complications in Hemodialysis Vascular Access

Access Type	Bleeding	Infection	Clotting
AV fistula or AV graft	Apply pressure to the needle puncture sites.	Prepare skin using best practices before cannulation. Typically 2% chlorhexidine is used, similar to central line skin preparation. Between hemodialysis sessions, the patient should wash the area with antibacterial soap and rinse with water.	Avoid constrictive devices such as blood pressure cuffs and tourniquets. Rotate needle insertion sites with each hemodialysis treatment. Assess for thrill and bruit.
Hemodialysis catheters (temporary and permanent)	Assess the access site every time you monitor vital signs.	Use aseptic technique to dress site and access catheter. Do not use catheters for blood sampling, IV fluids, or drug administration.	Place a heparin or heparin/saline dwell solution after hemodialysis treatment.

AV, Arteriovenous.

Temporary Vascular Access. Temporary access with special catheters can be used for patients requiring immediate HD. A catheter designed for HD may be inserted into the subclavian, internal jugular, or femoral vein. The lumens of these devices are much smaller than the permanent accesses, and more time (4 to 8 hours) is required to complete a dialysis session.

Subcutaneous devices may also be surgically inserted to provide temporary access for HD. Implanted beneath the skin, these devices are composed of two small metallic ports with attached catheters that are inserted into large central veins. The ports of subcutaneous devices have internal mechanisms that open when needles are inserted and close when needles are removed. Blood from one port flows from the body to the HD machine and returns to the body via the other port.

Hemodialysis Nursing Care. Many drugs are dialyzable (i.e., can be partially or completely removed from the blood during dialysis). Coordinate with the nephrology health care provider to assess the patient's drug regimen and determine which drugs should be held until after HD treatment. Table 63.12 lists common dialyzable drugs that should be given *after* rather than before HD. Consult the dialysis nurse or nephrologist to determine if antihypertensive drugs should be given before a scheduled dialysis treatment; some short-acting antihypertensives can contribute to hypotension during dialysis.

The time required to complete an HD treatment usually is at least 4 hours. During this time patients may use various distraction techniques to prevent boredom, such as reading, watching television or videos, visiting with friends or relatives, playing video games, or working puzzles. This time can be used also for brief health teaching opportunities.

Postdialysis Care. Closely monitor the patient immediately and for several hours after dialysis for any side effects from the treatment. Common problems include hypotension, headache, nausea, vomiting, dizziness, and muscle cramps.

Obtain vital signs and weight for comparison with predialysis measurements. Blood pressure and weight are expected to be reduced as a result of fluid removal. Hypotension may necessitate rehydration with IV fluids, such as normal saline. The patient's temperature may also be elevated because the dialysis machine warms the blood slightly. If he or she has a fever, sepsis may be present, and a blood sample is needed for culture and sensitivity.

The heparin or citrate required during HD increases the risk for excessive bleeding. All invasive procedures must be avoided for 4 to 6 hours after dialysis. Continually monitor the patient for hemorrhage during and for at least 1 hour after dialysis. See the Best Practice for Patient Safety & Quality Care: Caring for the Patient Undergoing Hemodialysis box.

Complications of Hemodialysis. Few adverse events occur during a 3- to 4-hour HD treatment under current practice protocols. Improved water treatment, more physiologic solutions, and improvements in HD equipment and procedures have significantly improved safe care for patients receiving this treatment. Complications during HD include hypotension, dialysis disequilibrium syndrome, cardiac events, and reactions to dialyzers (Norton et al., 2017b).

! NURSING SAFETY PRIORITY (QSEN)

Critical Rescue

Monitor the patient closely during dialysis to recognize hypotension, which is common. Heat transfer from warm solutions can result in vasodilation and a drop in blood pressure. When this occurs, reduce the temperature of the dialysate to 35°C (95°F). Fluid shifts from the plasma volume related to differences in electrolyte concentrations between HD solutions and blood also reduce blood pressure. Respond to modest declines in blood pressure by adjusting the rate of dialyzer blood flow and placing the patient in a legs-up (Trendelenburg) position. Respond to sustained or symptomatic hypotension by giving a fluid bolus of 100 to 250 mL of normal saline, albumin, or mannitol (if prescribed). A second bolus may be needed. If hypotension persists, new-onset myocardial injury or pericardial disease may be a contributing factor; respond by applying oxygen, reducing the blood flow, and notifying the primary health care provider urgently. Discontinue HD when hypotension continues despite two bolus infusions.

BEST PRACTICE FOR PATIENT SAFETY & QUALITY CARE (QSEN)

Caring for the Patient Undergoing Hemodialysis

- Weigh the patient before and after dialysis.
- Know the patient's dry weight.
- Discuss with the nephrology health care provider or pharmacist whether any of the patient's drugs should be withheld until after dialysis.
- Be aware of events that occurred during previous dialysis treatments.
- Measure blood pressure, pulse, respirations, and temperature.
- Assess for indications of orthostatic hypotension.
- Assess the vascular access site when taking vital signs and follow agency policy for central line care and dressing changes.
- Observe for bleeding at the vascular access site and other sites where skin integrity is disrupted because anticoagulants given during dialysis and the presence of uremia increase bleeding risk.
- Assess the patient's level of consciousness.
- Assess for headache, nausea, and vomiting.
- Assess serum laboratory tests to evaluate effectiveness of treatment in removing wastes and achieving desired outcomes (e.g., *fluid and electrolyte balance,* reduction of uremia).

TABLE 63.12 Examples of Dialyzable Drugs

Consult the pharmacist, nephrologist, or dialysis nurse to plan the best time to administer a drug based on the dialysis schedule.

Aminoglycosides
- Amikacin
- Gentamicin
- Tobramycin

Antituberculosis Agents
- Ethambutol
- Isoniazid

Antiviral and Antifungal Agents
- Acyclovir
- Ganciclovir
- Fluconazole

Cephalosporins
- Cefaclor
- Cefazolin
- Cefoxitin
- Ceftriaxone
- Cefuroxime
- Cefepime

Anticonvulsants
- Ethosuximide
- Gabapentin
- Phenobarbital

Penicillins
- Amoxicillin
- Ampicillin
- Dicloxacillin
- Penicillin G

Miscellaneous
- Aztreonam
- Cimetidine
- Vitamins
- Clavulanic acid
- Allopurinol
- Enalapril
- Aspirin

Dialysis disequilibrium syndrome may develop during HD or after HD has been completed. It is characterized by mental status changes and can include seizures or coma, although this severity of disequilibrium syndrome is rare with today's HD practice. A mild form of disequilibrium syndrome includes symptoms of nausea, vomiting, headaches, fatigue, and restlessness. It is thought to be the result of a rapid reduction in electrolytes and other particles. Reducing blood flow at the onset of symptoms can prevent this syndrome.

Cardiac events during HD are associated with underlying cardiovascular disease, especially left ventricular hypertrophy, coronary vascular disease, and a history of cardiac dysrhythmias. These conditions are described in Chapters 31, 32, and 35. Although cardiac arrest is a rare event, the setting should be equipped with an automatic defibrillator and staff or family trained in cardiopulmonary resuscitation. Often cardiac arrest is related to new-onset cardiac ischemia. This problem is managed in an acute care setting in which the presence of myocardial disease can be evaluated and cardiac treatment optimized.

Pericardial disease is a complication of patients with ESKD. Assess the patient's heart sounds for the presence of a pericardial rub before starting dialysis. Intensification of dialysis may be used to treat this complication. Other treatment might include NSAID use or surgery.

Reactions to dialyzers still occur, although more biocompatible membranes and careful attention to rinsing the dialyzer before use (to eliminate sterilizing agents) have reduced this adverse event during HD. Reactions occur during a "first-time" use of the filter and resemble an anaphylactic episode early during HD, with profound hypotension. (Chapter 18 describes anaphylactic reactions.) With suspected dialyzer reactions, do not return the blood to the patient, and discontinue HD. Corticosteroids may be used to treat the *immunity* reaction.

Other potential complications of HD require the nurse to monitor the level of consciousness and vital signs frequently during treatment and to slow or stop HD when symptoms occur. Hypoglycemia is a rare adverse HD event and more likely to occur when the patient has diabetes. It is managed by providing glucose and increasing dialysis glucose concentration in subsequent treatments. Hemorrhage can occur when needle dislodgment or circuit connections become loose and is amplified by anticoagulation used to maintain circuit patency. Some hemolysis occurs because of mechanical trauma to RBCs, contributing to anemia in the patient with CKD and, perhaps, to sensations of dyspnea or chest tightness.

Infectious diseases transmitted by blood transfusion are a serious complication of long-term HD. Two of the most serious blood-transmitted infections are hepatitis and human immune deficiency virus (HIV) infection. *Hepatitis B infection* and *hepatitis C infection* in patients with CKD have decreased because the use of erythropoietin-stimulating agents (ESAs) has reduced the need for blood transfusions to maintain RBC counts. Hepatitis is a problem because of the blood access and the risk for contamination during HD. The viruses can be transmitted through the use of contaminated needles or instruments, by entry of contaminated blood through open wounds in the skin or mucous membranes, or through transfusions with contaminated blood. Monitor all patients receiving HD for indications of hepatitis (see Chapter 53).

The risk for HIV transmission is reduced by the consistent practice of Standard Precautions, routine screening of donated blood for HIV, and decreased need for blood transfusions with CKD and ESKD. Patients who have been undergoing HD or who received frequent transfusions during the early to middle 1980s may have been infected at that time and are at risk for AIDS (HIV-III) (see Chapter 17).

PATIENT CENTERED CARE: OLDER ADULT CONSIDERATIONS (QSEN)

Adults over age 75 comprise one of the most rapidly increasing age-groups of dialysis patients. Patients should be educated about all aspects of dialysis care so that they can make an informed decision regarding dialysis initiation. In adults over age 80 with coronary artery disease in addition to other comorbid conditions, dialysis has not been shown to prolong life when compared with patients receiving more conservative treatments. Dialysis patients spend an average of 173 days per year in the hospital or at dialysis; nondialysis, medically treated patients spend an average of 16 days per year in the hospital (Himmelfarb & Ikizler, 2018).

Peritoneal Dialysis. Peritoneal dialysis (PD) allows exchanges of wastes, fluid, and electrolytes to occur in the peritoneal cavity. However, PD is slower than hemodialysis (HD), and more time is needed to achieve the same effect. Other disadvantages of PD are the protein loss in outflow fluid, risk for peritoneal injury, and potential discomfort from indwelling fluid. Advantages and complications are listed in Table 63.9. The use of PD is declining and accounts for less than 10% of the total dialysis population (Johnson et al., 2019).

Patient Selection. Most patients with CKD can select either HD or PD. For those who are unstable and those who cannot tolerate anticoagulation, PD is less hazardous than HD. For some patients, vascular access problems may eliminate HD as an option. At times a patient may use PD until a new arteriovenous (AV) fistula matures. PD is often the treatment of choice for older adults because it offers more flexibility if his or her status changes frequently.

PD *cannot* be performed if peritoneal adhesions are present or if extensive intra-abdominal surgery has been performed (Norton et al., 2017b). In these cases, the surface area of the peritoneal membrane is not sufficient for adequate dialysis exchange. Peritoneal membrane fibrosis may occur after repeated infection, which decreases membrane permeability.

Procedure. A siliconized rubber (Silastic) catheter is surgically placed into the abdominal cavity for infusion of dialysate (Fig. 63.8). Usually 1 to 2 L of dialysate is infused by gravity (*fill*) into the peritoneal space over a 10- to 20-minute period, according to the patient's tolerance. The fluid stays (*dwells*) in the cavity for a specified time prescribed for each patient individually by the nephrologist. It then flows out of the body (*drains*) by gravity into a drainage bag. The peritoneal outflow contains the dialysate and the excess water, electrolytes, and nitrogen-based waste products. The dialyzing fluid is called peritoneal *effluent* on outflow. The three phases of the process (infusion, or "fill"; dwell; and outflow, or drain) make up one PD exchange. The number and frequency of PD exchanges are prescribed by the physician, depending on symptoms and laboratory data.

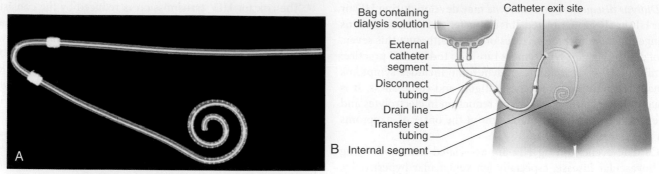

FIG. 63.8 Peritoneal dialysis catheter. (A) The actual Silastic peritoneal dialysis catheter. (B) Positioning of the Silastic catheter within the abdominal cavity. (A from Geary, D.F., & Schaefer, F. [2008]. *Comprehensive pediatric nephrology.* Philadelphia: Mosby.)

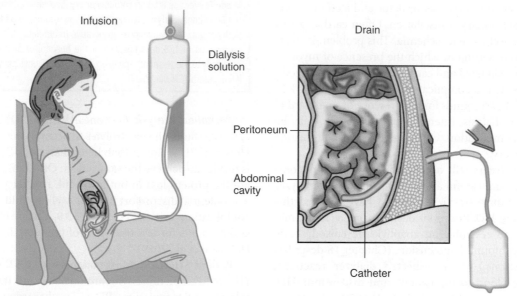

FIG. 63.9 Peritoneal dialysis exchange for control of fluids, electrolytes, nitrogenous wastes, blood pressure, and acid-base balance. The peritoneal membrane acts as the dialyzing membrane.

Process. PD occurs through diffusion and osmosis across the semipermeable peritoneal membrane and capillaries. The peritoneal membrane is large and porous. It allows particles and water to move from an area of higher concentration in the blood to an area of lower concentration in the dialyzing fluid (diffusion).

The peritoneal cavity is rich in capillaries and is a ready access to the blood supply. The fluid and waste products dialyzed from the patient move through the blood vessel walls, the interstitial tissues, and the peritoneal membrane and are removed when the dialyzing fluid is drained from the body.

PD efficiency is affected by many factors. Infection can cause scarring and reduce capillary blood flow. Vascular disease and decreased *perfusion* of the peritoneum reduce PD diffusion. For PD, water removal depends on the concentration of the dialysate. PD efficiency can be altered by the *tonicity* (i.e., number of particles per liter of fluid) of the dialysate. The dialysate concentration is prescribed on the basis of the patient's fluid status (Johnson et al., 2019).

Dialysate Additives. Heparin may be added to the dialysate to prevent clotting of the catheter or tubing. Usually intraperitoneal (IP) heparin is needed only after new catheter placement or if peritonitis occurs. IP heparin is not absorbed systemically and does not affect blood clotting.

Other agents that may be given in the dialysate include potassium and antibiotics. Commercially prepared dialysate does not contain potassium. Some patients need potassium added to the dialysate to prevent hypokalemia. Antibiotics may be given by the IP route when peritonitis is present or suspected. Potassium and antibiotics are not mixed in the same dialysate bag because interactions may reduce the antibiotic effect.

Types of Peritoneal Dialysis. Many types of PD are available, including continuous ambulatory PD, multiple-bag continuous ambulatory PD, automated PD, intermittent PD, and continuous-cycle PD. The type selected depends on the patient's ability and lifestyle. The two most commonly used types of PD are continuous ambulatory peritoneal dialysis and continuous cycling peritoneal dialysis.

Continuous ambulatory peritoneal dialysis (CAPD) is performed by the patient with the infusion of four 2-L exchanges of dialysate into the peritoneal cavity. Each time, the dialysate remains for 4 to 8 hours, and these exchanges occur 7 days a week (Figs. 63.9 to 63.11). During the dwell period, the patient can use a continuous connect system or disconnect and then reconnect at a later time. Most patients using PD long term prefer to complete exchanges overnight with an automated cycler (automatic peritoneal dialysis [APD]).

Automated peritoneal dialysis (APD) may be used in the acute care setting, the ambulatory care dialysis center, or the patient's home. APD uses a cycling machine for dialysate inflow, dwell, and outflow according to preset times and volumes. A warming chamber for dialysate is part of the machine (Fig. 63.12). The functions are programmed for the patient's specific needs. A typical prescription calls for 30-minute exchanges (10/10/10

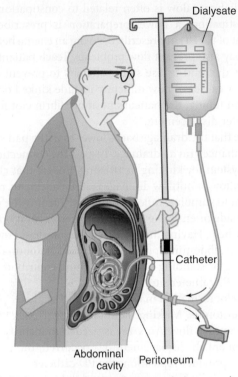

FIG. 63.10 Patient performing continuous ambulatory peritoneal dialysis (CAPD). Note that the patient can walk with this setup.

for inflow, dwell, and outflow) for a period of 8 to 10 hours. The machines have many safety monitors and alarms and are relatively simple to learn to use.

APD has advantages. It permits in-home dialysis during sleep, allowing the patient to be dialysis free during waking hours. The incidence of peritonitis is reduced with APD because fewer connections and disconnections are needed. Also, APD can be used to deliver larger volumes of dialysis solution for patients who need higher clearances.

Intermittent peritoneal dialysis (IPD) combines osmotic pressure gradients with true dialysis. The patient usually requires exchanges of 2 L of dialysate at 30- to 60-minute intervals, allowing 15 to 20 minutes of drain time. For most patients, 30 to 40 exchanges of 2 L three times weekly are needed. IPD treatments can be automated or manual.

Complications. Complications are possible with PD, but many can be prevented with meticulous care and appropriate patient education for self-management. Problems and complications are more common when evidence-based guidelines for catheter care are not followed.

Peritonitis is the major complication of PD, most commonly caused by connection site contamination. To prevent peritonitis, use meticulous sterile technique when caring for the PD catheter and when connecting and disconnecting dialysate bags. See the Best Practice for Patient Safety & Quality Care: Caring for the Patient With a Peritoneal Dialysis Catheter box.

Pain during the inflow of dialysate is common when patients are first started on PD therapy. Usually this pain no longer occurs after a week or two of PD. Cold dialysate increases discomfort. Warm the dialysate bags before instillation by using a heating pad to wrap the bag or by using the warming chamber of the automated cycling machine. *Microwave ovens are not recommended for warming dialysate.*

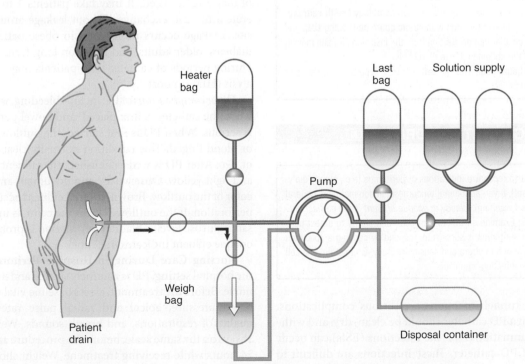

FIG. 63.11 Peritoneal dialysis machine circuit in automated peritoneal dialysis (APD).

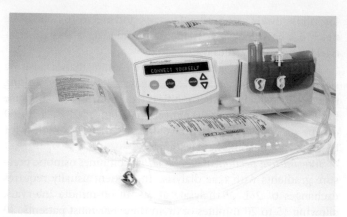

FIG. 63.12 Cycler machine for automated peritoneal dialysis at home. (Courtesy Baxter International, Inc., Deerfield, IL.)

BEST PRACTICE FOR PATIENT SAFETY & QUALITY CARE (QSEN)

Caring for the Patient With a Peritoneal Dialysis Catheter

- Mask yourself and your patient. Wash your hands.
- Put on sterile gloves. Remove the old dressing. Remove the contaminated gloves.
- Assess the area for signs of infection, such as swelling, redness, or discharge around the catheter site.
- Use aseptic technique:
  - Open the sterile field on a flat surface and place two precut 4 × 4–inch gauze pads on the field.
  - Place three cotton swabs soaked in povidone-iodine or other solution prescribed by the nephrology health care provider on the field. Put on sterile gloves.
  - Use cotton swabs to clean around the catheter site. Use a circular motion starting from the insertion site and moving away toward the abdomen. Repeat with all three swabs.
  - As an alternative (if recommended by the nephrology health care provider or clinic), cleanse the area with sterile gauze pads using soap and water. Use a circular motion starting from the insertion site and moving away toward the abdomen. Rinse thoroughly.
  - Apply precut gauze pads over the catheter site. Tape only the edges of the gauze pads.

! NURSING SAFETY PRIORITY (QSEN)

Action Alert

Monitor the patient to recognize indications of peritonitis (e.g., cloudy dialysate outflow (effluent), fever, abdominal tenderness, abdominal pain, general malaise, nausea, and vomiting). *Cloudy or opaque effluent is the earliest indication of peritonitis.* Examine all effluent for color and clarity to detect peritonitis early. When peritonitis is suspected, respond by sending a specimen of the dialysate outflow for culture and sensitivity study, Gram stain, and cell count to identify the infecting organism.

Exit site and tunnel infections are serious complications. The exit site from a PD catheter should be clean, dry, and without pain or inflammation. Exit-site infections (ESIs) can occur with any type of PD catheter. These infections are difficult to treat and can become chronic, leading to peritonitis, catheter failure, and hospitalization. Dialysate leakage and pulling or twisting of the catheter increase the risk for ESIs. A Gram stain and culture should be performed when exit sites have purulent drainage.

Tunnel infections occur in the path of the catheter from the skin to the cuff. Symptoms include redness, tenderness, and pain. ESIs are treated with antimicrobials. Deep cuff infections may require catheter removal.

Poor dialysate flow is often related to constipation. To prevent constipation, a bowel preparation is prescribed before placement of the PD. If prescribed, giving an enema before starting PD may also prevent flow problems. Teach patients to eat a high-fiber diet and to use stool softeners to prevent constipation. Other causes of flow difficulty include kinked or clamped connection tubing, the patient's position, fibrin clot formation, and catheter displacement.

Ensure that the drainage bag is lower than the patient's abdomen to enhance gravity drainage. Inspect the connection tubing and PD system for kinking or twisting. Ensure that clamps are open. If inflow or outflow drainage is still inadequate, reposition the patient to stimulate inflow or outflow. Turning the patient to the other side or ensuring that he or she is in good body alignment may help. Having the patient in a supine low-Fowler position reduces abdominal pressure. Increased abdominal pressure from sitting or standing or from coughing contributes to leakage at the PD catheter site.

Fibrin clot formation may occur after PD catheter placement or with peritonitis. Milking the tubing may dislodge the fibrin clot and improve flow. An x-ray is needed to identify PD catheter placement. If displacement has occurred, the nephrology health care provider repositions the PD catheter.

Dialysate leakage is seen as clear fluid coming from the catheter exit site. When dialysis is first started, small volumes of dialysate are used. It may take patients 1 to 2 weeks to tolerate a full 2-L exchange without leakage around the catheter site. Leakage occurs more often in obese patients, those with diabetes, older adults, and those on long-term steroid therapy. During periods of catheter leak, patients may require hemodialysis (HD) support.

Other complications of PD include bleeding, which is expected when the catheter is first placed, and bowel perforation, which is serious. When PD is first started, the outflow may be bloody or blood tinged. This condition normally clears within a week or two. After PD is well established, the effluent should be clear and light yellow. Observe for and document any change in the color of the outflow. Brown-colored effluent occurs with a bowel perforation. If the outflow is the same color as urine and has the same glucose level, a bladder perforation is probable. Cloudy or opaque effluent indicates infection.

Nursing Care During in-Hospital Peritoneal Dialysis. In the hospital setting, PD is routinely started and monitored by the nurse. Before the treatment, assess baseline vital signs, including blood pressure, apical and radial pulse rates, temperature, quality of respirations, and breath sounds. Weigh the patient, always on the same scale, before the procedure and at least every 24 hours while receiving treatment. Weight should be checked after a drain and before the next fill to monitor the patient's "dry weight." Baseline laboratory tests, such as electrolyte and glucose levels, are obtained before starting PD and repeated at least daily during the PD treatment.

In the hospital setting, especially with a new access, continually monitor the patient receiving PD fluid exchanges. Take and record vital signs every 15 to 30 minutes. Assess for respiratory distress, pain, or discomfort. Check the dressing around the catheter exit site every 30 minutes for wetness during the procedure. Monitor the prescribed dwell time and initiate outflow. Assess blood glucose levels in patients who absorb glucose.

Observe the outflow pattern (outflow should be a continuous stream after the clamp is completely open). Measure and record the total amount of outflow after each exchange. Maintain accurate inflow and outflow records when hourly PD exchanges are performed. When outflow is less than inflow, the difference is retained by the patient during dialysis and is counted as fluid intake. Weigh the patient daily to monitor fluid status.

NCLEX EXAMINATION CHALLENGE 63.5

Physiological Integrity

A client who performs continuous ambulatory peritoneal dialysis at home reports that the drainage (effluent) has become cloudy in the past 24 hours. What is the priority nursing action?

A. Remove the peritoneal catheter.

B. Notify the nephrology health care provider.

C. Obtain a sample of effluent for culture and sensitivity.

D. Teach the client that effluent should be clear or slightly yellow.

Kidney Transplantation. Dialysis and kidney transplant are life-sustaining *treatments* for end-stage kidney disease (ESKD). Kidney transplant is not considered a "cure." Each patient, in consultation with a nephrologist, determines which type of therapy is best suited to his or her physical condition and lifestyle. Approximately 17,107 kidney transplants take place annually in the United States. Just over 100,000 people are waiting for kidney transplants in the United States (National Kidney Foundation [NKF], 2019). The median wait time for a kidney transplant is 4 years (U.S. Renal Data System, 2019).

Candidate Selection Criteria. Candidates for transplantation have advanced kidney disease, have a reasonable life expectancy, and are medically and surgically fit to undergo the procedure. In the United States, patients can be added to the waiting list once the GFR is less than 20 mL/min/1.73 m². Absolute contraindications to transplant include active cancer, current infection, active psychiatric illness, active substance abuse, and nonadherence with dialysis or medical regimen (Himmelfarb & Ikizler, 2018).

Donors. Kidney donors may be living donors (related or unrelated to the patient), non–heart-beating donors (NHBDs), and cadaveric donors. The available kidneys are matched on the basis of tissue type similarity between the donor and the recipient. NHBDs are patients declared dead by cardiopulmonary criteria. Kidneys from NHBDs are removed (harvested) immediately after death in cases in which patients have previously given consent for organ donation. If immediate removal must be delayed, the organ is preserved by infusing a cool preservation solution into the abdominal aorta after death is declared and until surgery can be performed.

Organs from living donors have the highest rate of graft survival due to healthier donors, shorter cold ischemia times, and less ischemia-reperfusion injury. Patients who are able to find compatible kidney donors have shorter wait times for transplant. Donors must be healthy enough to undergo the procedure and be over the age of 18. Due to the benefits that have been shown, many transplant centers have relaxed their criteria and now accept donors with hypertension, obesity, and glucose intolerance, as well as a glomerular filtration rate (GFR) around the lower limits of the normal range (Himmelfarb & Ikizler, 2018). See Box 63.1.

Preoperative Care. Many issues related to patient health and the actual transplant procedure must be addressed before surgery.

Immunologic studies are needed because the major barrier to transplant success after a suitable donor kidney is available is the body's ability to reject "foreign" tissue. This immunologic process can attack the transplanted kidney and destroy it. For normal protective **immunity** to be overcome, tissue typing with human leukocyte antigen (HLA) studies and blood-typing are performed on all candidates. A donated kidney *must* come from a donor who is the same blood- type as the recipient. The HLAs are the main immunologic feature used to match transplant recipients with compatible donors. The more similar the antigens of the donor are to those of the recipient, the more likely the transplant will be successful, and rejection will be avoided (see Chapter 16).

Nursing actions before surgery include teaching about the procedure and care after surgery, in-depth patient assessment, coordination of diagnostic tests, and development of treatment plans. See Chapter 9 for more discussion of standard preoperative nursing care.

BOX 63.1 Never Ending Altruistic Donor Chain (NEAD)

Kidney transplants improve survival rates and lower costs compared with dialysis. The highest survival rates occur in living donor transplants (Himmelfarb & Ikizler, 2018). There are times when a patient needing a transplant has a willing donor who is not compatible and is not able to donate. Previously the patient would have had to wait until another donor was found, and the person who was willing to donate would have been denied. Fig. 63.13 shows an example of a paired exchange kidney donation, which is one option when a recipient has a donor that is not compatible.

Some transplant centers are now using Never Ending Altruistic Donor Chains (NEAD chains) that match donors with recipients. A NEAD chain begins with one nondirected donor. The nondirected donor gives to a person who has a willing but incompatible donor. That willing donor gives to the next person waiting with whom he or she is compatible, so that each living donor is giving to a stranger. The chain is kept going for as long as possible. For example, if a patient's spouse wanted to donate a kidney but was not compatible, the spouse would be matched with a compatible recipient and the patient would be matched with an acceptable donor. The NEAD chain allows for people to donate to help a specific person without having to be compatible. This simple initiative is improving countless lives (NKF, 2019).

The patient usually requires dialysis within 24 hours of the surgery and often receives a blood transfusion before surgery. Usually blood from the kidney donor is transfused into the recipient. This procedure increases graft survival of organs from living related donors (LRDs).

Operative Procedures. The donor nephrectomy procedure varies depending on whether the donor is a non–heart-beating donor (NHBD), cadaveric donor, or living donor. The NHBD or cadaveric donor nephrectomy is a sterile autopsy procedure performed in the operating room. All arterial and venous vessels and a long piece of ureter are preserved. After removal, the kidneys are preserved until time for implantation into the recipient. The technique for kidney removal from living donors is a laparoscopic procedure. Donors need postoperative nursing care and support for the psychological adjustment to loss of a body part.

Transplantation surgery usually takes several hours. The new kidney is placed in the right or left anterior iliac fossa (Fig. 63.14) instead of the usual kidney position. This placement allows easier connection of the ureter and the renal artery and vein. It also allows for easier kidney palpation. The recipient's own failed kidneys are not removed unless chronic kidney infection is present or, as in the case of polycystic kidney disease, the nonfunctioning, enlarged kidneys cause pain. After surgery, the patient is taken to the postanesthesia care unit and then, when stable, to a designated unit in the transplant center or to a critical care unit.

Postoperative Care. Care of the recipient after surgery requires nurses to be knowledgeable about the expected responses and potential complications. Nursing care includes ongoing physical assessment, especially evaluation of kidney function. The most common complications occurring in patients after kidney transplant are rejection and infection (Tran & Miniard, 2017). Drug therapy used to prevent tissue rejection reduces *immunity,* impairs healing, and increases the risk for infection.

Urologic management is essential to graft success. A urinary catheter is placed for accurate measurements of urine output and decompression of the bladder. Decompression prevents stretch on sutures and ureter attachment sites on the bladder.

Assess urine output at least hourly during the first 48 hours. An abrupt decrease in urine output (see Table 63.2) may indicate complications such as rejection, acute kidney injury (AKI), thrombosis, or obstruction. Examine the urine color. The urine is pink and bloody right after surgery and gradually returns to normal over several days to several weeks, depending on kidney function. Obtain daily urine specimens for urinalysis, glucose measurement, the presence of acetone, specific gravity measurement, and culture (if needed).

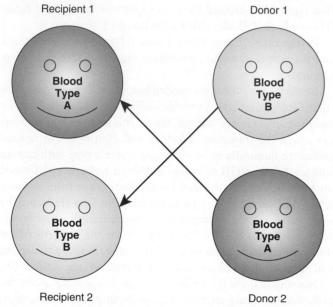

FIG. 63.13 Example of a paired exchange kidney donation. *Donor 1* is related to or acquainted with *recipient 1* and has agreed to donate a kidney but is not a blood-type or tissue-type match with *recipient 1.* *Donor 1* is compatible with *recipient 2* and agrees to donate a kidney to *recipient 2* if *donor 2* agrees to donate a kidney to *recipient 1* with confirmed compatibility to recipient 1.

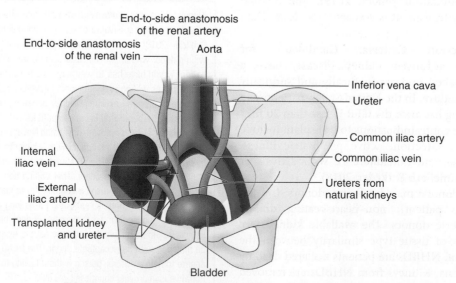

FIG. 63.14 Placement of a transplanted kidney in the right iliac fossa.

Occasionally, continuous bladder irrigation is prescribed to decrease blood clot formation, which could increase pressure in the bladder and endanger the graft. Perform routine catheter care, according to agency policy, to reduce catheter-associated urinary tract infection (CAUTI). The catheter is removed as soon as possible to avoid infection, usually 3 to 5 days after surgery. After surgery, the function of the transplanted kidney (graft) can result in either oliguria or diuresis. Oliguria may occur as a result of ischemia and acute kidney injury (AKI), rejection, or other complications. To increase urine output, the nephrology health care provider may prescribe diuretics and osmotic agents. Closely monitor the patient's fluid status because fluid overload can cause hypertension, heart failure (HF), and pulmonary edema. Evaluate his or her fluid status by weighing daily, measuring blood pressure every 2 to 4 hours, and measuring intake and output.

Instead of oliguria, the patient may have diuresis, especially with a kidney from a living related donor (LRD). Monitor intake and output and observe for disruptions of *fluid and electrolyte balance,* such as low potassium and sodium levels. Excessive diuresis may cause hypotension.

! NURSING SAFETY PRIORITY (QSEN)
Critical Rescue

Monitor the patient to recognize hypotension. If hypotension or excessive diuresis (e.g., unanticipated urine output 500 to 1000 mL greater than intake over 12 to 24 hours or other goal for intake and output) is present, respond by notifying the nephrology health care provider because hypotension reduces *perfusion* and oxygen to the new kidney, threatening graft survival.

Complications. Many complications are possible after kidney transplantation. Early detection and intervention improve the chances for graft survival.

Rejection is the most serious complication of transplantation and is the leading cause of graft loss. A reaction occurs between the tissues of the transplanted kidney and the antibodies and cytotoxic T-cells in the recipient's blood. These substances treat the new kidney as a foreign invader and cause tissue destruction, thrombosis, and eventual kidney necrosis.

The three types of rejection are hyperacute, acute, and chronic. Acute rejection is the most common type with kidney transplants. It is treated with increased immunosuppressive therapy and often can be reversed. Rejection is diagnosed by symptoms, a CT or renal scan, and kidney biopsy. Table 63.13 lists the features of the three types of rejection. Chapter 16 discusses their causes and treatment.

Ischemia from delayed transplantation following harvesting can contribute to acute kidney injury (AKI). Newly transplanted patients with AKI may need dialysis until adequate urine output returns and the blood urea nitrogen (BUN) and creatinine levels normalize. Biopsy can be used to determine if oliguria is the result of AKI or rejection.

Thrombosis of the major renal blood vessels may occur during the first 2 to 3 days after the transplant. A sudden decrease in urine output may signal impaired *perfusion* resulting from

TABLE 63.13 Comparison of Hyperacute, Acute, and Chronic Posttransplant Rejection

Hyperacute Rejection	Acute Rejection	Chronic Rejection
Onset		
Within 48 hr after surgery	1 wk to any time after surgery; occurs over days to weeks	Occurs gradually during a period of months to years
Signs and Symptoms		
Increased temperature	Oliguria or anuria	Gradual increase in BUN and serum creatinine levels
Increased blood pressure	Temperature over 100°F (37.8°C)	Fluid retention
Pain at transplant site	Increased blood pressure	Changes in serum electrolyte levels
	Enlarged, tender kidney	Fatigue
	Lethargy	
	Elevated serum creatinine, BUN, potassium levels	
	Fluid retention	
Treatment		
Immediate removal of the transplanted kidney	Increased doses of immunosuppressive drugs	Conservative management until dialysis required

BUN, Blood urea nitrogen.

thrombosis. Ultrasound of the kidney may show decreased or absent blood supply. Emergency surgery is required to prevent ischemic damage or graft loss.

Renal artery stenosis may result in hypertension. Other signs include a bruit over the artery anastomosis site and decreased kidney function. A CT or renal scan can quantify the *perfusion* to the kidney. The involved artery may be repaired surgically or by balloon angioplasty in the radiology department. The decision to perform a balloon repair is determined by the amount of healing time after the surgery.

Other vascular problems include vascular leakage or thrombosis, both of which require an emergency transplant nephrectomy.

Other complications may involve the surgical wound or urinary tract. Wound problems, such as hematomas, abscesses, and lymphoceles (cysts containing lymph fluid), increase the risk for infection and exert pressure on the new kidney. Infection from reduced *immunity* is a major cause of death in the transplant recipient (Tran & Miniard, 2017). Prevention of infection is essential. Strict aseptic technique and handwashing must be rigorously enforced. Transplant recipients may not have the usual symptoms of infection because of the immunosuppressive therapy. Low-grade fevers, mental status changes, and vague reports of discomfort may be the only symptoms before sepsis. Always consider the possibility of infection with any patient after a kidney transplant. Urinary tract complications include ureteral leakage, fistula, or obstruction; stone formation; bladder neck contracture; and graft rupture. Surgical intervention may be required.

Immunosuppressive Drug Therapy. The success of kidney transplantation depends on changing the patient's *immunity* response so the new kidney is not rejected as a foreign organ. Immunosuppressive drugs protect the transplanted organ. These drugs include corticosteroids, inhibitors of T-cell proliferation and activity (azathioprine, mycophenolic acid, cyclosporine, and tacrolimus), mTOR inhibitors (to disrupt stimulatory T-cell signals), and monoclonal antibodies. Chapter 16 discusses the mechanisms of action for these agents and the associated patient responses. Patients taking these drugs are at an increased risk for death from infection. Usually, the patient receives a period of high-dose (induction) therapy followed by lower-dose maintenance immunosuppressive therapy.

Some patients do not follow the maintenance regimen correctly and are at high risk for losing the transplanted kidney. Work with the patient to ensure adherence to the drug regimen.

Despite the complexity of drug regimens following kidney transplantation, 99% of recipients of living kidneys are alive at 1 year and 95% of deceased kidney recipients are alive at 1 year. At 4 years, kidney transplant recipients have an average 70% reduction in mortality compared with patients on dialysis (Himmelfarb & Ikizler, 2018)

Although rejection is uncommon with immunosuppressive therapy, kidney transplant recipients are at risk for cardiovascular disease (the most common cause of death among kidney transplant recipients), diabetes, cancer, and infections. Prevention and management of these complications are important to maintaining the health of the transplanted kidney and prolonging patient survival. Be aware that some patient groups, including African Americans, Hispanic Americans, and Native Americans, have a greater incidence of graft failure and systemic complications (especially cardiovascular disease) after transplantation.

> ### ! NURSING SAFETY PRIORITY (QSEN)
> **Action Alert**
>
> Teach patients and families about the importance of adhering to the antirejection drug regimen to prevent transplant rejection.

Care Coordination and Transition Management

Home Care Management. Because of the complex nature of CKD, its progressive course, and many treatment options, a case manager is helpful in planning, coordinating, and evaluating care. As kidney disease progresses, the patient is seen by a nephrologist or nephrology nurse practitioner regularly. Together with the registered dietitian nutritionist and social worker, evaluate the home environment and determine equipment needs before discharge. Once the patient is discharged, nephrology home care nurses direct care and monitor progress.

Provide health teaching about the diet in kidney disease and the progression of disease. As CKD approaches end-stage kidney disease (ESKD), treatment with hemodialysis (HD), peritoneal dialysis (PD), or transplantation is selected. For each form of treatment, the patient and partner must learn about the procedures and consider personal lifestyle, support systems, and

methods of coping. Decision making about treatment type or even whether to pursue treatment is difficult for patients and families. Provide information and emotional support to help patients with these decisions.

Teach patients who select hemodialysis (HD) about the machine and vascular access care. If in-home HD is selected, preparations are needed for the appropriate equipment, including a water-treatment system. A nephrology nurse is essential for a successful transition to at-home HD to teach the patient and monitor treatment and care. This nurse performs a home care visit before discharge to coordinate equipment setup. Family members must be available to respond to alarms during treatment. Nocturnal HD is a growing modality, and additional safety considerations must be addressed, including a plan for treatment discontinuation or generator backup during power outages. Regardless of whether the treatment occurs at home or in a center, promote independence through teaching and best practices in self-management.

The patient receiving PD needs extensive training in the procedure and help in obtaining equipment and the many supplies needed. A nephrology nurse assesses patients, monitors vital signs, assesses adherence with drug and diet regimens, and monitors for indications of peritonitis.

The nurse plays a vital role in the long-term care of the patient with a kidney transplant by facilitating acceptance and understanding of the antirejection drug regimen as a part of daily life. Carefully monitor patients for indications of graft rejection and for complications, such as infection. See the Focused Assessment: The Patient After Kidney Transplant box for care of the patient following kidney transplant.

Self-Management Education. Instruct patients and family members in all aspects of nutrition therapy, drug therapy, and complications. Teach them to report complications, such as fluid overload and infection. When a patient has a specific form of therapy, such as dialysis or transplantation, focus teaching on the chosen type of intervention. Assess the need for immunizations and request a prescription to administer needed ones before transplantation (Tran & Miniard, 2017).

Hemodialysis (HD) is the most complex form of therapy for the patient and family to understand. Even if patients receive HD in a dialysis center instead of at home, they are expected to have some knowledge of the process. Teach the patient or a family member to care for the vascular access and to report signs of infection and clotting. Teaching also includes instructing the patient to assess daily for a bruit and thrill in the vascular access. Those who plan to have in-home HD will need a partner. Both the patient and the partner must be taught the entire process of HD and must be able to perform it independently before the patient is discharged.

Peritoneal dialysis (PD) involves extensive health teaching for the patient and family. Emphasize sterile technique because peritonitis is the most common complication of PD. Instruct patients to report any symptoms of peritonitis, especially cloudy effluent and abdominal pain. If peritonitis develops, teach patients how to give themselves antibiotics by the intraperitoneal (IP) route. Stress the importance of completing the antibiotic regimen. Remind patients that repeated episodes of

FOCUSED ASSESSMENT

The Patient After Kidney Transplant

Assess cardiovascular and respiratory status, including:
- Vital signs, with special attention to blood pressure
- Presence of S_3 or pericardial friction rub
- Presence of chest pain
- Presence of edema (periorbital, pretibial, sacral)
- Jugular vein distention
- Presence of dyspnea
- Presence of crackles, beginning at the lung bases and extending upward

Assess nutritional status, including:
- Weight gain or loss
- Presence of anorexia, nausea, or vomiting

Assess kidney status, including:
- Amount, frequency, and appearance of urine (in nonanuric patients)
- Presence of bone pain
- Presence of hyperglycemia secondary to diabetes

Assess hematologic status, including:
- Presence of petechiae, purpura, ecchymosis
- Presence of fatigue or shortness of breath

Assess GI status, including:
- Presence of stomatitis
- Presence of melena

Assess integumentary status, including:
- Skin integrity
- Presence of pruritus
- Presence of skin discoloration

Assess neurologic status, including:
- Changes in mental status
- Presence of seizure activity
- Presence of sensory changes
- Presence of lower extremity weakness

Assess laboratory data, including:
- BUN
- Serum creatinine
- Creatinine clearance
- CBC
- Electrolytes

Assess psychosocial status, including:
- Presence of anxiety
- Presence of maladaptive behavior

BUN, Blood urea nitrogen; *CBC*, complete blood count.

peritonitis can reduce the effectiveness of PD, which may result in the transfer to HD.

The patient receiving a kidney transplant also needs extensive health teaching. Provide instruction about drug regimens, home monitoring, immunosuppression, symptoms of rejection, infection, and prescribed changes in the diet and activity level.

Psychosocial Preparation. In collaboration with the patient's mental health professional or counselor, provide psychosocial support for the patient and family. Help the patient adjust to the diagnosis of kidney failure and eventually accept the treatment regimens.

Many patients view dialysis as a cure instead of lifelong management. For many patients, reduction of uremic symptoms and improved *elimination* in the first weeks after starting dialysis treatment create a sense of well-being (the "honeymoon

period). They feel better physically, and their mood may be happy and hopeful. At this time they tend to overlook the discomfort and inconvenience of dialysis. Use this time to begin health teaching. Stress that although symptoms are reduced, they should not expect a complete return to the previous state of well-being before ESKD.

Many patients become discouraged during the first year of treatment. This mood state may last a few months to a year or longer. The difficulties of incorporating dialysis into daily life are staggering, and patients may become depressed as problems occur. They may struggle with the idea of having to be permanently dependent on a disruptive therapy. Patients may feel helpless and dependent. Some patients may deny the need for dialysis or may not adhere to drug therapy and diet restrictions. Monitor any behaviors that may contribute to nonadherence and suggest psychiatric referrals. Help the patient and family focus on the positive aspects of the treatments. Continue health education with patients as active participants and decision makers.

Most patients with CKD eventually enter a phase of acceptance or resignation. Each patient reacts differently. To make this long-term adaptation, he or she must adjust to continuous change. Concerns depend on the patient's health and specific treatment method.

After patients have accepted or become resigned to the chronic aspect of their disease, they usually attempt to return to their previous activities. However, resuming the previous level of activity may not be possible. Help patients develop realistic expectations that allow them to lead active, productive lives.

Health Care Resources. Professionals from many disciplines are resources for the patient with ESKD. Home care nurses monitor the patient's status and evaluate maintenance of the prescribed treatment regimen (HD or PD). Social services are often involved because of the complex process of applying for financial aid to pay for the required medical care. A physical therapist may be beneficial in helping to improve the patient's functional health. A registered dietitian nutritionist can help the patient and family members understand special dietary needs. A psychiatric evaluation may be needed if depressive symptoms are present. Pharmacists provide invaluable insight and teaching about drug therapy and adjustments to meet outcomes. Clergy and pastoral care specialists offer spiritual support.

Patients with CKD are routinely followed by a nephrologist. Organizations such as the National Kidney Foundation (NKF), the American Kidney Fund, and the American Association of Kidney Patients (AAKP) may be helpful to patients and families.

◆ **Evaluation: Evaluate Outcomes.** Evaluate the care of the patient with CKD based on the identified priority problems. The expected outcomes are that with appropriate management the patient should:
- Achieve and maintain appropriate fluid and electrolyte balance
- Maintain an adequate nutrition status
- Avoid infection at the vascular access site
- Use effective coping strategies
- Prevent or slow systemic complications of CKD, including osteodystrophy
- Report an absence of physical signs of anxiety or depression

❓ CLINICAL JUDGMENT CHALLENGE 63.1
Patient-Centered Care

The nurse is performing an assessment in the outpatient clinic on a 47-year-old male client who was diagnosed with stage 4 chronic kidney disease (CKD) 4 months ago. The client had an arteriovenous fistula implanted 2 months ago. He has been undergoing hemodialysis for the last 6 weeks. However, he reports missing the last two dialysis appointments because he was "just too tired to go." The client reports that he cannot afford his medications and that following his new diet is too hard and costly. Current assessment: temperature, 102.2°F; blood pressure, 188/90 mm Hg; respirations, 28 breaths/min; and heart rate, 89 beats/min. His oxygen saturation is 88% on room air, and crackles are noted in bibasilar lung fields. He reports feeling very anxious and states, "It's all my fault that this is happening." Current labs include potassium, 5.4 mEq/L; sodium, 142 mEq/L; magnesium, 2.1 mEq/L; and WBCs, 22,000 mm³.

1. **Recognize Cues:** What assessment information in this client situation is the most important and immediate concern for the nurse? (Hint: Identify the **relevant** information *first* to determine what is most important.)
2. **Analyze Cues:** What client conditions are consistent with the **most relevant** information? (Hint: Think about priority collaborative problems that support and contradict the information presented in this situation.)

3. **Prioritize Hypotheses:** Which possibilities or explanations are **most likely** to be present in this client situation? Which possibilities or explanations are the most serious? (Hint: Consider all possibilities and determine their urgency and risk for this client.)
4. **Generate Solutions:** What actions would most likely achieve the desired outcomes for this client? Which actions should be **avoided** or are **potentially harmful**? (Hint: Determine the desired outcomes first to decide which interventions are appropriate and those that should be avoided.)
5. **Take Action:** Which actions are the most appropriate and how should they be implemented? In what **priority order** should they be implemented? (Hint: Consider health teaching, documentation, requested health care provider orders or prescriptions, nursing skills, collaboration with or referral to health team members, etc.)
6. **Evaluate Outcomes:** What client assessment would indicate that the nurse's actions were **effective**? (Hint: Think about signs that would indicate an improvement, decline, or unchanged client condition.)

▌GET READY FOR THE NEXT-GENERATION NCLEX® EXAMINATION!

Key Points
Review these Key Points for each NCLEX Examination Client Needs Category.

Safe and Effective Care Environment

- Use sterile technique when initiating and providing kidney replacement therapy. **QSEN: Safety**
- Implement fall precautions and consider physical therapy referral for patients with CKD osteodystrophy to prevent fractures. **QSEN: Safety**
- Use skin protective measures to reduce injury and pressure injury in patients with CKD. **QSEN: Safety**
- Alert health care providers to patient assessments that indicate hypotension, dehydration, or hypovolemia to avoid inadequate kidney *perfusion*. **QSEN: Teamwork and Collaboration**
- Avoid taking blood pressure measurements or drawing blood from an arm with a vascular access. **QSEN: Safety**
- Do not use a kidney replacement vascular access device to give IV fluids. **QSEN: Safety**

Health Promotion and Maintenance

- Encourage patients with AKI, CKD, or end-stage kidney disease (ESKD) to follow fluid and dietary restrictions **QSEN: Evidence-Based Practice**
- Teach patients the expected side effects, any adverse reactions to prescribed drugs, and when to contact the prescriber. **QSEN: Safety**
- Teach patients using peritoneal dialysis the early signs and symptoms of peritonitis. **QSEN: Patient-Centered Care**
- Teach patients receiving immunosuppressive therapy for kidney transplantation to assess themselves daily for fever, general malaise, and nausea or vomiting, as well as changes in urine output and weight gain that indicate new fluid retention. **QSEN: Patient-Centered Care**

Psychosocial Integrity

- Allow patients to express concerns about the disruption of lifestyle and considerations for end-of-life care as a result of kidney failure. **QSEN: Patient-Centered Care**
- Use language and terminology that is understandable for the patient. **QSEN: Patient-Centered Care**
- Assess the patient for anxiety, depression, and nonacceptance of the diagnosis or treatment plan. **QSEN: Patient-Centered Care**
- Refer patients to community resources and support groups. **QSEN: Informatics**

Physiological Integrity

- Report immediately any condition that obstructs urine flow. **QSEN: Safety**
- Collaborate with the RDN to teach patients about dietary needs. **QSEN: Teamwork and Collaboration**
- Inform the primary health care provider immediately about hemodynamic instability, change in cognition, signs of infection, newly abnormal serum electrolytes, and urine output less than 0.5 mL/kg/hr for more than 2 to 4 hours (unless the patient is oliguric or anuric from ESKD). **QSEN: Teamwork and Collaboration**
- Teach patients in the early stages of CKD the symptoms of dehydration. **QSEN: Patient-Centered Care**
- Evaluate the patient's laboratory values, especially the metabolic panel, trends in serum creatinine, GFR, and albumin-to-creatinine ratio to assess the status of kidney problems, and communicate concerning changes to the interprofessional team. **QSEN: Teamwork and Collaboration**
- Teach patients in the later stages of CKD the indications of fluid overload and hyperkalemia. **QSEN: Patient-Centered Care**
- Avoid all invasive procedures in the 4 to 6 hours following hemodialysis. **QSEN: Evidence-Based Practice**

MASTERY QUESTIONS

1. Which client will the nurse identify as at risk for acute kidney injury? Select all that apply.
   A. 68-year-old male with diabetes mellitus
   B. 16-year-old male football player in preseason practice
   C. 27-year-old female recovering from shock following a car accident
   D. 52-year-old male with newly diagnosed hypertension
   E. 30-year-old female in intensive care receiving multiple intravenous antibiotics

2. The nurse is providing discharge teaching to a client recovering from kidney transplantation. Which client statement indicates understanding?
   A. "I can stop my medications when my kidney function returns to normal."
   B. "If my urine output decreases, I will increase my fluids."
   C. "The antirejection medications will be taken for life."
   D. "I will drink 8 ounces (236 mL) of water with my medications."

3. A client with a recently created vascular access for hemodialysis is being discharged. Which discharge teaching will the nurse include?
   A. Do not allow blood pressure measurements in the affected arm.
   B. Elevate the affected arm, allowing for total rest of the extremity.
   C. Assess for a bruit in the affected arm on a daily basis.
   D. Sleep on the affected side to protect the access device.

REFERENCES

Asterisk (*) indicates a classic or definitive work on this subject.

Brown, R. M., & Semler, M. W. (2019). Fluid management in sepsis. *Journal of Intensive Care Medicine, 34*(5), 364–373. https://doi.org/10.1177/0885066618784861.

Burchum, J., & Rosenthal, L. (2019). *Lehne's pharmacology for nursing care* (10th ed.). St. Louis: Elsevier.

Centers for Disease Control and Prevention. (2019). *Chronic kidney disease in the United States, 2019*. Atlanta, GA: US Department of Health and Human Services, Centers for Disease Control and Prevention.

Ferri, F. (2020). *Ferri's clinical advisor 2020, five books in one*. St Louis, MO: Elsevier.

Fuhrman, D. Y. -G. (2018). Acute kidney injury epidemiology, risk factors, and outcomes in critically ill patients 16–25 years of age treated in an adult intensive care unit. *Annals of Intensive Care*, 26–34.

Gilbert, S., & Weiner, D. (2018). *National kidney Foundation primer on kidney diseases* (7th ed.). St. Louis, MO: Elsevier.

Hain, D. (2015). Where's the evidence? Care coordination for adults with chronic kidney disease. *Nephrology Nursing Journal, 42*(1), 77–82.

Himmelfarb, J., & Ikizler, T. A. (2018). *Chronic kidney disease, dialysis and transplantation* (4th ed.). St. Louis: Elsevier.

Honicker, T., & Holt, K. (2016). Contrast-induced acute kidney injury: Comparison of preventive therapies. (2016). *Nephrology Nursing Journal, 43*(2), 109–116.

Jarvis, C., & Eckhardt, A. (2020). *Jarvis physical examinations and health assessment* (8th ed.). St. Louis, MO: Elsevier.

Johnson, R., Feehally, J., Floege, J., & Tonelli, M. (2019). *Comprehensive clinical nephrology* (6th ed.).

*Kidney Disease. (2012). *Improving Global outcomes (KDIGO) acute kidney injury work group. KDIGO clinical practice guideline for acute kidney injury. Kidney inter* (Vol. 2.) (pp. 1–138). https://kdigo.org/wp-content/uploads/2016/10/KDIGO-2012-AKI-Guideline-English.pdf.

Kidney Foundation of Canada. (2018). *Facing the Facts, 2018*. Retrieved from: https://www.kidney.ca/file/Facing-the-Facts-2018.pdf.

Lambert, P., Chasson, K., Horton, S., Petrin, C., Marshall, E., Bowdon, S., et al. (2017). Reducing acute kidney injury due to contrast material: How nurses can improve patient safety. *Critical Care Nurse, 37*(1), 13–26.

Lottaliany, M. B. (2018). Depression and chronic diseases: Co-occurrence and communality of risk factors. *Journal of Affective Disorders*, 461–468.

McCance, K., Huether, S., Brashers, V., & Rote, N. (2019). *Pathophysiology: The biologic basis for disease in adults and children* (8th ed.). St. Louis: Elsevier.

Moore, P. H. (2018). Management of acute kidney injury: Core Curriculum 2018. *American Journal of Kidney Diseases*, 136–148.

National Kidney Foundation. (2019). Organ Donation And Transplantation Statistics. Retrieved from National Kidney Foundation: https://www.kidney.org/news/newsroom/factsheets/Organ-Donation-and-Transplantation-Stats

Norton, J., Newman, M., Romancito, G., Mahooty, S., Kuracina, T., & Narva, A. (2017a). Improving outcomes for patients with chronic kidney disease: Part 1. *American Journal of Nursing, 117*(2), 22–32.

Norton, J., Newman, M., Romancito, G., Mahooty, S., Kuracina, T., & Narva, A. (2017b). Improving outcomes for patients with chronic kidney disease: Part 2. *American Journal of Nursing, 117*(3), 26–35.

Pagana, K., & Pagana, T. (2018). *Mosby's manual of diagnostic and laboratory tests* (6th ed.). St. Louis: Elsevier.

Pavkov, M. E., Harding, J. L., & Burrows, N. R. (2018). Trends in hospitalizations for acute kidney injury — United States, 2000–2014. *MMWR Morb Mortal Wkly Rep, 67*, 289–293. https://doi.org/10.15585/mmwr.mm6710a2external icon.

Ronco, C., Bellomo, R., Kellum, J., & Ricci, Z. (2019). *Critical care nephrology* (3rd ed.). St. Louis: Elsevier.

Schell-Chaple, H. (2017). Continuous renal replacement therapy update: An emphasis on safe and high-quality care. *AACN Advanced Critical Care, 28*(1), 31–40.

Tran, A., & Miniard, J. (2017). Preventing infection after renal transplantation. *Nursing, 74*(1), 57–60.

United States Renal Data System. (2019). *USRDS annual data report: Epidemiology of kidney disease in the United States.* Bethesda, MD:

National Institutes of Health, National Institute of Diabetes and Digestive and Kidney Diseases. 2019.

Woo, K. (2019). Hemodialysis access: Dialysis catheters. In A. P. Sidawy (Ed.), *Rutherford's vascular surgery and Endovascular therapy* (pp. 2315–2323). Philadelphia: Elsevier.

Assessment of the Reproductive System

Cherie R. Rebar

http://evolve.elsevier.com/Iggy/

LEARNING OUTCOMES

1. Collaborate with the interprofessional team to perform a complete reproductive assessment.
2. Prioritize evidence-based care for patients having diagnostic testing affecting the reproductive system and *sexuality.*
3. Teach evidence-based ways for adults to protect their reproductive system.
4. Explain physiologic aging changes of the reproductive system.
5. Implement nursing interventions to decrease the psychosocial impact caused by a reproductive problem.
6. Apply knowledge of anatomy and physiology, genetic risk, and principles of aging to perform a focused reproductive system assessment.
7. Use clinical judgment to document the reproductive assessment in the electronic health record.
8. Interpret assessment findings for patients with a suspected or actual reproductive problem.

KEY TERMS

amenorrhea Absence of menses.

circumcision Surgical removal of the prepuce or foreskin of the penis.

colposcopy Examination of the cervix and vagina using a colposcope, which allows three-dimensional magnification and intense illumination of epithelium with suspected disease. This procedure can locate the exact site of precancerous and malignant lesions for biopsy.

conization Removal of a cone-shaped sample of tissue.

digital 3D mammography (digital breast tomosynthesis) Breast imaging that allows the radiologist to visualize through layers or "slices" of breast tissue, similar to a CT scan.

dilation and curettage (D&C) Procedure in which tissue is removed from inside of the uterus due to abnormal bleeding or to remove pregnancy tissue after an abortion, miscarriage or childbirth.

human papillomavirus (HPV) test Test that can identify many high-risk types of HPV infection associated with the development of cervical cancer.

hysterosalpingogram an outpatient fluoroscopy procedure that uses an injection of a contrast medium to visualize the cervix, uterus, and fallopian tubes

hysteroscopy Procedure that uses a fiberoptic camera to visualize the uterus to diagnose and treat causes of abnormal bleeding.

laparoscopy Direct examination of the pelvic cavity through an endoscope.

libido Sex drive or desire.

mammography X-ray of the soft tissue of the breast.

orchitis An acute testicular inflammation resulting from trauma or infection.

Papanicolaou test (Pap test or Pap smear) A cytologic study that is effective in detecting. precancerous and cancerous cells within the female patient's cervix.

salpingitis Fallopian tube infection.

✳ **PRIORITY AND INTERRELATED CONCEPTS**

The priority concepts for this chapter are:
- *Infection*
- *Pain*

The interrelated concept for this chapter is:
- *Sexuality*

The nurse is often the first health care professional to assess the patient with a reproductive system health problem. These problems typically affect physical and psychosocial aspects of *sexuality* and are difficult for many people to discuss. Reproductive assessment should be part of every complete physical assessment. *Respect gender identity and differences in sexual orientation and practices.* A more detailed discussion of human *sexuality* is found in Chapter 1.

ANATOMY AND PHYSIOLOGY REVIEW

Structure and Function of the Female Reproductive System

The female reproductive system is located outside (external) and inside (internal) the body.

External Genitalia. The external female genitalia, or vulva, extends from the mons pubis to the anal opening. The mons pubis is a pad of fat that covers the symphysis pubis and protects it during coitus (sexual intercourse).

The labia majora are two vertical folds of adipose tissue that extend posteriorly from the mons pubis to the perineum. The size of the labia majora varies, depending on the amount of fatty tissue present. The skin over the labia majora is usually darker than the surrounding skin and is highly vascular. It protects inner vulval structures and enhances sexual arousal.

The labia majora surround two thinner, vertical folds of reddish epithelium called the *labia minora*. The labia minora are highly vascular and have a rich nerve supply. Emotional or physical stimulation induces marked swelling and sensitivity. Sebaceous glands in the labia minora lubricate the entrance to the vagina. The clitoris is a small, cylindric organ that is composed of erectile tissue with a high concentration of sensory nerve endings. During sexual arousal, the clitoris becomes larger and increases sensation.

The vestibule is a longitudinal area between the labia minora, the clitoris, and the vagina that contains Bartholin glands, the urethral meatus, the opening of the Skene (paraurethral) glands, the hymen, and the vaginal opening (Jarvis, 2020). The two Bartholin glands, located deeply toward the back on both sides of the vaginal opening, secrete lubrication fluid during sexual excitement. Their ductal openings are usually not visible.

The perineum is located between the vaginal opening and the anus. The skin of the perineum covers the muscles, fascia, and ligaments that support the pelvic structures.

Internal Genitalia. The internal female genitalia are shown in Fig. 64.1. The vagina is a hollow tube that extends from the vestibule to the uterus. Ovarian hormones (primarily estrogen) influence the amounts of glycogen and lubricating fluid secreted by the vaginal cells. The normal vaginal bacteria (flora) interact with the secretions to produce lactic acid and maintain an acidic pH (3.5 to 5.0) in the vagina. This acidity helps prevent infection in the vagina.

At the upper end of the vagina, the uterine cervix projects into a cup-shaped vault of thin vaginal tissue. The recessed pockets around the cervix permit palpation of the internal pelvic organs. The posterior area provides access into the peritoneal cavity for diagnostic or surgical purposes.

The *uterus* (or "womb") is a thick-walled, pear-shaped muscular organ attached to the upper end of the vagina. This inverted pear-shaped organ is located within the true pelvis, between the bladder and the rectum. The uterus is made up of the body and the cervix. The *cervix* is a short (1 inch [2.5 cm]), narrowed portion of the uterus and extends into the vagina. The surfaces of the cervix and the canal are the sites for Papanicolaou (Pap) testing. (See discussion later in this chapter.)

The *fallopian tubes* insert into the fundus of the uterus and extend laterally close to the ovaries. They provide a duct between the ovaries and the uterus for the passage of ova and sperm. In most cases, the ovum is fertilized in these tubes up to 72 hours after release.

The *ovaries* are a pair of almond-shaped organs located near the lateral walls of the upper pelvic cavity. These small organs develop and release ova, and produce estrogen and progesterone. Adequate amounts of these hormones are needed for normal female growth and development, and to maintain a pregnancy. Women are born with *oocytes,* which are germ cells involved in reproduction; these are finite in number and do not replenish throughout the lifespan. After menopause, the ovaries become smaller.

Breasts. The female breasts are a pair of mammary glands that develop in response to secretions from the hypothalamus, pituitary gland, and ovaries, and nourish an infant after birth.

Breast tissue is composed of a network of glandular and ductal tissue, fibrous tissue, and fat. The proportion of each component of breast tissue depends on genetic factors, nutrition, age, and obstetric history. The breasts are supported by ligaments that are attached to underlying muscles. They have abundant blood supply and lymph flow that drain from an extensive network toward the axillae (Fig. 64.2).

Structure and Function of the Male Reproductive System

The primary male hormone for sexual development and function is *testosterone.* Testosterone production is fairly constant in the adult male. Only a slight and gradual reduction of testosterone production occurs in the older adult male until he is in his 80s. Low testosterone levels decrease muscle mass, reduce skin elasticity, and lead to changes in sexual performance.

External Genitalia. The male reproductive system also consists of external and internal genitalia. The penis is an organ

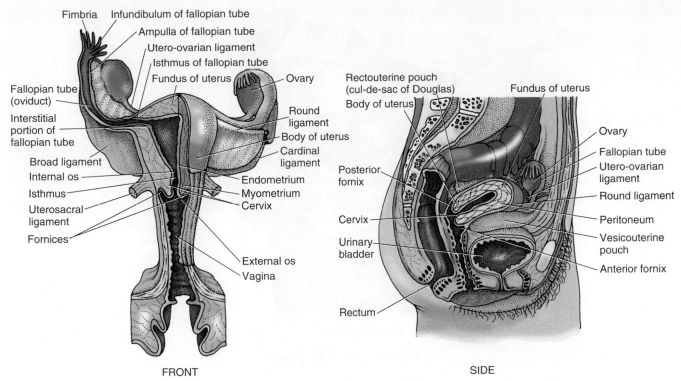

FIG. 64.1 Internal female genitalia.

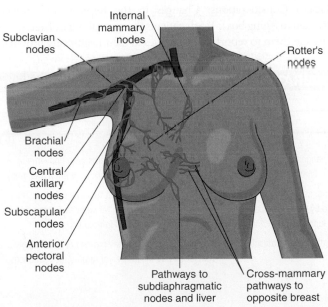

FIG. 64.2 Lymphatic drainage of the female breast.

for urination and intercourse consisting of the body or shaft and the glans penis (the distal end of the penis). The glans is the smooth end of the penis and contains the opening of the urethral meatus. Urine and semen both exit via the *urethra*. A continuation of skin covers the glans and folds to form the prepuce (foreskin). **Circumcision**, the surgical removal of the foreskin, is a common procedure performed in various parts of the world for cultural or religious reasons.

The scrotum is a thin-walled, fibromuscular pouch that is behind the penis and suspended below the pubic bone. This pouch protects the testes, epididymis, and vas deferens in a space that is slightly cooler than inside the abdominal cavity. The scrotal skin is darkly pigmented and contains sweat glands, sebaceous glands, and few hair follicles. It contracts with cold, exercise, tactile stimulation, and sexual excitement.

Internal Genitalia. The internal male genitalia are shown in Fig. 64.3. The major organs are the testes and prostate gland. The testes are a pair of oval organs located inside the scrotum that produce sperm and testosterone. Each testis is suspended in the scrotum by the spermatic cord, which provides blood, lymphatic, and nerve supply to the testis. Sympathetic nerve fibers are located on the arteries in the cord, and sympathetic and parasympathetic fibers are on the vas deferens. When the testes are damaged, these autonomic nerve fibers transmit signals of excruciating pain and a sensation of nausea.

The *epididymis* is the first portion of a ductal system that transports sperm from the testes to the urethra and is a site of sperm maturation. The *vas deferens,* or *ductus deferens,* is a firm, muscular tube that continues from the tail of each epididymis. The end of each vas deferens is a reservoir for sperm and tubular fluids. They merge with ducts from the seminal vesicle to form the ejaculatory ducts at the base of the prostate gland. Sperm from the vas deferens and secretions from the seminal vesicles move through the ejaculatory duct to mix with prostatic fluids in the prostatic urethra.

The *prostate gland* is a large accessory gland of the male reproductive system that can be palpated via the rectum. The gland

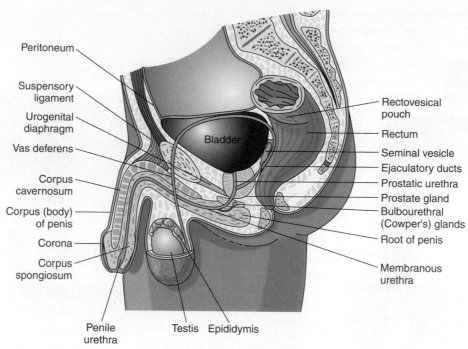

FIG. 64.3 Internal male genitalia.

secretes a milky alkaline fluid that adds bulk to the semen, enhances sperm movement, and neutralizes acidic vaginal secretions. Men older than 50 years commonly develop an enlarged prostate (benign prostatic hyperplasia [BPH]), which can cause problems such as overflow incontinence and nocturia (nighttime urination). Prostate function depends on adequate levels of testosterone.

Reproductive Changes Associated With Aging

Age brings changes to the function of the male and the female reproductive systems (see the Patient-Centered Care: Older Adult Health Considerations: Changes in the Reproductive System Related to Aging box). Teach patients the normal signs of aging, and remind them to report abnormalities to their health care provider.

PATIENT-CENTERED CARE: OLDER ADULT CONSIDERATIONS (QSEN)

Changes in the Reproductive System Related to Aging

Physiologic Change	Nursing Interventions	Rationales
Women		
Graying and thinning of the pubic hair Decreased size of the labia majora and clitoris	Discuss normal and expected changes (applies to all structures for both women and men).	Education helps prevent problems with body image (applies to all structures for both women and men).
Drying, smoothing, and thinning of the vaginal walls	Provide information about vaginal estrogen therapy (if desired and recommended by the health care provider) and water-soluble lubricants.	Education enables the patient to make informed decisions about the treatment of vaginal dryness, which can contribute to painful intercourse.
Decreased size of the uterus Atrophy of the endometrium Decreased size and marked convolution of the ovaries Loss of tone and elasticity of the pelvic ligaments and connective tissue	Teach Kegel exercises to strengthen pelvic muscles.	Strengthening exercises may prevent or reduce pelvic relaxation and incidences of urinary incontinence.
Increased flabbiness and fibrosis of the breasts, which hang lower on the chest wall; decreased erection of the nipples	Teach or reinforce the importance of breast self-awareness, and evidence-based recommendations for clinical breast examination and mammography based on the patient's age.	These methods can detect masses or other changes that may indicate the presence of cancer.
Men		
Graying and thinning of the pubic hair	Discuss normal and expected changes (applies to all structures for both women and men).	Education helps prevent problems with body image (applies to all structures for both women and men).
Increased drooping of the scrotum and loss of rugae	Teach or reinforce the importance of testicular self-examination (TSE).	TSE may detect changes that may indicate cancer.
Prostate enlargement, with an increased likelihood of urethral obstruction	Teach the signs of urethral obstruction and the importance of prostate cancer screening.	Education helps the patient detect enlargement or obstruction, which may indicate the presence of benign prostatic hyperplasia (BPH) or cancer.

Health Promotion and Maintenance

Many health problems of the reproductive system can be prevented through health promotion strategies and avoidance of risky lifestyle behaviors. For example, following evidence-based practices for routine preventive screenings, such as mammography and Pap tests, can detect cancer early so it can be treated with better chance for a cure. Sexually transmitted infections (STIs) and other reproductive infections can be avoided by using safer sex practices such as condoms or practicing abstinence. Teach patients about these health promotion strategies and the rationale for practicing them. Additional health promotion interventions are described under specific reproductive health problems within this unit.

ASSESSMENT: RECOGNIZE CUES

Establish a trusting relationship with the patient. Many patients find it difficult to share their reproductive history or concerns about *sexuality*. Provide information about why you are asking these questions, and how their answers can help inform the best approach to treatment. Respect their choice to refuse to answer questions if they state they do not wish to comment.

Patient History

Assess for chronic illnesses or surgeries that could affect reproductive function. Disorders that affect a woman's metabolism or nutrition can depress ovarian function and cause amenorrhea (absence of menses). Patients with diabetes mellitus may experience physiologic changes such as vaginal dryness or impotence. Chronic disorders of the nervous system, respiratory system, or cardiovascular system can alter the sexual response, as can psychiatric–mental health disorders.

Ask whether the patient has had infections. Pelvic inflammatory disease or a ruptured appendix followed by peritonitis in females can cause pelvic scarring and strictures or adhesions in the fallopian tubes. Salpingitis (uterine tube *infection*) is often caused by chlamydia, a sexually transmitted infection (STI), and can result in female infertility. A history of infections or prolonged fever in males may have damaged sperm production or caused obstruction of the seminal tract, which can cause infertility.

Ask whether the patient has been treated with radiation therapy, or had prolonged use of corticosteroids, internal or external estrogen, testosterone, or chemotherapy drugs. These can all lead to reproductive system dysfunction.

Ask about childhood conditions that could have an effect on the reproductive system. A history of mumps in men may cause orchitis (painful inflammation and swelling of the testes), which can lead to testicular atrophy and (uncommonly) sterility. A history of undescended testicles can contribute to male infertility. In women, a history of untreated sexually transmitted infections can lead to infertility.

Assess general health habits, such as sleep, exercise, and diet, as the amount of body fat may be related to ovarian dysfunction in females. Determine when patients have had their last screening for reproductive concerns. Ask females about the date and result of their most recent Pap test, breast self-examination, and vulvar self-examination. Determine when male patients older than 50 years had their last prostate examination and prostate-specific antigen (PSA) test.

Document any prescribed and over-the-counter drugs, including hormones or hormone replacement therapy, the patient is taking. Certain medications can affect the reproductive system, particularly in terms of libido (sex drive) or the male patient's ability to obtain and sustain an erection. Evidence demonstrates a higher risk for adverse effects associated with taking menopausal hormone therapy (MHT) in women over the age of 60 (Martin & Barbieri, 2020). Risks are lower in younger women yet still must be recognized, particularly in women who take combination therapy including estrogen and progesterone, as MHT has been associated with cardiovascular disease and cancer (Martin & Barbieri, 2020). Inquire whether the patient takes any vitamin, mineral, or herbal supplements, as any of these can affect reproductive function.

> ### 👤 PATIENT-CENTERED CARE: GENDER HEALTH CONSIDERATIONS (QSEN)
>
> Data about sexual activity are vital parts of the patient's history. Sexual orientation and gender identity should not be assumed. Patients who are lesbian, gay, bisexual, transgender, and queer/questioning (LGBTQ) are often not fully assessed by health care professionals due to lack of education on the part of the providers of care. These patients will feel more comfortable sharing information about their reproductive health and sexual activity when approached in a caring, nonjudgmental way. Chapter 1 describes interviewing techniques that are appropriate for LGBTQ patients. Chapter 68 in this unit discusses assessment and care of transgender patients in detail.

> ### 👤 PATIENT-CENTERED CARE: CULTURAL/ SPIRITUAL CONSIDERATIONS (QSEN)
>
> Cultural, religious, and spiritual beliefs and practices influence lifestyle and *sexuality*. These beliefs can influence specific sexual practices, the acceptable number of sexual partners, and philosophy of contraceptive use. Be sensitive to these differences by being nonjudgmental and supportive of the patient.

Nutrition History. A nutrition history is important when assessing the reproductive system. Fatigue and low libido may occur as a result of poor diet and anemia. The American Cancer Society (ACS) estimates that 70% of uterine corpus cancers are related to overweight or obesity and lack of physical activity, rendering them preventable if people made better nutrition choices (ACS, 2019b). Ask the patient to recall his or her dietary intake for a recent 24-hour period to assess quality of nutrition.

Assess the patient's height, weight, and body mass index (BMI). The patient may be hesitant to discuss eating habits such as bingeing, purging, restricting, or excessively exercising. Teach that a certain healthy level of body fat and weight is necessary for the onset of menses and the maintenance of regular menstrual cycles. Decreased body fat results in insufficient estrogen levels.

PATIENT-CENTERED CARE: GENDER HEALTH CONSIDERATIONS (QSEN)

Women have special nutrition needs. Those with heavy menstrual bleeding, particularly women who have intrauterine devices, may require iron supplements. Teach women about their body's need for calcium. Although adequate calcium intake throughout life is needed, it is especially important during and after menopause to help prevent osteoporosis caused by decreased estrogen production (see Chapter 45).

Social History. Assess for alcohol, tobacco, and illicit drug use. In males, libido, sperm production, and the ability to have or sustain an erection can be affected by these substances. Females may experience alteration or cessation of the menstrual cycle. Males and females who have chronically abused drugs and/or alcohol are at higher risk for development of cancer and infectious diseases (American Addiction Centers, 2020).

Family History and Genetic Risk. The family history helps determine the patient's risk for conditions that affect reproductive function. A delayed or early development of secondary sex characteristics may be a familial pattern.

The current age and health status of family members are important. Evidence of diseases or reproductive problems in family members (e.g., diabetes, endometriosis, reproductive cancer) can be helpful in understanding a patient's current health status, or risk for development of certain conditions. For example, daughters of women who were given diethylstilbestrol (DES) to control bleeding during pregnancy are at increased risk for fertility concerns, adverse pregnancy outcomes, reproductive cancers, and breast cancer (Hatch & Karam, 2020).

Specific *BRCA1* and *BRCA2* gene mutations increase the overall risk for breast or ovarian cancer (ACS, 2019d). Men with first-degree relatives (e.g., father, brother) with prostate cancer are at two to three times the risk for development of the disease than are men in the general population (American Society of Clinical Oncology, 2019).

Current Health Problems. Patients often seek medical attention due to pain, bleeding, discharge, or masses (see the Best Practice for Patient Safety & Quality Care: Assessing the Patient With Reproductive Health Problems box). *Pain* related to reproductive system disorders may be confused with symptoms of GI issues (e.g., abdominal discomfort) or urinary health problems (e.g., urinary frequency). Ask the patient to describe the nature of the pain, including its type, intensity, timing and location, duration, and relationship to menstrual, sexual, urinary, or GI function. Assess the factors that exacerbate (worsen) or relieve the pain. Ask about sleeping patterns and if pain or other symptoms affect the ability to get adequate rest.

Heavy menstrual *bleeding* or a lack thereof may concern the patient. The possibility of pregnancy in any sexually active woman with amenorrhea must be considered. Postmenopausal bleeding needs to be evaluated. Ask the patient to describe the amount and characteristics of any abnormal vaginal bleeding. Assess whether the bleeding occurs in relation to the menstrual cycle or menopause, intercourse, trauma, or strenuous

BEST PRACTICE FOR PATIENT SAFETY & QUALITY CARE (QSEN)

Assessing the Patient With Reproductive Health Problems

Patient Concern	Nursing Assessment
Pain	Type, intensity, and timing of pain
	Location and duration of pain
	Factors that relieve or worsen pain
	Relationship to menstrual, sexual, urinary, or GI function
	Relationship to sleeping and rest patterns
	Medications taken to address the pain
Bleeding	Presence or absence of bleeding
	Character and amount of bleeding
	Relationship of bleeding to events or other factors (e.g., menstrual cycle)
	Onset and duration of bleeding
	Presence of associated symptoms, such as pain
Discharge	Amount and character of discharge
	Frequency with which discharge is present (e.g., 1-2 days a month, all month)
	Presence of genital lesions, bleeding, itching, or pain
	Presence of symptoms or discharge in sexual partner
Masses	Location and characteristics of mass
	Presence of associated symptoms, such as pain
	Relationship to menstrual cycle

exercise. For male patients, ask about the presence of penile bleeding. Ask any patient who has abnormal bleeding about associated symptoms, such as *pain,* cramping or abdominal fullness, a change in bowel habits, urinary difficulties, and weight changes.

Discharge from the male or female reproductive tract can cause irritation of the surrounding tissues, itching, *pain,* embarrassment, and anxiety. Ask about the amount, color, consistency, odor, and chronicity of discharge that may be present from orifices used during sexual activity. Certain drugs (e.g., antibiotics) and clothing (e.g., tight clothing, synthetic underwear fabric) may cause or worsen genital discharge. Many types of discharge are caused by STIs or other *infection* (see Chapter 69).

Masses in the breasts, testes, or inguinal area must be evaluated. Ask if the patient can relate the changes in character or size of masses to menstrual cycles, heavy lifting, straining, or trauma. Ask about associated symptoms such as tenderness, heaviness, *pain,* dimpling, and tender lymph nodes.

Physical Assessment

Assessment of the Female Reproductive System. A Papanicolaou test (Pap test or Pap smear) should be scheduled between the patient's menstrual periods so the menstrual flow does not interfere with laboratory analysis. Teach women not to douche, use vaginal medications, powders, or deodorants, or have sexual intercourse for at least 24 hours before the test, because these may interfere with test interpretation.

The American Cancer Society (ACS, 2018) advises the following schedule for Pap testing:

- Women should begin having an annual Pap test at 21 years of age.
- Women between 21 and 29 years should have a Pap test every 3 years. Human papillomavirus (HPV) testing is not to be used for screening for this age group, although it can be used as part of a follow-up for an abnormal Pap result.
- Women between ages 30 and 65 years should have just the Pap test every 3 years.
- Women older than 65 years who have had regular cervical cancer testing with normal results in the past decade, and no serious cancers in the past 20 years, do not need further Pap testing.
- Women who have had a hysterectomy can discontinue Pap tests unless the hysterectomy was done to treat precervical or cervical cancer.
- Women with a history of cancer or precancer of the cervix should speak to their health care provider for individualized recommendations for Pap and HPV testing.

Canadian guidelines are similar. General Canadian recommendations include (Choosing Wisely Canada, 2019):

- Women should begin having an annual Pap test at 21 years of age.
- Women between 21 and 29 years who are sexually active should have a Pap test every 3 years.
- Women between ages 30 and 69 years should have a Pap test every 3 years.
- Women older than 70 years who have had three previous normal Pap tests do not need further Pap testing.
- Women with risk factors such as a history of cancer, precancerous cells in the cervix, or a weakened immune system should speak to their health care provider regarding Pap recommendations.

NCLEX EXAMINATION CHALLENGE 64.1

Health Promotion and Maintenance

A 68-year-old client who has had normal Pap results for 10 years and no history of cancer asks about scheduling a Pap smear. Which nursing response is appropriate?

A. "You will need a Pap test this year."
B. "You aren't due for a Pap test until next year."
C. "You do not need to have further Pap tests at this time."
D. "You do not need a Pap test unless you are sexually active."

The nurse generalist does not perform the comprehensive female or male reproductive examination. However, you should perform a focused physical assessment related to specific concerns of the patient. The health care provider conducts a more detailed gynecologic assessment as described in the following paragraphs; the nurse generalist often assists with the examination. The examination should be performed in a room that has adequate lighting for body inspection, has comfortable temperature, and ensures privacy. Immediately before the pelvic and breast examinations, ask the patient to empty her bladder and undress completely. Drape the patient adequately to provide as much privacy as possible throughout the examination. Remove drapes only over the region being examined and replace them after that area has been assessed. Mirrors can be used to facilitate teaching if the patient desires.

The health care provider may begin with assessing the breasts (see Chapter 65) before progressing to the abdomen and pelvic examination. The patient's arms should be at her sides or relaxed over her chest to allow better relaxation of the abdominal muscles. Assessment is conducted for symmetry, shape, skin color and temperature, and presence or absence of lesions or dimpling. Help the patient lie on her back while the health care provider performs palpation of the breast tissue (and then the abdomen). If the patient wishes to perform breast self-examinations at home, provide teaching (Chapter 65).

Inspection of the external female genitalia and the pelvic examination are usually performed at the end of a head-to-toe physical assessment. The patient may be more apprehensive about these portions of the examination than about any other part. *Pain* or lack of privacy during previous pelvic examinations may prevent the patient from relaxing. Stay with the patient and offer reassurance and compassion during this portion of the examination.

Assist the patient into the lithotomy position, continuously being mindful of draping for privacy. Assessment of external genitalia includes visualization of the mons pubis and vulva. Be aware that removal of pubic hair and/or piercings in this area may compromise tissue integrity and facilitate *infection.* In preparation for the internal genitalia examination, obtain a Graves speculum for most adult patients, or a Pederson speculum (which is narrower) for patients who are younger or postmenopausal; run warm water over it and apply a dime-sized amount of water-soluble gel lubricant (Jarvis, 2020). Teach that the plastic speculum makes a loud clicking sound when it locks and unlocks, so that this does not startle the patient (Jarvis, 2020).

Other than determining pregnancy or infertility, this portion of the examination is indicated to assess:

- Menstrual irregularities
- Unexplained abdominal or vaginal *pain*
- Vaginal discharge, itching, sores, or *infection*
- Rape trauma or other pelvic injury
- Physical changes in the vagina, cervix, and uterus

During the speculum examination, the health care provider palpates for symptomatic and asymptomatic abdominopelvic masses, which can be of reproductive, intestinal, or urinary tract origin. Gynecologic masses, such as ovarian masses, may be further differentiated from lesions on the body of the uterus during the bimanual portion of the pelvic examination. Several samples of cells from the cervix are obtained with a small brush or spatula during the Pap test, placed on a glass slide, and sent to the laboratory for examination. Nucleic acid amplification tests are collected to test for sexually transmitted infections, and samples for HPV testing are also obtained at this time. A bimanual examination will be performed by the health care provider to palpate the internal genitalia for location, size, mobility, and the presence of masses or tenderness (Jarvis, 2020). The health care provider may also perform a rectal examination, which can demonstrate external or internal hemorrhoids, fissures, or masses.

When the examination is complete, provide the patient with a towel to remove any residual water-soluble gel. Assist her to a sitting position, and provide privacy so that she can redress.

PATIENT-CENTERED CARE: CULTURAL/ SPIRITUAL CONSIDERATIONS (QSEN)

A patient's personal experiences, culture, and/or spiritual beliefs may influence thoughts about *sexuality*, which can affect his or her ability to enjoy a satisfactory sex life. These factors may include:

- Sexual trauma or abuse inflicted during childhood or adulthood
- Punishment for masturbation
- Psychological trauma
- Cultural influences
- Concerns about sexual partners or sexual lifestyle
- Use of alcohol or street drugs

Assessment of the Male Reproductive System. Unless a male patient seeks health care for a specific problem, the health care provider may not perform a reproductive assessment, depending on the setting and the age of the patient. Like women, men may be embarrassed and anxious when the reproductive system is assessed. The patient may be concerned about *pain,* the developmental stage of his genitalia, or the possibility of experiencing an erection during the examination. If he does have an erection, the examiner should assure him that this is a normal response to a tactile stimulus (touch) and should continue the examination unless the patient requests to stop the assessment.

Explain each step of the assessment procedure before it is performed. The patient needs to be reassured that the health care provider will stop and change the assessment plan or technique if requested. Provide nonjudgmental support and teach relaxation techniques that can be helpful to relieve pain, especially during the rectal examination to palpate the prostate gland.

Fears may affect the patient's satisfaction with *sexuality* or body image. He or she may also be concerned about the potential or actual reaction of family members to reproductive health problems (see the Best Practice for Patient Safety & Quality Care: Assessing the Patient with Reproductive Health Problems box). Use nonjudgmental listening to continue development of trust between yourself and the patient, allowing the patient to openly express feelings or concerns.

Provide privacy within a well-lit environment, and have the patient undress. As with the female patient, drape the male patient adequately to provide as much privacy as possible throughout the examination. Remove drapes only as needed for examination, and replace them after that area has been assessed.

The health care provider will conduct the physical examination, which may include a breast examination. Although men are less likely to have breast cancer than women, it is important to assess for this possibility, especially if the patient has been exposed to radiation, has a high level of estrogen, or has a family history of breast cancer (National Breast Cancer Foundation, 2019). The examination is performed by the health care provider in the same manner as for a female patient.

CLINICAL JUDGMENT CHALLENGE 64.1
Evidence-Based Practice; Patient-Centered Care

The nurse is taking a history on a 54-year-old male client who has come to the health care provider's office for an annual physical. The client reports being in good health other than "a couple of bumps in my left armpit." When asked about any pain in the left arm or breast area, the client states, "sometimes that side of my chest aches. I figure it's because I've worked out too hard."

1. **Recognize Cues:** What assessment information in this client situation is the most important and immediate concern for the nurse? (Hint: Identify the **relevant** information *first* to determine what is most important.)
2. **Analyze Cues:** What client conditions are consistent with the **most relevant** information? (Hint: Think about priority collaborative problems that support and contradict the information presented in this situation.)

An examination of the external genitalia includes visualization of the pubis, penis, and scrotum. Lesions or areas where tissue integrity is compromised can be identified during this portion of the examination. The health care provider will perform palpation to determine the presence of masses or *pain,* and a prostate examination. If a sexually transmitted infection is suspected, swabs may be obtained at this time by the provider. When the examination is complete, provide the patient with a towel to clean himself (if needed), and privacy while he redresses.

Psychosocial Assessment

Ask about sources of support, strengths, and coping reactions to illness or dysfunction. It is not uncommon for people with reproductive concerns to feel anxiety or fear. For patients who have few support systems in place, consider referral to community groups or social services that can be of assistance.

Diagnostic Assessment

Laboratory Assessment. The Laboratory Profile: Reproductive Assessment box summarizes important laboratory tests associated with reproductive function. The Pap test, a cytologic study, is effective in detecting precancerous and cancerous cells within the female patient's cervix.

The **human papillomavirus (HPV) test** performed on cells collected from the cervix can identify many high-risk types of HPV *infection* associated with development of cervical cancer. This test can be done at the same time as the Pap test for women at higher risk for HPV, or as a follow-up for those who have had an abnormal Pap test result. It does not replace the Pap test because it tests for viruses that can cause cell changes in the cervix that, if not treated, could lead to cancer. Women who have normal Pap test results and no HPV infection are at very low risk for developing cervical cancer. Conversely, women with an abnormal Pap test and a positive HPV test result are at higher risk if not treated.

Other types of laboratory testing include cytologic vaginal *cultures,* which can detect bacterial, viral, fungal, and parasitic disorders. Examination of cells from the vaginal walls can evaluate estrogen balance in female patients.

Serum levels of follicle-stimulating hormone (FSH), luteinizing hormone (LH), and prolactin are helpful in the diagnosis of male and female reproductive tract disorders. Serum testing

LABORATORY PROFILE

Reproductive Assessment

Test	Normal Range for Adults	Significance of Abnormal Findings
Serum Studies		
Follicle-stimulating hormone (FSH)	*Men:* 1.42-15.4 IU/L *Women:* • Follicular phase, 1.37-9.9 IU/L • Ovulatory peak, 6.17-17.2 IU/L • Luteal phase, 1.09-9.2 IU/L • Postmenopause, 19.3-100.6 IU/L Canadian: *Men:* 1.0-10.0 IU/L *Women:* • Follicular phase, 1.37-9.9 IU/L • Ovulatory peak, 6.17-17.2 IU/L • Luteal phase, 1.09-9.2 IU/L • Postmenopause, 40-250 IU/L	Decreased levels may indicate possible infertility, anorexia nervosa, hypothalamic failure, pituitary failure. Elevations may indicate possible ovarian or testicular dysgenesis.
Luteinizing hormone (LH)	*Men:* 1.24-7.8 IU/L *Women:* • Follicular phase, 1.68-15 IU/L • Ovulatory peak, 21.9-56.6 IU/L • Luteal phase, 0.61-16.3 IUL • Postmenopause, 14.2-52.3 IU/L Canadian: *Men:* 1.0-9.0 IU/L *Women:* • Follicular phase, 2.0-10.0 IU/L • Ovulatory peak, 15.0-65.0 IU/L • Luteal phase, 1.0-12.0 IU/L • Postmenopause, 12-65 IU/L	Decreased levels may indicate possible pituitary or hypothalamic failure, anorexia nervosa (and anovulation), or malnutrition. Elevations may indicate possible ovarian or testicular dysgenesis.
Prolactin	*Men:* 3-13 ng/mL *Women:* 3-27 ng/mL Pregnant women: 20-400 ng/mL	Decreased levels may indicate possible pituitary apoplexy or pituitary destruction from tumor. Elevations may indicate possible galactorrhea, hypothyroidism, anorexia nervosa, prolactin-secreting pituitary tumor, or amenorrhea or polycystic ovarian syndrome (in women).
Estradiol	*Men:* 10-50 pg/mL *Women:* • Follicular phase, 20-350 pg/mL • Midcycle, 150-750 pg/mL • Luteal phase, 30-450 pg/mL • Postmenopause, ≤20 pg/mL	Decreased levels may indicate possible pregnancy concerns or menopause (in women), hypopituitarism, or anorexia nervosa. Elevations may indicate possible adrenal, ovarian, or testicular tumor, or normal pregnancy development (in women).
Estriol (serum)	*Men:* N/A *Nonpregnant women:* N/A Canadian: Same	Same significance as levels of estradiol in women.
Progesterone	*Men:* 10-50 ng/dL *Women:* • Follicular phase, <50 ng/dL • Luteal phase, 300-2500 ng/dL • Postmenopausal, <40 ng/dL Canadian: *Men:* 0-1.3 nmol/L *Women:* • Follicular phase, 0.3-4.8 nmol/L • Luteal phase, 8.0-89.0 nmol/L • Postmenopausal, <1.27 nmol/L	Decreased levels in women may indicate possible preeclampsia, toxemia of pregnancy, threatened abortion, placental failure, fetal death, ovarian neoplasm, ovarian hypofunction, or amenorrhea. Elevations may indicate possible hyperadrenocorticalism or adrenocortical hyperplasia. In women, elevations indicate possible ovulation, pregnancy, or luteal cysts of the ovary.

Continued

LABORATORY PROFILE—CONT'D

Test	Normal Range for Adults	Significance of Abnormal Findings
Testosterone	*Men:* 280-1080 ng/dL *Women:* <70 ng/dL Canadian: *Men:* 275-875 ng/dL *Women:* 23-875 ng/dL	Decreased levels in men may indicate possible cryptorchidism, hypogonadism, trisomy 21, or orchidectomy. Increased levels in men may indicate possible testicular, extragonadal, or adrenocortical tumor, testosterone resistance syndrome, or hyperthyroidism. Elevations in women may indicate possible adrenal or ovarian tumor, polycystic ovaries, or idiopathic hirsutism.
Prostate-specific antigen	*Men:* • 0-2.5 ng/mL = low • 2.6-10 ng/mL = slightly to moderately elevated • 10-19.9 ng/mL = moderately elevated • 20 ng/mL = significantly elevated Canadian: *Men:* 0-4 ng/mL	Elevated levels in men may indicate prostatitis, benign prostatic hyperplasia, or prostate cancer.

1 mcg, 1 microgram or 1 millionth of a gram; *1 ng,* 1 nanogram or 1 billionth of a gram; *1 pg,* 1 picogram or 1 trillionth of a gram. *N/A,* Not applicable.

Data from Pagana, K.D., & Pagana, T.J. (2018). *Mosby's manual of diagnostic and laboratory tests* (6th ed.). St. Louis: Elsevier; and Pagana, K., Pagana, T., & Pike-MacDonald, S. (2019). *Mosby's Canadian manual of diagnostic and laboratory tests* (2nd ed.). Ontario, Canada, Elsevier.

can also detect estrogen, progesterone, and testosterone levels in men and women. Teach the patient that no nutrition restrictions are necessary before having these tests performed. See the Laboratory Profile: Reproductive Assessment box for normal values and the significance of abnormal findings.

Serologic studies detect antigen-antibody reactions that occur in response to foreign organisms. This form of diagnostic testing is helpful only after an **infection** has become well established. Serologic testing can be used in the evaluation of exposure to organisms causing syphilis, rubella, and herpes simplex virus type 2 (HSV2). Results may be read as *nonreactive, weakly reactive,* or *reactive.* A single titer is not as revealing as serial titers, which can detect the rise in antibody reactions as the body continues to fight the **infection.**

The *prostate-specific antigen (PSA)* test is used to screen for prostate cancer in men, and to monitor the disease after treatment. Although elevated PSA levels may be associated with prostate cancer, there is variance among health care providers in interpretation of results. Levels less than 2.5 to 4.0 ng/mL may be considered normal, depending on the resource used (Hoffman, 2020; Pagana & Pagana, 2018). Certain factors such as prostatitis, acute urinary retention, recent prostate biopsy, or transurethral resection of the prostate (TURP) can cause transient rises in PSA (Hoffman, 2020).

PATIENT-CENTERED CARE: CULTURAL/ SPIRITUAL CONSIDERATIONS QSEN

African-American men are 1.6 times as likely to develop prostate cancer and twice as likely to die from it than are white men (Research on Prostate Cancer in Men of African Ancestry, 2019). For this reason, teach African-American male patients to begin prostate cancer screening at age 40.

Imaging Assessment

Mammography. **Mammography** is an x-ray of the soft tissue of the breast. Mammograms assess differences in the density of breast tissue. They are especially helpful in evaluating poorly defined masses, multiple masses or nodules, nipple changes or discharge, skin changes, and ***pain.*** Mammography can detect many cancers that are not palpable by physical examination. However, false-positive and false-negative readings can occur (ACS, 2019c).

In young women's breasts, there is little difference in the density between normal glandular tissue and malignant tumors, which makes the mammogram less useful for evaluation of breast masses in these patients. For this reason, annual screening mammograms are not recommended for women younger than 40 years. In older women, it is not uncommon for the amount of fatty tissue to be higher, and the fatty tissue appears lighter than cancers. Cancer and cysts may have the same density. Cysts usually have smooth borders, and cancers often have starburst-shaped margins. Organizations such as the U.S. Preventive Services Task Force, the American Cancer Society (ACS), the American College of Obstetricians and Gynecologists (ACOG), and the American College of Physicians (ACP) have different guidelines on screening for breast cancer (Centers for Disease Control and Prevention, n.d.). Teach the patient to collaborate with her health care provider to determine the timing that is right for her to have a mammogram based on her age and risk factors.

No dietary restrictions are necessary before the mammogram. Remind the patient not to use creams, lotions, powders, or deodorant on the breasts or underarms before the study because these products may be visible on the mammogram and contribute to misdiagnosis. For women who come to their appointment and have used one of these products, provide washcloths and premoistened wipes to remove the residue. If there is any possibility that the patient is pregnant, the test should be rescheduled. Explain the purpose of the study and its anticipated discomforts. The technician or assistant provides a gown and privacy for the woman to undress above the waist. Allow the patient to express concerns about the mammogram and the presence of any lumps or breast changes that she has noticed.

When performing an analog (film) mammogram, a technician positions the patient next to the x-ray machine with one

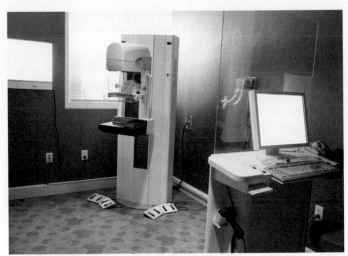

FIG. 64.4 System for digital 3D mammography, also known as digital breast tomosynthesis. (©iStock/JodiJacobson.)

breast exposed. A film plate and the platform of the machine are placed on opposite sides of the breast to be examined. The technician includes as much breast tissue as possible between the plates. The woman may experience some temporary discomfort when the breast is compressed (for about 30 seconds for each of two positions for each breast). The entire test takes less than 15 minutes. The patient usually is asked to wait until the films are reviewed in case a view needs to be repeated.

Digital imaging systems for mammography include direct radiography (DR), which is used most commonly in the United States, and computed radiography (CR). Digital mammography has been shown to have distinct advantages over analog mammography, including better resolution, the ability to detect subtle abnormalities by changing contrast and brightness of the image, and lower radiation dose (Venkataraman & Slanetz, 2020). Disadvantages include the cost of the overall system and associated higher-resolution monitors, compared to the cost of analog mammography (Venkataraman & Slanetz, 2020).

Digital 3D mammography (digital breast tomosynthesis) (Figs. 64.4 and 64.5) allows the radiologist to visualize through layers or "slices" of breast tissue, similar to a CT scan. Compared with conventional digital mammography, digital 3D mammography has been shown to increase cancer detection rates, although it does increase the radiation dose to the patient (Venkataraman & Slanetz, 2020).

Inform the patient when to expect the report of the results. Because this is a time when she may be anxious, teach or reinforce the importance of continued breast self-awareness and provide instructions as needed.

CT Scans. CT scans for reproductive system disorders involve the abdomen and the pelvis. Primary health care providers can detect and evaluate masses and identify lymphatic enlargement from metastasis. This scan can differentiate solid tissue masses from cystic or hemorrhagic structures.

MRI. MRI uses a magnetic field and radiofrequency energy to distinguish between normal and malignant tissues. MRI is used in addition to mammograms to assess for breast cancer in women who are at high risk, or for further diagnostic purposes for those who have already been diagnosed with breast cancer (ACS, 2019a). The use of MRI in evaluating patients with dense breast tissue may reduce the need for biopsy. MRI can also be used to detect pelvic tumors.

Ultrasonography. Ultrasonography (US) is a technique that is used to assess females for fibroids, cysts, ectopic pregnancy, and masses. It can be used to monitor the progress of tumor regression after medical treatment. US is also helpful in differentiating solid tumors from cysts in breast examinations. Prostate, scrotal, and rectal US can be used to detect abnormalities in these areas, such as prostate or testicular masses, varicoceles, or problems of the ejaculatory ducts, seminal vesicles and vas deferens (Pagana & Pagana, 2018).

For an external US of the abdomen, breast, or scrotum, the technician exposes the area and applies gel to the area to be scanned, which provides better transmission of sound waves from the transducer through the patient's skin. The transducer is moved in a linear pattern across the area being tested to outline and define soft-tissue masses and to differentiate tumor type, ascites, and encapsulated fluid.

For an internal *transvaginal* or *transrectal* scan, the transducer is covered with a condom-like sac onto which transmission gel has been placed. Teach the patient to report any allergies to latex, as the condom-like sac is often made of latex (Pagana & Pagana, 2018). The transducer is then inserted into the vagina or rectum as indicated. Women should have an empty bladder if they are having a transvaginal ultrasound. Patients having an internal ultrasound should be informed that they might feel some mild ***pain*** associated with pressure of the probe.

NCLEX EXAMINATION CHALLENGE 64.2

Physiological Integrity

A client has been scheduled for a transvaginal ultrasound. Which allergy does the nurse identify that should be **immediately** reported to the health care provider?

A. Eggs
B. Corn
C. Latex
D. Iodine

Hysterosalpingography. A **hysterosalpingogram** is an outpatient fluoroscopy procedure that uses an injection of a contrast medium to visualize the cervix, uterus, and fallopian tubes. This test is used to evaluate tubal anatomy and patency and is commonly done as part of an infertility evaluation, after placement of an internal contraception device, or after tubal ligation or tubal reversal (Lee & Kilcoyne, 2019). It can also

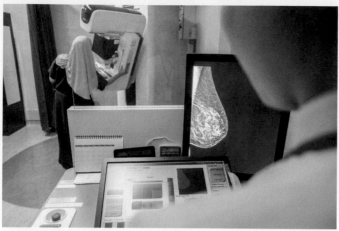

FIG. 64.5 Patient undergoing digital 3D mammography, also known as digital breast tomosynthesis. (©iStock/JohnnyGreig.)

be useful in evaluation of uterine problems such as fibroids, tumors, and fistulas. Assess the patient for pregnancy, vaginal bleeding, pelvic *infection* (even if taking antibiotics), and history of reaction to iodine, as these are all contraindications to this procedure.

The examination is best performed on days 6 to 11 from the patient's last menstrual cycle, which reduces the chance that the patient may be pregnant and helps to avoid menstruation (Lee & Kilcoyne, 2019). Teach that the procedure may cause some mild and self-limited pain, as well as a small amount of postprocedure bleeding; if cramping continues after the procedure, an NSAID can be used (Lee & Kilcoyne, 2019).

On the day of the examination, confirm the date of the patient's last menstrual period. Again, ask about allergies to iodine dye. The health care provider communicates benefits and risks of the procedure with the patient. As the nurse, you may witness the signed informed consent. Be aware that the patient may experience some nausea and vomiting, abdominal cramping, or faintness during the procedure. Provide support and assistance with relaxation techniques as needed.

After the patient is placed in lithotomy position, the health care provider will insert a speculum to view the cervix. Dye is injected through the cervix to fill and highlight the interior of the cervix, uterus, and fallopian tubes. If the fallopian tubes are patent, the contrast material spills into the peritoneal cavity. Usually only two or three views are obtained to show the path and distribution of the contrast medium.

As noted earlier, the patient may experience a small amount of vaginal bleeding and pelvic *pain* after the study, and should receive analgesic medications if prescribed. Inform her that she may also have referred pain to the shoulder because of irritation of the phrenic nerve. Provide a perineal pad after the test to prevent soiling of clothes as the dye drains from the cervix. Instruct the patient to contact the health care provider if bloody discharge continues for 4 days or longer and to immediately report any signs of *infection,* such as lower quadrant pain, fever, chills, malodorous discharge, or tachycardia.

Endoscopic Studies

Colposcopy. A colposcope allows three-dimensional magnification and intense illumination of tissue of the cervix, vagina, vulva, or anus (Feltmate & Feldman, 2020). Because it provides accurate site selection, this procedure can locate the exact site of precancerous and cancerous lesions for biopsy in preparation for early treatment. **Colposcopy** can also be used for further diagnosis after a woman has an abnormal Pap test result or has HPV (Feltmate & Feldman, 2020).

Teach the patient that she should not douche or use vaginal preparations for 24 to 48 hours before the test. This nearly painless procedure is better tolerated if it is explained in advance and if a picture of a colposcope is shown to the patient. Explain that the health care provider may take a biopsy specimen while performing colposcopy. The provider will obtain informed consent, and you, as the nurse, may witness this.

Provide the patient with a gown and privacy, and instruct her to undress from the waist down. Help the patient to assume the lithotomy position. The health care provider locates the cervix or vaginal site through a speculum, and a visual examination is performed. After 30 to 60 seconds, acetic acid is applied to the cervix to draw moisture from the tissue, which allows large or dense nuclei (e.g., metaplastic or dysplastic cells, or cells infected with HPV) to be visualized more easily. If no abnormalities are noted, other solutions composed of iodine, potassium iodine, and distilled water are applied to the cervix (Feltmate & Feldman, 2020), and cells with glycogen turn dark brown. The health care provider may use a green or blue filter to visualize differences between the abnormal vascularities and epithelium. During the procedure, a biopsy specimen can be taken if abnormal cells are seen. (See Cervical Biopsy section later in this chapter.)

After the procedure, allow the patient to rest for a few minutes, especially if she had a biopsy performed. Provide privacy and supplies to clean the perineum and a perineal pad to absorb dye or discharge. Inform the patient that she may wish to wear a menstrual pad because mild cramping, spotting, or dark or black-colored discharge (from medication applied to the cervix to reduce bleeding) may occur for several days. Remind the patient to take pain relievers as recommended by the health care provider but to avoid aspirin to decrease the chance of bleeding. The patient should be instructed to refrain from douching, using tampons, and having sexual intercourse for 1 week (or as instructed by the health care provider).

Dilation and Curettage. A **dilation and curettage** (D&C) is a procedure in which tissue is removed from inside of the uterus because of abnormal bleeding or to remove pregnancy tissue after an abortion, miscarriage, or childbirth. Done through a hysteroscope (see Hysteroscopy section later in this chapter), a type of endoscope, this procedure takes approximately 15 to 30 minutes. It is done with anesthesia before and during the procedure (ACOG, 2020).

Prior to the procedure, teach patients about the anesthesia that will be used, and assess for any prior adverse reactions to anesthesia. If prescribed, teach the patient about techniques or medication that is used before the procedure to begin dilating, or softening, the cervix. Ensure that patients have someone to drive them home after the procedure is over, and teach that mild spotting, light bleeding, and/or mild pain may occur. On the day of the procedure, the health care provider will obtain informed consent, and you may witness the patient signing this. Remind the patient to report heavy bleeding, fever, abdominal pain, or foul-smelling discharge to the health care provider right away. Also, teach the patient that her next menstrual cycle may occur earlier or later than the anticipated date (ACOG, 2020).

Laparoscopy. **Laparoscopy** is a direct examination of the pelvic cavity through an endoscope. This procedure can be used to rule out an ectopic pregnancy, evaluate ovarian disorders and pelvic masses, and aid in the diagnosis of infertility and unexplained pelvic *pain*. Laparoscopy is also used during surgical procedures such as:

- Tubal sterilization
- Ovarian biopsy
- Cyst aspiration
- Removal of endometriosis tissue or fibroids
- Lysis of adhesions around the fallopian tubes
- Retrieval of intrauterine devices that the patient cannot self retrieve

A laparoscopy is often preferred over laparotomy for minor surgical procedures because it is less costly, sometimes requires a shorter operative time, produces smaller scars, and lends itself to a faster recovery time without formation of adhesions (Sharp, 2019).

The surgeon describes benefits and risks of the procedure to the patient. Risks include complications associated with the use of anesthesia, postoperative shoulder pain from irritation of the phrenic nerve, effects of carbon dioxide gas and/or peritoneal stretching, irritation at the incision site, and the rare occurrence of infection or electrical burns. As the nurse, you may witness the patient signing the informed consent form. A laparoscopy can be performed with use of a regional or general anesthetic depending on the patient's risk factors related to anesthesia, the type of position the patient will be placed in during the procedure, and the anticipated length of procedural time (Joshi, 2019).

After the patient is anesthetized and placed in supine or dorsal lithotomy position, a urinary catheter is inserted to drain the bladder. The operating table is placed in slight Trendelenburg position to allow the intestines to fall away from the pelvis so that the pelvic viscera can be better visualized (Sharp, 2019). The cervix is held with a cannula to allow movement of the uterus during laparoscopy (Fig. 64.6). The surgeon inserts a

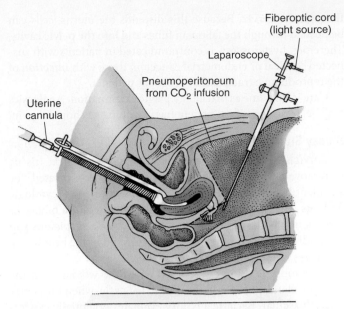

FIG. 64.6 Laparoscopy. *CO₂*, Carbon dioxide.

needle below the umbilicus to infuse carbon dioxide (CO_2) into the pelvic cavity, which distends the abdomen and permits better visualization of the organs. After the trocar and cannula are in place in the abdominal cavity, the surgeon removes the trocar and inserts the laparoscope. The surgeon can then visualize the pelvic cavity and reproductive organs. Further instrumentation is possible through one or more small incisions. The laparoscope is removed at the end of the procedure, and the abdomen is deflated. The small incision is closed with absorbable sutures and dressed with an adhesive bandage.

The patient is usually discharged on the day of the procedure. Incisional *pain* is managed by oral analgesics. The greatest discomfort is usually caused by referred shoulder pain. Most of these sensations disappear within 48 hours, depending on the extent of the procedure. Instruct the patient to change the small adhesive bandage as needed and to observe the incision for signs of *infection* or hematoma. Teach her to avoid strenuous activity for the first week after the procedure.

Hysteroscopy. **Hysteroscopy** is a procedure that uses a fiberoptic telescope to visualize the uterus to diagnose and treat causes of abnormal bleeding. The hysteroscope includes a fiberoptic camera that is inserted into the vagina to examine the cervix and uterus. Diagnostic hysteroscopy is used to diagnose new problems with the uterus or to confirm results from other tests. Hysteroscopy can also be used before or during other procedures (e.g., laparoscopy) for infertility and unexplained bleeding. The procedure is best performed in the proliferative stage to best visualize the uterine cavity (Bradley, 2020).

The health care provider informs the patient of benefits and risks associated with the procedure and obtains consent. You, as the nurse, may witness the patient signing the informed consent form. The preparation is the same as for a pelvic examination. After the patient is placed in lithotomy position, she may be anesthetized with a paracervical block before the cervix is dilated if the procedure will involve uterine biopsy (Bradley, 2020). The health care provider inserts the hysteroscope through the cervix. Because this distends the uterus, cells can be pushed through the fallopian tubes and into the pelvic cavity. Therefore, hysteroscopy is contraindicated in patients with suspected cervical or endometrial cancer, in those with *infection* of the reproductive tract, and in pregnant patients.

Care is the same as that after a pelvic examination. Analgesics may be prescribed if the patient has cramping or shoulder pain.

Biopsy Studies

Cervical Biopsy. In a cervical biopsy, cervical tissue is removed for cytologic study. A biopsy is indicated for an identifiable cervical lesion, regardless of the cytologic findings. The health care provider usually performs a biopsy in conjunction with colposcopy as a follow-up to a suspicious Pap test finding. The procedure may be performed in the health care provider's office setting.

The biopsy is usually scheduled when the woman is in the early proliferative phase of the menstrual cycle, when the cervix is least vascular. Because a biopsy evaluates potentially cancerous cells, your patient may be anxious and need time to discuss her feelings and fears. The use of relaxation techniques may address *pain*. Assist her into the lithotomy position, recognizing that further preparation depends on the type of procedure to be performed.

The health care provider may anesthetize the patient according to the needs of the chosen procedure. The type of anesthetic used for the procedure determines the type of immediate care that is needed after the procedure.

Several techniques can be used for a cervical biopsy. If a lesion is clearly visible, an endocervical curettage can be performed as an ambulatory care procedure and with little or no anesthetic. This tissue sample is immediately placed into a formalin solution. Conization (removal of a cone-shaped sample of tissue) and loop electrosurgical excision procedures (LEEPs) are procedures that can be done later if there is discrepancy between the Pap test and biopsy findings (Cooper & Menifee, 2020). Conization can be done as a cold-knife procedure, a laser excision, or an electrosurgical incision.

Discharge instructions can be found in the Patient and Family Education: Preparing for Self-Management: The Patient Recovering From Cervical Biopsy box.

PATIENT AND FAMILY EDUCATION: PREPARING FOR SELF-MANAGEMENT

The Patient Recovering From Cervical Biopsy

- Do not lift any heavy objects until the site is healed (about 2 weeks).
- Rest for 24 hours after the procedure.
- Report any excessive bleeding (more than that of a normal menstrual period) to your health care provider.
- Report signs of *infection* (fever, increased pain, foul-smelling drainage) to your health care provider.
- Do not douche, use tampons, or have vaginal intercourse until the site is healed (about 2 weeks).
- Keep the perineum clean and dry by using antiseptic solution rinses (as directed by your health care provider) and changing pads frequently.

Endometrial Biopsy. Both endometrial biopsy and aspiration are used to obtain cells directly from the lining of the uterus to assess for cancer of the endometrium. Biopsy helps assess menstrual disturbances (especially heavy bleeding) and infertility (corpus luteum dysfunction).

When menstrual disturbances are being evaluated, the biopsy is generally done in the immediate premenstrual period to provide an index of progesterone influence and ovulation. A biopsy performed in the second half of the menstrual cycle (about days 21 and 22) evaluates corpus luteum function and the presence or absence of a persistent secretory endometrium. Postmenopausal women may undergo biopsies at any time.

An endometrial biopsy is usually done as an office procedure with or without anesthesia. Menstrual data should be obtained from the patient and are included on the specimen request for the pathologist. Confirm that the patient is not pregnant, as this is an absolute contraindication for this procedure. Prepare the patient in the same way as you would for a pelvic examination. Tell her that she may experience some cramping when the cervix is dilated. Analgesia before the procedure and relaxation and breathing techniques during the procedure may be helpful to make her more comfortable. Some providers will prescribe an NSAID 30 to 60 minutes prior to the procedure to decrease cramping; others may administer a paracervical block or administer local anesthetic via intrauterine instillation (Del Priore, 2019).

After the uterus is measured and the cervix dilated, the health care provider inserts the curette or intrauterine cannula into the uterus. A portion of the endometrium is withdrawn using either the cuplike end of the curette or suction equipment and is placed into a formalin solution to be sent for histologic examination. It is at this time that the patient is most likely to have moderate cramping. Allow her to rest on the examining table until the cramping has subsided. Provide a perineal pad and a wipe to clean the perineum. Teach her that spotting may be present for 1 to 2 days but any signs of *infection* or excessive bleeding should be reported to the health care provider. Instruct the patient to avoid intercourse or douching until all discharge has ceased.

Breast Biopsy. All breast masses should be evaluated for the possibility of cancer. It is important to recognize that breast cancer can occur in both men and women; less than 1% of breast cancers occur in men (National Cancer Institute, 2019). Approximately 2620 men are diagnosed with breast cancer annually in the United States, and approximately 520 die from this condition yearly (ACS, 2020).

Fibrocystic lesions, fibroadenomas, and intraductal papillomas can be differentiated by biopsy. Any discharge from the breasts is examined histologically. Prior to the procedure, provide instructions to the patient based on the type of biopsy performed and the type of anesthesia that is to be used. The patient usually will receive a local anesthetic, and the tissue will either be aspirated through a large-bore needle (core-needle biopsy) or removed using a small incision to extract multiple samples of tissue.

Aspirated fluid from benign cysts may appear clear to dark green or brown. Bloody fluid suggests cancer. These specimens undergo histologic evaluation. If cancer is found, the tissue is evaluated for estrogen receptor analysis. Chapter 65 discusses types of breast cancer and their relationship to estrogen receptors.

Teach that discomfort after the procedure is usually mild and can be controlled with analgesics or the use of ice or heat, depending on the type and extent of the biopsy. Educate the patient about how to assess the area or incision for bleeding and edema. Teach the patient to wear a supportive bra continuously for 1 week after surgery or as recommended by their surgeon. Remind the patient that numbness around the biopsy site may last several weeks. If cancer is identified, provide emotional support and reinforce information about the importance of follow-up treatment options.

Prostate Biopsy. When prostate cancer is suspected, a biopsy must be performed. This can be done by transurethral biopsy, by inserting a needle through the area of skin between the anus and scrotum, or, most commonly, by transrectal biopsy. Preparation for the procedure depends on the technique used to puncture the gland. A urinalysis should be performed prior to the procedure; if the patient has a urinary tract infection (UTI), the procedure will need to be rescheduled after the UTI has been successfully treated (Benway & Andriole, 2020).

Because the purpose of this procedure is to evaluate prostate cells for cancer, allow the patient time to discuss fears. Some health care providers will prescribe an anxiolytic to address the patient's anxiety about the procedure (Benway & Andriole, 2020). Prophylactic antibiotics are usually prescribed to lower the incidence of postbiopsy bacteriuria (Benway & Andriole, 2020). Patients taking aspirin, warfarin, or other anticoagulants should talk with the health care provider about whether to continue taking these or withholding them prior to the procedure. The health care provider will discuss benefits and risks to the procedure; you may witness the patient signing the informed consent form.

Explain to the patient that he may experience some discomfort. Teach him about breathing and relaxation techniques that may be helpful to use during the procedure. Assist the patient who is undergoing transrectal biopsy into the side-lying position with his knees pulled up toward his chest. The health care provider will cleanse the area, apply gel, and then insert a thin ultrasound probe into the patient's rectum to anesthetize (if needed) and guide the biopsy needle into place. The biopsy specimen is collected over a 5- to 10-minute period. The patient may experience a brief, uncomfortable feeling each time the needle collects a sample.

After prostate biopsy, remind the patient that he may experience slight soreness, light rectal bleeding that is bright red for a few days, and moderate hematuria that should resolve in a few days (Benway & Andriole, 2020). Tell the patient that semen may be discolored red or rust for several weeks. Pain can be treated with over-the-counter acetaminophen. NSAIDs should be avoided due to the risk for bleeding. Teach the patient to contact the health care provider if he has fever, prolonged or heavy bleeding, worsening *pain,* swelling in the area of biopsy, and/or difficulty urinating. Rarely, sepsis can develop after a prostate biopsy, usually in patients who did not adhere to taking prophylactic antibiotics. Teach the patient to contact the health care provider immediately if he experiences fever, pain when urinating, or penile discharge.

GET READY FOR THE NEXT-GENERATION NCLEX® EXAMINATION!

Key Points
Review these Key Points for each NCLEX Examination Client Needs Category.

Safe and Effective Care Environment
- Teach women to report symptoms of *infection* or bleeding to their health care provider after endoscopic procedures and biopsies of the breast, cervix, and endometrium. **QSEN: Safety**
- Instruct men to report symptoms of *infection* to their health care provider after a transrectal biopsy of the prostate. **QSEN: Safety**

Health Promotion and Maintenance
- Encourage women to follow recommended guidelines for early detection of cervical cancer. **QSEN: Evidence-Based Practice**
- Assess and respect cultural preferences when discussing reproductive problems and health promotion practices. **QSEN: Patient-Centered Care**

Psychosocial Integrity
- Assess the patient's comfort level in discussing issues related to reproductive health and *sexuality.* **QSEN: Patient-Centered Care**
- Encourage patients to express feelings of anxiety related to genital examinations, reproductive testing, or changes in function. **QSEN: Patient-Centered Care**
- Provide privacy for patients undergoing examination or testing of the reproductive system. **Ethics**

Physiological Integrity
- Teach patients with *pain,* bleeding, discharge, masses, or changes in reproductive function to see their health care provider. **QSEN: Safety**
- Recognize age-related reproductive changes. **QSEN: Patient-Centered Care**
- Explain diagnostic procedures, restrictions, and follow-up care associated with testing and treatment. **QSEN: Evidence-Based Practice**

■ MASTERY QUESTIONS

1. A client has undergone a prostate biopsy. Which postprocedure symptom will the nurse teach the client to report **immediately** to the primary health care provider?
   A. Semen discoloration 5 days after biopsy
   B. Light rectal bleeding 2 days after procedure
   C. Tenderness at the site 1 day after biopsy
   D. Pain on urination 3 days after procedure

2. A client who is scheduled for a Pap smear reports having had sexual intercourse 1 day prior and douching afterward. What is the appropriate nursing action?
   A. Reschedule the Pap smear for another week
   B. Delay the procedure until later in the afternoon
   C. Help the client prepare for the procedure at this time
   D. Hold the procedure until the client's next menstrual cycle

REFERENCES

American Addiction Centers. (2020). What Role does drug abuse Play in the health of the reproductive system? Retrieved from https://americanaddictioncenters.org/health-complications-addiction/reproductive-system.

American Cancer Society (ACS). (2020). *Key statistics for breast cancer in men.* Retrieved from https://www.cancer.org/cancer/breast-cancer-in-men/about/key-statistics.html.

American Cancer Society (ACS). (2019a). *Breast MRI scans.* Retrieved from https://www.cancer.org/cancer/breast-cancer/screening-tests-and-early-detection/breast-mri-scans.html.

American Cancer Society (ACS). (2019b). *Cancer facts and figures 2019.* https://www.cancer.org/content/dam/cancer-org/research/cancer-facts-and-statistics/annual-cancer-facts-and-figures/2019/cancer-facts-and-figures-2019.pdf.

American Cancer Society (ACS). (2019c). *Limitations of mammograms.* Retrieved from https://www.cancer.org/cancer/breast-cancer/screening-tests-and-early-detection/mammograms/limitations-of-mammograms.html.

American Cancer Society (ACS). (2019d). *Testing for BRCA gene mutation.* Retrieved from https://www.cancer.org/cancer/breast-cancer/risk-and-prevention/genetic-testing.html.

American Cancer Society (ACS). (2018). *The American Cancer Society guidelines for the prevention and early detection of cervical cancer.* Retrieved from https://www.cancer.org/cancer/cervical-cancer/prevention-and-early-detection/cervical-cancer-screening-guidelines.html.

American College of Obstetricians and Gynecologists. (2020). *Dilation and curettage.* Retrieved from https://www.acog.org/patient-resources/faqs/special-procedures/dilation-and-curettage.

American Society of Clinical Oncology. (2019). *Prostate cancer: Risk factors and prevention.* Retrieved from https://www.cancer.net/cancer-types/prostate-cancer/risk-factors-and-prevention.

Benway, B., & Andriole, G. (2020). Prostate biopsy. In J. Richie (Ed.), *UpToDate.* Waltham, MA.

Bradley, L. (2020). Overview of hysteroscopy. In T. Falcone (Ed.), *UpToDate.* Waltham, MA.

Centers for Disease Control and Prevention. (n.d.). *Breast cancer screening guidelines for women.* Retrieved from https://www.cdc.gov/cancer/breast/pdf/breastcancerscreeningguidelines.pdf

Choosing Wisely Canada. (2019). *Pap tests: When you need them and when you don't.* Retrieved from https://choosingwiselycanada.org/pap-tests/.

Cooper, D., & Menifee, G. (2020). *Conization of cervix. StatPearls.* Treasure Island, FL: StatPearls Publishing.

Del Priore, G. (2019). Endometrial sampling procedures. In B. Goff (Ed.), *UpToDate.* Waltham, MA.

Feltmate, C., & Feldman, S. (2020). Colposcopy. In B. Goff (Ed.), *UpToDate.* Waltham, MA.

Hatch, E., & Karam, A. (2020). Outcome and follow-up of diethylstilbestrol (DES) exposed individuals. In V. Berghella, & B. Goff (Eds.), *UpToDate.* Waltham, MA.

Hoffman, R. (2020). Screening for prostate cancer. In J. Elmore, & M. O'Leary (Eds.), *UpToDate.* Waltham, MA.

Jarvis, C. (2020). *Physical examination & health assessment* (8th ed.). St. Louis: Saunders.

Joshi, G. (2019). Anesthesia for laparoscopic and abdominal robotic surgery in adults. In S. Jones (Ed.), *UpToDate.* Waltham, MA.

Lee, S., & Kilcoyne, A. (2019). Hysterosalpingography. In R. Barbieri (Ed.), *UpToDate.* Waltham, MA.

Martin, K., & Barbieri, R. (2020). Menopausal hormone therapy: Benefits and risks. In P. Snyder, & W. Crowley (Eds.), *UpToDate.* Waltham, MA.

National Breast Cancer Foundation. (2019). *Male breast cancer.* Retrieved from https://www.nationalbreastcancer.org/male-breast-cancer.

National Cancer Institute at the National Institutes of Health. (2019). *General information about male breast cancer.* www.cancer.gov/cancertopics/pdq/treatment/malebrcast/Patient/page1#Keypoint3.

Pagana, K. D., & Pagana, T. J. (2018). *Mosby's manual of diagnostic and laboratory tests* (6th ed.). St. Louis: Elsevier.

Research on Prostate Cancer in Men of African Ancestry: Defining the Roles of Genetics, Tumor Markers and Social Stress. (2019). *Respond: African American prostate cancer study.* Retrieved from http://respondstudy.org/Default.aspx.

Sharp, H. (2019). Overview of gynecologic laparoscopic surgery and non-umbilical entry sites. In T. Falcone (Ed.), *UpToDate.* Waltham, MA.

Venkataraman, S., & Slanetz, P. (2020). Breast imaging for cancer screening: Mammography and ultrasonography. In J. Elmore (Ed.), *UpToDate.* Waltham, MA.

65

Concepts of Care for Patients With Breast Disorders

Hannah M. Lopez, Cherie R. Rebar

http://evolve.elsevier.com/Iggy/

LEARNING OUTCOMES

1. Collaborate with the interprofessional team to coordinate high-quality care for patients with breast disorders.
2. Describe the three-pronged approach to early detection of breast masses: mammography, clinical breast examination (CBE), and breast self-awareness.
3. Describe factors that place a patient at high risk for breast cancer, and refer to the health care provider.
4. Implement nursing interventions to help patients cope with the psychosocial impact caused by a breast disorder.

5. Apply knowledge of anatomy, physiology, and pathophysiology to assess patients with breast disorders.
6. Use clinical judgment to analyze assessment findings and diagnostic data in the care of patients with breast disorders.
7. Prioritize evidence-based care for patients with a breast disorder associated with *cellular regulation*, *infection*, or *pain*.
8. Plan care coordination and transition management for patients with breast disorders.

KEY TERMS

adjuvant therapy Additional treatment following an initial surgical procedure; performed to help keep cancer from recurring.

atypical hyperplasia A proliferative breast disorder that is a change in the cellular structure of a cell but is not considered cancerous.

breast augmentation Surgery to increase or improve the size, shape, or symmetry of the breasts.

breast-conserving surgery Also known as *lumpectomy* or *partial mastectomy*; procedure in which the surgeon removes part of the breast that contains cancer and some normal tissue around it.

cysts Spaces filled with fluid lined by breast glandular cells.

ductal carcinoma in situ (DCIS) An early *noninvasive* form of breast cancer; in DCIS, cancer cells are located within the duct and have not invaded the surrounding fatty breast tissue.

fibroadenoma A well-defined solid mass of connective tissue that is unattached to the surrounding breast tissue and is usually discovered by the woman herself or during mammography.

fibrocystic changes (FCCs) A range of changes involving the lobules, ducts, and stromal tissues of the breast.

fibrosis Replacement of normal cells with connective tissue and collagen.

gynecomastia A benign ridge of glandular tissue within the male breast.

inflammatory breast cancer (IBC) Aggressive type of breast cancer characterized by diffuse erythema and edema (peau d'orange).

invasive ductal carcinoma The most common type of invasive breast cancer, in which the disease originates in the mammary ducts and breaks through the walls of the ducts into the surrounding breast tissue.

lobular carcinoma in situ (LCIS) A noninvasive disease in which the cells look like cancer cells and are contained within the lobules (milk-producing glands) of the breast; LCIS is less common than DCIS and is not thought to be a precursor of invasive cancer.

prophylactic mastectomy Preventive surgical removal of one or both breasts.

prophylactic oophorectomy Removal of the ovaries.

reduction mammoplasty Breast reduction surgery in which the surgeon removes excess breast tissue and then repositions the nipple and remaining skin flaps to produce the best cosmetic effect.

triple-negative breast cancer (TNBC) A type of breast cancer that lacks expression of the estrogen receptor (ER), progesterone receptor (PR), and human epidermal growth factor receptor 2 (HER2).

Changes in the breast tissue due to cellular regulation (in Chapter 1) can cause a great deal of anxiety for women, although many disorders of the breast are benign rather than malignant. A key nursing role is to assist patients by providing accurate information about benign breast disorders (BBDs) and breast cancer.

BENIGN BREAST DISORDERS

Benign breast disorders (BBDs) are very common, affecting more than one million women annually in the United States (Santen, 2018). Most women will experience some form of breast-related changes in their lifetime. Noncancerous changes to breast tissue can present as breast lumps, pain, and nipple changes (Mau, 2018). Table 65.1 highlights some common BBDs and the age at which these are likely to occur. BBDs are classified into three types of epithelial lesions: proliferative with atypia, proliferative without atypia, and nonproliferative. The risk of developing cancer from these breast changes varies.

PROLIFERATIVE BREAST LESION WITH ATYPIA: ATYPICAL HYPERPLASIA

Atypical hyperplasia (AH) is a proliferative breast disorder involving growth of breast cells that are abnormal. It is usually found as a result of a biopsy that was taken. AH, although not cancerous, does lead to an increased risk for development of breast cancer. The younger the woman is when diagnosed with AH, the higher the lifetime risk of developing cancer. The patient should be managed by a surgical oncologist or breast surgeon and should undergo yearly mammography and twice-yearly breast examinations (Sabel, 2018). Women with AH should be taught to stop taking oral contraceptives (under the supervision of their health care provider) and to avoid hormone replacement therapy (HRT) (Sabel, 2018). Surgical excision can also be considered as a treatment for AH.

PROLIFERATIVE BREAST LESION WITHOUT ATYPIA: FIBROADENOMA

Fibroadenomas are common benign tumors in women in their 20s and 30s, but they also may occur at any age (American Cancer Society [ACS], 2019d). A fibroadenoma is a well-defined solid mass of connective tissue that is unattached to the surrounding breast tissue and is usually discovered by the woman herself or during mammography. Although the immediate fear is that of breast cancer, these changes are generally not associated with an increased risk for such. On clinical examination, these tumors are oval, freely mobile, and rubbery, and vary in size.

Fibroadenomas may occur anywhere in the breast. The health care provider may request a breast ultrasound examination or may perform a needle aspiration to establish whether the lump is cystic (filled with fluid) or solid.

NONPROLIFERATIVE BREAST LESIONS: FIBROCYSTIC CHANGES (FCCS) AND CYSTS

Pathophysiology Review

Fibrocystic changes of the breast include a range of changes involving the lobules, ducts, and stromal tissues of the breast. Because these alterations affect at least half of women over the life span, they are referred to as fibrocystic changes (FCCs) (Fig. 65.1, normal breast tissue versus Fig. 65.2, FCCs) rather than *fibrocystic disease*. This condition most often occurs in premenopausal women between 20 and 50 years of age and is thought to be caused by an imbalance in the normal estrogen-to-progesterone ratio. Areas of fibrosis are made up of fibrous connective tissue (McCance et al., 2019). Typical symptoms include breast *pain* and firm, hard, tender lumps or swelling in the breasts, particularly before a woman's menstrual period. Having FCCs does not increase a woman's chance of developing breast cancer.

Cysts are spaces filled with fluid lined by breast glandular cells. They often enlarge in response to monthly hormonal changes, stretch the surrounding breast tissue, and become painful. Symptoms usually resolve after menstruation and then recur before the next menstrual period in a cyclic fashion. In postmenopausal women, symptoms often resolve because estrogen decreases. However, postmenopausal women on hormone

TABLE 65.1	Typical Presentation of Benign Breast Disorders	
Breast Disorder	**Description**	**Incidence**
Fibroadenoma	Most common benign lesion; solid mass of connective tissue that is unattached to the surrounding tissue	During teenage years into the 30s (most commonly)
Fibrocystic changes (FCCs)	Breast *pain* and tender lumps; the lumps are rubbery, ill defined, and commonly found in the upper outer quadrant of the breast	Onset late teens and 20s; usually subsides after menopause
Ductal ectasia	Hard, irregular mass or masses with nipple discharge, enlarged axillary nodes, redness, and edema; difficult to distinguish from cancer	Women approaching menopause
Intraductal papilloma	Mass in duct that results in bloody nipple discharge; mass is usually not palpable	Women 40-55 years of age

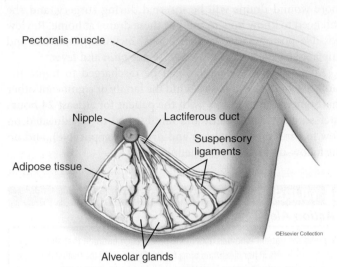

Pectoralis muscle

Nipple   Lactiferous duct

Suspensory
ligaments

Adipose tissue

Alveolar glands

Fig. 65.1 Normal breast. (© Elsevier Collection.)

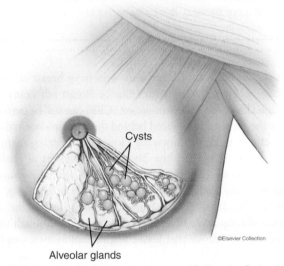

Cysts

Alveolar glands

Fig. 65.2 Breast with fibrocystic changes. (© Elsevier Collection.)

replacement therapy (HRT) may not have a significant reduction in symptoms.

Breast ultrasound is used to confirm the presence of a cyst. If a lump is very firm or has other features raising a concern for cancer, mammography is indicated. A needle biopsy or surgical biopsy may also be ordered. Biopsy may be indicated in these situations:

- No fluid is aspirated.
- The mammogram shows suspicious findings.
- A mass remains palpable after aspiration.
- The aspirated fluid reveals cancer cells.

❖ Interprofessional Collaborative Care

Management of FCCs focuses on the symptoms of the condition. Teach supportive measures for women with mild discomfort. The use of analgesics can address discomfort. Limiting salt intake before menses can help decrease swelling. Many women find relief with the reduction of dietary caffeine and other

stimulants. Teach patients that wearing a supportive bra, even to bed, can reduce pain by decreasing tension on the ligaments. Local application of ice or heat may provide temporary relief of pain. For a small number of women, draining the cysts by needle aspiration can help relieve painful symptoms.

In women with severe symptoms of FCCs, hormonal drugs such as oral contraceptives or selective estrogen receptor modulators (SERMs) may be prescribed to suppress oversecretion of estrogen. Diuretics may be prescribed to decrease premenstrual breast engorgement.

Encourage the patient to continue prescribed drug therapy and monitor the effectiveness of these interventions. Teach the patient to become familiar with the normal feel and texture of her breasts so she is aware of any ongoing changes.

> **! NURSING SAFETY PRIORITY** (QSEN)
>
> ### *Drug Alert*
>
> Explain to women the benefits and risks associated with hormonal drug therapy for FCCs. Risks include increased chance of thrombotic events (e.g., brain attack or blood clots), and risk of development of uterine cancer. Teach them to seek medical attention immediately if any signs or symptoms of these complications occur.

LARGE BREASTS

In Men

In men, a benign ridge of glandular tissue within the breast, caused by an increase in ratio of estrogen to androgen activity, is referred to as **gynecomastia** (Braunstein & Anawalt, 2019). It may be bilateral or unilateral, with a palpable mass of tissue at least 0.5 cm in diameter. Most men are asymptomatic, although some may report tenderness or sensitivity when clothing touches the nipple or the affected area.

Drugs such as spironolactone can cause gynecomastia; the first line of treatment is to discontinue any drugs that may contribute to this condition. If a medical condition such as hyperthyroidism or hypogonadism contributes to the condition, treatment of the underlying issue often helps to resolve gynecomastia. Selective estrogen receptor modulators (SERMs) such as tamoxifen, aromatase inhibitors, and androgens may also be used for treatment. Surgery can be considered for men who have unresolved gynecomastia where medical intervention does not resolve the condition.

In Women

Although Western society emphasizes large breasts as a positive attribute, women with excessive breast tissue may have health problems and experience *pain*. A woman with large breasts may have difficulty finding clothes that fit well and in which she feels attractive, or she may feel that her breast size is out of proportion to the rest of the body. Larger bras are expensive and may need to be specially ordered. The woman may have large dents in the shoulders from bra straps, and may develop a recurrent fungal *infection* under the breasts, especially in hot weather, because it is difficult to keep this area dry and exposed to air.

Backaches from the added weight of larger breasts are also common. If well-fitting bras do not help and obesity is not part of the problem, the alternative for this condition may be breast reduction surgery, called **reduction mammoplasty**. This procedure can be accomplished in several ways, depending on the breast position and shape prior to surgery. Sometimes the nipples can be left intact during surgery, and in other cases they may need to be moved for cosmetic reasons (Figs. 65.3, 65.4, and 65.5). Insurance usually covers the cost of reduction mammoplasty as long as health detriments are well documented by the health care provider.

The decision to have the procedure is usually made after years of living with the discomfort of excessive breast size. Allow the woman to verbalize her feelings. Provide appropriate preoperative teaching (as in Chapter 9). Nursing care after surgery is similar to that for the woman having reconstructive surgery. (See discussion of Breast Reconstruction in the Surgical Management section under Breast Cancer.)

SMALL BREASTS

Some women choose to have **breast augmentation** surgery to increase or improve the size, shape, or symmetry of their breasts. Most health insurers do not pay for this procedure, as it is usually considered cosmetic. Most surgeries involve the implantation of saline-filled or silicone prostheses. Some are constructed from the women's own tissue in much the same way as for reconstruction after mastectomy. *Saline* implants are filled with sterile saline and can be filled with the amount needed to get the shape and firmness the woman wants. If the implant shell leaks, the saline will be safely absorbed by the body. *Silicone* implants are filled with a silicone gel, which can leak into the breast and will not be absorbed. The plastic surgeon reviews the advantages and disadvantages of each implant or surgical option with the patient.

Before breast surgery, teach the patient to stop smoking (to promote healing); avoid aspirin and other NSAIDs; and avoid herbs that can cause bleeding during the procedure. One or more wound drains will be inserted during surgery, and she will need to know how to care for these drains at home. Review possible postoperative complications, including **infection** and implant leakage, which can cause severe **pain** and fever.

After surgery, the patient can be discharged to home the same day or the next day. Remind the family or significant other that someone should stay with the patient for at least 24 hours after surgery. The patient and family need to be educated on how to care for the incision and drains (if applicable), and on the follow-up care that is scheduled.

An important issue for patients who have breast augmentation surgery is breast cancer surveillance. Breast self-examination (BSE) and clinical breast examination (CBE) can still be performed because the prosthesis is placed behind the woman's normal breast tissue, actually pushing it forward. However, screening mammography may not be as sensitive because the amount of visualized breast tissue is decreased. Additional x-rays, called *implant displacement views*, may be used to examine the breast tissue more completely. Teach women desiring cosmetic breast augmentation about the differences in breast cancer screening. Although there is no conclusive evidence that breast augmentation increases breast

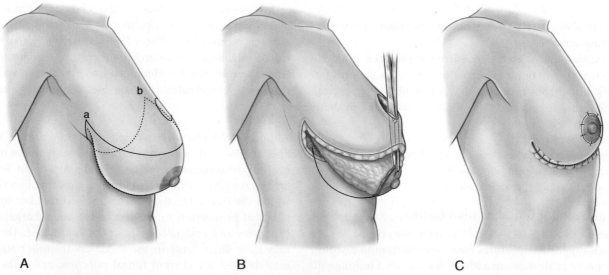

Fig. 65.3 Reduction mammoplasty: Passot technique of nipple transposition. (From Neligan P.C., & Buck D.W. [2020]. *Core procedures in plastic surgery* [2nd ed.]. Philadelphia: Elsevier.)

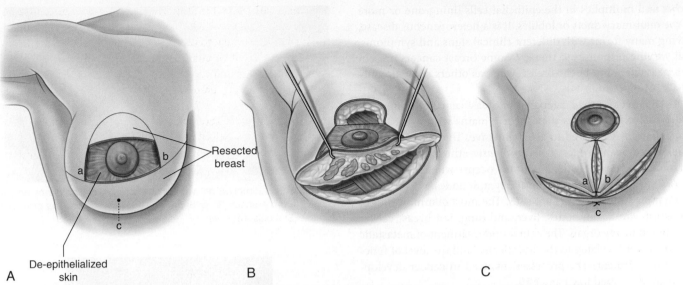

Fig. 65.4 Reduction mammoplasty: Strombeck horizontal bipedicle technique. (From Neligan P.C., & Buck D.W. [2020]. *Core procedures in plastic surgery* [2nd ed.]. Philadelphia: Elsevier.)

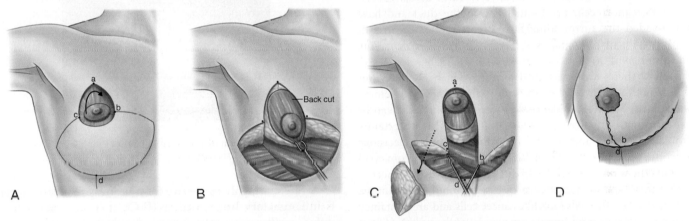

Fig. 65.5 Reduction mammoplasty: Superomedial pedicle with Wise pattern skin closure. (From Neligan P.C., & Buck D.W. [2020]. *Core procedures in plastic surgery* [2nd ed.]. Philadelphia: Elsevier.)

cancer risk, women must be informed that there is an increased risk for development of a rare form of non-Hodgkin lymphoma called breast implant–associated anaplastic large cell lymphoma (BIA-ALCL) (U.S. Food and Drug Administration, 2019).

BREAST INFLAMMATION AND INFECTION

Breast Abscess

Nonlactational breast abscesses can occur peripherally from the nipple, or in the vicinity of the areola. These types of infections are often found in patients 18 to 50 years old who have diabetes, clogged sweat glands, acne, or trauma to the area (American Society of Breast Surgeons Foundation, 2019). Risk factors that increase the chance for nonlactational breast abscesses include smoking, obesity, and nipple piercings. Common signs and symptoms include pain and swelling in the affected region. Treatment includes broad-spectrum antibiotics, ultrasound-guided aspiration, and/or incision and drainage (American Society of Breast Surgeons Foundation, 2019).

Mastitis

Mastitis—inflammation of the breast that may be accompanied by *infection* and *pain* (Dixon & Pariser, 2020)—is often associated with lactating and breast-feeding women; however, it can occur in women who are not lactating or breast-feeding. This condition is more common in women who smoke, and in women who have nipple piercings where bacteria can enter through a milk duct. Treatment options, depending on the specific type of mastitis, include antibiotic therapy, steroid therapy, or watchful waiting (Dixon & Pariser, 2020). Women with nonlactational mastitis have a higher risk of breast cancer than women without nonlactational mastitis (Chang et al., 2019).

✳ CELLULAR REGULATION CONCEPT EXEMPLAR: BREAST CANCER

Pathophysiology Review

Cancer is a common problem of impaired *cellular regulation.* Cancer of the breast begins as a single transformed cell that grows and multiplies in the epithelial cells lining one or more of the mammary ducts or lobules. It is a heterogeneous disease, having many forms with different clinical signs and symptoms, and varying responses to therapy. Some breast cancers present as a palpable lump in the breast, whereas others show up only on a mammogram.

There are two broad categories of breast cancer: noninvasive and invasive. As long as the cancer remains within the mammary duct, it is referred to as *noninvasive*. The more common type of breast cancer is classified as *invasive*; this type grows into surrounding breast tissue. *Metastasis* occurs when cancer cells spread beyond the breast tissue and lymph nodes, via the blood and lymph systems, to distant sites. The most common sites of metastasis are brain, bones, liver, and lung, but breast cancer can spread to any organ. The course and treatment of metastatic breast cancer is related to the site affected and the level of functional impairment. The processes involved in cancer development are described in Chapter 19.

Noninvasive (In Situ) Breast Cancers. Ductal carcinoma in situ (DCIS) is an early *noninvasive* form of breast cancer. In DCIS, cancer cells are located within the duct and have not invaded the surrounding fatty breast tissue. Because of more precise mammography screening and earlier detection, the number of women diagnosed with DCIS has increased. Currently there is no way to determine which DCIS lesions will progress to invasive cancer and which ones will remain unchanged; however, evidence does confirm that DCIS can be a precursor to invasive cancer (ACS, 2019c). This uncertainty can cause anxiety and conflict regarding treatment decisions in women diagnosed with DCIS. It is important to convey to patients the ways in which DCIS differs from invasive cancer.

Another type of noninvasive disease is lobular carcinoma in situ (LCIS). The cells look like cancer cells and are contained within the lobules (milk-producing glands) of the breast. LCIS is not considered cancer but does increase the patient's risk for developing invasive breast cancer (ACS, 2019e). It is usually diagnosed before menopause in women 40 to 50 years of age. Traditionally LCIS is treated with close observation only, but surgical excision is an option.

Invasive Breast Cancers. The most common type of invasive breast cancer is invasive ductal carcinoma. As the name implies, the disease originates in the mammary ducts and breaks through the walls of the ducts into the surrounding breast tissue. Once invasive, the cancer grows into the tissue around it in an irregular pattern. If a lump is present, it is felt as an irregular, poorly defined mass. As the tumor continues to grow, fibrosis (replacement of normal cells with connective tissue and collagen) develops around the cancer. This fibrosis may cause shortening of the Cooper ligaments and the resulting typical skin dimpling that is seen with more advanced disease (Fig. 65.6). Another sign, sometimes indicating late-stage breast cancer, is an edematous thickening and pitting of breast skin called *peau d'orange* (orange peel skin) (Fig. 65.7).

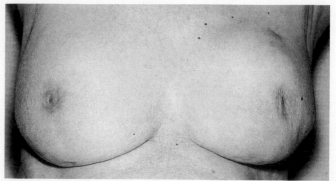

FIG. 65.6 Skin dimpling on a breast as a result of fibrosis or breast cancer. (From Mansel, R., & Bundred, N. [1995]. *Color atlas of breast disease.* St. Louis: Mosby.)

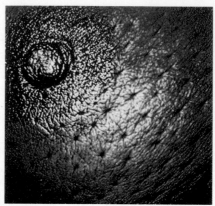

FIG. 65.7 Breast edema giving the skin an "orange peel" *(peau d'orange)* appearance. (From Gallager, H.S., Leis, H.P. Jr., Snyderman, R.K., & Urban, J.A. [1978]. *The breast.* St. Louis: Mosby.)

A rare but highly aggressive form of invasive breast cancer is inflammatory breast cancer (IBC). It is characterized by diffuse erythema and edema (peau d'orange). Patients typically report breast **pain** or a rapidly growing breast lump. Other common symptoms include a tender, firm, enlarged breast and breast itching. Because of its aggressive nature, IBC is usually diagnosed at a later stage than other types of breast cancer and is often harder to treat successfully (ACS, 2019f).

Other Types of Breast Cancer

Paget Disease. Paget disease of the nipple is a rare breast cancer that occurs in or around the nipple (Breastcancer.org, 2019). Although more common in women, it can also occur in men. It usually affects the nipple ducts, followed by the nipple surface, and then the areola, leaving the area scaly, red, and irritated (Breastcancer.org, 2019). It is critical to teach patients to see their health care provider if they have these symptoms, as people with Paget disease often have other types of breast cancer.

Triple-Negative Breast Cancer. Triple-negative breast cancer (TNBC) lacks expression of the estrogen receptor (ER), progesterone receptor (PR), and human epidermal growth factor receptor 2 (HER2) (Anders & Carey, 2020). This type of breast cancer grows rapidly and is often found in women with *BRCA* mutation who are premenopausal (Anders & Carey, 2020). African-American women are at higher risk for TNBC than women of other races (Anders & Carey, 2020).

PATIENT-CENTERED CARE: GENDER HEALTH CONSIDERATIONS (QSEN)

Male breast cancer is rare and accounts for less than 1% of all breast cancer cases (Attebery et al., 2020). Risk factors for male breast cancer include previous radiation, a family history of breast cancer (male or female), *BRCA1* and/or *BRCA2* mutation, diabetes, alcohol use and liver disease, testicular disorders, and obesity (ACS, 2020c).

Men usually present with a hard, painless, subareolar mass; gynecomastia may be present. Other symptoms include nipple discharge (often bloodstained), rash around the nipple, inverted nipple, ulceration or swelling of the chest, and possibly swollen lymph nodes. Because men usually do not suspect breast cancer, they often ignore the symptoms and postpone seeing their primary health care provider. As a result, many men are diagnosed at later stages than women. Treatment of breast cancer in men is the same as in women at a similar stage of disease.

PATIENT-CENTERED CARE: GENDER HEALTH CONSIDERATIONS (QSEN)

Genetic predisposition is a stronger risk factor for younger women than older women. Younger women frequently present with more aggressive forms of the disease; they are usually diagnosed at a later stage, have triple-negative breast cancer, and must receive more aggressive treatment. Screening tools can be less effective for this group because the breasts tend to be denser and mammographic recognition of breast cancer may be impaired in areas of dense tissue. Nurses should encourage women who have symptoms to seek evaluation and not watch and wait.

NCLEX EXAMINATION CHALLENGE 65.1

Health Promotion and Maintenance

When caring for four clients, which individual does the nurse identify as being at the **highest** risk for development of breast cancer?
A. 33-year-old male with gynecomastia and obesity
B. 45-year-old female whose mother has breast cancer
C. 60-year-old male whose father died from colon cancer
D. 72-year-old female who was treated for breast cancer 3 years ago

PATIENT-CENTERED CARE: CULTURAL/ SPIRITUAL CONSIDERATIONS (QSEN)

The rate of breast cancer in African-American women *younger than 60 years* is higher than for others in that age-group (Centers for Disease Control and Prevention [CDC], 2018). African-American women are also 40% more likely to die from breast cancer than white women (CDC, 2018). In their classic study, Ooi et al. (2011) found that American Indian, African-American, and Hispanic women were also likely to present with more aggressive breast cancer that is harder to treat, such as triple-negative breast cancer. African-American women have the highest risk for triple-negative breast cancer (Anders & Carey, 2019). These cultural disparities should be addressed with targeted interventions that are appropriate for specific cultural and ethnic groups. Nurses need to be culturally aware and competent to assist women to overcome barriers to care.

Incidence and Prevalence. One of every eight women in the United States will develop breast cancer in her lifetime (Howlader et al., 2020). It is the most common cancer diagnosis in women. Breast cancer is the second leading cause of cancer death in women aside from skin cancers (ACS, 2020a). Similar statistics can be found in Canada (Canadian Cancer Society [CCS], 2020). Early detection is the key to effective treatment and survival. The 5-year relative survival rate for localized breast cancer is 99%, whereas the rate drops to 86% when the cancer has spread to the regional lymph nodes, and to 27% for those with metastatic disease (ACS, 2020d). Metastatic cancer is not considered curable, but rather is treated as a chronic disease.

Etiology and Genetic Risk. Increased age is the primary risk factor for developing breast cancer in both women and men. Several other factors are known to increase the risk of developing breast cancer, such as family and genetic history, early menarche, and late menopause. These factors are not modifiable. Modifiable risk factors include, but are not limited to, postmenopausal obesity, physical inactivity, use of combined estrogen and progestin postmenopausal hormone replacement therapy (HRT), alcohol consumption, and lack of breast-feeding (ACS, 2019a).

According to the American Cancer Society (ACS, 2020b), breast cancer is often diagnosed late in the disease process for lesbian and bisexual women because of their fear of discrimination, negative experiences with health care professionals, and lack of health insurance. In addition, many women in these groups have no children or have a child after they are 30 years of age or older. Having several risk factors increases one's risk more than having a single risk factor. Table 65.2 lists major risk factors for breast cancer regardless of sexual orientation.

PATIENT-CENTERED CARE: GENETIC/ GENOMIC CONSIDERATIONS (QSEN)

Mutations in several genes, such as *BRCA1* and *BRCA2*, are related to hereditary breast cancer. People who have specific mutations in either one of these genes are at an increased risk for developing breast cancer and ovarian cancer. Encourage women to talk with a genetics counselor to carefully consider the benefits and potential consequences of genetic testing before these tests are done.

Health Promotion and Maintenance

The American Cancer Society (ACS) and the Canadian Cancer Society (CCS) establish evidence-based guidelines for breast cancer screening in women. Guidelines have not been recommended for screening men in the general population because breast cancer in men is so rare. Encourage men with a strong family history or known genetic mutations to discuss screening with their primary health care provider or request referral to a genetics counselor.

In addition to other screening and assessment methods the National Cancer Institute (n.d.) offers a Breast Cancer Risk Assessment Tool that can be used by a health care professional to estimate risk. Teach women that no single method for early detection of breast cancer is effective when used alone. The best approach for average-risk women is a screening mammogram, clinical breast examination (CBE), and breast self-awareness.

TABLE 65.2   Risk Factors for Breast Cancer

Factors	Comments
Female gender	Of all breast cancers, 99% occur in women.
Age >65 years	Risk increases across all ages until age 80 years.
Genetic factors	Inherited mutations of *BRCA1* and/or *BRCA2* increase risk.
History of a previous breast cancer	The risk for developing a cancer in the opposite breast is five times greater than for the average population at risk.
Breast density	Dense breasts contain more glandular and connective tissue, which increases the risk for developing breast cancer.
Atypical hyperplasia	Biopsy-confirmed atypical hyperplasia is a high relative risk.
Family history	Having a first-degree relative with breast or ovarian cancer increases risk.
Ionizing radiation	Women who received frequent low-level radiation exposure to the thorax have an increased risk, especially if the exposure occurred during periods of rapid breast formation or if there was high-dose radiation to the chest.
High postmenopausal bone density	High estrogen levels over time both strengthen bone and increase breast cancer risk.

Reproductive history
  Nulliparity *or*
  First child born after age 30 years
	Childless women have an increased risk, as do women who bear their first child at or after age 30.

Menstrual history
  Early menstruation (younger than 11 years) *or*
  Late menopause (at or older than 55 years) *or*
  Both
	The risk for breast cancer rises as the interval between menarche and menopause increases. Women who undergo bilateral oophorectomy before age 35 years have less risk for breast cancer than women who undergo natural menopause.

Recent oral contraceptive use	There is a slight increase in breast cancer risk in women taking oral contraceptives. The risk returns to normal 10 years after stopping the pill.
Recent hormone replacement therapy (HRT)	Use of HRT containing both estrogen and progestin increases risk; risk diminishes 5 years after discontinuation.
Obesity	Postmenopausal obesity (especially increased abdominal fat), increased body mass, insulin resistance, and hyperglycemia have been reported to be associated with an increased risk for breast cancer.
Other Risk Factors	
Alcohol consumption	Risk is dose dependent; consumption of 2-3 drinks per day is associated with a 20% increased risk; risk increases with increased consumption. This includes all forms of alcoholic beverages.
High socioeconomic status	Breast cancer incidence is greater in women of higher education and socioeconomic background. This relationship is possibly related to lifestyle differences, such as later age at first birth.
Jewish heritage	Women of Ashkenazi Jewish heritage have higher incidences of *BRCA1* and *BRCA2* genetic mutations.

Data from American Cancer Society. (2019). *Breast cancer facts & figures 2019-2020*. Atlanta: Author.

Mammography. In 2015 the American Cancer Society (ACS) updated its breast cancer screening guidelines, which now recommend that women at average risk of breast cancer begin annual screening mammography at age 45 up to age 54. Women ages 40 to 44 should have the choice to start annual mammograms after the risks and potential benefits have been explained. Women age 55 and older may switch to mammograms every 2 years, or continue annual screening mammograms if they choose to do so. Mammography should continue as long as a woman is in good health and has a life expectancy of at least 10 years (ACS, 2020a).

Canadian guidelines for mammography differ from those of the United States: no routine mammography screening is recommended until women reach 50 years of age. After 50, the recommended guidelines vary slightly across organizations but generally recommend that women after age 50 get a mammogram every 2 to 3 years until age 70 to 74 (CCS, 2020).

Breast Self-Awareness/Self-Examination. Data demonstrate that breast self-examination is not a meaningful screening tool for breast cancer (Komen, 2020). However, it is recommended that women increase breast self-awareness by becoming familiar with how their breasts look and feel so that they can report differences or abnormalities.

Teach a woman that lumps are not necessarily abnormal. For premenopausal women, lumps can come and go with the menstrual cycle. Most lumps that are detected and tested are not malignant.

Some women may want to practice regular breast self-examination (BSE) as a method for breast self-awareness. BSE should be presented as an option to women beginning in their early 20s. In addition to breast self-awareness, place emphasis on clinical breast examination (CBE) and mammogram for early detection of breast cancer. The combined approach is better than any single test. A woman who chooses to perform BSE should be taught the correct technique and have it reviewed by a health care provider during her CBE.

Use teaching models of normal and abnormal breasts when teaching BSE. Discuss the proper timing for BSE. Instruct premenopausal women to examine their breasts 1 week after the menstrual period. At this time, hormonal influence on breast tissue is decreased, so fluid retention and tenderness are reduced. Teach women whose breast tissue is no longer influenced by

BEST PRACTICE FOR PATIENT SAFETY & QUALITY CARE (QSEN)

Performing Breast Self-Examination

1. Lie on your back and place your right arm behind your head. Lying down spreads the breast tissue evenly over the chest wall, making it easier to feel all the breast tissue

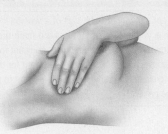

2. Use the finger pads of the three middle fingers on your left hand to feel for lumps in the right breast. Use overlapping dime-sized circular motions of the finger pads to feel the breast tissue

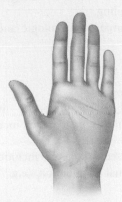

3. Use three different levels of pressure to feel all the breast tissue. Light pressure is needed to feel the tissue closest to the skin; medium pressure to feel a

little deeper, and firm pressure to feel the tissue closest to the chest and ribs. It is normal to feel a firm ridge in the lower curve of each breast.

4. Move around the breast in an up-and-down pattern, starting at an imaginary line drawn straight down your side from the underarm and moving across the breast to the middle of the chest bone (sternum or breastbone). Be sure to check the entire breast area, going down until you feel only ribs and up to the neck

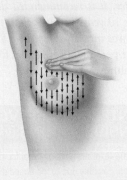

5. Repeat the examination on your left breast, putting your left arm behind your head and using the finger pads of your right hand to do the examination
6. While standing in front of a mirror with your hands pressing firmly down on your hips, look at your breasts for any changes in size, shape, contour, or dimpling, and look at your nipples and breast skin for redness or scaling. (Pressing down on the hips contracts the chest wall muscles and enhances any breast changes.)
7. Examine each underarm while sitting up or standing and with your arm only slightly raised so you can easily feel in this area. Raising your arm straight up tightens the tissue in this area and makes it harder to examine.

hormonal fluctuations, such as after a total hysterectomy or menopause, to pick a day each month to do BSE, such as the first day of the month. The BSE technique is similar for women and men. The Best Practice for Patient Safety & Quality Care: Performing Breast Self-Examination box describes the procedure for breast self-examination and may be used as a patient resource.

Clinical Breast Examination. Clinical breast examination (CBE) is typically performed by advanced practice nurses and other health care providers. It is recommended that the CBE be part of a periodic health assessment, at least every 3 years for women in their 20s and 30s and every year for asymptomatic women at least 40 years of age (National Comprehensive Cancer Network [NCCN], 2019). Teach patients what to expect during this examination. First, they will be asked to undress from the waist up. The health care provider inspects the breasts for abnormalities in size and shape and for skin and nipple changes. Then, using the pads of the fingers, the provider palpates the breasts for any lumps and, if present, whether such lumps are attached to the skin or deeper tissues. The area under both arms is also examined.

Remind the patient to report any breast changes she may have noted during a breast self-examination to the health care provider performing the clinical breast examination.

NCLEX EXAMINATION CHALLENGE 65.2

Health Promotion and Maintenance

When caring for a 28-year-old healthy client, how frequently does the nurse recommend a clinical breast examination (CBE)?

A. Every 3 years
B. At each annual physical
C. Not until age 30, as the risks are low
D. To begin at age 40 when risks increase

PATIENT-CENTERED CARE: OLDER ADULT CONSIDERATIONS (QSEN)

As women age, the breast tissue becomes flattened and elongated and is suspended loosely from the chest wall. On palpation, the breast tissue of the older woman has a finer, more granular feel than the lobular feel in a younger woman. The inframammary ridge may be more prominent as a result of atrophy of the breast tissue. Breast examination in older adults may be easier because of tissue atrophy and relaxation of the suspensory ligaments.

Options for High-Risk Women. Those with a personal history of breast cancer are at risk for developing a recurrence or a new breast cancer. Women with known *BRCA1* and/or *BRCA2* genetic mutation have a lifetime risk of developing breast cancer by age

70 of about 55% to 60% and 45%, respectively (National Breast Cancer Foundation, 2019). Women in this category usually practice *close surveillance* as a prevention option. It is a method of *secondary prevention* and is used to detect cancer early in the initial stages. In addition to annual mammography and clinical breast examination, high-risk women are recommended to have an annual breast MRI screening (ACS, 2019a). Close surveillance may begin as early as age 30 years, but evidence is limited regarding the best age at which to start screening. *For women with a high risk for breast cancer development due to family history such as cancer in a mother or sister, it is recommended that cancer screening begin at the age that is 10 years younger than the age at which the affected cancer patient was initially diagnosed.* Encourage high-risk women to discuss their personal preferences for close surveillance with their primary health care providers.

PATIENT-CENTERED CARE: VETERANS HEALTH CONSIDERATIONS (QSEN)

Research shows that female veterans have a higher incidence of breast cancer than the general population, possibly due to increased exposure to risk factors or to earlier detection (McDaniel et al., 2018). Encourage women veterans to have screening done per recommended guidelines due to this increased risk.

Other options currently available for reducing a woman's breast cancer risk are **prophylactic mastectomy** (preventive surgical removal of one or both breasts), **prophylactic oophorectomy** (removal of the ovaries), and chemopreventive drugs. Although each option significantly reduces the risk for breast cancer, no option completely eliminates it. Each option has its own risks and potentially serious complications.

Even though a woman may decide to have a prophylactic mastectomy, there is a small risk that breast cancer will develop in residual breast glandular tissue because no mastectomy reliably removes all mammary tissue. Women must also understand that breast reconstruction after a prophylactic mastectomy is very different from breast augmentation. It is a more complex surgical procedure with a greater potential for complications. The decision to have this type of surgery can be a very difficult one to make. Women may find it helpful to reach out to a breast cancer support organization and talk to someone who has been through a prophylactic mastectomy.

Women undergoing prophylactic oophorectomy will likely experience menopausal symptoms, although some estrogen remains in body fat tissue. Chemoprevention drugs, such as tamoxifen, reduce breast cancer recurrence but carry other risks such as blood clots and endometrial cancer (Boucher, 2018). Encourage women to carefully consider the benefits and risks of breast cancer risk–reducing options and discuss them with their health care provider.

❖ Interprofessional Collaborative Care

◆ Assessment: Recognize Cues

History. Early breast cancer often has no symptoms (ACS, 2019a). At other times, the history is taken after a mass has been discovered but before a diagnosis has been made. For some patients, the history may be obtained at the time they are seen for treatment of an identified cancer. The interview should focus on three major areas: risk factors, the breast mass, and health maintenance practices.

PATIENT-CENTERED CARE: CULTURAL/ SPIRITUAL CONSIDERATIONS (QSEN)

Some cultures do not allow men to be part of a woman's care, or allow only women to care for a woman. Other cultures are male predominant, and all decisions about female care are made by the significant man in her life, who may be a father, spouse, or oldest son. It is important for the health care provider and nurse to provide culturally sensitive care and to respect the beliefs and practices of the patient.

Ask specific information about personal and family histories of breast cancer. In addition to increasing the woman's own risk, these factors also affect any sisters' or daughters' risk and should be part of later counseling.

Ask about the woman's gynecologic and obstetric (if any) history, including:

- Age at menarche
- Age at menopause
- Symptoms of menopause
- Age at first child's birth (or nulliparity—having no children)
- Number of children and pregnancies, including miscarriages or terminations

Recognize that increased risk factors include:

- Prolonged hormonal stimulation (e.g., early menses, late menopause)
- Use of contraceptives
- Birth of the first child after 30 years of age

A history of the breast mass or lump can reveal the course of the disease and information related to health care–seeking practices and health-promoting behaviors. Ask the patient about how, when, and by whom the mass was discovered and the time between discovery and seeking care. The answer to this question reveals the need for discussion and teaching about health promotion practices, regardless of whether the mass proves to be cancerous. If there was a delay between discovery and seeing the health care provider, inquire what caused the delay. These questions are linked to the psychosocial assessment but also reveal the length of time that the mass has been untreated. Review with the patient which procedures have been performed to diagnose the problem and if they have noticed any other changes in their body within the past year. This information can help determine if there will be the likelihood of metastasis. Ask especially about the presence of joint and bone pain or cognitive changes.

Assess the use of alcohol intake because this is a factor that may increase breast cancer risk. Perform an in-depth medication review, including prescribed and over-the-counter (OTC) drugs that are used. Specifically ask about hormonal supplements, such as estrogen and natural or herbal substances that stimulate hormones, and birth control use. Estrogen can be taken orally, intravaginally, or via a transdermal patch. Document the type and form of hormones (birth control pills or patches, supplements) and length of use.

BEST PRACTICE FOR PATIENT SAFETY & QUALITY CARE (QSEN)

Assessing a Breast Mass

- Identify the location of the mass by using the "face of the clock" method.
- Describe the shape, size, and consistency of the mass.
- Assess whether the mass is fixed or movable.
- Note any skin changes around the mass, such as dimpling of the skin, increased vascularity, nipple retraction, nipple inversion, or skin ulceration.
- Assess the adjacent lymph nodes, both axillary and supraclavicular nodes.
- Ask patients if they experience *pain* or soreness in the area around the mass.

PATIENT-CENTERED CARE: GENDER HEALTH CONSIDERATIONS (QSEN)

Research about breast cancer and women who identify as lesbian or bisexual continues. Factors that are more likely to increase the risk of breast cancer in lesbian and bisexual women include nulliparity or increased age at birth of first child, use of oral contraceptives (ACS, 2020b), cigarette smoking, alcohol use, and obesity (Margolies, 2020). Lesbian and bisexual women may not seek regular care due to fear and distrust of culturally incompetent health care providers and/or health care access. Nurses' awareness and sensitivity to these issues help establish trust (Boehmer, 2018). Emphasize the importance of screening and early detection (Ceres et al., 2018). Assess the need for referrals to support organizations such as the National LGBT Cancer Network (2020).

Physical Assessment/Clinical Signs and Symptoms. Document any abnormal findings from the clinical breast examination. Describe specific information about a breast mass (as described in the Best Practice for Patient Safety & Quality Care: Assessing a Breast Mass box), such as location, using the "face of the clock" method; shape; size; consistency; and whether the mass is mobile or fixed to the surrounding tissue. Note any skin change, such as *peau d'orange*, redness and warmth, nipple retraction, or ulceration, which can indicate advanced disease. Document the location of any enlargements of axillary and supraclavicular lymph nodes. Evaluate for the presence of *pain* or tenderness in the affected breast.

Psychosocial Assessment. A breast cancer diagnosis is usually an unanticipated event in the life of a woman who feels physically well. It initiates a sudden and distressing transition into a potentially life-threatening illness. Feelings of fear, shock, and disbelief are predominant as a woman learns about the disease and faces numerous treatment decisions. Psychological distress is common at cancer diagnosis and at the various transitions of treatment. A previous history of mental illness, age, and life circumstances can contribute to increased psychological distress. Encourage expression of feelings, focusing on the human component of care (Mahon, 2017) and determine if a referral to a counselor would be helpful. There are also multiple community resources available for the person diagnosed with breast cancer. Talking with someone who has been through the experience is particularly helpful in dealing with the emotional aspects of the disease.

Assess the patient for concerns related to *sexuality*. Sexual dysfunction affects most breast cancer survivors in some way. Sometimes it is related to the loss of a breast and the threat to one's femininity, her image of herself, or how she perceives her partner's response. Lack of libido (sexual desire) related to hormonal changes, psychological distress, and anxiety are commonly experienced by women with breast cancer. If the patient does not discuss sexual concerns voluntarily, open the conversation in a nonthreatening, nonjudgmental way. Use resources that provide education about alternative expressions of intimacy and a focus on pleasure rather than performance. Refer the patient and her partner to counseling if appropriate.

Laboratory Assessment. The diagnosis of breast cancer relies on pathologic examination of tissue from the breast mass. After the diagnosis of cancer is established, laboratory tests, including pathologic study of the lymph nodes, help detect possible metastases. Elevated liver enzyme levels indicate possible liver metastases, and increased serum calcium and alkaline phosphatase levels could suggest bone metastases.

Imaging Assessment. Mammography is a sensitive screening tool for breast cancer. The uniqueness of this test results from its ability to reveal preclinical lesions (masses too small to be palpated manually). Most breast centers now use *digital mammography*, a system that is able to read, file, and transmit mammograms electronically. Patient preparation and the procedure for mammography are discussed in Chapter 64. Some women may voice concern about radiation exposure with mammograms. Reassure them that the dose is very small and the risk for harm from radiation is minimal.

Digital breast tomosynthesis is technology that is similar to mammography but uses three-dimensional images (see Chapter 64; Fig. 65.8). It is useful in evaluating dense breasts and is more accurate in women younger than 50. In the United States, currently it is covered by Medicare and most other major health insurances. This advanced technology is also available in Canada.

Ultrasonography of the breast is an additional diagnostic tool used to clarify findings on mammography. If the mammogram reveals a lesion, ultrasonography is helpful in differentiating a fluid-filled cyst from a solid mass. Mammography screening combined with ultrasound may be effective for detecting cancers in women with dense breasts, but currently it is not recommended for routine breast cancer screening as a stand-alone imaging tool (ACS, 2019a).

MRI is used for screening high-risk women and better examination of suspicious areas found on a mammogram (ACS, 2019a). It is more expensive than mammography. Most insurance companies will cover a portion of the cost if the woman is shown to be at high risk. Although higher-quality images are produced, there is concern about high costs and access to quality breast MRI services for high-risk women. Most major insurances will cover a portion of MRI costs for women shown to be at higher risk (ACS, 2019a).

If the patient has an invasive breast cancer, other imaging tests may be done to rule out metastases. Positron emission tomography (PET) scan, brain MRI, and CT scans of the chest, abdomen, and pelvis can reveal distant metastases.

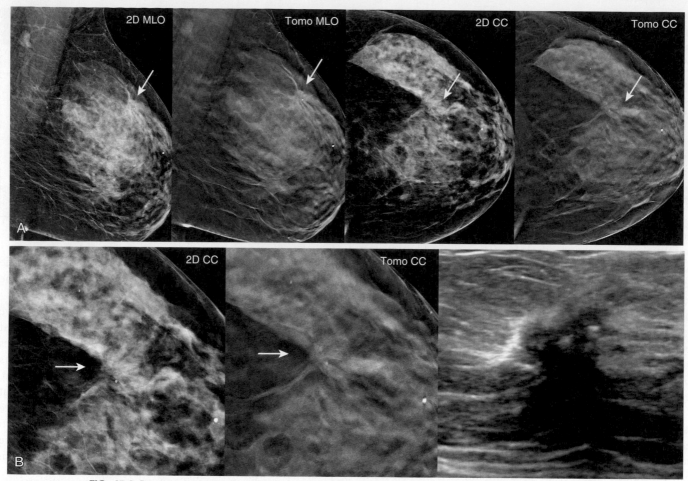

FIG. 65.8 Breast tomosynthesis. Architectural distortion (AD) seen on 2D and tomosynthesis screening mammography. **A,** Screening mammogram in a 50-year-old woman demonstrates an AD in the left upper outer breast *(arrows)*, which is better seen on tomosynthesis. **B,** Close-up craniocaudal views show the AD with associated microCa++ *(arrows)* to be very obvious on tomosynthesis. (From Philpotts, L.E., & Hooley, R.J. [2017]. *Breast tomosynthesis.* Philadelphia: Elsevier.)

Other Diagnostic Assessment. Although imaging techniques serve as tools for screening and more precise visualization of potential breast cancers, *breast biopsy (pathologic examination of the breast tissue) is the only definitive way to diagnose breast cancer* (see Chapter 64). Tissue samples are analyzed by a pathologist to determine the presence of breast cancer. If breast cancer is identified, it is classified according to the size and type of breast cancer, the histologic grade, and the type of receptors on the cells. These characteristics are used to guide treatment. For example, a small, noninvasive breast cancer may only be treated with lumpectomy and radiation, whereas a larger, aggressive tumor (one with a high histologic grade) may be treated with a mastectomy and chemotherapy, followed by radiation.

Cancer cells that contain estrogen receptors *(ER positive)* or progesterone receptors *(PR positive)* have a better prognosis and usually respond to hormonal therapy. If the type of breast cancer is *HER2 positive,* or one in which the *neu* gene is overexpressed, it may be treated successfully with trastuzumab, which is a HER2-positive breast cancer–specific *targeted therapy.*

Most women, even those with very small tumors, receive some sort of treatment in addition to surgery for breast cancer. Research has focused on ways to predict clinical outcomes so that low-risk women may avoid unnecessary treatments. Genomic tests, such as Oncotype DX and MammaPrint, have been developed to help predict clinical outcomes by analyzing genes in breast cancer tissue. Some health care providers use this information in addition to the pathologic analysis for guiding treatment decisions. These multigene tests have been shown to be accurate predictors of patient prognosis and response to therapy in breast cancer (National Comprehensive Cancer Network [NCCN] Guidelines, 2020).

◆ Analysis: Analyze Cues and Prioritize Hypotheses.

The priority collaborative problems for patients with breast cancer include:

1. Potential for cancer metastasis due to lack of, or inadequate, treatment
2. Potential for impaired coping due to breast cancer diagnosis and treatment

◆ Planning and Implementation: Generate Solutions and Take Action

Decreasing the Risk for Metastasis

Planning: Generate Solutions. The patient who is treated for breast cancer is expected to remain free of metastases or recurrence of disease, if possible. If cancer recurs, the patient will experience optimal health outcomes, including potential palliation and end-of-life care.

Interventions: Take Action. There are many surgical and nonsurgical options for breast cancer treatment. Because of the various options, the patient with breast cancer often faces difficult decisions. Although patients are living longer with metastatic disease, the 5-year survival rate remains low. Once cancer is diagnosed, the extent and location of breast cancer and metastases (if applicable) determine the overall treatment strategy. The emphasis of breast cancer treatment is on preventing or stopping the spread of tumor cells that lead to distant metastasis. Treatment is tailored specifically to each patient, taking into account other health problems and the patient's ability to tolerate a particular therapy.

Nonsurgical Management

Complementary and integrative health. Women with breast cancer often cope with distressing symptoms related to the disease itself or the side effects of treatment. Common symptoms associated with these treatments include *pain,* nausea/vomiting, hot flashes, anxiety, depression, and fatigue. Physical and emotional symptoms associated with breast cancer may be eased with the use of complementary and integrative therapy. Prayer is also widely used. Other types of therapies include guided imagery and massage. The most frequently used strategies are biologically based therapies such as vitamins, special cancer diets, and herbal therapy. Teach the patient that all ingested complementary agents potentially risk interaction with conventional drugs.

Encourage women to seek a practitioner with a certification or license for the specific type of integrative therapy intervention. In some states, a certification or license is required for acupuncture, chiropractic therapy, massage, and shiatsu. Some types of complementary and integrative therapy can be self-taught or done alone after a few sessions of instruction. Table 65.3 lists complementary and integrative therapies for specific symptoms associated with breast cancer and its treatments.

Although the use of complementary and integrative therapy can improve quality of life, its use does not alter the outcome of breast cancer, and it should not be used in place of standard treatment. Encourage patients who are interested in trying these therapies to check with their health care provider before using them. The website https://www.breastcancer.org/treatment/comp_med provides accurate information about complementary therapies and the extent to which they have been researched in breast cancer patients. Cost may be a factor in decision making because not all insurances provide coverage for complementary and integrative therapies. Remind the patient that it is important to disclose to the health care provider all treatments undertaken.

For patients with breast cancer at a stage for which surgery is the main treatment, follow-up with adjuvant (in addition to surgery) radiation, chemotherapy, hormone therapy, or targeted therapy is commonly prescribed. For those who cannot have surgery or whose cancer is too advanced, these therapies may be used to promote comfort (palliation). End-of-life care is discussed in Chapter 8.

Surgical Management. The management of early-stage breast cancer is surgery. A large tumor is sometimes treated

TABLE 65.3	**Common Complementary and Integrative Therapies Used by Patients With Breast Cancer**
Symptom	**Complementary and Integrative Therapy**
Physical	
Pain	Acupuncture, chiropractic therapy, hypnosis, massage, music, reiki, shiatsu
Nausea/vomiting	Acupuncture, aromatherapy, ginger, hypnosis, progressive muscle relaxation, shiatsu
Fatigue	Acupuncture, massage, meditation, reiki, tai chi, yoga
Hot flashes	Acupuncture, flaxseed, black cohosh. Use caution with all herbal and ingested supplements; there is no substantial data to support one treatment over others
Muscle tension	Aromatherapy, massage, shiatsu
Emotional	
Anxiety, stress, fear	Aromatherapy, guided imagery, hypnosis, journaling, massage, meditation, music therapy, progressive muscle relaxation, prayer, support groups, tai chi, yoga
Depression	Aromatherapy, yoga, journaling, progressive muscle relaxation

with chemotherapy, called neoadjuvant therapy, to shrink the tumor before it is surgically removed. An advantage of this therapy is that cancer can be removed by lumpectomy rather than mastectomy. This may provide less invasive surgery and a better cosmetic outcome for the patient.

Axillary lymph nodes are analyzed for the presence of cancer and staging purposes. Axillary lymph node dissection (ALND) is usually done when there are clinically positive nodes. Sentinel lymph node biopsy (SLNB) is a much less invasive approach and is recommended by guidelines for analyzing lymph nodes in early-stage breast cancers with low-to-moderate risk for lymph node involvement. In this method, the sentinel lymph node is identified during breast surgery by injecting the breast with radioisotope and/or dye that travels via lymphatic pathways to the sentinel lymph node. The nodes that take up the dye are removed and examined for the presence of cancer cells. It is believed that if cancer cells have traveled through the lymph channels, the cells will lodge in the sentinel nodes. Travel beyond these nodes to higher-level nodes may occur as a secondary event. Therefore the absence of cancer cells in the sentinel nodes is an indicator that no other nodes in the regional area are involved.

Preoperative care. Care of the patient facing surgery for breast cancer focuses on psychological preparation and preoperative teaching. Priority nursing interventions are directed toward relieving anxiety and providing information to increase patient knowledge. Include the spouse, partner, or other family member or significant other, who may be experiencing similar stress and confusion, in the health teaching unless the patient does not desire this or the patient's culture does not permit this approach.

Review the type of procedure planned. Use open-ended questions (e.g., "What type of surgery are you having? Can you explain what will happen?") to assess the patient's current level of knowledge. Provide postoperative information, including:

- The need for a drainage tube
- The location of the incision
- Mobility restrictions
- The length of the hospital stay (if any)
- General preoperative and postoperative information needed by any surgical patient (see Chapter 9)

Supplement teaching with written or digital materials for the patient and family. This information should include whom to call in case there are any complications or questions. Address body image issues and expectations before surgery to avoid misconceptions about appearance after surgery. If available, suggest that patients and their caregivers attend classes before surgery in an ambulatory care setting, such as a breast cancer center, to promote successful early discharge from the hospital. Programs that provide emotional support, information, and opportunities for discussion related to *sexuality,* body image, and preoperative and postoperative care enhance the recovery of the short-stay mastectomy patient.

Operative procedures. Types of breast surgeries are shown in Fig. 65.9. During breast-conserving surgery, also known as *lumpectomy* or *partial mastectomy,* the surgeon removes part of the breast that contains cancer and some normal tissue around it. The term *margins* refers to the distance between the tumor and the edge of the surrounding tissue. The desired outcome of breast-conserving surgery is to obtain *negative margins* in which no cancer cells extend to the edge of the tissue. Patients undergoing breast conserving surgery may have drainage tubes placed if the lump is large or if axillary node dissection is performed. Typically, radiation therapy follows to kill any residual tumor cells.

Breast-conserving procedures are usually performed in same-day surgical settings. The cosmetic results of these surgeries are good to excellent, and the psychological benefits of avoiding breast removal are significant for patients who choose this option.

Typically, indications for a mastectomy include multicentric disease (tumor is present in different quadrants of the breast), inability to have radiation therapy, presence of a large tumor in a small breast, genetic testing results, and patient preference. Mastectomy does not conserve the breast; the affected breast is completely removed. A total (simple) mastectomy is surgery to remove the whole breast that has cancer. A *modified radical mastectomy* removes the breast tissue, lymph nodes, and sometimes part of the underlying chest wall muscle. During this procedure, the surgeon places one or two drainage tubes, usually Jackson-Pratt (JP) drains, under the skin flaps and attaches the tubes to a small collection chamber. These collect any fluid that accumulates under the surgical area. Reconstruction can be performed at the same time as the mastectomy. Skin flaps or expanders may be used to create a breast mound at the time of the original procedure.

Postoperative care. The hospital stay after breast surgery is short, often same day or just overnight, and recovery is usually not complicated. After surgery, avoid using the affected arm for measuring blood pressure, giving injections, or drawing blood. If lymph nodes are removed, it is critical to prevent trauma to the affected arm. The patient returns from the postanesthesia

Breast-conserving Surgery
Lumpectomy

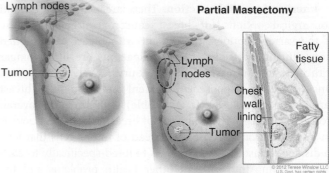

Partial Mastectomy

Breast-conserving surgery. Dotted lines show the area containing the tumor that is removed and some of the lymph nodes that may be removed.

Total (Simple) Mastectomy

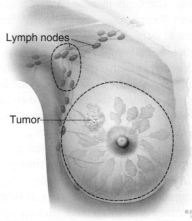

Total (simple) mastectomy. The dotted line shows where the entire breast is removed. Some lymph nodes under the arm may also be removed.

Modified Radical Mastectomy

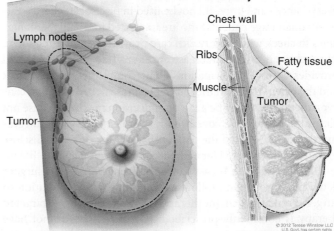

Modified radical mastectomy. The dotted line shows where the entire breast and some lymph nodes are removed. Part of the chest wall muscle may also be removed.

FIG. 65.9 Surgical treatment for breast cancer. (©2010 Terese Winslow. U.S. Govt. has certain rights.)

care unit (PACU) as soon as vital signs return to baseline levels and if no complications have occurred. Assess vital signs on a schedule of decreasing frequency, such as every 30 minutes for two times, every hour for two times, and then every 4 hours. During these checks, assess the dressing for bleeding.

When taking vital signs, monitor for the amount and color of drainage if drains are present. Document this within the intake and output section of the electronic health record.

NURSING SAFETY PRIORITY (QSEN)

Action Alert

To decrease the chance of surgical site *infection,* carefully observe the surgical wound after breast surgery for signs of swelling and infection throughout recovery. Assess the incision and flap of the postmastectomy patient for signs of bleeding, infection, and poor tissue perfusion. Drainage tubes are usually removed about 1 to 3 weeks after hospital discharge when the patient returns for an office visit. The drainage amount should be less than 30 mL in a 24-hour period. Inform the patient that tube removal may cause temporary *pain.* Provide or suggest analgesia before they are removed. Document all findings and report any abnormalities to the surgeon immediately.

Assess the patient's position to ensure that the drainage tubes or collection device is not pulled or kinked. The patient should have the head of the bed elevated at least 30 degrees, with the affected arm elevated on a pillow while awake. Keeping the affected arm elevated promotes lymphatic fluid return after removal of lymph nodes and channels. Provide other basic comfort measures, such as repositioning and analgesics as prescribed, on a regular basis until *pain* ceases. Patient controlled analgesia may be used for some patients for a short time, depending on the type of surgery that was performed.

Ambulation and a regular diet are resumed by the day after surgery. While the patient is walking, the arm on the affected side may need to be supported at first. Gradually the arm should be allowed to hang straight by the side. Encourage the patient to use good posture to prevent mobility issues. Beginning exercises that do not stress the incision can usually be started on the first day after surgery. These exercises include squeezing the affected hand around a soft, round object (a ball or rolled washcloth) and flexion/extension of the elbow. The progression to more strenuous exercises depends on the subsequent procedures planned (e.g., reconstruction) and the surgeon's directions. The patient can be discharged to home after safely ambulating and when surgical *pain* is under control. Common instructions for exercises after mastectomy are listed in the Patient and Family Education: Preparing for Self-Management: Postmastectomy Exercises box.

Breast reconstruction. Breast reconstruction after or during mastectomy for women is common with few complications. Patients consult with the plastic surgeon to discuss the type of reconstruction, timing of the procedure, and technique desired. Many women prefer reconstruction immediately after mastectomy using their own tissue (autogenous reconstruction). Breast reconstruction at the time of mastectomy, both autogenous and

PATIENT AND FAMILY EDUCATION: PREPARING FOR SELF-MANAGEMENT

Postmastectomy Exercises

The surgeon or physical therapist can provide additional stretches and exercises. Hold each stretch until you feel a gentle pulling. Exercises can be done standing, sitting or lying down.

Hand Wall Climbing
- Face the wall and put the palms of your hands flat against the wall at shoulder level.
- Flex your fingers so your hands slowly "walk" up the wall.
- Stop when your arms are fully extended.
- Slowly "walk" your hands back down the wall until they return to shoulder level.

Rope Turning
- Tie a rope to the knob of a closed door.
- Hold the other end of the rope and step back from the door until your arm is almost straight out in front of you.
- Swing the rope in a circle. Start with small circles and gradually increase to larger circles as you become more flexible.

Side Bends
- Sit in a chair.
- Clasp your hands together.
- Slowly raise your arms over your head and then gently bend to each side.

Shoulder Blade Squeeze
- Sit in chair. Do not rest your back against the chair.
- Place arms at side, elbows bent.
- Squeeze your shoulder blades together behind you. Do not lift your shoulders up toward your ears.

NCLEX EXAMINATION CHALLENGE 65.3

Physiological Integrity

The nurse has delegated care for a client with a radical left mastectomy for breast cancer to assistive personnel (AP). Which AP action requires nursing intervention? **Select all that apply.**
A. Obtains blood pressure via left arm
B. Reports client's pain level to the nurse
C. Applies gait belt prior to walking with the client
D. Records vital signs in the electronic health record
E. Assists client to administer patient-controlled analgesia

prosthetic, may lessen the psychological strain associated with undergoing a mastectomy. The surgeon should offer the option of breast reconstruction before surgery is performed.

Assess her attitude by asking about future plans for restoring appearance. Although reconstruction is not appropriate for some women and others may not be interested in it, the surgeon should discuss the indications and contraindications, advantages and disadvantages, and typical recovery. If immediate reconstruction is chosen, the breast surgeon should be aware of this before surgery so plans can be coordinated with those of the plastic surgeon.

Several procedures are available for restoring the appearance of the breast (Table 65.4). Reconstruction may begin during the

TABLE 65.4   Examples of Breast Reconstruction Procedures

Procedure	Description	Procedure	Description
Implantation	An implant matching the size of the other breast is placed under the muscle on the operative side to create a breast mound.	Flaps	A flap of skin, fat, and muscle is transferred from the donor site to the operative area. The flap contains an appropriate amount of fat to match the other breast and is similar in appearance to breast tissue. A blood supply is established by reanastomosis of vessels from the operative area to those with the flap when possible. A new nipple may be created with tissue from areas such as the labia or upper, inner thigh. Nipples can also be created by tattooing. Latissimus dorsi musculocutaneous flap Abdominal myocutaneous flap
Tissue expansion DIEP reconstruction (deep inferior epigastric perforator flap)	A tissue expander is placed under the muscle and gradually expanded with saline to stretch the overlying skin and create a pocket. After several weeks, the tissue expander is exchanged for an implant.		

original operative procedure or later in one to several stages. Common types of breast reconstruction are:

- Breast expanders (saline or silicone)
- Autologous reconstruction using the patient's own skin, fat, and muscle

Breast expanders are the most common method of breast reconstruction used in the United States. A tissue expander is a balloon-like device with a resealable metal port that is placed under the pectoralis muscle. A small amount of normal saline is injected intraoperatively into the expander to partially inflate it. The patient then receives additional weekly saline injections for about 6 to 8 weeks until the expander is fully inflated. When full

expansion is achieved, the tissue expander is then exchanged for a permanent implant during surgery in an ambulatory care center. The permanent implant is filled with either saline or silicone.

Autologous reconstruction using the patient's own skin, fat, and muscle is advantageous because the donor site tissue is similar in consistency to that of the natural breast. Therefore the results more closely resemble a real breast compared with implant reconstruction. Flap donor sites include the latissimus dorsi flap (back muscle); transverse rectus abdominis myocutaneous flap, known as the *TRAM flap* (abdominal muscle); and the gluteal flap (buttock muscle). Reconstruction of the nipple-areola complex is the last stage in the reconstruction of the breast.

BEST PRACTICE FOR PATIENT SAFETY & QUALITY CARE (QSEN)

Postoperative Care of the Patient After Breast Reconstruction

- Assess the incision and flap for signs of *infection* (excessive redness, drainage, odor) during dressing changes.
- Assess the incision and flap for signs of poor tissue perfusion (duskiness, decreased capillary refill) during dressing changes.
- Avoid pressure on the flap and suture lines by positioning the patient on her nonoperative side and avoiding tight clothing.
- Monitor and measure drainage in collection devices, such as for Jackson-Pratt (JP) drains.
- Teach the patient to return to her usual activity level gradually and to avoid heavy lifting.
- Remind the patient to avoid sleeping in the prone position.
- Teach the patient to avoid participation in contact sports or other activities that could cause trauma to the chest.
- Teach the patient to minimize pressure on the breast during sexual activity.
- Remind the patient to refrain from driving until advised by the surgeon.
- Remind the patient to ask at the 6-week postoperative visit when full activity can be resumed.
- Reassure the patient that optimal appearance may not occur for 3 to 6 months after surgery.
- If implants have been inserted, teach the proper method of breast massage to enhance expansion and prevent capsule formation (consult with the health care provider).
- Emphasize breast self-awareness; if the patient performs breast self-examination (BSE), review her technique.
- Remind the patient of the importance of clinical breast examination and follow-up surveillance by her health care provider.

Women who have had a mastectomy and breast reconstruction in one breast should have close-surveillance breast cancer screening in the contralateral (opposite) breast, including imaging with mammography or mammography and MRI. Mammography and MRI are not recommended to be done routinely in reconstructed breasts because most local recurrences of breast cancer in the residual tissue are palpable during clinical breast examination. Nursing care of the woman who has undergone breast reconstruction is outlined in the Best Practice for Patient Safety & Quality Care: Postoperative Care of the Patient After Breast Reconstruction box.

Refer the patient to the American Cancer Society's *Reach to Recovery* program. This program has trained breast cancer survivors who can help navigate the decisions needed when facing breast cancer. In this program, a volunteer who has had breast cancer visits the woman, offering information on breast forms, clothing, coping with breast cancer, and possible reconstructive options. For this intervention to be as helpful as possible, the volunteer should be about the same age as the patient and have experienced the same surgical procedure.

Adjuvant therapy. The decision to follow the original surgical procedure with additional treatment to help keep the cancer from recurring is known as *adjuvant therapy*. This decision is based on several factors:

- Stage of the disease
- Patient's age and menopausal and functional status
- Patient preferences
- Pathologic examination
- Hormone receptor (ER/PR) status
- HER2/neu status
- Presence of a known genetic predisposition

Adjuvant therapy for breast cancer consists of systemic chemotherapy, radiation therapy, or a combination of both. The purpose of radiation therapy is to reduce the risk for local recurrence of breast cancer. The goal of systemic therapy (with chemotherapy, hormone therapy, and targeted therapy) is to reduce the risk of recurrence (locally or at distant sites) and prevent cancer-related death. These drugs destroy breast cancer cells that may be present anywhere in the body. They are typically delivered after surgery for breast cancer, although neoadjuvant chemotherapy may be given to reduce the size of a tumor before surgery. Endocrine therapy may also be used as a chemoprevention option for high-risk women with a personal history of breast cancer.

Radiation therapy. Radiation therapy is administered after breast-conserving surgery to kill breast cancer cells that may remain near the site of the original tumor. This therapy can be delivered to the whole breast or to only part of the breast. Whole-breast irradiation is delivered by external beam radiation over a period of 5 to 6 weeks. Partial breast irradiation (PBI) is an option for women with early-stage breast cancer (Siefert et al., 2018). PBI is a convenient alternative to whole-breast radiation. Less time is needed for completion, and outcomes are comparable to those of whole-breast radiation. The advantage of this type of radiation is that it is delivered over a much shorter time interval, eliminating the need for weeks of treatment. The types of methods available for delivering PBI include the following:

- Brachytherapy is a form of treatment in which an external catheter is inserted at the lumpectomy cavity and surrounding margin, and radioactive seeds are inserted into a multi-catheter or balloon catheter device. Radiation is given over a period of 5 days. Ten treatments are given in total, with at least 6 hours between treatments.
- Intraoperative radiation therapy is the most accelerated form of PBI. It uses a high single dose of radiation delivered during the lumpectomy surgery.

Nursing care for the patient undergoing radiation therapy includes patient education and side effect management. Skin changes are a major side effect during this therapy (see Chapter 20). If brachytherapy is planned, instruct patients about the procedure. Assure them that they will be radioactive only while the radiation source is dwelling inside the breast tissue.

NURSING SAFETY PRIORITY (QSEN)

Action Alert

Teach women undergoing brachytherapy for breast cancer that radiation is contained in the temporary catheter and then removed prior to going home. The risk for others to be exposed to radiation is very small. Body fluids and items contacted by patients with brachytherapy are not radioactive. However, during the time that radiation is delivered, the patient will be alone in the room.

Drug therapy. The National Comprehensive Cancer Network (NCCN) provides a database of evidence-based practice and treatments for various cancers. *Chemotherapy* for breast cancer is a systemic treatment used to kill undetected breast cancer cells that may have left the original tumor and moved to more distant sites. Generalist nurses do not administer chemotherapy; consult your agency policies regarding the specific training and education that is needed to demonstrate and maintain competence in chemotherapy administration (Oncology Nursing Society, 2020).

Chemotherapy is recommended for treatment of invasive breast cancer after surgery (adjuvant chemotherapy). It may also be given before surgery to reduce the size of the tumor (neoadjuvant chemotherapy) and is most effective when combinations of more than one drug are used. Sometimes a patient needs to have a surgically implanted IV catheter before chemotherapy administration. Chemotherapy drugs are usually delivered in four to six cycles, with each period of treatment followed by a rest period to give the body time to recover from the adverse effects of the drugs. Each cycle is 2 to 3 weeks long. The total treatment time is 3 to 6 months, although treatment may be longer for advanced or HER2-positive breast cancer.

A common chemotherapy regimen for breast cancer treatment is doxorubicin, cyclophosphamide, and paclitaxel, which in the United States is also known as AC-T. If the patient is HER2 positive, a trastuzumab-based regimen will be used. In early-stage breast cancer, chemotherapy regimens lower the risk for breast cancer recurrence and death. In metastatic breast cancer, chemotherapy regimens reduce cancer size and slow the progression of disease.

Nurses who are qualified to give chemotherapy must be very proficient in the preparation and administration of these drugs and knowledgeable about various venous access devices. They must also be able to manage the distressing symptoms associated with side effects of these drugs. Chapter 20 discusses chemotherapy in more detail and general nursing management of alopecia, nausea and vomiting, mucositis, and bone marrow suppression.

Chemotherapy is unpleasant and expensive and can have life-threatening short-term and long-term side effects. Because more women are living longer with breast cancer, more long-term effects are emerging. For example, ovarian suppression from chemotherapy drugs can result in infertility, which can be devastating for some women of childbearing age.

NURSING SAFETY PRIORITY (QSEN)

Action Alert

Teach patients undergoing chemotherapy with doxorubicin and trastuzumab to be aware of cardiotoxic effects. Patients will have routine testing of their cardiac function and ejection fraction (EF) because this side effect is often asymptomatic (Morgan, 2020). Instruct them to report excessive fatigue, shortness of breath, chronic cough, and edema to the health care provider. This side effect can manifest years after treatment.

Targeted cancer therapies are drugs that target specific characteristics of cancer cells, such as a protein, an enzyme, or the formation of new blood vessels. The advantage of targeted therapy over traditional chemotherapy is that targeted therapy is less likely to harm normal, healthy cells and therefore it has fewer side effects. One of the first targeted therapies developed for breast cancer is the monoclonal antibody *trastuzumab.* This drug targets the *HER2/neu* gene product in breast cancer cells. Other targeted therapies are available.

Drugs that alter hormone levels may also be used in breast cancer prevention and treatment. The purpose of endocrine therapy is to reduce the estrogen available to breast tumors to stop or prevent their growth. *Premenopausal* women whose main estrogen source is the ovaries may benefit from drugs that inhibit estrogen synthesis. These drugs include leuprolide and goserelin, which suppress the hypothalamus from making luteinizing hormone–releasing hormone (LH-RH). When LH-RH is inhibited, the ovaries do not produce estrogen. Although the suppression of ovarian function decreases breast cancer risk, the drastic drop in estrogen causes significant menopausal symptoms. Therefore the decision to use these drugs is not made lightly.

Selective estrogen receptor modulators (SERMs), on the other hand, do not affect ovarian function. Rather, they block the effect of estrogen in women who have estrogen receptor (ER)–positive breast cancer (Burchum & Rosenthal, 2019). SERMs are also used as chemoprevention in women at high risk for breast cancer and in women with advanced breast cancer. For women with hormone receptor–positive breast cancer, tamoxifen reduces the chances of the cancer coming back by about half (ACS, 2019a). Common side effects of SERMs include hot flashes and weight gain. Rare but serious side effects of these drugs include endometrial cancer and thromboembolic events.

Aromatase inhibitors (AIs), such as letrozole and anastrozole, are used in *postmenopausal* women whose main source of estrogen is not the ovaries but, rather, body fat (Burchum & Rosenthal, 2019). AIs reduce estrogen levels by inhibiting the conversion of androgen to estrogen through the action of the enzyme *aromatase.* They are beneficial when given to postmenopausal women for up to 5 years. Newer research is recommending up to 10 years of tamoxifen or AI therapy to prevent recurrence (NCCN, 2020). A side effect of AIs, not seen with tamoxifen, is loss of bone density. Women taking AIs are candidates for bone-strengthening drugs and must be closely monitored for osteoporosis. Weight-bearing exercises and supplementation should be implemented into the daily routine.

Enhancing Coping Strategies

Planning: Generate Solutions. The patient who is treated for breast cancer will verbalize enhanced coping ability related to the diagnosis and treatment of the condition.

Interventions: Take Action. The patient with breast cancer may appear to have difficulty coping and experience anxiety related to the disease or treatment. The fear and uncertainty for the patient with breast cancer begin the moment a lump is discovered or when a mammogram reveals an abnormality. These feelings may be related to past experiences and personal associations with the disease. Assess the patient's situational perceptions. Allow the expression of feelings even if a diagnosis has not been established.

Assess the patient's need for knowledge. Some may want to read and discuss any available information. Provide accurate information and clarify any misinformation the patient may have received through the media, on the Internet, or from family and friends. If the mass has been diagnosed as cancer, many people feel a partial sense of relief to be dealing with a known entity. A feeling of shock or disbelief usually occurs. It is difficult to accept a diagnosis of cancer when one feels basically well. Patients and their families or significant others deal in individual ways with the mix of feelings. Adjust your approach to care as the patient's emotional state changes. The goal is to have the patient participate as an active partner in management of the disease.

An integral part of the plan to meet these emotional needs is the use of outside resources. For example, the patient who is worried in particular about the side effects of radiation therapy may benefit more from talking to someone who has undergone radiation than from talking to the nurse or primary health care provider. The American Cancer Society's "Reach to Recovery" program is just one community resource that connects breast cancer patients to a peer who has lived through the treatment the patient is facing. Be sure to assess her preference and place appropriate referrals.

Another helpful resource for patients who desire to receive care at one location is a full-service cancer center. Some agencies have all cancer services offered comprehensively in one location, including surgeon and provider services, counseling, nursing care, social services, nutrition services, rehabilitation, various therapies (including chemotherapy), and spiritual ministry. Obtaining all services in one familiar location can decrease the stress that the patient feels.

Care Coordination and Transition Management

Home Care Management. In collaboration with the case manager and members of the interprofessional health care team, make the appropriate referrals for care after discharge. Preoperative teaching and arrangements for home care management and referrals can be started before surgery or other treatment.

The patient who has undergone breast surgery can be discharged to the home setting unless other physical disabilities exist. Some are discharged the day after surgery with drains in place; some are discharged to home on the day of surgery. Older adults should not be sent home without a family member or friend who can stay with them for 1 to 2 days. These patients may need some assistance at home with drain care, dressings, and ADLs because of ***pain*** and impaired range of motion of the affected arm. See the Home Care Considerations: Patients Recovering From Breast Cancer Surgery box.

Teach patients that activities involving stretching or reaching for heavy objects should be avoided temporarily. This restriction can be discussed with a family member or significant other who can perform these tasks or place the objects within easy reach.

🏠 HOME CARE CONSIDERATIONS
Patients Recovering From Breast Cancer Surgery

Assess cardiovascular, respiratory, and urinary status:
- Vital signs
- Lung sounds
- Urine output patterns

Assess for ***pain*** and effectiveness of analgesics.

Assess dressing and incision site:
- Excess drainage
- Symptoms of ***infection***
- Wound healing
- Intact staples, sutures

Assess drain and site:
- Drainage around site and within drain reservoir
- Color and amount of drainage
- Symptoms of ***infection***

Review patient's recordings of drainage.

Evaluate patient's ability to care for and empty drain reservoir.

Assess status of affected extremity:
- Range of motion
- Ability to perform exercise regimen
- Lymphedema

Assess nutritional status:
- Food and fluid intake
- Presence of nausea and vomiting
- Bowel sounds

Assess functional ability:
- ADLs
- Mobility and ambulation

Assess home environment:
- Safety
- Structural barriers

Assess patient's compliance and knowledge of illness and treatment plan:
- Follow-up appointment with surgeon
- Symptoms to report to health care provider
- Hand and arm care guidelines

Self-Management Education. The teaching plan for the patient after surgery includes:
- Care of the incision and drainage device
- Exercises to regain full range of motion
- Measures to avoid lymphedema
- Measures to improve body image, coping, and self-esteem
- Information about interpersonal relationships and roles

See the Patient and Family Education: Preparing for Self-Management: Recovery From Breast Cancer Surgery box for additional important patient teaching.

Postoperative Mastectomy Teaching. Teach incisional care to the patient, family, and/or other caregiver. The patient may wear a light dressing to prevent irritation. Although swelling and redness of the scar itself are normal for the first few weeks, swelling, redness, increased heat, and tenderness of the surrounding area indicate ***infection*** and should be reported to the surgeon immediately. If a lymph node dissection was performed, instruct the patient to elevate the affected arm on a pillow and to use interventions to decrease risk of lymphedema. Encourage the patient to dress in comfortable street clothes at home, not pajamas, to further enhance a positive self-image.

PATIENT AND FAMILY EDUCATION: PREPARING FOR SELF-MANAGEMENT

Recovery From Breast Cancer Surgery

- There may be a dry gauze dressing over the incision when you leave the hospital. You may change this dressing if it becomes soiled.
- A small, dry dressing will be around the site where a drain is placed. Often there is some leakage of fluid around the drain. Check the gauze dressing for drainage and change it if it becomes soiled. Some leakage is normal, but if the dressing becomes soaked more than once a day, call your health care provider.
- You have been taught how to empty the reservoir from your drain and how to measure the volume of drainage. You should empty the reservoir twice a day and record the measurements.
- Drains are generally removed when drainage is less than 30 mL/day for 3 consecutive days.
- You may take sponge baths or tub baths, making certain that the area of the drain and incision stays dry. You may shower after the stitches, staples, and drains are removed.
- You can begin using your arm for normal activities, such as eating or combing your hair. Exercises involving the wrist, hand, and elbow, such as flexing your fingers, circular wrist motions, and touching your hand to your shoulder, are very good. You can usually resume more strenuous exercises after the drains have been removed.
- You can expect mild pain after surgery; but within 4 to 5 days, most patients have no need for pain medication or require medication only at bedtime.
- Numbness in the area of the surgery and along the inner side of the arm from the armpit to the elbow occurs in almost all patients owing to injury to the nerves. Patients have described sensations of heaviness, pain, tingling, burning, and "pins and needles." This is neuropathic pain, and short-acting analgesics may be given. These sensations may change over the next several months, becoming less and less noticeable, and may resolve entirely by the end of the first year following surgery.
- Pamphlets on exercises, hand and arm care, and general facts about breast cancer are available from your hospital or from a volunteer visitor of the local or national office on cancer or breast cancer. The American Cancer Society has volunteers who have had surgery similar to yours and are available to visit you.

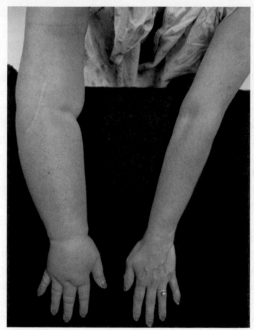

FIG. 65.10 Lymphedema of the arm. (From Song, D.H., & Neligan, P.C. [2018]. *Plastic surgery. Volume 4. Lower extremity, trunk, and burns* [4th ed.]. Philadelphia: Elsevier.)

Teach the patient to continue performing the exercises that began in the hospital. Active range-of-motion exercises should begin 1 week after surgery and should be continued after sutures and drains are removed. Emphasize that reaching and stretching exercises should continue only to the point of *pain* or pulling, never beyond that. Some YWCA locations have a free postmastectomy program that supports patients following breast cancer surgery.

Patients should be screened for mobility and provided education on exercises to perform after surgery. Referral to physical therapy prior to surgery allows for education and assessment to be done in a nonhurried environment. Additionally, if the patient is unable to raise her arm over her head, positioning for radiation therapy will be difficult.

Lymphedema (Fig. 65.10), an abnormal accumulation of protein fluid in the subcutaneous tissue of the affected limb after a mastectomy, is a commonly overlooked topic in health teaching. Risk factors include injury or *infection* of the extremity, obesity, presence of extensive axillary disease, and radiation treatment. Once lymphedema develops, it can be very difficult to manage, and *lifelong measures must be taken to prevent it*. Nurses play a vital role in educating patients about this complication. Teach patients, especially those who have had axillary lymph nodes removed, that measures to prevent lymphedema are lifelong and include avoiding trauma to the arm on the side of the mastectomy. Teach your patient to immediately report symptoms of lymphedema such as sensations of heaviness, aching, fatigue, numbness, tingling, and/or swelling in the affected arm, as well as swelling in the upper chest (Mehrara, 2020).

Nurses should not assume that women with lymphedema are disabled; they are able to live full lives within this limitation. A referral to a lymphedema specialist may be necessary for the patient to be fitted for a compression sleeve and/or glove, to be taught exercises and manual lymph drainage, and to discuss ways to modify daily activities to avoid worsening the problem. Management is directed toward measures that promote drainage of the affected arm.

! NURSING SAFETY PRIORITY (QSEN)

Action Alert

Teach the patient how to avoid *infection* and subsequent lymphedema of the affected arm after the mastectomy. Teach the importance of **avoiding** having blood pressure measurements taken on, having injections in, or having blood drawn from the arm on the side of the mastectomy, especially if lymph node dissection has occurred. Instruct the patient to wear a mitt when using the oven, wear gloves when gardening, and treat cuts and scrapes appropriately. If lymphedema occurs, early intervention provides the best chance for control.

Psychosocial Preparation. Concerns about appearance after surgery are common and are often a threat to the patient's self-concept as a woman. Before breast surgery, the woman and her partner can benefit from an explanation of the expected postoperative appearance. After a modified radical mastectomy, the chest wall is fairly smooth and has a horizontal incision from the axilla to the mid-chest area. After breast-conserving surgery, scars vary according to the amount of breast tissue removed. Emphasize that scars will fade and edema will lessen with time. Scars may be red and raised at first, but these features lessen in the first few months. After surgery, encourage the woman to look at her incision when she is ready. Do not push her to accept this body image change immediately.

Much of one's body image is a reflection of how others respond. Therefore the response of the patient's partner or family members to the surgery impacts the effect on self-esteem. These people may also need the support of the nurse. They may have concerns about their ability to accept the changes and need to discuss these feelings with an objective listener. They may also need help with communicating their feelings, both negative and positive, to their loved one. Involving them in teaching, if the patient desires, may also help reinforce learning and increase retention.

Discuss sexual concerns before discharge. Most surgeons recommend avoiding sexual intercourse for 4 to 6 weeks. Patients may prefer to lay a pillow over the surgical site or to wear a bra, camisole, or T-shirt to prevent contact with the surgical site during intercourse. He or she may be embarrassed to discuss the topic of *sexuality.* Be sensitive to possible concerns and approach the subject first.

For young women, issues related to childbearing may be a concern. Chemotherapy and radiation are considered serious teratogenic (birth defect–causing) agents. Advise sexually active patients receiving chemotherapy or radiotherapy to use birth control during therapy. The method and length of birth control should be discussed with the health care provider. Patients with hormone ER/PR–positive breast cancer need to avoid estrogen, including contraceptives.

Health Care Resources. Resources available to the patient after discharge include personal support and community programs. After discharge, the spouse or partner may need help in planning support for home responsibilities. This caregiver may be assuming additional duties at home and work, and may feel stressed. Discussing the need for ongoing emotional support is also beneficial to both the patient and caregiver. Leaving the hospital and appearing normal do not end the anxiety and fear. Identifying a support person with whom the patient or couple can explore these feelings and discussing the need to ventilate feelings enhance personal and family recovery.

Numerous support and educational resources are available to those diagnosed with breast cancer. Nurses must provide accurate and current information to patients who may have obtained inaccurate information from various outlets. There are over 3.8 million breast cancer survivors in the United States (ACS, 2019a), and many men and women are active in breast cancer support and advocacy organizations. National breast cancer organizations are accessible online, and many of them have local affiliates. Examples of such organizations are Susan G. Komen for the Cure, the National Breast Cancer Coalition, Sisters Network, and Young Survival Coalition. Local support organizations can be found and accessed through the health care provider, the local hospital, wellness centers, or home care agencies; by word of mouth; or by Internet search.

The American Cancer Society (ACS) is a comprehensive resource for information and support in the United States. Breastcancer.org provides evidence-based information in language a lay person can understand.

The Canadian Cancer Society offers information, resources, and support services for breast cancer patients and their families. The Breast Cancer Society of Canada conducts research on breast cancer in Canada.

Helping patients diagnosed with breast cancer to be active participants in their care, to find resources to help them cope, and to gain support with physical and emotional changes are priorities for the nurse and members of the interprofessional team.

◆ **Evaluation: Evaluate Outcomes.** Evaluate the care of the patient with breast cancer based on the identified priority patient problems. The expected outcomes include that the patient:

- Has no recurrence or metastasis of breast cancer after completion of treatment; if metastasis occurs, have optimal palliative and end-of-life care
- Reports adequately coping with the uncertainty of having breast cancer and its treatment

---

? CLINICAL JUDGMENT CHALLENGE 65.1

Safety

The telehealth nurse receives a call from a client who is home recovering from a right mastectomy 2 days prior. The client reports swelling in the right upper chest, and swelling in the right arm. When asked if she is in pain, the client says her right arm aches, but she is not in any other pain. She says she feels more fatigued each day following surgery, and just wants to know if this is normal.

1. **Recognize Cues:** What assessment information in this client situation is the most important and immediate concern for the nurse? (Hint: Identify the **relevant** information *first* to determine what is most important.)
2. **Analyze Cues:** What client conditions are consistent with the **most relevant** information? (Hint: Think about priority collaborative problems that support and contradict the information presented in this situation.)
3. **Prioritize Hypotheses:** Which possibilities or explanations are **most likely** to be present in this client situation? Which possibilities or explanations are the most serious? (Hint: Consider all possibilities and determine their urgency and risk for this client.)
4. **Generate Solutions:** What actions would most likely achieve the desired outcomes for this client? Which actions should be **avoided** or are **potentially harmful**? (Hint: Determine the desired outcomes first to decide which interventions are appropriate and those that should be avoided.)
5. **Take Action:** Which actions are the most appropriate and how should they be implemented? In what **priority order** should they be implemented? (Hint: Consider health teaching, documentation, requested health care provider orders or prescriptions, nursing skills, collaboration with or referral to health team members, etc.)
6. **Evaluate Outcomes:** What client assessment would indicate that the nurse's actions were **effective**? (Hint: Think about signs that would indicate an improvement, decline, or unchanged client condition.)

GET READY FOR THE NEXT-GENERATION NCLEX® EXAMINATION!

Key Points

Review these Key Points for each NCLEX Examination Client Needs Category.

Safe and Effective Care Environment

- Collaborate with the interprofessional health care team to reduce risk for lymphedema **QSEN: Safety; Teamwork and Collaboration**
- Notify the health care team that the arm of the surgical mastectomy side should not be used for blood pressures, blood drawing, IV therapy, or injections. **QSEN: Safety**

Health Promotion and Maintenance

- Identify and educate patients at high risk for breast cancer. **QSEN: Patient-Centered Care**
- Teach women the importance of breast self-awareness, and teach breast self-examination (BSE) to women who wish to learn. **QSEN: Patient-Centered Care**
- Encourage women to have a screening mammography and clinical breast examinations (CBE) according to recommended guidelines. **QSEN: Evidence-Based Practice**

- Observe for and report complications of breast surgery, especially *infection* and inadequate vascular perfusion. **QSEN: Safety**

Psychosocial Integrity

- Allow patients to express feelings about a cancer diagnosis and treatment on body image and *sexuality*. **QSEN: Patient-Centered Care**
- Teach women ways to minimize surgical area changes and enhance body image **QSEN: Patient-Centered Care**
- Provide support, education, and community referrals to the patient with breast cancer and their significant others. **QSEN: Patient-Centered Care**

Physiological Integrity

- Assess benign lumps as mobile and round or oval; assess possible malignant lumps as fixed and irregularly shaped. **Clinical Judgment**
- After breast surgery, assess vital signs, dressings, drainage tubes, amount of drainage, and return of arm and shoulder mobility. **Clinical Judgment**
- Teach self-management after breast surgery. **QSEN: Patient-Centered Care**

MASTERY QUESTIONS

1. Which nursing intervention is appropriate when caring for a female client who has undergone a mastectomy and will receive chemotherapy? **Select all that apply.**
   A. Encourage client to accept her new body image.
   B. Provide self-care resources to the primary caretaker.
   C. Teach client about birth control options that are available.
   D. Refer to support groups for people who have had mastectomy.
   E. Involve partner in discussions about sexuality if client desires.

2. Which assessment finding in a client who recently had a right mastectomy 2 days ago will the home health nurse report to the health care provider?
   A. Temperature of 99°F
   B. Tingling sensation in the right arm
   C. Impaired range of motion in the right arm
   D. Drainage of 20 mL collected over 24 hours

REFERENCES

Asterisk (*) indicates a classic or definitive work on this subject.

American Cancer Society (ACS). (2020a). *American Cancer Society recommendations for the early detection of breast cancer*. https://www.cancer.org/cancer/breast-cancer/screening-tests-and-early-detection/american-cancer-society-recommendations-for-the-early-detection-of-breast-cancer.html.

American Cancer Society (ACS). (2020b). *Cancer facts for lesbians and bisexual women*. https://www.cancer.org/healthy/find-cancer-early/womens-health/cancer-facts-for-lesbians-and-bisexual-women.html.

American Cancer Society (ACS). (2020c). *How common is breast cancer*. https://www.cancer.org/cancer/breast-cancer/about/how-common-is-breast-cancer.html.

American Cancer Society (ACS). (2020d). *Survival rates for breast cancer*. https://www.cancer.org/cancer/breast-cancer/understanding-a-breast-cancer-diagnosis/breast-cancer-survival-rates.html.

American Cancer Society (ACS). (2019a). *Breast cancer facts and figures 2019-2020*. https://www.cancer.org/content/dam/cancer-org/research/cancer-facts-and-statistics/breast-cancer-facts-and-figures/breast-cancer-facts-and-figures-2019-2020.pdf.

American Cancer Society (ACS). (2019b). *Cancer facts and figures*. 2019 https://www.cancer.org/content/dam/cancer-org/research/cancer-facts-and-statistics/annual-cancer-facts-and-figures/2019/cancer-facts-and-figures-2019.pdf.

American Cancer Society (ACS). (2019c). *Ductal carcinoma in situ (DCIS)*. https://www.cancer.org/cancer/breast-cancer/understanding-a-breast-cancer-diagnosis/types-of-breast-cancer/dcis.html.

American Cancer Society (ACS). (2019d). *Fibroadenomas of the breast*. https://www.cancer.org/cancer/breast-cancer/non-cancerous-breast-conditions/fibroadenomas-of-the-breast.html.

American Cancer Society (ACS). (2019e). *Lobular carcinoma in situ*. https://www.cancer.org/cancer/breast-cancer/non-cancerous-breast-conditions/lobular-carcinoma-in-situ.html.

American Cancer Society (ACS). (2019f). *Treatment of inflammatory breast cancer*. https://www.cancer.org/cancer/breast-cancer/treatment/treatment-of-inflammatory-breast-cancer.html.

American Cancer Society (ACS). (2017). *Breast cancer screening guideline*. https://www.cancer.org/research/infographics-gallery/breast-cancer-screening-guideline.html.

American Society of Breast Surgeons Foundation. (2019). *Breast abscess*. Retrieved from: https://breast360.org/topic/2017/01/01/breast-abscess/.

Anders, C., & Carey, L. (2020). ER/PR negative, HER2-negative (triple-negative) breast cancer. In D. Hayes, & H. Burstein (Eds.), *UpToDate*. Waltham, MA.

Attebery, L., Adams, J., & Weiss, M. (2020). *Male breast cancer*. Retrieved from: https://www.breastcancer.org/symptoms/types/male_bc.

Boehmer, U. (2018). LGBT populations' barrier to cancer care. *Seminars in Oncology Nursing, 34*(1), 21–29. https://doi.org/10.1016/j.soncn.2017.11.002.

Boucher, J. E. (2018). Chemoprevention: An Overview of Pharmacologic agents and nursing Considerations. *CJON, 22*(3), 350–353. https://doi.org/10.1188/18.CJON.350-353.

Braunstein, G., & Anawalt, B. (2019). *Clinical features, diagnosis, and evaluation of gynecomastia in adults*. In A. Matsumoso (Ed.). *UpToDate*. Waltham, MA.

Breastcancerorg. (2019). *Paget's disease of the nipple*. Retrieved from: https://www.breastcancer.org/symptoms/types/pagets.

Burchum, J. L. R., & Rosenthal, L. D. (2019). *Lehne's pharmacology for nursing care* (9th ed.). St. Louis: Elsevier.

Canadian Cancer Society. (2020). *Breast cancer statistics*. Retrieved from: https://www.cancer.ca/en/cancer-information/cancer-type/breast/statistics/?region=on.

Centers for Disease Control and Prevention (CDC). (2018). *Breast cancer rates among black women and white women*. Retrieved from: https://www.cdc.gov/cancer/dcpc/research/articles/breast_cancer_rates_women.htm.

Ceres, M., Quinn, G. P., Loscalzo, M., & Rice, D. (2018). Cancer screening considerations and cancer screening uptake for lesbian, gay, bisexual and transgender persons. *Seminars in Oncology Nursing, 34*(1), 37–51. https://doi.org/10.1016/j.soncn.2017.12.001.

Chang, C., Lin, M., & Yin, W. (2019). Risk of breast cancer in women with non-lactational mastitis. *Scientific Reports, 9*, 15587. https://doi.org/10.1038/s41598-019-52046-3.

Dixon, J., & Pariser, K. (2020). Nonlactational mastitis in adults. In Sexton, D. (Ed.), *UpToDate*. Waltham, MA.

Howlader, N., Noone, A., Krapcho, M., et al. (Eds.). (2020). *SEER cancer statistics review, 1975-2016*. Bethesda, MD: National Cancer Institute. https://seer.cancer.gov/csr/1975_2016/.

Komen, S. G. (2020). *Breast self-exam*. Retrieved from: https://ww5.komen.org/BreastCancer/BreastSelfExam.html.

Mahon, S. M. (2017). Genetics and Genomics: An Oncology nurse's Journey in practice. *CJON 2017, 21*(6), 715–721. https://doi.org/10.1188/17.CJON.715-721.

Margolies, S. (2020). *Lesbians and breast cancer risk*. National LGBT Cancer Network. Retrieved from: https://cancer-network.org/cancer-information/lesbians-and-cancer/lesbians-and-breast-cancer-risk/.

Mau, K. (2018). Benign breast diseases: An introduction for the advanced practice nurse. *CJON 2018, 22*(5), 493–495. https://doi.org/10.1188/18.CJON.493-495.

McCance, K., Huether, S., Brashers, V., & Rote, N. (2019). *Pathophysiology: The biologic basis for disease in adults and children* (8th ed.). St. Louis: Mosby.

McDaniel, J., et al. (2018). Breast cancer screening and outcomes: An ecological study of county-level female veteran population density and social vulnerability. *Journal of Military, Veteran, and Family Health, 4*(1). https://doi.org/10.3138/jmvfh.2017-0023.

Mehrara, B. (2020). Patient education: Lymphedema after cancer surgery (beyond the basics). In P. Ganz, & E. Bruera (Eds.), *UpToDate*. Waltham, MA.

Morgan, J. (2020). *Cardiotoxicity of trastuzumab and other HER-2 targeted agents*. In Hayes, D. (Ed.), *UpToDate*. Waltham, MA.

National Breast Cancer Foundation. (2019). *BRCA: The breast cancer gene*. Retrieved from: https://www.nationalbreastcancer.org/what-is-brca.

National Cancer Institute. (n.d). Breast Cancer Risk Assessment Tool. Bethesda, MD. Retrieved from: https://bcrisktool.cancer.gov/calculator.html.

National Comprehensive Cancer Network. (2020). *NCCN clinical practice guidelines in Oncology (NCCN Guidelines®)* [v 3 2017] Retrieved from: https://www.nccn.org/professionals/physician_gls/default.aspx.

National Comprehensive Cancer Network. (2019). *Breast cancer screening and diagnosis*. https://www.nccn.org/professionals/physician_gls/pdf/breast-screening.pdf.

National LGBT Cancer Network. (2020). https://cancer-network.org/.

Oncology Nursing Society. (2020). Which RN is competent in chemotherapy administration? https://voice.ons.org/news and views/which-rn-is-competent-in-chemotherapy-administration.

*Ooi, S., Martinez, M., & Li, C. (2011). Disparities in breast cancer characteristics and outcomes by race/ethnicity. *Breast Cancer Research and Treatment, 127*(3), 729–738.

Sabel, M. (2018). Overview of benign breast disease. In Chagpar, A. (Ed.), *UpToDate*. Waltham, MA.

Santen, R. J. (2018). Benign breast disease in women. In Feingold, K., Anawalt, B., Boyce, A. et al., (Eds.), *Endotext [Internet]*. South Dartmouth (MA): MDText.com, Inc.; 2000-. Available from: https://www.ncbi.nlm.nih.gov/books/NBK278994/.

Siefert, M. L., Fennie, K., & Knobf, M. T. (2018). Partial breast irradiation: A longitudinal study of symptoms and quality of life. *Clinical Journal of Oncology Nursing, 22*(6), 635–642. https://doi.org/10.1188/18.CJON.635-642.

U.S. Food and Drug Administration. (2019). *Questions and answers about breast implant-associated anaplastic large cell lymphoma (BIA-ALCL)*. https://www.fda.gov/medical-devices/breast-implants/questions-and-answers-about-breast-implant-associated-anaplastic-large-cell-lymphoma-bia-alcl.

66

Concepts of Care for Patients With Gynecologic Problems

Cherie R. Rebar

http://evolve.elsevier.com/Iggy/

LEARNING OUTCOMES

1. Collaborate with the interprofessional team to coordinate high-quality care for patients with a gynecologic problem.
2. Describe factors that place a patient at high risk for a gynecologic cancer, and refer to the health care provider.
3. Implement patient-centered nursing interventions to decrease the psychosocial impact of living with a gynecologic problem.
4. Apply knowledge of anatomy, physiology, and pathophysiology to assess patients with a gynecologic problem.
5. Use clinical judgment to analyze assessment findings and diagnostic data in the care of patients with a gynecologic problem.
6. Prioritize evidence-based care for patients with gynecologic problems affecting *elimination, infection, sexuality,* or *reproduction,* or that induce *pain.*
7. Plan care coordination and transition management for patients with a gynecologic problem.

KEY TERMS

anterior colporrhaphy Surgery for severe symptoms of cystocele in which the pelvic muscles are tightened for better bladder support.

bilateral salpingo-oophorectomy (BSO) Surgical removal of both fallopian tubes and both ovaries.

colposcopy Examination of the cervix and vagina using a colposcope, which allows three-dimensional magnification and intense illumination of epithelium with suspected disease. This procedure can locate the exact site of precancerous and malignant lesions for biopsy.

concurrent chemoradiation The use of chemotherapy and radiation together at the same time.

cystocele Protrusion of the bladder through the vaginal wall (urinary bladder prolapse).

dyspareunia Painful intercourse.

endometrial cancer Cancer of the inner uterine lining.

fibroid See *leiomyoma.*

leiomyoma Benign, slow-growing solid tumor of the uterine myometrium.

loop electrosurgical excision procedure (LEEP) Diagnostic procedure or treatment in which a thin loop-wire electrode that transmits a painless electrical current is used to cut away affected cervical cancer tissue.

myoma See *leiomyoma.*

myomectomy Removal of leiomyomas from the uterus.

pelvic organ prolapse (POP) Condition in which the sling of muscles and tendons that support the pelvic organs becomes weak and is no longer able to hold them in place.

posterior colporrhaphy Surgery to repair a rectocele by strengthening pelvic supports and reducing the bulging.

rectocele Protrusion of the rectum through a weakened vaginal wall (rectal prolapse).

stress urinary incontinence (SUI) Loss of urine during activities that increase intra-abdominal pressure, such as laughing, coughing, sneezing, or lifting heavy objects.

total hysterectomy Removal of the uterus and cervix; the procedure may be vaginal or abdominal.

uterine artery embolization Use of a percutaneous catheter by a radiologist, inserted through the femoral artery to inject polyvinyl alcohol pellets into the uterine artery. The resulting blockage starves the tumor of circulation, allowing it (or them) to shrink.

uterine fibroid embolization See *uterine artery embolization.*

uterine prolapse The most common kind of pelvic organ prolapse (POP); the downward displacement of the uterus into the vagina.

vulvovaginitis inflammation of the lower genital tract resulting from a disturbance of the balance of hormones and flora in the vagina and vulva.

✳ PRIORITY AND INTERRELATED CONCEPTS

The priority concepts for this chapter are:
- *Sexuality*
- *Infection*
- *Pain*

   The **Sexuality** concept exemplar for this chapter is Uterine Leiomyoma.

The interrelated concepts for this chapter are:
- *Elimination*
- *Reproduction*

Pain, vaginal discharge, abnormal bleeding, and urinary *elimination* problems are common gynecologic symptoms that are reported by adult women. These problems can impair her feelings about *sexuality* and intimacy with others, as well as *reproduction.* Because of the private nature of these concerns, women may be hesitant to seek medical attention. Create an open, nonjudgment, and therapeutic environment in which the patient can feel comfortable expressing her concerns. See Chapter 1 to review these concepts.

Nurses provide whole-person, patient-centered care to women across the lifespan. Sexual health is an important part of each woman's life, and the ability to discuss something this private allows the nurse and patient to work together to agree on a plan of care regardless of stage of life. Evidence shows that nurses must continue to learn more about entry-level competencies to provide this type of care, particularly for women who have cancer. (See the Evidence-Based Practice box.)

EVIDENCE-BASED PRACTICE (QSEN)

Sexual Health Care Provision in Cancer Nursing Care: A Systematic Review on the State of Evidence and Deriving International Competencies Chart for Cancer Nurses

Papadopoulou, C., Sime, C., Rooney, K., & Kotronoulas, G. (2019). Sexual health care provision in cancer nursing care: A systematic review on the state of evidence and deriving international competencies chart for cancer nurses. *International Journal of Nursing Studies, 100,* 103405.

The authors conducted a systematic review of research aligned with Preferred Reporting Items for Systematic Reviews and Meta-Analyses (PRISMA) guidelines for the evidence-based minimum set of items for report. An extensive literature review of nine databases, spanning from 2008 to 2018, yielded 31 unique studies to include in the review. Diverse research methods were represented in these studies, including randomized controlled trials, and single-arm before-and-after trials.

Evidence demonstrates that intrapersonal, interpersonal, societal, and organizational factors affect the nurse's professional confidence in providing sexual health care to women with cancer. The review demonstrated that this disconnect in care provision is often linked to the nurse's assumptions and prejudices about sexuality.

Level of Evidence: 1
The study was a systematic review, which is a strong source of evidence.

Implications for Research and Practice
As a result of this systematic review, a two-level chart was created to promote development of nurse competence. Containing competencies at the entry level and champion level, this educational approach can help nurses to be better prepared to provide sexual health care to women with cancer. In this chapter, a number of gynecologic cancers are covered; any patient with one of these disorders could benefit from nurse intervention to address *sexuality* concerns.

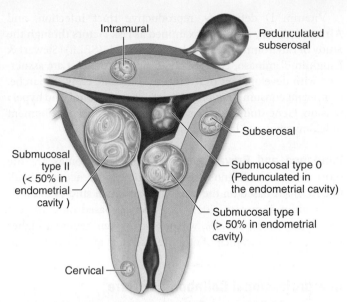

FIG. 66.1 Classification of uterine leiomyomas. (From Fielding, J.R., Brow, D.L., & Thrumond, A.S. [2011]. *Gynecologic Imaging.* Philadelphia: Elsevier.)

✳ SEXUALITY CONCEPT EXEMPLAR: UTERINE LEIOMYOMA

Pathophysiology Review

Leiomyomas, also called fibroids or myomas, are very commonly found in women. These are benign, slow-growing solid tumors of the uterine myometrium (muscle layer) that develop from excessive local growth of smooth muscle cells. The growth of leiomyomas may be related to stimulation by estrogen, progesterone, and growth hormone. They are classified according to their position in the layers of the uterus (Fig. 66.1) (Stewart & Laughlin-Tommaso, 2019) :

- *Intramural* leiomyomas are contained in the uterine wall within the myometrium.
- *Submucosal* leiomyomas protrude into the cavity of the uterus and can cause bleeding and disrupt pregnancy.
- *Subserosal* leiomyomas protrude through the outer surface of the uterine wall and may extend to the broad ligament, pressing other organs. These may have a broad or pedunculated base.

Although most fibroids develop within the uterine wall, a few may appear in the cervix, called *cervical* leiomyomas. Pedunculated leiomyomas are attached by a pedicle (stalk) to the outside of the uterus and occasionally break off and attach to other tissues (parasitic fibroids).

Etiology and Genetic Risk. The etiology of leiomyomas is not fully understood. Researchers continue to search for answers, recognizing that most are diagnosed at a peak time within a women's early 40s (McWilliams & Chennathukuzhi, 2017). The incidence of leiomyomas is two to three times greater in black women than white women, although again, the reason for this disparity is not known (Stewart & Laughlin-Tommaso, 2019).

Vitamin D deficiency, reproductive tract infection, and African ancestry are being examined as risk factors through the Study of Environment, Lifestyle, and Fibroids (SELF) (Stewart & Laughlin-Tommaso, 2019). Known risk factors that are associated with development of leiomyomas include early menarche, significant consumption of red meats, use of alcohol, and hypertension. Gene studies show a connection between development of leiomyomas and family history of such.

Incidence and Prevalence. Although leiomyomas are the most commonly diagnosed pelvic tumor, incidence is difficult to determine based on the lack of longitudinal studies (Stewart & Laughlin-Tommaso, 2019). Prevalence, based on a 10-year population study, is 9.6%, with black women having a higher prevalence than women of other races (Yu et al., 2018).

❖ Interprofessional Collaborative Care

◆ Assessment: Recognize Cues

History. Some women with fibroids do not experience *pain,* but others do. She may experience *dyspareunia* (painful intercourse) depending on the location of the leiomyoma. Acute discomfort may occur with twisting of the fibroid on its stalk. Many women with leiomyomas report painful menstruation, often with heavy flow and the presence of clots (Stewart & Laughlin-Tommaso, 2019).

The patient often seeks medical attention because of heavy vaginal bleeding. Ask about how many tampons or menstrual pads she uses in a day. Establish whether she has a predictable menstrual pattern, if she experienced intermenstrual bleeding (between periods), and if she has prolonged bleeding (periods that exceed the normal 5 to 6 days). Determine if she has a feeling of pelvic pressure and altered *elimination* patterns, including constipation and urinary frequency or retention. These symptoms result when the enlarged fibroid presses on other organs.

Physical Assessment/Signs and Symptoms. The patient may notice that her abdomen has increased in size. Assess the woman's abdomen for distention or enlargement. Abdominal, vaginal, and rectal examinations performed by the health care provider usually reveal the presence of a uterine enlargement. Further diagnostic procedures are needed to differentiate benign tumors from cancerous ones.

Psychosocial Assessment. Symptoms such as dyspareunia may significantly impact the patient's quality of life. A woman may fear that she has cancer or may have anxiety about abnormal bleeding or her failure to conceive. She may also be concerned if surgery is recommended if she desires to become pregnant in the future. Assess the woman's feelings and concerns. If hysterectomy is recommended, explore the significance of the loss of the uterus for the woman and her partner, including its effects on *sexuality* and *reproduction* plans.

Diagnostic Assessment. Laboratory testing is usually limited to a hematocrit (in the case of heavy bleeding), a thyroid-stimulating hormone (TSH) test (to rule out hypothyroidism), and a pregnancy test to determine whether pregnancy is the cause of the uterine enlargement. An endometrial biopsy may be performed to evaluate for endometrial cancer.

Transvaginal ultrasound (US), a procedure in which the ultrasound probe is placed into the vagina for visualization, is the diagnostic study of choice (Stewart & Laughlin-Tommaso, 2019). Saline infusion sonography, hysteroscopy, and MRI (which can differentiate between benign and malignant tumors) may also be ordered if the transvaginal ultrasounds results are inconclusive.

◆ Analysis: Analyze Cues and Prioritize Hypothesis. The priority collaborative problem for patients with uterine leiomyoma is:

- Potential for prolonged or heavy bleeding due to abnormal uterine growth

◆ Planning and Implementation: Generate Solutions and Take Action

Managing Bleeding

Planning: Expected Outcomes. The expected outcome for the patient with the diagnosis of uterine leiomyoma is that she will not experience or continue to experience heavy (severe) or prolonged bleeding following treatment.

Interventions. Asymptomatic leiomyomas may not require treatment. Leiomyomas in menopausal women usually shrink, so surgery may not be necessary. Management depends on the size and location of the tumor, as well as the woman's desire for future pregnancy. Women who want to become pregnant may be prescribed drug therapy or have a myomectomy procedure to remove the tumor. Uterine artery embolization, endometrial ablation, and hysterectomy are choices for women who no longer desire pregnancy.

Nonsurgical Management. If the woman has few symptoms or desires childbearing, the health care provider may recommend intermittent observation and examination. Mild leiomyoma symptoms can be managed with hormonal therapies. The choice of oral contraceptive is based on the woman's risk factors, co-occurring disorders, and personal symptoms associated with the leiomyoma (Stewart, 2020).

Myolysis is a laparoscopic thermal, radiofrequency, or cryoablation of leiomyoma tissue. Most women report an increased quality in life after this procedure, although it does bear risk of adhesion formation.

An alternative to surgery for the woman who does not desire pregnancy is **uterine artery embolization** (also called *uterine fibroid embolization [UFE]*) performed under local anesthesia, or with sedation if the patient requests it (van der Kooij & Hehenkamp, 2020). The interventional radiologist uses a percutaneous catheter inserted through the femoral artery to inject polyvinyl alcohol and gelatin-like pellets into the uterine artery. The uterine artery then carries these materials into the blood vessels that feed the leiomyoma. The resulting blockage starves the tumor of circulation, allowing it (or them) to shrink.

Common concerns reported following uterine artery embolization include pelvic pain, which is most severe in the first 24 hours, and vaginal discharge, which is self-limiting and can last for months (van der Kooij & Hehenkamp, 2020). Teach her to resume usual activities slowly and avoid strenuous activity until the surgeon recommends it. Most patients can return to work or daily routine within a week.

! NURSING SAFETY PRIORITY (QSEN)

Action Alert

After uterine artery embolization, the woman may have severe cramping within the first 24 hours owing to tissue necrosis. Cramping can last from a few days to 2 weeks. Patient-controlled analgesia (PCA) is often used before transition to oral pain medication. Remind the patient how to use PCA most effectively while hospitalized. If she experiences fever, nausea, and malaise with the pain (known as *postembolization syndrome*) or if severe pain or indication of **infection** is present (such as purulent vaginal drainage and fever), a continued hospital stay or readmission may be needed.

! NURSING SAFETY PRIORITY (QSEN)

Critical Rescue

Monitor for rare but potential complications of hysteroscopic surgery, which include:
- Fluid overload (fluid used to distend the uterine cavity can be absorbed)
- Embolism
- Hemorrhage
- Perforation of the uterus, bowel, or bladder and ureter injury
- Persistent increased menstrual bleeding
- Incomplete suppression of menstruation

   *Monitor for any indications of these problems and report signs and symptoms, such as severe **pain** and heavy bleeding, to the surgeon or Rapid Response Team immediately.*

Surgical Management. When possible, minimally invasive surgery (MIS) techniques are performed, such as a myomectomy, to prevent removing the uterus. If not, a hysterectomy is the procedure of choice.

Uterus-sparing surgeries. If the woman desires children, the surgeon may perform a laparoscopic or hysteroscopic myomectomy (the removal of leiomyomas from the uterus). Laparoscopic myomectomy, performed on an outpatient basis or with a 1-day hospital stay, is used to remove leiomyomas that are intramural or subserosal; hysteroscopic myomectomy is done to remove intracavity leiomyomas (Bradley, 2020). During this procedure, a laser may be used to remove the tumors. This MIS procedure is usually performed in the early phase of the menstrual cycle to minimize blood loss and avoid the possibility of interrupting an unsuspected pregnancy. A small percentage of leiomyomas recur after surgery. The health care provider, when obtaining informed consent, will share that scarring makes the uterus more likely to rupture during labor. Depending on the type of leiomyoma extracted, a planned cesarean delivery may be advised; other women can be offered a trial of labor.

Normal activities can resume as quickly as the woman is comfortable after the laparoscopic procedure. She can return to work, daily activities, and sexual activity whenever she is ready. Other nursing care is similar to that for a woman undergoing a hysterectomy, as discussed in the following paragraphs.

Hysterectomy. Leiomyomas are very common reason that a hysterectomy is performed. Hysterectomies may be performed abdominally, vaginally, or with laparoscopic or robotic assistance (Fig. 66.2) based on the patient's clinical reason for hysterectomy and the surgeon's area of technical expertise. Table 66.1 defines common terminology associated with common gynecologic surgeries.

Preoperative care. Preoperative teaching typically begins in the surgeon's office or surgical clinic. Explain procedures that routinely take place before surgery, including laboratory tests and expected drugs such as a prophylactic antibiotic. Depending on the type of surgical technique planned, teach about the need for turning, coughing, and deep-breathing exercises; incentive spirometry; early ambulation; and **pain** relief. (See Chapter 9 for a discussion of general patient care before surgery.) Correct any misperceptions about the effects of hysterectomy, such as association with masculinization and weight gain.

Psychological assessment is essential. Assess the significance of the surgery for the woman and her partner related to **sexuality** and **reproduction.** Many women relate their uterus to self-image, femininity, and/or sexuality. Although surgically induced menopause can contribute to a loss of libido and vaginal changes if the ovaries are also removed, teach the patient that vaginal estrogen cream, lubricants, and gentle dilation can help with these issues.

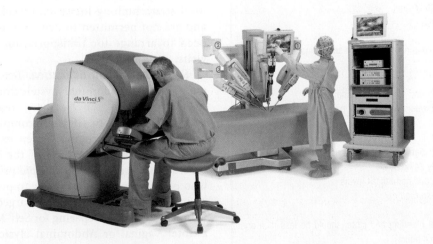

FIG. 66.2 Operating room layout for robotic surgery with da Vinci Robotic Surgery System. (©2016 Intuitive Surgical, Inc.)

Assess the patient's support system and recognize that she may fear rejection by her sexual partner. To be patient-centered, include the partner in all teaching sessions *unless this practice is not culturally acceptable or the patient prefers not to do so for other reasons*.

TABLE 66.1   Common Gynecologic Surgeries

Total Hysterectomy
- The entire uterus, including the cervix, is removed. The procedure may be performed via the vagina or abdominally, with laparoscopic or robotic assistance.

Supracervical Hysterectomy (Also Called "Subtotal" or "Partial" Hysterectomy)
- The upper part of the uterus is removed; however, the cervix is left in place. This procedure is performed laparoscopically or abdominally.

Salpingo-Oophorectomy (BSO)
- Fallopian tubes and ovaries are removed. This can be done on one side of the body, or both (termed *bilateral salpingo-oophorectomy*).
- If only the fallopian tubes are removed, it is a *salpingectomy*.
- If only the ovaries are removed, it is an *oophorectomy*.
- For patients at risk of ovarian or breast cancer who choose to have both ovaries removed (even if healthy) in order to decrease their risk of developing cancer, it is a *risk-reducing bilateral salpingo-oophorectomy*.

Radical Hysterectomy
- The uterus, cervix, adjacent lymph nodes, upper third of the vagina, and surrounding tissues (parametrium) are removed.

Data from American College of Obstetricians and Gynecologists. (2018). *Hysterectomy.* https://www.acog.org/Patients/FAQs/Hysterectomy.

 FOCUSED ASSESSMENT

Postoperative Nursing Care of the Patient After Open Total Abdominal Hysterectomy

Focus assessment on:
- Vital signs, including pain level
- Activity tolerance level
- Temperature and color of the skin
- Heart, lung, and bowel sounds
- Incision characteristics
  - Presence or absence of bleeding at the site (a small amount is normal)
  - Intactness of incision
  - Pain at site of incision
- Dressing and drains for color and amount of drainage
- Fluid intake (IVs until peristalsis returns and patient is tolerating oral intake)
- Urine output
  - Provide catheter care for patients with open surgery (catheter will be removed in approximately 24 hours)
- Red blood cell, hemoglobin, and hematocrit levels
- *For patients with vaginal hysterectomy:*
  - Perineal care
  - Perineal pads for vaginal bleeding and clots (should be less than one saturated perineal pad in 4 hours)

Operative procedures. Hysterectomy can be performed in several ways: vaginally, abdominally, laparoscopically, or via robotic-assisted laparoscopy. The choice of route is based on (Walters, 2020):
- Best approach to treatment of the underlying condition
- Risks and benefits of route
- The need (or lack thereof) to treat additional conditions
- Patient preference
- Surgeon's skill set, preference, and facility availability.

Postoperative care. Nursing care of the woman who has undergone a total abdominal hysterectomy is similar to that of any patient who has had laparoscopic or traditional open abdominal surgery. See the Focused Assessment: Postoperative Nursing Care of the Patient After Open Total Abdominal Hysterectomy box for specific information.

NCLEX EXAMINATION CHALLENGE 66.1

Physiological Integrity

The nurse is caring for a client who just had a laparoscopic total abdominal hysterectomy. Which assessment finding requires **immediate** nursing intervention?

A. Temperature of 99.2°F (37.3°C)
B. One saturated perineal pad per hour
C. Decreased bowel sounds in all quadrants
D. Report of pain level of 5 on a scale of 0 to 10

Care Coordination and Transition Management. Discharge teaching, including activity restrictions, depends on the type of surgical procedure performed.

Home Care Management. Patients who have *uterus-sparing surgeries* usually go home the same day of surgery or after a 1-day hospital stay. They usually experience less postprocedural **pain** and fewer complications than patients who have their uterus and cervix removed. See Chapter 9 for postoperative teaching points.

If the patient had a *laparoscopic hysterectomy,* few limitations in activity are needed. Teach patients who had a *vaginal hysterectomy* or *traditional open hysterectomy* to limit stair climbing for several weeks. If women live alone and are not permitted to drive for several weeks, they may need to arrange for transportation for follow-up surgical visits.

Self-Management Education. Teach the woman who has undergone an abdominal hysterectomy about the expected physical changes, any activity restrictions, diet, sexual activity, wound care (if any), complications, and the need for follow-up care. Some women experience abdominal or shoulder discomfort because of the introduction of carbon dioxide gas during a *laparoscopic* procedure. Teach patients who had a *vaginal* hysterectomy to promptly report excessive or increasing bleeding to their surgeon. See the Patient and Family Education: Preparing for Self-Management: Care After a Total Vaginal or Abdominal Hysterectomy box for more specific health teaching.

PATIENT AND FAMILY EDUCATION: PREPARING FOR SELF-MANAGEMENT

Care After a Total Vaginal or Abdominal Hysterectomy

Expected Physical Changes

- You will no longer have a period, although you may have some vaginal discharge for a few days after you go home.
- It will not be possible for you to become pregnant, and birth control methods are no longer needed. (Condoms should still be used to decrease the chance of getting a sexually transmitted infection [STI].)
- If your ovaries were removed, you may experience menopause symptoms such as hot flushes, night sweats, and vaginal dryness.
- It is normal to tire more easily and require more sleep and rest during the first few weeks after surgery.

Activity (Typically for Vaginal and Traditional Open Surgeries)

- Limit stair climbing to fewer than five times per day.
- Do not lift anything heavier than 5 to 10 lb.
- Gradually increase walking as exercise, but stop before you become fatigued.
- Avoid sitting position for extended periods. When you sit, do not cross your legs at the knees.
- Avoid strenuous activity and exercise for 2 to 6 weeks, depending on which type of surgical procedure was performed.
- Do not drive until your surgeon has told you that it's alright.

Sexual Activity

- Do not engage in sexual intercourse for 6 weeks or as prescribed by your surgeon.
- If you had a vaginal "repair" as part of your surgery, you may experience some tenderness or *pain* the first time you have intercourse because the vaginal walls are tighter. Careful intercourse and the use of water-based lubricants can help reduce this discomfort. It usually goes away with time and stretching of the vagina.

Complications

- Take your temperature twice each day for the first 3 days after surgery. Report fevers of over 100°F (38°C).
- Check any incisions daily for signs of infection (increasing redness, open areas, drainage that is thick or foul smelling, incision *pain*).

Symptoms to Report to Your Surgeon

- Increased vaginal drainage or change in drainage (bloodier, thicker, foul-smelling)
- Signs of infection at an incision site
- Temperature over 100°F (38°C)
- *Pain,* tenderness, redness, or swelling in your calves
- *Pain* or burning on urination

Health Care Resources. Loss of female reproductive organs causes many women to go through the grieving process. Psychological reactions can occur months to years after surgery, particularly if sexual functioning and libido are diminished. Intermittent sadness is normal, but continued feelings of low self-esteem or loss of interest or pleasure in usual activities and pastimes is not expected and should be evaluated.

If desired and culturally appropriate, refer the woman to a religious or spiritual leader, or a community support group, to discuss feelings of sadness. Women identified as being at high risk for psychological problems may need long-term follow-up care or referral to a mental health counselor or clinical psychologist, particularly if they exhibit symptoms of depression.

◆ **Evaluation: Evaluate Outcomes.** Evaluate the care of the patient with leiomyomas on the basis of the identified priority problem. The expected outcomes are that she:

- Has relief of bleeding after effective management

PELVIC ORGAN PROLAPSE

Pathophysiology Review

The pelvic organs are supported by a sling of muscles and tendons, which sometimes become weak and no longer able to hold an organ in place. Uterine prolapse, the most common type of pelvic organ prolapse (POP), can be caused by neuromuscular damage of childbirth; increased intra-abdominal pressure related to pregnancy, obesity, or physical exertion; or weakening of pelvic support caused by decreased estrogen. The stages of uterine prolapse are described by the degree of descent of the uterus through the pelvic floor.

Whenever the uterus is displaced, other structures such as the bladder, rectum, and small intestine can protrude through the vaginal walls (Fig. 66.3). A cystocele is a protrusion of the bladder through the vaginal wall (urinary bladder prolapse), which can lead to stress urinary incontinence (SUI) and urinary tract infections (UTIs). A rectocele is a protrusion of the rectum through a weakened vaginal wall (rectal prolapse).

❖ Interprofessional Collaborative Care

◆ **Assessment: Recognize Cues.** Patients with suspected uterine prolapse may report a feeling of "something falling out," dyspareunia, backache, and/or heaviness or pressure in the pelvis. A pelvic examination performed by the health care provider may reveal a protrusion of the cervix or anterior vaginal wall when the woman is asked to bear down. Listen to her concerns and note signs of anxiety or depression from having long-term symptoms.

Ask the patient whether she has urinary *elimination* problems, such as difficulty emptying her bladder, urinary frequency and urgency, a urinary tract *infection* (UTI), or stress urinary incontinence (SUI) (loss of urine during activities that increase intra-abdominal pressure, such as laughing, coughing, sneezing, or lifting heavy objects). These symptoms may be associated with a cystocele (bladder prolapse).

Diagnostic assessment methods performed by the health care provider may include (Fashokun & Rogers, 2020):

- Speculum and bimanual examination
- Rectovaginal examination
- Pelvic floor muscle testing—accomplished by palpating through the vagina or rectum to determine pelvic floor strength
- Pelvic Organ Prolapse Quantification (POP-Q) system assessment—a staging system that helps to guide surgical planning (if needed)

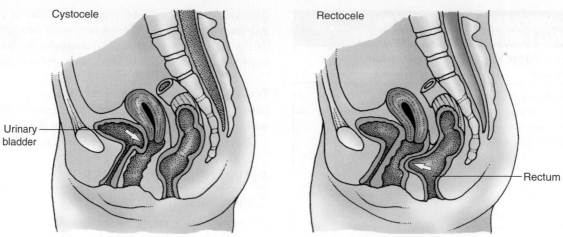

FIG. 66.3 In cystocele, the urinary bladder is displaced downward, causing bulging of the anterior vaginal wall. In rectocele, the rectum is displaced, causing bulging of the posterior vaginal wall.

The health care provider may also order a perineal ultrasound and/or a postvoid residual urine volume (PRUV) test.

◆ **Interventions: Take Action.** Interventions are based on the degree of the POP. Conservative treatment is preferred over surgical treatment when possible.

Nonsurgical Management. Teach women to improve pelvic support and tone by doing pelvic floor muscle exercises (PFMEs, or Kegel exercises). Space-filling devices such a vaginal pessary can be worn to elevate the uterine prolapse. Women with bladder symptoms may benefit from bladder training and attention to complete emptying. Management of a rectocele focuses on promoting bowel *elimination.* The primary health care provider usually prescribes a high-fiber diet, stool softeners, and laxatives.

Surgical Management. Various surgical approaches may be considered for severe symptoms of POP, with preference given to the least invasive approach. Most women with symptomatic POP are treated with a reconstructive procedure, which may or may not include hysterectomy (Jelovsek, 2020). Synthetic mesh is often used in transabdominal POP repair; mesh intended for *transvaginal* surgical repair was discontinued in the United States in 2019 because of complications associated with this procedure (Trabuco & Gebhart, 2020; U.S. Food and Drug Administration [FDA], 2019). Follow preoperative assessment processes as in Chapter 9.

Teach patients who have just had the mesh procedure to avoid strenuous exercise, heavy lifting, and sexual intercourse for 6 weeks. After 6 weeks, the patient may gradually begin to return to regular activities but must be educated about prevention of increasing intra-abdominal pressure (e.g., constipation, weight lifting, cigarette smoking) for a minimum of 3 months to allow proper healing and prevent POP recurrence.

If caring for a patient who previously underwent a transvaginal mesh procedure prior to discontinuation of this product, advise her to see her health care provider if she has any concerns or complications. There is no additional action that is needed, unless complications have arisen since the time of implantation (FDA, 2019).

Alternatives to minimally invasive surgery (MIS) are open surgical techniques. An **anterior colporrhaphy** (anterior repair) tightens the pelvic muscles for better *bladder* support, and is usually performed only after the patient has unsuccessfully tried conservative management and continues to have bothersome symptoms. This procedure is usually deferred until the woman no longer wishes to have children. Teach the patient to adhere to preoperative teaching (as in Chapter 9) and to consult her surgeon about the possible use of transvaginal estrogen prior to the procedure, which helps to maximize vaginal mucosal thickening (Mahajan, 2020).

A vaginal surgical approach is used and may be done as a laparoscopic-assisted procedure. Nursing care for a woman undergoing an anterior repair is similar to that for a woman undergoing a vaginal hysterectomy.

After surgery, the woman will have a urinary catheter in place for approximately 24 hours. Provide appropriate catheter care, and follow other postoperative care recommendations as in Chapter 9. Instruct the patient in how to splint her abdomen to protect sutures, and teach her to limit activities. She should *avoid lifting anything heavier than 5 lb (2.27 kg), strenuous exercises, straining with bowel movements, and sexual intercourse for up to 6 weeks* (Mahajan, 2020). If she is prescribed postoperative vaginal estrogen, teach her how to administer this. Tell the woman to notify her surgeon if she has signs of *infection,* such as fever, persistent *pain,* or purulent, foul-smelling discharge, and to be sure to keep her follow-up appointment after surgery.

Although there are a number of approaches to managing posterior vaginal defects, traditional posterior colporrhaphy, which reduces *rectal* bulging, is used most commonly. If both a cystocele and a rectocele are present, an *anterior and posterior colporrhaphy* (A&P repair) is performed. In this case, the woman may return from surgery with a urinary catheter in place to keep the surgical area clean and dry.

The nursing care after a posterior repair is similar to that after any rectal surgery. After surgery, a low-residue (low-fiber) diet is usually prescribed to decrease bowel movements and allow time for the incision to heal. Instruct the patient to avoid straining when she does have a bowel movement so she does not put pressure on the suture line. Bowel movements are often painful, and she may need pain medication before having a stool. Provide sitz baths or delegate this activity to assistive personnel (AP) to relieve the woman's *pain*; this is a task that the AP can easily perform, and he or she can then report outcomes back to you. Health teaching for the patient undergoing a posterior repair is similar to that for the patient undergoing an anterior repair.

NCLEX EXAMINATION CHALLENGE 66.2

Safe and Effective Care Environment

A client is scheduled for a transvaginal surgical repair this morning. Which assessment finding requires **immediate** nursing intervention?

A. Notation of surgery type with mesh
B. Expression of fear prior to procedure
C. Blood pressure 140/92 mm Hg, P 88, R 20, T 98.8°F
D. Client request for caregiver to come to PACU

ENDOMETRIAL CANCER

Pathophysiology Review

Cancer can affect any organ in the reproductive tract. This chapter covers very common gynecologic cancers. Endometrial cancer (cancer of the uterine lining) is the most common gynecologic malignancy; its incidence continues to rise in the United States, with an estimated 65,620 new cases diagnosed annually (American Cancer Society [ACS], 2020b).

Endometrial cancer grows slowly in most cases, and early symptoms of vaginal bleeding generally lead to prompt evaluation and treatment. As a result, this type of cancer has a generally favorable prognosis. *Adenocarcinoma* of the endometrium is the most common type of uterine cancer. Abnormal uterine bleeding (AUB) is the most common symptom, resulting from estrogen exposure that leads to endometrial hyperplasia (McCance et al., 2019).

The initial growth of the cancer is within the uterine cavity, followed by extension into the myometrium and the cervix. Staging reflects the location of the cancer and whether it has spread. Categorized by histology, type I uterine tumors (the most common) result from endometrial hyperplasia (described above). Type II, which reflect 10% of endometrial cancers, are likely to invade the uterine muscle and metastasize (McCance et al., 2019).

Endometrial cancer is strongly associated with conditions causing prolonged exposure to estrogen without the protective effects of progesterone. Although most cases of endometrial cancer do not involve a genetic predisposition, it is more common in families that have gene mutations for hereditary nonpolyposis colon cancer (HNPCC) (McCance et al., 2019). Other risk factors are listed in Table 66.2.

❖ Interprofessional Collaborative Care

◆ Assessment: Recognize Cues. *The main symptom of endometrial cancer is abnormal uterine bleeding [AUB], especially postmenopausal bleeding. Ask the patient how many tampons or menstrual pads she uses each day. Some women also have a watery, bloody vaginal discharge or low back, low pelvis, or abdominal pain (caused by pressure of the enlarged uterus). Ask the patient to describe the exact location and intensity of her discomfort. A pelvic examination performed by the health care provider may reveal the presence of a palpable uterine mass or uterine polyp. The uterus is enlarged if the cancer is advanced.*

Several laboratory tests are used to determine the overall condition of the woman with possible or confirmed endometrial cancer. A complete blood count may shows anemia due to heavy bleeding. Serum tumor markers to assess for metastasis include CA 125 (cancer antigen 125) and alpha fetoprotein (AFP), both of which may be elevated when ovarian cancer is present (Pagana & Pagana, 2018). A human chorionic gonadotropin (hCG) level may be obtained to rule out pregnancy before treatment for cancer begins.

Transvaginal ultrasound and *endometrial biopsy* are the gold standard diagnostic tests to determine the presence of endometrial thickening and cancer. Saline may be infused during the

---

TABLE 66.2 Risk Factors for Endometrial Cancer

- Early menarche or late menopause
- Use of estrogen after menopause
- Use of birth control pills or tamoxifen
- Use of an intrauterine device (IUD)
- Nulliparity
- History of type 2 diabetes, polycystic ovarian syndrome (PCOS), breast or ovarian cancer, or endometrial hyperplasia
- Treatment of the pelvis with radiation therapy
- Obesity; especially if body mass index at age 18 was high

Data from American Cancer Society. (2019). *Endometrial cancer risk factors.* https://www.cancer.org/cancer/endometrial-cancer/causes-risks-prevention/risk-factors.html; Katz, A. (2019). Obesity-related cancer in women: A clinical review. *American Journal of Nursing, 119*(8), 34-40; and McCance, K., Huether, S., Brashers, V., & Rote, N. (2019). *Pathophysiology: The biologic basis for disease in adults and children* (8th ed.). St. Louis: Mosby.

ultrasound to improve the image of the uterine cavity. This allows for careful evaluation of the uterine cavity and any small lesions that may be missed on other diagnostic tests (Feldman, 2020).

Other diagnostic tests to determine the patient's overall health status and the presence of metastasis (cancer spread) include (Campos & Cohn, 2020; Feldman, 2020):

- Dilation and curettage (when the patient cannot tolerate an endometrial biopsy)
- Hysteroscopy (for better visualization of the endometrial cavity)
- Chest x-ray
- Whole-body imaging of chest, abdomen, and pelvis (CT, MRI, positron emission tomography [PET], or combined PET/CT can be used)
- Liver and bone scans to assess for distant metastasis

During the diagnostic phase, the woman may express fears and concerns about having the disease and the effect on her *sexuality* and/or *reproduction.* After the diagnosis is confirmed, she may express disbelief, anger, depression, anxiety, or withdrawal behaviors. Assess these emotional reactions, and encourage the patient to discuss her feelings. Ask her about how she copes with other stressful events, and assess her support systems.

◆ **Interventions: Take Action.** Surgical removal and cancer staging of the tumor with adjacent lymph nodes are the most important interventions for endometrial cancer. Cancer staging is often done using minimally invasive techniques, such as laparoscopic or robotic-assisted procedures.

Nonsurgical Management. Nonsurgical interventions (radiation therapy and chemotherapy) are typically used after surgery and depend on the surgical staging.

Radiation Therapy. The oncologist may prescribe radiation therapy to be delivered by external beam and/or brachytherapy depending on stage and grade.

The purpose of *brachytherapy* is to prevent disease recurrence. This procedure is used for women who have had their uterus and cervix removed (ACS, 2019). The upper part of the vagina is treated when a cylinder is placed inside it by the radiologist. In high-dose-rate (HDR) brachytherapy, each treatment takes about 10 to 20 minutes. While the radioactive implant is in place, radiation is emitted that can affect other people, so others will not be in the room. Inform the patient that she is restricted to bedrest during the treatment session to prevent dislodgment of the radioactive source. At the completion of treatment, the woman may go home the same day. There are no restrictions for the woman to stay away from her family or the public between treatments. Depending on the oncologist's determination, treatments may be given weekly or daily for at least three doses (ACS, 2019).

The Best Practice for Patient Safety & Quality Care: Health Teaching for the Patient Having Brachytherapy for Gynecologic Cancer box lists additional health teaching for the patient having brachytherapy for gynecologic cancer.

BEST PRACTICE FOR PATIENT SAFETY & QUALITY CARE (QSEN)

Health Teaching for the Patient Having Brachytherapy for Gynecologic Cancer

Teach the patient to report any of these signs and symptoms to the health care provider immediately:
- Heavy vaginal bleeding
- Urethral burning for more than 24 hours
- Blood in the urine
- Extreme fatigue
- Severe diarrhea
- Fever over 100°F (38°C)
- Abdominal *pain*

External beam radiation therapy (*EBRT*) may be used to treat any stage of endometrial cancer in combination with surgery, brachytherapy, and/or chemotherapy. The treatment is given on an ambulatory care basis usually 5 days a week for 4 to 6 weeks, with each session taking less than 30 minutes (ACS, 2019). Tissue around the tumor and pelvic wall nodes also is treated. *Teach the patient to monitor for signs of skin breakdown, especially in the perineal area; to avoid sunbathing; and to avoid washing the markings outlining the treatment site.*

Reactions to radiation therapy vary. Some women feel "radioactive" or "unclean" after treatments and may exhibit withdrawal behaviors. Reassure them by correcting any misconceptions. Chapter 20 discusses nursing care of patients receiving radiation therapy in more detail.

Drug Therapy. Multiagent *chemotherapy* is used as palliative treatment in advanced and recurrent disease when it has spread to distant parts of the body, but it is not always effective (Campos & Cohn, 2020). For that reason, it is important to also consider other methods of palliative care (see Chapter 8).

A common side effect of chemotherapy used to treat endometrial cancer is alopecia (hair loss). Remind the patient of this possibility before treatment starts. Chapter 20 describes chemotherapy and general nursing care during treatment.

Complementary and Integrative Health. Every woman experiences cancer differently. Many complementary and integrative therapies have evidence of benefit in decreasing the side effects of drug therapy and boosting the immune system. Provide your patient with information that will help her make informed, evidence-based decisions. Encourage her to check with her oncologist and/or pharmacist because some integrative therapies can be harmful or interfere with cancer treatment. Current evidence-based information is available at the American Cancer Society (www.cancer.org) and Canadian Cancer Society (www.cancer.ca) websites about mind-body therapies, healing touch, herbs, vitamins, nutrition, and biologic therapies.

Surgical Management. The most common surgical procedure to address endometrial cancer involves the removal of the uterus, fallopian tubes, and ovaries (total hysterectomy and bilateral salpingo-oophorectomy [BSO]). Laparoscopy or robotic-assisted surgery is preferred when the disease is confined to the uterus (Cohn, 2020), as these surgeries are usually less expensive and have fewer complications and shorter hospital stays. If minimally invasive surgery is not possible, laparotomy can be considered. Vaginal or abdominal hysterectomy are also options.

Care Coordination and Transition Management. Home care after surgery for endometrial cancer is the same as that after a hysterectomy. Patients who are receiving chemotherapy or radiation therapy are treated on an ambulatory care basis. Most women are surprised by the fatigue caused by radiation and chemotherapy. Help the patient and her family plan daily activities around treatment requirements so that she can effectively pace herself.

High doses of radiation cause sterility, and vaginal shrinkage can occur. Vaginal dilators can be used with water-soluble lubricants for 10 minutes three to four times weekly until sexual activity resumes, generally within 4 weeks (ACS, 2020c).

Often patients experience emotional crises because of the physical effects of cancer treatments. Radical hysterectomy may be seen as mutilating. Both radiation and chemotherapy have side effects that change physical appearance and body image. Women may have a grief reaction to these changes. The feelings of loss depend on the visibility of the loss and the perception or reality of loss of function. Help the patient adapt to the body changes. Using a calm and accepting approach, encourage self-management as soon as her physical condition is stable.

Encourage patients and their families to discuss their feelings. Refer to support services such as a certified hospital chaplain or other spiritual leader, social worker, or counselor. In the United States, local American Cancer Society chapters provide written materials about endometrial cancer and information about local support groups. Each province in Canada also has a division of the Canadian Cancer Society (www.cancer.ca).

Death can occur with or without treatment. The goal is for the patient to meet and exceed the 5-year survival mark without a recurrence of disease. If the tumor recurs and cure is not likely, the woman and her family need to consider hospice care and whether she can be cared for in the home. If nursing care is needed at home, the hospital nurse or case manager makes referrals to a home health care agency. A referral to a social services agency may be needed if the patient needs financial assistance for treatment and long-term follow-up.

OVARIAN CANCER

Pathophysiology Review

Ovarian cancer is the leading cause of gynecologic cancer death, and the second most common type of gynecologic cancer (Chen & Berek, 2019). Most ovarian cancers are epithelial tumors that grow on the surface of the ovaries. These tumors grow rapidly, spread quickly, and are often bilateral. Tumor cells spread by direct extension into nearby organs and through blood and lymph circulation to distant sites (McCance et al., 2019). Free-floating cancer cells also spread through the abdomen to seed new sites, usually accompanied by ascites (abdominal fluid).

Ovarian cancer seems to be disordered growth in response to excessive exposure to estrogen. This would explain the

TABLE 66.3	Risk Factors for Ovarian Cancer

- Middle to older age
- *BRCA1* or *BRCA2* gene mutations
- Infertility
- Difficulty getting pregnant
- Nulliparity
- History of endometriosis
- History of breast, uterine, or colorectal (colon) cancer (especially Lynch syndrome, hereditary nonpolyposis colorectal cancer [HNPCC])
- Of Eastern European or Ashkenazi Jewish background

Data from Centers for Disease Control and Prevention (CDC). (2019). What are the risk factors for ovarian cancer? https://www.cdc.gov/cancer/ovarian/basic_info/risk_factors.htm; and Lu, K., & Schmeler, K. (2020). Lynch syndrome (Hereditary nonpolyposis colorectal cancer): Screening and prevention of endometrial and ovarian cancer. In *UpToDate*. Goff, B. (Ed.). Waltham, MA.

protective effects of pregnancies and oral contraceptive use, both of which interrupt the monthly estrogen exposure.

Risk factors include older age, obesity, nulliparity, use of estrogen alone (without progesterone), and certain infertility diagnoses (ACS, 2020a; Centers for Disease Control and Prevention [CDC], 2019b). Women with genetic mutations of *BRCA1* or *BRCA2* are at higher risk (National Ovarian Cancer Coalition, 2020a). Of these, some choose to have a *risk-reducing bilateral salpingo-oophorectomy* (BSO) (see Table 66.1) to prevent ovarian cancer. For many years, the use of talcum powder was associated with development of ovarian cancer; the most current research shows that this correlation is not statistically significant (O'Brien et al., 2020). Table 66.3 lists known and suspected risk factors for ovarian cancer.

Formerly, it was thought that ovarian cancer was a "silent" disease where symptoms did not present until the late stages of the disease. Evidence now shows that common symptoms of bloating, urinary urgency or frequency, difficulty eating, feeling full, and pelvic pain are often experienced very early (Chen & Berek, 2019). Caught early, ovarian cancer is treatable in the early stages (ACS, 2020a). However, many women do not seek care because they associate those and other vague symptoms (weight gain, constipation, bloating) with menopause (Bohnenkamp et al., 2019). Survival rates are low, therefore, because it is often not detected until its late stages (ACS, 2020a).

❖ Interprofessional Collaborative Care

◆ **Assessment: Recognize Cues.** As a matter of prevention, it is important for nurses to teach women to *"think ovarian"* even at the onset of vague abdominal and GI symptoms. Most women with ovarian cancer have had mild symptoms for several months but may have thought they were caused by normal perimenopausal changes or stress. They may report abdominal **pain** or swelling or have vague GI disturbances such as indigestion and gas. Ask the patient if she has had urinary frequency or incontinence, unexpected weight loss, and/or vaginal bleeding.

Complications of advanced metastatic cancer include (Chen & Berek, 2019):

- Pleural effusion
- Venous thromboembolism (VTE)
- Bowel obstruction

On pelvic examination, an abdominal mass may not be palpable until it reaches a size of 4 to 6 inches (10 to 15 cm). Any enlarged ovary found after menopause should be evaluated as though it were malignant.

A cancer antigen test, *CA 125,* measures the presence of damaged endometrial and uterine tissue in the blood. It may be elevated if ovarian cancer is present, but it can also be elevated in patients with endometriosis, fibroids, pelvic inflammatory disease, pregnancy, and even menses (Pagana & Pagana, 2018). It is also useful for monitoring a patient's progress during and after treatment. Abdominal and pelvic CT scans or MRI is most commonly used to evaluate for metastasis. A chest x-ray is obtained to evaluate for the presence of pleural effusion, metastases, and mediastinal lymphadenopathy (Chen & Berek, 2019). A liver profile may be ordered if there is ascites.

The woman with ovarian cancer has concerns similar to those described for the patient with other gynecologic cancers. Because the cancer is often diagnosed in an advanced stage, thoughts of death and dying, menopause, and loss of fertility may come as a shock.

NCLEX EXAMINATION CHALLENGE 66.3

Psychosocial Integrity

The nurse is preparing a client for surgery related to ovarian cancer. When the client states, "I'm just going to die anyway; why do I even need this surgery?" what is the appropriate nursing response?

A. "We don't know that you will die from this."
B. "Are you thinking of canceling the surgery?"
C. "Ovarian cancer has an unfavorable prognosis."
D. "If the condition is fatal, hospice can provide care."

◆ **Interventions: Take Action.** Nursing care of the patient with ovarian cancer is similar to that for the patient with endometrial or cervical cancer. The options for treatment depend on the extent of the cancer and usually include surgery first, followed by chemotherapy. Radiation may be used for treatment of metastasis, but is not used often for ovarian cancer alone as a treatment method (National Ovarian Cancer Coalition, 2020b).

Diagnosis depends on findings during surgical exploration and diagnostic testing. A total abdominal hysterectomy, bilateral salpingo-oophorectomy (BSO; removal of the ovaries and fallopian tubes), and pelvic and para-aortic lymph node dissection are usually performed. Tumors are staged during surgery. Very large tumors that cannot be removed are debulked (reduced). These procedures can be performed via laparoscopic technique or robotic-assisted laparoscopy to decrease recovery time, minimize *pain,* and reduce postoperative complications.

Nursing care of the patient is similar to that for any patient having abdominal surgery (see Chapter 9). As for any patient after abdominal surgery, assess vital signs and *pain* and maintain catheters and drains. Teach her the importance of antiembolism stockings, incentive spirometry, and early ambulation. Evaluate for respiratory or urinary *infection.* Assess vital signs and monitor the quantity and quality of urine output.

After removing and staging ovarian cancer, *chemotherapy* is used often. See Chapter 20 for care of the patient with cancer for more information. Chemotherapeutic agents may be given IV and/or intraperitoneally. Intraperitoneal (IP) therapy is described in Chapter 15.

Care Coordination and Transition Management. Teach patients discharged to home to avoid tampons, douches, and sexual intercourse for at least 6 weeks or as instructed by the surgeon. Remind them to keep their follow-up surgical appointment and to follow the surgeon's other recommendations about resuming usual activities.

Refer patients and their families to Gilda's Club within their local demographic (e.g., www.gildasclubnyc.org) and the National Ovarian Cancer Coalition (NOCC) (www.ovarian.org) for more information and support groups. In Canada, Ovarian Cancer Canada (www.ovariancanada.org) is available for the same purpose.

Ovarian cancer has a high recurrence rate. After recurrence, the cancer is treatable but no longer curable. A once-daily oral pill, Zejula (niraparib), is now approved for *maintenance therapy,* which is a type of treatment given after a favorable response to chemotherapy to keep ovarian cancer from recurring (GSK, 2020). If the patient refuses maintenance therapy, or if maintenance therapy is unsuccessful, the patient may deny symptoms at first or express feelings of anger and grief. The patient and family are often fearful of the outcome. Provide encouragement and support during this difficult time and refer to grief counseling, spiritual leaders (if desired), and community support groups. For patients with advanced metastatic disease, collaborate with members of the interprofessional team for possible referral to hospice. Chapter 8 discusses end-of-life care.

CERVICAL CANCER

Pathophysiology Review

The uterine cervix is covered with squamous cells on the outer cervix and columnar (glandular) cells that line the endocervical canal. Papanicolaou (Pap) tests sample cells from both areas as a screening test for cervical cancer. The squamocolumnar junction is the *transformation zone* where most cell abnormalities occur. The adolescent has more columnar cells exposed on the outer cervix, which may be one reason that she is more vulnerable to sexually transmitted infections (STIs) and human immune deficiency virus (HIV). In contrast, in the menopausal woman the squamocolumnar junction may be higher up in the endocervical canal, making it difficult to sample for a Pap test.

Premalignant changes are classified on a continuum from cervical intraepithelial neoplasia (dysplasia) to cervical carcinoma in situ (where the full epithelial thickness of the cervix is involved) to invasive carcinoma (McCance & Huether, 2019).

Most cervical cancers arise from the squamous cells on the outside of the cervix. The other cancers arise from the mucus-secreting glandular cells (adenocarcinoma) in the endocervical canal. The disease spreads by direct extension to the vaginal mucosa, lower uterine segment, parametrium, pelvic wall, bladder, and bowel. Metastasis is usually confined to the pelvis, but distant spread can occur through lymphatic spread and the circulation to the liver, lungs, or bones.

TABLE 66.4 Risk Factors for Cervical Cancer
• Infection with human papillomavirus (HPV)
• Infection with chlamydia
• Smoking
• Being immunocompromised (e.g., having HIV, or taking immunosuppressant drugs for an autoimmune condition)
• Multiparity (multiple births)
• Obesity
• Women whose mothers took diethylstilbestrol (DES; a hormone to prevent miscarriage) between 1940 and 1971
• Long-term use of oral contraceptives
• Use of an intrauterine device (IUD)
• Having multiple full-term pregnancies
• Having a first full-term pregnancy earlier than age 17
• Having a family history of cervical cancer

Data from Centers for Disease Control and Prevention (CDC). (2020). *Risk factors for cervical cancer*. https://www.cancer.org/cancer/cervical-cancer/causes-risks-prevention/risk-factors.html; and Katz, A. (2019). Obesity-related cancer in women: A clinical review. *American Journal of Nursing, 119*(8), 34-40.

Human papillomavirus *infection* (HPV) is the most common type of sexually transmitted infection (STI) in the United States (CDC, 2019a). Almost all women will have HPV sometime in their life, but not all types lead to cancer. Most cases of cervical cancer are caused by certain types of HPV. The high-risk HPV types 16 and 18 are responsible for 70% of cervical cancers (World Health Organization [WHO], 2019). They impair the tumor-suppressor gene and cause most of the cervical cancers. The unrestricted tissue growth can spread, becoming invasive and metastatic (McCance et al., 2019). Risk factors for cervical cancer are listed in Table 66.4. Teach patients how to reduce their risk of sexual exposure to HPV by being immunized with an HPV vaccine, and using condoms during sexual intimacy.

Health Promotion and Maintenance

Girls and young women should be immunized with one of the HPV vaccines:

- *Gardasil* (available in Canada)—available for ages 9 through 26
- *Gardasil 9* (available in the United States and Canada)—available for ages 9 to 26; can be administered until age 45
- *Cervarix* (available in Canada)—available for ages 9 through 25

In addition to being immunized, women should be taught to follow the U.S. Preventive Services Task Force recommendations on Papanicolaou (Pap) tests and HPV testing (U.S. Preventive Services Task Force, 2018). See Chapter 69 for a thorough discussion of the importance of HPV vaccination; Pap and HPV testing recommendations; and associated patient teaching.

Canadian guidelines for cervical cancer screening were last established in 2013, as of this writing. These recommend no screening for women age 19 years and younger, or older than 70 years (if she has had three negative Pap tests over the past 10 years) (Canadian Task Force on Preventive Health Care, 2013). For women ages 20 to 24, no routine screening is recommended. For women ages 25 to 69, screening is recommended every 3 years.

❖ Interprofessional Collaborative Care

◆ Assessment: Recognize Cues

Physical Assessment/Signs and Symptoms. The patient who has preinvasive cancer is often asymptomatic. The classic symptoms of invasive cancer include painless vaginal bleeding, which may be irregular or heavy, and bleeding after sexual intercourse. As the cancer grows, bleeding increases in frequency, duration, and amount and may become continuous. Other symptoms may include pelvic or back pain, hematuria, hematochezia, or vaginal passage of stool or urine, which accompanies advanced disease (Frumovitz, 2020).

A physical examination may not reveal any abnormalities regarding early preinvasive cervical cancer. The internal pelvic examination may identify late-stage disease.

❓ CLINICAL JUDGMENT CHALLENGE 66.1

Safety; Patient-Centered Care

A 39-year-old female client reports that she has heavy menstrual periods that have been irregular in nature for the last couple of years. For the last 3 months, the frequency of the periods has increased, and she has noticed that she has begun bleeding after sexual intercourse. She says she wants to have a hysterectomy so that she will not bleed anymore, because she had a friend who had that procedure and is very happy not having periods.

1. **Recognize Cues:** What assessment information in this client situation is the most important and immediate concern for the nurse? (Hint: Identify the **relevant** information *first* to determine what is most important.)
2. **Analyze Cues:** What client conditions are consistent with the **most relevant** information? (Hint: Think about priority collaborative problems that support and contradict the information presented in this situation.)
3. **Prioritize Hypotheses:** Which possibilities or explanations are **most likely** to be present in this client situation? Which possibilities or explanations are the most serious? (Hint: Consider all possibilities and determine their urgency and risk for this client.)
4. **Generate Solutions:** What actions would most likely achieve the desired outcomes for this client? Which actions should be **avoided** or are **potentially harmful**? (Hint: Determine the desired outcomes first to decide which interventions are appropriate and those that should be avoided.)
5. **Take Action:** Which actions are the most appropriate and how should they be implemented? In what **priority order** should they be implemented? (Hint: Consider health teaching, documentation, requested health care provider orders or prescriptions, nursing skills, collaboration with or referral to health team members, etc.)
6. **Evaluate Outcomes:** What client assessment would indicate that the nurse's actions were **effective**? (Hint: Think about signs that would indicate an improvement, decline, or unchanged client condition.)

Diagnostic Assessment. Taken during the Pap test, an *HPV-typing DNA test* of the cervical sample can determine the presence of one or more high-risk types (CDC, 2020e; Emory Winship Cancer Institute, 2020). The health care provider may perform a colposcopic examination to view the transformation zone. Colposcopy is a procedure in which application of an acetic acid solution is applied to the cervix. The cervix is then examined under magnification with a bright filter light that enhances the visualization of the characteristics of dysplasia or cancer. If abnormal tissue is recognized, multiple biopsies of the cervical tissue are performed.

If atypical glandular cells are suspected, the health care provider may perform a cervical biopsy in the form of a punch biopsy, a cone biopsy, or *endocervical curettage* (scraping of the endocervix wall) as well. Inform her that a small amount of bleeding is expected for several days after this procedure, and that she should not douche, use tampons, or have sexual intercourse for at least a week.

◆ **Interventions: Take Action.** Interventions for the woman with cervical cancer are similar to those for endometrial cancer: surgery, which is possibly followed by radiation and chemotherapy for late-stage disease.

Nonsurgical Management. Radiation therapy can be used to treat certain stages of cervical cancer, or cervical cancer that has spread to other organs. Brachytherapy and external beam radiation therapy (EBRT) are the two types used.

A combination of chemotherapy and radiation, referred to as *concurrent chemoradiation,* may also be used. This treatment modality has been shown to be effective because the chemotherapy enhances the effect of the radiation. See Chapter 20 for more information about the general nursing care for the patient on chemotherapy and radiation.

Surgical Management. Choice of surgical management approach is dependent on the patient's overall health, desire for future childbearing, tumor size and stage, cancer cell type, degree of lymph node involvement, and patient preference.

The loop electrosurgical excision procedure (LEEP) is short (10 to 30 minutes) and is performed in a health care provider's office or an ambulatory care setting with a local anesthetic injected into the cervix. A thin loop-wire electrode that transmits a painless electrical current is used to cut away affected tissue. LEEP (Fig. 66.4) is both a diagnostic procedure and a treatment because it provides a specimen that can be examined by a pathologist to ensure that the lesion was completely removed. Spotting (very scant bleeding) and slight *pain* after the procedure is common. Teach patients to adhere for 3 weeks, or the time frame recommended by the health care provider, to the restrictions listed in the Patient and Family Education: Preparing for Self-Management: Care After Local Cervical Ablation Therapies box.

Laser surgery is also an office procedure done under local anesthesia to address early cancers. A laser beam is directed through the vagina to vaporize abnormal cells. A small amount of bleeding occurs with the procedure, and the woman may have a slight vaginal discharge. Healing occurs in 6 to 12 weeks. A disadvantage of this procedure is that no specimen is available for study.

PATIENT AND FAMILY EDUCATION: PREPARING FOR SELF-MANAGEMENT

Care After Local Cervical Ablation Therapies

- Refrain from sexual intercourse.
- Do not use tampons.
- Do not douche.
- Take showers rather than tub baths.
- Avoid lifting heavy objects.
- Report any heavy vaginal bleeding, foul-smelling drainage, or fever.

Cryosurgery involves freezing of the cancer, causing subsequent necrosis. The procedure is usually painless, although some women have slight cramping after it. Teach the patient that she will have heavy, watery brown discharge for several weeks after the procedure. Instruct her to follow the restrictions in the Patient and Family Education: Preparing for Self-Management: Care After Local Cervical Ablation Therapies box.

In cases of microinvasive cancer, a *conization* can remove the affected tissue while still preserving fertility. This procedure is done when the lesion cannot be visualized by colposcopic examination. A cone-shaped area of cervix is removed surgically and sent to the laboratory to determine the extent of the cancer. Potential complications from this procedure include hemorrhage and uterine perforation. Long-term follow-up care is needed because new cancers can develop.

For women who may wish to become pregnant in the future, a *radical trachelectomy* can be done. Going through the vagina or abdomen (sometimes laparoscopically), the cervix and upper part of the vagina are removed, leaving the body of the uterus intact (ACS, 2020d). A "purse-string" stitch is made, which then functions as an artificial opening of the cervix, and close lymph nodes are removed. This procedure can help some women to carry a pregnancy to term and deliver by cesarean section, although the risk of miscarriage still exists (ACS, 2016b).

A *total hysterectomy* may be performed as treatment of microinvasive cancer if the woman does not wish to become pregnant in the future. A laparoscopic approach is commonly used, although evidence shows that women who have the open approach have a lesser chance of recurrence of cancer, and live longer lives (ACS, 2020d). Lymph node dissection can be performed at the same time, if needed. Care for patients undergoing hysterectomy is discussed in the Sexuality Concept Exemplar: Uterine Leiomyoma section earlier in this chapter.

Care Coordination and Transition Management. As with all patients who have undergone treatment, provide discharge teaching that is congruent with the procedure used. Refer to psychosocial support as needed, and encourage the patient to keep all follow-up appointments.

VULVOVAGINITIS

Pathophysiology Review

Vaginal discharge and itching are two common problems experienced by most women at some time in their lives. Vaginal infections may be transmitted sexually and nonsexually. Gonorrhea, syphilis, chlamydia, and herpes simplex virus infections are sexually transmitted infections (STIs) discussed in Chapter 69.

Vulvovaginitis is inflammation of the lower genital tract resulting from a disturbance of the balance of hormones and flora in the vagina and vulva. It may be characterized by itching, change in vaginal discharge, odor, or lesions. Pediculosis pubis, known as crab lice or "crabs," and scabies are parasitic infections of the vulvar skin that are *sexually* transmitted. The most common causes of *nonsexually* transmitted infections include (U.S. National Library of Medicine, 2020):

- Infections
  - Yeast infections

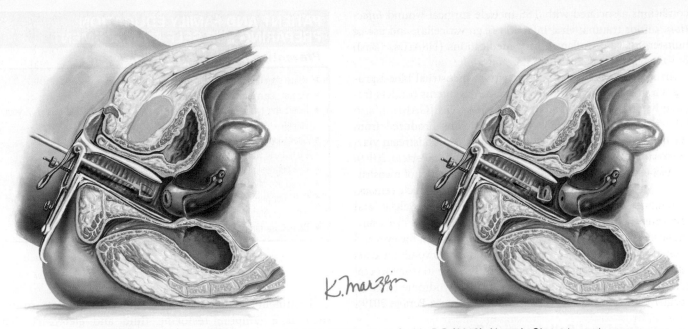

FIG. 66.4 Loop electrosurgical excision procedure (LEEP). (From Smith, R.P. [2018]. *Netter's Obstetrics and Gynecology* [3rd ed.]. Philadelphia: Elsevier.)

- Chemicals
  - Spermicide
  - Vaginal sponges
  - Feminine hygiene sprays
  - Bubble baths and soaps
  - Use of new or different laundry detergent
- Other causes
  - Wearing tight-fitting clothing
  - Wiping from back to front, introducing bacteria from stool into the vagina

Some women may have an *itch-scratch-itch cycle*, in which the itching leads to scratching, which causes excoriation that then must heal. As healing takes place, itching occurs again. If the cycle is not interrupted, the chronic scratching may lead to the white, thickened skin of lichen planus. This dry, leathery skin cracks easily, increasing the risk for *infection.*

❖ Interprofessional Collaborative Care

Assess for vulvovaginitis by asking questions about the symptoms, assisting with a pelvic examination, and obtaining vaginal smears for laboratory testing. Ask if the patient is experiencing an itching or burning sensation, erythema (redness), edema, and/or superficial skin ulcers. Use a nonjudgmental approach and provide reassurance during the assessment because the patient may be embarrassed or afraid to discuss her symptoms. Encourage her to talk about her problem and its effect on *sexuality.*

Interventions for vulvovaginitis depend on the specific vaginal *infection.* Proper health habits can benefit treatment. Instruct the patient to get enough rest and sleep, observe good dietary habits, exercise regularly, and use good personal hygiene. Teach her about how to manage the condition and prevent further infections per the instructions in the Patient and Family Education: Preparing for Self-Management: Prevention of Vulvovaginitis box.

Cold compresses can be recommended, as can a lukewarm sitz bath for 5 to 10 minutes several times a day. Topical drugs such as estrogens and lidocaine may be prescribed to relieve

---

PATIENT AND FAMILY EDUCATION: PREPARING FOR SELF-MANAGEMENT
Prevention of Vulvovaginitis

- Wear cotton underwear.
- Avoid wearing tight clothing, such as pantyhose or tight jeans, because it can cause chafing. You can also get hot and sweaty, which can increase the risk for *infection.*
- Always wipe front to back after having a bowel movement or urinating.
- Use fragrance-free laundry detergent.
- During a bath or shower, cleanse inner labial mucosa with water, not soap.
- Do not douche or use feminine hygiene sprays.
- Choose other methods of contraception instead of spermicide or vaginal sponges, which can irritate the condition
- If your sexual partner has an *infection* of the sex organs, do not have intercourse with him or her until he or she has been treated.
- You are more likely to get an *infection* if you are pregnant, have diabetes, take oral contraceptive drugs, or are menopausal.
- Practice vulvar self-examination monthly.
- If irritation is due to a yeast infection, fully take the prescribed drug treatment as ordered by the primary health care provider.

---

itching. Encourage the patient to wear breathable fabrics such as cotton and to avoid irritants or allergens in products such as laundry detergents or bath products.

Treatment of pediculosis and scabies is used if needed and includes:

- Applying a topical pediculicide to the affected area as prescribed
- Cleaning affected clothes, bedding, and towels
- Disinfecting the home environment (Lice cannot live for more than 24 hours away from the body.)

TOXIC SHOCK SYNDROME
Pathophysiology Review

Toxic shock syndrome (TSS) can result from leaving a tampon, contraceptive sponge, or diaphragm in the vagina. Other conditions associated with TSS include surgical wound *infection,* minor trauma, viral infection (e.g., varicella), and use of nonsteroidal anti-inflammatory medications (NSAIDs) (Bush & Vazquez-Pertejo, 2019). *TSS can be fatal.*

In infection related to menstruation, menstrual blood provides a growth medium for *Staphylococcus aureus* (or, less frequently, group A beta-hemolytic *Streptococcus* [GABHS], also known as *Streptococcus pyogenes*). Exotoxins produced from the bacteria cross the vaginal mucosa to the bloodstream via a mucosal break or via the uterus (Bush & Vazquez-Pertejo, 2019).

TSS usually develops within 5 days after the onset of menstruation. Most common symptoms include fever (which remains elevated despite treatment), diffuse macular rash, myalgias, and hypotension. The rash associated with TSS often looks like a sunburn, and patients often develop broken capillaries in the eyes and skin. TSS due to *Staphylococcus aureus* also causes vomiting, diarrhea, thrombocytopenia, and confusion; TSS due to streptococcal infection can cause acute respiratory distress syndrome (ARDS), coagulopathy, and hepatic damage (Bush & Vazquez-Pertejo, 2019).

❖ Interprofessional Collaborative Care

Educate all women on prevention of TSS as covered in the Patient and Family Education: Preparing for Self-Management: Prevention of Toxic Shock Syndrome box.

PATIENT AND FAMILY EDUCATION: PREPARING FOR SELF-MANAGEMENT
Prevention of Toxic Shock Syndrome

- Wash your hands before inserting a tampon.
- Do not use a tampon if it is dirty.
- Insert the tampon carefully to avoid injuring the delicate tissue in your vagina.
- Change your tampon every 3 to 6 hours.
- Do not use superabsorbent tampons.
- Use perineal pads ("sanitary napkins") (instead of tampons) at night.
- Avoid use of insertable contraceptive devices
- Call your primary health care provider if you experience a sudden onset of high temperature, vomiting, or diarrhea.
- Do not use tampons at all if you have had toxic shock syndrome.

Treatment includes removal of the *infection* source, such as a tampon; restoring fluid and electrolyte balance; administering drugs to manage hypotension; and IV antibiotics. Other measures may include transfusions to reverse low platelet counts and corticosteroids to treat skin changes.

GET READY FOR THE NEXT-GENERATION NCLEX® EXAMINATION!

Key Points
Review these Key Points for each NCLEX Examination Client Needs Category.

Safe and Effective Care Environment
- Collaborate with the interprofessional team when planning care for patients with gynecologic problems. **QSEN: Teamwork and Collaboration**
- Perform a focused physical assessment for patients reporting gynecologic problems. **QSEN: Patient-Centered Care**
- Remind patients wanting to use complementary and integrative therapies to check with their health care provider first. **QSEN: Safety**
- Teach patients receiving external beam radiation therapy how to preserve skin integrity. **QSEN: Safety**

Health Promotion and Maintenance
- Teach women to follow the American Cancer Society's screening guidelines for prevention and early detection of gynecologic cancers. **QSEN: Evidence-Based Practice**
- Teach women methods of practicing safer sex to prevent *infection* of the reproductive tract. **QSEN: Evidence-Based Practice**
- Teach women at risk for gynecologic cancer to be screened and to follow early detection guidelines. **QSEN: Evidence-Based Practice**
- Teach women methods to prevent toxic shock syndrome (TSS). **QSEN: Safety**

Psychosocial Integrity
- Explain all tests, procedures, and treatments, especially if they cause *pain.* **Ethics**
- Assess patient's understanding regarding the fact that some procedures related to reproductive problems cause infertility. **Ethics**
- Assess the patient's anxiety before surgery and allow expression of feelings of fear or grief. **QSEN: Patient-Centered Care**
- Assess the patient's reaction to the possible loss of *reproduction* ability, and concerns about *sexuality* and changes in body image. **QSEN: Patient-Centered Care**
- Refer patients with gynecologic cancer to resources that can provide support. **QSEN: Patient-Centered Care**

Physiological Integrity
- Coordinate postoperative care for women having gynecologic surgery. **QSEN: Teamwork and Collaboration**
- Provide self-care health teaching for the woman who had gynecologic surgery. **QSEN: Patient-Centered Care**
- When caring for a patient who has a radioactive implant, use best safety practices. **QSEN: Evidence-Based Practices**
- Observe for and report complications after surgery, including *infection, pain,* and *elimination* problems. **Clinical Judgment**
- Assess for and report symptoms associated with toxic shock syndrome. **Clinical Judgment**

MASTERY QUESTIONS

1. What teaching will the nurse provide to a 30-year-old female client who has never been sexually active about decreasing her risk of developing cervical cancer? **Select all that apply.**
   A. "You cannot lower the risk for cervical cancer."
   B. "You cannot receive the Gardasil-9 immunization."
   C. "Use condoms when you plan to be sexually intimate."
   D. "Over-the-counter contraceptive methods can be used to prevent HPV."
   E. "Having an annual Pap test will decrease your chances of cervical cancer."

2. The nurse has provided teaching to a client with vulvovaginitis. Which client statement indicates that nursing intervention is required? **Select all that apply.**
   A. "I will wipe from the front to the back."
   B. "I will wash with fragranced soap to prevent odor."
   C. "I am going to the store now to buy cotton underwear."
   D. "I will use fragrance-free laundry detergents in the future."
   E. "I am going to take all of the medicine the provider prescribed."

REFERENCES

Asterisk (*) indicates a classic or definitive work on this subject.

American Cancer Society (ACS). (2019). *Radiation therapy for endometrial cancer.* Retrieved from https://www.cancer.org/cancer/endometrial-cancer/treating/radiation.html.

American Cancer Society (ACS). (2020a). *About ovarian cancer.* Retrieved from https://www.cancer.org/cancer/ovarian-cancer/about/what-is-ovarian-cancer.html.

American Cancer Society (ACS). (2020b). *Key statistics for endometrial cancer.* Retrieved from https://www.cancer.org/cancer/endometrial-cancer/about/key-statistics.html.

American Cancer Society (ACS). (2020c). *Radiation therapy can affect the sex life of females with cancer.* Retrieved from http://www.cancer.org/treatment/treatments-and-side-effects/physical-side-effects/fertility-and-sexual-side-effects/sexuality-for-women-with-cancer/pelvic-radiation.html.

American Cancer Society (ACS). (2020d). *Surgery for cervical cancer.* Retrieved from https://www.cancer.org/cancer/cervical-cancer/treating/surgery.html.

American Cancer Society (ACS). (2020e). *The HPV DNA test.* Retrieved from https://www.cancer.org/cancer/cervical-cancer/prevention-and-early-detection/hpv-test.html.

Bohnenkamp, S., McClurg, E., & Bohnenkamp, Z. (2019). What medical-surgical nurses need to know about caring for patients with epithelial ovarian cancer: Part I. *Medsurg Nursing, 28*(5), 334–338.

Bradley, L. (2020). Uterine fibroids (leiomyomas): Hysteroscopic myomectomy. In T. Falcone (Ed.), *UpToDate.* Waltham, MA.

Bush, L., & Vazquez-Pertejo, M. (2019). *Toxic shock syndrome.* https://www.merckmanuals.com/professional/infectious-diseases/gram-positive-cocci/toxic-shock-syndrome-tss.

Campos, S., & Cohn, D. (2020). Treatment of metastatic endometrial cancer. In B. Goff, & D. Dizon (Eds.), *UpToDate.* Waltham, MA.

*Canadian Task Force on Preventive Health Care. (2013). Cervical Cancer: Summary of recommendations for clinical and policy-makers. Retrieved from https://canadiantaskforce.ca/guidelines/published-guidelines/cervical-cancer/.

Centers for Disease Control and Prevention (CDC). (2019a). *Genital HPV infection: Fact sheet.* www.cdc.gov/std/hpv/stdfact-hpv.htm.

Centers for Disease Control and Prevention (CDC). (2019b). What are the risk factors for ovarian cancer? Retrieved from https://www.cdc.gov/cancer/ovarian/basic_info/risk_factors.htm.

Chen, L., & Berek, J. (2019). Epithelial carcinoma of the ovary, fallopian tube, and peritoneum: Clinical features and diagnosis. In B. Goff, & D. Dizon (Eds.), *UpToDate.* Waltham, MA.

Cohn, D. (2020). Endometrial carcinoma: Staging and surgical treatment. In B. Goff (Ed.), *UpToDate.* Waltham, MA.

Emory Winship Cancer Institute. (2020). *HPV DNA test.* https://www.cancerquest.org/patients/detection-and-diagnosis/hpv-dna-test.

Fashokun, T., & Rogers, R. (2020). Pelvic organ prolapse in women: Diagnostic evaluation. In L. Brubaker (Ed.), *UpToDate.* Waltham, MA.

Feldman, S. (2020). Overview of evaluation of the endometrium for malignant or premalignant disease. In D. Levine, & B. Goff (Eds.), *UpToDate.* Waltham, MA.

Frumovitz, M. (2020). Invasive cervical cancer: Epidemiology, risk factors, clinical manifestations, and diagnosis. In B. Goff, & D. Dizon (Eds.), *UpToDate.* Waltham, MA.

GSK. (2020). *Benefits of Zejula.* https://www.zejula.com/en/benefits-of-ZEJULA.

Jelovsek, J. (2020). Pelvic organ prolapse in women: Choosing a primary surgical procedure. In L. Brubaker (Ed.), *UpToDate.* Waltham, MA.

Johnson, C., George, M., & Fader, A. (2017). Distress screening: Evaluating a protocol for gynecologic cancer survivors. *Clinical Journal of Oncology Nursing, 21*(3), 353–361.

Mahajan, S. (2020). Pelvic organ prolapse in women: Surgical repair of anterior vaginal wall prolapse. In L. Brubaker (Ed.), *UpToDate.* Waltham, MA.

McCance, K., Huether, S., Brashers, V., & Rote, N. (2019). *Pathophysiology: The biologic basis for disease in adults and children* (8th ed.). St. Louis: Mosby.

McWilliams, M., & Chennathukuzhi, V. (2017). Recent advances in uterine fibroid etiology. *Seminars in Reproductive Medicine, 35*(2), 181–189.

National Ovarian Cancer Coalition (NOCC). (2020a). Do I have a genetic predisposition to ovarian cancer? Retrieved from http://ovarian.org/about-ovarian-cancer/am-i-at-risk/do-i-have-a-genetic-predisposition

National Ovarian Cancer Coalition. (2020b). *Radiation.* Retrieved from http://ovarian.org/about-ovarian-cancer/treatment/14-iii.

O'Brien, K., et al. (2020). Association of powder use in the genital area with risk of ovarian cancer. *Journal of the American Medical Association, 323*(1), 49–59.

Pagana, K. D., & Pagana, T. J. (2018). *Mosby's manual of diagnostic and laboratory tests* (6th ed.). St. Louis: Mosby.

Stewart, E. (2020). Uterine fibroids (leiomyomas): Treatment overview. In R. Barbieri (Ed.), *UpToDate*. Waltham, MA.

Stewart, E., & Laughlin-Tommaso, S. (2019). Uterine Fibroids: Epidemiology, clinical features, diagnosis, and natural history. In R. Barbieri, & D. Levine (Eds.), *UpToDate*. Waltham, MA.

Trabuco, J., & Gebhart, E. (2020). Transvaginal synthetic mesh: Complications and risk factors. In K. Brubaker (Ed.), *UoToDate*. Waltham, MA.

U.S. Food and Drug Administration (FDA). (2019). *Urogynecologic surgical mesh implants*. Retrieved from https://www.fda.gov/medical-devices/implants-and-prosthetics/urogynecologic-surgical-mesh-implants.

U.S. National Library of Medicine. (2020). Vulvovaginitis. Retrieved from https://medlineplus.gov/ency/article/000897.htm.

U.S. Preventive Services Task Force. (2018). *Cervical cancer: Screening.* Retrieved from. https://www.uspreventiveservicestaskforce.org/uspstf/recommendation/cervical-cancer-screening.

van der Kooij, S., & Hehenkamp, W. (2020). Uterine leiomyomas (fibroids): Treatment with uterine artery embolization. In D. Levine, & R. Barbieri (Eds.), *UpToDate*. Waltham, MA.

Walters, M. (2020). Choosing a route of hysterectomy for benign uterus disease. In H. Sharp (Ed.), *UpToDate*. Waltham, MA.

World Health Organization (WHO). (2019). *Human papillomavirus (HPV) and cervical cancer*. Retrieved from https://www.who.int/news-room/fact-sheets/detail/human-papillomavirus-(hpv)-and-cervical-cancer.

Yu, O., et al. (2018). A US population-based study of uterine fibroid diagnosis incidence, trends, and prevalence: 2005 to 2014. *American Journal of Obstetrics and Gynecology, 219*(6), 591.e1–591.e8.

67

Concepts of Care for Patients With Male Reproductive Problems

Cherie R. Rebar

http://evolve.elsevier.com/Iggy/

LEARNING OUTCOMES

1. Collaborate with the interprofessional team to coordinate high-quality care for patients with a male reproductive problem.
2. Describe factors that place a patient at high risk for a male reproductive cancer, and refer to the health care provider.
3. Implement patient-centered nursing interventions to decrease the psychosocial impact of living with a male reproductive problem.
4. Apply knowledge of anatomy, physiology, and pathophysiology to assess patients with a male reproductive problem.
5. Use clinical judgment to analyze assessment findings and diagnostic data in the care of patients with a male reproductive problem.
6. Prioritize evidence-based care for patients with a male reproductive problem affecting *elimination, infection, cellular regulation, sexuality,* or *reproduction.*
7. Plan care coordination and transition management for patients with a male reproductive problem.

KEY TERMS

active surveillance (AS) Observation for cancer without immediate active treatment.

azoospermia The absence of living sperm in the semen.

bilateral orchiectomy The surgical removal of both testes, typically performed as palliative surgery in patients with prostate cancer. It is not intended to cure the prostate cancer but to arrest its spread by removing testosterone.

cryptorchidism Failure of the testes to descend into the scrotum.

erectile dysfunction (ED) The inability to achieve or maintain a penile erection sufficient for sexual intercourse.

gynecomastia Abnormal enlargement of the breasts in men.

hematuria Blood in the urine.

hydronephrosis Abnormal enlargement of the kidney caused by a blockage of urine lower in the tract and filling of the kidney with urine.

hydroureter Abnormal distention of the ureter.

hyperplasia Growth that causes tissue to increase in size by increasing the number of cells; abnormal overgrowth of tissue.

libido Sexual desire.

lower urinary tract symptoms (LUTS) Symptoms that occur as a result of prostatic hyperplasia, such as urinary retention and overflow incontinence, or urinary leaking.

nocturia The need to urinate excessively at night. Also called *nocturnal polyuria.*

oligospermia Low sperm count.

orchiectomy The surgical removal of one or both testes.

overflow urinary incontinence The involuntary loss of urine when the bladder is overdistended. In males, urine "leaks" around an enlarged prostate, causing dribbling.

prostate artery embolization A procedure in which the interventional radiologist threads a small vascular catheter into the prostate's arteries and injects particles blocking some of the blood flow to shrink the prostate gland.

prostate-specific antigen (PSA) A glycoprotein produced solely by the prostate.

prostatitis Inflammation and possible infection of the prostate.

radiation proctitis Rectal mucosa inflammation that results from external beam radiation therapy.

retrograde ejaculation A condition where semen flows backward into the bladder so only a small amount will be ejaculated from the penis; usually is a result of nerve damage during surgery.

transurethral resection of the prostate (TURP) The traditional "closed" surgical procedure for removal of the prostate. In this procedure, the surgeon inserts a resectoscope (an instrument similar to a cystoscope, but with a cutting and cauterizing loop) through the urethra. The enlarged portion of the prostate gland is then resected in small pieces.

tumescence Swelling; vascular congestion in erectile tissue.

✳ **PRIORITY AND INTERRELATED CONCEPTS**

The priority concepts for this chapter are:
- *Elimination*
- *Cellular Regulation*
- *Infection*

The **Elimination** concept exemplar for this chapter is Benign Prostatic Hyperplasia.

The **Cellular Regulation** concept exemplar for this chapter is Prostate Cancer.

The interrelated concepts for this chapter are:
- *Sexuality*
- *Reproduction*

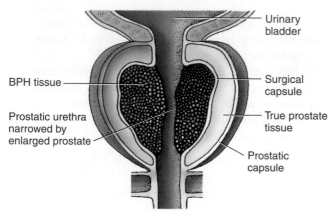

FIG. 67.1 Benign prostatic hyperplasia (BPH) grows inward, causing narrowing of the urethra.

The nurse's role in caring for men with reproductive problems is to be open, supportive, and nonjudgmental. Male reproductive problems are very personal and can range from short-term infections to long-term health care problems that require end-of-life care. These conditions can affect the human need for *sexuality, elimination,* and *reproduction,* all of which can impact the man's physiological and psychosocial sense of well-bring. See Chapter 1 for a review of the nursing concepts applied in this chapter.

✳ ELIMINATION CONCEPT EXEMPLAR: BENIGN PROSTATIC HYPERPLASIA

Pathophysiology Review

With aging and increased dihydrotestosterone (DHT) levels, the glandular units in the prostate undergo nodular tissue hyperplasia (an increase in the number of cells; an abnormal overgrowth of tissue). This altered tissue promotes local inflammation by attracting cytokines and other substances (McCance et al., 2019).

As the prostate gland enlarges, it extends upward into the bladder and inward, causing bladder outlet obstruction (BOO) (Fig. 67.1). In response, urinary *elimination* is affected in several ways, causing lower urinary tract symptoms (LUTS)—an umbrella term that includes problems such as urinary retention, urinary leaking, or incontinence. First, the detrusor (bladder) muscle thickens to help urine push past the enlarged prostate gland (McCance

et al., 2019). In spite of the bladder muscle change, the patient has increased residual urine (stasis) and chronic urinary retention. The increased volume of residual urine often causes overflow urinary incontinence, in which the urine "leaks" around the enlarged prostate, causing dribbling. Urinary stasis can also result in urinary tract infections and bladder calculi (stones).

In a few patients the prostate becomes very large and the man cannot void (acute urinary retention [AUR]). The patient with this problem requires *emergent* care. In other patients, chronic urinary retention may result in a backup of urine and cause a gradual, abnormal distention of the ureters (hydroureter) and enlargement of the kidneys (hydronephrosis) if benign prostatic hyperplasia (BPH) is not treated. These urinary *elimination* problems can lead to chronic kidney disease as described in Chapter 63.

Etiology and Genetic Risk. BPH is a very common male health problem, but the exact cause is unclear. Its relationship to aging is the only known factor (McCance et al., 2019). Other unmodifiable risk factors include (McVary, 2019):
- Race—Black men younger than 65 need treatment earlier than white men; also, LUTS is more common in black men than white men.
- Genetic susceptibility—Variants in the *GATA3* gene have been associated with development of BPH/LUTS.
- Family history of cancer—Men with a family history of bladder cancer (not prostate cancer) are at higher risk to develop BPH. Modifiable risk factors include (McVary, 2019):
- Obesity and metabolic syndrome—Obesity, glucose intolerance, dyslipidemia, and hypertension are associated with higher risk for development of BPH.
- Beverage consumption—Coffee and caffeine intake have been associated with an increase in risk for progression of existing BPH.

Incidence and Prevalence. Benign prostatic hyperplasia affects 40% to 50% of men between the ages of 51 and 60, and over 80% of men older than 80 years (McVary, 2019).

Health Promotion and Maintenance. Teach men that BPH is a common occurrence and that sexual frequency does not cause this condition. Current evidence does not show that there are absolute specific actions that prevent the development of BPH; however, teach men that addressing modifiable risk factors can improve their overall health.

❖ Interprofessional Collaborative Care

◆ Assessment: Recognize Cues

History. When taking a history, several standardized assessment tools are used to help the health care provider determine the severity of lower urinary tract symptoms (LUTS) associated with prostatic enlargement. One of the most commonly used assessments is the International Prostate Symptom Score (I-PSS) (Fig. 67.2). This tool incorporates the American Urological Association Symptom Index (AUA-SI) as questions 1 through 7 and asks an eighth question about the implication of the patient's urinary symptoms on quality of life.

International Prostate Symptom Score (I-PSS)

Patient Name:_____ Date of Birth:_____ Date Completed_____

In the past month:	Not at All	Less Than 1 in 5 Times	Less Than Half the Time	About Half the Time	More Than Half the Time	Almost Always	Your Score
1. Incomplete Emptying How often have you had the sensation of not emptying your bladder?	0	1	2	3	4	5	
2. Frequency How often have you had to urinate less than every 2 hours?	0	1	2	3	4	5	
3. Intermittency How often have you found you stopped and started again several times when you urinated?	0	1	2	3	4	5	
4. Urgency How often have you found it difficult to postpone urination?	0	1	2	3	4	5	
5. Weak Stream How often have you had a weak urinary stream?	0	1	2	3	4	5	
6. Straining How often have you had to strain to start urination?	0	1	2	3	4	5	
	None	**1 Time**	**2 Times**	**3 Times**	**4 Times**	**5 Times**	
7. Nocturia How many times do you typically get up at night to urinate?	0	1	2	3	4	5	
Total I-PSS Score							

Score: 1-7: Mild   8-19: Moderate   20-35: Severe

Quality of Life Due to Urinary Symptoms	Delighted	Pleased	Mostly Satisfied	Mixed	Mostly Dissatisfied	Unhappy	Terrible
If you were to spend the rest of your life with your urinary condition just the way it is now, how would you feel about that?	0	1	2	3	4	5	6

FIG. 67.2 The International Prostate Symptom Score (I-PSS). (Adapted from the American Urological Association Practice Guidelines Committee. [2003]. Guideline on the management of benign prostatic hyperplasia [BPH]. *Journal of Urology, 170*[2 Pt 1], 530–547.)

Continued

About the I-PSS

The International Prostate Symptom Score (I-PSS) is based on the answers to seven questions concerning urinary symptoms and one question concerning quality of life. Each question concerning urinary symptoms allows the patient to choose one out of six answers indicating increasing severity of the particular symptom. The answers are assigned points from 0 to 5. The total score can therefore range from 0 to 35 (asymptomatic to very symptomatic).

The questions refer to the following urinary symptoms:

Questions	Symptom
1	Incomplete emptying
2	Frequency
3	Intermittency
4	Urgency
5	Weak Stream
6	Straining
7	Nocturia

Question 8 refers to the patient's perceived quality of life.

The first seven questions of the I-PSS are identical to the questions appearing on the American Urological Association (AUA) Symptom Index, which currently categorizes symptoms as follows:

Mild (symptom score less than or equal to 7)
Moderate (symptom score range 8 to 19)
Severe (symptom score range 20 to 35)

The International Scientific Committee (SCI), under the patronage of the World Health Organization (WHO) and the International Union Against Cancer (UICC), recommends the use of only a single question to assess the quality of life. The answers to this question range from "delighted" to "terrible," or 0 to 6. Although this single question may or may not capture the global impact of benign prostatic hyperplasia (BPH) symptoms or quality of life, it may serve as a valuable starting point for a doctor-patient conversation.

The SCI has agreed to use the symptom index for BPH, which has been developed by the AUA Measurement Committee, as the official worldwide symptoms assessment tool for patients suffering from prostatism.

The SCI recommends that physicians consider the following components for a basic diagnostic workup: history; physical examination; appropriate labs such as U/A, creatinine, etc.; and DRE or other evaluation to rule out prostate cancer.

FIG. 67.2 Cont'd

Most patients complete the questions as a self-administered tool because it is available in many languages. If the patient cannot read, or does not wish to read, the nurse or health care provider can ask the questions to complete the assessment.

Physical Assessment/Signs and Symptoms. Ask about the patient's current urinary *elimination* pattern, and ask if it has changed recently. Assess for urinary frequency and urgency. Determine the number of times the patient awakens during the night to void (nocturia). Also assess for:

- Difficulty in starting (hesitancy) and continuing urination
- Reduced force and size of the urinary stream ("weak" stream)
- Sensation of incomplete bladder emptying
- Straining to begin urination
- Postvoid (after voiding) dribbling or leaking

The patient is also at risk to develop an *infection* or other bladder problem. Ask whether the patient has had hematuria (blood in the urine) when starting the urine stream or at the end of voiding. BPH is a common cause of hematuria in older men due to *infection.*

Remind the patient to void before the physical examination. Inspect and palpate the abdomen. If the patient has a sense of urgency when gentle pressure is applied, the bladder may be distended. Patients with obesity are best assessed by percussion (done by the health care provider) or bedside ultrasound bladder scanner rather than by inspection or palpation.

Prepare the patient for the prostate gland examination, which will be conducted by the health care provider. Tell him that he may feel the urge to urinate as the prostate is palpated. Because the prostate is close to the rectal wall, it is easily examined by *digital rectal examination* (DRE). If needed, help the patient bend over the examination table or assume a side-lying fetal position, whichever is the easiest position for him. The health care provider assesses for size and consistency of the prostate. BPH presents as a uniform, elastic, nontender enlargement; whereas cancer of the prostate gland feels like a stony-hard nodule. Advise the patient that after the prostate gland is palpated, it may be massaged to obtain a fluid sample for examination to rule out prostatitis (inflammation and possible **infection** of the prostate), a common problem that can occur with BPH. If the patient has bacterial prostatitis, he is treated with broad-spectrum antibiotic therapy to prevent the spread of infection (McCance et al., 2019).

Psychosocial Assessment. Patients who have nocturia and other LUTS may be frustrated or depressed as a result of interrupted sleep and ongoing visits to the bathroom. Assess the effect of sleep interruptions on the patient's mood and mental status. Ask him about the impact of symptoms on **sexuality** and libido (sexual desire).

Postvoid dribbling and overflow incontinence may cause embarrassment and prevent the patient from socializing or leaving the home. For some patients, this social isolation can affect quality of life and lead to clinical depression and/or severe anxiety. Provide time for the patient to express his feelings about these concerns.

Laboratory Assessment. A *urinalysis* and *urine culture* are typically obtained to diagnose urinary tract infection and microscopic hematuria. If **infection** is present, the urinalysis measures the number of white blood cells (WBCs).

Other laboratory studies that may be performed include:

- A *complete blood count* (CBC) to evaluate any evidence of systemic infection (elevated WBCs) or anemia (decreased red blood cells [RBCs]) from hematuria.
- *Blood urea nitrogen* (BUN) and *serum creatinine* levels to evaluate renal function (both are usually elevated with kidney disease).
- A *prostate-specific antigen* (PSA) test for screening purposes (the most commonly used and valuable test for early detection of prostate cancer [Kantoff et al., 2020]).
- A *serum acid phosphatase* level if metastatic prostate cancer is suspected (this is typically elevated in patients who have prostate cancer that has metastasized).
- A biopsy, which may be performed if life expectancy is greater than 5 to 10 years, and if needed to confirm a histologic diagnosis; usually transrectal ultrasound (TRUS) or MRI is performed first (Kantoff et al., 2020); see Other Diagnostic Assessment (next section).
- *Culture and sensitivity* of prostatic fluid (if expressed during the examination).

Other Diagnostic Assessment. Imaging studies that are typically performed are *transrectal ultrasound (TRUS)* (more common in the United States) and *MRI* (more common in other countries) (Kantoff et al., 2020). The patient having a TRUS lies on his side while the transducer is inserted into the rectum for viewing the prostate and surrounding structures. A tissue biopsy may also be done during this procedure.

In some cases, cystoscopy may be ordered to view the interior of the bladder, the bladder neck, and the urethra. This procedure is used to study the presence and effect of bladder neck obstruction and is usually done in an ambulatory care setting. Residual urine can also be measured when the cystoscope is inserted. See Chapter 60 for a detailed description of *cystoscopy* and the nursing care needed for patients having this procedure.

Residual urine may be determined by *bladder ultrasound* immediately after the patient voids. *Urodynamic pressure-flow studies* can be helpful in determining if there is urine blockage or weakness of the detrusor muscle.

◆ **Analysis: Analyze Cues and Prioritize Hypotheses.** The priority collaborative problems for the patient with benign prostatic hyperplasia (BPH) are:

1. Urinary retention due to bladder outlet obstruction (BOO)
2. Decreased self-esteem due to overflow urinary incontinence and possible sexual dysfunction

---

❓ CLINICAL JUDGMENT CHALLENGE 67.1

Evidence-Based Practice; Patient-Centered Care

A 61-year-old male client presents to the emergency department reporting that he has not fully urinated other than dribbling in the past 13 hours. He reports difficulty emptying his bladder and having an intermittent urinary stream for the past several months. He also admits to rising two to three times nightly to urinate. He states that he usually has no pain on urination, but does report increasing abdominal discomfort today after being unable to urinate.

1. **Recognize Cues:** What assessment information in this client situation is the most important and immediate concern for the nurse? (Hint: Identify the **relevant** information *first* to determine what is most important.)
2. **Analyze Cues:** What client conditions are consistent with the **most relevant** information? (Hint: Think about priority collaborative problems that support and contradict the information presented in this situation.)
3. **Prioritize Hypotheses:** Which possibilities or explanations are **most likely** to be present in this client situation? Which possibilities or explanations are the most serious? (Hint: Consider all possibilities and determine their urgency and risk for this client.)
4. **Generate Solutions:** What actions would most likely achieve the desired outcomes for this client? Which actions should be **avoided** or are **potentially harmful**? (Hint: Determine the desired outcomes first to decide which interventions are appropriate and those that should be avoided.)
5. **Take Action:** Which actions are the most appropriate and how should they be implemented? In what **priority order** should they be implemented? (Hint: Consider health teaching, documentation, requested health care provider orders or prescriptions, nursing skills, collaboration with or referral to health team members, etc.)
6. **Evaluate Outcomes:** What client assessment would indicate that the nurse's actions were **effective**? (Hint: Think about signs that would indicate an improvement, decline, or unchanged client condition.)

◆ Planning and Implementation: Generate Solutions and Take Action

Improving Urinary Elimination

Planning: Generate Solutions. The patient with BPH is expected to have a normal urinary *elimination* pattern without lower urinary tract symptoms (LUTS) or *infection.*

Interventions: Take Action. Treatment for BPH ranges from careful monitoring to surgery, depending on the degree of impairment the patient is experiencing. If the patient is not experiencing complications or discomfort, behavioral modification may be recommended. Patients with symptomatic BPH are usually first treated with nonsurgical interventions, such as drug therapy.

Nonsurgical Management

Behavioral modification. Teach patients with BPH to avoid drinking large amounts of fluid in a short time, especially before going out or at bedtime (Cunningham & Kadmon, 2019). Caffeine and alcohol consumption should be limited, as these have a diuretic effect. Caution patients to avoid drugs that can cause urinary retention, especially anticholinergics, antihistamines, antipsychotics, and muscle relaxants (Cunningham & Kadmon, 2019). *Emphasize the importance of telling any health care provider about the diagnosis of BPH so these drugs are not prescribed.*

Drug therapy. *Alpha₁-adrenergic antagonists,* which act to relax smooth muscle in the bladder neck, and *5-alpha-reductase inhibitors* (5-ARIs), which act to reduce prostate size, are often prescribed in combination, as evidence shows that they work better in combination (Burchum & Rosenthal, 2019). See the Common Examples of Drug Therapy: Drug Therapy Used to Treat Benign Prostatic Hyperplasia (BPH) box for an overview of drug therapy used to treat BPH.

The most effective drug therapy approach used for many patients is a combination of a 5-ARI drug and an alpha₁-adrenergic antagonist. Two commonly prescribed drug regimens include finasteride and doxazosin, and dutasteride and tamsulosin.

💊 COMMON EXAMPLES OF DRUG THERAPY

Drug Therapy Used to Treat Benign Prostatic Hyperplasia (BPH)

Drug Category	Selected Nursing Implications
Alpha₁-Adrenergic Antagonists Common examples of alpha₁-adrenergic antagonists: • Alfuzosin • Doxazosin • Prazosin • Tamsulosin • Silodosin	Monitor blood pressure, and teach to move slowly from sitting to standing; *orthostatic hypotension can occur.* Monitor for side effects such as ongoing dizziness, headache and weakness; *these side effects may require dose reduction or discontinuation of the drug.* Teach patient to report taking this drug to all health care providers; *Alpha₁-adrenergic antagonists can increase or decrease the side effects of other drugs such as beta blockers, calcium channel blockers, or medications used to treat erectile dysfunction (ED).*
5-Alpha-Reductase Inhibitors Common examples of 5-alpha-reductase inhibitors: • Dutasteride • Finasteride	Monitor blood pressure, and teach to move slowly from sitting to standing; *orthostatic hypotension can occur.* Teach about possible side effect of gynecomastia; *men taking a 5-alpha-reductase inhibitor are three times more likely to develop this condition.* Teach about the increased risk for development of prostate cancer; *men taking a 5-alpha-reductase inhibitor are at higher risk for development of prostate cancer.* Teach to keep medications stored away from pregnant women or women who may become pregnant; *these drugs are teratogenic and can be absorbed through the skin; therefore, pregnant women should not touch dutasteride nor finasteride.* Teach patients taking dutasteride to take the capsule with a full glass of water, and to refrain from opening the capsule to sprinkle on food; *dutasteride irritates oropharyngeal mucosa.*
Erectogenic • Tadalafil	Teach that this drug is usually given to treat erectile dysfunction, but can also be used to improve lower urinary tract symptoms (LUTS); *the patient needs to know the mechanism of action as it relates to treatment of BPH and LUTS.* Teach that the duration of action is up to 36 hours, and to avoid taking more than once daily; *this duration of action is much longer than that of most phosphodiesterase-5 (PDE5) inhibitor medications that the patient may have used in the past, which have only a 4-hour duration of action.* Teach to refrain from taking this drug with grapefruit juice or grapefruits. *Drinking grapefruit juice or eating grapefruit while taking tadalafil can increase the amount of drug in the body.*

Other information taken from Burchum, J.L.R., & Rosenthal, L.D. (2016). *Lehne's pharmacology for nursing care* (9th ed.). St. Louis: Elsevier. Data from Hagberg, K., et al. (2017). Risk of gynecomastia and breast cancer associated with the use of 5-alpha reductase inhibitors for benign prostatic hyperplasia. *Clinical Epidemiology, 9,* 83-91.

> **! NURSING SAFETY PRIORITY** (QSEN)
>
> **Drug Alert**
>
> Remind patients taking a 5-ARI for BPH that they may need to take it for as long as 6 months before improvement is noticed. Remind them to keep all follow-up appointments for laboratory testing, because liver damage can occur. Teach about possible side effects including erectile dysfunction (ED), decreased libido, and dizziness due to orthostatic hypotension. *Remind them to change positions carefully and slowly!*

> **! NURSING SAFETY PRIORITY** (QSEN)
>
> **Drug Alert**
>
> Teach patients taking a 5-ARI to keep these drugs stored away from pregnant women or women who may become pregnant. These drugs are absorbed through the skin, and are teratogenic.

> **! NURSING SAFETY PRIORITY** (QSEN)
>
> **Drug Alert**
>
> If giving alpha blockers in an inpatient setting, assess for orthostatic (postural) hypotension, tachycardia, and syncope ("blackout"), especially after the first dose is given to older men. If the patient is taking the drug at home, *teach him to be careful when changing position and to report any weakness, light-headedness, or dizziness to the health care provider immediately.* Bedtime dosing may decrease the risk for problems related to hypotension.

Other drugs may be helpful in managing specific urinary symptoms. For example, low-dose oral desmopressin, a synthetic antidiuretic analog, has been used successfully for nocturia (Burchum & Rosenthal, 2019).

Complementary and integrative health. Saw palmetto *(Serenoa repens)* has been shown in some studies to be useful in treating BPH. However, other studies have demonstrated no benefit, or benefit that is similar to placebo effect. Remind patients who are interested in taking saw palmetto to talk with their health care provider before taking this herb because of potential interactions with prescribed drugs such as anticoagulants and NSAIDs. Side effects of saw palmetto are rare, and are usually limited to mild nausea and headache (Burchum & Rosenthal, 2019).

Other nonsurgical interventions. Frequent sexual intercourse can reduce obstructive symptoms because it causes the release of prostatic fluid. This approach is helpful for the man whose obstructive symptoms result from an enlarged prostate with a large amount of retained prostatic fluid.

If drug therapy or other measures are not helpful in relieving urinary symptoms, several noninvasive techniques are available to shrink or destroy excess prostate tissue. The minimally invasive **prostate artery embolization** is performed by an interventional radiologist (IR) who threads a small vascular catheter into an artery in the wrist or groin. An arteriogram (dye injected in the blood vessels) allows the IR to see the vessels that feed the prostate, into which particles are injected to reduce some of the blood flow. In turn, this shrinks the prostate gland. This procedure has a low side effect profile for development of incontinence or erectile dysfunction (ED), so it is preferred by many patients. Local anesthesia is used rather than general anesthesia (Abt et al., 2018), which allows a typical discharge from the hospital in as little as 3 hours after the procedure. Select other procedures that treat BPH are included in Table 67.1.

All of these minimally invasive treatments use local or regional anesthesia. Some, but not all, require an indwelling urinary catheter for a short period after the procedure. They are also associated with less risk for complications such as intraoperative bleeding and erectile dysfunction when compared with traditional surgical approaches. Patients can return to their usual activities in a short time as prescribed by their provider.

Surgical Management. For patients who are not candidates for nonsurgical management or are not interested in medication or other less invasive options, surgery may be performed. Some or all of these criteria indicate the need for surgery:

- Acute urinary retention (AUR) due to obstruction
- Chronic urinary tract infections secondary to residual urine in the bladder
- Hematuria
- Hydronephrosis
- Persistent pain with decrease in urine flow

If a lesser invasive procedure is not indicated or desired, the historical gold standard surgery has been a **transurethral resection of the prostate (TURP)**, in which the enlarged part of the prostate is removed through an endoscopic instrument. A similar procedure is the transurethral incision of the prostate (TUIP) in which small cuts are made into the prostate to relieve pressure on the urethra. This alternate technique is used for smaller prostates.

The holmium laser enucleation of the prostate (HoLEP) procedure, laparoscopic prostatic adenomectomy, and robotic-assisted simple prostatectomy (RASP) are safer minimally invasive surgeries (MISs) that may be performed for BPH. Open, laparoscopic, or robotic-assisted simple prostatectomy (entire prostate removal) may also be considered (see discussion of Surgical Management in the section Cellular Regulation Concept Exemplar: Prostate Cancer). Very little blood is lost during these procedures, and patient recovery is faster than that for the more traditional TURP.

Preoperative care. When planning surgical interventions, the patient's general physical condition, the size of the prostate gland, and the man's preferences are considered. The patient may have fears and misconceptions about prostate surgery, such as believing that automatic loss of sexual functioning or permanent incontinence will occur. Assess the patient's anxiety, correct any misconceptions about the surgery, and provide accurate information to him and his family. Regardless of the type of surgery to be performed, reinforce information about anesthesia (see Chapter 9). Remind patients taking anticoagulants that the drugs will be discontinued several days prior to the TURP or

TABLE 67.1	Other Procedures Used to Treat Benign Prostatic Hyperplasia (BPH)	
Procedure	**Description**	**Nursing Implications**
Photoselective vaporization (PVP)—GreenLight Laser Therapy	Laser energy is used to vaporize the prostate tissue	Teach: • A catheter will be in place following the procedure, and removed in a day. • Retrograde ejaculation may occur.
Transurethral needle ablation (TUNA)	Low radiofrequency energy is used to shrink the prostate	Teach: • The patient will need someone to drive him home from the procedure. • A catheter will be in place following the procedure, and removed in several days. • Take the full course of antibiotics prescribed to prevent a urinary tract infection (UTI) from the catheter.
Transurethral microwave therapy (TUMT)	An antenna is inserted through the penis toward the prostate to deliver a dose of microwave energy that heats and destroys prostate tissue	Teach: • A urinary catheter will be needed after the procedure for approximately 1 week. • It may take up to several months to experience the best procedural benefit, as this is dependent on how long the body needs to absorb the overgrown prostate that has been destroyed • Have continued digital rectal examinations (DREs) and screenings for prostate cancer annually, even after the procedure.
Transurethral electro-vaporization of the prostate (TUEVAP)	Involves the use of a *roller ball* to heat the prostate tissue, reducing it to vapor	Teach: • Avoid heavy lifting; avoid straining when having a bowel movement. • Drink 8 cups of water daily. • It may take several months before fully normal urination occurs, although the stream will likely be stronger right after the procedure.
Transurethral water vapor therapy (Rezum)	A radiofrequency current is applied to an *inductive coil heater,* which produces water vapor that is delivered to the transition zone of the prostate; this produces necrosis in targeted cell tissue (Westwood et al., 2018)	Teach: • Dysuria, hematuria, hematospermia, and urgency may last several weeks, and usually resolve. • A favorable change will begin in about 2 weeks following the procedure, with full benefit noticed around 3 months postprocedure.
Urolift	A delivery device is placed through the obstructed urethra; small implants are placed to lift and hold the enlarged prostate tissue, which increases the urethral opening (NeoTract, 2020).	Teach: • Relief will be felt in as little as 2 weeks. • Dysuria, hematuria, and urgency may be experienced postprocedure; these usually resolve in 2-4 weeks.

open prostate surgery to prevent postoperative bleeding. Other general preoperative care is described in Chapter 9.

The patient may have other medical problems that increase the risk for complications of general anesthesia and may be advised to have spinal anesthesia. Because the patient is conscious during spinal anesthesia, it is easier to assess for hyponatremia (low serum sodium), fluid overload, and water intoxication, which can result from large-volume bladder irrigations.

After a TURP, all patients have an indwelling urethral catheter. *Be sure that they know that they will feel the urge to void while the catheter is in place.* Tell the patient that he will likely have traction on the catheter that may cause discomfort, and reassure him that analgesics will be prescribed to relieve pain. Explain that it is normal for the urine to be blood-tinged after surgery. Small blood clots and tissue debris may pass while the catheter is in place and immediately after it is removed. Some patients also have continuous bladder irrigation (CBI), depending on the procedure performed.

Operative procedures. The traditional TURP is a "closed" surgery. To perform the procedure, the surgeon inserts a resectoscope (an instrument similar to a cystoscope, but with a cutting and cauterizing loop) through the urethra. The enlarged portion of the prostate gland is then removed in small pieces (prostate chips). The estimated blood loss during TURP is less than 500 mL (Schreiber, 2017). A fibrinolytic inhibitor such as tranexamic acid may be used during surgery to prevent bleeding and excess clotting. This does not prevent the need for blood transfusions, nor is it effective in increasing hemoglobin levels, after surgery. However, it does assist in preventing perioperative blood loss (Mina & Garcia-Perdomo, 2018; Qian-Qian et al., 2019).

The disadvantage of a TURP is that only small pieces of the gland are removed. Remaining prostate tissue may continue to grow and cause urinary obstruction, requiring additional TURPs. Urethral trauma from the resectoscope with resulting urethral strictures is also possible.

Postoperative care. During any surgical procedure for BPH, a urinary catheter is placed into the bladder. Traction is often applied on the catheter by pulling it taut and taping it to the patient's abdomen or thigh. If the catheter is taped to the patient's thigh, instruct him to keep his leg straight. The patient who had a TURP may have a catheter and continuous bladder irrigation (CBI) in place for several days. For the CBI, a three-way urinary catheter is used to allow drainage of urine and inflow of a

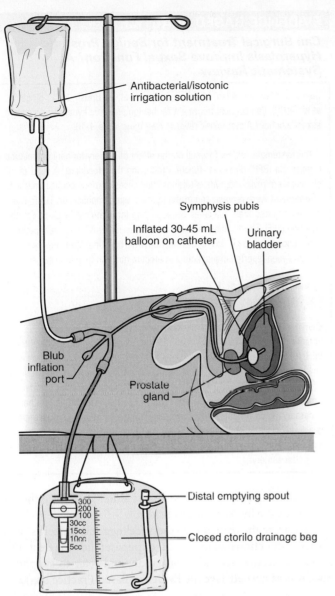

Antibacterial/isotonic irrigation solution

Symphysis pubis

Inflated 30-45 mL balloon on catheter

Urinary bladder

Blub inflation port

Prostate gland

Distal emptying spout

Closed sterile drainage bag

FIG. 67.3 Continuous bladder irrigation system after a TURP. *TURP,* Transurethral resection of the prostate.

bladder irrigating solution (Fig. 67.3). Be sure to maintain the flow of the irrigant to keep the urine clear. When measuring the fluid in the urinary drainage bag, subtract the amount of irrigating solution that was used, to determine actual urinary output.

NCLEX EXAMINATION CHALLENGE 67.1

Physiological Integrity

A client has continuous bladder irrigation after surgery yesterday. The amount of bladder irrigating solution that has infused over the past 12 hours is 1100 mL. The amount of fluid in the urinary drainage bag is 1950 mL. The nurse records that the client had _____ mL urinary output in the past 12 hours.
Fill in the blank.

Remind the patient that because of the urinary catheter's large diameter and the pressure of the retention balloon on the internal sphincter of the bladder, he will feel the urge to void continuously. This is a normal sensation, not a surgical complication. Advise

BEST PRACTICE FOR PATIENT SAFETY & QUALITY CARE (QSEN)

Care of the Patient After Transurethral Resection of the Prostate

- Monitor the patient closely for signs of *infection.* Older men undergoing prostate surgery often also have underlying chronic diseases (e.g., cardio-vascular disease, chronic lung disease, diabetes).
- Help the patient out of the bed to the chair as soon as permitted to prevent complications of immobility. Provide assistance, especially for patients with underlying changes in the musculoskeletal system (e.g., decreased range of motion, stiffness in joints). These patients are at *high risk* for falls.
- Assess the patient's pain every 2 to 4 hours and intervene as needed to control pain.
- Provide a safe environment for the patient. Anticipate a temporary change in mental status for the older patient in the immediate postoperative period as a result of anesthetics and unfamiliar surroundings. Reorient the patient frequently. Keep catheter tubes secure.
- Maintain the rate of the continuous bladder irrigation to ensure clear urine without clots and bleeding.
- Use normal saline solution (which is isotonic) for the intermittent bladder irrigant unless otherwise prescribed.
- Monitor and document the color, consistency, and amount of urine output.
- Check the drainage tubing frequently for external obstructions (e.g., kinks) and internal obstructions (e.g., blood clots, decreased output).
- Assess the patient for reports of severe bladder spasms with decreased urinary output, which may indicate obstruction.
- If the urinary catheter is obstructed, irrigate it per agency or surgeon protocol.
- Notify the surgeon immediately if the obstruction does not resolve by hand irrigation or if the urinary return looks like ketchup.

PATIENT-CENTERED CARE: OLDER ADULT CONSIDERATIONS (QSEN)

When caring for older men who may become confused after surgery, reorient them frequently and remind them not to pull on the catheter. If the patient is restless or "picks" at tubes, provide a familiar object such as a family picture for him to hold for distraction and a feeling of security. Do not restrain the patient unless all other alternatives have failed.

! NURSING SAFETY PRIORITY (QSEN)

Critical Rescue

Monitor the patient for the rare, yet critical, complication of TURP syndrome. If irrigation fluid is over-absorbed into the body in addition to blood transfusions and bleeding, stress can be placed on the heart. Signs and symptoms include headache, dizziness, and/or shortness of breath; the patient is likely to also have hypertension, bradycardia, and an altered level of consciousness. ECG findings include wide QRS, elevated ST, and inverted T wave (Schreiber, 2017). Notify the surgeon immediately, as the patient will likely need intensive care while diuresing.

him not to try to void around the catheter, which causes the bladder muscles to contract and may result in painful spasms.

The Best Practice for Patient Safety & Quality Care: Care of the Patient After Transurethral Resection of the Prostate box summarizes the nursing care for patients having a TURP.

! NURSING SAFETY PRIORITY (QSEN)
Critical Rescue

After a TURP, monitor the patient's urine output every 2 to 4 hours and vital signs (including pain assessment) every 4 hours for the first postoperative day or according to agency or surgeon protocol. Assess for postoperative bleeding. *Patients who undergo a TURP are at risk for severe bleeding or hemorrhage after surgery. Although rare, bleeding is most likely within the first 24 hours.* Bladder spasms or movement may trigger fresh bleeding from previously controlled vessels. This bleeding may be arterial or venous, but venous bleeding is more common.

! NURSING SAFETY PRIORITY (QSEN)
Critical Rescue

If *arterial* bleeding occurs, the urinary drainage is bright red or ketchup-like with numerous clots. *Notify the surgeon immediately and irrigate the catheter with normal saline solution per surgeon or hospital protocol.* Surgical intervention may be needed to clear the bladder of clots and stop bleeding.

If the bleeding is *venous,* the urine output is burgundy, with or without any change in vital signs. *Inform the surgeon of any bleeding.* Closely monitor the patient's hemoglobin (Hgb) and hematocrit (Hct) levels for anemia as a result of blood loss.

Observe for other possible but uncommon complications of TURP, such as **infection** and incontinence. Teach the patient that sexual function should not be affected after surgery but that retrograde ejaculation is possible, wherein semen flows backward into the bladder so only a small amount will be ejaculated from the penis.

NCLEX EXAMINATION CHALLENGE 67.2
Physiological Integrity

The nurse notes bright red urinary drainage from a client who had a transurethral resection of the prostate (TURP) with continuous bladder irrigation yesterday. What is the appropriate **initial** nursing action?

A. Calculate intake and output.
B. Monitor hemoglobin and hematocrit.
C. Increase the rate of the bladder irrigation.
D. Document findings in the electronic health record.

Improving Self-Esteem
Planning: Generate Solutions. The expected outcome is that the patient will experience improved self-esteem through incontinence management and avoidance of sexual dysfunction.

Interventions: Take Action. The patient with BPH typically has frequent urges to void and may have overflow incontinence at times because of urinary retention. Teach him to keep the surrounding area clean and dry to prevent skin breakdown. Remind him to toilet when he feels the urge and, if needed, to wear a small absorbent pad to prevent undergarment soiling. Involve the patient's sexual partner, if the patient agrees, in teaching about the cause of the incontinence and any prescribed

EVIDENCE-BASED PRACTICE (QSEN)
Can Surgical Treatment for Benign Prostatic Hyperplasia Improve Sexual Function? A Systematic Review

Soans, J., Vazirian-Zadeh, M., Kum, F., Dhariwal, R., Breish, M.O., Singh, S., et al. (2019). Can surgical treatment for benign prostatic hyperplasia improve sexual function? A systematic review. *The Aging Male,* 1-10.

This systematic review focused on the effect of surgery for benign prostatic hyperplasia (BPH) on sexual function following the procedure. A total of 16 studies were reviewed, with a total of 2087 cases. Various surgical methods of treatment were represented in the studies, with emphasis on TURP. Most studies reported their outcomes based on the International Index of Erectile Function (IIEF). The findings revealed that in the majority of studies, patients experienced no changes in erectile function (from baseline) after surgery. Some patients even reported improvement in erectile function following surgery.

Level of Evidence: 1
A systematic review was performed.

Commentary: Implications for Practice and Research
Erectile dysfunction is a known risk of any operative procedure that treats BPH. It is important that patients know the risks and benefits associated with any procedure. The surgeon will cover these with the patient when obtaining informed consent, which the nurse can witness. If at any time the patient expresses further concern or fear, the nurse can listen to the patient and, if necessary, place the patient back in touch with the surgeon for clarification. It is also important for the nurse to be aware of the evidence available demonstrating that most men experience no changes in erectile function (from baseline) after surgery.

treatment. Once the patient is treated either with drug therapy or surgery, the incontinence subsides.

Encourage the patient to express feelings and concerns about sexual dysfunction that may occur or persist following treatment. Provide objective, factual information, and refer to supportive resources as needed. (see the Evidence-Based Practice box).

Care Coordination and Transition Management. The patient with benign prostatic hyperplasia (BPH) is typically managed at home. Patients who have surgery are also discharged to their home or other setting from where they were admitted.

Home Care Management. Depending on the procedure performed, some patients may be discharged with a urinary catheter in place for a short period of time. Teach patients not to take a bath or swim, to prevent a urinary tract **infection** while the catheter is in place. When the urinary catheter is removed, the patient may experience burning on urination and some urinary frequency, dribbling, and leakage. Reassure him that these symptoms are normal and will decrease. Instruct him to increase fluid intake to at least 2000 to 2500 mL daily, which helps decrease dysuria and keep the urine clear. *Be aware that an older patient who has renal disease or who is at risk for heart failure may not be able to tolerate this much fluid.*

Self-Management Education. Some patients, especially those who have had a TURP, may have temporary loss of control of urination or a dribbling of the urine. Reassure the patient that these symptoms are almost always temporary and will resolve. Also remind him that *reproduction* ability should not be affected by surgery.

Help the patient and his family find ways to keep his clothing dry until sphincter control returns. Instruct him to contract and relax his sphincter frequently to re-establish urinary *elimination* control (Kegel exercises). External urinary (condom) catheters are not used except in extreme cases because they may give the patient a false sense of security and delay urinary control.

Health Care Resources. Patients being managed for BPH usually do not require extensive follow-up care or health care resources. Older men may need one or two visits from a home health care agency to ensure that they are not experiencing postsurgical complications and can provide safe self-care.

Teach patients to have follow-up care as recommended by the surgeon. After prostatic surgery, some men experience a return of LUTS and/or erectile dysfunction, which can decrease their quality of life.

◆ **Evaluation: Evaluate Outcomes.** Evaluate the care of the patient with BPH based on the identified priority patient problem. The primary expected outcome is that the patient will:
- Have improved urinary *elimination* as a result of appropriate and effective interprofessional management
- Experience improved self-esteem as a result of effective BPH management

✴ CELLULAR REGULATION CONCEPT EXEMPLAR: PROSTATE CANCER

Pathophysiology Review

Testosterone and dihydrotestosterone (DHT) are the major androgens (male hormones) in the adult male. Testosterone is produced by the testis and circulates in the blood. DHT is a testosterone derivative in the prostate gland. In some patients, the prostate grows very rapidly, leading to noncancerous high-grade prostatic intraepithelial neoplasia (PIN). This impairment of *cellular regulation* causes men to be at a higher risk for developing prostate cancer than men who do not have that growth pattern.

Many prostate tumors are androgen sensitive (McCance et al., 2019). Most are adenocarcinomas and arise from epithelial cells located in the posterior lobe or outer portion of the gland (Fig. 67.4).

Of all malignancies, prostate cancer is one of the slowest growing, and it metastasizes in a predictable pattern. Common sites of metastasis are the nearby lymph nodes, and bones (McCance et al., 2019), although it can also metastasize to the lungs or liver. The bones of the pelvis, sacrum, and lumbar spine are most often affected. Chapter 19 describes staging categories of localized and advanced cancers.

Etiology and Genetic Risk. Advanced age is the leading risk factor for development of prostate cancer (Centers for Disease Control and Prevention [CDC], 2019). The risk increases for men who have a first-degree relative (father, brother, son) with the disease, and for African-American men (CDC, 2019).

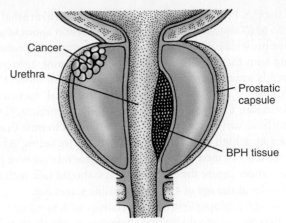

FIG. 67.4 Prostate gland with cancer and benign prostatic hyperplasia (BPH). Note that cancer normally arises in the periphery of the gland, whereas BPH occurs in the center of the gland.

👤 PATIENT-CENTERED CARE: CULTURAL/ SPIRITUAL CONSIDERATIONS (QSEN)

Prostate cancer affects African Americans more often than other ethnic/racial groups (McCance et al., 2019). Males of African descent who live in the Caribbean have the highest mortality rates in the world (McCance et al., 2019). Mortality is increasing in Asia as well as in Central and Eastern European countries, whereas it has decreased in Australia, Canada, Italy, Norway, the United Kingdom, and the United States (McCance et al., 2019). Be aware of epidemiologic factors to best teach your patient.

Studies are ongoing regarding what role, if any, that diet has in the risk for development of prostate cancer, or the progression once it has been diagnosed. The hypothesis for the current Men's Eating and Living (MEAL) Study is that consuming more fruits and vegetables (versus animal fat) will slow the progression of aggressive prostate cancer.

👤 PATIENT-CENTERED CARE: GENETIC/ GENOMIC CONSIDERATIONS (QSEN)

Many gene mutations play a role in various types of prostate cancer. Some men with the most aggressive prostate cancers have *BRCA2* mutations similar to those women who have *BRCA2*-associated breast and ovarian cancers. The most common genetic factor that increases the risk for prostate cancer is a mutation in the glutathione *S*-transferase *(GSTP1)* gene. This gene is normally part of the pathway that helps to protect against carcinogen damage (McCance et al., 2019).

Incidence and Prevalence. Prostate cancer is the most commonly diagnosed nonskin cancer in men in the United States (McCance et al., 2019). If found and treated early, has a nearly 100% cure rate. Men older than 65 years have the greatest risk for the disease (McCance et al., 2019), with the average age at diagnosis being 66 (American Cancer Society, 2019a). In the United States, one in every nine men will be diagnosed with prostate cancer in his lifetime (American Cancer Society, 2020).

Health Promotion and Maintenance. Teach men about the most current evidence-based guidelines for prostate cancer screening and early detection. The current recommendations from the U.S. Preventive Services Task Force (2018) are that men aged 55 to 69 should make an informed decision about whether to have prostate cancer screening. This is best accomplished by talking with their health care provider. This same agency recommends against screening for men age 70 and older. Other organizations such as the American Urological Association, the American College of Physicians, and the American Cancer Society have varying guidelines. It is important to note that:

- Men at a high risk for prostate cancer, including African Americans or men who have a first-degree relative with prostate cancer before the age of 65 years, should talk with their provider at the age of 45 about possible screening.
- Men with multiple first-degree relatives with prostate cancer at an early age should discuss screening at age 40 (American Cancer Society, 2010).

Although a family history of prostate cancer cannot be changed, certain nutritional habits can be modified to possibly decrease the risk for the disease. First, teach men to eat a healthy, balanced diet, including decreasing animal fat (e.g., red meat) and the intake of dairy product (Sartor, 2020). Also reinforce the need to increase fruits and vegetables—especially tomatoes, which are high in lycopene (Sartor, 2020). Soy contains phytoestrogens that are thought to be helpful in reducing the risk for prostate cancer (Sartor, 2020).

❖ Interprofessional Collaborative Care

◆ Assessment: Recognize Cues

History. Assess the patient's age, race/ethnicity, and family history of prostate cancer. Ask about his nutritional habits, especially focusing on the intake of red meat and dairy products as a source of concern. Recognize that in early prostate cancer, there are often no signs or symptoms experienced by the patient.

Assess whether the patient has existing or new problems with urinary *elimination.* Take a drug history to determine if he is taking any medication that could affect voiding. The first symptoms that the man may notice and report are related to bladder outlet obstruction (BOO), such as difficulty in starting urination, frequent bladder infections, and urinary retention. Ask about urinary frequency, hematuria (blood in the urine), and nocturia. Ask if he has had any pain during intercourse, especially when ejaculating. Inquire if he has had or currently has any other pain (particularly bone pain in the hips and legs), a symptom associated with advanced prostate cancer. Ask him if he has had any recent unexpected weight loss.

Take a sexual history for recent changes in *sexuality,* including libido or function. Ask about current or previous sexually transmitted infections, penile discharge, or scrotal pain or swelling.

Physical Assessment/Signs and Symptoms. Most *early* cancers are diagnosed while the patient is having a routine physical examination or is being treated for benign prostatic hyperplasia (BPH). Gross blood in the urine (hematuria) is a common sign of *late* prostate cancer. Pain in the pelvis, hips, spine, or ribs, and swollen nodes indicate advanced disease that has spread. Take and record the patient's weight because unexpected weight loss is also common when the disease is advanced.

Prepare the patient for a digital rectal examination (DRE) by the health care provider. A prostate that is stony hard and with palpable irregularities or indurations is suspected to be malignant.

Psychosocial Assessment. A diagnosis of any type of cancer causes fear and anxiety for most people. Some men, particularly African Americans, develop the disease in their 40s and 50s (Richie, 2020) when they are putting their children through college, looking toward retirement in the coming years, and/or enjoying their middle years. Assess the reaction of the patient and family to the diagnosis. Men may describe their feelings as shock, fear, or anger, or a combination of these. Expect that patients usually go through the grieving process and may be in denial or depressed. Determine what support systems they have, such as family, friends, spiritual leaders, or community group support, to help them through diagnosis, treatment, and recovery.

One of the biggest concerns the patient may have is his ability for sexual function after cancer treatment. Tell him that function will depend on the type of treatment he has. Common surgical techniques used today do not involve cutting the perineal nerves that are needed for an erection. A dry climax may occur if the prostate is removed because it produces most of the fluid in the ejaculate. Refer the patient to his surgeon (urologist), sex therapist, or intimacy counselor if available.

Laboratory Assessment. Prostate-specific antigen (PSA) is a glycoprotein produced by the prostate. If the patient and health care provider have agreed to screening, *PSA analysis can be used as a screening test for prostate cancer. Because other prostate problems also increase the PSA level, it is not specifically diagnostic for cancer.* However, it is commonly used in an effort to detect cancer early (Kantoff et al., 2020). If the test is performed, the specimen should be drawn before the DRE because the examination can cause an increase in PSA as a result of prostate irritation.

Most authoritative sources agree that the normal blood level of PSA in men younger than 50 years is less than 2.5 ng/mL. PSA levels increase to as high as 6.5 ng/mL when men reach their 70s (Pagana & Pagana, 2018). *African-American men between the ages of 50 and 59 have a slighter higher normal value than men who are Caucasian or Asian, but the reason for this difference is not known.* However, levels greater than 4 ng/mL have been noted in more than 80% of men with prostate cancer (Pagana & Pagana, 2018).

An elevated PSA level should decrease a few days after a prostatectomy for cancer. An increase in the PSA level several weeks after surgery may indicate that the disease has recurred (Pagana & Pagana, 2018).

Because PSA is not absolutely specific to prostate cancer, another blood test, *early prostate cancer antigen (EPCA-2),* may be a serum marker for prostate cancer. It can reveal changes in the prostate gland early and is a very sensitive test.

Other Diagnostic Assessment. After assessments by DRE and PSA, most patients have a *transrectal ultrasound (TRUS)* of the prostate in an ambulatory care or imaging setting. Before the procedure, the health care provider uses lidocaine jelly on the ultrasound probe and/or injects lidocaine into the prostate gland to promote patient comfort. The provider inserts a small probe into the rectum and obtains a view of the prostate using sound waves. If prostate cancer is suspected, a *biopsy* is usually performed at that time to obtain an accurate diagnosis.

TABLE 67.2 Prostate Cancer Staging

Stage	Description	Metastasis
0	No evidence of a primary tumor	N/A
I	Tumor not detectable by digital rectal examination (DRE); cannot be seen on imaging studies	No
II	Tumor detected by DRE; present only in prostate	No
III	Tumor extends outside of prostate and possibly to seminal vesicles	No
IV	Tumor has spread to tissues near prostate and beyond seminal vesicles, such as bladder or pelvis wall	Yes

Adapted from Prostate Conditions Education Council. (2020). https://www.prostateconditions.org/images/about/Tumor_Chart.jpg; and American Cancer Association. (2019). https://www.cancer.org/cancer/prostate-cancer/detection-diagnosis-staging/staging.html.

! NURSING SAFETY PRIORITY (QSEN)

Action Alert

After a transrectal ultrasound with biopsy, instruct the patient about possible complications, although rare, including hematuria with clots, signs of *infection,* and perineal pain. Teach him to report fever, chills, bloody urine, and any difficulty voiding. Advise him to avoid strenuous physical activity and to drink plenty of fluids, especially in the first 24 hours after the procedure. Teach him that a small amount of bleeding turning the urine pink is expected during this time. However, bright red bleeding should be reported to the health care provider immediately.

After prostate cancer is diagnosed, the patient has additional imaging and blood studies to determine the extent of the disease. Common tests include lymph node biopsy, CT of the pelvis and abdomen, and MRI to assess the status of the pelvic and para-aortic lymph nodes. A radionuclide bone scan may be performed to detect metastatic bone disease. An enlarged liver or abnormal liver function study results indicate possible liver metastasis.

Patients with advanced prostate cancer often have *elevated levels of serum acid phosphatase.* Most men with bone metastasis have *elevated serum alkaline phosphatase* levels and severe pain.

As with any cancer, accurate staging and grading of prostate tumors guide monitoring and treatment planning during the course of the disease. Based on diagnostic assessment results, the cancer is staged, which can help to guide treatment choices. Table 67.2 shows how prostate cancer is staged.

◆ **Analysis: Analyze Cues and Prioritize Hypotheses.** The priority collaborative problem for the patient with prostate cancer is:
1. Potential for cancer metastasis due to lack of, or inadequate, treatment

◆ **Planning and Implementation: Generate Solutions and Take Action**

Preventing Metastasis

Planning: Generate Solutions. The patient with prostate cancer is expected to remain free of metastases or recurrence of disease, if possible. If cancer recurs, the patient will experience optimal health outcomes, including potential palliation and end-of-life care.

Interventions: Take Action. Patients are faced with several treatment options. A urologist and an oncologist usually collaborate to help patients make the best decision.

Active Surveillance. Because prostate cancer is slow growing with late metastasis, older men who are asymptomatic and have other illnesses may choose observation without immediate active treatment, especially if the cancer is at an early stage. This option is known as active surveillance (AS). This form of treatment involves initial surveillance with active treatment only if the symptoms become bothersome. The average time from diagnosis to start of treatment is up to 10 years. During the AS period, men are monitored at regular intervals through DRE and PSA testing. Factors that are considered in choosing AS include potential side effects of treatment (e.g., urinary incontinence, erectile dysfunction), estimated life expectancy, the presence of comorbid medical conditions, and the risk for increased morbidity and mortality from not seeking active treatment.

Patients who have very early–stage cancer of the prostate who choose AS require close follow-up by their primary health care provider. If obstruction occurs, a transurethral resection of the prostate (TURP) may be done. The care of patients having this procedure is described in the discussion of Surgical Management in the section Elimination Concept Exemplar: Benign Prostatic Hyperplasia.

Specific management is based on the extent of the disease and the patient's physical condition. The patient may undergo surgery for a biopsy (if not previously done), staging and removal of the tumor, or palliation to control the spread of disease or relieve distressing symptoms. As with AS, the health care provider and patient must weigh the benefits of treatment against potential adverse effects such as incontinence and erectile dysfunction (ED).

Nonsurgical Management. Nonsurgical management may be an adjunct to surgery or alternative intervention if the cancer is widespread or the patient's condition or age prevents surgery. Available modalities include radiation therapy, hormone therapy, and chemotherapy (less often).

Radiation therapy. External or internal radiation therapy may be used in the treatment of prostate cancer or as salvage treatments when cancer recurs. It may also be done for palliation of the patient's symptoms.

External beam radiation therapy (EBRT) comes from a source outside the body. Patients are usually treated 5 days a week for a minimum of several weeks. EBRT can also be used to relieve pain from bone metastasis. Three-dimensional conformal radiation therapy (3D-CRT) can more accurately target prostate tissue and reduce damage to nearby organs and tissue. An advanced type of 3D-CRT radiation is *intensity-modulated radiation therapy,* which provides very high doses to the prostate. It is the most commonly used type of external beam radiation therapy for prostate cancer (American Cancer Society, 2019b).

Teach patients that external beam radiation causes ED in many men well after the treatment is completed. Remind the

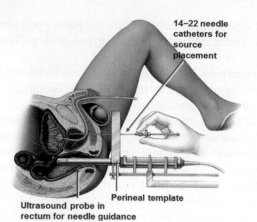

14–22 needle
catheters for
source
placement

Perineal template

Ultrasound probe in
rectum for needle guidance

FIG. 67.5 Patient position and vital component of prostate brachytherapy with transrectal ultrasound guidance. (From Stish, B.J., Davis, B.J., Mynderse, L.A., Deufel, C.L., & Choo, R. [2017]. Brachytherapy in the management of prostate cancer. *Surgical Oncology Clinics of North America, 26*[3], 491–513. https://doi.org/10.1016/j.soc.2017.01.008.)

patient that other complications from EBRT include urinary frequency, diarrhea, and *acute radiation cystitis*, which causes persistent pain and hematuria. Symptoms are usually mild to moderate and subside 6 weeks after treatment, although there is a rare chance that this will not go away. Teach the patient to avoid caffeine and continue drinking plenty of water and other fluids.

Radiation proctitis may also develop but is less likely with 3D-CRT. Radiation that has irritated the rectum can cause urgency and cramping, which leads to rectal leakage (American Cancer Society, 2019b). Teach him to report these symptoms to the health care provider. Like cystitis, this problem usually resolves 4 to 6 weeks after the treatment stops, although in rare cases it is permanent. If proctitis occurs, teach patients to limit spicy or fatty foods, caffeine, and dairy products.

Low-dose brachytherapy is a type of internal radiation (Fig. 67.5) that is delivered by implanting low-dose radiation "seeds" (the size of a grain of rice) directly into the prostate gland. This treatment involves transrectal ultrasound, CT scans, or MRI, which are used to guide implantation of the seeds. These procedures are usually done on an ambulatory care basis under spinal or general anesthesia, and are the most cost-effective treatment for early-stage prostate cancer. Reassure the patient that the dose of radiation is low and that the radiation will not pose a hazard to him or others. Teach him that ED, urinary incontinence, and rectal problems do occur in a small percentage of cases. Fatigue is also common and may last for several months after the treatment stops. Chapter 20 describes general nursing care for patients having radiation therapy.

Drug therapy. Drug therapy may consist of either hormone therapy (androgen deprivation therapy [ADT]) or chemotherapy. Because most prostate tumors are hormone dependent, patients with extensive tumors or those with metastatic disease may be managed by androgen deprivation. *Luteinizing hormone–releasing hormone (LHRH) agonists* or antiandrogens can be used.

LHRH agonists available in the United States include leuprolide, goserelin, histrelin, and triptorelin. These drugs first stimulate the pituitary gland to release luteinizing hormone (LH). After about 3 weeks, the pituitary gland is depleted of LH, which reduces testosterone production by the testes (Burchum & Rosenthal, 2019). Leuprolide is used most commonly for advanced prostate cancer with the goal of palliation (Burchum & Rosenthal, 2019).

! NURSING SAFETY PRIORITY (QSEN)

Drug Alert

Teach patients taking LHRH agonists that side effects include "hot flashes," which usually decrease as treatment progresses. The subsequent reduction in testosterone may contribute to erectile dysfunction and decreased **libido** (desire to have sex). Some men also develop **gynecomastia** (abnormal enlargement of the breasts in men.). These drugs can also increase the patient's risk for osteoporosis and fractures. Teach the patient to take calcium and vitamin D and to engage in regular weight-bearing exercise. Bisphosphonates can be prescribed to prevent bone fractures.

Antiandrogen drugs, also known as *androgen deprivation therapy (ADT),* work differently in that they block the body's ability to use the available androgens (Burchum & Rosenthal, 2019). These drugs are the major treatment for metastatic disease. Examples include flutamide, bicalutamide, and nilutamide. They inhibit tumor progression by blocking the uptake of testicular and adrenal androgens at the prostate tumor site. Patients should be taught to follow closely with their health care provider and to undergo all laboratory testing as prescribed. These medications increase the risk for liver toxicity. Regular liver functions tests will be ordered at baseline, monthly during the first 4 months, and periodically thereafter (Burchum & Rosenthal, 2019).

Antiandrogens may be used alone or in combination with LHRH agonists for total or maximal androgen blockade (hormone ablation).

Systemic *chemotherapy* may be an option for patients whose cancer has spread and for whom other therapies have not worked. For example, small cell prostate cancer is rare and is more responsive to chemotherapy than to hormone therapy. The goal of therapy is not curative; it is to slow the cancer's growth so that the patient experiences a better quality of life. Chapter 20 describes general nursing care for patients receiving chemotherapy.

Surgical Management. Surgery is the most common intervention for a cure. Minimally invasive surgery (MIS) or, less commonly, an open surgical technique for radical prostatectomy (prostate removal) can be performed. A **bilateral orchiectomy** (removal of both testicles) is another palliative surgery that slows the spread of cancer by removing the main source of testosterone.

Preoperative care. Preoperative care depends on the type of surgery that will be done. Minimally invasive surgery (MIS) is most appropriate for localized prostate cancer and is used as a curative intervention. The most common procedure is the *laparoscopic radical prostatectomy (LRP),* often done with robotic assistance. Other procedures include transrectal high-intensity focused ultrasound (HIFU) and cryotherapy.

Patients who qualify for LRP must have a PSA less than 10 ng/mL and have had no previous hormone therapy or abdominal surgeries. Remind the patient that the advantages of this procedure over open surgery include:

- Decreased hospital stay (1 to 2 days)
- Minimal bleeding
- Smaller or no incisions and less scarring
- Less postoperative discomfort
- Decreased time for urinary catheter placement (usually removed on third postoperative day)
- Fewer complications
- Faster recovery and return to usual activities
- Nerve-sparing advantages

For the patient undergoing an *open* radical prostatectomy, provide preoperative care as for any patient having surgery (see Chapter 9).

Operative procedures. For the *LRP procedure,* the patient is placed in lithotomy positioning with steep Trendelenburg. The urologist makes one or more small punctures or incisions into the abdomen. A laparoscope with a camera on the end is inserted through one of the incisions while other instruments are inserted into the other incisions. The robotic system may be used to control the movement of the instruments by a remote device. The prostate is removed along with nearby lymph nodes, but perineal nerves are not affected.

The *open* radical prostatectomy can be performed via several surgical approaches, depending on the patient's desired outcomes and the staging of the disease. The perineal and retropubic (nerve-sparing) approaches are most commonly used. The surgeon removes the entire prostate gland along with the prostatic capsule, the cuff at the bladder neck, the seminal vesicles, and the regional lymph nodes. The remaining urethra is connected to the bladder neck. The removal of tissue at the bladder neck allows the seminal fluid to travel upward into the bladder rather than down the urethral tract, resulting in retrograde ejaculation.

Postoperative care. Provide postoperative care of the patient after *open* radical prostatectomy as summarized in the Best Practice for Patient Safety & Quality Care: Care of the Patient After an Open Radical Prostatectomy box. Nursing interventions include all the typical care for a patient undergoing major surgery. Maintaining hydration, caring for wound drains (open procedure), managing pain, and preventing pulmonary complications are important aspects of nursing care. (See general postoperative care in Chapter 9.)

Assess the patient's pain level and monitor the effectiveness of pain management with opioids given as patient-controlled analgesia (PCA), a common method of delivery during the first 24 hours after surgery. Administer a stool softener if needed to prevent possible constipation from the drugs.

The patient has an indwelling urinary catheter to straight drainage to promote urinary **elimination.** Monitor intake and output every shift and record or delegate this activity to assistive personnel (AP), as this is a task that is within an AP's scope that can effectively and quickly be reported back to the nurse. An antispasmodic may be prescribed to decrease bladder spasm induced by the indwelling urinary catheter. The time for

BEST PRACTICE FOR PATIENT SAFETY & QUALITY CARE (QSEN)

Care of the Patient After an Open Radical Prostatectomy

- Encourage the patient to use patient-controlled analgesia (PCA) as needed.
- Help the patient get out of bed into a chair on the night of surgery and ambulate by the next day.
- Maintain the sequential compression device until the patient begins to ambulate.
- Monitor the patient for venous thromboembolism and pulmonary embolus.
- Keep an accurate record of intake and output, including drainage from a Jackson-Pratt or other drainage device.
- Keep the urinary meatus clean using soap and water.
- Avoid rectal procedures or treatments.
- Teach the patient how to care for the urinary catheter because he may be discharged with the catheter in place.
- Teach the patient how to use a leg bag.
- Emphasize the importance of not straining during a bowel movement yet to avoid suppositories or enemas.
- Remind the patient about the importance of follow-up appointments with the surgeon and oncologist to monitor progress.

catheter removal depends on the type of procedure that is performed and overall patient condition. Those who undergo the laparoscopic prostatectomy usually have the catheter in place until the third postoperative day. Those who had open surgical procedures use the catheter for 7 to 10 days or longer.

Ambulation should begin no later than the day after surgery. Provide assistance in walking the patient when he first gets out of bed. Assess for scrotal or penile swelling from the disrupted pelvic lymph flow. If this occurs, elevate the scrotum and penis and apply ice to the area intermittently for the first 24 to 48 hours.

Many patients who have the minimally invasive techniques are discharged 1 to 2 days after surgery and can resume usual activities in about a week or two. Those who have open procedures are discharged in 2 to 3 days or longer, depending on their progress.

Remind patients that common potential long-term complications of open radical prostatectomy are erectile dysfunction (ED) and urinary incontinence. For ED, drugs such as sildenafil may be effective. *Urge incontinence* may occur because the internal and external sphincters of the bladder lie close to the prostate gland and are often damaged during the surgery. Kegel perineal exercises may reduce the severity of urinary incontinence after radical prostatectomy. Teach the patient to contract and relax the perineal and gluteal muscles in several ways. For one of the exercises, teach him to:

1. Tighten the perineal muscles for 3 to 5 seconds as if to prevent voiding, and then relax
2. Bear down (but not to strain) as if having a bowel movement
3. Relax and repeat the exercise

Show him how to inhale through pursed lips while tightening the perineal muscles and how to exhale when he relaxes. He may also sit on the toilet with the knees apart while voiding and start and stop the stream several times.

Care Coordination and Transition Management. Interprofessional collaborative care of the man with prostate cancer should include his partner, if he agrees. The diagnosis and treatment of cancer greatly affect couples who survive the disease. Recognize that the patient and partner have specific physical and psychosocial needs that should be addressed before hospital discharge, and management should continue in the community setting.

Patients with prostate cancer may require care in a wide variety of settings at any stage of the disease process: at the hospital, the radiation therapy department, the oncologist's office, or home. Specific interventions depend on which treatment the patient had or if he had a combination of treatments. Regardless of treatment, coordination to effectively manage transitions in care is essential. This section focuses on the needs of those who had a *radical prostatectomy*.

Home Care Management. Discharge planning and health teaching start early, even before surgery. A patient can better plan home care management when he knows what to expect. Collaborate with the case manager to coordinate the efforts of various health care providers, surgical unit nursing staff, and possibly a home nurse. *As specified by The Joint Commission and other accrediting agencies, continuity of care is essential when caring for this patient because he may need weeks or months of therapies.*

Self-Management Education. An important area of teaching for the patient going home is urinary catheter care. An indwelling urinary catheter may be in place for 3 days for the patient who had an LRP, or up to several weeks for the patient who underwent an open radical prostatectomy. Teach him and his partner how to care for the catheter, use a leg bag, and identify signs and symptoms of **infection** and other complications. See the Patient and Family Education: Preparing for Self-Management: Urinary Catheter Care at Home box.

Encourage the patient to walk short distances. Lifting may be restricted to no more than a milk jug for up to 6 weeks if an open procedure was done. Remind him to maintain an upright position and not to walk bent or flexed. Vigorous exercise such as running or jumping should be avoided for at least 6 weeks and then gradually introduced. By contrast, patients having the minimally invasive laparoscopic surgery can usually return to work or usual activities in about a week.

Teach the patient not to strain to defecate. A stool softener may be prescribed to reduce the need for straining. If an opioid is prescribed for pain management, encourage the patient to drink adequate water to prevent constipation.

If the patient had an *open* radical prostatectomy, teach him to adhere to the surgeon's recommendation for when he can first shower and to continue showering for the first 2 to 3 weeks rather than soak in a bathtub. Patients who had a *laparoscopic* procedure can usually shower in 1 to 2 days. Teach them to remove the small bandage but leave the wound closure tape in place and allow it to fall off naturally in about a week. Show patients how to inspect the incision or puncture site(s) daily for signs of **infection.** Remind them to keep all follow-up appointments. PSA blood tests are performed 6 weeks after surgery and then every 4 to 6 months to monitor progress.

Health Care Resources. Refer the patient and partner to agencies or support groups such as the American Cancer Society's *Man-to-Man* program to help cope with prostate cancer. This program provides one-on-one education, personal visits, educational presentations, and the opportunity to engage in open and candid discussions. Another prostate cancer support group is *Us TOO International* (https://www.ustoo.org/Support-Group-Near-You) sponsored by the Prostate Cancer Education and Support Network. This group provides education and support with national and international chapters. Information can also be obtained from the Prostate Cancer Foundation (www.prostatecancerfoundation.org) or the National Alliance of State Prostate Cancer Coalitions (www.naspcc.org). In Canada, the Canadian Cancer Society (www.prostatecancer.ca) is dedicated to research and support for this disease. Other personal and community support services such as spiritual leaders or churches, synagogues, or mosques are also important to many patients.

For same-sex couples surviving prostate cancer, *Malecare* (http://malecare.org) is an excellent resource. This nonprofit organization provides support groups for gay and bisexual men and their partners.

Some men have erectile dysfunction (ED) for the first 3 to 18 months after a prostatectomy. Refer them to a specialist who can help with this problem. (ED is discussed later in this chapter.) Refer patients with urinary incontinence to a urologist who specializes in this area. Chapter 61 discusses incontinence management in detail.

◆ **Evaluation: Evaluate Outcomes.** Evaluate the care of the patient with prostate cancer based on the identified priority patient problem. The primary expected outcome is that the patient with prostate cancer is expected to remain free of metastases or recurrence of disease, if possible. If cancer recurs, the patient will experience optimal health outcomes, including potential palliation and end-of-life care.

PATIENT AND FAMILY EDUCATION: PREPARING FOR SELF-MANAGEMENT

Urinary Catheter Care at Home

- Once a day, gently wash the first few inches of the catheter, starting at the penis and washing outward with mild soap and water.
- Rinse and dry the catheter well.
- If you have not been circumcised, push the foreskin back to clean the catheter site; when finished, push the foreskin forward.
- Change the drainage bag at least once a week as needed:
  - Hold the catheter with one hand and the tubing with the other hand and twist in opposite directions to disconnect.
  - Place the end of the catheter in a clean container to catch leakage of urine.
  - Remove the rubber cap from the tubing of the leg bag or clean drainage bag.
  - Clean the end of the new tubing with alcohol swabs.
  - Insert the end of the new tubing into the catheter and twist to connect securely.
  - Clean the drainage bag just removed by pouring a solution of one part vinegar to two parts water through the tubing and bag. Rinse well with water and allow the bag to dry.

TESTICULAR CANCER

Pathophysiology Review

Testicular cancer, which can occur in one or both testicles, is a rare cancer that most often affects men between 20 and 35 years of age but can affect men of any age. It usually strikes men at a productive time of life and thus has significant economic, social, and psychological impact on the patient and his family and/or partner. With early detection by testicular self-examination (TSE) (see the Patient and Family Education: Preparing for Self-Management: Testicular Self-Examination box and Fig. 67.6) and treatment, testicular cancer has a greater than 95% cure rate (McCance et al., 2019).

Primary testicular cancers fall into two major groups:

- Germ cell tumors (GCTs) arising from the sperm-producing cells (account for most testicular cancers)
- Non–germ cell tumors arising from the stromal, interstitial, or Leydig cells that produce testosterone (account for a very small percentage of testicular cancers)

Testicular germ cell tumors are classified into two broad categories: germ cell tumors (GCTs) and others (Table 67.3). The most common type of testicular tumor is *seminoma*. Patients with seminomas have the most favorable prognoses because the tumors are usually localized, metastasize late, and respond to treatment. They often are diagnosed when they are still confined to the testicles and retroperitoneal lymph nodes.

The risk for testicular tumors is higher in males who have an undescended testis (cryptorchidism); human immune deficiency virus (HIV) infection or acquired immune deficiency syndrome (AIDS [HIV-III]); frequent use of marijuana; or history of testicular cancer (McCance et al., 2019; Michaelson & Oh, 2020).

PATIENT-CENTERED CARE: GENETIC/GENOMIC CONSIDERATIONS (QSEN)

Men are at a higher risk for testicular cancer if they have a family history of the disease (Michaelson & Oh, 2020). The incidence is higher among identical twins, brothers, and other close male relatives. Caucasian men are at a higher risk for testicular cancer than men of other races or ethnicities (Michaelson & Oh, 2020). The reason for these differences is not known.

PATIENT AND FAMILY EDUCATION: PREPARING FOR SELF-MANAGEMENT

Testicular Self-Examination

- Examine your testicles monthly immediately after a bath or a shower, when your scrotal skin is relaxed.
- Examine each testicle by gently rolling it between your thumbs and fingers. Testicular tumors tend to appear deep in the center of the testicle.
- Look and feel for any lumps; smooth rounded masses; or any change in the size, shape, or consistency of the testes.
- Report any lump or swelling to your primary health care provider as soon as possible.

Synchronous bilateral testicular cancer is extremely rare; many men have metastatic disease versus those who experience primary testicular cancer (in one testicle) (Campobasso et al., 2017).

❖ Interprofessional Collaborative Care

◆ Assessment: Recognize Cues

History. When taking a history from a patient with a suspected testicular tumor, assess for risk factors including a history or presence of an undescended testis and a family history of testicular cancer.

The most common report is a painless, hard swelling or enlargement of the testicle, although a small portion of patients do report pain. Patients with testicular pain, lymph node swelling, bone pain, abdominal masses or aching, sudden hydrocele (fluid in the scrotum), or gynecomastia may have metastatic disease. Determine and document how long any signs and symptoms have been present.

Questions about sexuality and ***reproduction*** are important. If the man has one healthy testis, he can function sexually. If he has a retroperitoneal lymph node dissection (RPLND) or chemotherapy, he may become sterile because of treatment effects on the sperm-producing cells or surgical trauma to the sympathetic nervous system resulting in retrograde ejaculation. Therefore, collect information regarding whether the patient is sexually active, whether he wishes to have children in the future, and if so, if he would be interested in learning about sperm storage in a sperm bank.

Physical Assessment/Signs and Symptoms. The testes, lymph nodes, and abdomen should be examined thoroughly. Patients may feel embarrassed about having this examination. Provide privacy and explain the procedure to the patient. Inspect the testicles for swelling or a lump that the patient reports is painless. A health care provider will palpate the testes for lumps and swelling that are not visible.

Psychosocial Assessment. Because testicular cancer and its treatment can lead to sexual dysfunction, pay close attention to the psychosocial aspects of the disease. ***Sexuality*** is likely to be a prime concern for any patient, yet it may be even concerning for younger men who may have a fear of not being able to perform sexually, or father children. Assess the man's support systems, and refer to community support resources as necessary.

TABLE 67.3 Classification of Testicular Tumors

Germ Cell Tumors (GCTS)	Non–Germ Cell Tumors	Mixed Tumors
- Seminomas - Classic - Spermatocytic - Nonseminomas - Embryonal carcinoma - Yolk sac carcinoma - Choriocarcinoma - Teratoma	- Leydig cell - Sertoli cell - Granulosa cell - Thecal cell	- Teratocarcinoma - Other

Adapted from McCance, K., Huether, S., Brashers, V., & Rote, N. (2019). *Pathophysiology: The biologic basis for disease in adults and children* (8th ed.). St. Louis: Mosby.

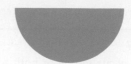
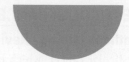

Monthly Self-Exam

HOW TO PERFORM A MONTHLY SELF EXAM.

Always perform monthly self-exams and ask your doctor for a testicular exam at your annual appointment, or sports physical.

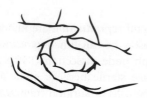

One.
Cup one testicle at a time using both hands.
This is best performed during or after a warm shower.

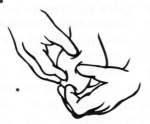

Two.
Examine by rolling the testicle between thumb and fingers.
Use slight pressure.

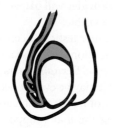

Three.
Familiarize yourself with the spermatic cord and epididymis.
The tube like structures connected on the back side of each testicle.

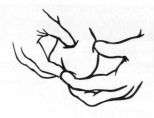

Four.
Feel for lumps, changes in size, or irregularities.
It is normal for one testis to be slightly larger than the other.

KNOW THE FACTS ABOUT TESTICULAR CANCER
•• *Leading cancer in men 15-44*
•• *Early detection is key*
•• *Every hour a male is diagnosed*
•• *Every day a life is lost*

RISK FACTORS
•• *Undescended testicles (cryptorchidism)*
•• *Family history*
•• *Personal history of TC*
•• *Intratubular germ cell neoplasia*

SIGNS & SYMPTOMS
•• *A painless lump, change in size or any irregularity*
•• *Pain or discomfort in the scrotum or testicle*
•• *A dull ache or sense of pressure in the lower abdomen, back or groin*

ADVANCED SIGNS
•• *Significant weight loss*
•• *Back and/or abdominal pain*
•• *Chest pain, coughing or difficulty breathing*
•• *Headaches*
•• *Enlarged lymph nodes in abdomen and/or neck*

 Testicular Cancer Awareness Foundation

Awareness •• Support •• Survivorship

FIG. 67.6 Monthly self-examination of testicles. (Courtesy of Testicular Cancer Awareness Foundation.)

PATIENT AND FAMILY EDUCATION: PREPARING FOR SELF-MANAGEMENT

Sperm Banking

- You may want to investigate sperm storage (called "cryopreservation") in a sperm bank as a way to preserve your sperm for future use.
- No one knows how long sperm can be stored successfully, but pregnancies have resulted from sperm stored for longer than 40 years (Szell et al., 2013).
- Check with the sperm bank to see how much it charges to process and store your sperm and whether you must pay when the service is provided.
- Investigate whether your health insurance company will reimburse you for sperm collection and storage.

Diagnostic Assessment. Common serum tumor markers and other diagnostic methods that are used when formulating a diagnosis of testicular cancer are:

- Alpha fetoprotein (AFP)
- Beta human chorionic gonadotropin (hCG)
- Lactate dehydrogenase (LDH)
- Scrotal ultrasound
- Chest x-ray
- CT of the chest (if metastasis is suspected)
- CT scan of the abdomen and pelvis
- MRI of the brain (if metastasis is suspected)

◆ **Interventions: Take Action.** The incidence of oligospermia (low sperm count) and azoospermia (absence of living sperm) is common in patients diagnosed with testicular cancer. In the pretreatment phase, review the normal reproductive function, as well as possible effects of cancer and its treatment on reproductive function. Explore with the patient various reproductive options if desired (see the Patient and Family Education: Preparing for Self-Management: Sperm Banking box). A sperm bank facility provides comprehensive information on semen collection, storage of semen, the storage contract, costs, and the insemination process.

Nonsurgical Management. Chemotherapy or radiation therapy may be used depending on the tumor staging, whether surgery is performed, and based on the degree of adherence to treatment that is anticipated (Oh, 2020). The specific treatment, including frequency, cycling, and duration, will vary from patient to patient, depending on the extent of the disease and the protocol being followed. Chapter 20 discusses the general nursing care for the patient receiving chemotherapy.

Surgical Management. Surgery is the main treatment for testicular cancer. For localized disease, the surgeon performs a unilateral orchiectomy to remove the affected testicle, which is usually curative (Oh, 2020).

Preoperative Care. Like most patients with cancer, the man with testicular cancer may be very apprehensive. Offer support and reinforce the teaching provided by the surgeon. Teach the patient and his family or partner about what to expect after surgery.

Operative Procedures. Most patients with seminoma have only one surgery to remove the diseased testicle through the groin (inguinal) for a cure. A frozen section of the tumor is examined to confirm the type and stage of the cancer. A saline-filled silicone prosthesis may be surgically implanted into the scrotum at the time of the orchiectomy or later if the patient desires. This type of reconstructive surgery gives the appearance of having two testes. With one functioning testicle, the man is still able to achieve an erection for sexual intercourse.

Some men have more advanced disease or tumor types that are more aggressive. The preferred method to address this is laparoscopic retroperitoneal lymph node dissection (RPLND), which is a minimally invasive surgery (MIS). This technique is much shorter than the traditional open surgical approach, which is much more complicated and requires more postoperative hospital recovery time. In laparoscopic RPLND, very small skin incisions in the abdomen are made by a laparoscope, through which the nodes are dissected for examination. Bleeding, postoperative pain, and postoperative complications are minimized. The patient who has had laparoscopic RPLND can still achieve an erection, yet if there has been nerve damage during surgery, he may experience retrograde ejaculation. Newer nerve-sparing surgeries have shown to be very successful when performed by experienced surgeons (American Cancer Society, 2018). Research continues on robotic-assisted laparoscopic RPLND (R-RPLND) regarding whether it is superior to laparoscopic RPLND (Schwen et al., 2018).

Postoperative Care. Nursing care for the patient after surgery depends on the type of surgical procedure that was performed and the extent of the disease process. The patient is usually hospitalized for multiple days after an *open* radical retroperitoneal lymph node dissection. The patient having the laparoscopic procedure may have a urinary catheter in place following the procedure, which is removed before discharge 1 to 2 days later. Refer to Chapter 9 for general postoperative care.

NCLEX EXAMINATION CHALLENGE 67.3

Physiological Integrity

Which assessment finding will the nurse report to the health care provider for a client who had an orchiectomy and laparoscopic radical retroperitoneal lymph node dissection this morning?

A. BP 130/80 mm Hg, T 98.9°F, R 16, P 70
B. Urinary catheter draining clear yellow urine
C. Expresses fearfulness of inability to perform sexually
D. Reports pain of 9 on a 0-10 scale after receiving pain medication

Care Coordination and Transition Management. After an open *orchiectomy,* the patient is discharged without a dressing on the inguinal incision (as long as there is no wound complication). A scrotal support may be needed for several days. He may want to wear a dry dressing to prevent clothing from rubbing on the sutures and causing irritation. Tell him that the sutures will be removed in the health care provider's office 7 to 10 days after surgery.

Patients who also had an *open* RPLND recover even more slowly. They should not lift anything over 15 lb (6.8 kg), should avoid stair climbing, and should not drive a car for several weeks. Be sure that bathroom facilities are on the first floor of the house where he can easily access them.

Teach the patient who had a laparoscopic procedure that he will be able to resume most of his usual activities within 1 week after discharge. He can take a shower 1 or 2 days after surgery, but be sure that he does not remove the wound closure tape. These strips of tape will loosen and fall off about a week after surgery.

> ### ! NURSING SAFETY PRIORITY (QSEN)
> *Action Alert*
>
> For the patient who has undergone testicular surgery, emphasize the importance of scheduling a follow-up visit with the surgeon to examine the incision for proper healing. Instruct him to notify the surgeon immediately if chills, fever, vomiting, increasing incisional pain, drainage, or dehiscence of the incision occurs. These signs and symptoms may indicate **infection** for which antibiotics are needed.

Explain the importance of performing monthly testicular self-examination (TSE) on the remaining testis and scheduling follow-up examinations with the health care provider. The patient who has had testicular cancer should be seen regularly by his health care provider for follow-up care and testing.

For the patient who has reproductive concerns, refer to the American Society for Reproductive Medicine (www.reproductivefacts.org) or RESOLVE: The National Infertility Association (www.resolve.org).

ERECTILE DYSFUNCTION

Pathophysiology Review

Erectile dysfunction (ED), also known as *impotence,* is the inability to achieve or maintain an erection for sexual intercourse. It affects millions of men throughout the world. There are two major types of ED: organic and psychogenic.

Organic ED is a gradual deterioration of function. The man may first notice diminishing firmness and a decrease in frequency of erections. Causes include (McCance et al., 2019; Schreiber, 2019):

- Vascular, endocrine, or neurologic disease
- Chronic disease (e.g., diabetes mellitus, renal failure)
- Penile disease or trauma
- Surgery or pharmaceutical therapies
- Obesity
- Psychological conditions

If the patient has episodes of ED, it usually has a *psychogenic* cause. Men with this type of ED usually still have normal nocturnal (nighttime) and morning erections. Onset is usually sudden and follows a period of high stress.

❖ Interprofessional Collaborative Care

The health care provider will attempt to determine the cause of the ED through a variety of diagnostic tests. These may include evaluating glycated hemoglobin, a lipid panel for cardiac risk factors, thyroid-stimulating hormone (TSH) to rule out thyroid disease, and serum total testosterone (Khera, 2020a). Doppler ultrasonography can be used to determine blood flow to the penis. Treatment depends on the underlying cause, and may include (Khera, 2020b):

- Lifestyle modifications (e.g., smoking cessation, weight loss, management of hypertension)
- Management of medications that may cause ED (e.g., antidepressants)
- Penile self-injection with prostaglandin E1
- Phosphodiesterase-5 (PDE5) drug therapy
- Psychotherapy
- Testosterone and PDE5 drug therapy (for men with hypogonadism)
- Surgery (prosthesis)
- Vacuum-assisted erection devices
  See Table 67.4 for select treatment options for ED.

> ### ! NURSING SAFETY PRIORITY (QSEN)
> *Drug Alert*
>
> Instruct patients taking PDE-5 inhibitors to abstain from alcohol before sexual intercourse because it could impair the ability to have an erection. Common side effects of these drugs include dyspepsia (heartburn), headaches, facial flushing, and stuffy nose. If more than one pill a day is being taken, leg and back cramps, nausea, and vomiting also may occur. *Teach men who take nitrates to avoid PDE-5 inhibitors because the vasodilation effects can cause a profound hypotension and reduce blood flow to vital organs* (Burchum & Rosenthal, 2019).

VASECTOMY

Vasectomy is the most effective mode of male contraception. It involves interruption or occlusion of each vas deferens (Viera, 2019). The preferred procedure is the "no-scalpel" vasectomy, performed with local anesthetic (without epinephrine) in an outpatient setting.

Teach the patient to leave the bandaging in place for at least 48 hours post-procedure, and to apply an ice pack intermittently to the scrotum for 24 to 48 hours to minimize pain and swelling. Remind the patient that mild pain, swelling, and bruising are normal, however, for the first few days. Teach him to report increasing pain, incisional bleeding, increased swelling, or fever to the health care provider (Viera, 2019).

The patient is usually instructed by the health care provider to rest for 1 to 2 days, and then he can return to light work. Heavy lifting, sports, and sexual intercourse should be avoided for at least 1 week. Teach the patient and partner to use an alternate form of contraception until a 3-month follow-up. At that time, a semen analysis will be performed to determine if the procedure was effective.

Although this procedure is performed with the intention of permanent sterilization, vasectomy can be reversed microsurgically in approximately 50% to 70% of cases (Viera, 2019).

OTHER CONDITIONS AFFECTING THE MALE REPRODUCTIVE SYSTEM

Other conditions that can affect the male reproductive system include inflammation, infection, swelling, trauma, and torsion. Table 67.5 lists select examples of these common conditions with nursing implications.

TABLE 67.4 Select Treatment Options for Erectile Dysfunction

Procedure	Description	Nursing Implications
Phosphodiesterase-5 (PDE5) inhibitors (drug therapy)	Work by relaxing the smooth muscles in the corpora cavernosa so blood flow to the penis is increased. The veins exiting the corpora are compressed, limiting outward blood flow and resulting in penile **tumescence** (swelling).	Teach: • Any PDE5 drug can lower blood pressure; teach to be aware of safety precautions before taking the drug. • When taking avanafil, sexual stimulation is needed within 15 minutes to promote an erection. Take pill about 15 minutes before intercourse. • When taking sildenafil or vardenafil, sexual stimulation is needed within ½ to 1 hour to promote the erection. Take pill about 1 hour before intercourse. • When taking tadalafil, an erection can be stimulated over several hours; take pill at least 2 hours before intercourse. Effects can last up to 36 hours. • When taking any PDE5 drug, refrain from eating grapefruit or drinking grapefruit juice.
Penile injections	Self-injection into the shaft of the penis. Patient uses an insulin syringe with prostaglandin E1.	Teach: • Use a condom due to increased risk for infection created at injection site. • Ibuprofen can be used to treat penile pain.
Penile prostheses	Semirigid or inflatable options. • Semirigid option results in permanent erection. • Inflatable option involves placement of two hollow cylinders in the corpora cavernosa, and a saline reservoir. Use of a pump moves the saline from behind the cylinders to the front of the eates an erection.	Teach: • Report any signs of infection immediately to the health care provider.
Vacuum-assisted erection device	A cylinder is placed over the penis, sitting firmly against the body. Using a pump, a vacuum is created to draw blood into the penis to maintain an erection. A rubber ring (tension band) is placed around the base of the penis to maintain the erection, and the cylinder is removed.	Teach: • Do not apply vacuum for more than 30 minutes • The vacuum device can be used in tandem with PDE5 inhibitors

TABLE 67.5 Select Conditions Affecting the Male Reproductive System

Condition Type	Examples of Condition	Description	Signs and Symptoms	Nursing Implications
"Cele"	Hydrocele	Swelling in the scrotum where fluid has collected around one or both testicles	Painless testicle swelling; often the sensation is described as "heaviness" of the scrotum	Teach: • Treatment is usually not needed unless the condition becomes painful or too large for comfort; at that time, surgery may be recommended. • If pain does occur, acetaminophen or ibuprofen can be taken. • Report any changes involving pain, fever, redness, or swelling.
	Spermatocele	A cyst that develops in the epididymis; usually is painless	Is usually asymptomatic; sometimes there is pain and/or heaviness in the affected testicle	Teach: • Treatment is usually not needed unless the condition becomes painful or too large for comfort; at that time, surgery may be recommended. • If pain does occur, acetaminophen or ibuprofen can be taken.
	Varicocele	Vein enlargement inside the scrotum (usually on the left side), which can cause low sperm production	Is often asymptomatic; pain, if experienced, may be dull or sharp, and worsens with activity and throughout the day	Teach: • Treatment is usually not needed unless the condition becomes painful or too large for comfort; at that time, surgery may be recommended, particularly if the condition has left the patient infertile.

Continued

Condition Type	Examples of Condition	Description	Signs and Symptoms	Nursing Implications
Emergent	Paraphimosis	The foreskin (of an uncircumcised male) cannot be pulled over the penis tip, resulting in the foreskin becoming stuck, impeding blood flow to the penile tip and lymphatic drainage	Enlargement and congestion of glans and foreskin, with a band of constrictive tissue that prevents moving the foreskin forward over the penile tip (glans)	Teach: • This is a *urologic emergency;* seek emergency care immediately. • Treatment can be manual or surgical in nature. • Topical antibiotic ointment may be prescribed following reduction of the paraphimosis; this should be applied as directed. • The foreskin should not be retracted for a week following reduction.
	Priapism		Persistent, painful erection (usually >4 hr) not associated with sexual stimulation; is common in patients with sickle cell disease, and can be caused by certain drugs	Recognize: • Treatment varies depending on underlying cause; medical therapy involves injection of a sympathomimetic drug into the penis, with or without aspiration of blood to decompress the corpora. Surgical intervention includes placement of a shunt. • Patients with sickle cell disease may require additional treatment including a simple red blood cell transfusion. Monitor: • Patients with sickle cell disease should receive venous thromboembolism prophylaxis. • See Chapter 9 for postoperative procedures.
	Testicular torsion	Twisting of the spermatic cord that results in ischemia from decreased arterial inflow and venous outflow obstruction; can occur spontaneously or as a result of trauma	Nausea Vomiting Lower abdominal pain A tender mass or knot above the testis	Teach: • This is a *urologic emergency;* seek emergency care immediately. Damage may be irreversible after 8 hours. • Surgery is usually performed urgently; manual detorsion is attempted if surgery is not available immediately Monitor: • See Chapter 9 for postoperative procedures.
Infection	Epididymitis	Inflammation or infection of the epididymis; often caused by *Neisseria gonorrhoeae* or *Chlamydia trachomatis* in men under 35; in older men, it often occurs in association with obstructive uropathy from benign prostatic hyperplasia (BPH)	Localized testicular pain Tenderness and swelling on palpation of the epididymis May have scrotal erythema	Teach: • Take the full course of antibiotics, even if you begin to feel better. • Ibuprofen can be used for pain. • Elevate the scrotum and apply ice intermittently. • Refrain from sexual intercourse until treatment is completed. • Always use a condom when engaging in sexual intercourse. • Report development of fever, chills, and/or lower urinary tract symptoms (LUTS) to the health care provider right away.
	Phimosis	Tightness that results in the inability to retract the foreskin	Swelling and pain at the head of the penis, causing difficulty in retraction of the foreskin Is often associated with hygienic concerns (neglecting to replace the foreskin after cleaning, intercourse, or urination), or body piercing of the glans or foreskin	Teach: • Proper hygiene is important. • Topical corticosteroids may be prescribed. • Circumcision may be recommended by the health care provider.

Information adapted from Bragg, B., & Leslie, S. (2019). *Paraphimosis.* StatPearls Publishing, LLC. Treasure Island, FL; Deveci, S. (2019). Priapism. Evaluation of acute scrotal pain in adults. In *UpToDate,* O'Leary, M. (Ed.). Waltham, MA; Eyre, R. (2020). Evaluation of acute scrotal pain in adults. In *UpToDate,* O'Leary, M. (Ed.). Waltham, MA; Eyre, R. (2020). Evaluation of nonacute scrotal conditions in adults. In *UpToDate,* O'Leary, M. (Ed.). Waltham, MA; Field, J. et al. (2019). Priapism and erectile dysfunction in sickle cell disease. In *UpToDate,* Mahoney, D., & Vichinsky, E. (Eds.). Waltham, MA.

GET READY FOR THE NEXT-GENERATION NCLEX® EXAMINATION!

Key Points

Review these Key Points for each NCLEX Examination Client Needs Category.

Safe and Effective Care Environment

- Perform a focused physical assessment for patients reporting lumps or swelling in their genital area; inspect and palpate bladder and scrotum. **QSEN: Safety**
- Teach patients to not lift more than 15 lb (6.8 kg) after open prostate surgery. **QSEN: Safety**
- Teach patients to report signs of *infection* when caring for a urinary catheter in the home. **QSEN: Safety**

Health Promotion and Maintenance

- Teach patients to eat a well-balanced diet including fish, fruits, and vegetables to help prevent prostate cancer. **QSEN: Evidence-Based Practice**
- Teach men at risk for prostate cancer to be screened and follow early detection guidelines. **QSEN: Evidence-Based Practice**
- Teach men how to perform testicular self-examination **QSEN: Evidence-Based Practice**
- Teach men who are uncircumcised about the importance of keeping the penis clean to prevent penile cancer. **QSEN: Evidence-Based Practice**

Psychosocial Integrity

- Assess the patient's understanding regarding the fact that some procedures and drugs related to reproductive problems cause temporary or permanent erectile dysfunction and/or incontinence. **Ethics**
- Assess the patient's anxiety before surgery and allow expression of feelings of fear or grief. **QSEN: Patient-Centered Care**
- Assess the patient's reaction to the possible loss of *reproduction* ability, and concerns about *sexuality* and changes in body image. **QSEN: Patient-Centered Care**
- Teach patients with male reproductive cancer about resources available to provide support. **QSEN: Patient-Centered Care**

Physiological Integrity

- Remind patients wanting to use complementary and integrative therapies to check with their health care provider first. **QSEN: Safety**
- Maintain traction on the urinary catheter and continuous bladder irrigation after a TURP. **QSEN: Safety**
- Observe for and report complications after surgery, including *infection,* severe pain, urinary infection, *elimination* problems, bloody urine with clots, and/or erectile dysfunction. **Clinical Judgment**
- Teach patients with BPH to avoid drugs that can cause urinary retention. **QSEN: Evidence-Based Practice**
- Teach patients about hormone therapies used to treat prostate cancer. **QSEN: Evidence-Based Practice**
- Teach patients with a urinary catheter how to properly care for it at home. **QSEN: Safety**

MASTERY QUESTIONS

1. The nurse is teaching a client with erectile dysfunction about taking sildenafil to achieve an erection. Which client statement demonstrates an understanding of this drug?
   A. "I can have sex up to 8 hours after taking the drug."
   B. "I might get a headache or stuffy nose when this drug is used."
   C. "Taking this with a drink or two of alcohol will enhance my performance."
   D. "If one pill doesn't work, it is acceptable for me to quickly take another pill."

2. A client with a history of BPH calls the telehealth nurse reporting the sudden onset of testicular pain after moving heavy furniture. What is the appropriate nursing response?
   A. "Taking ibuprofen may help alleviate the pain."
   B. "Please go to your closest emergency department right away."
   C. "This is a common reaction when performing labor; the pain will go away."
   D. "Your BPH is probably giving you difficulty because you were moving furniture."

REFERENCES

Asterisk (*) indicates a classic or definitive work on this subject.

Abt, D., et al. (2018). Comparison of prostatic artery embolisation (PAE) versus transurethral resection of the prostate (TURP) for benign prostatic hyperplasia: Randomised, open label, non-inferiority trial. *British Medical Journal [BMJ]*, *361*, k2338.

*American Cancer Society (ACS). (2010). *American Cancer Society guideline for the early detection of prostate cancer: Update 2010.* Retrieved from https://onlinelibrary.wiley.com/doi/full/10.3322/caac.20066.

American Cancer Society (ACS). (2018). *Surgery for testicular cancer.* Retrieved from https://www.cancer.org/cancer/testicular-cancer/treating/surgery.html.

American Cancer Society (ACS). (2019a). *About prostate cancer.* Retrieved from https://www.cancer.org/content/dam/CRC/PDF/Public/8793.00.pdf.

American Cancer Society (ACS). (2019b). *Radiation therapy for prostate cancer.* Retrieved from https://www.cancer.org/cancer/prostate-cancer/treating/radiation-therapy.html.

American Cancer Society (ACS). (2020). *Key statistics for prostate cancer.* Retrieved from https://www.cancer.org/cancer/prostate-cancer/about/key-statistics.html.

Burchum, J. L. R., & Rosenthal, L. D. (2016). *Lehne's pharmacology for nursing care* (9th ed.). St. Louis: Elsevier.

Campobasso, D., Ferretti, S., & Frattini, A. (2017). Synchronous bilateral testis cancer: Clinical and oncological management. *Contemporary Oncology*, *21*(1), 70–76.

Centers for Disease Control and Prevention. (2019). *Who is at risk for prostate cancer?* Retrieved from https://www.cdc.gov/cancer/prostate/basic_info/risk_factors.htm.

Cunningham, G., & Kadmon, D. (2019). Medical treatment of benign prostatic hyperplasia. In M. O'Leary (Ed.), *UpToDate*. Waltham, MA.

Hagberg, K., et al. (2017). Risk of gynecomastia and breast cancer associated with the use of 5-alpha reductase inhibitors for benign prostatic hyperplasia. *Clinical Epidemiology*, *9*, 83–91.

Kantoff, P., Taplin, M., & Smith, J. (2020). Clinical presentation and diagnosis of prostate cancer. In N. Vogelzang, W. Lee, & J. Richie (Eds.), *UpToDate*. Waltham, MA.

Khera, M. (2020a). Evaluation of male sexual dysfunction. In P. Snyder, A. Matsumoto, & M. O'Leary (Eds.), *UpToDate*. Waltham, MA.

Khera, M. (2020b). Treatment of male sexual dysfunction. In P. Snyder, & M. O'Leary (Eds.), *UpToDate*. Waltham, MA.

McCance, K., Huether, S., Brashers, V., & Rote, N. (2019). *Pathophysiology: The biologic basis for disease in adults and children* (8th ed.). St. Louis: Elsevier.

McVary, K. (2019). Epidemiology and pathophysiology of benign prostatic hyperplasia. In M. O'Leary (Ed.), *UpToDate*. Waltham, MA.

Michaelson, M., & Oh, W. (2020). Epidemiology of and risk factors for testicular germ cell tumors. In P. Kantoff (Ed.), *UpToDate*. Waltham, MA.

Mina, S., & Garcia-Perdomo, H. (2018). Effectiveness of tranexamic acid for decreasing bleeding in prostate surgery: A systematic review and meta-analysis. *Central European Journal of Urology*, *71*(1), 72–77.

Neotract. (2020). *What is urolift?* https://www.urolift.com/what-is-urolift?.

Oh, W. (2020). Overview of the treatment of testicular germ cell tumors. In P. Kantoff (Ed.), *UpToDate*. Waltham, MA.

Pagana, K. D., & Pagana, T. J. (2018). *Mosby's manual of diagnostic and laboratory tests* (6th ed.). St. Louis: Mosby.

Qian-Qian, M., et al. (2019). Tranexamic acid is beneficial for reducing perioperative blood loss in transurethral resection of the prostate. *Experimental and Therapeutic Medicine*, *17*(1), 943–947.

Richie, J. (2020). Active surveillance for men with clinically localized prostate cancer. In N. Vogelzang & J. Richard (Eds.). *UpToDate*, Waltham, MA.

Sartor, A. (2020). Risk factors for prostate cancer. In N. Vogelzang, et al. (Ed.), *UpToDate*. Waltham, MA.

Schreiber, M. (2017). Postoperative nursing considerations: Transurethral resection of the prostate. *Medsurg Nursing*, *26*(6), 419–422.

Schreiber, M. (2019). Erectile dysfunction. *MedSurg Nursing*, *28*(5), 327–330.

Schwen, Z., Gupta, M., & Pierorazio, P. (2018). A review of outcomes and technique for the robotic-assisted laparoscopic retroperitoneal lymph node dissection for testicular cancer. *Advances in Urology*, *214680*, 1–7. https://doi.org/10.1155/2018/2146080.

Szell, A., et al. (2013). Live births from frozen human semen stored for 40 years. *Journal of Assisted Reproduction and Genetics*, *30*(6), 743–744.

U.S. Preventive Services Task Force. (2018). Final recommendation statement: *Prostate cancer: Screening*. Retrieved from https://www.uspreventiveservicestaskforce.org/Page/Document/RecommendationStatementFinal/prostate-cancer-screening.

Viera, A. (2019). Vasectomy. In M. O'Leary (Ed.), *UpToDate*. Waltham, MA.

Westwood, J., et al. (2018). Rezum: A new transurethral water vapour therapy for benign prostatic hyperplasia. *Therapeutic Advances in Urology*, *10*(11), 327–333.

68

Concepts of Care for Transgender Patients

Donna D. Ignatavicius, Stephanie M. Fox

http://evolve.elsevier.com/Iggy/

LEARNING OUTCOMES

1. Collaborate with the interprofessional team to provide evidence-based care to transgender patients.
2. Explain the role of the nurse in providing high-quality care and minimizing **health care disparities** for transgender patients.
3. Discuss how to use culturally sensitive terminology when providing care for transgender patients.
4. Identify appropriate health care resources for transgender patients.
5. Identify major sources of stress that contribute to transgender health issues.
6. Prioritize evidence-based care for patients having male-to-female or female-to-male genital surgery, or feminizing or masculinizing genital surgery.
7. Develop a health teaching plan for transgender patients who take hormone therapy and/or have gender-affirming surgery.

KEY TERMS

female-to-male (FtM) An adjective to describe people who were born with anatomically female parts but identify as and/or live as male; FtM persons are also referred to as *transmen*.

gender dysphoria Emotional or psychological distress caused by an incongruence between one's natal (birth) sex and gender identity.

gender identity A person's inner sense of being a male, a female, or an alternative gender (e.g., genderqueer); not related to *reproduction* anatomy.

gender-affirming surgery (GAS) A group of surgical procedures that change primary and/or secondary sex characteristics to affirm a person's gender identity; also called *gender reassignment surgery (GRS)* or *gender-confirming surgery*.

LGBTQ An acronym referring to lesbian, gay, bisexual, transgender, and queer/questioning individuals (people who do not feel they belong in any other subgroup).

LGBTQIA+ An acronym referring to lesbian, gay, bisexual, transgender, queer, intersex, and asexual people, as well as those who identify with other sexualities, sexes, and genders not included in the acronym.

male-to-female (MtF) An adjective to describe people who were born with anatomically male parts but identify as and/or live as female; MtF persons are also known as *transwomen*.

sex A person's genital anatomy present at birth; also called *biological* or *natal sex*.

transgender An adjective that describes persons who self-identify as the opposite gender or a gender that does not match their natal sex.

※ PRIORITY AND INTERRELATED CONCEPTS

The priority concepts for this chapter are:
- *Patient-Centered Care*
- *Health Care Disparities*

The interrelated concepts for this chapter are:
- *Sexuality*
- *Reproduction*

The American Nurses Association (ANA) Code of Ethics states that the nurse practices with compassion and respect for the dignity and worth of every patient (ANA, 2015). The Institute of Medicine (IOM; now the National Academies of Sciences, Engineering, and Medicine) and the Quality and Safety Education for Nurses (QSEN) Institute further have identified the need for nurses to be competent in *patient-centered care* (see Chapter 1). This competency ensures that nurses provide care with sensitivity and respect for diverse patients, even if those patients have values and preferences different from their own (ANA, 2015). Diversity is often discussed as ethnicity and race, but other cultural aspects such as sexual orientation and gender identity are part of the diverse human experience.

People of minority sexual and gender identities are often grouped under one umbrella population category described by the acronym **LGBTQ**—lesbian, gay, bisexual, transgender, and queer/questioning individuals (people who do not feel they belong in any other subgroup). Another similar acronym used is **LGBTQIA+**, encompassing lesbian, gay, bisexual, transgender, queer, intersex, and asexual people, as well as those who identify as other sexualities, sexes, and genders not included in the acronym. Some literature includes only the letters "LGBT." These evolving labels are misleading regarding people who identify as transgender. The grouping of *sexuality* (sexual attraction and behavior) and gender identity (the sense of self as male, female, a blend of both, or neither) (Human Rights Campaign, 2020) suggests that these two concepts are related or dependent on one another, but they are very different. *LGB* refers to specific sexual orientation. However, transgender people may identify as heterosexual, homosexual, bisexual, or neither.

Nurses and other health care professionals should not assume that transgender patients have the same experiences or health care needs as those who identify as lesbian, gay, or bisexual; this misconception leads to inequality in care. Since 2016, people in the sexual and gender minorities have been designated (for research purposes) as populations who experience differences in access to or availability of appropriate health care services, called **health care disparities** (IOM, 2011; Margolies & Brown, 2019). It is important for the nurse to remember that members of these populations are extremely diverse and represent many ethnicities, religions, and socioeconomic statuses (Landry, 2017) and that care must be personalized according to each individual.

PATIENT-CENTERED TERMINOLOGY

Commonly, gender is categorized with one of two terms: *male* and *female*. For the majority of people, these descriptors are accurate. However, some people do not clearly fit into either category and may define themselves as *transgender*. Identifying oneself as transgender is not a choice or lifestyle, but rather an inner sense of being born in the wrong body. When transgender people pursue ways of making their physical body and appearance affirm their gender identity, their interaction with the health care system requires knowledge, respect, compassion, and specialized **patient-centered care.**

Use of appropriate terminology is essential to demonstrating respect. Of utmost importance is the distinction between gender and sex. Gender, also known as **gender identity,** describes a person's inner sense of being a male, a female, an alternative gender (e.g., genderqueer), or neither (Human Rights Campaign, 2020) and is not related to **reproduction** anatomy. **Sex,** also known as *biological* or *natal sex*, refers to a person's genital anatomy present, designated, or assigned at birth.

When babies are born, the gender of the child is determined by the genitalia present, but there is no way of knowing the child's true sense of gender. Transgender people report feeling a mismatch between their gender identity and natal sex, often extending back into early childhood. The sense of gender and feelings toward maleness or femaleness can develop in children as early as age 2 years and is usually present in most people during the early elementary years. When this incongruence occurs, the person can experience **gender dysphoria,** or the emotional or psychological distress caused by an incongruence between one's natal (birth) sex and gender identity. Some people who have gender dysphoria may seek interventions to transition to the identified gender.

The term *transgender* is often used as an umbrella description for all people whose gender identity and presentation do not conform to social expectations. In this text, **transgender** describes people who self-identify as the opposite gender or a gender that does not match their natal sex (Rosendale et al., 2018). For proper usage, the term *transgender* should be used only in adjective form. For example, a patient "is transgender," "identifies as transgender," or "is a transgender patient." Note that "transgender" never ends in "-ed." The term *transgender* should not be used as a noun, and a patient should never be described as "*a transgender.*"

The most recent data on the transgender population indicate that there are approximately 1 to 1.4 million adults in the United States who identify as transgender (Flores et al., 2016; Meerwijk & Sevelius, 2017). Most scholars suggest that the prevalence is much higher, and more research is needed to collect accurate demographic data for this population.

An aging term that is less commonly used is *transsexual,* which originated from the medical and psychological communities (GLAAD, 2020). This term has historically been used to describe a person who has modified his or her natal body to match the appropriate gender identity, through cosmetic, hormonal, or surgical means. In some populations, this term is considered offensive (The Trevor Project, 2020). *As with other terms, use terminology **only** if the patient identifies as such.* If used, the word "transsexual" is an adjective. People who were born with anatomically male parts but identify as and/or live as female are known as **male-to-female (MtF)**. Male-to-female people are also known as "transwomen," with the gender descriptor indicating the current-lived gender identity. Conversely, "transmen" are natal females who identify as and/or live as men. They are described as **female-to-male (FtM)**.

Transgender people are sometimes inaccurately described as "transvestites" or "cross-dressers," often in a judgmental or negative manner. These terms should **not** be used unless the patient identifies as such. It is also important to note that people who practice *transvestism* or *cross-dressing* (dressing as a member of the opposite sex at chosen times, while living in public as the natal gender) should not be confused with people who are transgender.

Other terms, such as *tranny, he-she,* or *shemale,* are inappropriate, offensive, and hurtful. These terms and other negative comments should *never* be used.

A patient may self-identify with certain terms or choose not to be defined at all. Become familiar with appropriate terms and concepts, but do not force definitions on your patients. *Instead, if you are unsure how to address patients, during your nursing assessment ask them how they define their gender identity* (Margolies & Brown, 2019) *and what terms they prefer to be used.*

TRANSGENDER HEALTH ISSUES

Transgender people (also referred to as *transpeople*) encounter frequent discrimination and are faced with numerous stressful situations related to their identity. Sources of stress such as job discrimination and bias-related harassment can have an impact on patients' physical and psychological health. In the most recent large-scale national survey on discrimination, the majority of transgender people had experienced mistreatment in the workplace (James et al., 2016). Also, approximately one-third of transgender respondents reported loss of job or denial of promotion because of their transgender identity (James et al., 2016). Loss of income may result in homelessness, with one in five transgender people reporting homelessness at one point in their lives (National Center for Transgender Equality, 2020). In some cases, they may turn to sex work (prostitution) as a mechanism for survival (James et al., 2016). Only a small subset of primarily MtF transgender people engage in sex work, which can expose them to human immune deficiency virus (HIV) and sexually transmitted infection (STI).

Transgender people are also vulnerable to bias-related violence and verbal harassment, including threats and intimidation. In the most recent national survey, 45% of transgender people had been physically attacked at least once in the past year, with 16% reporting four or more physical attacks (James et al., 2016). Nearly half of transgender people experience sexual assault in their lifetime, with 10% experiencing a sexual assault in the previous year (James et al., 2016). MtF people are more likely to experience physical violence and discrimination than nontranswomen; the likelihood of harassment is even greater for transwomen of color (James et al., 2016). Factors that increase this risk for violence include poverty, homelessness, and sex work.

Having an identity that puts a person at risk for violence and mistreatment can lead to emotional distress, particularly if the person has been victimized directly. Transgender people who have experienced traumatic situations may demonstrate symptoms of posttraumatic stress disorder (PTSD) and/or depression. Risks for psychological distress are even higher for transgender people living in poverty and those with disabilities. They may turn to a variety of coping strategies to deal with distress, some of which can negatively affect physical health. In a large-scale national survey, 29% of transgender people reported illicit drug use in the previous month and 27% reported binge-drinking in the previous month (James et al., 2016). Most important, major life stressors, emotional distress, and lack of resources can lead to suicidal ideation or suicide attempts when all other methods of coping have failed. In a sample of over 27,000 transgender adults in all 50 states in the United States, 40% reported at least one suicide attempt in their lifetime (James et al., 2016). Data support similar trends in Canada, reflecting the fact that individual, systemic, and structural factors affect the complexity of suicide among people who are transgender (Bauer & Scheim, 2015; McNeil et al., 2017).

Stress and Transgender Health

Several risk factors for poor health outcomes have been identified in the transgender population, with greater risks for those who have housing and economic instability, lower educational status, and lack of family support (James et al., 2016). Transgender people have additional sources of stress when attempting to access health care, such as lack of health insurance due to unemployment and lack of knowledge of health care professionals. This barrier to health care—one of many **health care disparities**—causes them to postpone acute as well as preventive medical care. For people who are insured, coverage for health care related to gender transition, such as hormone use and surgery, is often denied.

When transgender people gain access to health care, they are often fearful and anxious about the providers and setting. In particular, they may be hesitant to disclose their transgender status because of fear of discrimination or ridicule. They may also fear that this information will be documented in health records and shared with family members. This reluctance is increased if they have had previous negative experiences with primary health care providers. One national survey found that 33% of transgender adults who saw a primary health care provider in the previous year had a negative experience, including being refused treatment or receiving verbal abuse (James et al., 2016). Male-to-female transgender people were more likely to encounter discrimination and avoid health care because of these experiences (James et al., 2016). Another study demonstrated that transgender people of racial/ethnic minorities experienced negative health care experiences related to race/ethnicity as well as gender identity (Howard et al., 2019). A primary concern of this population is that health care providers do not understand the transgender experience (Halloran, 2015). Even with providers who seem tolerant and caring with transgender patients, there is still a risk for patients overhearing jokes in the hallway and defamatory comments. Consequently, up to 25% of transgender people may not seek necessary medical care owing to a fear of mistreatment (James et al., 2016), which again leads to **health care disparities.**

When health care professionals do not have knowledge about the needs of the population (James et al., 2016), transgender patients are put in a position of acting as their own health care experts, which can limit the quality of their care. Although most transgender patients generally expect their providers to have some level of knowledge or know where to seek answers, a majority of them find that they have to teach their providers. When they encounter primary health care providers who are unfamiliar with the specific health care needs of their population, patient confidence can diminish drastically and affect desire for future health care.

Although transgender patients may encounter health care professionals who do not understand or who overlook their gender identity, some may encounter those who over-focus on it. Although it is important to be generally knowledgeable about a patient's gender status and understand how it may affect health care needs, this factor is not always relevant for every health problem. For example, transgender patients with fractures or influenza do not need to be questioned extensively about their gender identity. Although there are instances in which the presenting problems require transgender-specific care, many other instances require the same health care that all patients receive. At these times, most transgender patients prefer to be treated as any other patient. Use sound clinical judgment to decide if gender identity impacts patient assessment and care at each encounter.

Transgender Aging

Many nurses are not knowledgeable about culturally competent care of older adults or the LGBTQ population. Estimates have indicated that there are between 217,000 and 700,000 transgender adults who are 65 or older in the United States (Dragon et al., 2017). Many of them lived through the acquired immune deficiency syndrome (AIDS [HIV-III]) crisis of the 1980s and experienced the loss of friends at an early age when life expectancy was much lower; this generation is now included in today's population of older adults (Pfeifer, 2019). Up to 60% of respondents to a 2018 survey of LGBT adults age 45 years and older expressed concerns with neglect, abuse, and harassment in long-term care agencies (Houghton, 2018, in Pfeifer, 2019). This is compelling evidence that nurses need to understand how to meet the special needs of aging transgender people. They may have avoided seeking health care due to fear of ridicule and social stigma. Many of these people may not have had an opportunity to seek gender-affirming hormones or surgeries and feel isolated or alone.

Older transgender adults may be at greater risk for health problems because they may have used ineffective coping strategies such as heavy drinking and smoking for a longer period of time compared with their younger counterparts (Kraus & Duhamel, 2018). This population has been shown to face greater risks for disability, anxiety, depression, victimization, and stigma in comparison with older adults who are not transgender (Johnson et al., 2018).

As a result of these factors, older transgender patients often do not trust health care professionals or the health care system. They may fear staff mistreatment, abuse and neglect, and discrimination, especially when admitted to an acute or long-term care facility. Advocate for older transgender patients and support their gender identity and right to dignity and respect. Seek and refer to long-term care agencies that hire LGBT staff, advertise LGBT friendliness, and display welcoming signs online and inside the facility (Pfeifer, 2019) (see Fig. 68.1). Reassure all patients that they are safe, which is a primary component of culturally competent care (Kraus & Duhamel, 2018).

The Need to Improve Transgender Health Care

During the past few years, several national documents have been published by the U.S. Department of Health and Human Services and private health care organizations that call for improvement in LGBTQ health care to reduce **health care disparities.** These important publications include:

- *Healthy People 2020* and *Healthy People 2030*
- The Institute of Medicine of the National Academies (now the National Academies of Sciences, Engineering, and Medicine) report on LGBT health
- The Joint Commission (TJC) Field Guide for care of LGBT patients
- World Professional Association for Transgender Health (WPATH) Standards of Care (SOC)

The U.S. Department of Health and Human Services' *Healthy People 2010* publication did *not* include the need to improve health care for LGBT people. As a result of this omission, a companion document was developed by the Gay and Lesbian

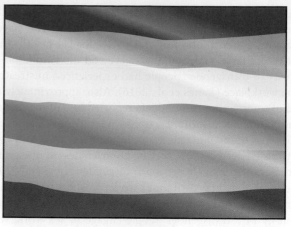

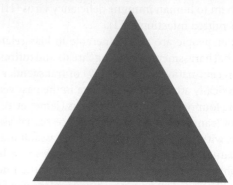

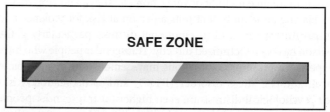

FIG. 68.1 The Safe Zone—rainbow or pink triangle signs welcome LGBTQ patients in a health care agency.

Medical Association (GLMA) to address special health care needs of this population across the life span. Ten common health problems affecting the LGBT group were identified, including cancer, nutrition and weight, and sexually transmitted infection (STI).

The *Healthy People 2020* agenda added objectives for improving the health of LGBT people, including the need to recognize and address the special health needs of transgender patients of all ages. *Healthy People 2030* continues to focus on these objectives. Select proposed objectives include increasing national surveys that collect data on or for transgender populations, and increasing health questions about sexual orientation and gender identity that could improve patient outcomes (Office of Disease Prevention and Health Promotion, 2020).

The IOM LGBT health report calls for the need for more research to identify the special health care concerns of LGBT people of all ages. To help meet this outcome, the document outlined the need to collect more demographic data to better

BEST PRACTICE FOR PATIENT SAFETY & QUALITY CARE (QSEN)

The Joint Commission Recommendations for Creating a Safe, Welcoming Environment for LGBTQ Patients

- Post the *Patients' Bill of Rights* and nondiscrimination policies in a visible place.
- Make waiting rooms inclusive for LGBTQ patients and families, such as posting *Safe Zone*, rainbow, or pink triangle signs.
- Designate unisex or single-stall restrooms.
- Ensure that visitation policies are equitable for families of LGBTQ patients.
- Avoid assumptions about any patient's sexual orientation and gender identity.
- Include gender-neutral language on all medical forms and documents (e.g., "partnered" in addition to married, single, or divorced categories).
- Do not limit gender options on medical forms to "male" and "female."
- Reflect the patient's choice of terminology in communication and documentation.
- Provide information on special health concerns for LGBTQ patients.
- Become knowledgeable about LGBTQ health needs and care.
- Refer LGBTQ patients to qualified health care professionals as needed.
- Provide community resources for LGBTQ information and support as needed.

Adapted from The Joint Commission (TJC). (2011). *Advancing effective communication, cultural competence, and patient- and family-centered care for the lesbian, gay, bisexual, and transgender community.* www.jointcommission.org/lgbt.

TABLE 68.1 Core Principles for Health Care Professionals Who Care for Transgender Patients

- Become knowledgeable about the health care needs of transgender and other gender-nonconforming people.
- Become knowledgeable about the treatment options for transgender patients and required follow-up care.
- Do not assume that all transgender patients are the same; treat each one as an individual and develop an individualized plan of care.
- Demonstrate respect for patients with nonconforming gender identities.
- Provide culturally sensitive care and use appropriate terminology that affirms the patient's gender identity.
- Facilitate patient access to appropriate and knowledgeable health care providers.
- Seek informed consent before providing treatment.
- Offer continuity of care or refer patients for ongoing quality health care.
- Advocate for patients within their families and communities.

Data from Coleman, E., et al. (2012). Standards of care for the health of transsexual, transgender, and gender-nonconforming people, Version 7, *International Journal of Transgenderism, 13*(4), 165–232. DOI: 10.1080/15532739.2011.700873; and Makadon, H., Goldhammer, H., & Davis, J. (2015). *Fenway guide to lesbian, gay, bisexual, and transgender health* (2nd ed.). Philadelphia, PA: American College of Physicians.

identify this population. LGBTQ people need to feel safe when disclosing this very personal information.

In 2011, the World Professional Association for Transgender Health (WPATH) updated its Standards of Care (Coleman et al., 2012). As of this writing, the 2011 edition of the Standards of Care (SOC) remains the most current. The SOC document outlines core principles that nurses and other health care professionals should follow when caring for transgender patients (Table 68.1).

Also in 2011, The Joint Commission (TJC) published a similar document recommending ways for health care agencies to create a welcoming and safe environment for LGBT patients. In response to growing attention to the need for cultural competence for all health care professionals and to provide high-quality health care for sexual and gender minority patients, TJC published a classic field guide for health care agencies to improve LGBT patient care (TJC, 2011). The Best Practice for Patient Safety & Quality Care: The Joint Commission Recommendations for Creating a Safe, Welcoming Environment for LGBTQ Patients box lists the recommendations for health care agencies in designing a safe environment for this population.

Fig. 68.1 shows an example of a "safe zone" image that should be used to reassure these patients that they are in a safe place where they can receive respectful and knowledgeable high-quality care.

Further resources for creating an inclusive environment for LGBT patients can be found through the National LGBT Health Education Center, a program of the Fenway Institute. Part of the Fenway Health, this organization's mission is "to enhance well-being of the LGBTQIA+ community and all people in [their] neighborhoods and beyond through access to the highest quality health care, education, research, and advocacy" (Fenway Health, 2020).

❖ Interprofessional Collaborative Care

◆ **Assessment: Recognize Cues.** As with any patient, ask during the nursing history and physical assessment how he or she prefers to be addressed. For example, for nontransgender patients, some people may use a nickname or their middle name and prefer to be addressed as such. For transgender patients, it is not uncommon for driver's licenses, insurance cards, and other forms of identification to retain their birth names (and by extension, birth sex) because it can be difficult to change this information, particularly if a person is in the process of transitioning. Therefore nurses may receive patient documentation with misleading patient data, such as health care record listing a male name and birth sex while caring for a patient who presents as female in appearance. It can be offensive and embarrassing for the patient who clearly identifies as female to be called "Mister" or "sir" or by the male birth name. Not only does it communicate disrespect, it also signals to the patient that she may receive inadequate care or that the environment is unsafe.

In addition to preferred names, correct pronoun usage is also important. Each patient has his or her own pronoun preference. A MtF patient may visit a clinic during lunch hour at work. Because the patient has not disclosed the transgender identity at work, this patient maintains male dress and demeanor at the office. Although the patient may identify as female and live as female at home, the patient may request the nurse to use male pronouns (he, him, his) to match the patient's current presentation and may not disclose the transgender identity to the nurse. Conversely, even though the patient presents at the time as male, the patient may ask the nurse to use female pronouns (she, her, hers) because the patient identifies with a female gender identity.

In general, use pronouns that match the patient's physical presentation and dress unless the patient requests otherwise. Even though the biologic sex may not match, patients presenting as female should be addressed as female, and patients presenting as male should be addressed as male. With changing clothing styles and trends, do not rely on clothing cues alone. However, it is most appropriate to address a patient as male whose birth sex is listed as female yet presents in traditionally male attire, facial hair, and a men's hairstyle. Understandably, the clinical setting can be fast paced, and nurses may encounter multiple patients at a time; however, taking time to use clinical judgment is important. Appropriately interacting with a transgender patient can sometimes mean the difference between the patient continuing to seek health care or not.

In some cases you might notice that patients may not identify as male or female and prefer not to use male or female pronouns. These patients often feel that the binary gender system in which a person must fit clearly into one category or the other is too limiting. Although this is a small subset of the transgender population, it is important to be aware of this subculture in case you encounter a patient who does not identify with a specific gender. Some patients may request the use of gender-neutral pronouns, or they may use these pronouns in the nurse's presence. Some examples of gender-neutral pronouns are "they/them/their/theirs/themself," "sie/hir/hirs/hirself," and "zie/zir/zirs/zirself" (University of Southern California, 2020).

Getting used to addressing the patient by the correct name or pronoun can take some time. Occasionally, nurses recognize the cues and know their patient's preferred name or pronoun, but accidentally say the wrong one. Transgender patients encounter this situation often and typically anticipate an occasional error. When this error occurs, simply self-correct and continue with care rather than make a prolonged apology. Focusing too much on the error may make the patient more uncomfortable because more attention has been drawn to the situation. Most transgender patients, particularly those who live full time in their gender-affirming role, wish to be treated like any other patient.

History. Transgender people who experience gender dysphoria (discomfort with one's natal sex) may have had one or more of these interventions (Coleman et al., 2012):

- Changes in gender expression that may involve living part-time or full-time in another gender role
- Psychotherapy to explore gender identity and expression, improve body image, or strengthen coping mechanisms
- Hormone therapy to feminize or masculinize the body
- Surgery to change primary and/or secondary sex characteristics (e.g., the breasts/chest, facial features, internal and/or external genitalia)

During the health history, inquire about which interventions the patient has had, if any, or if there are plans to have them in the future. Ask about current use of *drug therapy,* including hormones, and other feminizing or masculinizing agents, including silicone injections. These medications are usually prescribed by endocrinologists or other specialists in transgender health care, but some patients may obtain them from nonmedical sources, including the Internet.

Exogenous hormone therapy can cause adverse health problems and requires careful patient monitoring, including laboratory testing. Estrogen therapy can increase health risks such as increased blood clotting causing venous thromboembolism (VTE), elevated blood glucose, hypertension, estrogen-dependent cancers, and fluid retention. Smoking and obesity increase these risks. The risks also increase with higher doses of the medication. Ask the patient about a history of these problems.

Inquire about the patient's *surgical history.* For the MtF patient, ask about breast surgery and any surgical changes to the genitalia, such as a penectomy (removal of the penis), orchiectomy (removal of one or both testes), and vaginoplasty (creation of a vagina). The MtF patient still has a prostate gland. For older patients, ask about any problems with prostate health problems, such as urinary dribbling and retention. For the FtM patient, ask whether a hysterectomy, bilateral salpingo-oophorectomy (BSO), mastectomy, phalloplasty (creation of a penis), and/or scrotoplasty (creation of a scrotum) was performed.

Keep in mind that health insurance usually does not cover the cost of the transition process and patients may seek alternative care. Hormones may be obtained illegally or from countries that do not have quality controls for medication. "Gray market pharmacies," secondary wholesalers that are unauthorized by drug manufacturers, offer many of these products at significantly higher costs. Other products can also be purchased through venues that are not regulated. The risk for hepatitis C and silicone complications increases significantly when products are obtained through these channels. Ask patients about the use of these alternatives as a part of their transition process.

Physical Assessment. Be sure to review the patient's health record carefully before performing a physical assessment. To help increase the patient's comfort with examinations and the purpose of the assessment, explain why the information or examination is important to their health care. Be culturally sensitive, nonjudgmental, and respectful during the assessment. Recognize that transgender patients may be young, middle-age, or older adults.

When assessing transgender patients, be aware that they may be in varying stages of transition. Some patients present with no obvious physical signs that they are in the process of transitioning. Others have had gender-confirming surgery such that their new appearance matches their gender identity. Realize that a transgender patient's genitalia may not match his or her physical appearance.

Psychosocial Assessment. If gender and/or *sexuality* are relevant to the patient's presenting health problem, ask specific questions to determine how these factors may impact care. Again, it is helpful to share with patients why this information is relevant to their treatment. Reassure patients that their responses are confidential and will not be shared with any family, friends, or significant others without the patient's permission. However, evidence of abuse must be reported as mandated by law. Appropriate screening questions about psychosocial functioning related to gender and *sexuality* include:

- Are you experiencing any challenges, concerns, or anxiety related to your sexuality?

- Related to your gender, how do you identify?
- Are you experiencing sadness, depression, or thoughts of hurting yourself?
- Have you experienced violence or discrimination in your personal or work life?
- Are you currently being seen by a counselor or psychologist related to your sexuality and gender identity? If so, would you wish to share the reason?

If the responses to these questions indicate that the patient has potential or actual mental health concerns, consult with the primary health care provider for further evaluation by a qualified mental health care professional, such as a licensed counselor or clinical psychologist.

◆ **Interventions: Take Action.** Nurses may care for transgender patients of any age who are transitioning or have completed gender confirmation. They may care for them for health problems related to their transition process or for problems that are unrelated to the patient's *sexuality* or gender identity. In general, care for transgender patients with most health problems is the same as for any other patient. However, some interventions such as hormone therapy may affect nursing assessment and care. As a leader in health care, advocate for transgender patients and provide health teaching to promote their health. Encourage them to include their partner, if desired, in discussions about the transition process.

Nonsurgical Management. The primary nonsurgical interventions for transgender patients include drug (hormone) therapy, counseling about *reproduction* and reproductive health, and vocal therapy. The type of intervention depends on whether the patient is transitioning from male to female (MtF) or from female to male (FtM).

Drug Therapy. Drug therapy may be started after completing a psychosocial assessment by a qualified mental health care professional and informed consent has been obtained. According to WPATH's most recent Standards of Care (Coleman et al., 2012), the criteria for gender-affirming hormonal therapy include:

- Continuing and well-documented gender dysphoria
- Patient ability to make a fully informed decision and give consent to treatment
- Patient older than 18 years
- Well-controlled existing medical or mental health problems, if any

Feminizing Drug Therapy. Patients transitioning from male to female (MtF) typically take a combination of estrogen therapy and androgen-reducing medications to achieve feminizing effects. Expected physical changes from *estrogen therapy* are listed in Table 68.2. Additional measures to eliminate facial hair may be needed, such as laser treatment or electrolysis (Ettner et al., 2016). Aesthetic fillers and neurotoxins are also used to achieve facial changes (Ginsberg, 2017).

Because oral estrogen can increase the risk for venous thromboembolism (VTE), transdermal estrogen or injectable estradiol is preferred for use in transgender patients. Progesterone may also be prescribed to be used during a portion of each month (Burchum & Rosenthal, 2019).

TABLE 68.2 Feminizing Drug Therapy for MtF Patients: Expected Changes

- Breast tissue development
- Reduced or absent sperm count and ejaculatory fluid
- Reduced muscle mass
- Change in emotions
- Change in sweat and odor patterns
- Decreased testicular size
- Reduced erectile function
- Decreased libido (sex drive)
- Decreased body hair growth
- Softening of skin

! NURSING SAFETY PRIORITY (QSEN)

Drug Alert

Before the first dose of transdermal estrogen, teach the patient to apply the patch to an area that is hairless to ensure good contact with the skin. When changing to a new patch, wash any excess drug and adhesive from the skin where the previous patch was applied.

Teach patients taking any form of estrogen about side effects such as headache, breast tenderness, nausea/vomiting, and weight gain (often due to fluid retention) or loss. Tell them to report increased feelings of anxiety or depression to their primary health care provider. Estrogens can also cause estrogen-dependent cancers, hypertension (due to fluid retention), venous thromboembolism (VTE) such as deep vein thrombosis (DVT), and gallbladder disease. Teach patients to follow up with their primary health care provider to monitor for these potential adverse drug effects.

NCLEX EXAMINATION CHALLENGE 68.1

Physiological Integrity

The nurse provides health teaching for a transgender woman receiving estrogen therapy. Which statement by the client indicates a **need for further teaching**?

A. "I'll call my doctor if I have any redness or swelling in my legs."
B. "I'll have less hair on my body after taking this drug."
C. "I know that the drug will make my breasts bigger."
D. "I think I will have more sex drive when taking this drug."

In addition to estrogen therapy, androgen-reducing agents (also called androgen blockers or antiandrogens) are often given to block the effects of testosterone, including (Burchum & Rosenthal, 2019; Deutsch, 2016):

- Spironolactone (the most commonly used androgen blocker), a low-cost diuretic that also inhibits testosterone secretion and androgen binding to androgen receptors
- 5-alpha-reductase inhibitors (e.g., finasteride and dutasteride), drugs typically used to treat benign prostatic hyperplasia (BPH) (These drugs block the conversion of testosterone to a more active ingredient to decrease the hair loss associated with estrogen therapy and shrink prostate tissue.)

! NURSING SAFETY PRIORITY (QSEN)

Drug Alert

Teach patients taking *spironolactone* to monitor their blood pressure for hypotension. Remind them to expect polyuria and possible polydipsia. Periodic laboratory tests to assess for hyperkalemia may be needed for patients with renal insufficiency (Burchum & Rosenthal, 2019; Deutsch, 2016). Remind those patients that increased serum potassium can cause cardiac dysrhythmias and skeletal muscle spasticity.

Common side effects of finasteride and other *5-alpha reductase inhibitors* include dizziness, cold sweats, and chills. These symptoms typically decrease over time. If patients continue to have them, instruct them to contact their health care provider.

Masculinizing Drug Therapy. Testosterone is the primary drug used for achieving masculinizing effects in transgender people transitioning from female to male; however, much of the available drug converts to estrogen in the body. This drug can be taken orally, transdermally (topical gel or patch), or parenterally (IM). Buccal and implantable forms of testosterone are also available. Oral testosterone is the least effective form of the drug. Depo-Testosterone, the most common IM preparation, is usually started at a low dose and increased every 1 to 2 weeks (Burchum & Rosenthal, 2019). Teach patients the importance of not sharing needles to prevent bloodborne diseases such as hepatitis C.

Testosterone gel and the testosterone patch are topical forms that are more expensive than other testosterone preparations but may provide more consistent (although slower) results. A newer topical form of the drug, testosterone axillary gel, can be applied to the armpits to increase serum testosterone levels. For all topical testosterone preparations, be sure that the patient washes his hands between applications and covers the area with clothing.

Expected effects of testosterone therapy are listed in Table 68.3. Teach the patient taking testosterone that some of these changes take up to a year to occur. If menses does not stop in the first few months of drug therapy, the patient may be placed on progesterone until the testosterone becomes effective.

Common undesirable effects of testosterone therapy include edema, acne, seborrhea (oily skin), headaches, weight gain,

TABLE 68.3 Masculinizing Drug Therapy for FtM Patients: Expected Changes

- Voice deepening
- Body hair growth (hirsutism), but possibly hairline recession and male pattern baldness
- Increased muscle mass
- Increased libido
- Increased aggression
- Vaginal dryness
- Clitoral growth
- Redistribution of fat
- Cessation of menses

and possible psychosis. Before taking this medication, the patient must be screened for a history of liver and heart disease. Testosterone therapy can cause increased liver enzymes, increased low-density lipoproteins (LDLs, or "bad" cholesterol), and decreased high-density lipoproteins (HDLs, or "good" cholesterol). Increased blood glucose and decreased clotting factors can also occur when taking the drug. Teach patients that these changes can lead to diabetes, heart disease, and stroke. Remind patients that they need to follow up with their health care providers for careful monitoring for these complications, including having extensive diagnostic and laboratory testing.

Reproductive Health Options. Using feminizing or masculinizing hormone therapy affects reproductive health, especially fertility. Ensure that patients know their options for **reproduction,** if desired, *before* transition begins. MtF patients may want to consider sperm banking before drug therapy or gender-confirming surgery if they desire to have a biologic child. FtM patients may want to consider oocyte (egg) or embryo freezing. These frozen gametes or embryos could be implanted in a surrogate woman to become pregnant and carry to birth. Inform patients that these options are expensive, but are still available to them. Be sure to include the patient's partner, if the patient desires, in discussions related to reproductive options.

Voice and Communication Therapy. Communication is an essential aspect of human behavior and gender expression. Voice deepening for transgender people who are transitioning from female to male is accomplished by taking masculinizing hormones, such as testosterone. However, feminizing hormones have no effect on the adult MtF voice.

MtF patients may undergo surgery to change the voice (Schwarz et al., 2017). Others may seek assistance from a voice and communication specialist to help them modify certain vocal characteristics, such as pitch and intonation. Vocal therapy can assist in management of gender dysphoria and be a positive step in the transition process. Remind patients to seek a speech-language pathologist (SLP) who is knowledgeable in transgender health, and has specialized training in assessment and development of vocal health and therapy for transgender patients.

The purpose of vocal therapy is to help patients adapt their voice and communication such that it is authentic and reflects their gender identity. The SLP should take the patient's communication preferences and style into consideration as part of the assessment process to develop an individualized treatment plan. Vocal therapy can also be completed after surgery.

Surgical Management. Many transgender people are satisfied with their gender identity, role, and self-expression without surgery. Surgery, particularly procedures that affect the external or internal genitalia, is usually the last and most carefully considered option for transitioning from one's natal sex to one's inner gender identity. These procedures are often referred to as **gender-affirming surgery (GAS)** but are also known as gender-confirming surgery or gender reassignment surgery. The patient may have a number of surgeries that change primary and/or secondary sex characteristics to confirm a person's gender identity. These procedures achieve either feminizing or masculinizing effects. Regardless of the procedure(s) performed, the nurse collaborates with the patient, family, and health care team to promote positive outcomes for the transition process.

Gender-affirming surgeries are procedures that alter anatomically healthy structures. Not all surgeons feel comfortable in performing procedures that could "harm" transgender patients. However, these procedures help treat gender dysphoria. Some patients elect to undergo the full range of surgeries, whereas others choose to have only some or none of them, typically because of the profound medical expense.

Surgeries that remove or create breasts are often referred to as "top surgery." Genital surgeries "below the waist," often called "bottom surgery," are the most invasive procedures. The criteria for genital surgery depend on the type of surgery being requested. For example, most surgeons (usually urologists or plastic surgeons) require 12 months of hormone therapy plus one or two referrals from qualified psychotherapists for MtF patients who desire an orchiectomy. The same requirements may be needed for FtM patients who desire a hysterectomy (uterus removal) and bilateral salpingo-oophorectomy (BSO), or removal of both fallopian tubes and ovaries.

The psychotherapist assesses the patient's readiness for genital surgery and hormone therapy, including a discussion of risks and out-of-pocket costs. The patient's support system is assessed to ensure that the patient makes the best possible decision and achieves the desired outcomes.

For MtF patients requesting a vaginoplasty (creation of a vagina) or FtM patients desiring a phalloplasty (creation of a penis), the required criteria include 12 continuous months of living in a gender role that is congruent with the patient's gender identity. Prior to any surgical procedure, the surgeon ensures that coexisting medical health problems are well managed and monitored. The patient is advised to discontinue all hormonal therapy at least 2 weeks prior to surgery (Ettner et al., 2016). Current evidence shows that GAS is associated with multiple, significant psychological benefits for those who had gender dysphoria (Wernick et al., 2019) despite other evidence showing prosthesis complications in up to one-third of patients (Rooker et al., 2019).

Feminizing Surgeries for MtF Patients. Feminizing surgeries are performed for MtF patients to create a functional and/or aesthetic (cosmetic) female anatomy, including:

- *Breast/chest surgeries,* such as breast augmentation (mammoplasty to increase breast tissue)
- Other surgeries, such as *facial feminizing surgery* (to achieve feminine facial contour); liposuction (fatty tissue removal), often from the waist or abdominal area; *vocal feminizing surgery*; and other body-contouring procedures
- *Genital surgeries,* such as partial penectomy (removal of the penis), orchiectomy (removal of the testes), vaginoplasty and labiaplasty/vulvoplasty (creation of a vagina and labia/vulva), and clitoroplasty (creation of a clitoris)

Breast augmentation creates breast tissue for the MtF patient through the use of silicone gel-filled implants or saline implants. Although not a prerequisite, it is recommended that MtF patients take feminizing hormones for 12 months before surgery for the best results. Feminizing breast augmentation procedures require small incisions and are therefore usually performed as same-day surgeries. Teach patients that they may have swelling, soreness, and mild bruising for several weeks after surgery, but complications are rare (Ettner et al., 2016).

Voice feminizing surgery, such as reduction thyroid chondroplasty, is performed to decrease the size of the "Adam's apple" (Schwarz et al., 2017). This procedure is performed through a bronchoscope for cosmetic purposes. Nursing care of the patient having a bronchoscopy is discussed in Chapter 24.

The most common *genital surgeries* for MtF patients are bilateral *orchiectomy* to remove the testes and vaginoplasty with partial penectomy. Orchiectomy procedures and associated nursing care are the same for the transgender patient as they are for other natal males (see Chapter 67 for a detailed discussion).

A *vaginoplasty* is the construction of a neovagina (new vagina), usually with inverted penile tissue (obtained during a partial penectomy) and scrotal, skin, or colon graft. This complex surgical procedure also usually includes creating a clitoris and labia (clitoro-labioplasty) using scrotal or penile tissue and skin grafts.

Preoperative Care. In addition to the required criteria to qualify for a vaginoplasty (also called *transvaginal surgery*), the transgender patient is medically evaluated like any other presurgical patient. Patients who have poorly controlled diabetes with vascular complications, coronary artery disease, or other systemic disease that limits functional ability are not candidates for major gender-affirming surgery. Chapter 9 describes general preoperative care for any patient.

The surgeon explains the options for selected procedures, postoperative care expectations, and potential for complications after surgery. Postoperative recovery for transvaginal surgery takes a long time and has a high complication rate. As seen after any surgery, patients with obesity have a higher incidence of surgical infection and often have problems with adequate ventilation (breathing) and ambulation (see Chapter 9).

Written and verbal preoperative instructions are provided by the surgeon, including optional methods of body hair removal. A bowel preparation may be started 24 hours before surgery and may include a clear liquid diet, laxatives, and sodium phosphate/saline enemas. Increased fluids are recommended until the patient goes to bed the night before surgery because the bowel preparation can be very dehydrating. Antimicrobials are typically given on the day of surgery to minimize the risk for infection.

Some surgeons require that the patient take supplements to prevent bruising and promote tissue healing, such as vitamin C. Patients who are very thin are encouraged to eat a high-protein diet. A powdered protein supplement with arginine (an amino acid) may also be prescribed to promote wound healing.

Patients undergo a number of laboratory tests to ensure that they are healthy before surgery. Adequate hemoglobin and hematocrit (H&H) levels are especially important because some blood is lost during surgery. For patients who have low H&H levels, an erythropoietin such as epoetin alfa or IM testosterone with iron is given. Most patients choose testosterone because it is a lower-cost drug.

Operative Procedures. Because surgery requires multiple procedures to create a female anatomy, the patient is on the operating table for many hours. The surgery may be performed in a hospital or specialized center for transgender surgeries. After general or epidural anesthesia is administered, the patient is placed in a lithotomy position (feet in stirrups) for the procedure. Epidural anesthesia is preferred for patients with asthma or obesity. The patient is transferred to the postanesthesia care unit (PACU) with a perineal dressing and packing, Jackson-Pratt drain, and indwelling urinary catheter.

Postoperative Care. Provide general postoperative care as described in Chapter 9. In addition, starting immediately after surgery, to decrease pain and bruising apply an ice pack to the perineum for 20 minutes every hour and continue for the first postoperative week (Deutsch, 2016). Monitor the patient's pain level carefully and offer analgesia as needed. *Genital surgery is very painful because there is a high concentration of nerve endings in the perineum.*

Although not a common postoperative complication, monitor the patient for bleeding. Observe the surgical dressing and surrounding area for oozing or bright red blood. Always look under the patient in case blood has pooled there. Report and document any indication of active bleeding immediately to the surgeon and keep the patient in bed.

> ## ❗ NURSING SAFETY PRIORITY (QSEN)
>
> ### Action Alert
>
> Patients are in a lithotomy position for an extended period during surgery. After surgery, monitor lower extremity neurovascular status and encourage the patient to move the legs often during the first 24 hours after surgery to help prevent compartment syndrome. Report and document any unexpected findings, such as continued numbness, inability to move the lower legs or feet, or leg pain and swelling. Patients who had epidural anesthesia are not able to move their legs for several hours after surgery until the effect of the drug diminishes.

All patients stay in the hospital for at least 1 night after genital surgery, but some patients may stay much longer, depending on the number and complexity of the surgical procedures. Patients who have the inverted skin flap technique for a *vaginoplasty* usually remain on bedrest for at least 4 to 5 days with a dilator or gauze packing in the neovagina. Subcutaneous fractionized heparin is given during this time to prevent venous thromboembolism (VTE) (Ettner et al., 2016).

After the bedrest period, the dilator or gauze packing is removed to allow the patient to ambulate. The patient is taught how to cleanse the new vagina with an antiseptic solution and given careful instructions on how to follow the strict dilator protocol. Other postoperative instructions are listed in the Best Practice for Patient Safety & Quality Care: Postoperative Teaching for Patients Who Have a Vaginoplasty box (Deutsch, 2016).

The Jackson Pratt drain is removed when drainage is less than 15 to 20 mL in a 24-hour period. About 7 to 10 days after surgery, the surgical pressure dressing and external sutures are removed. The urinary catheter is removed between postoperative days 7 and 12. Early removal can cause urinary retention, but prolonged placement can lead to catheter-associated urinary tract infection (CAUTI).

Patients should continue follow-up visits with their primary health care provider for signs and symptoms of complications. One of the worst complications is a vaginal-rectal fistula, which

> ## BEST PRACTICE FOR PATIENT SAFETY & QUALITY CARE (QSEN)
>
> ### Postoperative Teaching for Patients Who Have a Vaginoplasty
>
> - Resume taking showers after the first postoperative follow-up visit.
> - Do not take baths (submerged in water) for 8 weeks after surgery.
> - Avoid strenuous activities for at least 6 weeks.
> - Avoid swimming or bike riding for 3 months.
> - Expect minimal vaginal bleeding/spotting and/or a brownish-yellow drainage for 6 to 8 weeks; use a soap and water douche to minimize these problems.
> - Avoid tobacco or smoking for at least a month after surgery to promote healing.
> - Take stool softeners as prescribed to help prevent constipation.
> - Take acetaminophen as prescribed for pain control at home.
> - Carefully follow the prescribed individualized dilator protocol.
> - Do not have sexual intercourse until at least 3 months after surgery.

is caused by rectal perforation during surgery. Teach patients to report any leakage of stool into the vagina immediately to their surgeon. The treatment for this complication is a temporary colostomy and fistula wound management for many months. Other surgical complications of vaginoplasty are listed in Table 68.4.

Some MtF patients are not satisfied with the quality of the results of feminizing surgeries. For example, the neovagina may not be functional for sexual intercourse. Some patients request another surgery to achieve more satisfying results.

> ## NCLEX EXAMINATION CHALLENGE 68.2
>
> ### Physiological Integrity
>
> The nurse is caring for a client who had a vaginoplasty yesterday. Which assessment finding will the nurse report to the health care provider?
> A. Perineal pain
> B. Lower extremity swelling
> C. Constipation
> D. Urinary retention

Masculinizing Surgeries for FtM Patients. Masculinizing surgeries are performed for FtM patients to create a functional and/or aesthetic male anatomy, including:

- Breast/chest surgeries, usually a bilateral mastectomy (removal of both breasts) and chest reconstruction and contouring
- Genital surgeries, such as a hysterectomy and bilateral BSO, vaginectomy (removal of the vagina), phalloplasty (creation of an average-size male penis) with ureteroplasty (creation of a urethra) or metoidioplasty (creation of a small penis using hormone-enhanced clitoral tissue), and scrotoplasty (creation of a scrotum) with insertion of testicular prostheses
- Other surgeries, such as liposuction, pectoral muscle implants, and other facial or body-contouring procedures

Care of transgender patients having a mastectomy, hysterectomy, and bilateral salpingo-oophorectomy (BSO) is similar

TABLE 68.4 Postoperative Complications of Vaginoplasty Surgery

Most Serious Complications

- Vaginal-rectal fistula
- Rectal perforation
- Lower extremity compartment syndrome
- Bleeding (early but rare)

Other Complications

- Surgical wound infection
- Urinary leakage/incontinence
- Chronic urinary tract infections
- Urinary meatus stenosis (late but rare)
- Vaginal stenosis
- Vaginal collapse
- Labial hematoma
- Inadequate vaginal length or width
- Lack of sensation
- Lack of sexual pleasure

to care for any patient having these procedures as described elsewhere in this text. Some FtM patients are not satisfied with the results of mastectomy and chest reconstruction due to complications, which can include scarring, nipple-areola misplacement or size, and contour abnormalities (Deutsch, 2016). As an alternative to breast surgery, use of a binder to constrict and hide the breasts may be preferred (Ettner et al., 2016). Remind the patient that long-term use of a binder can result in lax or drooping breast tissue. If the patient has not had previous abdominal surgery, a laparoscopic procedure is preferred for the hysterectomy and BSO surgery.

Procedures to create a male anatomy for FtM patients are not performed as often as for MtF patients who desire a female anatomy. Phalloplasties are the most difficult reconstructive genital surgeries to perform and usually require several stages. Skin flaps from the radial forearm, anterior lateral thigh, or back are used to create the penis. Fat grafts may be needed to increase penile girth, and buccal mucosal tissue may be used to create the urethra. A penile prosthesis or implant is not inserted until months after surgery when the initial surgical healing has occurred.

Complications from phalloplasty include:

- Urethral complications
- Bleeding
- Wound infections
- Donor graft site scarring or loss
- Rectal injury

In addition to these physical problems, the patient may not be satisfied with the results of the surgery, such as an inadequate length of the penis. For these reasons, many FtM patients do not have this procedure and prefer to have only a laparoscopic hysterectomy and BSO.

Care Coordination and Transition Management. Transgender patients often take hormone therapy for many years. Teach them that ongoing follow-up with a qualified health care professional is needed to maintain health and detect any complications, such as diabetes or cardiovascular problems, as early as possible.

Long-term follow-up with the surgeon after gender-affirming surgery is essential to detect and treat the frequent complications that occur. Assess the patient's support systems and coping strategies, including financial status and health insurance benefits. Collaborate with the case manager to ensure a smooth transition into the community, including the possible need for any ongoing mental health counseling or therapy.

Urogenital care is also needed for patients who have gender-affirming surgery. FtM patients usually do not have a vaginectomy and therefore may experience vaginal atrophy causing itching and burning. Recommend that they seek gynecologic care to treat this problem, although the examination can be physically and emotionally painful.

MtF patients may need counseling about *sexuality*, genital hygiene, and prevention of sexually transmitted diseases. They are also at a high risk for frequent urinary tract infections as a result of a shortened urethra and urinary incontinence if they have had genital surgery. Teach patients the importance of having follow-up care for these problems.

Preventive health care screenings for transgender patients are also important. The MtF patient requires prostate health care screenings that natal males need. Mammograms are also recommended to monitor for early signs of cancer in the augmented breast. FtM patients who have not undergone a hysterectomy and BSO need gynecologic care to minimize risk for cervical and ovarian cancer, as well as mammograms if the breasts have not been removed.

A number of community resources and organizations are available for transgender support and information, such as:

- National Coalition for LGBT Health (https://healthlgbt.org/)
- Advocacy and Services for LGBT Elders (www.sageusa.org)
- Transgender Health Information Program (http://www.phsa.ca/our-services/programs-services/trans-care-bc)
- University of California San Francisco Center of Excellence for Transgender Health (www.transhealth.ucsf.edu)
- Vancouver Coastal Health Transgender Health Program (http://www.vch.ca/locations-services/result?res_id=1342)
- Canadian Professional Association for Transgender Health (www.cpath.ca)
- World Professional Association for Transgender Health (www.wpath.org)

❓ CLINICAL JUDGMENT CHALLENGE 68.1

Evidence-Based Practice; Patient-Centered Care

A client who is well-known to the nurse has come to see the primary care provider. The client, a natal sex female, asks the nurse to be addressed by the name "Marc" but to keep the name "Michelle" on the electronic health record. While bringing the history up-to-date and asking the reason for today's visit, the nurse notices that the client makes only intermittent eye contact. The client responds, "I want to talk with the provider about hormones."

1. **Recognize Cues:** What assessment information in this client situation is the most important and immediate concern for the nurse? (Hint: Identify the **relevant** information *first* to determine what is most important.)
2. **Analyze Cues:** What client conditions are consistent with the **most relevant** information? (Hint: Think about priority collaborative problems that support and contradict the information presented in this situation.)
3. **Prioritize Hypotheses:** Which possibilities or explanations are **most likely** to be present in this client situation? Which possibilities or explanations are

the most serious? (Hint: Consider all possibilities and determine their urgency and risk for this client.)
4. **Generate Solutions:** What actions would most likely achieve the desired outcomes for this client? Which actions should be **avoided** or are **potentially harmful**? (Hint: Determine the desired outcomes first to decide which interventions are appropriate and those that should be avoided.)
5. **Take Action:** Which actions are the most appropriate and how should they be implemented? In what **priority order** should they be implemented? (Hint: Consider health teaching, documentation, requested health care provider orders or prescriptions, nursing skills, collaboration with or referral to health team members, etc.)
6. **Evaluate Outcomes:** What client assessment would indicate that the nurse's actions were **effective**? (Hint: Think about signs that would indicate an improvement, decline, or unchanged client condition.)

GET READY FOR THE NEXT-GENERATION NCLEX® EXAMINATION!

Key Points

Review these Key Points for each NCLEX Examination Client Needs Category.

Safe and Effective Care Environment

- Depending on identified health care needs, collaborate with multiple members of the interprofessional team when caring for the transgender patient. **QSEN: Teamwork and Interprofessional Collaboration**
- Monitor for expected, side, and adverse effects of hormone therapy, including effects on *sexuality* and *reproduction*, as described in Tables 68.2 and 68.3. **QSEN: Safety**

Health Promotion and Maintenance

- Advocate for the transgender patient who may be distrustful of health care professionals and fearful when seeking care. **QSEN: Patient-Centered Care**
- Refer the transgender patient and partner, as appropriate, to local and national resources for information and support. **QSEN: Patient-Centered Care**

Psychosocial Integrity

- Use culturally sensitive and accurate language and pronouns when communicating with transgender patients. **QSEN: Patient-Centered Care**
- Provide *patient-centered care* for the transgender patient with dignity and respect. **Ethics**
- Be aware that transgender people may experience gender dysphoria. **QSEN: Patient-Centered Care**
- Assess transgender patients for sources of stress that can lead to health issues. **Clinical Judgment**
- Be aware that transgender patients may experience *health care disparities* due to lack of insurance or other circumstances. **QSEN: Patient-Centered Care**

Physiological Integrity

- Recognize that patients receiving hormone therapy need periodic laboratory testing to monitor for adverse drug events and complications. **QSEN: Evidence-Based Practice**
- Provide thorough preoperative and postoperative care for patients having gender affirming surgery. **QSEN: Evidence-Based Practice**
- Monitor for potentially life-threatening complications of vaginoplasty, such as fistula development, bleeding, and wound infection after surgery (see Table 68.4). **Clinical Judgment**

MASTERY QUESTIONS

1. The nurse is caring for a client who reports beginning to transition from male to female. Which nursing action is appropriate regarding pronoun use?
   A. Ask the patient which pronouns are preferred and use those.
   B. Implement use of "he/him" pronouns as the client's natal sex is male.
   C. Use "Miss" or" Mrs.," since the client has begun the transition to female.
   D. Document that male or female pronouns are appropriate to use at this time.

2. Which nursing action decreases the risk for health care disparities for transgender clients? **Select all that apply.**
   A. Refer to the client's identification card for name.
   B. Determine gender identity based on clothing worn.
   C. Seek to understand the experience of the transgender client.
   D. Apologize several times if the wrong name is used for the client.
   E. On meeting the client, ask what name and which pronouns are desired.
   F. Explain how the health history and assessment are affected by gender identity.

REFERENCES

Asterisk (*) indicates a classic or definitive work on this subject.

*American Nurses Association (ANA). (2015). *Code of ethics for nurses*. Washington, DC: Author.

*Bauer, G. R., & Scheim, A. I. (2015). *Transgender people in Ontario, Canada: Statistics from the Trans PULSE Project to inform human rights policy*. London, ON: Canadian Institute of Health Research.

Burchum, J. L. R., & Rosenthal, L. D. (2019). *Lehne's pharmacology for nursing care* (10th ed.). St. Louis: Elsevier.

*Coleman, E., Bockting, W., Botzer, M., Cohen-Kettenis, P., DeCuypere, G., Fladman, J., et al. (2012). Standards of care for the health of transsexual, transgender, and gender-nonconforming people (Version 7). *International Journal of Transgenderism, 13*, 165–232.

Deutsch, M. B. (2016). *Guidelines for the primary and gender-affirming care of transgender and gender nonbinary people*. Center of Excellence for Transgender Health. University of California San Francisco. http://transhealth.ucsf.edu/trans?page=guidelines-home.

Dragon, C. N., Guerino, P., Ewald, E., & Laffan, A. M. (2017). Transgender Medicare beneficiaries and chronic conditions: Exploring fee-for-service claims data. *LGBT Health, 4*(6), 404–411.

Ettner, R., Monstrey, S., & Coleman, E. (2016). *Principles of transgender medicine and surgeries* (2nd ed.). New York: NY: Routledge.

Fenway Health. (2020). *Your care, your community*. https://fenwayhealth.org/about/history/.

Flores, A. R., Herman, J. L., Gates, G. J., & Brown, T. N. T. (2016). *How many adults identify as transgender in the United States?* Los Angeles, CA: The Williams Institute. https://williamsinstitute.law.ucla.edu/publications/trans-adults-united-states/.

Ginsberg, B. (2017). Dermatologic care of the transgender patient. *International Journal of Women's Dermatology, 3*(1), 65–67.

GLAAD. (2020). *GLAAD media reference guide: Transgender*. https://www.glaad.org/reference/transgender.

Halloran, L. (2015). Caring for transgender patients. *The Journal for Nurse Practitioners, 11*(9), 915–916.

Houghton, A. (2018). *Maintaining dignity: Understanding and responding to the challenges facing older LGBT Americans*. Washington, DC: AARP Research. https://doi.org/10.26419/res.00217.001. March 2018.

Howard, S., et al. (2019). Healthcare experiences of transgender people of color. *Journal of General Internal Medicine, 34*(10), 2068–2074.

Human Rights Campaign. (2020). *Sexual orientation and gender identity definitions*. https://www.hrc.org/resources/sexual-orientation-and-gender-identity-terminology-and-definitions.

*Institute of Medicine (IOM). (2015). *The health of LGBT people: Building a foundation for better understanding*. Washington, DC: National Academies Press.

James, S. E., Herman, J. L., Rankin, S., Keisling, M., Mottet, L., & Anafi, M. (2016). *The report of the 2015 U.S. transgender survey*. Washington, DC: National Center for Transgender Equality.

Johnson, K., et al. (2018). Gay and gray session: An interdisciplinary approach to transgender aging. *American Journal of Geriatric Psychiatry, 6*(7), 719–738.

Kraus, S., & Duhamel, K. V. (2018). Culturally competent care for older LGBTQ patients. *Nursing, 48*(8), 48–53.

Landry, J. (2017). Delivering culturally sensitive care to LGBTQI patients. *The Journal for Nurse Practitioners, 13*(5), 342–347.

Margolies, L., & Brown, C. G. (2019). Increasing cultural competence with LGBTQ patients. *Nursing, 49*(6), 34–40.

McNeill, J., Ellis, S., & Eccles, S. (2017). Suicide in trans populations: A systematic review of prevalence and correlates. *Psychology of Sexual Orientation*. https://doi.org/10.1037/sgd0000235.

Meerwijk, K. E., & Sevelius, J. M. (2017). Transgender population size in the United States: A meta-regression of population-based probability samples. *American Journal of Public Health, 107*(2), 1–8.

National Center for Transgender Equality. (2020). *Issues: Housing and homelessness*. Retrieved from https://transequality.org/issues/housing-homelessness.

Office of Disease Prevention and Health Promotion. (2020). *Healthy people 2030 Framework*.

Pfeifer, G. (2019). Panel convened to discuss end-of-life care concerns in the LGBT community. *American Journal of Nursing, 119*(9), 14.

Rooker, S., et al. (2019). The rise of the neophallus: A systematic review of penile prosthetic outcomes and complications in gender-affirming surgery. *The Journal of Sexual Medicine, 16*(5), 661–672.

Rosendale, N., Goldman, S., Ortiz, G. M., & Haber, L. A. (2018). Acute clinical care for transgender patients: A review. *JAMA Internal Medicine, 178*(11), 1535–1542.

Schwarz, K., et al. (2017). Laryngeal surgical treatment in transgender women: A systematic review and meta-analysis. *The Laryngoscope, 127*, 2596–2603.

*The Joint Commission (TJC). (2011). *Advancing effective communication, cultural competence, and patient- and family-centered care for the lesbian, gay, bisexual, and transgender community*. www.jointcommission.org/lgbt.

The Trevor Project. (2020). *Trans + gender identity*. https://www.thetrevorproject.org/trvr_support_center/trans-gender-identity/.

University of Southern California. (2020). Gender neutral pronouns. https://lgbtrc.usc.edu/trans/transgender/pronouns/

Wernick, J., et al. (2019). A systematic review of the psychological benefits of gender-affirming surgery. *Urologic Clinics, 46*(4), 475–486.

69

Concepts of Care for Patients With Sexually Transmitted Infections

Cherie R. Rebar

http://evolve.elsevier.com/Iggy/

LEARNING OUTCOMES

1. Collaborate with the interprofessional team to coordinate high-quality care for patients with sexually transmitted infections (STIs).
2. Provide a safe, private environment for patients when assessing and discussing STIs.
3. Teach evidence-based ways for adults to protect themselves from acquiring a sexually transmitted **infection.**
4. Teach patients with STIs and their partners self-care measures, including the role of expedited partner therapy.
5. Implement nursing interventions to help patients cope with the psychosocial impact caused by an STI and/or **reproduction** concern associated with an STI.

6. Apply knowledge of anatomy, physiology, and pathophysiology to assess patients with STIs.
7. Use clinical judgment to analyze assessment findings and diagnostic data in the care of patients with STIs.
8. Plan care coordination and transition management for patients with STIs.
9. Describe **health care disparities** associated with the incidence and management of STIs.
10. Maintain patient confidentiality and privacy related to STIs.
11. Respect patients' personal values and beliefs regarding **sexuality.**

KEY TERMS

chancre The ulcer that is the first sign of syphilis. It develops at the site of entry (inoculation) of the organism, usually 3 weeks after exposure. The lesion may be found on any area of the skin or mucous membranes but occurs most often on the genitalia, lips, nipples, and hands and in the oral cavity, anus, and rectum.

dyspareunia Painful sexual intercourse.

dysuria Painful urination.

endometritis Endometrial infection.

expedited partner therapy (EPT) The practice of treating sexual partners of patients diagnosed with chlamydia infection or gonorrhea by providing prescriptions or medication to the patient, which they can take to their partner(s), without the primary health care provider examining the partner(s). Also called *patient-delivered partner therapy.*

genital herpes (GH) An acute, recurring incurable viral disease of the genitalia caused by the herpes simplex virus and transmitted through contact with an infected person.

pelvic inflammatory disease (PID) An acute syndrome resulting in tenderness in the Fallopian tubes and ovaries (adnexa) and, typically, dull pelvic pain.

safer sex practices Interventions that reduce the risk of nonintact skin or mucous membranes coming in contact with infected body fluids and blood, such as using a condom.

salpingitis Fallopian tube infection.

sexually transmitted disease (STD) Term used by the Centers for Disease Control and Prevention for sexually transmitted infection.

sexually transmitted infection (STI) Infectious organisms that have been passed from one person to another through intimate contact.

syphilis A complex sexually transmitted disease that can become systemic and cause serious complications and even death.

INTRODUCTION TO SEXUALLY TRANSMITTED INFECTIONS

Infectious organisms that have been passed from one person to another through intimate contact—usually oral, vaginal, or anal intercourse—are considered sexually transmitted infections (STIs). Some organisms that cause these diseases are transmitted only through sexual contact. Others are transmitted also by parenteral exposure to infected blood, fecal oral transmission, intrauterine transmission to the fetus, and perinatal transmission from mother to neonate. The term sexually transmitted disease (STD) is used by the Centers for Disease Control and Prevention (CDC, 2020b). The CDC provides best practice guidelines for treatment of STIs (CDC, 2015). This includes information, treatment standards, and counseling recommendations to help decrease the spread of these diseases and their complications.

The reported numbers of cases of STIs are influenced by improved diagnostic techniques, increased knowledge about organisms that can be sexually transmitted, and changes in *sexuality* (see Chapter 1) and sexual practices. Other factors such as an increasing population, cultural practices, political and economic policies, incidences of sexual abuse and human trafficking, and international travel and migration also affect the prevalence of STIs.

The prevalence of STIs is a major public health concern worldwide. People at greatest risk for acquiring an STI include those who (American College of Obstetricians and Gynecologists, 2017; U.S. Department of Health and Human Services, 2020a):
- Have more than one sexual partner (especially anonymous partners)
- Have had more than one sexual partner in the past
- Engage in sexual activity with someone who has an STI
- Have a history of having an STI
- Use intravenous drugs
- Have or had a partner who uses (used) intravenous drugs
- Engage in anal, vaginal, or oral sex without a condom
- Have sex while using drugs or alcohol

There are populations that are more affected than others, and a key nursing role is to ensure that all people are equally assessed for, and educated about, STIs. It is important to not assume that certain groups are less vulnerable than others, as sexual practices and knowledge about self-protection vary greatly.

One of the greatest factors associated with STI prevalence is the interest in *sexuality,* sexual behaviors, and intimacy in the American culture. The stigma of STIs in the United States has been associated with higher rates of these infections compared with rates in other developed countries. The prevalence of STIs is also affected by changing human physiology patterns such as earlier onset of menarche, comorbidities associated with human immune deficiency virus (HIV) and diabetes, and *health care disparities* (see Chapter 1). Misuse of substances has also been identified as a significant risk factor because of the effects that drugs have on decision making and risk-taking behavior.

STIs cause complications that can contribute to severe physical and emotional pain, including infertility, ectopic pregnancy, cancer, and death. Some of the most common complications caused by sexually transmitted organisms are listed in Table 69.1.

Certain types of STIs must be reported to local health authorities. Check requirements in your state, and communicate incidences of reportable STIs accordingly (see the Ethical/Legal Considerations: Reporting Sexually Transmitted Infections [STIs] box).

Nurses in all environments of care have a responsibility to recognize patients who are at risk for or who have STIs, possibly while being treated for another unrelated health problem. Sexual issues, particularly those involving suspected or actual STIs, are sensitive, personal, and sometimes controversial. As a patient advocate, demonstrate a nonjudgmental attitude when caring for people who have concerns related to *sexuality.* Providing confidentiality and privacy is essential for patients to receive correct information, make informed decisions, and obtain evidence-based care.

Recognize that 88% of victims of human trafficking have had to seek medical care at some point (The Joint Commission, 2019). In any clinical setting, you are in a key position to identify and assist victims. Signs of trafficking can be found in Chapter 10. Best practices for identifying and caring for people who may need assistance include (The Joint Commission, 2019):

- Interviewing the patient without the presence of a partner or other person who accompanies them
- Providing professional interpreters, if needed; never rely on the partner or others to speak for the patient
- Collaborating with social workers, sexual assault nurse examiners (SANEs), and other members of the interprofessional team, as indicated
- Ensuring that documentation is consistent if there are concerns regarding trafficking

PATIENT-CENTERED CARE: GENDER HEALTH CONSIDERATIONS (QSEN)

Because of the very vascular and large surface area of the mucous membranes of the vagina, women are more easily infected with STIs and are at greater risk for STI-related health problems than are men. Women are also more vulnerable to infections because of the exposure of cervical basal epithelium cells. Lesbian women who exclusively have had sex with women have a *lower* risk for STIs than women who have had sex with men (Molin et al., 2016). Transgender women have a *higher* rate of HIV infection (Neumann et al., 2017; Raiford et al., 2016) than others.

Changing social relationships later in life affect risk for exposure to STIs. Women who are no longer concerned with pregnancy may be at risk for STIs if they do not use barrier methods. Physiologic changes experienced by postmenopausal women such as mucosal tears from vaginal atrophy increase risk.

Women have more asymptomatic infections, which may delay diagnosis and treatment. Many infectious organisms reside in the cervical os and cause little change in vaginal discharge or vulvar tissue, so women are not aware that they are infected. This delay increases the risk for complications, including ascending infections that may cause reproductive organ damage and illness. Embarrassment, denial, or fear about STIs may further delay treatment, increasing the potential for serious complications.

Health Promotion and Maintenance

A *Healthy People 2020* objective is to reduce sustained domestic transmission of primary and secondary syphilis (U.S. Department of Health and Human Services, 2020b) (Table 69.2). *Healthy People 2030,* in development at the time of publication, also contains proposed objectives to reduce syphilis specifically in women, as well as to reduce congenital syphilis (U.S. Department of Health and Human Services, 2019). One of the primary tools for prevention of sexually transmitted infections (STIs), including syphilis, is education. All people, regardless of age, natal gender, gender identity, ethnicity, socioeconomic status, education level, or sexual orientation, are susceptible to these diseases. Health literacy, motivation, and perceived risk can affect the health status of any patient. Do not assume that a person is not sexually active because of age, education, marital status, profession, culture, or religion.

STIs are largely preventable through safer sex practices. Discuss prevention methods, including safer sex, with all patients who are or may become sexually active. **Safer sex**

TABLE 69.1 Complications Caused by Sexually Transmitted Organisms

Complication	Causative Organisms
Salpingitis, infertility, and ectopic pregnancy	*Neisseria gonorrhoeae* *Chlamydia trachomatis* *Mycoplasma hominis* *Ureaplasma urealyticum*
Puerperal infection	*N. gonorrhoeae* *C. trachomatis*
Perinatal infection	Hepatitis B virus HIV Human papillomavirus *N. gonorrhoeae* *C. trachomatis* Herpes simplex virus *Treponema pallidum* Cytomegalovirus Group B streptococci
Cancer of genital area	Human papillomavirus
Male urethritis	*M. hominis* Herpes simplex virus *N. gonorrhoeae* *C. trachomatis* *U. urealyticum*
Vulvovaginitis	Herpes simplex virus *Trichomonas vaginalis* Bacterial vaginosis *Candida albicans*
Cervicitis	*N. gonorrhoeae* *C. trachomatis* Herpes simplex virus
Proctitis	*N. gonorrhoeae* *C. trachomatis* Herpes simplex virus *Campylobacter jejuni* *Shigella* species *Entamoeba histolytica*
Hepatitis	*T. pallidum* Hepatitis A, hepatitis B, and hepatitis C viruses
Dermatitis	*Sarcoptes scabiei* *Phthirus pubis*
Genital ulceration or warts	*C. trachomatis* Herpes simplex virus Human papillomavirus *T. pallidum* *Haemophilus ducreyi* *Calymmatobacterium granulomatis*

practices are those that reduce the risk for nonintact skin or mucous membranes coming in contact with infected body fluids and blood. These practices include:

- Using a latex or polyurethane condom for genital and anal intercourse
- Using a condom or latex barrier (dental dam) over the genitals or anus during oral-genital or oral-anal sexual contact

TABLE 69.2 Meeting *Healthy People 2020* Objectives and Targets for Improvement: Sexually Transmitted Infections/Diseases

- Reduce the proportion of adolescents and young adults with *Chlamydia trachomatis* infections
- Increase the proportion of sexually active females aged 24 years and under enrolled in Medicaid plans who are screened for genital *Chlamydia* infections during the measurement year
- Increase the proportion of sexually active females aged 24 years and younger enrolled in commercial health insurance plans who are screened for genital *Chlamydia* infections during the measurement year
- Reduce gonorrhea rates
- Reduce sustained domestic transmission of primary and secondary syphilis
- Reduce the proportion of females with human papillomavirus (HPV) infection
- Reduce the proportion of young adults with genital herpes due to herpes simplex type 2

Data from https://www.healthypeople.gov/2020/topics-objectives/topic/sexually-transmitted-diseases/objectives.

- Wearing gloves for finger or hand contact with the vagina or rectum
- Practicing abstinence
- Practicing mutual monogamy
- Decreasing the number of sexual partners

GENITAL HERPES

Pathophysiology Review

Genital herpes (GH) is an acute, recurring, common viral disease. Although preventative and therapeutic vaccines are still under investigation, at this time, GH is still considered incurable (American Sexual Health Association, 2020). Two serotypes of herpes simplex virus (HSV) affect the genitalia: type 1 (HSV-1) and type 2 (HSV-2) (McCance et al., 2019). Most *nongenital* lesions such as cold sores are caused by HSV-1, transmitted via oral-oral contact. Historically, HSV-2 caused most of the genital lesions. However, either type can produce oral or genital lesions through oral-genital or genital-genital contact with an infected person. HSV-2 recurs and sheds asymptomatically more often than HSV-1. Many people with GH have not been diagnosed because they have mild symptoms and shed the virus intermittently.

The incubation period of genital herpes is 2 to 20 days (average is 1 week). Many people do not have symptoms during the primary outbreak. The virus remains dormant and recurs periodically, even if the patient is asymptomatic. Recurrences are not caused by reinfection; they are related to *viral shedding, and the patient is infectious*. Long-term complications of GH include the risk for neonatal transmission and an increased risk for acquiring HIV **infection** (McCance et al., 2019).

HSV-1 is highest in prevalence among Mexican Americans, and HSV-2 is highest in prevalence among non-Hispanic blacks (National Center for Health Statistics [NCHS], 2018). The

FOCUSED ASSESSMENT

The Patient With a Sexually Transmitted Infection

Assess history of present illness:
- Chief concern
- Time of onset
- Symptoms by quality and quantity, precipitating and palliative factors
- Any treatments taken (self-prescribed or over-the-counter products), and whether they have been helpful

Assess past medical history:
- Major health problems, including any history of STIs, PID, or immunosuppression
- Surgeries: obstetric and gynecologic; circumcision

Assess current health status:
- Menstrual history for irregularities
- Sexual history:
  - Type and frequency of sexual activity
  - Number of lifetime and past 6 months sexual contacts/partners, or monogamous
  - Sexual orientation
  - Contraception history
- Medications
- Allergies
- Lifestyle risks: drugs, alcohol, tobacco

Assess preventive health care practices:
- Papanicolaou (Pap) tests
- Regular STI screening
- Use of barrier contraceptives to prevent STIs and/or pregnancy

Assess physical examination findings:
- Vital signs
- Oropharyngeal findings
- Abdominal findings
- Genital or pelvic findings
- Anorectal findings

Assess laboratory data:
- Urinalysis
- Hematology
- ESR or CRP if PID is being considered
- Cervical, urethral, oral, rectal specimens
- Lesion samples for microbiology and virology
- Pregnancy testing

CRP, C-reactive protein; *ESR*, erythrocyte sedimentation rate; *PID*, pelvic inflammatory disease; *STI*, sexually transmitted infection.

overall prevalence of HSV-1 and HSV-2 in the United States has continued to decrease over time since 2000 (NCHS, 2018).

❖ Interprofessional Collaborative Care

◆ **Assessment: Recognize Cues.** The diagnosis of GH is based on the patient's history and physical examination (see the Focused Assessment: The Patient With a Sexually Transmitted Infection box).

Ask the patient if he or she felt itching or a tingling sensation in the skin 1 to 2 days before the outbreak, known as the *prodrome*. These sensations are usually followed by the appearance of **vesicles** (blisters) in a typical cluster on the vulva (Fig. 69.1), vagina, cervix, scrotum, penis (Fig. 69.2), or perianal region at the site of inoculation. The blisters rupture spontaneously in a

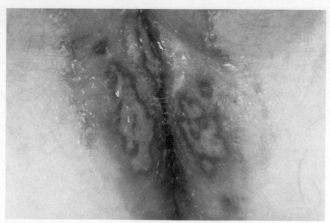

FIG. 69.1 Herpes simplex virus type 2 (HSV-2) infection; blisters on the vulva. (From Jarvis, C. [2020]. *Physical examination and health assessment* [8th ed.]. St. Louis: Elsevier.)

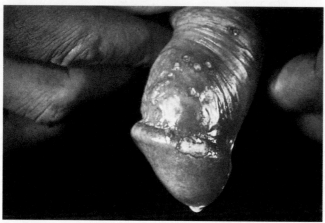

FIG. 69.2 Herpes simplex virus type 2 (HSV-2) infection; blisters on the penis. (From Jarvis, C. [2020]. *Physical examination and health assessment* [8th ed.]. St. Louis: Elsevier.)

day or two and leave ulcerations that can become extensive and cause *pain.*

Assess for other symptoms such as headaches, fever, general malaise, and swelling of inguinal lymph nodes. Ask if urination is painful. External dysuria is a painful symptom when urine passes over the eroded areas. Patients with urinary retention may need to be catheterized. Lesions resolve within 2 to 6 weeks. After the lesions heal, the virus remains in a dormant state in the sacral nerve ganglia.

Periodically the virus activates, and symptoms recur. These recurrences can be triggered by stress, fever, sunburn, poor nutrition, menses, and sexual activity. Provide anticipatory guidance regarding stressor management to prevent outbreaks.

GH is usually confirmed through a viral culture or polymerase chain reaction (PCR) assays of the lesions (Albrecht, 2018). Fluid from inside the blister obtained within 48 hours of the first outbreak will yield the most reliable results because accuracy decreases as the blisters begin to heal. Direct fluorescent antibody can also be used. Serology testing, which is glycoprotein G antibody based, can identify the HSV type,

BEST PRACTICE FOR PATIENT SAFETY & QUALITY CARE

Care of or Self-Management for the Patient With Genital Herpes (GH)

- Administer oral analgesics as prescribed.
- Apply local anesthetic sprays or ointments as prescribed.
- Apply ice packs or warm compresses to lesions.
- Administer sitz baths three or four times a day.
- Encourage increase in fluid intake to replace fluid lost through open lesions.
- Encourage frequent urination.
- Pour water over genitalia while voiding or encourage voiding while standing in a shower.
- Catheterize as necessary and prescribed.
- Encourage genital hygiene, and teach to keep the skin clean and dry.
- Wear gloves when applying ointments or making any direct contact with lesions.
- Wash hands thoroughly after contact with lesions
- Launder towels that have had direct contact with lesions.
- Teach avoidance of sexual activity when lesions are present.
- Teach use of latex or polyurethane condoms during all sexual exposures.
- Teach about the use, side effects, and risks versus benefits of antiviral agents.
- Encourage discussion of the diagnosis of GH with current and new partners.

either 1 or 2. Antibodies may take up to 12 weeks to develop, so false-negative results can occur if testing is performed too soon after the initial infection (Albrecht, 2018).

◆ **Interventions: Take Action.** The desired outcomes of treatment for patients infected with GH are to decrease *pain* from ulcerations, promote healing without secondary infection, decrease viral shedding, and prevent *infection* transmission (see the Best Practice for Patient Safety & Quality Care: Care of or Self-Management for the Patient With Genital Herpes [GH] box).

Drug Therapy. Antiviral drugs are used to treat GH. The drugs decrease the severity, promote healing, and decrease the frequency of recurrent outbreaks, but do not cure the *infection.*

Drug therapy should be offered to anyone with an initial outbreak of GH regardless of the severity of the symptoms. The CDC (2015) recommends treatment with acyclovir, famciclovir, or valacyclovir. Intravenous acyclovir and hospitalization may be indicated for patients with severe HSV and possibly fatal infections, such as disseminated (systemic) disease or encephalitis (brain infection) (Albrecht, 2019).

Dosage and length of treatment differ and can be discussed between the patient and health care provider. Intermittent therapy for recurrent outbreaks is most beneficial if it is started within 1 day of the appearance of lesions or during the period of itching or tingling before lesions appear. Daily antiviral therapy (called *chronic suppressive therapy*) can also be offered to patients (Albrecht, 2019; Burchum & Rosenthal, 2019). Suppression reduces recurrences in most patients, but it does not prevent viral shedding, even when symptoms are absent. Encourage patients on chronic suppressive therapy to follow up at least annually with their provider.

Self-Management Education. Nursing interventions focus on *pain* control by treatment of the underlying problem, and patient education. Teach about the *infection,* modes of sexual transmission, potential for recurrent episodes, and correct use and possible side effects of antiviral therapy. Clear discussion about sexual activity, including whether the patient has new or multiple partners, is an essential component of the nurse's intervention.

Assess the patient's and partner's emotional responses to the diagnosis of GH. Many people are initially shocked and need reassurance that they can manage the disease. Patients who are infected may have feelings of disbelief, uncleanness, isolation, and loneliness. They may be angry at their partner(s) for transmitting the *infection* or fear rejection because they have it. Help patients cope with the diagnosis by being nonjudgmental, sensitive, and supportive during assessments and interventions. Encourage social support and refer patients to support groups (e.g., local support groups of the Herpes Resource Center [http://www.ashasexualhealth.org/stdsstis/herpes/]) and therapists. Symptomatic care may include oral analgesics, topical anesthetics, sitz baths, and increased oral fluid intake. People who have tested serology positive for HSV-1 or HSV-2 but have never had GH symptoms should be counseled with the same information as those who have symptoms.

! NURSING SAFETY PRIORITY (QSEN)

Action Alert

Remind patients to abstain from sexual activity while GH lesions are present. Sexual activity can cause *pain,* and likelihood of viral transmission is higher. Urge condom use during all sexual encounters because of the increased risk for HSV transmission from viral shedding, which can occur even when lesions are not present. Teach the patient how to properly use condoms (see the Patient and Family Education: Preparing for Self-Management: Use of Condoms box).

PATIENT AND FAMILY EDUCATION: PREPARING FOR SELF-MANAGEMENT

Use of Condoms

- Use latex or polyurethane condoms; avoid natural membrane condoms as they provide much less protection.
- Use a new condom with every sexual encounter (including oral, vaginal, and anal).
- Internal condoms ("female condoms")—polyurethane or nitrile sheaths in the vagina—are thought to be somewhat protective against STIs, but have not been studied as closely as traditional male condoms (Hoke et al., 2020).
- Condoms can break during sexual intercourse. If a condom breaks, replace it immediately.
- Keep condoms (especially latex) in a cool, dry place, out of direct sunlight.
- Do not use condoms that are in damaged packages or are brittle or discolored.
- Always handle a condom with care to avoid damaging it with fingernails, teeth, or other sharp objects.
- Put condoms on before any genital contact. Hold the condom by the tip and unroll it on the penis. Leave a space at the tip to collect semen.
- Ensure that lubricant, if used, is water based and washes away with water. Oil-based products damage latex condoms.
- Use of spermicide (nonoxynol-9) with condoms, either lubricated condoms or vaginal application, has *not* been proven to be more or less effective against STIs than use without spermicide. Nonoxynol-9 may increase risk for transmission of HIV in women during vaginal and anal intercourse, so its use is discouraged (Bartz, 2019; World Health Organization, 2020).
- After ejaculation, withdraw the erect penis carefully, holding the condom at the base of the penis to prevent the condom from slipping off.
- Never use a condom more than once.

STI, Sexually transmitted infection.
Modified from Centers for Disease Control and Prevention (CDC). (2015). Sexually transmitted diseases treatment guidelines, 2015. *Morbidity and Mortality Weekly Report Recommendations and Reports, 64*(RR-3), 1-137.

SYPHILIS

Pathophysiology Review

Syphilis is a complex sexually transmitted **infection** (STI) that can become systemic and cause serious complications, including death. The causative organism is a spirochete called *Treponema pallidum.* The infection is usually transmitted by sexual contact and blood exposure, but transmission can occur through close body contact such as touching or kissing where there are open lesions (e.g., on the breast, genitals, or lips, or in the oral cavity) (Hicks & Clement, 2020a).

Untreated syphilis is divided into two categories—early and late—and progresses through four stages: primary (localized chancre), secondary (systemic illness), early latent (seropositive yet without symptoms), and tertiary (symptomatic infection). Neurosyphilis can occur at any time in any stage; patients with this form of the disease may experience meningitis, vision or hearing loss, and brain and spinal cord dysfunction.

The appearance of an ulcer called a chancre is the first sign of primary syphilis (Fig. 69.3). It develops at the site of entry (inoculation) of the organism from 12 days to 12 weeks days after exposure (3 weeks is average) (McCance et al., 2019). Chancres may be found on any area of the skin or mucous membranes but occur most often on the genitalia (Hicks & Clement, 2020a).

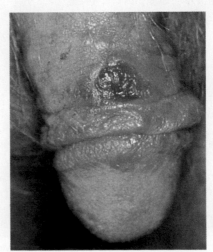

FIG. 69.3 Syphilitic chancre on the penis. (From Jarvis, C. [2020]. *Physical examination and health assessment* [8th ed.]. St. Louis: Elsevier.)

During this highly infectious stage, the chancre begins as a small papule, approximately 1 to 2 cm in diameter with a raised margin (Hicks & Clement, 2020a). Within 3 to 7 days, it breaks down into its typical appearance: a painless, indurated, smooth, weeping lesion. Regional lymph nodes enlarge, feel firm, and are not painful. Without treatment, the chancre usually disappears within 3 to 6 weeks (Hicks & Clement, 2020a). However, the organism spreads throughout the body, and the patient is still infectious.

Secondary syphilis develops in approximately 25% of untreated infected persons within a few months (Hicks & Clement, 2020a). During this stage, syphilis is a systemic disease because the spirochetes circulate throughout the bloodstream. Commonly mistaken for influenza, signs and symptoms include malaise, low-grade fever, headache, muscular aches, sore throat, hoarseness, generalized adenopathy, joint pain, and a generalized rash (McCance et al., 2020a). There is no typical appearance of this rash, but it usually appears on the palm, soles, trunk, and mucous membranes. It can appear as diffuse macules (reddish brown), papules (usually less than 5 mm) or pustules, scaly psoriasis-like lesions (Fig. 69.4), or gray-white wartlike lesions (condylomata lata). *All of these lesions are highly contagious and should not be touched without gloves.* Patchy alopecia on the scalp or facial hair (missing part of the eyebrow, "moth-eaten" appearance) is another symptom. The rash subsides without treatment in 4 to 12 weeks (McCance et al., 2019), and the patient enters the early latent stage, during which he or she is seropositive but asymptomatic. The stage may last as little as a year, or as long as a lifetime (McCance et al., 2019).

Tertiary, or late, syphilis is uncommon because of the widespread availability of antibiotics (McCance et al., 2019). If experienced, this occurs after a highly variable period, from 4 to 20 years. This stage develops in untreated cases and can mimic other conditions because any organ system can be affected. Signs and symptoms of late syphilis include (McCance et al., 2019):

- Cardiovascular infection with *T. pallidum,* which may cause aneurysms, heart valve insufficiencies, and heart failure
- Neurosyphilis, including progressive dementia and locomotor ataxia
- Gummatous syphilis (uncommon) lesions on the skin, bones, or internal organs

👤 PATIENT-CENTERED CARE: CULTURAL/ SPIRITUAL CONSIDERATIONS (QSEN)

Health care disparities exist between racial and ethnic groups in the incidence of primary and secondary syphilis. In recent reports from the CDC (2020b, 2018c), the prevalence of syphilis was highest among blacks and Native Hawaiians/Other Pacific Islanders (NHOPI). The reason for these differences is unclear, but access to high-quality health care is thought to be a factor (CDC, 2018b).

👤 PATIENT-CENTERED CARE: GENDER HEALTH CONSIDERATIONS (QSEN)

Identify unique needs regarding sexual health and prevention and treatment of STIs for lesbian, gay, bisexual, transgender, and questioning (LGBTQ) patients. Discrimination, **health care disparities,** and health care provider lack of understanding can greatly affect the health status of this population (Fenway Health, 2020). People who identify as LGBTQ may have difficulty finding health care providers who ask about and address their particular needs, risks, and concerns. Taking a health history that provides opportunity for the patient to identify sexual orientation, gender identity, and sexual activity is crucial.

Especially among transgender people, opportunities for health assessment may be avoided by the patient or missed by the provider because of fears of being misunderstood or inadequately prepared to give or receive appropriate care. Chapter 1 describes recommendations for communicating with this population. Chapter 68 discusses the special health care needs of transgender patients.

👤 PATIENT-CENTERED CARE: GENDER HEALTH CONSIDERATIONS (QSEN)

Gay, bisexual, and other men who have sex with men (MSM) are at greatest risk for contracting primary and secondary syphilis and made up 79.6% of cases of these diseases in 2017 (CDC, 2018b). Assuming that gay men or lesbian women have sex only with same-gender partners or similarly assuming that heterosexual patients never have sexual encounters with partners of the same sex limits the accuracy of the nurse's risk assessment.

❖ Interprofessional Collaborative Care

◆ **Assessment: Recognize Cues.** Assessment of the patient with signs and symptoms of syphilis begins with gathering a history about ulcers or rash. Take a sexual history and conduct a risk assessment to include whether previous testing or treatment for syphilis or other STDs has ever been done (see the Focused Assessment: The Patient With a Sexually Transmitted Infection box). Ask about allergic reactions to drugs, especially penicillin. A woman may report inguinal lymph node enlargement resulting from a chancre in the vagina or cervix that is not easily visible to her. She may report a history of contact with a male partner who had an ulcer

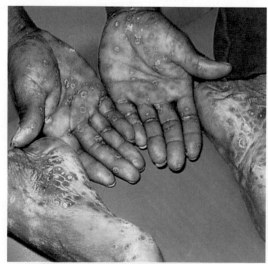

FIG. 69.4 Palmar and plantar secondary syphilis. (From Morse, S., Ballard, R., Holmes, K., & Moreland, A. [2003]. *Atlas of sexually transmitted diseases and AIDS* [3rd ed.]. Edinburgh: Mosby.)

that she noticed during a sexual encounter. Men usually discover the chancre on the penis or scrotum.

Conduct a physical examination, including inspection and palpation. *Wear gloves while palpating any lesions because of the highly contagious treponemes that are present.* Observe for and document rashes of any type because of the variable presentation of secondary syphilis.

The health care provider will obtain a specimen of the chancre for examination under a darkfield microscope. Diagnosis of primary or secondary syphilis is confirmed if *T. pallidum* is present.

Nontreponemal blood tests include the *Venereal Disease Research Laboratory (VDRL)* serum test, the more sensitive *rapid plasma reagin (RPR)* test, and the *toluidine red unheated serum test (TRUST)*. These tests are based on an antibody-antigen reaction that determines the presence and amount of antibodies produced by the body in response to an **infection** by *T. pallidum*. False-positive and false-negative results are a downfall of these types of tests.

Treponemal tests detect antibodies directed against treponemal antigens; they are more reliable than nontreponemal tests (Hicks & Clement, 2020a). These include:

- Fluorescent treponemal antibody absorption (FTA-ABS) test
- Microhemagglutination test for antibodies to *T. pallidum* (MHA-TP)
- *T. pallidum* particle agglutination assay (TPPA)
- *T. pallidum* enzyme immunoassay (TP-EIA)
- Chemiluminescence immunoassay (CIA)

Patients who are shown to be reactive to one of these nontreponemal tests will have this positive result for their entire life, even after treatment. This may be surprising news for a patient who denies a history of or does not know that he or she had syphilis. Use therapeutic communication skills and a nonjudgmental attitude to objectively discuss this finding.

◆ Interventions: Take Action

Drug Therapy. Interprofessional collaborative care includes drug therapy and health teaching to resolve the **infection** and prevent transmission to others. Benzathine penicillin G given IM as a single dose at the time of the initial visit with the health care provider is the evidence-based treatment for primary, secondary, and early latent syphilis (CDC, 2015). Patients in the latent stage receive weekly treatment for a longer time (CDC, 2015). A different regimen, found in the CDC's *2015 STD Treatment Guidelines,* is recommended for patients who are pregnant or have HIV.

! NURSING SAFETY PRIORITY (QSEN)

Drug Alert

Allergic reactions to benzathine penicillin G can occur. Monitor for allergic signs and symptoms (e.g., rash, edema, shortness of breath, chest tightness, anxiety). Penicillin desensitization is recommended for penicillin-allergic patients. *Keep all patients at the health care agency for at least 30 minutes after they have received the antibiotic so signs and symptoms of an allergic reaction can be detected and treated. The most severe reaction is anaphylaxis. Treatment should be available and implemented immediately if symptoms occur.* Chapter 18 describes the management of drug allergies in detail.

The *Jarisch-Herxheimer reaction* may also follow antibiotic therapy for syphilis. This reaction is caused by the rapid release of products from the disruption of the cells of the organism. Symptoms include fever, generalized aches, rigors, vasodilation, diaphoresis, hypotension, and worsening of any rash that was present. These symptoms are usually benign and begin within 24 hours after therapy, and are treated symptomatically with analgesics and antipyretics (Hicks & Clement, 2020b).

Self-Management Education. To provide teaching, choose a setting that offers privacy and encourages open discussion. Discuss the importance of partner notification and treatment, including the risk for reinfection if the partner goes untreated. All sexual partners must be prophylactically treated as soon as possible, preferably within 90 days of the syphilis diagnosis.

Inform the patient that the disease will be reported to the local health authority and that all information will be held in strict confidence. Urge the patient to keep follow-up appointments. For primary and secondary syphilis, drug therapy is provided at the first visit, which may suggest to the patient that no further visits are indicated or important. Remind the patient that follow-up for self and partner(s) is critical, and that sexual abstinence is recommended until full treatment is complete. After the initial antibiotic, the CDC recommends follow-up evaluation, including blood tests at 6, 12, and 24 months. Repeat treatment may be needed if the patient does not respond to the initial antibiotic.

The emotional responses to syphilis vary and may include feelings of fear, depression, guilt, and anxiety. Patients may experience guilt if they have infected others or anger if a partner has infected them. If further psychosocial interventions are needed, encourage the patient to discuss these feelings or refer him or her to other resources such as psychotherapy, self-help support groups, or STI/STD clinics.

NCLEX EXAMINATION CHALLENGE 69.1

Physiological Integrity

The nurse is caring for a client who has just been diagnosed with primary syphilis. Which client statement reflects that teaching has been effective?
Select all that apply.
A. "I can resume having intercourse right after this injection."
B. "At least this infection is not as serious as gonorrhea or chlamydia."
C. "I'm afraid, but I'm going to tell my partners about my diagnosis."
D. "After my treatment, I still need several follow-up appointments."
E. "I can take acetaminophen if I get a fever and chills after this shot."
F. "I am going to wait here in the clinic 30 minutes after treatment."

CONDYLOMATA ACUMINATA (GENITAL WARTS)

Pathophysiology Review

Condylomata acuminata (genital warts) are caused by certain types of *human papillomavirus (HPV)*. Genital warts are a very common viral disease that is sexually transmitted and often coexist with other infections. Most of these infections

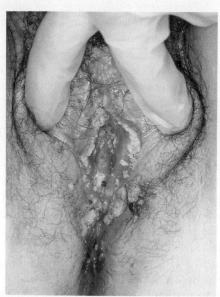

FIG. 69.5 Genital warts on the vulva. (From Jarvis, C. [2020]. *Physical examination and health assessment* [8th ed.]. St. Louis: Elsevier.)

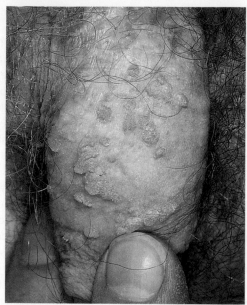

FIG. 69.6 Genital warts on the penis. (From Jarvis, C. [2020]. *Physical examination and health assessment* [8th ed.]. St. Louis: Elsevier.)

originate from HPV types 6 and 11, which cause 90% of genital warts (Palefsky, 2019). HPV types 16, 18, 31, 33, 45, 52, and 58 are associated with precancerous or dysplastic lesions, as well as cervical, vulvar, vaginal, and anal cancers (Merck Sharp & Dohme Corp., 2019). HPV infection has been established as the primary risk factor for development of cervical cancer. Evidence shows that HPV can also cause cancer of the penis and the oropharynx (throat, tongue, and tonsils) (CDC, 2019). High-risk HPV (strains that cause cancer) *infection* may coexist with low-risk HPV (strains that cause warts). The presence of one strain increases the risk for acquiring other strains.

❖ Interprofessional Collaborative Care

◆ Assessment: Recognize Cues.
The diagnosis of condylomata acuminata is made by examination of the lesions. They are initially small, papillary growths that are white or resemble the color of the patient's skin (Figs. 69.5 and 69.6) and may grow into large cauliflower-like masses (Fig. 69.7). Multiple warts usually occur in the same area. Bleeding may occur if the wart is disturbed. Warts may disappear or resolve on their own without treatment. They may occur once or recur at the original site. Warts can occur on the external or internal surfaces of the genitalia, including the mucosal surfaces of the vagina and urethra. Screening for HPV and dysplasia of the cervix is done by obtaining cervical specimens for Papanicolaou (Pap) and HPV DNA testing.

Identifying high-risk strains of HPV and correlating with abnormal Pap smear findings are the standard of care (CDC, 2015). The diagnosis should include consideration of condyloma lata (which occurs in secondary syphilis) because STIs frequently coexist. Blood tests, an HIV test, and cultures for chlamydia and gonorrhea infections are done. If a wartlike lesion bleeds easily, appears infected, is atypical, or persists, a biopsy of the lesion is performed to rule out other pathologic problems such as cancer. A biopsy of warts that are seen on the cervix should be performed before any treatment to eradicate them.

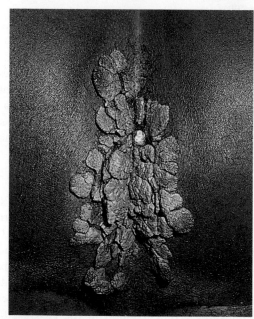

FIG. 69.7 Perianal condylomata acuminata. (From Morse, S., Ballard, R., Holmes, K., & Moreland, A. [2003]. *Atlas of sexually transmitted diseases and AIDS* [3rd ed.]. Edinburgh: Mosby.)

◆ Interventions: Take Action.
The outcome of treatment is to remove the warts. No current therapy eliminates the HPV *infection,* and recurrences after treatment are likely. It is not known whether removal of visible warts decreases the risk for disease transmission.

Nonsurgical Management. Patients may be prescribed cryodestructive therapies such as podophyllotoxin, podophyllum resin, or trichloroacetic acid (TCA) as personally applied topical applications for treatment of warts (Carusi, 2019). Immune-mediated therapies include imiquimod (topical), sinecatechins (topical), and interferons (available as a topical treatment, as well as through IM and subcutaneous injections). Patients taking imiquimod should be taught to minimize exposure to the sun and tanning beds, wear protective clothing, and use sunscreen, as this medication increases sensitivity to ultraviolet radiation (Burchum & Rosenthal, 2019). These treatments are less expensive than those performed in the health care provider's office, but they take longer for healing. *Teach patients that over-the-counter (OTC) wart treatments should not be used on genital tissue.*

Surgical Management. Surgical excision, cryoablation, laser ablation, electrocautery, and ultrasonic aspiration are treatment options that the health care provider can perform (Carusi, 2019). Extensive warts have been treated with carbon dioxide laser procedures, intralesion interferon injections, and surgical removal (CDC, 2015). The choice of treatment is based on the patient's individualized presentation, including number, size, and location of warts; preference of the patient; cost; adverse effects; the skills of the clinician; and treatment availability.

Self-Management Education. The priority nursing intervention is patient and sexual partner education about the mode of transmission, incubation period, treatment, and complications, especially the association with various types of cancer. Teach about local care for postsurgical lesions or patient-applied treatment for self-management.

> **! NURSING SAFETY PRIORITY (QSEN)**
>
> ***Drug Alert***
>
> Teach patients that, after treatment with podophyllotoxin, podophyllum resin, or trichloroacetic acid (TCA), they may experience **pain,** bleeding, or discharge from the site or sloughing of parts of warts. Teach to keep the area clean and dry, and to be alert for any signs or symptoms of further **infection** or side effects of the treatment.

Inform patients that recurrence is likely, especially in the first 3 months, and that repeated treatments may be needed. Urge all patients to have complete STI testing, since exposure to one STI increases the risk for contracting another. Sexual partners should also be evaluated and offered treatment if warts are present. Teach patients to avoid intimate sexual contact until external lesions are healed, and to use condoms to help reduce transmission even after warts have been treated (see the Patient and Family Education: Preparing for Self-Management: Use of Condoms box). Teach women to follow the U.S. Preventive Services Task Force (2018) recommendations on Pap and HPV testing:

- If 21 to 29 years old, get a Pap test every 3 years.
- If 30 to 65 years old, get:
  - A Pap test every 3 years, or
  - An HPV test every 5 years, or
  - A Pap test and HPV test together (called co-testing) every 5 years
- If older than 65, ask the health care provider whether Pap tests and HPV tests can be stopped.

Vaccination to protect patients against HPV is one of the most important interventions available, especially for MSM and immunocompromised young adults (CDC, 2015). Teach

TABLE 69.3 Human Papillomavirus (HPV) Vaccines

Vaccination	HPV Type	Gender and Age Recommended
Gardasil (available in Canada)	6, 11 16, 18	Males 9-26 yr Females 9-26 yr
Gardasil 9 (available in Canada and the United States)	6, 11, 16, 18, 31, 33, 45, 52, 58	Males and females 9-26 yr (can be administered up to age 45 yr)
Cervarix (available in Canada)	16, 18	Males 9-25 yr Females 9-25 yr

aFrom Merck. (2019). https://www.gardasil9.com/about-gardasil9/schedule/.
bFrom FDA.gov. https://www.fda.gov/media/78013/download.

patients about the various vaccinations available (Table 69.3), and encourage them to be immunized.

CHLAMYDIA INFECTION

Pathophysiology Review

Chlamydia trachomatis is an intracellular bacterium and the causative agent of cervicitis (in women), urethritis, and proctitis. It invades the epithelial tissues in the reproductive tract. The incubation period ranges from 1 to 3 weeks, but the pathogen may be present in the genital tract for months without producing symptoms.

C. trachomatis is reportable to local health departments in all states. In the United States, it is the most frequently reported bacterial sexually transmitted **infection** (CDC, 2018a; CDC, 2016). Diagnosed cases continue to increase yearly, which reflects more sensitive screening tests and increased public health efforts to screen high-risk people. Because it is frequently asymptomatic, the estimated incidence is approximately double what is reported.

> **👤 PATIENT-CENTERED CARE: CULTURAL/ SPIRITUAL CONSIDERATIONS (QSEN)**
>
> Significant **health care disparities** exist between racial/ethnic groups. Prevalence among non-Hispanic blacks is 5.6 times greater than the prevalence among non-Hispanic whites (CDC, 2018a). There is also a high prevalence of rectal and pharyngeal chlamydial **infection** among men who have sex with men (MSM) (CDC, 2018a).

❖ Interprofessional Collaborative Care

◆ **Assessment: Recognize Cues.** As with all interviews concerning *sexuality,* use a nonjudgmental approach and provide privacy and confidentiality. Obtain a complete history, including a genitourinary system review, psychosocial history, and sexual history (see the Focused Assessment: The Patient With a Sexually Transmitted Infection box). In particular, ask about:

- Presence of symptoms, including vaginal or urethral discharge, dysuria (painful urination), pelvic **pain,** and any irregular bleeding (for women)

- A history of sexually transmitted diseases (STIs)
- Whether current or past sexual partners have had symptoms or a history of STIs
- Whether the patient has had a new partner, or multiple sexual partners
- Whether the patient or a current or recent partner has had unprotected intercourse

Evidence shows that incidence is higher among black, Native Alaskan, and American Indian populations (U.S. Department of Health and Human Services, Indian Health Services, U.S. Centers for Disease Control and Prevention, 2015).

PATIENT-CENTERED CARE: GENDER HEALTH CONSIDERATIONS QSEN

Ask men about about dysuria, frequent urination, or discharge, which may indicate urethritis. He may report a mucoid discharge that is more watery and less copious than what is expected with a gonorrheal discharge. Some men have the discharge only in the morning on arising. Complications of untreated chlamydia in men include epididymitis, prostatitis, infertility, and Reiter syndrome, a type of connective tissue disease.

Men may report penile discharge, urinary frequency, and dysuria. In contrast, many women have no symptoms. Those with symptoms may report mucopurulent vaginal discharge (typically yellow and opaque), urinary frequency, and abdominal discomfort or *pain.* Cervical bleeding, from infected, fragile tissue, may present as spotting or bleeding between menses and frequently after intercourse. Complications of *infection* with chlamydia include salpingitis (inflammation of the fallopian tubes), pelvic inflammatory disease (PID), and *reproduction* problems including infertility, ectopic pregnancy, and complications with a newborn that is delivered. These health problems are discussed in detail in maternal-child textbooks.

Diagnosis is made by sampling cells from the endocervix, urethra, or both, easily obtained with a swab. Because chlamydiae can reproduce only inside cells, cervical (or host) cells that harbor the organism (or parts of it) are required in the sample. Tissue culture obtained from the cervical os during the female pelvic examination or from male urethral examination obtained by swabbing has been replaced by genetic tests. Nucleic acid amplification tests (NAATs) are the most common method of detecting chlamydia in endocervical samples, urethral swabs, and urine. Samples can be obtained by swab by the examining clinician or by a patient-collected swab or urine specimen. Retesting after 3 months is advised in order to detect repeat *infection* (CDC, 2015; Johnson-Mallard et al., 2018).

All sexually active women 25 years old or younger and all women older than 25 years with a new partner, multiple partners, or a partner with an STI should be screened annually for chlamydia (CDC, 2018a). Routine screening is not recommended for men; however, screening should be done for sexually active younger men, especially those who have sex with men (MSM) (CDC, 2018a).

◆ Interventions: Take Action

Drug Therapy. The treatment of choice for chlamydia infections is azithromycin (usually given in a single dose at the time of the initial visit with the health care provider) or doxycycline. The one-dose course, although more expensive, is preferred because of the ease in completing the treatment. Directly observing the patient taking the medication in the health care setting will assure you of adherence. Alternative treatments that are prescribed for patients with allergies to these drugs include erythromycin, ofloxacin, and levofloxacin (CDC, 2015).

Sexual partners should be treated and tested for other STIs. Expedited partner therapy (EPT), or patient-delivered partner therapy, shows signs of reducing chlamydia *infection* rates (CDC, 2015). Expedited partner therapy (EPT) involves treating sexual partners of patients diagnosed with chlamydia infection or gonorrhea by providing prescriptions or medication to the patient, which they can take to their partner(s), without the partner(s) having to be examined by a provider of care. Evidence shows that when the patient gives the drug to their partner(s), rates of infection decrease, and more partners report receiving treatment (CDC, 2015).

Self-Management Education. As with all STI diagnoses, patient and partner education is a crucial nursing intervention geared toward effectively treating the condition and reducing the risk of reinfection. Teach about:

- The sexual mode of transmission
- The incubation period
- The high possibility of asymptomatic infections and the usual symptoms, if present
- The need for antibiotic treatment of *infection* and the need to complete all medications, even if feeling better
- The need for abstinence from sexual intercourse until the patient and partner(s) have all completed treatment (7 days from the start of treatment, including if treated with the single-dose regimen)
- The need for women to be rescreened for reinfection 3 to 12 months after treatment because of the high risk for PID; also, the fact that there is less evidence of the need for rescreening of treated men, but it should be considered
- The need to return for evaluation if symptoms recur or new symptoms develop (most recurrences are reinfections from a new or untreated partner)
- Complications of untreated or inadequately treated *infection,* which may include PID, infertility, ectopic pregnancy, or newborn complications

GONORRHEA

Pathophysiology Review

Gonorrhea is a sexually transmitted bacterial *infection* caused by *Neisseria gonorrhoeae,* a gram-negative intracellular diplococcus. It is transmitted by direct sexual contact with mucosal surfaces (vaginal intercourse, orogenital contact, or anogenital contact) (McCance et al., 2019).

The first symptoms of gonorrhea may appear within a week after sexual contact with an infected person. The disease can be present without symptoms and can be transmitted or progress without warning. In women, ascending spread of the organism can cause pelvic infection (pelvic inflammatory disease [PID]), **endometritis** (endometrial infection), **salpingitis** (fallopian tube infection), and pelvic peritonitis. In men, gonorrhea can cause epididymitis, which can lead to infertility if left untreated.

❖ Interprofessional Collaborative Care

◆ Assessment: Recognize Cues.
Establish a trusting relationship and use a nonjudgmental approach to gather complete information. A complete history includes a review of the genitourinary system, and colleting a sexual history. Sites of sexual exposure or intercourse should be elicited, because gonorrhea can affect the genitals, rectum, and throat. Assess for allergies to antibiotics.

The *infection* can be asymptomatic in both men and women, but women have asymptomatic, or "silent," infections more often than do men. If symptoms are present, men usually notice dysuria and a penile discharge that can be either profuse yellowish-green fluid or scant clear fluid. The urethra, epididymis, seminal vesicles, and prostate can become infected. Men seek curative treatment sooner, usually because they have symptoms, and thereby avoid some of the serious complications.

Women may report a change in vaginal discharge (yellow, green, profuse, odorous), urinary frequency, or dysuria. The cervix and urethra are the most common sites of *infection*.

Anal signs and symptoms may include itching and irritation, rectal bleeding or diarrhea, and painful bowel movements. Assess the mouth for a reddened throat, ulcerated lips, tender gingivae, and lesions in the throat. Fig. 69.8 shows common sites of gonococcal infections.

Fever may be a sign of an ascending (PID or epididymitis) or systemic (disseminated gonococcal) *infection.* Symptoms often include joint pain of the shoulder, wrist, and lower extremities, and a rash of several days' duration (Schweon, 2019).

Clinical symptoms of gonorrhea can resemble those of chlamydia *infection* and need to be differentiated. Nucleic acid amplification tests (NAATs) are the most common type of testing for the initial microbiologic diagnosis of gonorrhea; culture is also used when antibiotic resistance is suspected (Ghanem, 2020). During examination, the health care provider can swab the male urethra or female cervix to obtain specimens. Patient-collected urine or vaginal swabs can also be used to diagnose both gonorrhea and chlamydia infections, allowing for testing without a full examination.

All patients with gonorrhea should be tested for syphilis, chlamydia, hepatitis B and hepatitis C, and HIV infection and, if possible, examined for HSV and HPV because they may have been exposed to these STIs as well. Sexual partners who have been exposed in the past 30 days should be examined, and specimens should be obtained.

◆ Interventions: Take Action.
Uncomplicated gonorrhea is treated with antibiotics. Chlamydia *infection*, which is four times more common, is frequently found in patients with gonorrhea. Because of this, patients treated for gonorrhea should also be managed with drugs that treat chlamydia infection.

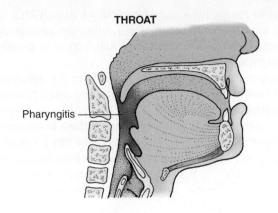

THROAT

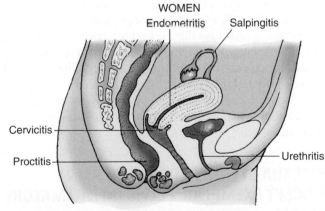

PELVIC/GENITAL

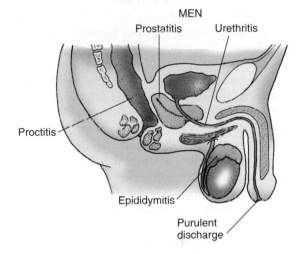

FIG. 69.8 Areas of involvement of gonorrhea in men and women.

Drug Therapy. Drug therapy recommended by the CDC is IM ceftriaxone *plus* oral azithromycin in a single dose at the time of the initial visit with the health care provider *or* oral doxycycline for a longer period of time to treat a presumed co-infection with chlamydia (unless a negative chlamydia result has been obtained). These combinations seem to be effective for all mucosal gonorrheal infections; treatment failure is rare (CDC, 2015). A test-of-cure is not required for treatment of uncomplicated urogenital or rectal gonorrhea treated with ceftriaxone and azithromycin; patients with oropharyngeal gonorrhea treated with any alternative treatment should be advised to return for a test-of-cure in 14 days (CDC, 2015). Advise any patient to return for a follow-up examination if symptoms persist after treatment. Reinfection is usually the cause of these symptoms.

Sexual partners must be education about the *infection* and treated (not just evaluated) to prevent reinfection. Because the best treatment for gonorrhea is injected ceftriaxone, expedited partner therapy (EPT) is not effective. If there is concern that the partner may not come to a health care facility for treatment, providing oral cefixime as an alternative has been recommended by the CDC (2015). Because of the potential for resistance of gonorrhea to cefixime, a test-of-cure is recommended after treatment is completed.

Gonorrhea *infection* can become disseminated, requiring hospitalization and IV or IM ceftriaxone. If symptoms resolve within 24 to 48 hours, the patient may be discharged to home to continue cefixime as oral antibiotic therapy while recovering (CDC, 2015).

Self-Management Education. Teach the patient about transmission and treatment of gonorrhea. Explain that the use of medication to treat chlamydia *infection* at the same time is important, as the likelihood of co-infection is high. Discuss the possibility of reinfection, including the risk for pelvic inflammatory disease (PID) (see discussion of PID later in this chapter). Instruct patients to abstain from sexual activity until the antibiotic therapy is completed and they no longer have symptoms. Reinforce the need for use of condoms at all times. Explain that gonorrhea is a reportable disease.

Patients with gonorrhea (or any other STI) may have feelings of fear or guilt. They may be concerned that they have contracted other STIs or consider the disease a religious or spiritual punishment for their sexual behaviors. Such feelings can impair relationships with intimate partners. Encourage patients to express their feelings and offer other information and professional resources to help them understand their diagnosis and treatment. Ensure privacy during your discussion and maintain confidentiality of personal health information.

✳ SEXUALITY, INFECTION, AND PAIN CONCEPT EXEMPLAR: PELVIC INFLAMMATORY DISEASE

Pathophysiology Review

Pelvic inflammatory disease (PID) is an acute syndrome resulting in tenderness in the tubes and ovaries (adnexa) and, typically, dull pelvic *pain.* Some women experience only mild discomfort or menstrual irregularity, whereas others have acute *pain,* which can affect their gait (Table 69.4). Others experience no symptoms at all (i.e., so-called "silent" or "subclinical" PID).

This infectious process involves movement of organisms from the endocervix upward through the uterine cavity into the fallopian tubes. Usually multiple pathogens are involved in the development of PID. Sexually transmitted organisms are most often responsible, especially *C. trachomatis, N. gonorrhoeae,*

TABLE 69.4   Diagnostic Criteria for Pelvic Inflammatory Disease (PID)

Minimum Criteria for Initiating Empiric Treatment for Pelvic Inflammatory Disease

- Sexually active woman and at risk for sexually transmitted infections (STIs)
- Pelvic or lower abdominal pain
- Cervical motion, uterine, or adnexal tenderness on examination
- No other cause for illness can be found (e.g., appendicitis)

Additional Criteria to Increase the Specificity of the Diagnosis of PID

- Oral temperature >101°F (>38.3°C)
- Abnormal cervical or vaginal mucopurulent discharge, or cervical friability
- Abundance of white blood cells (WBCs) on saline microscopy of vaginal secretions
- Laboratory documentation of cervical infection with *Neisseria gonorrhoeae* or *Chlamydia trachomatis*

Definitive Criteria for Diagnosing PID, Warranted in Selected Cases

- Histopathologic evidence of endometritis on endometrial biopsy
- Transvaginal sonography or MRI techniques showing thickened, fluid-filled tubes with or without free pelvic fluid or tubo-ovarian complex, or Doppler studies suggesting pelvic infection
- Laparoscopic abnormalities consistent with PID

Modified from Centers for Disease Control and Prevention (CDC). (2015). Sexually transmitted diseases treatment guidelines, 2015. *Morbidity and Mortality Weekly Report Recommendations and Reports, 64*(RR-3), 1-137; and Ross, J., & Chacko, M. (2020). Pelvic inflammatory disease: Clinical manifestations and diagnosis. In *UpToDate,* Marrozzo, J. (Ed.). Waltham, MA.

---

and *Mycoplasma genitalium* (Ross & Chacko, 2020). Bacterial vaginosis has also been shown to be a causative agent (Ross & Chacko, 2020).

The spread of *infection* to other organs and tissues of the upper genital tract occurs from direct contact with mucosal surfaces or through the fimbriated ends of the tubes to the ovaries, parametrium, and peritoneal cavity (Fig. 69.9). This may involve one or more pelvic structures, including the uterus, fallopian tubes, and adjacent pelvic structures. The most common site is the fallopian tube (salpingitis). Complications of PID include chronic pelvic pain, infertility, risk for ectopic pregnancy, and tubo-ovarian abscess (TOA), a serious short-term condition requiring hospitalization in which an inflammatory mass arises on the fallopian tube, ovary, and/or other pelvic organs (CDC, 2017). These complications are discussed in maternal-newborn textbooks. Perihepatitis—inflammation of the liver capsule and peritoneal surfaces of the anterior right upper quadrant—occurs in 10% of women with acute PID (Ross & Chacko, 2020). This condition is characterized by right upper quadrant pain with a pleuritic component (often the right shoulder) (Ross & Chacko, 2020).

Infections can be spread during sexual intercourse, during childbirth (including the postpartum period), and after abortion. *Sepsis and death can occur, especially if treatment is delayed or inadequate.*

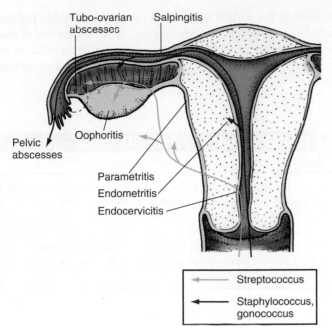

FIG. 69.9 The spread of pelvic inflammatory disease.

❖ Interprofessional Collaborative Care
◆ Assessment: Recognize Cues

History. Obtain a complete history of the symptoms with menstrual, obstetric, sexual, and family history. Inquire about any history of previous episodes of pelvic inflammatory disease (PID) or other sexually transmitted infections (see Focused Assessment: The Patient With A Sexually Transmitted Infection). Assess for contraceptive use, a history of reproductive surgery, and other risk factors previously discussed. Ask the patient if sexual abuse has occurred. If so, encourage her to discuss what happened and whether she was seen by a health care provider.

Many of the same factors that place women at risk for STIs also place them at risk for PID. Risk factors for sexually active women include (CDC, 2017):

- Being younger than 26 years old
- Having a new sexual partner, or having multiple sexual partners
- Having a sexual partner who has other concurrent sexual partners
- Practicing inconsistent use of condoms
- Having a history of PID
- Having a concurrent chlamydial or gonococcal *infection,* or having bacterial vaginosis
- Practicing vaginal douching
- Having a history of sexually transmitted diseases (STIs)
- Having had an intrauterine device (IUD) placed within the previous 3 weeks (this is noted as a small risk)

Physical Assessment/Signs and Symptoms. One of the most frequent symptoms of PID is lower abdominal or pelvic *pain.* Conduct a complete pain assessment. Other symptoms include irregular vaginal bleeding (spotting or bleeding between periods), dysuria (painful urination), an increase or change in vaginal discharge, **dyspareunia** (painful sexual intercourse), malaise, fever, and chills.

Observe whether the patient has pain with movement. She may bend forward to guard her abdomen. She may find it difficult to independently get on the examination table or stretcher. Assess for lower abdominal tenderness, possibly with rigidity or rebound tenderness. A pelvic examination by the health care provider may reveal yellow or green cervical discharge and a reddened or friable cervix (a cervix that bleeds easily). Criteria for accurate diagnosis of PID are listed in Table 69.4. The diagnosis of PID is based on health history, physical assessment, and laboratory tests. Imaging studies and laparoscopy are not generally used to make the diagnosis.

❓ CLINICAL JUDGMENT CHALLENGE 69.1
Patient-Centered Care; Evidence-Based Practice

The nurse is caring for a 19-year-old female client who reports lower abdominal *pain,* a low-grade fever, and burning on urination. She states that she "must have gotten the flu" from a co-worker, and "probably has a urinary tract infection." On assessment, the client states that she became sexually active for the first time 6 months ago, and has noticed recently that intercourse is uncomfortable. When a pelvic examination is recommended by the health care provider, the client states she does not understand why she needs that type of assessment when she is certain she has a urinary tract infection (UTI) and influenza. She asks for a prescription to treat these conditions, and says she does not want to have the pelvic examination.

1. **Recognize Cues:** What assessment information in this client situation is the most important and immediate concern for the nurse? (Hint: Identify the **relevant** information *first* to determine what is most important.)
2. **Analyze Cues:** What client conditions are consistent with the **most relevant** information? (Hint: Think about priority collaborative problems that support and contradict the information presented in this situation.)
3. **Prioritize Hypotheses:** Which possibilities or explanations are **most likely** to be present in this client situation? Which possibilities or explanations are the most serious? (Hint: Consider all possibilities and determine their urgency and risk for this client.)
4. **Generate Solutions:** What actions would most likely achieve the desired outcomes for this client? Which actions should be **avoided** or are **potentially harmful**? (Hint: Determine the desired outcomes first to decide which interventions are appropriate and those that should be avoided.)
5. **Take Action:** Which actions are the most appropriate and how should they be implemented? In what **priority order** should they be implemented? (Hint: Consider health teaching, documentation, requested health care provider orders or prescriptions, nursing skills, collaboration with or referral to health team members, etc.)
6. **Evaluate Outcomes:** What client assessment would indicate that the nurse's actions were **effective**? (Hint: Think about signs that would indicate an improvement, decline, or unchanged client condition.)

Psychosocial Assessment. The woman who has symptoms of PID may be anxious and fearful of the examination and unknown diagnosis. She may need reassurance and support during the examination because of pelvic *pain.* Explain what is taking place in real time to help promote understanding.

Because PID is often associated with an STI, the woman may feel embarrassed or uncomfortable discussing symptoms or history. Use a nonjudgmental approach and encourage expression of feelings and concerns. Assessing the patient's ability to follow through with the interprofessional collaborative plan of care is essential in deciding whether hospitalization should be considered.

Laboratory Assessment. The health care provider obtains specimens from the cervix, urethra, and rectum to determine the presence of *N. gonorrhoeae* or *C. trachomatis.* The white blood cell (WBC) count may be elevated but is not specific for PID. A sensitive test that detects human chorionic gonadotropin (hCG) in urine or blood should be performed to determine whether the patient is pregnant (Pagana & Pagana, 2018). Microscopic examination of vaginal discharge is done to evaluate for the presence of WBCs.

Other Diagnostic Assessment. Abdominal *ultrasonography* may be used to determine the presence of appendicitis and tubo-ovarian abscesses (TOAs) that need to be ruled out when the diagnosis of PID is made. Ultrasound can be used to visualize the upper genital tract. CT or MRI can be helpful in determining if there is gastrointestinal pathology (Ross & Chacko, 2020).

◆ **Analysis: Analyze Cues and Prioritize Hypotheses.** The priority collaborative problem for a patient with pelvic inflammatory disease (PID) is:

1. *Infection* due to invasion of pelvic organs by sexually transmitted pathogens

◆ **Planning and Implementation: Generate Solutions and Take Action**

Managing Infection and Pain

Planning: Expected Outcomes. The patient with PID is expected to have the *infection* resolved, be free of abdominal *pain,* and prevent reinfection.

Interventions. Interprofessional collaborative care includes antibiotic therapy and self-management measures. Uncomplicated PID is usually treated on an ambulatory care basis. The CDC recommends oral and/or parenteral antibiotics for PID (CDC, 2015). The CDC (2015) recommends hospitalization for the patient with PID if:

- A surgical emergency (e.g., appendicitis) has not been excluded as a diagnosis
- The patient is pregnant
- She cannot follow or tolerate treatment as an outpatient
- There is severe illness, nausea and vomiting, or high fever
- A tubo-ovarian abscess (TOA) has been diagnosed
- There has been no clinical response to earlier oral antimicrobial treatment

Inpatient therapy involves a combination of several IV antibiotics until the woman shows signs of improvement (e.g., decreased pelvic tenderness for at least 24 hours). Then oral antibiotics are continued at home until the course of treatment has lasted 14 days.

Antibiotic therapy relieves *pain* by destroying the pathogens and decreasing the inflammation caused by *infection.* Other measures to treat pain include taking mild analgesics and applying heat to the lower abdomen or back. As with any infection,

encourage the patient to increase the intake of fluids and eat nutritious foods that promote healing. Teach the patient to rest in semi-Fowler position and encourage limited ambulation to promote gravity drainage of the infection that may help relieve *pain.*

⚠ NURSING SAFETY PRIORITY (QSEN)

Action Alert

Instruct women who are being treated for PID on an ambulatory care basis to avoid sexual intercourse for the full course of antibiotic treatment and until their symptoms have resolved. Teach them to check their temperature twice daily, and to report an increase in temperature to their health care provider. Remind them to be seen by the health care provider within 72 hours from starting antibiotic treatment and then 1 and 2 weeks from the time of the initial diagnosis.

Laparoscopy can confirm the presence of PID, but it is uncommonly performed for this purpose (Ross & Chacko, 2020). It is more frequently performed if the patient has not responded to outpatient treatment and the health care provider is considering alternative causes for symptoms, or if the patient's symptoms are not improving or are worsening after 72 hours of inpatient treatment (Ross & Chacko, 2020). Before surgery, provide information about the procedure. After surgery, the care of the woman with PID is similar to that of any patient after laparoscopic abdominal surgery. One difference is that she may have a wound drain for drainage of abscess fluid if an abscess was removed during the procedure. Observe, measure, and record wound drainage every 4 to 8 hours as requested.

Care Coordination and Transition Management. Establish an atmosphere of trust that encourages the woman to return frequently, if needed, for education or reassurance. Teach the patient with PID to see her health care provider for follow-up to assess for complications and to confirm that the *infection* has resolved. If the woman is hospitalized, collaborate with the case manager or discharge planner before she is discharged to home.

Home Care Management. Parenteral antibiotic therapy may be given at home, but usually the health care provider changes the treatment regimen to oral antibiotics before hospital discharge. Home care for the patient who had laparoscopic surgery is discussed in Chapter 9.

Self-Management Education. Patient teaching focuses on providing information about PID, identifying symptoms of persistent or recurrent *infection* (persistent pelvic *pain,* dysmenorrhea, low backache, fever), and teaching about the importance of completion of treatment, rest, and healthy nutrition. Teach specifically about oral antibiotic therapy (see the Patient and Family Education: Preparing for Self-Management: Oral Antibiotic Therapy for Sexually Transmitted Infections box).

PATIENT AND FAMILY EDUCATION: PREPARING FOR SELF-MANAGEMENT

Oral Antibiotic Therapy for Sexually Transmitted Infections

- Take medicine for the number of times a day that it is prescribed and until it is completed, even if you begin to feel better.
- Take your antibiotics on an empty stomach unless your health care provider instructs you to take them with food.
- Do not take antacids containing calcium, magnesium, or aluminum, such as Tums, Maalox, or Mylanta, with your antibiotics. They may decrease the effectiveness of the antibiotic.
- Your sexual partner must be treated if you have a sexually transmitted infection (STI). Expedited partner therapy is one way to ensure that partners are treated.
- Do not have sex until after you and your partner complete your antibiotic therapy. Wait 7 days to resume intimacy if treatment was delivered in one dose.
- Drink at least 8 to 10 glasses of fluid a day while taking your antibiotics.
- Be sure to return for your follow-up appointment after completing your antibiotic treatment.
- Call if you have any questions or concerns.

NCLEX EXAMINATION CHALLENGE 69.2

Physiological Integrity

Which teaching will the nurse provide to a client who has been prescribed antibiotics for pelvic inflammatory disease (PID)? **Select all that apply.**

A. "Finish all of the prescribed drug even if you begin to feel better."
B. "If you feel nauseated from the antibiotics, take a dose of Tums or Maalox."
C. "Take antibiotics with food to decrease the chance of stomach irritation."
D. "You may resume intercourse once you have been on the antibiotic for 48 hours."
E. "You will need to return to see the health care provider after finishing drug therapy."

Teach the patient to contact her sexual partner(s) for examination and treatment. All sexual partners should be treated for gonorrhea and chlamydia *infection* regardless of whether they have symptoms. Remind the patient about follow-up care, and counsel her about the complications that can occur after an occurrence of PID, including recurrence, chronic pelvic *pain*, ectopic pregnancy, and infertility.

Discuss contraception and the patient's feelings about this. Teach about the use of condoms that can provide contraception and decrease the risk for future episodes of PID. Help the patient understand that having sexual intercourse with multiple partners increases the risk for recurrent episodes. Douching has also been suggested as a risky behavior for development of PID and/or infection with chlamydia or *N. gonorrhoeae*.

Psychosocial concerns may require counseling. A patient who has PID may exhibit a variety of feelings (guilt, disgust, anger) about having a condition that may have been transmitted to her sexually. These feelings may affect her relationship with significant others and future sexual partners. She may also have concerns about future fertility if PID has damaged or scarred the fallopian tubes and other reproductive organs. Provide nonjudgmental emotional support and allow time for her to discuss her feelings. Collaborate with a mental health care provider as a longer-term method of support for the patient.

Health Care Resources. The cost of antibiotics for patients with PID and other STIs may be a concern for those who are uninsured, underinsured, or impoverished. Ask the patient directly if she has the ability to pay for the drug and her follow-up visits, regardless of her apparent financial status. Collaborate with the case manager or social worker, as these professionals can help to locate free or reduced-cost drugs and community resources for women who cannot afford them.

If infertility is a result of PID, the patient may need referral to a clinic specializing in infertility treatment and counseling. She can also contact infertility support groups, which exist in many local communities.

◆ **Evaluation: Evaluate Outcomes.** Evaluate the care of the patient with PID based on the identified priority patient problem(s). The expected outcomes include that the patient should:

- Show evidence that the *infection* has resolved
- Report or demonstrate that *pain* is relieved or reduced and that she feels more comfortable
- Articulate a plan for ensuring treatment of her partner, obtaining antibiotics, and returning for follow-up care

▎ GET READY FOR THE NEXT-GENERATION NCLEX® EXAMINATION!

Key Points

Review these Key Points for each NCLEX Examination Client Needs Category.

Safe and Effective Care Environment

- Use gloves when examining genitalia and oral or skin lesions. **QSEN: Safety**

Health Promotion and Maintenance

- Teach to refrain from sexual intercourse during treatment for sexually transmitted *infection* (STI). **QSEN: Safety**
- Assume that all adult patients may be sexually active, regardless of age or stage of life. **QSEN: Patient-Centered Care**

- Educate people who are most vulnerable about risk for STIs. **QSEN: Safety**
- Teach about the availability of expedited partner therapy. **QSEN: Evidence-Based Practice**
- Encourage adults who are sexually active to use condoms. **QSEN: Evidence-Based Practice**
- Teach sexually active adults to have STI screenings at least annually. **QSEN: Safety**
- Respect the sexual choices and practices of all patients. **QSEN: Patient-Centered Care**

Psychosocial Integrity

- Maintain patient and partner confidentiality and privacy at all times. **QSEN: Patient-Centered Care**
- Treat all patients, regardless of diagnosis, gender identity, or sexual orientation, with respect. **QSEN: Patient-Centered Care**
- Provide privacy for patients undergoing examination or testing for STIs. **QSEN: Patient-Centered Care**
- Encourage expression of feelings regarding a diagnosis of STI. **QSEN: Patient-Centered Care**
- Refer patients newly diagnosed with an STI to local resources and support groups. **QSEN: Teamwork and Collaboration**

Physiological Integrity

- Assess patients with an STI using best practice guidelines. **QSEN: Evidence-Based Practice**

- Recognize that some STIs progress in stages and over various periods of time. **QSEN: Evidence-Based Practice**
- Understand that patients without symptoms may still be infected with an STI. **QSEN: Evidence-Based Practice**
- Teach about the importance of completing the entire antiinfective drug regimen, even when feeling better. **QSEN: Evidence-Based Practice**
- Teach the expected side effects of and possible adverse reactions to prescribed drugs. **QSEN: Safety**
- Teach about the short-term and long-term complications of STIs. **QSEN: Safety**
- Encourage all patients who have an STI to inform their sexual partner(s). **QSEN: Safety**

▌ MASTERY QUESTIONS

1. The nurse hears a patient tell her partner that condoms with spermicide are important to protect themselves from sexually transmitted infections (STIs). What is the appropriate nursing response?
   A. Teach that spermicide has not been shown to be effective in STI prevention.
   B. Do nothing because the nurse should not be listening to the client's conversation.
   C. Educate that spermicide must be used with water-based lubricant to be effective.
   D. Affirm that spermicide helps to block transfer of sexually transmitted organisms.

2. The nurse is caring for a 33-year-old female client who has been intimate with women and men. What teaching will the nurse provide regarding the Gardisil 9 vaccine?
   A. "Patients older than 26 cannot receive an HPV vaccine."
   B. "You will need three doses of the vaccine instead of two."
   C. "I will give you a single dose and you will be protected from future HPV."
   D. "HPV vaccines must be administered to people who have never had intercourse."

REFERENCES

Albrecht, M. (2018). Epidemiology, clinical manifestations, and diagnosis of genital herpes simplex virus infection. In M. Hirsch (Ed.), *UpToDate*. Waltham, MA.

Albrecht, M. (2019). Treatment of genital herpes simplex infection. In M. Hirsch (Ed.), *UpToDate*. Waltham, MA.

American College of Obstetricians and Gynecologists. (2017). *How to prevent sexually transmitted infections (STIs)*. https://www.acog.org/Patients/FAQs/How-to-Prevent-Sexually-Transmitted-Infections-STIs?IsMobileSet=false#risk.

American Sexual Health Association. (2020). *Diagnosing and managing genital herpes*. http://www.ashasexualhealth.org/?s=herpes.

Barrow, R., Ahmed, F., Bolan, G., & Workowski, K. (2020). Recommendations for providing quality sexually transmitted diseases clinical services, 2020. *Morbidity and Mortality Weekly Report Recommendations and Reports*, 68(No. RR-5), 1–20.

Bartz, D. (2019). Pericoital contraception: Diaphragm, cervical cap, spermicide, and sponge. In C. Schreiber (Ed.), *UpToDate*. Waltham, MA.

Burchum, J. L. R., & Rosenthal, L. D. (2019). *Lehne's pharmacology for nursing care* (10th ed.). St. Louis: Elsevier.

Carusi, D. (2019). Condylomata acuminate (anogenital warts): Treatment of vulvar and vaginal warts. In R. Barbieri (Ed.), *UpToDate*. Waltham, MA.

Centers for Disease Control and Prevention (CDC). (2015). Sexually transmitted diseases treatment guidelines, 2015. *Morbidity and Mortality Weekly Report Recommendations and Reports*, 64(RR–3), 1–137.

Centers for Disease Control and Prevention. (2016). *Chlamydia – CDC fact sheet*. https://www.cdc.gov/std/chlamydia/stdfact-chlamydia-detailed.htm.

Centers for Disease Control and Prevention. (2017). *Pelvic inflammatory disease (PID) – CDC fact sheet*. https://www.cdc.gov/std/pid/stdfact-pid-detailed.htm.

Centers for Disease Control and Prevention. (2018a). *Sexually transmitted disease surveillance, 2017*. Atlanta, GA: Department of Health and Human Services.

Centers for Disease Control and Prevention. (2018b). *STDs in racial and ethnic minorities*. https://www.cdc.gov/std/stats17/minorities.htm.

Centers for Disease Control and Prevention. (2018c). Syphilis. https://www.cdc.gov/std/stats17/syphilis.htm.

Centers for Disease Control and Prevention. (2019). *Genital HPV infection – fact sheet*. https://www.cdc.gov/std/hpv/stdfact-hpv.htm.

Centers for Disease Control and Prevention. (2020a). *2020 national notifiable conditions*. https://wwwn.cdc.gov/nndss/conditions/notifiable/2019/.

Centers for Disease Control and Prevention. (2020b). *Sexually transmitted diseases*. https://www.cdc.gov/std/default.htm.

Fenway Health. (2020). *The national LGBT health education Center*. https://fenwayhealth.org/the-fenway-institute/education/the-national-lgbt-health-education-center/.

Ghanem, K. (2020). Clinical manifestations and diagnosis of Neisseria gonorrhoeae infection in adults and adolescents. In J. Marrazzo (Ed.), *UpToDate*. Waltham, MA.

Hicks, C., & Clement, M. (2020a). Syphilis: Epidemiology, pathophysiology, and clinical manifestations in patients without HIV. In J. Marrazzo (Ed.), *UpToDate*. Waltham, MA.

Hicks, C., & Clement, M. (2020b). Syphilis: Treatment and monitoring. In J. Marrazzo (Ed.), *UpToDate*. Waltham, MA.

Hoke, T., et al. (2020). Female condoms. In C. Schreiber (Ed.), *UpToDate*. Waltham, MA.

Johnson-Mallard, V., et al. (2018). Managing sexually transmitted infections: Beyond the 2015 guidelines. *The Nurse Practitioner Journal, 43*(8), 28–34.

McCance, K., Huether, S., Brashers, V., & Rote, N. (2019). *Pathophysiology: The biologic basis for disease in adults and children* (8th ed.). St. Louis: Elsevier.

Merck Sharp & Dohme Corp. (2019). Why 9 HPV types? https://www.merckvaccines.com/Products/Gardasil9/hpv-types.

Molin, S. B., De Blasio, B. F., & Olsen, A. O. (2016). Is the risk for sexually transmissible infections (STI) lower among women with exclusively female sexual partners compared with women with male partners? A retrospective study based on attendees at a Norwegian STI clinic from 2004 to 2014. *Sexual Health, 13*(3), 257–264.

National Center for Health Statistics (NCHS). (2018). *Data brief number 304*. https://www.cdc.gov/nchs/products/databriefs/db304.htm#hsv1_prevalence_by_race_comparision.

Neumann, M., Finlayson, T., Pitt, N., & Keatley, J. (2017). Comprehensive HIV prevention for transgender persons. *American Journal of Public Health, 107*(2), 207–212.

Pagana, K. D., & Pagana, T. J. (2018). *Mosby's manual of diagnostic and laboratory tests* (6th ed.). St. Louis: Elsevier.

Palefsky, J. (2019). Human papillomavirus infections: Epidemiology and disease associations. In M. Hirsch (Ed.), *UpToDate*. Waltham, MA.

Raiford, J., Hall, G., Taylor, R., Bimbi, D., & Parsons, J. (2016). The role of structural barriers in risky sexual behavior, victimization, and readiness to change HIV/STI-related risk behavior among transgender women. *AIDS Behaviors, 20*(10), 2212–2221.

Ross, J., & Chacko, M. (2020). Pelvic inflammatory disease: Clinical manifestations and diagnosis. In J. Marrazzo (Ed.), *UpToDate*. Waltham, MA.

Schweon, S. (2019). Disseminated gonococcal infection. *Nursing2019, 49*(3), 15–16.

The Joint Commission. (2019). *Why clinicians struggle with identifying human trafficking victims*. https://www.jointcommission.org/resources/news-and-multimedia/blogs/dateline-tjc/2019/06/why-clinicians-struggle-with-identifying-human-trafficking-victims/.

U.S. Department of Health and Human Services, Indian Health Service, US Centers for Disease Control and Prevention (2015). *2015 Indian health surveillance report: Sexually transmitted diseases*. https://www.cdc.gov/std/stats/ihs/18IHS-DEDP102_REPORT_STD_M_508.pdf.

U.S. Department of Health and Human Services. (2019). *Proposed objectives for inclusion in Healthy People 2030*. https://www.healthypeople.gov/sites/default/files/ObjectivesPublicComment508_1.17.19.pdf

U.S. Department of Health and Human Services. (2020a). *HIV and sexually transmitted diseases (STDs)*. https://aidsinfo.nih.gov/understanding-hiv-aids/fact-sheets/26/98/hiv-and-sexually-transmitted-diseases--stds-.

U.S. Department of Health and Human Services (USDHHS), Office of Disease Prevention and Health Promotion. (2020b). *Healthy people 2020*. https://www.healthypeople.gov/.

U.S. Preventive Services Task Force. (2018). *Cervical cancer: Screening*. https://www.uspreventiveservicestaskforce.org/uspstf/recommendation/cervical-cancer-screening.

World Health Organization. (2020). *Nonoxynol-9 ineffective in preventing HIV infection*. https://www.who.int/mediacentre/news/notes/release55/en/.

Chapter 1
1. B, E
2. A, D, E

Chapter 2
1. A, B, C, E
2. A, B, C, D, E

Chapter 3
1. A, C, F
2. A
3. B

Chapter 4
1. A, B, C, D, E
2. C
3. B

Chapter 5
1. A
2. A

Chapter 6
1. A
2. C
3. D
4. B, F

Chapter 7
1. C
2. A, C, E
3. C

Chapter 8
1. D
2. A, B, D, F

Chapter 9
1. B
2. C, D
3. A, C, D, E
4. A
5. A
6. A
7. C, D, E

Chapter 10
1. D
2. B, E
3. C

Chapter 11
1. A, D, E
2. D
3. A, B, C, D, E, F, G

Chapter 12
1. B
2. A, C, D
3. A, B, C, D, F, G

Chapter 13
1. A
2. A, D, F
3. C
4. D
5. C
6. C

Chapter 14
1. C
2. D
3. C, D

Chapter 15
1. C
2. B

Chapter 16
1. D
2. C
3. C, D

Chapter 17
1. C
2. C
3. A
4. C
5. B, F, G
6. B

Chapter 18
1. A, E
2. C

Chapter 19
1. C
2. A, D, E, F
3. C, D, G

Chapter 20
1. A
2. B, C, F
3. B
4. B
5. C, D, E

Chapter 21
1. A, B, D
2. A, B, C, D, E

Chapter 22
1. B, C, D
2. D

Chapter 23
1. C
2. A, C, D, E
3. D
4. C

Chapter 24
1. C, F, G
2. B
3. D

Chapter 25
1. D, F, H
2. C
3. D
4. B, C

Chapter 26
1. A
2. B, C, G, H
3. D
4. B

Chapter 27
1. C
2. B
3. A
4. D, F, G
5. B

Chapter 28
1. C
2. B
3. A, G

Chapter 29
1. B
2. A, C, D
3. C
4. A

Chapter 30
1. A, D, E, G
2. C
3. B

Chapter 31
1. C
2. D
3. C, D, B, A, E

Chapter 32
1. B, C, E, F
2. B
3. C
4. B

Chapter 33
1. C, D, E
2. A
3. D
4. C
5. A, D, E

Chapter 34
1. A, B, D, E, H
2. C
3. D
4. B, C

Chapter 35
1. A, C, D, E
2. B, D, F
3. A

Chapter 36
1. D
2. A, C, E
3. A

Chapter 37
1. C
2. A, C, E
3. C
4. C

Chapter 38
1. A, B, D, E
2. A
3. D

Chapter 39
1. A, F
2. C
3. A, C, D, E
4. B, C, D, E, F

Chapter 40
1. B, C, D, E, F
2. C
3. A

Chapter 41
1. A
2. B
3. C
4. B

Chapter 42
1. D
2. A
3. B, C, D, E
4. C
5. C

Chapter 43
1. D
2. A, C, D
3. A, C, E

Chapter 44
1. A, B, C, D, E, F
2. C

Chapter 45
1. A, B, C, F
2. C
3. C

Chapter 46
1. B, C, D
2. A, B, D, E
3. C
4. A, D, F

Chapter 47
1. A, B, C, D
2. B, C, E
3. D
4. C

Chapter 48
1. A, B, E, G
2. C
3. A, D, E

Chapter 49
1. B
2. A
3. A, E
4. B, F
5. B
6. D, F

Chapter 50
1. B, C, E
2. A

Chapter 51
1. A, B, C, D, E, F
2. A
3. C

Chapter 52
1. B, C
2. A, B, C, D, E
3. A

Chapter 53
1. A, B, C, D, E
2. A, C
3. C, D

Chapter 54
1. C
2. A, B, C, E, F

Chapter 55
1. 40.0
2. B
3. A, B, C, E, F

Chapter 56
1. A
2. B

Chapter 57
1. A, B, F
2. C
3. B
4. C

Chapter 58
1. C, D
2. A
3. C

Chapter 59
1. B, C, D, E, G
2. D
3. A
4. B
5. B

Chapter 60
1. A, C, D
2. B, C, E, F
3. B, C, D, E
4. A

Chapter 61
1. A
2. C, D, E, F
3. A
4. C

Chapter 62
1. A, B, D, F
2. B
3. A

Chapter 63
1. B
2. B, C, E
3. B
4. A
5. C

Chapter 64
1. C
2. C
3. A, B, D

Chapter 65
1. B
2. A
3. A, E

Chapter 66
1. B
2. A
3. B

Chapter 67
1. 850 mL.
2. C
3. D

Chapter 68
1. D
2. B

Chapter 69
1. C, D, E, F
2. A, E

MASTERY QUESTIONS ANSWER KEY

Chapter 1
1. A
2. A, D, E

Chapter 2
1. C
2. D
3. D

Chapter 3
1. A, B, D, F
2. A

Chapter 4
1. D
2. A, B, C, D, E

Chapter 5
1. A
2. B

Chapter 6
1. C
2. A, B, F, G
3. A
4. B, D

Chapter 7
1. A, D, F
2. C

Chapter 8
1. B
2. B

Chapter 9
1. A, C, D
2. B

Chapter 10
1. A
2. A

Chapter 11
1. B
2. D

Chapter 12
1. D
2. C

Chapter 13
1. A, D
2. D
3. B
4. B

Chapter 14
1. A
2. C

Chapter 15
1. D
2. C

Chapter 16
1. A, B, C, F
2. C
3. A

Chapter 17
1. B
2. D
3. A
4. D

Chapter 18
1. B, C, G
2. C
3. B

Chapter 19
1. B
2. D
3. C, D

Chapter 20
1. B
2. A, D, E
3. B

Chapter 21
1. A, B, C, D, E
2. B

Chapter 22
1. B, C
2. A, C, E

Chapter 23
1. C
2. D
3. C

Chapter 24
1. C
2. A

Chapter 25
1. D
2. A
3. C

Chapter 26
1. D
2. C
3. D
4. B, D, F

Chapter 27
1. B
2. C
3. A
4. A, B, E, F
5. B

Chapter 28
1. B
2. C
3. B, C, D, E

Chapter 29
1. D
2. C, D, G
3. A, C, E, F

Chapter 30
1. A, C, E, F
2. A
3. B

Chapter 31
1. B
2. D
3. C

Chapter 32
1. A, B, C, D, E
2. C
3. A

Chapter 33
1. D
2. B
3. B

Chapter 34
1. D
2. A
3. A, C, D

Chapter 35
1. A, D, E, F
2. C
3. A
4. B

Chapter 36
1. B
2. D
3. C

Chapter 37
1. A, C, E
2. D
3. A, F

Chapter 38
1. C
2. B

Chapter 39
1. D
2. A, B, C, D
3. A, B, C, D, E

Chapter 40
1. D
2. B
3. D

Chapter 41
1. A, D, E
2. D

Chapter 42
1. A, B, C
2. A, C, D, E

Chapter 43
1. A
2. A, B, D, E
3. D

Chapter 44
1. A, B, C, D, E
2. D

Chapter 45
1. A
2. A, B

Chapter 46
1. A
2. D
3. B, D, E

Chapter 47
1. B
2. C
3. B, C, D, E

Chapter 48
1. C, D
2. A, B, D, E

Chapter 49
1. A, B, D
2. A, B, D
3. B

Chapter 50
1. B
2. A, B, D, E

Chapter 51
1. A, D, E
2. C

Chapter 52
1. B
2. C

Chapter 53
1. A, C
2. C

Chapter 54
1. D
2. A, B, C, D, E

Chapter 55
1. A
2. A, C, E

Chapter 56
1. C
2. B

Chapter 57
1. C
2. A
3. A, B, C, D, E, F
4. D

Chapter 58
1. A
2. B, E, G
3. C

Chapter 59
1. A, C
2. C
3. B, C
4. D
5. B

Chapter 60
1. A
2. B
3. B, D, F
4. D

Chapter 61
1. B, C, D, G
2. C, E, F, G
3. D
4. D

Chapter 62
1. B
2. B
3. A, D, E, F

Chapter 63
1. B, C, E
2. C
3. A

Chapter 64
1. D
2. A
3. D

Chapter 65
1. B, C, D, E
2. B

Chapter 66
1. B, C
2. B

Chapter 67
1. B
2. B

Chapter 68
1. A
2. C, E, F

Chapter 69
1. A
2. B
